D1568632

Signs and Symptoms

Applied Pathologic Physiology
and
Clinical Interpretation

Fifth Edition

Contributors

Richard D. Aach

Elisha Atkins

Robert Stanley Blacklow

Francis I. Catlin

William F. Collins

William H. Daughaday

Leon M. Edelstein

George L. Engel

Richard H. Freyberg

Joseph H. Galicich

Robert Goldstein

Helen Goodell

Lawrence E. Hinkle, Jr.

H. H. Hyland

Harold Jeghers

E. Charles Kunkle

William M. Landau

Bernard S. Lipman

Daniel S. Lukas

Cyril Mitchell MacBryde

Edward Massie

James E. McGuigan

Roger S. Mitchell

James L. O'Leary

Robert Paine

Alan D. Perlmutter

Malcolm L. Peterson

John A. Pierce

Robert D. Reinecke

Edward H. Reinhard

Leon Schiff

Henry Alfred Schroeder

Arthur L. Shapiro

William M. Sherman

John R. Smith

Othmar C. Solnitzky

Eugene Anson Stead, Jr.

Richard W. Vilter

Harold G. Wolff

SIGNS AND SYMPTOMS

Applied Pathologic Physiology
and Clinical Interpretation

Edited by

Cyril Mitchell MacBryde, A.B., M.D., F.A.C.P.

*Associate Professor of Clinical Medicine, Washington
University School of Medicine; Assistant Physician, The
Barnes Hospital, St. Louis, Missouri*

and

Robert Stanley Blacklow, A.B., M.D.

*Assistant Professor of Medicine, Assistant to the Dean,
Member of the Faculty of Medicine, Harvard Medical
School; Senior Associate in Medicine, Peter Bent
Brigham Hospital, Boston, Massachusetts*

FIFTH EDITION
with 241 Figures and 4 Color Plates

J. B. Lippincott Company
Philadelphia • Toronto

Fifth Edition

Distributed in Great Britain by
Blackwell Scientific Publications
Oxford · London · Edinburgh

ISBN–0–397–52046–8

Library of Congress Number 77-109949

Printed in the United States of America

3   5   4

Contributors

Richard D. Aach, M.D.

Assistant Professor of Internal Medicine, Washington University School of Medicine; Assistant Physician, Barnes Hospital, St. Louis.

Elisha Atkins, A.B., M.D.

Professor of Medicine, Yale University School of Medicine; Attending Physician, Yale-New Haven Hospital, New Haven, Connecticut; Attending Physician, West Haven Veterans Administration Hospital.

Robert Stanley Blacklow, A.B., M.D.

Assistant Professor of Medicine, Assistant to the Dean, Member of the Faculty of Medicine, Harvard Medical School; Senior Associate in Medicine, Peter Bent Brigham Hospital, Boston.

Francis I. Catlin, M.D.

Associate Professor of Otolaryngology, Johns Hopkins University School of Medicine, Baltimore.

William F. Collins, B.S., M.D.

Professor and Chairman of Neurological Surgery, Yale University School of Medicine; Neurosurgeon-in-Chief, Yale-New Haven Medical Center; Consultant in Neurosurgery, West Haven Veterans Administration Hospital.

William H. Daughaday, A.B., M.D.

Professor of Medicine, Director of the Metabolism Division, Washington University School of Medicine; Associate Physician, Barnes Hospital, St. Louis.

Leon M. Edelstein, B.A., M.D.

Clinical Assistant Professor of Pathology, University of Massachusetts School of Medicine; Assistant Pathologist, St. Vincent Hospital, Worcester; Research Fellow, Department of Dermatology, Tufts University School of Medicine, Boston.

George L. Engel, M.D.

Professor of Psychiatry and Professor of Medicine, University of Rochester School of Medicine, Rochester, New York.

Richard H. Freyberg, M.D.

Clinical Professor of Medicine, Emeritus, Cornell University Medical College; Consultant, Department of Rheumatic Diseases, Hospital for Special Surgery, New York Hospital-Cornell Medical Center, New York.

Joseph H. Galicich, A.B., M.D.

Assistant Professor of Neurological Surgery, Yale University School of Medicine; Attending Neurosurgeon, Yale-New Haven Medical Center; Attending Neurosurgeon, West Haven Veterans Administration Hospital.

Robert Goldstein, A.B., M.D.

Professor of Medicine and Acting Chairman, Department of Medicine, New York Medical College; Attending Physician, Flower and Fifth Avenue Hospitals; Visiting Physician, Metropolitan Hospital and Bird S. Coler Hospital, New York.

Helen Goodell, B.S.

Research Fellow, Emeritus, Cornell University Medical College, New York; Research Consultant, Westchester Division, New York Hospital, White Plains, N. Y.

Lawrence E. Hinkle, Jr., M.D.

Associate Professor of Medicine, and Associate Professor of Medicine in Psychiatry, Director of the Division of Human Ecology, New York Hospital-Cornell Medical Center, New York.

H. H. Hyland, M.D., F.R.C.P. (London), F.R.C.P. (Canada)

Formerly Associate Professor of Medicine (in Charge of Neurology), University of Toronto; Consulting Physician, Toronto General Hospital, Wellesley Hospital, Sunnybrook (D.V.A.) Hospital and Queen Elizabeth Hospital, Toronto.

Harold Jeghers, M.D.

Professor of Medicine, Tufts University School of Medicine, Boston, Massachusetts; Professor of Medicine, Emeritus, New Jersey College of Medicine, Newark; Medical Director, St. Vincent Hospital, Worcester, Massachusetts.

E. Charles Kunkle, M.D.

Associate Neurologist, Maine Medical Center, Portland, Maine; Formerly Professor of Neurology, Duke University School of Medicine, Durham, North Carolina.

William M. Landau, M.D.

Professor and Head, Department of Neurology, Washington University School of Medicine; Neurologist-in-Chief, Barnes Hospital, St. Louis.

Bernard S. Lipman, A.B., M.D., F.A.C.P., F.A.C.C.

Associate Professor of Clinical Medicine, Emory University Medical School; Director of Heart Station, St. Joseph Hospital; Co-Director of Glenville Giddings Cardiac Clinic, St. Joseph Hospital; Visiting Physician and Consultant Cardiologist, Grady Memorial Hospital; Area Consultant in Cardiology to the Veterans Administration, Atlanta, Georgia.

Daniel S. Lukas, A.B., M.D.

Associate Professor of Medicine, Cornell University Medical College; Director, Cardiopulmonary Laboratory, and Associate Attending Physician, New York Hospital-Cornell Medical Center, New York.

Cyril Mitchell MacBryde, A.B., M.D., F.A.C.P.

Associate Professor of Clinical Medicine, Washington University School of Medicine; Assistant Physician, Barnes Hospital, St. Louis.

James E. McGuigan, M.D.

Professor of Medicine, and Chief, Division of Gastroenterology, University of Florida College of Medicine, Gainesville, Florida.

Edward Massie, A.B., M.D., F.A.C.P., F.A.C.C.

Professor of Clinical Medicine, Washington University School of Medicine; Director of Heart Station, Barnes Hospital; Consultant to Heart Station, Jewish Hospital; Assistant Physician, Barnes Hospital; Senior Attending Physician, Jewish Hospital, St. Louis.

Roger S. Mitchell, B.A., M.D.

Head, Division of Pulmonary Disease, University of Colorado School of Medicine; Director, Webb-Waring Institute for Medical Research; Consultant to Veterans Administration Hospital, Denver; Consultant to Fitzsimmons General Hospital, Denver.

James L. O'Leary, M.D.

Professor of Neurology, Washington University School of Medicine; Associate Neurologist, Barnes Hospital, St. Louis.

Robert Paine, M.D.

Associate Professor of Clinical Medicine, Washington University School of Medicine; Assistant Physician, Barnes Hospital; Chief of Medical Service, St. Luke's Hospital, St. Louis.

Alan D. Perlmutter, M.D.

Clinical Associate in Surgery, Harvard Medical School; Director of the Urology Clinic and Associate in Surgery (Urology), Children's Hospital Medical Center, Boston.

Malcolm L. Peterson, M.D., Ph.D.

Associate Professor of Medicine, Johns Hopkins University School of Medicine; Associate Professor of Medical Care and Hospitals, Johns Hopkins School of Hygiene and Public Health; Director, Health Services Research and Development Center, Johns Hopkins Medical Institutions, Baltimore.

John A. Pierce, M.D.

Associate Professor of Medicine; Director, Division of Pulmonary Diseases, Washington University School of Medicine; Assistant Physician, Barnes Hospital, St. Louis.

Robert D. Reinecke, A.B., M.D.

Professor and Chairman, Department of Ophthalmology, Albany Medical College of Union University; Chairman, Department of Ophthalmology, Albany Medical Center Hospital, Albany, New York.

Edward H. Reinhard, M.D., F.A.C.P.

Professor of Medicine, Washington University School of Medicine; Director, Private Medical Service, Barnes Hospital; Associate Physician, Barnes Hospital; Consultant in Oncology to the Mallinckrodt Institute of Radiology, St. Louis.

Leon Schiff, Ph.D., M.D.

Professor of Medicine, University of Cincinnati College of Medicine; Director, Gastric Laboratory, Cincinnati General Hospital.

Henry Alfred Schroeder, A.B., M.A., M.D., F.A.C.P.

Professor of Physiology, Dartmouth Medical School, Hanover, New Hampshire; Director of Research, Brattleboro Memorial Hospital, Brattleboro, Vermont.

Arthur L. Shapiro, M.D.

Clinical Professor of Dermatology, The Chicago Medical School; Associate Attending Physician in Dermatology, Mount Sinai Hospital; Consultant in Dermatology, Jackson Park Hospital, and South Chicago Community Hospital, Chicago.

William M. Sherman, M.D.

Resident in Internal Medicine, St. Louis University School of Medicine, St. Louis University Group of Hospitals; Formerly Fellow in Cardiology, St. Luke's Hospital, St. Louis.

John R. Smith, A.B., A.M., M.D.

Professor of Medicine, Chief, Cardiovascular Division, Washington University School of Medicine; Associate Physician, Barnes Hospital, St. Louis.

Othmar C. Solnitzky, A.M., Ph.D., M.D.

Professor of Anatomy, Georgetown University School of Medicine, Washington, D. C.

Eugene Anson Stead, Jr., B.S., M.D.

Professor of Medicine, Duke University School of Medicine, Durham, North Carolina.

Richard W. Vilter, A.B., M.D.

Professor of Medicine and Director, Department of Internal Medicine, University of Cincinnati; Director of Medical Services, Cincinnati General Hospital and Holmes Hospital.

*Harold G. Wolff, A.M., M.D.

Professor of Medicine (Neurology), Cornell University Medical College; Attending Physician, New York Hospital, New York.

* Deceased

Preface to the Fifth Edition

Since the first slim preliminary volume appeared in 1944 preceding the first edition of this book (1947), there have been major changes in medical education, both in undergraduate and postgraduate phases. There is hardly a medical school that has not recently or is not at present engaged in major revision of its curriculum. Longer residency training programs are common; the practicing physician is increasingly interested in continuing education, and medical centers offer frequent refresher courses. We are ever more aware of the dramatic and explosive progress in all the sciences basic to medicine. The mass of information has become so vast that it has become impossible to teach or to learn during medical school years more than a basic core of knowledge. Medical curricula have become more eclectic; a critical approach to the acquisition of knowledge is a highly important part of the process of medical education. To recognize what is true, what is of value, or even what is relevant, is often difficult because judgments change as knowledge expands.

These remarks define some of the major problems of medical education today. Medical curricula both in medical schools and in continuing medical education should provide knowledge that can grow. The approach should help the student learn today, and provide him with views and concepts that will prepare him to learn effectively tomorrow.

The general goal of medical education now is the same as it was a decade or a century ago, even though our means of attaining it are different. This goal is that of understanding both normal and disturbed physiologic processes, and to use this insight for the benefit of man. It is our belief that this book can be highly useful not only in furnishing a large amount of "core" information, but also in showing gaps in our knowledge and directions for new exploration. The reader should be stimulated toward further study and toward developing attitudes and approaches needed for continuing education.

Signs and Symptoms continues to use the same format; are we failing to "change with the times"? We believe not. This book continues to approach diagnosis as the physician must when studying patients. Signs and symptoms are the basic parameters of medical diagnosis and are the final common pathways for the expression of disease. As our knowledge of the mechanism of a disease process unfolds, the significance of its signs and symptoms becomes clear. The evidences of illness do not change much over the centuries, but our insight into what these evidences represent does change greatly. A book that approaches medicine in this fashion will of necessity need frequent revisions in order to remain up-to-date concerning current views among developing and changing interpretations of the mechanisms of disease processes, and their interrelationships to the manifestations of disease. The development of our recent understanding of the pathophysiology of the signs and symptoms of gout and hyperuricemia bears witness to this in dramatic fashion.

This book is dedicated to the proposition that the physician with the most insight into the processes of illness is best equipped to aid the patient. We are concerned with *understanding the processes* which result in manifestations of the disabilities and derangements of disease. In each chapter, a major sign or symptom is analyzed and the operations and interrelationships of the various factors in its causation are considered, and wherever possible are clarified and logically related. The gap between the "preclinical" and "clinical" approaches that unfortunately does exist in the minds of many medical students, teachers, and practicing physicians is deplorable and artificial. The medical student studying human biology must be able to see the relationship between the normal and the abnormal. The subject material needed for learning applied pathologic physiology and normal physiology, brought together and integrated in a fashion which recapitulates the steps in the process of thinking by which a physician reaches a diagnosis—by an analysis and an interpretation of symptoms and signs, —often must be drawn from lectures, books, original articles, and other sources, often fragmented and scattered. Since, by necessity, the major emphasis is on *technique* of history-taking and physical examination in the traditional introductory course "Examination of the Patient," this course has failed to provide the needed synthesis of the preclinical and the clinical. In this book we have attempted to synthesize and integrate the available relevant information and to make it useful in the explanation of how and why certain signs and symptoms develop. An intelligent approach to a patient with jaundice must involve knowledge of the regional anatomy, physiology, and biochemistry of bilirubin. A discussion of pain similarly must integrate many areas. Medical students are now seeing patients at the beginning of the first year in medical school, and in this way anatomy, physiology, and biochemistry are being made to come alive. In this book the chief aim in the treatment of every subject discussed is the development of understanding and insight into disturbed mechanisms resulting in abnormal clinical evidence. For these reasons, we believe that the need for such a book as *Signs and Symptoms* is even more pressing today than it was when the first edition appeared.

This volume is of multiple authorship, deriving breadth, depth, and strength from the varied talents and special interests of 39 contributors doing research, teaching, and serving patients in 21 different medical centers. Fresh insight into many fields is introduced by 15 authors who are contributors to this book for the first time.

This new volume has been expanded to include five important subject areas not analyzed in previous editions. The new areas included in this edition consider the pathophysiology of: (1) loss of vision; (2) problems of communication (speech, hearing); (3) signs and symptoms associated with renal tract disorders; (4) signs and symptoms associated with anemia; (5) conversion symptoms. The latter chapter discusses how psychologic disturbances may produce actual symptoms and signs, a field of which all physicians are becoming increasingly aware.

Much effort has been devoted to properly interrelate the various parts of the book and to present in general an integrated approach and a similar logical systematic treatment of each subject. The 40 chapters are parts of an interconnected whole, not an assemblage of unrelated monographs. An outline heads each chapter. Liberal use is made of illustrations, diagrams, and tables. Thorough reference lists follow each chapter, specific reference numbers being employed throughout the text to encourage exploration of original medical literature. It is our hope that the newly available knowledge and concepts that have been included in this fifth edition have been synthesized with older facts and hypotheses in a manner that will excite the interest of and be useful to both medical students and graduate physicians.

The editors are deeply grateful to Anita Koehler MacBryde, who has been infinitely patient during her husband's labors and has rendered valuable and devoted assistance in many phases of editing.

To Mr. J. Stuart Freeman, Jr. (Production Editor, Medical Department of the Lippincott Company) go special thanks for constructive and efficient cooperation.

Finally, the editors and all who have contributed to this volume express gratitude to those who have found in this book a work which integrates the preclinical sciences with clinical medicine. We trust that this thoroughly revised and considerably enlarged fifth edition will prove to be increasingly useful to practicing physicians, to teachers and students of medicine, and to all who labor to understand and relieve the diseases of man.

CYRIL MITCHELL MACBRYDE

ROBERT STANLEY BLACKLOW

Preface to the First Edition

How convenient it would be for the physician if the new patient were able to announce: "I have a gastrointestinal disturbance," or, "My trouble is nephritis." A perusal of the usual textbooks of diagnosis or of medicine would lead one to believe this might be the case, for the chapters consider "infectious diseases," "intoxications," "deficiency diseases," "metabolic diseases," "respiratory diseases" and so on, in rigorous order, as though every sick person carried his presumptive diagnosis labeled on his chest. Where in such textbooks can the doctor seek help when the patient confronts him complaining, for example, of severe epigastric pain, or of headache, or of jaundice?

One must admit that monographic development of the complete picture of a disease is an important means of medical education, but there are serious defects in a system which encourages us to force the ailing person into a compartment, no matter how poorly it may fit him. It is widely recognized by experienced clinicians that a skillfully taken history, with a careful analysis of the chief complaints and of the course of the illness, will more frequently than not indicate the probable diagnosis, even before a physical examination is made or any laboratory tests are performed. A master diagnostician I know says: "Let me take the history and I will accept any good intern's word on the physical findings." In other words, even today the accomplished physician can learn more in the majority of cases from what his patient says, and the way he says it, than from any other avenue of inquiry. If one doubts this, let him remember that pain in one of its thousands of guises is by far the most common presenting symptom. How handicapped we would be if the patient could not tell us that he had pain, or where it was, or its nature, or duration, or radiation!

A useful aid in the interpretation of symptoms consists in grouping them together to form quickly recognizable complexes or syndromes. Every medical student learns that "dermatitis, diarrhea and dementia" means pellagra, and that "tremor, tumor and tachycardia" indicates hyperthyroidism. The veriest medical tyro knows that a chill, a pain in the chest and rusty sputum could hardly signify anything but pneumonia. Little medical rhymes, hallowed by word-of-mouth transmission to successive medical generations, honor *ileus*, "the symptom-complex known throughout the nation, characterized by pain, vomiting, tympanites and obstipation," and epilepsy, "the aura, the cry, the fall, the fits, the tonus, the clonus, the involuntary defecation." Indelibly stamped in many a physician's mind lies *"Charcot's triad"* of INSular (multiple or disseminated) sclerosis: Intention tremor, Nystagmus and Scanning speech. Frequently, however, in the commonly recognized syndromes very little is understood as to the actual origin or mechanism of production of the primary symptoms and signs. Thus these tricks, these aids to memory, lull us into a false complacency, based too often upon very little real knowledge.

The physician today has many techniques available to assist him in making accurate diagnoses. He can peer into the recesses of the body: bronchoscopy, gastroscopy, thoracoscopy, peritoneoscopy, cystoscopy; he can study the shadows cast by the body's parts upon the x-ray film: simple x-ray, laminography, kymography, cholecystography, encephalography, gastroenterography, pyelography, bronchography; he can remove blood or lymph or abnormal fluid accumulations for physical and chemical analysis; he can remove bits of tissue from the surfaces or the cavities of the body and study them under the microscope and in the chemical and physiologic laboratory; the action potential, the very currents of life itself, he can record and analyze in the electroencephalogram and the electrocardiogram. However, without an understanding of the meaning of symptoms, how useless are these refined diagnostic techniques. They are but tools which are only as valuable as the mind which directs them. The informed mind will understand the meaning of the specific type of mucosal defect seen through the bronchoscope in relation to the patient's symptom of hemoptysis. The high icterus index observed in the laboratory study of a patient's serum has significance of one type if associated with recurrent attacks of right upper quadrant pain, but of another when found in association with a shrinking liver during pregnancy.

No mechanical measures can take the place of careful consideration of the patient's complaints. No device, be it ever so clever mechanically, electrically or chemically, can serve as a substitute in the art of medicine for the informed mind of the physician. The physician's ability as a diagnostician will determine the nature and the efficacy of the treatment he chooses to employ. His ability to diagnose will depend in only a minor degree upon his ability to use special technical

measures. He must know when to use them, which tests to select, and how to interpret the physical findings, as well as the special laboratory tests. The physician's judgment in these matters will depend largely upon his ability to analyze and interpret symptoms.

This book attempts, so far as present knowledge permits, to give the basis for analysis and interpretation of some of the commonest symptoms which bring patients to the physician. Emphasis is placed upon the pathologic physiology of the symptom, while its correlation with other symptoms and with physical and laboratory evidence is considered as important, but secondary in the diagnostic method. Our knowledge concerning many of these symptoms is incomplete, but it is rapidly expanding. Although the final word often cannot be said, critical and analytical thinking in the manner followed in these chapters should prove productive for us all: patient, practitioner, professor and student.

CYRIL MITCHELL MACBRYDE

Contents

Signs and Symptoms

Applied Pathologic Physiology
and
Clinical Interpretation

Fifth Edition

1

The Study of Symptoms

CYRIL M. MacBRYDE and ROBERT S. BLACKLOW

Definitions. As broadly and generally employed, the word *symptom* is used to name any manifestation of disease. Strictly speaking, symptoms are subjective, apparent only to the affected person. *Signs* are detectable by another person and sometimes by the patient himself. Pain and itching are symptoms; jaundice, swollen joints, cardiac murmurs, etc., are physical signs. Some phenomena, like fever, are both signs and symptoms. In this chapter the word symptom is often used to denote any evidence of disturbed physiology perceived by the patient or the physician.

PATIENT AND PHYSICIAN: THE INTERVIEW

The patient comes to the physician because he has a problem and wants help. The problem may be a simple one requiring only a health survey for school, employment, insurance, or for personal information, and the patient may have no complaints. Nevertheless, the physician may discover in the course of such an examination one or more signs or symptoms of significance. In this book we are concerned primarily with the study of the patient who presents himself with a *disturbing sign or symptom*. The *aim* of studying the patient's signs and symptoms must be kept in mind constantly: the purpose of analyzing the history carefully and of evaluating the physical findings thoughtfully is to determine the *pathophysiologic processes* involved. When these processes are understood, clinical interpretation may be attempted and diagnosis may be possible. A sign or a symptom occurring in any person is not an isolated phenomenon: it may have multiple interrelationships including causes, associated phenomena, and effects. There may be interrelationships evidencing various types of disturbed physiology, and there is always a subjective, psychological component, sometimes of minor but often of major importance. The responses of the patient to his disorder, his reactions to it, and understanding of it are essential and often deeply revealing parts of the history.

Each illness has an emotional component, sometimes slight, sometimes amounting to an emotional crisis. The eventual health and well-being of the patient depend not only on his physical but also on his emotional recovery. From the very outset of the patient-physician relationship, at the beginning of

1

the first interview, it is important to recognize that, no matter what the problem may be, every person has particular needs according to his individual personality. The patient should, by the physician's approach, be given reason to know at once that the doctor is interested in him as a person as well as in his disease. The patient has the right to expect kindness and humane consideration, as well as professional competence.

The physician, as he starts to converse with his patient and elicits the story of the illness, becomes engaged in the most intensely personal experience in medicine. With the account of complaints and medical problems may be yielded up embarrassing confidences and more or less pertinent information about past frustrations, present anxieties, and hopes for the future.

The young and inexperienced physician is often apt to neglect or to feel scorn for emotional and psychological manifestations unless they constitute well-defined and therefore "interesting" neuroses and psychoses. The physician who fails to utilize opportunities to consider and evaluate subjective aspects of the illness and confines his efforts unduly to objective data is not studying the patient as a whole and may be misled into inaccurate or incomplete conclusions and solutions.

To derive the fullest possible potential from the history, the physician must become skilled in eliciting the patient's story. Securing a meaningful history requires an interpersonal relationship, involving give-and-take co-operation between two strangers about one's intimate problems. With the patient distressed and distracted, the physician sometimes inexpert or inexperienced, and time pressing, it is small wonder that many histories are inadequate. Since amassing laboratory data requires much less skill and experience than the ability to evaluate signs and symptoms, technical approaches are often overemphasized in the diagnostic work-up.

The technical and the scientific aspects of medicine can be learned largely through reading and study; not so the arts and the skills required in the interpersonal parts of the patient-physician relationship. The clinical ability to secure a good history is an art developed by imitation of accomplished preceptors and by practice and experience.

The accumulation, classification, and mathematical manipulation of great masses of technical data, with mechanical analysis of itemized information, can yield quickly, in this age of marvelous computer machines, answers formerly obscure or requiring much time.

Some of our contemporaries expect that computer machines will largely replace the mental processes heretofore required in diagnosis.[14] Such hopes are doomed to disappointment because of misunderstanding of the meaning of *diagnosis*. True diagnosis means *understanding thoroughly*, and necessarily involves human relationships: those of the person with his disease, with other persons, etc. These subtle and complex aspects of human problems can not be programmed for computer analysis.[15] Machines can yield highly useful data based upon masses of other data fed into them.[16] Human understanding of human problems is possible only through human thought.

One must not confuse the accumulation and the interpretation of technical data (no matter how clever and helpful or even decisive) with the development of true insight into human problems.

The patient's attitude toward the physician should be analyzed as the history is being obtained. It will depend on his background and on elements in the present situation, including responses to the appearance, the attitude, the actions, and the words of the physician. Excessive hopes or dependence must be forestalled. Insufficient trust in the doctor or anger or secretiveness may defeat the patient's objective in seeking medical help. The skillful physician guides the patient's attitude into desirable channels.

The physician's attitude toward the patient requires self-study. His thought processes will be influenced by those of the patient. His emotions will respond to those of the patient and he must be aware of and evaluate his own emotional resonances. The physician must direct his own attitudes, words, and actions into a pattern most apt to promote the patient's welfare. Certain ingredients are taken for granted in a good physician: medical knowledge and self-confidence based upon competence, emotional self-control in the face of stress, dignity, kindness, graciousness and good manners. The patient usually becomes aware of these quickly, even during a first interview.

In addition to these characteristics, other important qualities required of the physician who is skillful in interviewing are: interest, acceptance, warmth, and flexibility.

The physician's concern for his patient is conveyed by his actions, rather than by a statement. Confidence and co-operation of the patient are not secured by saying "Trust me. I am trying to help you." It is best not to handicap oneself with such a bald, obvious, and superfluous remark, which may give the patient pause and make him distrustful. Proceed with the job at hand; the patient by his own observations will soon know whether the physician cares about him and his problem.

In the art of interviewing there is no substitute for genuine interest not only in the patient's problems but in the patient as a person. In trying to obtain a truly valuable history the physician will do well to keep these points in mind:

1. Interest springing from the desire to understand and to help is evident to the patient; as a rule, the patient responds by answering questions and telling his story so as to assist the doctor as much as possible. Frequently, realization that the doctor really cares about him as a person, not just as "a case" of illness, will remind the patient of aspects of his problem and lead to illumination of facets of the situation of great diagnostic importance.

2. Acceptance of the patient is essential. The physician must not reveal moral judgments he may have or his own emotional responses in regard to attitudes or behavior or statements of his patient. This does not necessarily imply approval, but the physician must be tolerant and understanding. The physician must be objective in evaluating the patient's story. In addition, he should convey to the patient his belief that the patient also is trying his best to be objective.

3. Warmth and Empathy. No one can ever actually share the experiences of another person, but the effort to do so always brings one person closer to another. The physician who can combine sensitive insight and understanding (without over-sympathizing or sentimentalizing) with a sensible objective approach to the patient's problem usually will win the patient's friendship and confidence quickly.

4. Flexibility. The topics selected and the direction of the inquiry stem naturally (at least in the beginning) from the patient's presenting complaints. As the story is developed, the picture of the present illness will emerge. Then past history, family history, and other related subjects will be explored. This is the usual course along which the interviewer gently guides his patient in order to secure a coherent history, which may be recorded in some logical order. However, the physician will find often that adherence to a rigid pattern is a handicap and that the apparent wanderings of the patient's talk may be highly revealing. Frequently, what at first seems to be only a bypath will be found to be the main highway.

Sometimes the topics that the patient avoids are the most significant ones. If he shies away, changes the subject, becomes irritated, anxious or confused, the interviewer may explore a more neutral area for a while, returning to the sensitive topic more productively later.

Therefore, the expert interviewer must be flexible and prepared to allow the patient to vary the order in which topics are discussed. The interviewer may learn much by allowing the subject to run on freely with his story: he will observe what the patient wants to emphasize and thus may learn what seems to be important to the patient, or what his motives are.

The responses of the physician must be flexible, natural, and appropriate. As a rule, the medical interview is serious business, but the physician tries to keep it upon a constructive, optimistic level. He should respond with hopeful reassurance to the depressed patient, but not with excessive cheerfulness. To the patient who is anxious or fearful he should offer some basis for confidence and courage. If the patient is ill at ease, angry, or suspicious, the physician may establish more relaxed and friendly co-operative relations by discussing briefly a mutual interest, or by inquiring into the possible causes for the patient's disquieting attitude before continuing the study of his medical problems.

The accomplished physician develops a technic in securing the history, and his technic must vary from patient to patient and according to circumstances. Knowledge of medicine and an understanding of human beings are limitless fields of endeavor; the physician's skill in obtaining the patient's story and interpreting it will grow in proportion to his progress in these very complex fields.

ANALYZING AND INTERPRETING SYMPTOMS

IMPORTANCE OF THE HISTORY

Symptoms are apt to appear some time before striking physical signs of disease are evident and before laboratory tests are useful in detecting disordered physiology. For this reason, and because a careful, detailed, properly analyzed and interpreted history usually leads the physician more directly toward the correct conclusion than any other diagnostic method, one should never neglect to elicit an accurate and sufficiently detailed history.

Persons vary greatly in their abilities to observe and describe their symptoms; intelligence, education, and verbal proficiency differ so much that eliciting a lucid and coherent account demands flexibility and adaptability. Routine or mechanical recording of data does not constitute a medical history. The emotional status of the patient colors his story; his background and environment always will condition his responses to stimuli as well as his efforts to describe such responses. Evaluation and perception of the patient as a person proceed simultaneously with the process of learning about his immediate symptoms.

So productive of insight, so apparently simple, so truly complex: "taking the history" involves analysis and interpretation and requires the highest order of medical skill.

"Of all the technical aids which increase the doctor's power of observation, none comes even close in value to the skillful use of spoken words—the words of the doctor and the words of the patient. Throughout all of medicine, use of words is still the main diagnostic technic."[1]

PATIENT QUESTIONNAIRE

There is no doubt that a detailed printed history form to be filled in by the patient can be of great assistance under certain circumstances. When time permits and the patient is not acutely ill, and for use in screening for disease, in health surveys, etc., such a record of medical history may help to prevent omission of significant data and may save the physician much time.[7,16]

It might be suggested that such a multipaged questionnaire be presented to the patient *after* the initial history is obtained by the physician, if and when the intellectual, physical, and emotional status of the subject encourage such a method of assembling information. Such a detailed health record would then be very useful for later more incisive or pertinent inquiry by the physician.

However, when the patient's complaint is urgent or he is emotionally disturbed, as is usually the case in illness, he must of course not be confronted with a routine printed form or by a clerk or physician following any routine method of approach to his problem. The approach must vary appropriately with the problem and with the person affected.

No impersonal inquiry into the patient's complaints, no mechanical system, no tabular compilation with check marks or crosses or pressed buttons or electronic computers can substitute in diagnosis or care of the patient for personal interest and acquaintance by the physician with each individual, unique human being, and with his particular problem.

TIME WITH THE PATIENT

The most successful physician in the field of diagnosis is often simply he who devotes sufficient *effort* and *time* to discussion of the patient's problems with the patient himself.

Too often the physician fails to take full advantage of the phase of his work which is frequently the most productive: *repeated* conversation with and examination of his patient. The first history and physical examination usually can be substantially and significantly supplemented later, especially after there has been establishment of rapport (a good, friendly, co-operative relationship) directed toward solving the patient's problems.

Important points in the history and in the physical examination are frequently elicited only after patient and physician have gotten to know each other and have learned to work together.

In a time study of the activities of two medical interns on a university service in a teaching hospital[8] it was found that, "contrary to some expectation, a very small amount of the intern's time was spent with patients"! The authors very properly regard their teaching program as "similar in philosophy, design and standards of performance to that at any other prominent university teaching hospital in the United States." It is pointed out that no definite conclusions or recommendations can be evolved from this limited pilot study. However, "results of this study stimulate questions concerning postgraduate programs. . . ." Among these questions were: "Do attending physicians sufficiently encourage interns to broaden their experience of patient-doctor contact? When does the doctor in training learn how to relate himself to patients?"[8]

TECHNICAL VS. CLINICAL METHODS

It seems that at present we are going through a prolonged phase of overemphasis in both undergraduate and in postgraduate medical teaching upon mechanical and laboratory assessment of patients. There is danger that physicians will be more concerned with the study of diseases than the study of patients. There is now excessive involvement of the doctor-in-training in technical matters, with insufficient emphasis on the learning of clinical skills—especially the skill of "getting a good history"—of really communicating with patients. Students of medical education have proposed steps that should be heeded to bring about a halt in the decline of clinical tradition.[12]

There should be no conflict (although at present there is much) between the two approaches. Certainly we need all of the help that laboratory science and that time and labor-saving machines and computers can render us in understanding man's diseases, but we must use all of our new scientific knowledge plus all available clinical acumen in the service of the patient.

Without scientific knowledge, a compassionate wish to serve mankind's health is meaningless. However, scientific knowledge without wisdom is like a powerful rocket without a guidance system. Scientific knowledge is more readily taught, whereas the application of knowledge at the bedside is largely a function of judgment and wisdom inherent in or personally developed by the individual physician. With the paradox of increasing scientific knowledge, but narrower and narrower specialty interests of physician-investigators, to combine the science and the art of medicine at the bedside, to weigh the evidence, and to decide wisely are ever more difficult, but increasingly necessary efforts.

Physicians must have technical skills and make maximum intelligent use of them and of the great multiplicity of laboratory procedures now available in the study of the ill person, but not excessive and maldirected use.

One reason that doctors tend to become better technicians but poorer true physicians is that it is much more difficult and takes much more time to deal with the *patient + disease* than with the *disease* only. The true physician devotes sufficient time and applies his best efforts not just to assembling information, not just to recording data, not just to determining what the disease is, but equally to each of these problems: how is this particular person affected? (physically, emotionally, mentally, socially, etc.); also—what relief can be offered? (not just physically, but in *all the ways he is affected* and needs help).

Those who intend to develop superior ability in the art of diagnosis must be prepared to spend many hours learning how to talk with patients and how to obtain not just adequate but highly significant, truly rewarding medical histories.

CONDUCT OF THE INTERVIEW

Satisfactory use of the physician's abilities or of the information available from the patient cannot be made under adverse conditions. A private room should be available. No third person should be present. Neither patient nor physician should feel under pressure to be elsewhere or otherwise employed.

Time and skill are required in obtaining an informative and sufficiently complete history. The physician must not hurry, nor must he seem hurried. All his attention must be devoted to the patient, who must feel that the doctor is interested, sympathetic, and eager to help. The interview should be uninterrupted and conducted in privacy and quiet. The purpose is to get the patient to talk, so that the doctor can listen and learn. The doctor says only enough to keep the patient's story going. Each statement of the patient must be considered in relation to the aid it may furnish in understanding his chief complaints or symptoms. The patient may not present the story of his difficulties well, or in logical order: he may use misleading words in describing his symptoms; he may omit important relevant information. All of these defects may be corrected if the physician *asks the proper questions*—not merely to fill in spaces on a printed form, but to develop the story. It is best to let the patient tell his story in his own words whenever possible. Many patients will present a coherent and concise description of the development of the presenting symptoms. When, however, the patient wanders, or when important facts are omitted, pointed questions are necessary. Care must be taken that the answer is not implied in the question—that the questions are not leading.

There are two essentially contrasting techniques in taking a history; they have two different objectives. The first may be termed the *cross-examination technique*:—"Do you have pain? Where? How long does it last? Is it sharp, dull, constant, or colicky? Does it radiate? Where does it radiate?" This technique has as its objective the accurate identification of the hallmarks of organic disease.

The second is the *listening technique*, which enables the patient to relate his experiences in terms of his own values and concerns. It often allows the physician to understand more clearly the meaning of the illness to the patient and helps in understanding the patient as a person. Permitting the patient to relate freely what is uppermost in his mind encourages him to verbalize the experiences that are, to him, of the greatest emotional significance. In describing his symptoms in detail, the patient transfers to the physician the material that has been the focus of his anxiety. In a very real sense, his anxieties then become the doctor's problem rather than his own. These two techniques are not wholly separate; frequently, they overlap and merge; always, they supplement each other in an understanding of the disease and of the person.

The most successful histories combine skillful use of both interrogation and listening, and for every patient and every problem the proportion and the pattern of use of the two techniques must be appropriately varied. Filling in or following a printed form cannot fulfill the requirements of a good history.

Often patients are confused about anatomic terms: to some, "the stomach" includes the whole abdomen; to others, any discomfort in the back is located in "the kidneys." Descriptions of sensations are often misleading. "Pain" is employed to include almost any kind of discomfort, such as itching, aching, smarting and burning, as well as true pain. "Dizziness" may mean vertigo or faintness. One must not simply put down the patient's words; one must make certain of *what he means*. For example, a patient may complain of pain in his heart, but inquiry may reveal that the discomfort is epigastric—not related to exertion, but relieved by food, thus suggesting not heart disease but peptic ulcer. Sometimes the patient complains of alternating constipation and diarrhea, but the fact may be omitted that diarrhea never occurs unless a cathartic is taken. The patient may present symptoms of goiter and nervousness, but may not yield the information, until after careful questioning, that the goiter had been present for years and had not increased in size, and that the nervous symptoms came on after recent marital difficulties. Careful cross-questioning is often necessary in the process of analyzing the patient's symptoms. Sometimes the physician will have to pursue a symptom, and often he may have difficulty in getting the patient to decide which one or two of his complaints are the most distressing. For example, he may have to elicit more data about progressive weight loss, unemphasized by the patient, and may devote less attention to the patient's favorite topic of insomnia.

Often the entire analysis of the symptom is not possible on the basis of the patient's story alone, and important information is obtainable from the spouse or another member of the family, or from friends. Usually it is best to obtain the patient's story first and privately, then the spouse's or other person's story, also privately. Either may be inhibited by the presence of the other. Frequently additional information from a spouse or another associate is of special help in relationship to fatigue and to nervous symptoms. For example, the cause of backache and exhaustion in one woman seemed obscure until her husband came in to report that she had stubbornly insisted on painting the fence, a job she said he had been neglecting. Her real difficulty was emotional, not physical; her nervous symptoms were due to domestic problems.

Thus symptoms may be considered as primary, when directly related to the basic cause, or secondary or even tertiary, when more remotely related. In the instance just cited, the backache was not a primary symptom: it did not indicate disease present in the back. It was secondary to an emotional situation. A young man had visual difficulty; various lenses were tried before it was discovered that he had an unequal but bilateral proptosis; the latter was found to be associated with hyperthyroidism. A man had pains in the arms and the legs characteristic of peripheral neuritis; the neuritis was found to be due to thiamine deficiency; the thiamine deficiency seemed to result from alcoholism. One might stop here, but the alcoholism was not the final diagnosis—

it was a *symptom* of an underlying severe neurosis. Not until one had traced through the steps in the pathologic physiology, from the tertiary symptom neuritis → thiamine deficiency → alcoholism → psychic disorder, did one have a true *diagnosis*, the result of "understanding through" or thoroughly.

The physical examination will be performed with greater curiosity and perception and any necessary laboratory studies can be directed much more intelligently after a careful, complete and exact history is obtained. Physical findings or the lack of them become points of great interest and significance when they are considered in relation to points in the history. The hurried physician is apt to hope that the laboratory will give him the diagnosis and may be tempted to skimp on the history to save the time, the effort, and the thought it requires. However, sufficient time and effort to get a clear story are usually well repaid, whereas the hours, the work, and the expense devoted to unnecessary laboratory tests are notorious.

The trouble with most histories is, first, that they are too short and, second, that they are taken without pursuing the main points far enough and completely enough. Printed history forms can lead to bad habits and shallowness of inquiry. Perhaps a blank page and an untrammeled interest and curiosity are better. Probably best of all is to take only brief notes while listening to the patient; writing is distracting to patient and physician—the written summary can be put down later. One must not feel that, because he has a printed blank to fill out, questions must be asked routinely, always in the same order. The spaces on the blank are useful reminders, but the nature of the patient's trouble and the informed mind of the physician must govern the course of the questioning and the development of the story. Skill must be used in excluding extraneous material, while care is necessary at the same time to obtain as much as possible of the information that will prove helpful.

As a rule, organic disorders cause clearcut symptoms, whereas emotional or nervous disorders are apt to be presented by the patient as a number of poorly defined, apparently unrelated complaints. That is, they seem to be unrelated until one discovers the nervous trouble responsible for the various symptoms, such as headache, indigestion, and insomnia.

Sometimes the patient is too ill or too excited to give or to be bothered with giving a complete history. The most essential facts then are obtained from him as quickly as possible, or from a companion or a relative. Later the complete story may be obtained.

EACH PATIENT UNIQUE

The most successful medical study requires a properly balanced, scientific-humanistic, interrelated approach to the study of each patient and his problems. The investigation should include appropriate psychological, physical, laboratory, quantitative, and mechanical assessment, plus full consideration of the special features that make every single clinical study unique—different in some aspects from every other, although possibly also similar in many ways. The physician must attempt to acquire as much information as possible about the affected individual, because in every case there are special peculiarities in the *constitution* of the subject which personalize his disease and differentiate it from the same disease in other patients. His specific constitution will consist of interrelated psychic and somatic elements.

Not only his inborn constitution, but all elements of his environment will color his symptoms: training, education, experiences, etc.

The clinician will understand that illness is related to the *patient as a whole* and to his *life history* in its entirety, not just to his medical history (past diseases). One should learn about *positive aspects* of the patient's life: aims, ambitions, accomplishments, pleasures, recreations. Knowledge of constructive factors brings insight and provides material for assisting the patient. Often it is of tremendous help to the physician to visit the *patient's home* and to get to know his immediate family. Thus, one may be able to integrate his sickness into his life history: to relate it to his home, his job, his parents, spouse, children, his economic and social problems, etc.

After decades of emphasis upon specialization and the development of technical skills, with a great decline in the practice of family medicine and with almost the disappearance of "house calls" (preferable name would be "home visits"), medicine has gained much; but it has lost much in the understanding and care of the individual sick person.

It seems today that we may be on the threshold of a new era. Medical educators are becoming interested in family and community medicine; the use of preceptorships with practicing physicians is being rediscovered; Family Practice is being revived as a worthy profession; even home visits may become respectable again.

One can learn much in this broader approach to obtaining a medical history, not only about symptoms of obvious psychological origin, but about disorders usually considered as primarily physical.

Many conditions are influenced greatly by various tensions or frustrations and by the attitudes of others (whether the patient is pitied, loved, feared, or respected, etc.). Often one may discover by investigating the home or place and type of work that there are environmental aspects of importance in regard to home or neighborhood or working conditions: light, heat and cold, dust, noise, stairs to climb, etc. Knowledge concerning ability to secure rest, or interest or engagement in hobbies or cultural activities may prove to be valuable.

PSYCHE AND SOMA

In the study of each sign or symptom, or in the formulation of a complete concept of an illness as it involves the particular person, evaluation of the psychological aspects are necessary, as well as thorough consideration of the primarily physical elements. For example, in some cases of vascular hypertension, or of headache, or of peptic ulcer, or of dermatitis, psychological factors may prove to be most important, whereas in other cases physical causes and effects may predominate. In each disorder there are various combinations of these elements, even though the presenting symptoms or chief complaints at first may seem highly similar as they occur in various persons.

Modern psychosomatic concepts of health and illness have taught us that there is close interrelation, even integration, between psyche and soma. At times more attention must be paid to one aspect than the other, but in man neither aspect should be dealt with alone. Realization of the variety of aspects but the basic unity of each person is the essence of modern medicine's attempt to study each person *individually* and as *a whole*, as a unique, complex, but integrated entity.

CHIEF COMPLAINTS AND PRESENT ILLNESS

Every symptom (or sign) has a beginning or onset. Each symptom has its course—a

life, so to speak, of its own. It may subside and disappear or it may develop and flourish. It is always a product of the organism that produces it, and its character depends upon the specific nature of that individual person.

The physician strives to ascertain and understand the interrelationships between the person and his illness. The involved individual, not only in a sense produces his own special variation of signs and symptoms, but responds in his own particular way—physically, emotionally, and intellectually.

Eliciting the story of the onset of a sign or symptom and of the patient's responses requires the highest degree of medical expertise. The physician who aspires to excel as a diagnostician reflects his competence largely by the quality of the histories that he pursues, plumbs, and unravels.

Information concerning the onset and the course of development of the patient's symptom (or sign), its nature, quality, duration, intermittent or cyclic character, etc., helps in analysis of the true nature of the symptom. Such an analysis of one or more chief presenting complaints constitutes the part of the medical history usually recorded under the heading of *present illness*. "The complaints of the patient—fragmentary expressions of the underlying disease—should be used as *leads* . . . [which] can be followed to the actual seat of disease."[2] The present illness should be described by the patient in detail, and where parts are missing, or helpful information is lacking, the physician should get the patient to fill in, round out, or dig deeper to obtain as full a story as possible.

Symptoms are not always what they seem. Was the black stool accompanied by abdominal pain or preceded by indigestion? Or, perhaps, was it preceded by the taking of bismuth powders? Was the pain in the left chest and the left arm really precipitated by exertion, or only by motion of the left shoulder? Is the shortness of breath caused only by exertion, or does it occur at rest and result from nervous tension and hyperpnea? Is the blood really coughed up in a case of suspected hemoptysis, or does it come from the nose, the pharynx, or the mouth? In suspected jaundice, has the patient been taking atabrine, or could it be carotinemia? Often the fact that back pain is at its worst on rising in the morning suggests that the patient sleeps on an excessively soft mattress and consequently has back strain, whereas pain increasing during the day suggests postural or arthritic factors related to occupation. Getting all such related details may prevent one from being led astray and may sharply narrow the diagnostic possibilities.

Symptoms must be interpreted. One must determine not only what the symptom is, but what part it plays in the patient's life —*how it affects him.* Does the nausea interfere with taking regular meals, does it come at night, has it caused weight loss? Does the dyspnea get worse with exercise or recumbency? Has it led to loss of a job?

When the symptoms suggest involvement particularly of one organ or system, one should attempt to determine whether or not any of the other possible symptoms associated with disorders of that system or organ have been present. For example, if polyuria has suggested possible diabetes, one should inquire concerning polydipsia, polyphagia, weakness, fatigue, weight loss, etc. Or if costovertebral pain has suggested renal or ureteral disease, one should find out whether there has been pain referred to the genital region, or dysuria, frequency, hematuria, etc.

A typical day or a typical attack should be described. The physician thus may learn much about the time of occurrence, the precipitating factors, correlation with the day's activities, times of recurrence, factors that give relief, and other informative phenomena related to the symptom.

In recording the history, one should first list the chief complaints in the order of their severity, noting the duration of each.

Often the duration, or time of onset, or some periodicity of attacks or intervals of relief will furnish important clues. "My headaches began about 2 years ago, a few weeks after my mother died." Follow the clue—note that the patient is linking the symptom to psychic trauma. "My asthma came on in the summer, went away while we were in the mountains, but came back on the desert ranch." Possibly due to allergy to ragweed and to horse dander? "The dermatitis started on a Sunday; it gets better during the week but usually flares up on Sundays." Possibly due to dyes in the ink of Sunday rotogravure or color sections?

"I've had this heart murmur since childhood. My heart never bothered me. My fever came on a few days after I had that tooth pulled three weeks ago." Look for petechiae. Get a blood culture. Very likely subacute bacterial endocarditis.

One should take up each symptom or sign or complaint in order, following its course throughout the present illness. Even when the physician is unable to get the patient to give an orderly account, the written record should be ordered, consecutive, compact, and complete but not verbose.

The evolution of one or several signs and symptoms constitutes the *clinical course* of the illness. Characteristics of the clinical course are apt to be highly significant in diagnosis.

ASSOCIATION OF SYMPTOMS: SYNDROMES

Certain disorders in physiology are characterized by the association of two or more related symptoms or signs. Investigation of either symptom will then lead to a further understanding of the related complaints and of the basic disease. For example, it is useful to know that a convulsion was preceded by carpopedal spasm, for that suggests hypocalcemia, whereas a convulsion preceded by hunger and perspiration suggests hypoglycemia. Likewise, vomiting accompanied by right lower abdominal pain and muscle spasm may indicate appendicitis, whereas vomiting with headache and failing vision leads one to suspect increased intracranial pressure.

One must be alert to recognize characteristic groupings of certain signs and symptoms (syndromes). Often the anatomical location of the cause may be suggested (e.g.: scalenus anticus s., Horner's s., Meniere's s.) or the organ or tissue or system involved (Banti's s., Cushing's s.) or the etiology (Korsakoff's s., Plummer-Vinson s.), etc.

It is important, however, not merely to learn by rote, for instance, that sore tongue, pallor, digestive disorders, and numbness in the extremities suggest pernicious anemia, but to try to understand as thoroughly as possible *how* these symptoms happen to be related and *why* the disease process results in these particular manifestations.

PATIENT'S ATTITUDE TOWARD HIS SYMPTOMS

Much can be learned from the manner and the method used by the patient in telling his story. If he is obviously oversensitive and apprehensive, the interpretation of his complaints must usually differ from that of similar complaints of a calm and unemotional person. If he is exaggerating or minimizing his symptoms, evaluation must be correspondingly adjusted, and motives must be sought. While the physician is taking the history he has an excellent chance to form preliminary impressions of the patient's personality.

Only rarely can a sick person present a relatively objective account of the illness. More often than not, the patient's presentation of his story to the physician is colored by (1) *emotional reaction* or (2) *motivation*. Among frequently encountered **emotional states** are: *fear*, which sometimes operates to limit information, sometimes leads to excessive emphasis and elaboration; *embarrassment*, usually leading to fragmentary or misleading statements; *anger*, resentment, or rebellion at being ill, which often causes the afflicted person to blame others in his family, his employer, his physician, or some element in his environment. Anger is often the expression of guilt feelings; sometimes anger is used as a cover for or defense reaction against anxiety or fear.

Among **motives,** one must consider first the usual one—the patient tries in his own way (which may be misguided) *to assist* the physician, because he wants relief. One must consider the patient's self-diagnosis, but beware of accepting it uncritically. For example, beware of the patient who has "just a little cough"—it may be tuberculosis; or "just a little constipation"—it may be rectal carcinoma. Second, consider motives that might lead *to overemphasis* or malingering: compensation neuroses, etc. Third, remember motives leading *to discounting* of the importance of symptoms: ambition, religious faith wrongly employed, etc. A Christian Scientist, a man of 50, collapsed and died after having repeated tarry stools. Autopsy revealed a deep chronic duodenal ulcer. His sister said he had had epigastric pain relieved by food for years, but he would never admit it. We should teach everyone that it is admirable not to exaggerate symptoms, but it is foolish to be reticent or to conceal clues. A symptom that may seem minor to the patient could prove important in the development of the diagnostic picture.

Symptoms as Buffers. Usually diagnosis of an illness and removal of its cause is a welcome contribution to the patient's general health. One must realize, however, that in many chronic illnesses the handicap comes to play an essential part in the patient's life —so important sometimes that he may not gracefully part with it. For example, a man who for years had suffered with peptic ulcer was dramatically cured by gastrectomy and for the first time in years was free of pain. Surprisingly, instead of being happy he became depressed and attempted suicide. It became evident that his stomach symptoms had served as a crutch, buffer, or excuse to spare him from stress or unpleasant situations. His symptoms were gone and so was his protection.[1] Therefore we must consider: *what does this symptom mean to this patient?*

EVOLUTION OF SYMPTOMS

Not only must the presenting symptom or symptoms be clearly understood, but they must be followed in their *development* from the onset to the date the history is obtained. Data should be sought indicating any alteration or *change* in the symptom. Has the pain changed its location? Has it changed in severity or nature? Is it now accompanied by any new phenomena? Was it first in the epigastrium and relieved by food or alkali, but now not so relieved? Did the ankle edema at first disappear upon recumbency, but does it now persist all night?

The course, or evolution of each sign or symptom forming the clinical picture of the present illness should be traced so that the significance of alterations may be considered in regard to possible changes in the pathologic physiology.

ELABORATION OF THE HISTORY

Every effort should be made to get a good history at the first interview. Later, further study of the patient's story may prove to be important. Often a useful procedure is repetition or elaboration or further cross-questioning concerning certain points in the history after some information is obtained from the physical examination or the laboratory tests. For example, a patient who has very dry or thickened skin will be questioned further about loss of energy, sensitivity to cold, drowsiness, and other symptoms that may be due to hypothyroidism. Or, if leukocytosis is revealed, further evidence of possible infection may be sought. Or, if a cardiac murmur is discovered, inquiry is pursued concerning previous episodes of joint soreness, or febrile illness.

PAST HISTORY

The history of previous illnesses and health problems should be reviewed, and in some instances fully explored, particularly when information *of help in understanding the present complaint* is elicited. No listing of "measles, mumps, whooping cough, and chickenpox in childhood" is sufficient if, in the history of a man with edema, the information is omitted that he had scarlet fever and albuminuria as a child. Inquiry concerning trauma may be pursued, particularly if joint pain or back pain is the chief symptom. A careful analysis of the diet and inquiry concerning appetite, diarrhea, vomiting, or digestive disorders are indicated when weight loss is prominent.

ENVIRONMENTAL HAZARDS

Adverse reactions to *natural* elements in the environment formerly constituted a large part of medical histories: heat, cold, microorganisms, etc.; today in our urban, industrialized society many illnesses are caused by *man-made* machines, pollutants, chemicals, and drugs.

VOLUNTARY USE

Persons in the United States consume vast quantities of drugs, only a small fraction of which are prescribed by physicians. Among the substances most commonly used with druglike actions, but not usually thought of as drugs, are alcohol, tobacco, coffee, tea, and cola drinks.

Alcohol and tobacco, both used chronically by a large percentage of our population, cause many disturbing symptoms and sometimes serious disease.

Aspirin is the drug most widely employed, and although generally considered safe, it not infrequently has unpleasant or dangerous effects. Self-medication with easily-purchased *over-the-counter pharmaceuticals* is nearly universal, involving practically every man, woman, and child. Types of medications commonly ingested include preparations containing vitamins, iron, various "health foods," analgesics, soporifics, stimulants, laxatives, etc. In addition to those ingested are those applied externally, such as ointments, lotions, douches, etc., against eye irritation, dandruff, dermatitis, for feminine hygiene, etc.

Another vast field involving exposure of a large proportion of our population to chemicals is that of *cosmetics:* perfumes, powders, hair dyes, and bleaches, creams and lotions, rouges, nail applications, antiperspirants, deodorants, etc. The incidence of adverse reactions to these is high.

Another tremendous class of chemicals to which everyone is exposed includes *soaps*, detergents, and other household cleansing agents.

So far we have been discussing drugs and chemicals *voluntarily* employed which may or may not be *beneficial* but are often *harmful*.

INVOLUNTARY EXPOSURE

Practically everyone is today exposed to many chemicals, involuntarily and usually without his knowledge. Even the experts are just beginning to realize the ubiquity of the contaminations of the environment, the high degrees of pollution often present, and the severity of the health hazards.

Industry. In many industries the worker is subjected to psychological, physical, or chemical hazards. The physician should be educated about what these may be so that he can evaluate the part they play in many medical histories.

The General Public. Unwittingly man is involuntarily "medicating" himself in many ways. We cannot discuss here in detail the various kinds of chemical threats to which human beings are increasingly subjecting themselves. However, we are concerned here with the medical history, and it is highly important to emphasize that many signs and symptoms may be due to man-created environmental constituents of perilous significance.

In the health history of every person, in present illness or past, there may be pertinent data. Did the conjunctivitis occur after swimming in contaminated water? Did the bronchitis, asthma, or pneumonia begin during exposure to "smog"?

We are brought in contact with or ingest chemicals **sprayed upon plants** or **put into soil.** DDT, among others, constitutes a real danger. Fertilizers may be hazardous.

In the commercial processing of foods various chemicals are often **added as preservatives,** or to affect taste, color, texture, etc. More studies are needed to determine which may be harmless and which are hazardous.

A widespread threat of which many are unaware is the dissemination already taking place of **radioactive nuclear material** from "atom bomb" explosions. Not only in Nagasaki or Hiroshima have human beings and animals absorbed appreciable quantities of such materials. Many of us now have radioactive iodine in our thyroid glands and radioactive strontium in our bones and teeth.

Chemical **pollutants** of air and water and soil have already greatly damaged and increasingly threatened human and animal life. Sources of deleterious material include industrial wastes, human sewage, automobile exhausts, etc.

Excess Technology. Man's technological skills have exceeded his judgment and wisdom. Man himself and his world are being despoiled by his *own products.* In a society largely controlled by technologists, the ability to accomplish a material, physical, mechanical, or chemical feat is considered a mandate. "We can do it, therefore we *must* do it." It should be obvious that such a philosophy is wrong. Knowledge and technologic skills should not alone control actions. Desirability or undesirability of *consequences* should be the paramount consideration. Judgment and wisdom should control and direct technology.

Our technologists today are usually mistakenly called "scientists"—they are not, because science is a branch of knowledge and does not consist of material manipulation and manufacture. Science does not consist of technology; it utilizes technology. Now, let us relate these considerations to the field of medicine.

Too Many Drugs. Medical "scientists" (mostly technologists) have created a vast variety of drugs. Many have become highly useful; a few are truly essential. *The great majority could be dispensed with*, without serious handicaps to the physician or detriment to the health of our people. Reduction in the tremendous number of drugs would improve the practice of medicine, avoid the exposure of patients to many hazards, and save vast amounts of money and wasted effort. Physicians would not be compelled to learn the comparative merits and dangers of perhaps some 40 different antibiotics (or analgesics, or diuretics, etc.), nor would pharmacies have to stock them. All drugs would be much less expensive if pharmaceutical companies were spared the astronomical expense involved in their promotion.

PRESCRIPTION DRUGS

Prescription drugs constitute only a small part of all the medications people are exposed to (and a tiny fraction of the combined exposure to all sorts of chemicals), but here physicians do exert limited control. Physicians write prescriptions, but there are many slips between pen and lips. Physicians can make mistakes; unwittingly and innocently, it is inevitable also that every physician will sometimes advise medications to which certain persons will have unpredictable adverse responses. Also, many persons may be concerned with getting the drug from the pharmacy into the patient, and there is a possibility of error at every juncture. Even when the correct drug arrives at the patient's bedside, he may take (or be given) an excessive amount, or by some mischance he may get a wrong drug by mistake.

With the already tremendous and rapidly increasing therapeutic and diagnostic drug and chemical armamentarium at our disposal, no past history is complete without a history of present and past medications and a record of any *bad effects* from such agents. Even the most commonly used drugs, such as aspirin, quinidine, digitalis, the thiazides and hormonal agents such as thyroid, insulin, corticosteroids, and oral contraceptives, to name only a few, under certain conditions carry considerable risk to the patient. Drugs can be standardized, but patients cannot. Individual idiosyncrasy or hypersensitivity to many chemicals and drugs is quite common. The high frequency of untoward effects in private practice often has been reported.

Less well-known are the chances of drug reaction during a closely supervised period of hospitalization in a university teaching situation. In one of the leading teaching hospitals, a record was kept of adverse responses attributed to widely accepted and well-intentioned diagnostic and therapeutic measures.[13] Every patient admitted to the medical service (1,014 in all) over an eight-month period was included in the study. Twenty per cent of patients had some untoward reaction. Forty-five per cent of the adverse episodes were minor, 20 per cent major, and the balance moderate. Overall, there was a 5 per cent incidence of major (life-threatening) occurrences attibutable to diagnostic or therapeutic procedures. One-half of all the untoward episodes were reactions to drugs used in treatment. Adverse responses observed were (in order of frequency) of the types indicated and due to the drugs specified: pencillin (allergic); antineoplastic agents (toxic); insulin (hypoglycemic); steroids and ACTH; sedatives; anticoagulants; and digitalis (toxic).

FLEXIBILITY OF TECHNIQUE:
ADAPT TO EACH PATIENT

The process of taking the history of past illnesses, as of present disease, should not be pointless and rigidly systematic, but pointed and varied, adapted to each person and his individual problems, so as to draw out the maximum amount of pertinent information.

FAMILY HISTORY

It is not sufficient to ask if there are any known familial diseases. Such a vague and general question is usually answered in the negative. If a patient has symptoms suggesting thyrotoxicosis, one is especially interested in and must inquire specifically about the occurrence of goiter or nervous troubles in the family. Or if migraine is suspected, one inquires particularly about headaches, epilepsy, and allergic or nervous disorders. When a growth or developmental problem is being studied, these characteristics of the close relatives are investigated. When an infectious disease, such as tuberculosis, is suspected, one should learn whether or not the patient could have been exposed to a relative suffering from it. If there is a question of allergic disease, inquiry is made concerning hay fever, hives, asthma, and other allergic manifestations in the family. In other words, every effort should be made by *specific inquiry* to determine whether or not the family history will yield data helpful in understanding the patient's problems. Many disorders have genetic patterns, and the possibility of such conditions should be kept in mind, so that clues are sought in the family history. When an hereditary trait is suspected, a diagram of the pedigree may clarify the nature of the disease.

MARITAL HISTORY

Often much may be learned by inquiry concerning domestic and sexual happiness, compatibility, the emotional tone of the home, the health of the spouse, the number of children, pregnancies, and miscarriages, housing conditions, diet, infections within the family, and family problems affecting husband, wife, or children.

SOCIAL HISTORY

In certain instances, especially of nervous or emotional disorders, the social history is of great importance. It may also bear important relationships to the understanding of obviously organic disease. For example, it is important to know about the excessive use of tobacco by a patient with toxic loss of vision, or about alcoholism in a patient with vitamin deficiencies or jaundice, or about what caused the poor food habits (possible food faddism, or economic problems, etc.), when malnutrition or vitamin deficiency is suspected, or about the emotional factors that may precipitate attacks of angina pectoris or peptic ulcer symptoms.

Persons who are disadvantaged or frustrated economically, educationally, or socially are more subject to many types of disorders, both psychological and physical. Full information about the personal social history is of great importance in understanding illness.

Information is obtained about the patient's education, home and family life, compatibility with siblings and parents, compatibility of parents, possible "broken" home, living conditions, economic status, ambitions and interests, area (urban or rural), country and climate of residence, business, work and social life, recreations, sex experiences, habits, and all of the personal factors that may assist the physician in understanding him more completely *as an individual.*

When sympathetically obtained and skillfully developed, such knowledge often is most important in revealing the origin and the nature of the patient's difficulties.

SEX PROBLEMS

Sexual aberrations seem to be much more common in recent years. Not only psychological disorders, but physical illness of certain types is apt to occur in persons with sexual maladjustment or with guilt syndromes.

DRUGS (ADDICTION)

Widespread use of drugs with habituation is more prevalent recently. Bizarre behavior, accidents, suicides, psychological disorders and physical illness of certain kinds is more common among those involved. Among the drugs commonly implicated are marijuana, LSD, amphetamines, barbiturates, and heroin. Alcohol, although not usually considered to be a drug, causes similar problems.

OCCUPATIONAL HISTORY

Certain occupations expose persons to particular hazards, such as physical injury, muscular or joint strain, nervous tension, viruses, bacteria, fungi, animal infections or animal products, dusts, gases, chemicals, noise, heat, cold, abnormal lighting conditions, unhygienic surroundings, and the possible presence of infected insects. It often is necessary to know what kind of work the patient does and under what conditions. Not only the physical conditions of the work itself, but relationships with employers and fellow workers may be important in determining, for example, whether irritability, headache, undue fatigue, tremor, or increasing inefficiency and inaccuracy may be a result of work problems.

The occupations of children likewise should be studied. School progress and conditions and play habits and environment may be related to the patient's symptoms.

INTERPRETING SYMPTOMS

The History as a Guide to Other Studies. The history largely consists of an analysis of the presenting symptom or symptoms and of the associated information that may be pertinent. The next step usually employed in the diagnostic method is the physical examination, and thereafter certain laboratory procedures may be utilized. The physician who pursues as far as possible the logical processes of reasoning based upon and initiated by his analysis of the symptoms often finds that he can understand the pathologic physiology leading to the complaints, even with no data but the history. Thinking through as far as possible toward a diagnosis and writing down preliminary *diagnostic impressions*, arranged in order of probability or possibility at the end of the history, are useful clinical exercises.

Do Physical Examinations with Curiosity. Such a practice enables one to perform the *physical examination* with *discrimination and curiosity*, not as a routine requirement. For example, if symptoms have suggested a blood dyscrasia, particular attention is paid to the skin color, the mouth and the tongue, and to the lymph nodes and the spleen; or, if the patient has had arthritis or rheumatism, the heart, the extremities, the joints, the phalanges, and the tonsils are studied with special care.

Guided Studies. When certain diagnostic possibilities are under consideration, the choice of certain *special studies, tests,* and *laboratory procedures* is logical. *Purpose, discrimination,* and a *guided curiosity* depending upon the problem and the data yielded by the history and physical examination should direct the choice of special tests and laboratory studies. Other irrelevant studies may be omitted, and time, expense, discomfort, and possible untoward effects may be avoided. Thus, if epigastric distress relieved by food is present, gastroscopy, gastric analysis, and x-ray studies of the gastrointestinal tract may promptly yield the diagnosis. Or if pain that may originate in the ureter is present, a urinalysis and an x-ray may at once give positive evidence of a kidney stone.

Omit Useless Tests. Interpretation of symptoms leads the clinician to choose valuable laboratory tests, but to avoid compilation of useless data. He will secure blood sugar tests in diabetes, but not a sugar tolerance test. He will avoid bone marrow puncture or liver biopsy puncture if the hematologic or hepatic diagnostic pictures are already clear. The wise doctor will protect his patient from even slight dangers or small pains or minimal expenses unless possible gains warrant them. He will not order a battery of tests in the hope that his shotgun diagnostic method will accidentally score a bull's-eye.

BASIC PATHOPHYSIOLOGY

Chief Groups. As he attempts to interpret the signs and symptoms in each study of a patient, the physician will find his diagnostic impressions falling into one or more of four large groups on the basis of the chief types of pathophysiology involved. These groups are:

Neuroses and Psychoses
Psychosomatic Diseases
Pathophysiologic Diseases (Functional Disorders) without Visible Pathology
Organic Diseases

There are many interrelationships and overlappings between these groups; that is, each is not clearly distinct from the other. Also, any one person's problems may fit well into several of the categories, although his principal disorder may lie clearly in one group. Thus, the main problem may be pulmonary tuberculosis, but a neurosis also may cause serious symptoms; or an illness with early characteristics of a neurosis may be complicated by the development of a peptic ulcer.

It is highly useful to the physician engaged in the process of interpreting signs and symptoms to keep in mind these basic types of disease processes. Each is discussed briefly below.

Neuroses

Studies[3,4] have shown that from 30 to 40 per cent of persons consulting internists and diagnosticians have psychoneuroses. These psychoneuroses may cause many of the symptoms discussed in the various chapters in this book: chest pain, backache, headache, malnutrition, obesity, nervousness, fatigue, to name just a few.

Psychological problems may occur alone or may simulate organic disease, or be interrelated with true organic disease. Emotional illness can provoke symptoms duplicating those of somatic disorders; it can even produce definite somatic lesions. Physical illness can, of course, beget many emotional and psychological responses. This vast field is discussed in the chapter on Conversion Symptoms.

It is not possible, nor is it advisable, for the doctor to refer all such patients to psychiatrists. Often the mechanism of production of the symptom can be elucidated and the patient can be relieved through simple measures by the general physician. Careful history with proper interpretation of symptoms will reveal which patients are to be included in this large group with "functional" or "nervous" symptoms.

Psychosomatic Disease

In recent years there has been ample demonstration that not only functional "nervous" symptoms may result from emotional or psychic disorders, but that organic disease may be so caused. *Psychosomatic illness* is common, and the more familiar the physician is with the two-way interplay of mental and emotional factors with body physiology and even with body structure, the better he will be able to interpret signs and symptoms.

Psychosomatic interrelationships are considered in all the chapters of this book, because they are important in the study of every sign and every symptom, in every complaint of every patient. In the chapter on Conversion Symptoms, the pathophysiology involved is discussed.

Pathophysiologic Diseases (Functional Disorders) Without Visible Pathology

Many illnesses are attributed to "functional" abnormalities, which usually means that there is disturbed physiology but there is no known structural defect involved in the etiology. Physical or structural derangements as understood in the past were those visible through the microscope. Today we are aware that absence or excess of certain chemical entities, or abnormalities in the chemical configuration of many substances, can account for a number of diseases. Although not visible to the eye, these defects are detected and measured by other tests. They are, in a sense, therefore physical and structural.

Whether we should include such chemical abnormalities in the categories of "organic" disease has been a problem, depending upon the meaning implied by the word "organic." If we mean by this word the old concept of a visible change in a tissue, these disorders are not organic. If, instead, we mean *structural*, including chemical composition of body constituents, chemical disorders are thus included as *organic* as contrasted with *functional*. We should adopt a different word; "organic" bears echoes of body organs Structural seems a better term to carry the concept we intend.

Whether there is ultimately any disorder of function without a causative structural defect remains uncertain. As our knowledge increases, there is a steady dwindling in the number of disturbances still considered "functional" (without known material origin). Even various psychological illnesses are believed to have chemical etiologies.

Organic Disease

Possibly 60 per cent of patients may be expected to have an organic basis for their symptoms. As one diagnostician has sagely pointed out,[4] *clinical-pathologic conferences* offer excellent training in the differential diagnosis of fatal diseases with an anatomic substratum, but there are many organic illnesses which are functional and nonfatal, and the clinician must be interested in these. He must be concerned not only in the diagnosis of anatomic disease, but in pathophysiologic disorders without visible causes, and also in the personal and emotional problems of victims of disease. Study of differential diagnosis based upon autopsies[5] is recommended highly, but one must keep in mind that, fortunately, a large percentage of the clinician's practice will have similar symptoms with much less dire implications.

It has been estimated that "about 55 per cent of all internal diseases can be diagnosed from aspect and history alone, an additional 20 per cent by physical examination and another 20 per cent by laboratory tests. The rest of the patients remain undiagnosed, regardless of whether they get well or die."[4]

SUMMARY

First the physician finds out what the signs and symptoms are (the patient's complaints) and traces their evolution through the clinical course of the presenting illness. He must determine their true character, not accept uncritically what the patient or someone else thinks they are. He must *analyze* the signs and symptoms to ascertain the pathophysiologic processes involved.

Interpretation of signs and symptoms involves aid secured from all parts of the history, from the physical examination and from laboratory studies and special tests.

Interpretation may be faulty if based upon inaccurate or incomplete information. Therefore, analysis of the symptom or symptoms must precede interpretation. With a good history the physician, by virtue of his knowledge of the mechanisms of disease, of pathologic physiology, and of the causation of signs and symptoms, may arrive at a tentative conclusion concerning the malady present.

The **physical examination** can be done with curiosity and true interest when guided by a perceptive history. Examination so conducted is much more productive of significant information. There should be no such thing as a *routine* physical examination.

The choice of **laboratory studies** and **special tests** should be guided by the particular indications of each individual patient's history. Indiscriminate tests are wasteful and hazardous to the patient. Only studies that offer hope of giving *pertinent* data should be done. The diagnostic study must be guided throughout by consideration of the pathophysiologic processes believed to be likely causes of the patient's complaints. Unrelated physical findings or laboratory data of interesting or important nature may be discovered, but one's primary aim should be the detection of the cause of the symptoms. Thus may we progress in the understanding of disease and in the development of means to relieve or cure it.

CONCLUSION

Since so much depends upon it, the history, with its careful analysis of the patient's symptoms, deserves the physician's utmost attention and effort. Many believe that obtaining a good history requires practice of the greatest art in medicine.[6] The editors of this book are convinced that eliciting a good history *and interpreting it* certainly constitute the greatest of the medical arts.

REFERENCES

1. Bird, B.: Talking With Patients, Philadelphia, Lippincott, 1955.
2. Cabot, R. C.: Differential Diagnosis, Philadelphia, Saunders, 1915.
3. Allan, F. N., and Kaufman, M.: Nervous factors in general practice, J.A.M.A. 138:1135, 1948.
4. Bauer, J.: Differential Diagnosis of Internal Diseases, New York, Grune, 1955.
5. Harvey, A. McG., and Bordley, J.: Differential Diagnosis, Philadelphia, Saunders, 1955
6. Platt, R.: Two essays on the practice of medicine, Lancet, 2:305, 1947.
7. Forkner, C. E.: Record of medical history, Arch. Intern. Med. 106:22, 1960.
8. Payson, H. E., Gaenslen, E. C., and Stargardter, F. L.: Time study of an internship on a university medical service, New Eng. J. Med. 264:439, 1961.
9. Wittkower, E. D., and White, K. L.: Bedside manners, Brit. Med. J. 1:1432, 1954.
10. Meares, A.: The Medical Interview, Springfield, Ill., Thomas, 1958.
11. Stevenson, I.: Medical History Taking, New York, Hoeber-Harper, 1960.
12. Ruesch, J.: Declining clinical tradition, J.A.M.A. 182:110, 1962.
13. Schimmel, E. M.: The hazards of hospitalization, Ann. Intern. Med. 60:100, 1964.
14. Barnett, G. O.: Computers in patient care, New Eng. J. Med. 279:1321, 1968.
15. Jacquez, J. (ed.): The Diagnostic Process, Ann Arbor, Mich., Malloy Lithographing, Inc., 1964.
16. Wilson, J., and Jungner, G.: Principles and Practice of Screening for Disease, New York, Columbia Univ. Press, 1968.

2

Growth and Sex Development

WILLIAM H. DAUGHADAY

The human organism develops from a single cell to a sexually mature person of adult stature in a period of 16 to 20 years. In view of the extraordinary complexity of the processes involved, derangement in normal growth and development provides one of the most sensitive manifestations of disease in childhood.

BODY SIZE

GENETIC ENDOWMENT

The fertilized ovum contains within it all the programmed information required for embryonic growth and postnatal development. While it is legitimate to focus attention on the nucleus of the cell as the storehouse of genetic information, cytoplasmic influences should not be completely overlooked. It is known that mitochondria contain DNA which participates in the regulation of protein synthesis independent of the nucleus. It is therefore possible that cytoplasmic changes may prove important in subsequent growth.

The bulk of the genetic information of the human being resides in 46 chromosomes. The correct number was recognized by Tijo and Levan in 1956. As shown in Figure 2-1, the chromosomes can be matched depending on their size and the position of the centromere into 22 pairs common to both male and female human cells and an additional set of sex chromosomes. In the female there are two relatively large X chromosomes. In the normal male there is one X chromosome and a very short Y chromosome with its centromere near one end of the chromosome (acrocentric).

For the purpose of this discussion, the many detrimental mutations which impair normal growth by producing overt disease will be disregarded. There remain many other gene mutations which affect stature without impairing health or inducing deformity. While the existence of such hereditary influences are widely accepted by the general public, the number of factors involved and the manner in which growth is determined remains very much of a mystery. More is known of the participation of the sex chromosomes in the regulation of growth than of the autosomes because of the various effects of differences in number of the X and Y chromosomes which have been encountered.

In the early embryo both X chromosomes of the female participate equally in cellular regulation but after the 16th day to the 18th day of fetal life, one of the two X chromosomes exists in a condensed form which can be recognized in a heterochromatic bead (chromatin body) just inside the nuclear membrane (Fig. 2-2). This sex chromosome plays a restricted role in determining ribonucleic acid synthesis and thereby influencing cellular processes. The X chromosome of the chromatin body is also characterized by the fact that its DNA is replicated late in the process of cell division. If more than two X chromosomes are present, the maximum number of observed sex chromatin bodies is one less than the total number of X chromosomes. Once the choice has

been made between one or the other X chromosomes for full metabolic participation in any given cell line, this choice remains fixed for all subsequent cell divisions of that line. While the choice between normal X chromosomes appears to be random, there is a beneficial bias for abnormal X chromosomes to be selected for formation of sex chromatin bodies.

It is incorrect to consider the DNA condensed in the chromatin body as devoid of function. Persons with only a single X chromosome are phenotypically female but have only a streak representing the gonad. They

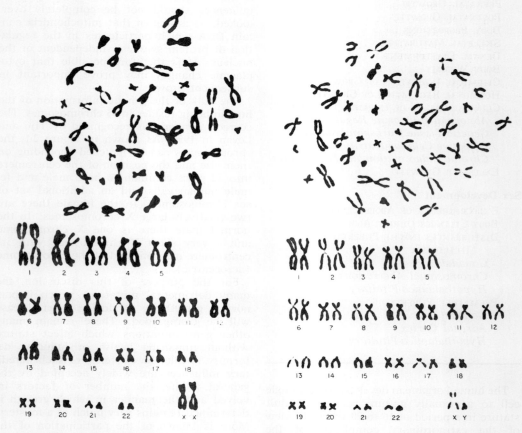

FIG. 2-1. (*Left*) Appearance of the chromosomes of a dividing human cell at metaphase. Each chromosome is longitudinally doubled, the chromatids (potential daughter chromosomes) been held together at their respective centromeres. (*Bottom*) Karyotype of a normal human female showing twenty-two pairs of autosomes and an XX sex chromosome constitution. This was constructed from the preparation above by sorting and matching homologous pairs of chromosomes.

(*Right*) Chromosomes of a dividing human cell at metaphase; from a male. (*Bottom*) The chromosome constitution of a normal human male containing 22 pairs of autosomes and an XY sex chromosome complex. (Barr, M. L., and Carr, D. H.: Canad. M.A.J., 83:979)

ing repeated measurements on the same child. Replotting the data on the basis of years from the peak height velocity indicates the general uniformity of pattern of pubertal growth. The shaded areas in Figures 2-5 and 2-6 have been constructed from longitudinal data with normalization of the age of puberty.

BODY PROPORTIONS

In addition to measurement of height, it is frequently informative to make other simple measurements. These include: 1) span (from finger tip to finger tip); 2) lower segment (top of symphysis pubis to the floor); 3) upper segment (difference between total height and lower segment); 4) circumference of head; 5) circumference of chest; 6) circumference of abdomen. In Tables 2-1 and 2-2 are given the average normal measurements for females and males from birth to age 20 years as compiled by Wilkins from data of Shelton and Engelbach for Caucasian Americans.

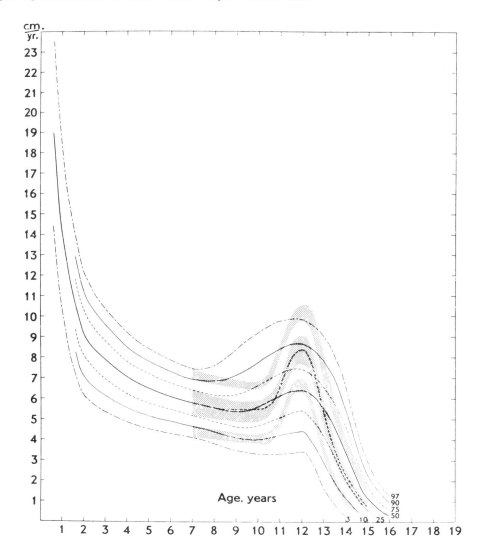

FIG. 2-6. Whole year velocity standards for height of British girls. The shaded areas represent typical curves for children whose peak velocity occurs at the average time. (Reprinted by permission from Tanner, J. M., Whitehouse, R. H., and Takaishi, M.: Arch. Dis. Child. 41:454, 1966)

TABLE 2-1. NORMAL MEASUREMENTS IN RELATION TO AGE (MALE)*†

AGE	HEIGHT	WEIGHT	SPAN	UPPER MEAS.	LOWER MEAS.	RATIO U/L	HEAD	CHEST	ABDO- MEN
Birth	20.2	7.4	19.1	12.7	7.5	1.69	13.9	13.8	13.4
1 Mo.	21.9	10.4	21.1	13.7	8.2	1.67	15.2	14.3	13.8
2 Mos.	23.1	12.0	22.0	14.4	8.7	1.65	16.0	15.6	15.2
3 "	24.1	13.6	23.0	15.0	9.1	1.65	16.6	16.4	16.0
4 "	25.0	15.0	24.0	15.5	9.5	1.63	17.0	16.9	16.5
5 "	25.7	15.8	24.4	15.9	9.8	1.62	17.4	17.2	16.8
6 "	26.4	17.3	25.4	16.3	10.1	1.61	17.7	17.5	17.1
7 "	27.1	18.0	25.9	16.6	10.4	1.61	17.9	17.7	17.3
8 "	27.6	18.7	26.4	16.9	10.7	1.58	18.1	17.9	17.5
9 "	28.1	19.4	26.9	17.2	10.9	1.58	18.2	18.0	17.6
10 "	28.6	20.0	27.3	17.4	11.2	1.55	18.4	18.2	17.7
11 "	29.1	20.7	27.8	17.6	11.5	1.53	18.5	18.3	17.8
12 "	29.5	21.4	28.3	17.9	11.6	1.54	18.6	18.5	17.9
15 "	30.7	22.7	29.3	18.5	12.2	1.52	18.9	18.8	18.2
18 "	31.9	24.6	30.8	19.2	12.7	1.51	19.1	19.1	18.5
21 "	32.9	25.9	31.8	19.6	13.3	1.47	19.3	19.4	18.7
24 "	33.9	27.2	32.7	20.0	13.9	1.44	19.4	19.7	18.9
30 "	35.7	29.2	34.2	20.8	14.9	1.40	19.6	20.2	19.2
36 "	37.3	32.0	36.2	21.3	16.0	1.33	19.8	20.6	19.5
42 "	38.8	34.0	37.7	22.0	16.8	1.31	20.0	21.0	19.8
48 "	40.2	35.5	38.8	22.5	17.7	1.27	20.1	21.4	20.0
54 "	41.5	37.7	40.3	22.9	18.6	1.23	20.3	21.7	20.2
60 "	42.7	39.3	41.4	23.4	19.3	1.21	20.4	22.1	20.4
5½ Yrs.	43.9	41.9	42.9	23.7	20.2	1.17	20.4	22.4	20.6
6 "	45.0	43.9	44.0	24.0	21.0	1.14	20.5	22.7	20.9
6½ "	46.1	45.9	45.1	24.3	21.8	1.11	20.5	23.0	21.1
7 "	47.2	48.1	46.2	24.7	22.5	1.10	20.6	23.3	21.3
7½ "	48.2	50.4	47.3	24.9	23.3	1.07	20.7	23.7	21.5
8 "	49.2	52.8	48.6	25.3	23.9	1.06	20.7	24.0	21.8
8½ "	50.2	55.3	49.8	25.7	24.5	1.05	20.8	24.3	22.0
9 "	51.2	58.0	51.0	26.0	25.2	1.03	20.9	24.6	22.3
9½ "	52.2	61.0	52.2	26.4	25.8	1.02	20.9	25.0	22.5
10 "	53.2	64.3	53.4	26.8	26.4	1.02	21.0	25.3	22.8
10½ "	54.2	67.7	54.5	27.1	27.1	1.00	21.0	25.7	23.0
11 "	55.2	71.2	55.6	27.5	27.7	0.99	21.1	26.1	23.3
11½ "	56.2	74.7	56.7	27.9	28.3	0.99	21.2	26.6	23.6
12 "	57.1	78.3	57.9	28.3	28.8	0.98	21.2	27.0	23.9
12½ "	58.0	82.0	59.1	28.7	29.3	0.98	21.3	27.5	24.2
13 "	58.9	85.8	60.2	29.1	29.8	0.98	21.4	28.0	24.6
13½ "	59.8	89.8	61.3	29.5	30.3	0.97	21.5	28.6	25.0
14 "	60.7	92.0	61.9	29.9	30.8	0.97	21.6	29.1	25.4
14½ "	61.6	96.5	63.0	30.3	31.3	0.97	21.7	29.7	25.9
15 "	62.4	101.4	64.1	30.7	31.7	0.97	21.8	30.3	26.4
15½ "	63.2	103.9	64.7	31.1	32.1	0.97	21.9	31.0	26.8
16 "	64.0	109.0	65.8	31.5	32.5	0.07	22.0	31.7	27.2
16½ "	64.7	111.7	66.4	31.9	32.8	0.97	22.1	32.3	27.5
17 "	65.4	117.7	67.5	32.2	33.2	0.97	22.2	32.9	27.8
17½ "	66.0	121.0	68.1	32.5	33.5	0.97	22.3	33.3	28.0
18 "	66.6	124.4	68.6	32.8	33.8	0.97	22.4	33.7	28.2
18½ "	67.1	127.8	69.2	33.2	33.9	0.98	22.4	34.1	28.4
19 "	67.5	131.4	69.8	33.4	34.1	0.98	22.5	34.4	28.5
19½ "	67.8	135.0	70.4	33.6	34.2	0.98	22.5	34.6	28.6
20 "	68.0	135.0	70.4	33.7	34.3	0.98	22.5	34.7	28.7

* From Williams, R. H.: Textbook of Endocrinology, ed. 4, Philadelphia, Saunders, 1968.
† Dimensions are in inches and weight in pounds.

TABLE 2-2. NORMAL MEASUREMENTS IN RELATION TO AGE (FEMALE)*†

AGE	HEIGHT	WEIGHT	SPAN	UPPER MEAS.	LOWER MEAS.	RATIO U/L	HEAD	CHEST	ABDO-MEN
Birth	19.9	7.5	19.0	12.6	7.3	1.73	13.6	13.6	13.2
1 Mo.	21.5	9.7	20.5	13.5	8.0	1.69	14.9	14.1	13.6
2 Mos.	22.7	11.2	21.4	14.2	8.5	1.67	15.7	15.3	15.0
3 "	23.7	12.7	22.4	14.8	8.9	1.66	16.3	16.0	15.7
4 "	24.6	14.1	23.3	15.2	9.4	1.62	16.7	16.5	16.2
5 "	25.3	15.5	24.3	15.6	9.7	1.61	17.1	16.8	16.5
6 "	26.0	16.2	24.8	16.0	10.0	1.60	17.3	17.0	16.8
7 "	26.6	16.9	25.3	16.3	10.3	1.58	17.5	17.2	17.0
8 "	27.1	17.6	25.8	16.6	10.5	1.58	17.7	17.4	17.2
9 "	27.6	18.2	26.2	16.8	10.8	1.56	17.8	17.6	17.3
10 "	28.1	18.8	26.7	17.0	11.1	1.53	18.0	17.8	17.4
11 "	28.6	19.5	27.2	17.3	11.3	1.53	18.1	17.9	17.5
12 "	29.0	20.1	27.7	17.5	11.5	1.52	18.2	18.1	17.6
15 "	30.2	21.3	28.7	18.1	12.1	1.50	18.5	18.4	17.9
18 "	31.4	23.2	30.1	18.7	12.7	1.47	18.7	18.7	18.2
21 "	32.4	24.4	31.1	19.2	13.2	1.45	18.9	19.0	18.4
24 "	33.4	25.7	32.1	19.6	13.8	1.42	19.0	19.2	18.6
30 "	35.1	27.7	33.6	20.4	14.7	1.39	19.2	19.6	18.9
36 "	36.7	29.8	35.1	20.9	15.8	1.32	19.4	20.0	19.1
42 "	38.2	31.9	36.6	21.5	16.7	1.29	19.6	20.4	19.3
48 "	39.6	34.0	38.1	22.0	17.6	1.25	19.7	20.7	19.5
54 "	40.9	36.2	39.7	22.4	18.5	1.21	19.9	21.0	19.7
60 "	42.2	37.7	40.7	22.9	19.3	1.19	20.0	21.4	19.9
5½ Yrs.	43.4	40.2	42.3	23.2	20.2	1.15	20.1	21.7	20.0
6 "	44.6	42.0	43.3	23.7	20.9	1.13	20.1	22.0	20.2
6½ "	45.7	44.0	44.4	24.1	21.6	1.12	20.2	22.3	20.4
7 "	46.8	47.2	46.0	24.4	22.4	1.09	20.3	22.7	20.5
7½ "	47.9	49.5	47.1	24.7	23.2	1.06	20.3	23.0	20.7
8 "	48.9	52.0	48.2	25.0	23.9	1.05	20.4	23.4	20.8
8½ "	49.9	54.6	49.3	25.4	24.5	1.04	20.5	23.8	21.0
9 "	50.9	57.4	50.4	25.7	25.2	1.02	20.5	24.2	21.2
9½ "	51.9	60.7	51.5	26.1	25.8	1.01	20.6	24.6	21.5
10 "	53.0	63.6	52.6	26.7	26.3	1.01	20.7	25.0	21.8
10½ "	54.1	67.2	53.7	27.2	26.9	1.01	20.8	25.5	22.1
11 "	55.3	72.4	55.3	27.7	27.6	1.00	20.9	26.1	22.4
11½ "	56.5	76.2	56.3	28.2	28.3	1.00	20.9	26.6	22.8
12 "	57.6	80.6	57.5	28.7	28.9	0.99	21.0	27.1	23.2
12½ "	58.7	85.1	58.5	29.2	29.5	0.99	21.1	27.6	23.6
13 "	59.7	90.0	59.7	29.7	30.0	0.99	21.2	28.1	23.9
13½ "	60.6	95.4	60.8	30.3	30.3	1.00	21.3	28.5	24.2
14 "	61.4	101.4	61.3	30.6	30.8	0.99	21.4	28.9	24.5
14½ "	62.0	104.5	62.4	30.9	31.1	0.99	21.5	29.3	24.7
15 "	62.5	107.7	63.0	31.2	31.3	1.00	21.6	29.6	24.8
15½ "	62.9	110.9	63.6	31.4	31.5	1.00	21.7	29.9	25.0
16 "	63.2	110.9	63.6	31.6	31.6	1.00	21.7	30.1	25.1
16½ "	63.5	114.2	64.2	31.8	31.7	1.00	21.8	30.3	25.2
17 "	63.7	114.2	64.2	31.9	31.8	1.00	21.8	30.5	25.3
17½ "	63.9	117.5	64.8	32.0	31.9	1.00	21.8	30.7	25.4
18 "	64.0	117.5	64.8	32.1	31.9	1.01	21.9	30.8	25.5
18½ "	64.0	117.5	64.8	32.1	31.9	1.01	21.9	30.8	25.5
19 "	64.0	117.5	64.8	32.1	31.9	1.01	21.9	30.9	25.6
19½ "	64.0	117.5	64.8	32.1	31.9	1.01	21.9	30.9	25.6
20 "	64.0	117.5	64.8	32.1	31.9	1.01	21.9	31.0	25.7

* From Williams, R. H.: Textbook of Endocrinology, ed. 4, Philadelphia, Saunders, 1968.
† Dimensions are in inches and weight in pounds.

The most useful measurement of body proportions is the ratio of the upper to the lower segment of the body (U:L). At birth the trunk is relatively long and therefore the ratio is approximately 1.7:1. Normally, this ratio falls with age so that after 10 or 11 years the two body segments are approximately equal. A number ·of characteristic changes in the ratio of body segments can be recognized in disease. In congenital hypothyroidism the body proportions remain infantile, with a failure of the U:L ratio to fall. In hypogonadism the absence of sex hormones permits continued epiphysial growth of extremities, so the U:L ratio is less than 1. A somewhat similar pattern in growth exists in Marfan's syndrome despite the occurrence of puberty. It should be remembered that the norms for the U:L ratio have been obtained from Caucasian individuals. A relatively greater lower segment length and span breadth is found normally in many Negroes.

Abnormalities in body proportions can be anticipated in congenital or acquired diseases which affect either the extremities or the spine. In achondroplasia the predominant effect is shortening of the extremities, while in Morquio's disease the primary growth disturbance is in the spine.

SKELETAL MATURATION

Skeletal growth is the result of cartilage proliferation and the conversion of cartilage into bone. Growth ceases with the obliteration of the cartilage proliferation which occurs at the epiphysial plates. Primary centers of ossification are established in utero; secondary centers of ossification develop after birth. The sequence in time of appearance of the secondary centers of ossification is fairly predictable, as is also the order of the fusion of the epiphysial and diaphysial centers of calcification (Fig. 2-7). X-rays of the bones of growing children have long been used to estimate the relative maturity of any single subject as compared to certain population norms. The method which is

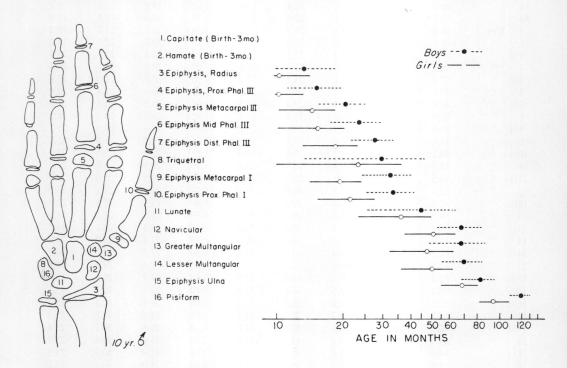

FIG. 2-7. Diagrammatic representation of hand and wrist of a 10-year-old boy. The circles on the accompanying chart represent the average age at the time of ossification of the individual bones. The bars represent one standard deviation from the mean. (Data obtained from Greulich and Pyle, after Parker, M. L., and Daughaday, W. H.: The Pituitary in Disorders of Growth, Chicago, Year Book Medical Publishers, Inc., 1962)

most practical in clinical practice is to examine the hands and wrists by radiography.
The films are then compared to an atlas of
representative films accumulated from longitudinal studies of a relatively small group
of normal children. The commonly used
standards of Gruelich and Pyle were derived
from study on California children who were
primarily Caucasian. Their relevance to
other populations and other social settings
can be questioned. The actual interpretation
of the films is seldom uniform and may be
influenced by subjective judgments such as
the relative importance attached to carpal
ossification centers as compared to the characteristics of the phalangeal epiphyses. The
method is of limited value in the early
months of life where more reliable information can be obtained by examination of the
knees. A more elaborate system of interpretation of radiographs has been recommended
by Tanner and Whitehouse based on a scor-
ing system for each bone in the hand and
wrist. Norms have been established for this
grading system for a relatively large population of British children with varied social
backgrounds. These norms would appear to
be at least one year behind the Greulich and
Pyle standards.

In 10 per cent of cases there may be
asymmetry of skeletal maturation between
the two sides of the body or maturation in
the hands and wrist may not be representative of the maturation in epiphysial centers
in other parts of the body. Bilateral examination of all epiphysial centers would lead
to a greater reliability in estimating bone
maturation, but the increased expense and
the greater radiation exposure negate the
practicality of this approach.

Bone maturation is expressed as "bone
age" by matching the individual's radiographs with age standards. Wilkins has proposed a useful method of comparing bone
age with height age and other developmental
parameters. As shown in Figure 2-8 a plot
is made of the developmental age versus the
chronologic age of the subject. The developmental age is defined as the age at which
the average child achieves the growth parameter in question such as height, weight,
bone maturity, mental development, etc. In
this way it is easy to detect whether specific
alterations of one or more parameters is occurring. For instance, in hypothyroidism the
bone age is more markedly retarded than
height while in hypopituitarism both height

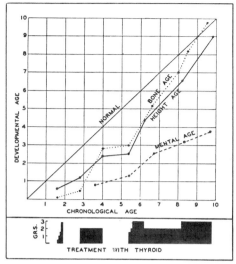

FIG. 2-8. Chart illustrates mehod of following and comparing growth and development. Chronologic age is plotted horizontally and developmental age is plotted
vertically. The patient's "height age" indicates that he has the height of an average
child of the same sex of the age specified.
Such a chart permits a comparison of the
rate of growth with that of osseous and
mental development.

The case shown is a cretin whose thyroid
medication was omitted during two periods
because of failure of the parents to cooperate. The resulting retardation in growth
and development are shown. By this
method of charting, inadequate treatment
sometimes is detected by a lag in growth
and development, even when other signs of
deficiency are not obvious. (Wilkins, L.:
The Diagnosis and Treatment of Endocrine
Disorders in Childhood and Adolescence,
ed. 2, Springfield, Thomas, 1957)

age and bone age are proportionately retarded.

The physician is frequently called upon to
make a prediction concerning the future
growth of a child. Some indication is provided by the percentile position on the height
attainment charts. A better prediction is possible when the degree of bone maturation is
also considered. The tables of Bayley and
Pinneau were constructed from longitudinal
studies of a relatively few children and indicate the percentage of mature stature
reached at any given bone age. Separate
tables are provided for boys and girls and
the tables are further subdivided for children whose bone age is retarded, parallel, or

TABLE 2-3. CHRONOLOGY OF DENTITION*

							ROOT
	TOOTH		FIRST EVIDENCE	CROWN	ERUPTION	ROOT	RESORP-
			OF CALCIFICATION	COMPLETED		COMPLETED	TION
	Name	Number					BEGINS
DECIDUOUS TEETH	Lower central incisors	L. I.	5th month in utero	4 mos.	6-8 mos.	1½-2 yrs.	5-6 yrs.
	Upper incisors Lower lateral	U.I. & II	5th month in utero	5 mos.	8-10 mos.	1½-2 yrs.	5-6 yrs.
	incisors	L. II	5th month in utero	5 mos.	10-14 mos.	1½-2 yrs.	5-6 yrs.
	Canines (cuspids)	III	6th month in utero	9 mos.	16-20 mos.	2½-3 yrs.	6-7 yrs.
	First molars	IV	5th month in utero	6 mos.	12-16 mos.	2-2½ yrs.	4-5 yrs.
	Second molars	V	6th month in utero	10-12 mos.	20-30 mos.	3 yrs.	4-5 yrs.
UPPER JAW	Central incisor	1	3-4 mos.	4-5 yrs.	7-8 yrs.	10 yrs.	
	Lateral incisor	2	1 yr.	4-5 yrs.	8-9 yrs.	11 yrs.	
	Canine (cuspid)	3	4-5 mos.	6-7 yrs.	11-12 yrs.	13-15 yrs.	
	First bicuspid	4	1½-1¾ yrs.	5-6 yrs.	10-11 yrs.	12-13 yrs.	
	Second bicuspid	5	2-2¼ yrs.	6-7 yrs.	10-12 yrs.	12-14 yrs.	
	First molar	6	At birth	2½-3 yrs.	6-7 yrs.	0-10 yrs.	
	Second molar	7	2½-3 yrs.	7-8 yrs.	12-14 yrs.	14-16 yrs.	
	Third molar	8	7-9 yrs.	12-16 yrs.	17-30 yrs.	18-25 yrs.	
LOWER JAW	Central incisor	1	3-4 mos.	4-5 yrs.	6-7 yrs.	9 yrs.	
	Lateral incisor	2	3-4 mos.	4-5 yrs.	7-8 yrs.	10 yrs.	
	Canine (cuspid)	3	4-5 mos.	6-7 yrs.	10-11 yrs.	12-14 yrs.	
	First bicuspid	4	1¾-2 yrs.	5-6 yrs.	10-12 yrs.	12-13 yrs.	
	Second bicuspid	5	2¼-2½ yrs.	6-7 yrs.	11-12 yrs.	13-14 yrs.	
	First molar	6	At birth	2½-3 yrs.	6-7 yrs.	9-10 yrs.	
	Second molar	7	2½-3 yrs.	7-8 yrs.	12-13 yrs.	14-15 yrs.	
	Third molar	8	8-10 yrs.	12-16 yrs.	17-30 yrs.	18-25 yrs.	

(PERMANENT TEETH label spans Upper Jaw and Lower Jaw sections)

* Holt and McIntosh: Pediatrics, ed. 12, New York, Appleton-Century-Crofts.

advanced as compared to chronological age. In many cases these tables are useful in reassuring concerned parents of short children with delayed maturation and parents of tall children who are advanced in their skeletal maturity that final height will not be grossly abnormal.

DENTAL DEVELOPMENT

The development, eruption, and shedding of deciduous teeth and the formation and eruption of permanent teeth follow a regular sequence which is given in Table 2-3. Those disease processes which accelerate or retard bony development such as thyroid deficiency or pituitary deficiency often similarly affect dental development.

BODY WEIGHT

The measurement of body weight is a common procedure in any medical examination. The parameter is a less useful one than height in the assessment of growth but it does provide an indication of the nutritional state of the subject. If the weight is greater than predicted for height and general build, it is usually assumed that the subject is overweight, possibly obese, and when the weight is below the predicted value, reduced fat depots are assumed. The limitations of weight as an indication of body composition should be recognized from common experience. Many well-muscled athletes exceed the normal standards of weight and many older persons with atrophied muscles may have disproportionately large fatty depots, despite "normal" weight.

To provide more accurate measurements of the growth of individual constituents of the body, special methods are required which are not generally available clinically. Measurement of total body density can be performed by weighing in water or by displacement of gases. Knowing the density of fat and the density of "lean body mass" it is possible to calculate the relative contribution of each. An ingenious method for determining the metabolically active cellular mass is by measuring the body content of potassium 40. This isotope is naturally radioactive and emits gamma radiation with a characteristic spectrum which allows it to be distinguished from other radioactive atoms contained in the body. Because potassium is such an important and relatively uniformly distributed atom of intracellular water, its measurement in a total body counter provides an index of the cellular metabolic mass.

Although these methods require special, cumbersome and expensive instrumentation and rarely are applicable to clinical problems, the results of such measurements have provided information of interest concerning human growth. The rise in lean body mass as a function of age is shown in Figure 2-9. The rise in lean body mass is progressive throughout the growing period for both males and females. The period of growth is essentially completed between 14 and 16 years in girls but persists beyond age 17 in boys.

The pattern of growth of fatty tissues is considerably different in males and females. This is most clearly shown when the percentage of fat is plotted as a function of age, Figure 2-10. In boys, relative fattiness increases during the prepubertal years and then falls after puberty. In females, there is no fall in proportion of body fat occurring with puberty; relative fattiness increases after puberty.

Because of the importance of measurements of body fat in health and nutrition surveys, simpler methods have been sought. Because about half the body fat is deposited under the skin, measuring the thickness of skin folds has been advanced as a technique to estimate adiposity or obesity. Special calipers have been devised which exert a defined pressure over a standard area. A number of studies have attempted to correlate skin fold thickness of different parts of the body with relative body fat content. Some have challenged the use of the triceps skin fold and have measured several skin

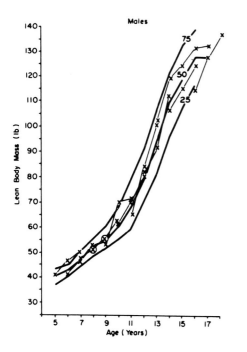
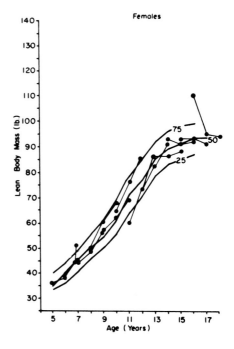

FIG. 2-9. Lean body mass as a function of age. Males are presented on the left and females on the right. The heavy lines described the 25, 50 and 75 percentiles from the 1963 sample. The thin lines plot a series of three annual values for individual children ranked as 50 percentile for their age from the 1965 sample. A circled point represents two children with the same value. Estimates made on basis of multiple regression equations of Cheek by Rauh and Schumsky. (Reprinted by permission from Cheek, D. B.: Human Growth, Energy and Intelligence, Philadelphia, Lea & Febiger, 1968, p. 246)

areas. Unfortunately, these methods have not been standardized sufficiently for general use but such information is accumulating.

For further discussion of body fat and body weight see Chapter 37 on Obesity.

CHEMICAL INDICATION OF GROWTH

A number of chemical measurements provide useful information concerning the growth of certain tissues. One such measurement is the determination of urinary hydroxyproline. The urine contains small amounts of free hydroxyproline and much larger quantities of hydroxyproline present as oligopeptides. Only very small amounts of larger hydroxyproline containing peptides are present in the urine. All urinary hydroxyproline is derived from collagen catabolism. In the adult, the major site of

collagen breakdown is in the skeleton and is related to the remodeling of bone. In growing children a certain fraction of newly synthesized collagen is lost from the connective tissue before it can be incorporated into mature insoluble collagen. Some of the cleavage products of enzymatic action on collagen resist further peptidase digestion and appear in the urine as hydroxyproline containing peptides.

Normally, total urinary hydroxyproline rises progressively during childhood with peak excretions noted at the time of puberty (Fig. 2-11). Much lower values are found in adults. When growth is impaired, urinary hydroxyproline falls. When the cause of the growth failure is eliminated the excretion of hydroxyproline returns to normal. This parameter has been of particular use in the study of the effects of growth hormone in

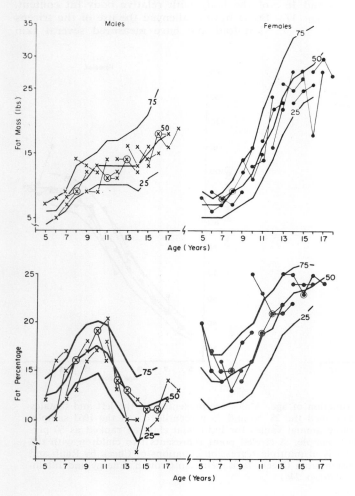

FIG. 2-10. Changes in body fat as a function of age. Fat mass is presented above and fat percentage below. Males are presented on the left and females on the right. The heavy lines described the 25, 50 and 75 percentiles from the 1963 sample. The thin lines plot a series of three annual values for individual children ranked as 50 percentile for their age from the 1965 sample. A circled point represents two children with the same value. (Reprinted by permission from Cheek, D. B.: Human Growth, Energy and Intelligence, Philadelphia, Lea & Febiger, 1968, p. 247)

treatment of dwarfism. The measurement can not be directly equated with net growth of connective tissue, because some of the highest levels are encountered in disease states associated with rapid bone turnover, e.g. Paget's disease or hyperparathyroidism, in which no net accretion of collagen is occurring.

Another chemical parameter of body composition is the measurement of urinary creatinine. This constituent of urine is derived entirely from muscle creatine, or, more likely, its phosphorylated derivative. Nearly all body creatine is located within muscles and the rate of conversion of creatine to creatinine is a relatively constant 2 per cent per day. It is evident therefore that urinary creatinine provides a reasonable estimate of total muscle mass. By correlating urine creatinine with total calculated muscle mass, Cheek concluded that one gram of urine creatinine was equivalent to about 20 Kg. of muscle mass. The measurement of urinary creatinine has two general applications which are based on these considerations. The constancy of urinary creatinine from day to day provides a reasonable indication of the completeness of urine collection. Comparison of the excretion of individuals of different size may be achieved by expressing the urinary excretion of a given constituent per gram of creatinine. For instance, the excretion of urinary 17-hydroxy-corticosteroids when expressed per gram of creatinine is relatively constant during the growing years.

HORMONAL REGULATION OF GROWTH

Normal growth is dependent on the secretion of several key hormones. The most important of these is the **pituitary growth hormone.** We now know that this hormone is a single chain polypeptide of 188 amino acids. The somatotrophic cells of the pituitary synthesize the hormone and store it in large characteristic granules. The release of the hormone from the pituitary is regulated by a hypothalamic neurohumor, the growth hormone releasing factor, which enters the hypothalamico-pituitary portal system of the veins in the region of the median eminence and is transported to the adenohypophysis.

Plasma growth hormone levels remain elevated in the early days of life but after several weeks plasma levels are about the same level as in older children. There is no clearly recognizable difference between growth hormone levels of rapidly growing children and those of adults without net somatic growth. Again, most investigators have not found any striking change at the time of puberty. These fragmentary observations can not be considered definitive because of the inconstant and episodic nature of growth hormone secretion. It is known that a number of factors such as hypoglycemia, exercise, amino acid loads, and even psychic stress can elevate plasma growth hormone. The instability of plasma growth hormone makes it difficult to assess the total production of hormone in any human subject. More accurate appraisals by recourse

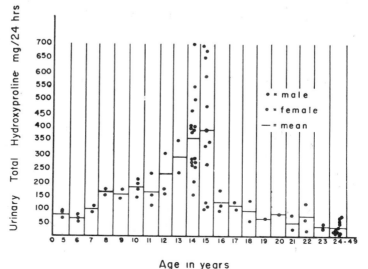

FIG. 2-11. Twenty-four hour urinary total hydroxyproline excretion by 80 normal subjects from 5 to 49 years of age on an ad lib. diet. (Reprinted by permission from Jones, C. R. et al.: Urinary hydroxyproline excretion in normal children and adolescents, Proc. Soc. Exp. Biol. Med. 115:85, 1964)

TABLE 2-4

A FUNCTIONAL CLASSIFICATION
OF GROWTH IMPAIRMENT

1. *Abnormal Endocrine Regulation*
   Decreased Growth Hormone Activity
      Secondary (hypothalamic)
         hyposomatotropism
      Primary (pituitary) hyposomatotropism
         Genetic—monohormonal
         Sporadic mono- or polyhormonal
      Impaired sulfation factor activation
   Hypothyroidism
   Hypoinsulinism
   Hyperadrenal corticism

2. *Tissue Unresponsiveness—Genetic Factors*
   Chromosomal Imbalance
      Monosomy X and other X chromosome
         deficits
      Trisomy 21—Down's syndrome
   General tissue unresponsiveness
      Racial—pygmies
      Familial short stature
   Specific genetic disorders of bone and
      cartilage

3. *Tissue Unresponsiveness—Nutritional Factors*
   Major nutriments
   Vitamins
   Minerals
   Oxygen

4. *Chronic Inflammation and Toxic States*

to repetitive or continuous sampling techniques have been used in investigations.

Growth hormone exerts multiple effects in the body other than augmenting growth, such as promoting lipolysis, and antagonizing the action of insulin. These effects are difficult to relate to the anabolic effect of the hormone. It is the promotion of protein synthesis which is of obvious importance in a consideration of human growth. The exact mechanism of this action on many tissues remains obscure because it has been extremely difficult to reproduce the effects observed in vivo by the direct addition of growth hormone in vitro. My laboratory has presented evidence that growth hormone acts on skeletal tissue by induction of a secondary mediator. The presence of this mediator in plasma is most conveniently measured by its ability to stimulate the uptake of sulfate by cartilage from hypophysectomized rats in vitro and has been called "sulfation factor". The concentration of this factor is low in pituitary dwarfism and is elevated in acromegaly.

Dependence on growth hormone for continued normal growth becomes evident within the first year of life. Thereafter through the years of childhood the role of growth hormone is vital. While the cessation of skeletal growth can be attributed to closure of the epiphyses, it is also evident that soft tissues and viscera also cease to grow at maturity. Since we find that growth hormone persists in the plasma of adults, we can speculate that the tissues may lose their responsiveness. If so, such resistance is only relative, because visceral growth resumes with the elevated plasma growth hormone concentrations characteristic of active acromegaly.

CLINICAL CAUSES OF IMPAIRED GROWTH

Many classifications of growth failure which have been proposed have often been so inclusive that they are of relatively little use in considering individual cases. The classification presented in Table 2-4 is an attempt to divide growth failure into four major physiologic types: (1) abnormal endocrine regulation; (2) inherent defects of cellular responsiveness; (3) nutritional causes of cellular unresponsiveness; (4) cellular unresponsiveness due to inflammatory and toxic states.

Abnormal Endocrine Regulation. Deficiency of growth hormone production is the most important endocrine cause of growth failure. In some cases this is the result of destructive lesions of the hypothalamus with decrease in the production of the growth hormone releasing factor. It is likely that in many cases the hyposomatotropism occurring with supracellar cysts is the result of hypothalamic insufficiency rather than direct destruction of the pituitary. Other tumors and inflammatory conditions may act similarly. Unfortunately, direct techniques for distinguishing secondary from primary hyposomatotropism have not yet been developed.

There is great interest in the possibility that emotional disturbances may act on the hypothalamus to produce secondary hyposomatotropism. Seriously disturbed children who have been reared in an environment of deprivation of parental affection may exhibit impaired growth. In the more severe examples of this syndrome a pecular disturbance of appetite may develop in which these children eat all available food, even garbage. Absorption of food may be impaired by a functional malabsorption syndrome. It is difficult to attribute the growth failure to nutritional deficiency because of the absence of specific signs and the maintenance of fairly adequate adipose depots. Characteristically when these children are removed from the bad home environment and placed in more secure surroundings they exhibit a characteristic makeup type of growth spurt. The suggestion has been made that the growth failure of the maternal deprivation syndrome is the result of functional hyposomatotropism. It has been difficult to establish this hypothesis because some of these children when tested in the hospital have normal plasma growth hormone responses to provocative stimuli. Unanswered is the question whether responsiveness might not have been impaired if the test could be performed in the home environment.

Primary (pituitary) hyposomatotropism can be the result of a homozygous state for a specific gene. The pituitary dysfunction is limited to an inability to secrete growth hormone. All other pituitary hormones are secreted in near normal concentrations. The non-hereditary form of primary hyposomatotropism can also be monohormonal but more often is polyhormonal. The pathologic lesion may be limited to an unexplained reduction of pituitary somatotrophic cells, but in other cases a neoplastic, infiltrative or infectious process can be recognized.

In congenital growth hormone deficiency the growth rate slows within the first year of life (Figure 2-12). Thereafter it continues at about one-third to one-half the normal rate. Because of the frequent failure of puberty to occur, epiphysial closure often does not occur and slow growth persists through the third and fourth decades. Body proportions remain appropriate for height, and bone age is proportionately retarded as compared to height age. Subcutaneous "baby" fat is retained in childhood and fine radiating facial wrinkles are found in adults. The voice is often high pitched and squeaky. Dentition is usually retarded but intelligence is normal.

Dwarfism may result from the failure of growth hormone to induce the secondary mediator, sulfation factor. Familial cases described by Laron with the physical features of hyposomatotropism have normal or high growth hormone concentrations in plasma, but a low plasma sulfation factor, which does not rise following growth hormone treatment. Laron suggested that these

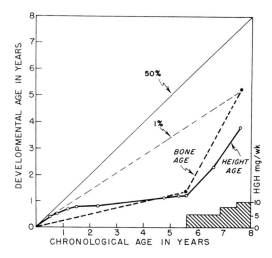

Fig. 2-12. Developmental chart for a boy with hypopituitary dwarfism. Before growth hormone treatment his height was below the first percentile curve. Note the excellent growth following human growth hormone administration. (From Daughaday and Parker: Pituitary in disorders of growth, Disease-a-Month, 1962: 1–47)

children secrete an abnomal growth hormone, but this has not been established.

The thyroid gland is second only to the pituitary in the regulation of growth. In the rat, at least, some of the growth failure of hypothyroidism is the result of a depletion of pituitary somatotrophic cells. While some hypothyroid children fail to exhibit rises of plasma growth hormone following provocative stimuli, others have perfectly normal responses. It is likely that the direct cellular effects of thyroid hormone deficiency are paramount in many. In congenital hypothyroidism or cretinism, growth failure occurs in the early months of life. Bone maturation is retarded much more than height. These children are pale, dry-skinned, and puffy. Umbilical hernias are common. The cry is hoarse. Feeding is poor and constipation is common. A prolongation of physiologic jaundice of the newborn is an important clue.

When hypothyroidism occurs later in childhood, growth is also impaired but the clinical findings are less dramatic and may be overlooked. Intelligence is normal. Again bone age is retarded out of proportion to height. Infrequently, premature puberty with inappropriate lactation occurs in girls with juvenile hypothyroidism.

Before adequate treatment of diabetes mellitus, growth impairment was a common feature of the disease. It is likely that **insulin** is necessary at the cellular level for growth hormone to exert its effects. Also, uncontrolled diabetes leads to caloric and other nutritional deficits. Fortunately, growth impairment due to diabetes is not encountered when medical care is adequate.

Hyperadrenalcorticism is a most important cause of growth failure. Fortunately, spontaneous Cushing's syndrome is rare in childhood but iatrogenic Cushing's syndrome occurs whenever corticosteroids are administered for long periods of time. In addition to the inhibition of growth, corticosteroids may lead to facial and truncal obesity, atrophy of skin, muscle, and bone, diabetes and lowered resistance to infection. Although large doses of corticosteroids block growth hormone release by the pituitary in response to provocative stimuli, this may not be a significant factor in children receiving usual therapeutic doses of corticosteroids. It has been shown that even when growth hormone is administered to children receiving corticosteroids, nitrogen retention is minimal and normal growth is not restored. In addition, plasma growth hormone responses to hypoglycemia are not consistently depressed in children receiving the usual doses of corticosteroids. From these observations it would appear that the major factor responsible for growth impairment in children receiving corticosteroid therapy is not an inhibition of the secretion of growth hormone but a refractoriness of tissues to growth hormone.

Genetic Tissue Unresponsiveness. Genetic factors are important in determining the responsiveness of tissues to circulating hormonal regulation. The polygenic control of growth has already been mentioned earlier in this chapter. Impairment in growth can be the result of imbalance of gene dosage due to chromosomal abnormalities or due to gene substitutions at appropriate sites. **Monosomy X** (Turner's syndrome) with karyotype 45 XO is the most common type of chromosomal imbalance seen with short stature and can be easily recognized by the stigmata of the condition evident in Figure 2-3. Facial and body proportions often are less abnormal in cases of mosaicism where some of the cells contain the normal XX constitution and other cells contain only a single X chromosome or an abbreviated X chromosome. It is important to recognize that the presenting clinical findings of these children in the prepubertal years may be limited to short stature. A carefully performed cytologic examination of the buccal smear usually will show a decreased percentage of sex chromatin bodies or the chromatin body may be abnormal in size. Definite diagnosis requires chromosomal analysis. It is usually sufficient to study the chromosomes derived from circulating lymphocytes but in more difficult cases of mosaicism examination of fibroblasts and other cells may be required.

Abnormalities in the normal diploid number of other chromosomes generally produces impaired growth associated with gross maldevelopment of the brain and other organs. The only condition that is apt to be seen in the physician's office is trisomy 21. There are 47 chromosomes. The clinical condition is called Down's syndrome (mongoloidism). Again the physical signs indicate disproportions in the growth process and should lead one away from a consideration of endocrine deficiencies.

The general responsiveness of tissues to hormonal regulation of growth is determined by multiple genes. In the pygmies of Africa, selection has concentrated several of the specific genes which *decrease the responsiveness* to growth hormone. These people have normal amounts of circulating growth hormone and normal growth hormone responses to provocative stimuli. In addition, it has been established that the concentration of sulfation factor in the serum is essentially normal. The finding of subnormal responses of plasma insulin to arginine and glucose administration is similar to that occurring in growth hormone deficiency. Administered human growth hormone did not lower plasma urea and increase insulin response to provocative stimuli. Although these observations were carried out under the most difficult field conditions, they do suggest subnormal responses to endogenous and exogenous hormones when compared to other racial groups.

It is likely that certain types of familial short stature may be attributed to a similar refractoriness to growth hormone, although studies of this problem are still fragmentary. Growth hormone treatment does not induce a sustained increase in growth velocity when administered in the same dose that induces remarkable increments in patients with pituitary dwarfism. It is possible that when larger supplies of growth hormone become available, larger doses of hormone may successfully stimulate growth in such children.

Lastly, consideration should briefly be given to the many genetic disorders of bone and cartilage which limit the response to hormonal stimulation. Most familiar to physicians in this class is achrondroplasia with its short extremities and deformed skull. In the differential diagnosis of growth impairment these cases seldom present problems because of their evident distortions of body proportions and the characteristic radiographic findings.

Defective Cellular Nutrition. In many cases no primary abnormality in hormonal regulators or genetic defects in cellular responsiveness exist, but growth impairment is the result of a failure to provide the proper nutriments required for the synthesis of cellular constituents. Dietary deficiencies of calories, essential amino acids, vitamins, or essential minerals almost without exception produce growth impairment as one feature of the deficiency condition. The growth deficiency in these situations seldom presents specific characteristics. Recently there have been a number of reports from the Middle East that zinc deficiency can lead to growth deficiency and hypogonadism. The suggestion was made that pituitary deficiency was responsible for growth failure in zinc deficiency, but further studies indicate that the defect is at the cellular level.

Growth deficiency is a common finding in patients with congenital heart disease. The disturbance is attributable to the failure of provision of oxygen to the tissues. Following correction of the cardiac defect by appropriate surgical operation a period of accelerated "catch-up" growth often occurs.

Chronic Inflammation and Toxic States. A fall in growth velocity often provides an early indication of significant chronic disease. This is particularly evident in the collagen disease group such as juvenile rheumatoid arthritis or the nonspecific inflammatory states such as regional enteritis or ulcerative colitis. Growth impairment is also a characteristic response to a number of chronic infections. This is particularly evident if predisposing factors such as cystic fibrosis or defective immune mechanisms are operative.

Growth failure is commonly observed in a number of chronic metabolic conditions such as the glycogenoses, defects in intermediary amino acid metabolism, and chronic renal disease. In renal tubular acidosis and azotemia the growth failure is usually associated with clinical or radiographic signs of osteitis fibrosa or osteomalacia.

EXCESSIVE GROWTH

When somatic growth exceeds two standard deviations of the mean, excessive growth can be considered to exist. Most cases of excessive tallness are attributable to augmented nutrition, to an excess of anabolic hormones, or to increased tissue responsiveness.

Forbes has pointed out that obese children are of two general types. The first is associated with increased height, increased lean body mass as well as total fat, and increased bone maturation. The second type of childhood obesity is unassociated with these changes in the non-fatty tissues. It is not known whether the increased growth of the first type is determined by nutritional factors, but its recognition is important for parental counseling.

Increased body growth as a result of excessive growth hormone secretion is infrequent. Pituitary gigantism resulting from an eosinophilic adenoma of the pituitary is a rare and dramatic syndrome which can be diagnosed with confidence using radioimmunoassay of plasma growth hormone. It is possible that in the future a more detailed study of children with excessive growth will reveal additional cases of mild functional hypersomatotropism. More sophisticated techniques for comparing total growth hormone secretion in persons of normal and of excessive stature are required.

Sexual precocity leads to an acceleration of growth and a greater increase in bone maturation. Therefore, children with sexual precocity are taller than their peers during the early years of their precocity. Following epiphysial closure they are overtaken in stature by their normal peers and will be of short final stature.

Most cases of excessive stature are the result of increased tissue responsiveness to normal nutritional and hormonal factors. A family history of tall stature in one or both parents can usually be obtained. Parents bring tall girls to the physician in hope that growth can be curtailed. Unfortunately, after the pubertal growth spurt is underway, little benefit results from hormonal treatment. If the bone age is less than 11 years and the predicted height is in excess of 70 inches, there is a possibility of some control of eventual height with moderately high doses of estrogens. I have employed the sequential estrogen-progestin preparations such as those utilized for fertility control in these girls. The initial response is an acceleration of growth but final height can be decreased by 1 to 3 inches. Following cessation of sex hormone administration, menses usually appear promptly. It is still unknown how frequently disturbed menstruation or other complications are associated with this therapy. The risks are not justified unless the projected height is likely to be a major psychologic and social barrier.

An unusual form of excessive growth has been reported in certain cases of mental deficiency and cerebral damage. It has not been possible to demonstrate excess growth hormone levels in these cases of cerebral gigantism. The mechanism of the accelerated growth remains a mystery and the validity of the syndrome remains open to question.

SEX DEVELOPMENT

Endocrinology of Adolescence

At birth the gonads of both male and female infants show evidence of stimulation

and secretory activity. Gonadal stimulation is largely the result of fetal pituitary secretion, but small amounts of placental gonadotropin may pass the placental barrier and enter fetal rather than maternal circulation. The period of gonadal stimulation is short-lived and regression takes place soon after birth. Thereafter, the gonads remain in a functionally dormant state until puberty. To be sure, small concentrations of both FSH and LH have been detected in plasma of prepubertal children with sensitive radioimmunoassay but urinary gonadotropins are undetectable by bioassay.

The basic change in the pubertal process must lie in the hypothalamus. For reasons which are still largely unknown, the hypothalamus begins to secrete increased amounts of the releasing factors for the gonadotropic hormones into the hypothalamic-pituitary portal system. It has been suggested that even in the prepubertal state there is a feedback system of regulatory control acting between pituitary and gonad. The event of puberty might result from a rise in the threshold of the hypothalamic centers which are sensing the concentration of gonadal steroids. With less feedback inhibition the

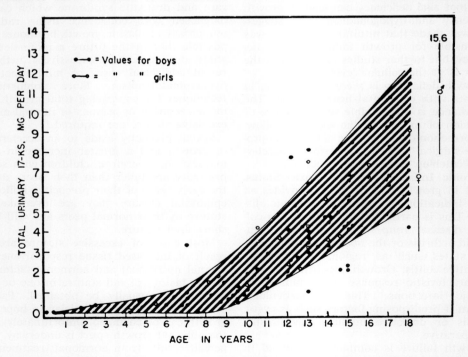

Fig. 2-13. Excretion of 17-ketosteroids in children. (From Wilkins, L.: The Diagnosis and Treatment of Endocrine Disorders in Childhood and Adolescence. Springfield, Illinois, Charles C Thomas, 1965, p. 65)

TABLE 2-5. AVERAGE APPROXIMATE AGE AND SEQUENCE OF APPEARANCE OF SEXUAL
CHARACTERISTICS IN BOTH SEXES*

AGE, YEARS	BOYS	GIRLS
9-10		Growth of bony pelvis. Budding of nipples.
10-11	First growth of testes and penis.	Budding of breasts. Pubic hair.
11-12	Prostatic activity.	Changes in vaginal epithelium and the smear. Growth of external and internal genitalia. Pigmentation of nipples. Mammae filling in.
12-13	Pubic hair.	
13-14	Rapid growth of testes and penis. Subareolar node of nipples.	Axillary hair. Menarche (average 13½ yrs., range 9-17 yrs.). Menstruation may be anovulatory for first few years.
14-15	Axillary hair. Down on upper lip. Voice change.	Earliest normal pregnancies.
15-16	Mature spermatozoa (average 15 yrs., range 11¼-17 yrs.).	Acne. Deepening of voice.
16-17	Facial and body hair. Acne.	Arrest of skeletal growth.
21	Arrest of skeletal growth.	

* From Wilkins, L.: The Diagnosis and Treatment of Endocrine Disorders in Childhood and Adolescence, ed. 3, Springfield, Thomas, 1966. (after Seckel).

release of gonadotropins is promoted. While this view has many attractive features it does not explain the relatively low levels of gonadotropins in young children with gonadal agenesis.

Another aspect of hypothalamic function is important in the understanding of puberty. There is a fundamental difference in the functional organization of the male and female hypothalamus which is established in fetal or neonatal life. In the postpubertal male the secretion of pituitary gonadotropic hormones is relatively constant. In the postpubertal female there is a recurring pattern of sudden outpouring of luteinizing hormone and to a certain extent of follicle-stimulating hormone, resulting in ovulation. More uniform secretion occurs throughout the remainder of the ovarian cycle. Although the sudden discharge of gonadotropins may be partially dependent on a rising concentration of ovarian hormones, the basic capacity to respond in this manner is not present in the male hypothalamic-pituitary system. Experimental studies in lower species have established that the fundamental difference between the male and female pattern is determined by the presence or absence of androgens at a critical period of fetal or neonatal life. Androgens convert the potential for cyclic

secretory responses to a continuous pattern.

The pubertal rise in gonadotropin titers stimulates the growth and secretion of the gonads. Not only do gonadal steroids promote the development of secondary sexual characters, but they induce characteristic metabolic and psychic effects. Some of the effects of gonadal steroids on secondary sexual characters are indirectly mediated in the female. The development of axillary and pubic hair is not normally the result of ovarian hormones, but is a consequence of adrenal androgen secretion. In the prepubertal state the adrenal gland secretes only small amounts of the potentially androgenic 17-ketosteroids. At puberty a change in adrenal enzyme composition occurs, possibly as a result of estrogen action, so that the secretion of 17-ketosteroids increases greatly (Figure 2-13). The androgenic activity derived from these steroids by hepatic metabolism gives rise in normal girls to axillary and pubic hair, occasional acne and slight lowering of the voice.

The effects of estrogens on the breast are partially indirect. In hypophysectomized animals estrogens by themselves have little ability to stimulate mammogenesis. In intact animals they act on the hypothalamic-pituitary system to promote the secretion of prolactin and thereby play a major role

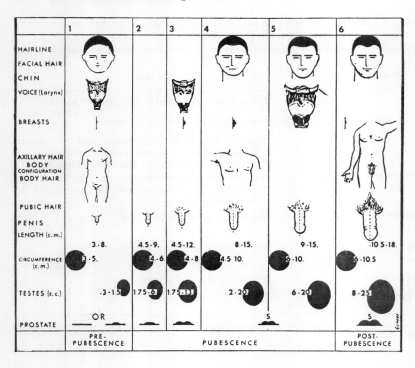

FIG. 2-14. Stages of sexual development and maturation. (Schonfeld, Wm. A.: Primary and secondary sexual characteristics, Am. J. Dis. Child. 65:535)

in mammogenesis as well as lactation. It is likely that in man, mammogenesis is similarly controlled.

BODY CHANGES DURING ADOLESCENCE

The sequential stages of puberty in boys follow one another in a predictable pattern in the vast majority of cases. They are given in Table 2-5 and Figure 2-14. The first change detectable in boys is an increase in the size and firmness of the testis, due to gonadotropic stimulation. At this time Leydig cells, which had disappeared from the testis soon after birth, reappear and take up their role as producers of testosterone. Penile development and scrotal development soon follow. Finally, the pubic hair becomes noticeable and scrotal skin becomes corrugated. It is important to recognize that pubic hair precedes the development of axillary hair by a year or two and axillary hair precedes the development of beard growth by an equal period of time. The complete male escutcheon is not achieved until late in adolescence. During the most rapid phase of pubertal development there is normally limited proliferation of the male breast. Usually this escapes notice. Occasionally it is prominent enough to cause embarrassment and must be distinguished from pathologic gynecomastia

resulting from Klinefelter's syndrome (a buccal smear will show sex chromatin bodies, and chromosomal studies will demonstrate an XXY pattern) or from adrenal or testicular tumors.

Associated with the changes in primary and secondary sexual characteristics many other bodily changes occur. Linear growth velocity increases markedly (Figures 2-5 & 2-6) and there is an acceleration of the process of epiphysial closure. In boys there is a disproportionate increase in muscle mass and muscle strength. Body fat increases in absolute amounts during and immediately after puberty in adolescent boys, yet the percentage of body fat actually falls (Fig. 2-10).

Pubertal changes in girls also follow a predictable sequence (Table 2-5). Mammary budding is followed by the appearance of the first wisps of pubic hair which is followed by evident estrogenic effects on vaginal epithelium and uterine size. Menstruation usually develops about a year and one half after the first indication of puberty.

The changes in bodily composition at puberty in girls primarily involve the sudden disposition of body fat about hips, in the breast, and quite generally throughout the body. The pubertal growth spurt is less pro-

FIG. 2-15. (Schonfeld, Wm. A.: Primary and secondary sexual characteristics, Am. J. Dis. Child. 65:535)

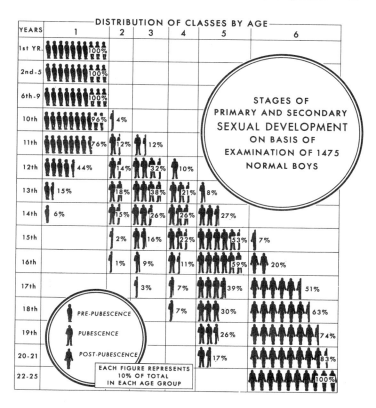

nounced in girls than in boys, and the increase in lean body mass is much less accelerated during puberty.

Time of Occurrence of Puberty. The factors which determine the age of puberty are still poorly understood. Nutritional, climatic, and racial influences have been recognized. Even in a single population under the same general environmental conditions there may be great variability in the time of onset of the pubertal changes. In some cases distinct familial patterns of puberty development are recognized. Often the timing of puberty seems more closely correlated with other parameters of maturity than with calendar age. Children with advanced skeletal maturation and advanced height attainment tend to enter puberty at an earlier age, while poorly developed children with retarded bone maturation may be several years behind their peers at the onset of their puberty. The fact that many children with constitutionally delayed maturation have delayed pubertal growth spurt leads to exaggerated differences in height evident in peer groups from 12 to 15 years of age. These striking differences tend to decrease later in life.

Some indication of the variability of timing of normal puberty in boys is given in Figure 2-15. This chart shows that normal puberty may commence any time in a wide range between the ages of 10 and 14 years. In unusual cases as compared with the average it may start quite early or quite late without being considered truly abnormal. Recognition of the important information set forth in this chart is of great assistance in counseling parents of children with minor disturbances of the timing of puberty.

The onset of puberty of girls precedes that of boys by about 2 years. The average age of peak velocity of growth occurs at about 12 years in girls and 14 years in boys. The average age of menarche is a useful milestone for determining secular and geographical trends. In the United States this is now about 12.7 years. The variability of the age of onset of puberty and the age of menarche in girls is equal to that in boys but is seldom of as great concern to parents as the deviations from the average which occur in boys.

TABLE 2-6. A PHYSIOLOGIC CLASSIFICATION
OF SEXUAL PRECOCITY

INDEPENDENT OF GONADOTROPIN SECRETION	GONADOTROPIN-DEPENDENT
Gonadal (interstitial cell tumors of boys, tumors and cysts involving granulosa or thecal cells in girls)	*Primary pituitary hypergonadotropism* (not yet recognized)
Adrenal Defective steroidal hydroxylations (adrenogenital syndrome) Adrenal tumors	*Premature gonadotropic secretion secondary to hypothalamic dysfunction* With hypothalamic gross pathology (tumor, encephalitis, trauma, etc.) Without hypothalamic structural change (idiopathic, familial, Albright's polyostotic fibrous dysplasia)
Exogenous sex steroid intake	*Ectopic gonadotropin production*

DISTURBANCE IN THE PUBERTAL MECHANISM

Delayed Puberty. Frequently physicians see children who have not shown pubertal changes by the 14th or 15th birthday. Fortunately, most of these children will eventually enter a spontaneous puberty. A history of delayed puberty in one or both parents with a comparable delay in height and skeletal maturation is reassuring. Malnutrition and chronic illness are important causes of delayed puberty. When none of these factors seem to be operative, serious consideration must be given to the possibility of endocrine disorders.

The physician should first determine whether the defect resides primarily **in the gonads.** Failure to find scrotal testes in boys suggests, but by no means establishes, primary hypogonadism as a cause of the pubertal failure. In such boys the measurement of urinary gonadotropins has been used in the past to help establish the normality of gonadotropic stimulation, but this difficult and inaccurate measurement will soon be replaced by measurements of plasma follicle-stimulating (FSH) and interstititial cell stimulating (LH or ICSH) hormone. The presence of elevated concentrations of these hormones is indicative of gonadal failure. Decreased concentrations of these hormones

does not necessarily mean that the gonads are capable of responding to tropic hormones because the pituitary phase of puberty may be delayed in some persons with gonadal causes of sexual infantilism.

When doubt exists concerning the adequacy of the gonads, the administration of chorionic gonadotropin (2,000 I.U., two to three times a week for 8 weeks), will lead to unequivocal enlargement of the responsive testis and somatic evidence of testosterone production. In certain cases this procedure seems to be therapeutic as well as diagnostic in that the pubertal mechanism seems to follow shortly. It has been impossible to establish the validity of this clinical impression because some of these boys would have entered puberty spontaneously in the absence of gonadotropin administration. If there is little or no response to gonadotropin, gonadal inadequacy may be diagnosed.

In the presence of gonadal causes of sexual infantilism the physician should consider developmental abnormalities of gonads related to **sex chromosomal aberrations.** A buccal smear may be sufficient to establish gonadal dysgenesis, but more elaborate chromosomal studies are required to define more complicated conditions. It is estimated that X chromosome abnormalities may account for as many as 40 to 50 percent of cases of sexual infantilism in girls.

Hypothalamico-pituitary causes of failure of sexual development must be considered when levels of pituitary gonadotropins are low and the gonads are responsive to exogenous gonadotropins. The hypogonadotropism can be temporary (delayed puberty) or permanent (hypogonadotropic eunuchoidism). The deficiency of gonadotropic hormones need not be associated with deficiencies of other pituitary hormones. In the absence of recognizable gross pathology, it is often impossible to determine whether hypogonadotropism is due to a disturbance in pituitary or in hypothalamic function. An increased gonadotropin concentration in the plasma following the administration of clomaphine argues for a functional rather than an organic disease of the pituitary.

The bodily changes of hypogonadism may or may not be evident in persons with delayed puberty. When bone maturation is normal, the delay in appearance of the sex hormones permits continued growth of the long bones and leads to the increase in ratio of the lower bodily segment to total height and increase in span which we recognize as characteristic of eunuchoidism. However, in constitutional growth retardation and in growth retardation secondary to malnutrition or chronic illness, the body proportions are not disturbed and the normal pattern of growth evolves, but at a retarded rate.

PREMATURE PUBERTY

The initiation of puberty before the age of 8 years in girls and 10 years in boys is distinctly abnormal and deserves medical inquiry. It is frequently difficult to determine whether the sexual precocity will evolve into complete sexual maturity. The physiologic approach to these children is given in Table 2-6. The first major question which must be answered is whether the **production of gonadal hormones** is independent of gonadotropic production. Valuable information is provided by the physical examination. If a testicular or ovarian neoplasm is the source of the precocious production of sex steroids the tumor may present with a detectable mass. In boys this is usually a carcinoma but in girls benign cystic or solid tumors of the ovary are more common; they usually can be detected by thorough gynecologic examination. If the gonads are not the source of the sex hormones they will be found to be atrophic (e.g. with adrenocortical hyperplasia or tumor).

Laboratory tests can assist in the study of these children by providing primary evidence of overproduction of the sex hormone in question (plasma or urine testosterone, urinary estrogen) or secondary evidence of production (prostatic acid phosphatase elevation in males, estrogenic transformation of the vaginal mucosa in girls). Plasma and urine gonadotropic hormones will be low.

Dysfunction of the adrenal associated with excessive production of 17-ketosteroids is an important cause of isosexual precocity in boys and heterosexual precocity in girls. Signs of excess androgen production are detected at birth or soon thereafter in most cases. The gonads are small except in the rare conditions in which adrenal rest cells are present in the testis and respond to the high level of circulating corticotropin. In all but very young children with adrenocortical hypersecretion the urinary excretion of 17-ketosteroids and of pregnanetriol are elevated. Space does not here permit a more complete description of the different varieties of adrenal dysfunction associated with virilization. The reader should consult a textbook of endocrinology for a description of the clinical characteristics and diagnoses of this group of diseases.

The adrenal cortex can give rise to adenomas and carcinomas that are associated with virilism. Such cases are recognized by high levels of 17-ketosteroids which do not fall following corticosteroid administration. Very rarely adrenal cortical tumors give rise to estrogenic hormones. Usually a mass lesion is not difficult to demonstrate in these cases.

It is important in evaluating children with sexual precocity to consider the possibility of an exogenous source of sex hormones. Breast development and menstrual bleeding have been reported in little girls who ingest contraceptive and other estrogenic medications obtained from the mother's supply. Short boys may have received androgenic therapy to stimulate growth without the parents being aware of the nature of the medication.

Sexual precocity which is dependent on the premature release of gonadotropic hormones by the pituitary is caused by **hypothalamic dysfunction.** In about 40 percent of boys and 10 percent of girls with premature gonadotropin secretion a recognizable disease process of the hypothalamus can be detected. Tumors of the corpora mammillaria or the posterior region of the hypothalamus are most apt to result in premature puberty, whereas tumors of the anterior hypothalamus often lead to hypogonadism. While pinealomas have received much attention as a cause of premature puberty, other types of hypothalamic tumors also can lead to the syndrome. Demonstration of these tumors requires air encephalographic or angiographic studies. Diffuse disease such as encephalitis can also lead to premature puberty.

In most cases of premature puberty no clinical evidence of organic hypothalamic disease can be detected and the cases can be classified as functional or idiopathic. This does not mean that structural changes do not exist in the hypothalamus, because few of these individuals have come to postmortem examination and even fewer have been subjected to detailed study of the hypothalamus by modern methods. There is a rare familial type of premature puberty which is associated with an X-linked dominant pattern of transmission.

In rare cases, gonadotropins of extrahypophysial origin can lead to sexual precocity. Most frequently this phenomenon occurs with production of chorionic gonadotropin by teratomas or chorioepitheliomas. Of great interest but of infrequent occurrence is the development of sexual precocity in boys who have hepatomas secreting gonadotropin (probably of chorionic type). In adults the ectopic production of gonadotropic hormones has been associated with lung tumors but this type of tumor has not occurred in children.

Partial Pubertal Syndromes. In certain cases the sequence of pubertal events may be abnormal. In premature pubarche, girls occasionally develop pubic hair and some increase in skeletal growth and maturation without other evidences of puberty. Except as a cause of parental alarm the syndrome is of little significance. Urinary 17-ketosteroids are only slightly elevated for the age and the other features of puberty develop after one or more years. This syndrome appears to be due to premature secretion of adrenal androgens.

Of more significance are cases of **selective gonadotropic deficiency** in which there is a deficiency of only one gonadotropic hormone. Isolated *follicle-stimulating hormone deficiency* in the male leads to aspermia without abnormal Leydig cell function. In the female with isolated FSH deficit both estrogen production and sexual maturation will be absent.

Luteinizing hormone deficiency in males leads to decreased testosterone production with little impairment in spermatogenesis (fertile eunuch). Functional luteinizing hormone deficiency is commonly encountered in girls and leads to delayed appearance of menses and subsequent failure of ovulation. Nutritional and psychic factors frequently are involved in selective luteinizing hormone deficiency. Ovulation often follows clomaphine therapy.

Unresponsiveness of certain tissues to sex hormones may exist and distort pubertal development. In **testicular feminization** complete refractoriness to the effects of testosterone is present and the genotypic male develops into a phenotypic female lacking pubic and axillary hair and possessing labial testes. In less dramatic situations the growth of facial, axillary, or pubic hair may not develop during puberty. Absence of facial hair is a racial characteristic of American Indians.

Increased sensitivity to mammogenic hormones may lead to mammary development long in advance of actual puberty and of the other physiological and anatomical evidences of puberty. This condition has been called premature *thelarche*. The possible role of pituitary prolactin in the genesis of this syndrome has not been studied.

BIBLIOGRAPHY

Bayley, N., and Pinneau, S. R.: Tables for predicting adult height from the skeletal age: revised for use with the Greulich-Pyle hand standards, J. Pediat. 40:423–441, 1952.

Brasel, J. A., and Blizzard, R. M.: The Influence of the Endocrine Glands upon Growth and Development *in* Textbook of Endocrinology. Williams, R. H., ed., Ed. 4, W. B. Saunders Co., Philadelphia, 1968.

Cheek, D. B.: Human Growth, Energy, and Intelligence, Lea and Febiger, Philadelphia, 1968.

Cheek, D. B.: Cellular growth, hormones, nutrition time, Pediatrics 41:30–46, 1968.

Cheek, D. B., and Cooke, R. E.: Growth and growth retardation, Ann. Rev. Med. 15:357–382, 1964.

Daughaday, W. H.: The Adenohypophysis *in* Textbook of Endocrinology, Williams, R. H., ed., Ed. 4, W. B. Saunders Co., Philadelphia, 1968.

Daughaday, W. H., and Kipnis, D. M.: The growth-promoting and anti-insulin actions of somatotropin, Rec. Prog. Hormone Res. 22:49–99, 1966.

Daughaday, W. H., and Parker, M. L.: The pituitary in disorders of growth. Disease-a-Month. 1962: 1–47, 1962.

Ferguson-Smith, M. A.: Karyotype-phenotype correlations in gonadal dysgenesis and their bearing on the pathogenesis of malformations, J. Med. Genet. 2:142–155, 1965.

Ferrier, P., Shepard, T. H., and Smith, E. K.: Growth disturbances and values for hormone excretion in various forms of precocious sexual development, Pediatrics 28:258–275, 1961.

Forbes, G. B.: Toward a new dimension in human growth, Pediatrics 36:825–835, 1965.

Greulich, W. W., and Pyle, S. I.: Radiographic Atlas of Skeletal Development of the Hand and Wrist, Ed. 2, Stanford University Press, Stanford, 1959.

Heald, F. P., Daugela, M., and Brunschuyler, P.: Physiology of adolescence, New Eng. J. Med. 268:192–198, 243–252, 299–306, 1963.

Hook, E. B., and Reynolds, J. W.: Cerebral gigantism: endocrinological and clinical observations of six patients including a congenital giant, concordant monozygotic twins and a child who achieved adult gigantic size, J. Pediat. 70:900, 1967.

Jones, R. C., Bergman, M. W., Kittner, P. J., and Pigman, W. W.: Urinary hydroxyproline excretion in normal children and adolescents, Proc. Soc. Exp. Biol. Med. 115:85–87, 1964.

Laron, Z., Pertzelan, A., and Karp, M.: Pituitary dwarfism with high serum levels of growth hormone, Israel J. Med. Sci. 4:883–894, 1968.

Merimee, T. J., Rimoin, D. L., Cavalli-Sforza, L. C., Rabinowitz, D., and McKusick, V. A.: Metabolic effects of human growth hormone in the African pygmy, Lancet, II: 194–195, 1968.

Parker, M. L., Hammond, J. H., and Daughaday, W. H.: The arginine provocative test: an aid in the diagnosis of hyposomatotropism, J. Clin. Endocr. 27: 1129–1136, 1967.

Mellman, W. J., Bongiovanni, A. M., and Hope, J. W.: The diagnostic usefulness of skeletal maturation in an endocrine clinic, Pediatrics 23: 530–544, 1959.

Pertzelman, A., Adam, A., and Laron, Z.: Genetic aspects of pituitary dwarfism due to absence or biological inactivity of growth hormone, Israel J. Med. Sci. 4: 895–900, 1968.

Powell, G. F., Brasel, J. A., and Blizzard, R. M.: Emotional deprivation and growth retardation simulating idiopathic hypopituitarism, I. Clinical evaluation of the syndrome, New Eng. J. Med. 276: 1271–1278, 1967.

Rimoin, D. L., Merimee, T. J., and McKusick, V. A.: Growth hormone deficiency in man: an isolated, recessively inherited defect, Science, 152: 1635–1637, 1966.

Tanner, J. M., Whitehouse, R. H., and Takaishi, M.: Standards from birth to maturity for height, weight, height velocity and weight velocity, British Children, 1965. Arch. Dis. Child. Part I. 41: 454–471, 1966. Arch. Dis. Child. Part II. 41: 613–635, 1966.

Tanner, J. M.: Growth at Adolescence, Ed. 2, Blackwell Scientific Publications Ltd., Oxford, 1962.

Van Wyk, J. J., and Grumbach, M. M.: Disorders of Sex Differentiation, *in* Textbook of Endocrinology, Ed. 4, Williams, R. H., ed., W. B. Saunders Co., Philadelphia, 1968.

Whitelaw, M. J.: Experiences in treating excessive height in girls with cyclic oestradiol valerate, Acta Endocr. 54: 473–484, 1967.

Wilkins, L.: The Diagnosis and Treatment of Endocrine Disorders in Childhood and Adolescence, Charles C Thomas, Springfield, Illinois, 1965.

3

Pain

GEORGE L. ENGEL

CLINICAL CHARACTERISTICS OF PAIN

REQUIREMENTS FOR PAIN

Pain, without doubt, is the most common and compelling symptom for which patients consult physicians. In one general medical clinic, 75 percent of those attending had pain.[1] In the mind of the average patient pain is *the* cardinal manifestation of illness. Indeed, some patients do not even regard themselves as ill if they are not in pain; a painless swelling, for example, may be disregarded because "it didn't hurt." For the physician the interpretation of pain constitutes a difficult diagnostic procedure, in which success rests on a clear comprehension of what pain is and how it comes about.

What is pain? At first glance the answer seems obvious enough. Every reader can at once refer to his own personal experience and be sure that he "knows" what pain is. Yet difficulties arise the moment he attempts to define pain in words.[2,3,4] Perhaps before attempting to do so, it would be wise to consider the following clinical facts about pain:

1. **Pain is a private, subjective experience, information about which can come only from the sufferer.** Although one may sometimes be able to deduce from behavior that a person is in pain, and even where the pain is located, details of the pain experience are contingent upon what the sufferer is able and willing to report. Hence the clinical diagnosis as well as the scientific investigation of pain must take into account the psychological processes governing how subjective experiences are communicated.

2. **Pain is not a pure sensation.** It is always mixed with other bodily sensations such as pressure, stretch, pull, squeeze, touch, heat, or cold. Indeed, clinical observation justifies the view that pain often is a quality that is added to other sensations. The reader need only consider how he decides that a particular body sensation is painful; for example, the sensation accompanying an intestinal cramp, sitting in an awkward position, or slowly pressing the point of a pencil into the palm of the hand. Each involves a complex of sensations which, if intense enough, may ultimately be designated as painful by some and merely as uncomfortable by others.

3. **Generally speaking pain correlates with the intensity of stimulation.** The more intense the stimulation, the more likely is the sensation to be experienced as painful. Further, this likelihood increases sharply as a stimulus approaches the threshold for injury; that is, as it becomes a noxious stimulus. Yet it is also a clinical fact that pain may be absent in the presence of injury and present in the absence of injury. *Thus, tissue injury is neither a necessary nor a sufficient condition for pain.*

4. If body sensations tend to be felt as pain when the stimulus becomes intense enough, what quality distinguishes the new sensation?

Again, introspection and clinical experience reveal that **pain includes an affective quality of suffering, discomfort, distress, misery, torture, and punishment.** One suffers with pain, is afflicted with pain, is racked by pain, is tormented by pain. In contrast to other sensory experiences, pain hardly ever is neutral. Even the prospect of pain characteristically evokes aversive responses. Yet clinical observation shows that there can also be an element of pleasure or satisfaction in the suffering of pain. Indeed there are circumstances under which pain may be welcomed, and some persons knowingly or unknowingly solicit pain. *Thus, pain includes an unpleasant affective quality but can also be made to yield pleasure.*

5. **Only those parts of the body which have an afferent nerve supply belonging to the dorsal root system (or their analogues in the cranial nerves) can give rise to pain.** Interrupting such nerve supply renders the part insensitive to peripheral stimulation. Yet spontaneous pain may be referred to an amputated or denervated limb (phantom pain), and purely psychological means (suggestion, hypnosis, conversion) may render a heretofore painful stimulus painless, or a painless stimulus, painful. Thus, *stimulation of peripheral receptors and the intactness of the peripheral nerve supply is neither a necessary nor a sufficient condition for pain.*

6. **Both consciousness and attention are necessary for the experience of pain.** Pain may be ameliorated or eliminated by drugs or other factors which reduce consciousness, as well as by various circumstances that distract attention, as suggestion, placebo, hypnosis, or intense preoccupation. Conversely, pain may develop or intensify when attention is drawn to it. A soldier in combat may not be aware of the pain of a wound until after the action has ceased.

7. **Psychological factors significantly influence how and when pain is experienced and reported.** A body sensation is less likely to be experienced and/or reported as pain when it is familiar, understood, and known to be benign than when it is new, strange, and anxiety-provoking. For some persons pain is a sign of weakness, to be hidden; for others it is a claim to special attention. For some it is an intolerable threat, which must be relieved at once; for others a deserved punishment, which must be endured. For some, pain and suffering is a way of life, for others, an unwelcome intruder.

8. **Social and cultural influences modify how different peoples react to and report pain.** In some cultures stoicism and self-control are virtues, whereas in others, public expression of pain enjoys wide cultural approval. In some cultures pain has primarily health and medical implications, in others pain has magical and religious implications.

A Definition of Pain

On the basis of these eight clinical characteristics of pain, the following definition is proposed:

Pain is a basically unpleasant sensation referred to the body which represents the suffering induced by the psychic perception of real, threatened, or phantasied injury.

This defines pain as a psychological experience involving the concepts of injury and suffering, but not contingent on actual physical injury. The *idea* of injury as well as the *need to suffer* may lead to pain, just as may a real lesion or injury. Similarly, the need not to suffer or not to accept the fact of injury may render a "painful" injury painless. Hence, at the clinical level, the report of pain first must be analyzed in the psychological terms of attention, consciousness, feeling, cognition, language, and behavior, from which certain inferences may then be drawn concerning underlying neural processes mediating the experience. *The clinician never deals directly with pain, per se, he deals with the patient's statements about his pain.*

The term **perception** is critical for this definition. Perception involves comprehending something new by assimilating it with the sum of one's previous knowledge and experience. Pain as experienced and reported involves in essence an interpretation of the sensory input in terms of what has gone before. The end result, the perception that it is pain (rather than some other sensation) and that it has a particular character, is clearly subject to the influences of the individual's current and past psychological experience. It is this assimilation which accounts for the fact that the same stimulus may be experienced and reported differently by different persons, or by the same person at different times; that actual injury is neither necessary nor sufficient for a sensation to be felt as pain; that pain may occur without input; that pain and suffering may acquire pleasurable or satisfying qualities. In brief, pain is not a perceptual fact until and unless psychological processing of underlying physical events in the nervous system has taken place.

Injury occupies a central position in this definition. Not only is injury the most reliable means of inducing pain, but aversive and protective responses are regular reactions to pain and serve to limit the effects of a noxious stimulus. Actually the stimulus threshold for pain is lower than that required to produce injury.[5] Hence, pain may be felt *before* actual injury takes place. Thus, not only may pain mean that injury has taken place, it may also warn that injury *might* take place. In this way pain plays a critical role in learning what environmental circumstances may be injurious and how they are to be avoided. Psychologically speaking, the organism learns not what is injurious, but what is painful. This is the basis of aversive conditioning. Melzack showed that dogs raised in isolation from birth to maturity had markedly elevated thresholds for avoidance responses to electric shock, nose-burning, and pin pricks.[6] They behaved as if they knew neither what was painful nor what might be injurious nor how to avoid such stimuli. Evidently the development of the higher neural and psychic systems whereby the organism learns to appreciate and avoid what might be injurious requires experience with pain early in life. By virtue of such superordinate systems to avoid injury, pain not only signals that the intensity of a stimulus is approaching the threshold of injury, it also indicates that such stimulus is currently present or that it *might* be present in the immediate future. *Thus, pain may indicate actual injury, a threat of injury, or some special meaning of injury to the individual, whereas absence of pain may convey the message "no injury," sometimes even when injury is actually present. Further, pain may come to symbolize injury, even in the absence of peripheral stimulation, if and when it serves the psychic need of the individual for it to do so.* In this way one may suffer pain when, for example, guilt imposes a need for punishment and atonement (see Chapter 30).

NEURAL ORGANIZATION SERVING PAIN

Recent years have seen much progress in our knowledge of the neural organization involved in pain; so much so that modern neurophysiological theory much more adequately accounts for the clinical phenomenology of pain than did classical theory. For more than a century the field had been dominated by the doctrine of "specific energies of nerve fibers" as enunciated by Johannes Muller in 1838. In essence, this held that for each sensation there is a specific receptor, a specific nerve, and a specific central locus of appreciation. Goldscheider (1881) proposed four primary sensations from skin—namely, touch, heat, cold, and pain— and subsequently claims were made for the existence of specific receptors and pathways for each sensation.[7,8] Since then it has been customary to believe that pain occurs when a "pain" stimulus impinges on "pain" receptors and is transmitted centrally along "pain" fibers and "pain" pathways to a "pain center" in the brain. Such a "telephone" model of a fixed direct-line communication system between the periphery and brain is not only inconsistent with modern neurophysiologic data, but also involves a fallacious psychologic assumption. To ascribe the quality "pain" to receptors, fibers, or tracts implies that their stimulation must always elicit pain and only pain, and that pain must always originate in the periphery. Further, such a model confuses sensation, a psychologic experience, with physiologic function. The clinical data already cited clearly cast doubt on the validity of any such assumption.

To overcome the deficiencies of classical theory, Melzack and his associates have proposed a theory in which the cortex controls afferent input in terms of its meaning to the individual **(Gate Control Theory)**.[9,10,11] When an input, whether coming from the body, the environment, or from the mind (fantasy), is interpreted as signifying injury, the movement of impulses to the areas of the brain mediating avoidance and internal adjustment is facilitated, and the total complex of pain as behavior and subjective experience is elicited. This theory involves four neural components:

1. **A modulating (gating) spinal cord system,** which controls the amount of input transmitted from receptors and peripheral fibers through the dorsal-horn transmission (or T) cells, which project to the ascending fibers in the anterolateral cord.

2. **A sensory discriminative system** whereby incoming stimuli are localized in space and time and along an intensity continuum.

3. **A motivational-affective (action) system,** which contributes the quality of unpleasantness, mobilizes internal defenses, and drives the organism into action aimed at stopping the distress.

4. **A central control (cognitive) system,** which evaluates and analyzes input in terms of past experience, probability of outcome, and symbolic meaning. It regulates response and behavior through facilitating or inhibit-

ing influences on the discriminative and motivational systems, as well as on input through the gate control system.

RECEPTORS AND AFFERENT FIBERS

Two basic kinds of receptor organs serving body sensory function can be distinguished, free nerve endings and specialized corpuscular receptors.[12,13] They differ in their capacity to transduce mechanical, thermal, and chemical energy into electrical impulses. The corpuscular endings are mainly responsive to various forms of deformation (mechanical energy), including vibration (Pacinian corpuscles). Free nerve endings on the other hand are sensitive to all the physical modalities, but different endings differ in their sensitivity as well as thresholds to different stimuli. Some are excited best by strong mechanical stimulation, others by both mechanical and thermal stimulation; some respond only to high temperatures, others to low temperatures, and still others to changes in temperature.[14] A small minority of free nerve endings respond only at levels of stimulation where actual tissue injury is imminent. Such receptors characteristically show continued or delayed firing even after the original physical stimulus has been discontinued. Thus, receptors show physiological response specificity as well as a continuous range of threshold responses.

Chemical substances formed in tissues in response to injury may increase the sensitivity of some receptors.[15,16] These include histamine from mast cells, 5-hydroxytryptamine (serotonin) from disintegrating platelets, acetylcholine, and peptides of the bradykinin group. The kinins have algesic effects in exceedingly small quantities, well within the range of naturally occurring biological agents, suggesting that they are specific chemical mediators for receptors activated by injury.[16] Since kinin formation takes place after a latency period of 15 to 30 seconds following an injury and does not reach a peak for another 10 to 15 seconds, their effect on threshold could well contribute to the continued or delayed firing of high threshold receptors, as noted previously.

The axons serving the receptors vary in size. Most corpuscular receptors are served by the larger fibers (A beta). Different free nerve endings are served by different-sized fibers, ranging from the large (A beta) and medium to small (A gamma-delta) fibers, to the smallest (C) fibers. Fiber size correlates with conduction velocity and threshold. The larger fibers are the most rapidly conducting and have the lowest threshold. The smallest fibers are the slowest conducting and have the highest threshold. The larger fibers belong to the phylogenetically newer sensory systems, which ascend with few relays to posterior thalamus and project to the somesthetic cortex. The smaller fibers belong to the phylogenetically older sensory systems. They have shorter ascending pathways with multiple relays terminating variously in the reticular formation of the medulla and tegmentum, or in the intralaminar nuclei of the thalamus.[17]

The distribution of receptors and fibers is important to the understanding of the nature of sensory information derived from the periphery. The surface of the body, including orificial mucous membranes, is the most extensively innervated. The basic supply of skin and mucous membrane is in the form of networks of free nerve endings, the so-called dermal-nerve networks, each of which is derived from several terminal fibers forming an interweaving arborization, although without fusion between axons of neighboring nerves.[18] Thus, stimulation at any point always invokes impulses flowing up several nerve fibers to the cells of the dorsal root ganglia. In hairy skin, such networks surround the hair follicle. A wide spectrum of fiber sizes is involved in these networks, from the large A beta to the small C fibers. Specialized endings, sensitive to pressure, served by large fibers, lie below the ridged epidermis of palms and soles, in mucocutaneous regions, and in the deeper layers of the skin and subcutaneously.

The cornea is served by networks of free terminals derived from fibers of the A gamma-delta and C fiber range. Contrary to earlier opinions, sensations other than pain can be elicited from the cornea.[19]

Except for the muscle spindle and the proprioceptors of joint capsules and tendons, all other innervated deep structures, visceral as well as somatic, are served by free nerve endings of fine fibers of the A delta and C range. These are much more sparsely distributed than in skin. Especially important are the *paravascular* fibers, which are under 6 μ in diameter. These run parallel with small blood vessels down to the level of capillaries, terminating as free nerve endings. They are peripheral axons of dorsal root ganglia and are to be distinguished from the perivascular plexus, which is composed of sympathetic vasomotor fibers. They may accompany autonomic nerves, but do not synapse in the autonomic ganglia. Lim believes the *paravascular* nerve endings to be primarily chemoreceptors, responding to the chemical products of injury, notably the kinins.[20]

Afferent nerves have a definite segmental distribution, each dorsal root serving a particular segment. On the surface of the body these are topographically distributed as the cutaneous dermatomes, which overlap somewhat with each other and slightly cross the midline. For deeper somatic structures, as muscles, tendons, and fascia, the distribution of afferents corresponds with the motor innervation. The segmental innervation of the viscera derives from levels of embryologic origin rather than from the actual anatomical location. The visceral afferents run centripetally in the sympathetic and parasympathetic nerves, pass through the ganglia without synapse, and reach the posterior roots via the rami communicantes. The afferents from such structures as the heart, aorta, biliary ducts, and upper gastrointestinal tract pass through sympathetic ganglia, those from trachea and bronchi traverse the vagi, and those from lower bowel, urinary bladder, uterine cervix, and prostate traverse the parasympathetic rami of the sacral nerves.[21]

SPINAL CORD GATE CONTROL SYSTEM[9,10,11]

The dorsal horn transmission cells (T-cells), which receive and transmit rostrally the impulses from small fiber activity, are subject to modulating influences by the cells of the substantia gelatinosa that surround them. Melzack has delineated this as a gating mechanism regulating inflow from the periphery. Through this arrangement activity of the phylogenetically newer large fiber system can inhibit inflow from small fibers. Input through the large fiber system, by virtue of its more rapid conduction and fewer synaptic delays, reaches higher connections first, and hence can give rise to downflowing impulses to the substantia gelatinosa cells, which *inhibit* further transmission of small fiber impulses (a negative feedback). On the other hand, small fiber impulses reaching the substantia gelatinosa *facilitate* the transmission of later-arriving small fiber impulses (a positive feedback). Thus, transmission of small fiber activity through T-cells depends upon the relative balance of activity in small versus large fibers reaching the cord. When peripheral stimulation induces predominantly large fiber activity (e.g., gently stroking the skin), central transmission of concomitant small fiber activity through the T-cells is inhibited by downflowing impulses and the gate is closed; when peripheral stimulation increases the amount of small fiber relative to large fiber activity (e.g., scraping the skin), T-cell transmission is facilitated and the gate is opened wider to more small fiber activity. Since large fiber receptors generally have the lower thresholds, gentle stimulation tends to close the gate, more intense stimulation to open it. This may explain the ameliorating effects of gently rubbing a painful part.

As we shall see later, there are other modulating influences on the gate which involve both affective and cognitive processes and are mediated by the action and central control systems.

The contrasting effects of small and large fiber activity on the gate control mechanism and the relative segregation of fibers by size within the cord draws attention to differing functional properties related to fiber size. The larger fibers prove to be distributed more into the *sensory discriminative system*, the smaller fibers into the *motivational affective (action) system*. The sensory discriminative system dominates as long as the small fiber inflow is not too great. When small fiber activity reaches a critical intensity, as monitored centrally, the motivational-affective system is activated, at which point pain experience and response enter the picture.[9,10,11] The interrelationships of these two systems and their role in pain will now be considered.

SENSORY-DISCRIMINATIVE SYSTEM[9,10,11]

The sensory-discriminative system is constituted of those medium to larger-sized myelinated fibers that reach the ventral nucleus of the thalamus and project to the somesthetic area of the cortex. It is served in part by two main tracts, the dorsal column-medial lemniscal and the neospinothalamic. The first, phylogenetically the most recently developed, arises from the large A-beta fibers, which ascend in the dorsal column to their first relay in the cuneate and gracile nuclei, from whence they pass upward in the medial lemniscus and terminate in the ventrobasal complex of the thalamus, others joining the way, the neospinothalamic, originating mainly in A gamma-delta fibers, projects from the T-cells of the dorsal horn, crosses in the ventral white commissure of the cord and ascends in the anterolateral column, some fibers terminating in the posterior nuclear complex of the thalamus, others joining the medial lemniscus to terminate in the ventro-basal complex of the thalamus. The latter sends projections to the second sensory area of the cortex and probably makes the larger contribution to sensory-discriminative function.

The sensory-discriminative system is organized along precise topographic lines and shows high fidelity in following alterations in the spatial, temporal, and intensity properties of the input. This is strikingly so with respect to the larger fiber input of the lemniscal system, but much less so with that input of the neospinothalamic tract, which terminates in the posterior thalamic nuclei.[22] Various studies indicate exquisite preservation of specificity throughout the lemniscal system (Mountcastle). Thus, any given cell of the ventrobasal complex of the thalamus may be activated by one form of peripheral mechanical stimulation but not by another. In addition, as an impulse ascends from a single locus in the periphery, the receptive fields in the dorsal column nuclei, thalamus, and sensory cortex grow progressively larger as one proceeds rostrally. Conversely, a single recording locus in thalamus and cortex can be activated from a relatively large but circumscribed area of the cortex. Mountcastle proposes that information concerning spatial, temporal, and intensity relationships is extracted from the profile of activity in this large population of cells which is activated from a discrete peripheral locus.[22]

In contrast, that segment of the neospinothalamic tract which terminates in the posterior nuclei complex of the thalamus has much less specificity.[22] Thus, a given cell in the thalamus may be responsive not only to a variety of modalities of stimulation, but such unit cell responses may be evoked from distantly separated parts of the body. Since aversive functions may also be elicited from this region of the thalamus, it is possible that this part of the system discriminates the quality of "hurting," whereas the lemniscal system discriminates temporal, spatial, and intensity dimensions.[23,24] This view receives some support from the observation that surgical lesions in the ventrobasal nuclei of the thalamus of patients with intractable pain may produce profound deficit in sensory discrimination without relieving pain, whereas lesions in posterior nuclei give pain relief without interfering with sensibility.[25,26]

MOTIVATIONAL AFFECTIVE (ACTION) SYSTEM[9,10,11]

The obvious role of pain in protecting the organism from injury warrants close attention to the neural system concerned with avoidance behavior. There is reason to believe that the reticular core of the brain stem and the medial thalamus form part of this complex. These structures receive projections from the phylogenetically older ascending tracts originating in the small myelinated and unmyelinated fibers (A gamma-delta, C range). In contrast to the discriminative system, this paramedial ascending system has numerous relays, and neither it nor the structures with which it connects are organized to provide discrete spatial or temporal information. A striking feature of the paramedial ascending system is its strategic relation to the limbic system and associated structures via reciprocal interconnections in the midbrain central gray. Limbic system structures are known to play an important role in aversive drives and similar pain-related behavior, including the flight-fight and conservation-withdrawal patterns (see Chapter 29).

Intimately related to the brain areas involved in aversive behavior are also regions involved in approach (reward) and pleasure responses.[27] In general, low-level stimulation elicits approach responses, and intense stimulation evokes avoidance responses. Most important for the thesis being developed is that complex excitatory and inhibitory interactions among these areas make it possible for aversive responses to noxious stimuli to be blocked by stimulation of reward areas, while approach responses may be blocked by stimulation of avoidance areas.[28,29] Many years ago Pavlov showed that if painful electric shocks or burns are used as the conditioning stimulus for feeding, dogs eventually respond to the presentation of such painful stimuli as signals for food and show not even the most subtle signs of pain. Yet they respond appropriately to other painful stimuli.[30]

The paramedial reticular and limbic systems are constantly receiving inflow from enteroceptive and exteroceptive systems as well as from elsewhere in the nervous system. On what basis are aversive rather than approach mechanisms triggered? Melzack proposes that these systems function as a *central intensity monitor*.[9,10,11] This function may be served by cells in the medial brain stem which show summation and prolonged afterdischarge in relation to input from spatially separated and temporally dispersed units.[31] Such summation would transform discrete spatial and temporal information into intensity information and could be a measure of total T-cell output after it has undergone modulation by the dorsal horn gate control system. Beyond a certain intensity level (it is suggested) the output of these monitoring cells activates areas underlying negative affect and aversive drive.

CENTRAL CONTROL (COGNITIVE) SYSTEM[9,10,11]

Pain so far has been considered in terms of its sensory and affective components and the neural system serving each. Still to be accounted for are the central control factors determining how and whether the sensory input is perceived and/or the action system controlled. How do such factors as memory, attention, past experience, anticipation, and the symbolic meaning of pain determine when and how pain is experienced, responded to, and reported? These processes presumably are served by neocortical functions. It is now well established that forebrain structures, through corticofugal influences, can act on both the sensory discriminative and the motivational-affective systems. As already discussed, descending inhibitory influences exerted at the dorsal horn cells can affect the gate control system so that input is modulated before it even reaches either the discriminative or the motivational system. Extensive interconnection among sensory and associational cortical areas and reticular and limbic structures provide a means of mediating between cognitive activities and the motivational affective features of pain. Such relationships may account for the effect of prefrontal lobotomy or certain drugs in reducing the suffering of pain without eliminating pain; or for conversion or hypnotically induced pain, in which the *idea* of injury, but no actual injury, is implicated.

The central control system also serves to evaluate the input in terms of present and past experience and to modulate it *before* it activates the discriminative or motivational systems. In this way a "painful" injury may be rendered "painless" during the heat of battle or sport, or the "pain" of disease successfully denied; in brief, perception as "pain" does not take place. This is rendered possible by the rapid conduction properties of the pathways reaching the cortex, permitting information carried by them to undergo analysis, interact with other sensory input, and activate memory stores and preset response strategies so that the activation of central control processes can be begun *before* the pain response has developed (for example, the decision whether or not to drop or put down gently a hot teacup). Subsequent pain behavior then undergoes integration and modification in terms of the continuous monitoring of the central control system.

PAIN AND PSYCHOLOGIC DEVELOPMENT

Pain is not simply the expression of a biological system concerned with protecting the body from injury. As suffering it also contributes to moral and ethical values and plays a major role in the regulation of behavior and interpersonal relationships. It is a means whereby attributes of the environment are judged as safe or dangerous, as well as an instrument whereby power and control may be exercised. In the course of development, pain becomes complexly related in the mind to such polarities as good-bad, love-hate, innocence-guilt, reward-punishment, and victory-defeat. The learning processes involved in the development of such values for most part take place in childhood and presumably are represented in the *central control (cognitive) system*, which provides the memory traces influencing whether and under what circumstances pain and suffering may be felt.

Among the earliest functions of pain in infancy is its contribution to the process of differentiation of the body from the environment and the formation of a body image. When the baby first bites too hard on his own finger he is learning that what hurts is part of his own body. Szasz suggests that this early psychic equation may contribute to a later use of pain as a means of denying the loss of a body part (e.g., phantom pain after amputation).[4]

Early pain experiences also form the basis for numerous conditioning experiences, which determine the readiness to feel pain or be relieved of pain under some circumstances and not under others. The familiar sequence of the pain of minor injuries disappearing as the child is comforted by the mother underlies the magical belief that mother's display of affection is what makes the pain go away. (Mother kisses the pain away.) This has its counterpart in the amelioration of pain often felt by patients as soon as the physician concerns himself with relief of their suffering (the placebo effect).

The regular association of pain with punishment forms the basis for the relationship between pain and feelings of guilt. For the child, pain is inflicted when one is bad. It is an easy step from this to the notion that pain signifies guilt, often expressed by patients as "What have I done to deserve such pain (suffering)?" By the same token pain may also be utilized to expiate feelings of guilt. The development of such an association is especially likely to occur in children whose early relationships were marked by frequent painful punishments followed by contrite reconciliations. For such children suffering pain may come to represent a necessary condition for both the alleviation of guilt and the reconciliation with a loved one. In this way pain and suffering may anticipate pleasure, and some patients may suffer pain rather than feel guilt (the "pain-prone" patient, see Chapter 30).

The child also is not long in discovering the association between pain and aggression and power. He soon realizes that he too can impose his will on others by inflicting or threatening to inflict pain. But he also learns that he may control his own aggression by threatening himself with pain. This provides an intrapsychic method of controlling aggression, since an aggressive act may be forestalled by avoidance of pain rather than by experiencing pain (see Chapter 30).

From such considerations it is easy to see that certain conditions early in life may predispose to the use of pain to meet psychological needs later in life. By exhibiting suffering and pain one may influence the behavior of others, while pain may also constitute a means to relieve guilt or to control aggression. When such psychic determinants are strong enough, the readiness to feel pain may be greatly enhanced, and pain may be experienced with little or even no afferent input from peripheral receptors (see Chapter 30–Conversion).

CLINICAL INTERPRETATION OF PAIN

THE CLINICAL IMPLICATIONS OF THE REPORT OF "PAIN" OR "NO PAIN"

The compelling issue for the physician is to explain why a patient is complaining of pain. Sometimes, paradoxically, he must also explain why a patient is *not* complaining of pain. This emphasis on the patient's *report* of pain or no pain, rather than on pain, per se, identifies in operational terms the data upon which the physician depends for his evaluation of pain.

A report of pain may reflect any one, or combination, of the following:

1. The presence of local tissue injury or of a peripheral stimulus approaching the threshold of tissue injury.
2. A local afferent input which has become associated in the mind with the threat of injury or disease, so that a sensation not previously felt as painful is felt and reported as pain (e.g., a vague abdominal sensation reported as pain by a patient fearful of cancer).
3. Peripheral or central nervous system damage that interferes with the normal modulation (gating) of small fiber afferent input (e.g., the neuralgias, causalgia, and "central" pain).
4. An unconscious psychological need to suffer or to be punished or to assume the role of a sufferer, a pain previously associated with physical trauma or the infliction of punishment being taken as the paradigm of suffering (e.g., conversion).
5. A conscious and deliberate attempt to deceive others for personal gain (malingering).

On the other hand a **report of no pain** may indicate the following:

1. No injury or tissue damage or no peripheral stimulation approaching the threshold of tissue damage.
2. Receptors or pathways are damaged and incapable of transmitting impulses centrally.
3. The tissue or structure involved in a pathological process has no afferent nerve supply capable of transmitting impulses into the dorsal root system (e.g., lung parenchyma).
4. The chemical or physical properties of a given pathological process are not such as to activate the receptors, fibers, or ascending connections of the dorsal root system (e.g., acute lymphadenitis is painful; the lymphadenopathy of lymphoma is not).
5. The patient's level of consciousness or attention is insufficient to interpret the quality of the sensory experience or to report it as pain.
6. Psychological factors are influencing the patient to reject notions of injury or suffering; hence, body sensations are not experienced as pain.
7. Psychological or social factors are influencing the patient not to report that he is suffering pain, a simulation of health.

PROFILE OF PAIN

The characteristics of pain as experienced and reported are the product of both physiologic and psychologic determinants. The physiologic determinants include the nature of the physical stimuli impinging on receptors, the response characteristics of receptors and afferent fibers, the level of consciousness, and the capability of the sensory-discriminative systems to analyze the input. Psychological determinants include such factors as the meaning of the somaesthetic experience in terms of suffering, the influences of past experience and social-cultural forces, the setting and the psychologic circumstances of the individual at the time, the patient's level of attention, and his capability to communicate verbally. The effects of such factors are by no means random. On the contrary, they endow pain experiences with a sufficient degree of predictability that the physician is able to reconstruct from the patient's verbal account the nature of the underlying physiologic and psychologic processes responsible for the pain. It is precisely for this reason that a firm grasp of physiologic and psychologic principles is essential for the diagnostic process.[33]

The profile of pain involves six dimensions, which reflect the influence of the underlying physiologic and psychologic processes. The characterization of any pain experience requires exploration of all these dimensions. They include:

   1. Topographic aspects—the bodily location
   2. Quantitative aspects—intensity
   3. Temporal aspects—chronology
   4. Qualitative aspects—descriptive language
   5. Associated physiologic aspects—spontaneous physiologic processes that aggravate or alleviate the pain
   6. Behavioral and psychologic aspects—behavior induced by or associated with the pain and the psychologic meaning of pain.

Topographic Aspects (Location)

Pain is always assigned a body location, a function of the sensory discriminative system. Structures with the most extensive innervation are the most fully represented centrally in the body image and are the sites of the most precisely localized pain.

Superficial somatic structures, such as skin and subcutaneous tissue, fascia and fibrous tissue encasing the limbs and trunk (e.g., intercostal fascia and parietal pleura), and periosteum, ligaments and tendon sheaths situated subcutaneously, all are relatively richly supplied with receptors and fibers of widely ranging threshold and size (A beta, gamma, delta, and C). Hence, pain resulting from stimulation of these regions is likely to be relatively well localized.

Deeper somatic structures and *viscera* are more sparsely innervated, for the most part by small fibers (A delta, C) that do not have direct connection with the sensory-discriminative system. Afferent activity from these areas therefore gives rise to pain that is more diffuse and poorly localized. Further, pain from the deeper structure is not necessarily felt in its actual topographic location, but is referred according to the spinal segmental distribution of its innervation. Thus pain from the heart is not felt precordially but in the distribution of T_{1-3}. Such reference of pain to somatic areas of like dermatomal origin is thought to be due to the convergence of afferents from both deep and superficial structures on the same pool of cells in the posterior horn. Since the main contribution to the sensory discriminative system arises from the larger fibers innervating more superficial structures, input from the viscera and other deep structures is felt as arising from these more familiar somatic segments. Occasionally, visceral disease may also be associated with segmental cutaneous hyperesthesia and hyperalgesia. This may be explained in terms of the facilitating effect of small fiber activity from the affected viscus lowering the threshold of T-cells to simultaneous small fiber activity from the skin.

Since the afferent supply of individual viscera generally enters the cord through several adjacent roots, pain of visceral origin usually is felt somewhere within the segmental distribution of several roots. Sometimes it may be felt as well within the zone of immediately neighboring roots. For example, the sensory supply of *the heart* is served mainly by the first three thoracic roots (T_{1-3}), with the predominant inflow from left.[21] The most common sites of pain from myocardial ischemia include behind the sternum, the left pectoral region and shoulder, along the inner aspect of the left arm to the elbow, and occasionally in the back, usually in the midline or just to the left. All of these are within the distribution of T_{1-3}. However, pain may also be felt on the right side, or behind the lower sternum and even substernally (T_{4-5}), as well as down the inner side of the forearm to the fourth and fifth fingers (C8). It may even be felt in the neck, throat, lower jaw, or ear, suggesting spread to the lower and then upper cervical segments and even to the sensory roots of the Vth and Xth cranial nerves.

Clinical experience also demonstrates that *past* or *concurrent* painful processes involving neighboring or overlapping segments may enhance the tendency to feel the pain in spinal segments shared by both distributions, sometimes resulting in an atypical location of the pain. Thus anginal pain may be referred to the right arm in a patient with a recent fracture or to the epigastrium in a patient with duodenal ulcer.

Pain from deep structures, and especially from the viscera, is commonly reported as *radiating*, that is, it is felt to extend in some direction from some primary focus. Cardiac pain, for example, may be described as beginning retrosternally and "radiating" to the left shoulder and down the inner side of the left arm; gallbladder pain may be felt to originate in the right hypochondrium and to radiate to the angle of the scapula. Radiations are generally within the segmental innervation of the affected organ. They probably reflect the recruitment by the developing pathological process of additional receptors so that more spinal segments become involved. Patterns of radiation with different disorders have a relatively high degree of consistency, and hence are of diagnostic value. Occasionally pain may radiate toward the focus of the disease rather than away from it (inverse radiation). Thus, the pain of angina pectoris may sometimes begin in the hypogastrium and radiate upward; or it may radiate from the fingers, wrist, forearm, elbow, or arm of one or both sides to the sternum.[35]

When pain originates from actual involvement of a nerve root or trunk its distribution typically follows, quite exactly, the afferent distribution of the root or nerve. Thus, a herniated intervertebral disc compressing the fifth lumbar root (L5) gives pain that extends down the lateral thigh and legs and is felt deeply as well as superficially.

The locations of pain personally experienced or observed in someone else presumably are recorded centrally as part of the body image. Such pain memories provide the basis for conversion or for malingered pain, the location of which is determined by the meaning of the pain to the sufferer, not by the nature of the afferent innervation of the painful body region. Thus, conversion (or malingered) "heart" pain is more likely to be located in the region of the left nipple than retrosternally or in the left arm. However, when the symptom is modelled on a painful disorder previously experienced by the patient (e.g., an injury or a coronary attack) its location may more closely approximate the usual distribution (see Chapter 30–Conversion Symptoms).

Quantitative Aspects (Intensity)

Patients report intensity of pain in such terms as slight, mild, bearable, severe, or unbearable, or excruciating, but it is virtually impossible to know to what extent the report corresponds with the actual experience. Many factors influence how patients report the severity of pain; but often enough to be of diagnostic value there is a good correlation between the intensity of the noxious stimulation and the severity of the pain reported. This reflects a direct relationship between pain intensity and the amount or concentration of small fiber activity transmitted through dorsal horn cells to activate the central intensity monitor of the action system. Yet, as is well-known in clinical practice, there are many exceptions to this general principle.

1. **Reduction in the level of consciousness** at the time of the pain or in the interval before the pain is reported may yield a much muted account of its severity. Shock, prolonged syncope, or delirium may sometimes account for instances of coronary occlusion, dissecting aneurysm, or subarachnoid hemorrhage with little or no pain.

2. **Attention or distraction** may alter appreciation of pain severity significantly. Pain developing when the patient is alone often is reported as more intense than that developing when concerned persons are available. Relative isolation or sensory restriction, as may occur with a patient immobilized in a body cast, may heighten awareness of pain, especially when chronic.[36] When pain is not too severe or too sudden in its development, even mild distraction, such as music, or having the patient concentrate on something else may ameliorate the pain.[37] Patients instructed preoperatively to take a deep breath from time to time, with the explanation that it will relax tense abdominal muscles, have been found to require much less narcotic for pain relief postoperatively than do patients not so instructed.[38] Simply having ward personnel inquire at frequent intervals about the pain of postoperative patients may enhance the effects of placebo.[39] Here the reduction of anxiety also plays a role.

3. **Expectation, fear, and intolerance of suffering** may influence the severity of the pain reported. In their desperation not to suffer, certain patients may report almost any pain as unbearable, in effect a plea for

help. Some patients show a progressive moderation in their report of pain severity as they gain confidence in the physician or are relieved of anxiety.

4. **A need to suffer or to assume the role of a sufferer,** sometimes determined by unconscious guilt and a wish for expiation and sometimes used as a means to influence or control others, may result in reports of pain of great severity. When the need to suffer is based on guilt, the patient may appear surprisingly composed despite the complaint of very severe pain.[32] Patients utilizing the role of sufferer, consciously or unconsciously, often exhibit more pain in the presence of persons important to them.

5. **A need to appear as strong, tough, and stoical or a wish to overcome the fear of serious illness or death** may lead some patients to minimize pain or deny it altogether. Such attitudes of stoicism and silent suffering are fostered by some cultures and religions, whereas others encourage a public display to bring family and professional support and sympathy.[40] The more pronounced the patient's need to be strong and in command, the more likely is he successfully to block perception of pain, a true psychic denial. Such patients may even fail to remember previous hospitalizations or operations. Coronary patients with such personality features may not report pain or may attempt to deny serious implications by using other terms or by ascribing their symptoms to "indigestion". Only after recovery may they acknowledge that the pain actually had been intense.[41]

6. **Apprehension about the doctor's intentions** may lead some patients, especially children, to claim that pain is inconsequential or absent. Concern about surgery or disagreeable diagnostic procedures, a wish to go home, or a hope to please the doctor all may encourage such deceptive reports.

7. **Intrinsic variations in the neurobiologic system serving pain** may be responsible for some individual differences in response to noxious stimuli. Rare cases of congenital insensitivity (or indifference) to pain have been reported.[3] In one case postmortem study revealed absence of small neurons in the dorsal ganglia, lack of small fibers in the dorsal roots, and absence of the shorter ascending pathway (dorsolateral fasciculus, Lissauer's tract).[42] These children typically suffer numerous injuries and trophic disturbances.

8. Excessively severe pain in response to relatively minor stimulation is typical of **peripheral or central nervous system lesions,** which interfere with the gate control mechanism, permitting relatively unopposed small fiber activity. Post-herpetic neuralgia and causalgia are typical examples.[43]

9. The severity of **conversion pain** bears no relationship to any concurrent afferent stimulus. More important is the severity of suffering required to satisfy the need for punishment and atonement (Chapter 30– Conversion Symptoms).

From the practical point of view it is not always possible to clarify at the bedside all of the factors contributing to a patient's estimate of pain severity. Yet on occasion one encounters patients among whom the evaluation of the severity of the pain is crucial for diagnosis, yet whose report of pain appears at variance with other clinical findings. Under such circumstances it is valuable to be able quickly to demonstrate the patient's typical manner of responding to a painful stimulus. Libman has introduced a simple and practical test for this purpose.[35] It involves first pressing the thumb firmly against the tip of the mastoid bone and then slipping the finger forward and pushing hard upward against the styloid process. Pressure on the normal mastoid bone causes no pain and therefore serves as a control. Pressure in the direction of the styloid process is reported as painful by some individuals and not by others. The sensitive point is thought to be a branch of the greater auricular nerve. The test is carried out quickly and without giving the patient any information as to its objective. Some patients, referred to as "hyposensitive," manifest no outward sign of feeling pain in spite of firm pressure and when asked what they felt, say "nothing," "only pressure," "a little pain," or "it hurt only when you pressed real hard." At the other extreme are the "hypersensitive" patients who report the experience as extremely painful, often flinching, grimacing, wincing, or crying out even before maximum pressure has been exerted. They may continue to complain of pain or to rub the site for some minutes. Some even report mastoid pressure as painful. The "normal" response falls somewhere between these two extremes. About 15 to 20 per cent of the population may be classified as "hyposensitive" and about the same percentage as "hypersensitive." The proportion of "hyposensitives" is higher among men, especially men engaged in hazardous occupations and sports or members of certain ethnic groups (e.g., Indians). Women, on the other hand, include a higher percentage of "hypersensitives."[35,44]

The response of a patient to the Libman test can be very valuable in guiding the physician in his interpretation of the patient's report of pain severity. Thus, one can be assured of the reliability of a report of only mild pain by a patient whose response to styloid pressure is normal or "hypersensitive," and of severe pain by a patient with a "normal" or a "hyposensitive" response. In both instances it is likely that the pain report corresponds to the intensity of the input. But when a patient reporting excruciating pain also overreacts to styloid pressure, or one reporting little or no pain shows a hyposensitive response, then more careful scrutiny of the various factors determining intensity must be carried out. Of interest is Libman's observation that "hyposensitive" patients may show unusual locations or radiations of pain or may complain of sensations other than pain, such as pressure, squeezing, crowding, fullness, burning, numbness, prickling, or tingling. They also are more likely to develop autonomic disturbances, such as sweating, nausea, weakness, or syncope on occasions when pain would be the expected symptom.[35]

In the clinical evaluation of pain severity it is also helpful to have the patient compare his pain to pains experienced in the past, such as toothaches, injuries or labor pains. He may also be asked to measure the severity of his pain against the worst pain he ever experienced. The degree to which a pain interferes with everyday activity provides another index whereby pain intensity can be gauged.

Temporal Aspects

The temporal sequence of a pain often accurately reflects the capability of the sensory-discriminative system to identify the spatiotemporal characteristics of the afferent input. For the most part the rate of rise and fall of a pain corresponds with the rate of stimulation and recruitment of receptors. A sudden prick or a blow will provoke a pain that reaches a peak within a fraction of a second and declines in a few seconds, only to resume in lesser intensity and persist for several minutes longer. This sequence reflects the sudden recruitment of receptors responding to mechanical energy (pressure, stretching, deformation), followed by the for-

mation of chemical products of injury which stimulate chemoreceptors. The stretching of an inflamed pleura during inspiration evokes a volley of impulses felt as a sharp pain with each breath. The rhythmic peristaltic waves of a hollow viscus attempting to expel its contents against resistance, as with labor, renal colic, or intestinal obstruction, yields a characteristic sequence of pain which mounts in intensity over the course of 10 to 20 seconds, is maintained for a minute or so, and then subsides, only to recur within a few minutes. Here one can readily visualize the recruitment of mechanical receptors responding as the region proximal to the obstruction is stretched with each successive peristaltic wave. Similarly may be visualized the throbbing character of the pain associated with arteritis or an abscess, in which the rhythmic stretch and relaxation with each systolic pulse of the sensitive arterial wall or of the tensely swollen inflammatory mass governs the pattern of afferent impulses.

The elaboration at the site of tissue injury of kinins and other chemical substances which lower receptor thresholds accounts for the steady pain and the exquisite tenderness typically associated with trauma and acute inflammation.[16] Such a mechanism probably also explains how structures ordinarily insensitive to pain, such as the mucosa of the gastrointestinal tract, may give rise to a steady pain when inflamed.[45]

Other irritating chemical substances, such as gastric juice, pancreatic enzymes, and bile, coming in contact with naked nerve terminals in the peritoneum or bed of the pancreas, are responsible for pain that mounts in intensity over a matter of minutes and is sustained for hours. The metabolic products of muscle ischemia act in a similar way to produce a pain that is sustained as long as they are present.

The point in time at which a pain begins to recede, whether minutes, hours, or days, may reflect the duration of activity of the responsible pathological process, a change in its character, or damage to the receptors or afferent nerves involved. The duration of the pain of angina pectoris, usually a matter of minutes, correlates with the period of myocardial ischemia, whereas that of coronary occlusion, a matter of hours, is limited by the onset of anoxic necrosis of the involved heart muscle and its afferent nerve supply. Reduction in the level of consciousness may also bring pain to an end, such as by analgesic or tranquilizing drug, or favorable psychological influences, including placebo effects.

Pain associated with nerve or root injury often shows a characteristic delay of a second or so between the onset of stimulation and the appreciation of the pain, followed by a sustained afterpain (hyperpathia). Such nerve damage interferes chiefly with the fast-conducting large myelinated fibers, leaving the slower small fiber activity unopposed by the normal gate control mechanism.[43]

The temporal characteristics of pain determined mainly by psychological factors, such as conversion and malingering, usually are not in keeping with temporal response patterns ordinarily associated with peripheral afferent activity. Rather they correspond more with the patient's idiosyncratic notion of what the pain should be like. Only when the conversion or malingered pain is based on a painful illness previously experienced by the patient himself are the time parameters likely to approximate those of an organically induced pain.

Qualitative Aspects (Descriptive Language)

In eliciting descriptions of pain it is important that the physician not bias the patient's account by proposing descriptive terms before the patient has been encouraged to use his own terms. Indeed, at times patients are describing sensations other than pain, such as pressure, tingling, or fullness, and the clinical picture is only confused if the physician refers to these as "pain." Sometimes the sensation is actually a somatic delusion (see Chapter 30).

The limiting factor in pain description is the patient's verbal capacity. One must accept the fact that some persons simply lack the vocabulary and fluency to report much beyond the fact that they are in pain. However, in evaluating the report of a patient who is unable to describe his pain, it is wise to inquire about *other* pain experiences, for one may then discover that it is the pain that is "indescribable," rather than the patient who is incapable of describing pain.

As a subjective experience, ultimately inaccessible to consensual validation, the available language for pain is limited. Some of the terms of widest currency reflect spatiotemporal characteristics, such as sharp, dull, throbbing, aching, and lightning. Often a pain is described in terms of some commonly familiar painful experience, such as a toothache, a burn, a bruise, a sting, a cramp, or an electric shock. Such descriptions are usually also within the range of the personal experi-

ence of the physician and hence effectively convey a picture of the patient's pain. Or the description may be in terms of a pain previously experienced by the patient, such as labor pain, ulcer pain, or migraine, a very informative description when the disorder referred to has been documented.

Very often patients make use of simile, often involving themes of violence.[1,46] They speak of pain as "like a knife sticking in there," "like somebody hitting you," "like being burnt with a red-hot poker," or "like having the skin peeled off." Such similes demonstrate the intimate psychological association between pain and aggression. For some patients they merely constitute the most lucid way of describing how the pain feels and are related in a quite matter of fact tone of voice. Other patients use such expressions in a dramatic way to impress upon the doctor the intensity of their suffering or the desperateness of their need for help. Usually such dramatic presentations also reflect the presence of powerful underlying aggressive and self-punitive impulses. Their use is more prevalent among members of cultures that foster public display of suffering and dramatic appeals for help, as well as among patients with hysterical personality features. The latter are especially likely to exhibit conversion symptoms. Hence a dramatic pain presentation justifies looking for other evidence for conversion as the explanation of the pain (see Chapter 30).

Careful analyses of the similes used by patients to describe pain often reveal that they accurately convey the temporospatial characteristics of an underlying somatic process. For example, a patient with a herniated intervertebral disc said of his pain, "It was like a dog would bite you," and then, "As if somebody lit a match and went down the back of the leg with it." Further questioning made it clear that he used the imagery of a dog biting into his thigh to describe how the pain would grab him and hang on, that is, the sudden onset and the ensuing muscle spasm. The lighted match simile described the radiation of burning pain along the root distribution. Had these vivid terms referred to conversion pains, the other imagery offered in elaboration would have been more consistent with their symbolic meaning to the patient rather than with known physiological processes.

Some pains simply are not capable of being described in words because they do not correspond with any previous experience or fantasy. Pain that originates from injured nerves (e.g., neuralgia, causalgia) or from lesions involving the mediating system (e.g., "central" pain) is especially likely to defy description. Patients may use terms such as burning, tingling, knotting, cramping, boring, gnawing, or crushing, but above all they emphasize that the sensation is like nothing ever before experienced. This is understandable for when an area innervated by a damaged nerve is stimulated the afferent input pattern does not correspond with any input ever before experienced; it conveys information about the stimulus that is meaningless in terms of any past experience. The patient, accustomed to reporting a skin sensation in terms of the stimulus ("You're pricking me," "a pinch," "touch with cotton") finds that a familiar stimulus is yielding a completely unfamiliar sensation, the only consistent feature of which is that it is disagreeable.[43,47]

Associated Physiologic Aspects

Body activities and physiologic processes serve to modify pain by increasing or decreasing afferent activity. Such relationships are helpful in identifying the site and nature of the pathologic process responsible for the pain.

1. **Skin.** Any modality of stimulation, including light contact of clothing, may intensify pain originating from the skin. On the other hand, gentle stimulation, such as stroking, warmth, or vibration, in adjacent uninvolved areas may reduce the pain, presumably through the inhibitory action of large fiber activity on small fiber transmission through the T-cells. Cooling may reduce pain of inflammatory origin, whereas dependency, which increases engorgment, may increase it. Cutaneous hyperesthesia and hyperalgesia may be referred from visceral disease or nerve lesions.

Similar influences operate in pain originating in the sensitive mucous membranes of the nose and throat, conjuctiva, and anal and urogenital orifices.

2. **Subcutaneous structures.** Pressure or tension, and dependency in the case of inflammatory lesions, are the main influences increasing pain.

3. **Skeletal muscle** pain is intensified by use of the muscle as well as by mechanical forces such as pressure. The sudden movements of coughing, sneezing, or laughing, will increase pain coming from abdominal and trunk musculature. When pain is due to ischemia, as is characteristic of intermittent claudication, there is a direct relationship between the degree of circulatory insufficiency and muscle work. The interval between the beginning of muscle contraction and the onset of pain depends on how long it takes for hypoxic products of muscle metabolism to accumulate and exceed the threshold of receptor response. Hence pain from an ischemic muscle builds up with use of the muscle and subsides with rest.

4. **Movable skeletal parts, including bones, joints, bursae, and tendons** give rise to pain when the structure is used and relief when rested.

5. **Nerve and root** pain is intensified by any movement or posture that impinges on the involved nerve or root. Sudden increases in intraspinal pressure produced by coughing, sneezing, or straining typically exacerbate root pain.

6. **Peripheral nerve or plexus** disorders give rise to pain that is intensified by stimulation of receptors within peripheral distribution of the damaged nerve. Any contact of the skin or pressure on deeper structures may be excruciating, although there may be a quite noticeable delay between the effective stimulus and the onset of the pain. Cold is very poorly tolerated, whereas warmth may ameliorate the pain. Pain may also sometimes be induced by stimulation of receptor zones that feed impulses into the same spinal segment. Sometimes there are trigger points, the slightest contact with which will provoke an intense paroxysm of pain; this is characteristic of trigeminal and glossopharyngeal neuralgia.

7. **Lesions of cord, bulb, pons, thalamus or the second sensory area of the cortex** may give rise to pain which often characteristically appears as unprovoked paroxysms, but may also be steady and exacerbated by mild stimulation in the area of the body served by the damaged neural system (e.g., the lightning pains of tabes dorsalis, the thalamic syndrome).[21]

8. **Pain arising from arteries,** as with arteritis, migraine, and vascular headaches, increases with systolic impulse. Hence any process associated with increased systolic or pulse pressure, such as exercise, fever, alcohol, or bending over may intensify the throbbing pain.[49]

9. **Intracranial masses** which put pain-sensitive structures under tension are sensitive to processes which suddenly displace intracranial structures. Thus pain may be increased by jarring the head, jogging, or

sudden alterations in intracranial pressure, as with coughing or sneezing.[49]

10. **Pain from pleura,** as well as from **trachea,** correlates with respiratory movements.

11. **Heart pain,** a consequence of muscle ischemia, correlates with metabolic demand. Hence, with coronary insufficiency (angina pectoris) pain may develop when the work of the heart is increased, as with exertion or emotion, and subside with rest and composure.

12. **Pain from mediastinum** may be influenced by the activity of neighboring moving parts, esophagus (swallowing), musculoskeletal structures (movement), aorta (increased systolic thrust).

13. **Pain from the gastrointestinal tract** tends to increase with peristaltic activity, particularly if there is any obstruction to forward progress. Hence it is increased with ingestion and may lessen with fasting, or upon emptying the involved segment (vomiting or bowel movement). When hollow viscera are distended, body positions or movements that increase intra-abdominal pressure may intensify the pain, whereas positions that reduce pressure or support the structure may ease the pain. The patient with an acutely distended gallbladder may slightly flex his trunk and support his right hypochondrium with his hand. Pain secondary to the effect of gastric acid on esophagus, stomach, or duodenum correlates with pH; hence, it is relieved by the presence of food or other neutralizing material in the stomach and intensified when the stomach is empty and secreting acid.

14. **Viscera with capsules, such as liver, kidneys, spleen, and pancreas,** may give rise to pain when swollen. The pain increases with compression of the tense organ, as may occur with increased intra-abdominal pressure. Patients achieve some relief by assuming postures that decrease pressure on the organ. With pain arising from a tense swollen kidney (or distended renal pelvis) the patient flexes his trunk and tilts away from the involved side; with pancreatic pain, he may sit or lie with his knees drawn up to the chest.[50]

15. **Irritation of the parietal peritoneum,** local or generalized, yields pain that is intensified by any movement of the inflamed area. This may include movements of the trunk, respiratory movements, or movements of the underlying organ.

16. When pain is determined by psycho-logical needs to any significant extent, correlation with physiological influences may be obscured or even absent altogether, as is typically the case with conversion pain or malingering. Indeed, such lack of correlation is one criterion suggestive of conversion (see Chapter 30).

Behavioral and Psychological Aspects

Much behavior exhibited by the person in pain constitutes trial-and-error efforts at relief. These may include rest, movement, change in posture, increased or decreased food intake, attempts to regurgitate, eructate, or urinate, and the use of heat, cold, massage, compresses, pressure, or self-medication. For the most part, patients first utilize measures that they have found effective with other pains. Some, they quickly discover, make matters worse, whereas others have no effect. When nothing relieves the pain the patient may persist in quite irrational and even dangerous activities; patients with acute myocardial infarction, for example, have been known to do pushups in a vain attempt to terminate the pain!

Some pain behavior is aimed at soliciting help. Here the setting and personal style, as well as cultural influences, determine the pattern of behavior manifested.[3] The behavior of individuals for whom the pain is profoundly disturbing is primarily determined by their desperate need to be relieved of the pain. They may exaggerate the pain or be loudly insistent in their demand for relief. Others, those who take pride in their stoicism, may display little or no pain behavior. Some patients, those for whom suffering serves important psychological ends, behave as if they are more concerned with how others respond to them as sufferers than they are with the relief of pain. They include persons with deep underlying feelings of guilt and masochism or with intense aggressive impulses. Such persons are likely to invite injury or to suffer pain as a conversion symptom[32,51] (see Chapter 30).

Relationships between behavior and relief or exacerbation of pain must be interpreted with care, for patients are quick to ascribe significance to what may be merely coincidence. It is not uncommon, for example, for a patient to report that his pain was improved or made worse by the medication when in fact the change reflected the natural progress of the underlying disorder, or perhaps the relief of anxiety or the intensification of anger or guilt.

TABLE 3-1. PAIN PROFILE IN RELATION TO SOURCE OF INPUT

	LOCATION	INTENSITY	TEMPORAL ASPECTS	DESCRIPTION	ASSOCIATED PHYSIOLOGIC ASPECTS	BEHAVIOR
SUPERFICIAL SOMATIC	Surface; well localized	Basically correlated with intensity of stimulation	Correlates with tempo of input and extent of after-discharge	In terms of familiar surface injuries; mainly determined by spatial-temporal intensity dimensions	Intensified by contact; alleviated by gentle stimulation in adjacent areas	Guarding of involved area; application of warmth, cold, soothing agent, counter irritation
DEEP SOMATIC	Segmental; deep; poorly localized; radiates; referred to surface	Basically correlated with intensity of stimulation	Correlates with tempo of input and extent of after-discharge	Vague, aching, sharp, boring, pounding; mainly determined by spatial-temporal intensity dimensions	Intensified by movement, compression, pulsation, (artery); alleviated by inactivity	Avoidance of movement, pressure; awkward movement due to protective spasm
VISCERAL	Segmental; deep; poorly localized; radiates; referred to surface	Basically correlated with intensity of stimulation	Correlates with tempo of input and extent of after-discharge	Griping, cramping, aching, squeezing, crushing, stabbing, burning; mainly determined by spatial-temporal intensity dimensions	Intensified by motor activity or compression of involved viscus, correlates with secretory or motor rhythms of involved viscus	Trial and error behavior to relieve pain, based on physiological concomitants, previous experience, psychic factors
NEUROGENIC	Within neural distribution; surface or deep; radiates	Excessive response to stimulation	No correlation with input	Indescribable; unlike any naturally occurring pain; unusual combination of painful sensations	Provoked by any peripheral stimulation in involved zone; trigger points "spontaneous" paroxysms	Vigilant guarding of involved part—apprehensive concern
PSYCHOGENIC	According to body image or appropriate to fantasy; surface or deep; well or poorly localized; may radiate	Variable; correlates with psychic needs for suffering, intensity of guilt, aggression, depression; inconsistent with severity of concurrent organic process	Variable; correlates with individual notions of injury, suffering, or disease	Vivid psychic imagery; correlates with notions of suffering, punishment, torture; variable; inconsistent; elaborated; spatial-temporal intensity dimensions vague or inconsistent with organic processes	Inconsistent or no correlation with physiological processes	Emphasis on suffering; discrepancy between appearance and intensity of pain reported; distractible; background of violence or aggression; sadistic or masochistic attitudes: guilt. Importance of pain in past or current relationships; prominence of pain in family; pain seen as punishment; response to loss

Acute pain is likely to provoke anxiety and a general arousal reaction with the concomitant physiological changes of the flight-fight pattern (see Chapter 29). Vasodepressor syncope may develop and progress to vascular collapse and shock.[52] Occasionally a patient in pain reacts with an outburst of anger. With some patients this is an expression of helpless frustration; with others it indicates the presence of underlying aggressive conflicts, which may be psychic determinants of the pain. With more chronic pain, feelings of guilt and depression become more prominent. When pain is severe and of long standing its significance as a warning signal loses its meaning and the patient may become totally absorbed in his world of suffering.

CLASSIFICATION OF PAIN ACCORDING TO SOURCE (TABLE 3-1)

Although appreciating that the experience of pain is ultimately psychological and personal, the clinician must, for purposes of diagnosis, identify and evaluate in each case the relative importance of the sources of input underlying the pain. These may conveniently be classified as "peripheral," "neurogenic," and "psychogenic."

Peripheral sources include all afferent input originating from receptors of the dorsal root system. These may be subdivided into *superficial somatic, deep somatic,* and *visceral.*

"Neurogenic" refers to input so modified by damage to the peripheral or central nervous system that it is experienced as pain. Such pain may result from abnormal processing of normal afferent activity or from paroxysmal activity originating within the nervous system itself.

"Psychogenic" sources include fantasies, wishes, needs, or impulses involving ideas of injury, punishment, atonement, or suffering, which contribute to pain through such psychic mechanisms as symbolization (conversion) or simulation (malingering) (see Chapter 30–Conversion Symptoms).

REFERENCES

1. Devine, R., and Merskey, H.: The description of pain in psychiatric and general medical patients, J. Psychosom. Res. 9:311, 1965.
2. Merskey, H., and Spear, F. G.: Pain, Psychological and Psychiatric Aspects, Baltimore, Williams & Wilkins, 1967.
3. Sternbach, R.: Pain, A Psychophysiological Inquiry, New York, Academic Press, 1968.
4. Szasz, T.: Pain and Pleasure. A Study of Bodily Feelings, New York, Basic Books, 1957.
5. Hardy, H. D., Wolff, H. G., and Goodell, H.: Pain Sensations and Reactions, Baltimore, Williams & Wilkins, 1952.
6. Melzack, R.: Effects of early experience on behavior: experimental and conceptual considerations, in Hoch, P. H., and Zubin, J. (eds.): Psychopathology of Perception, pp. 271-300, Grune and Stratton, 1965.
7. Goldscheider, A.: Die Lehre von den specifischen Energeen der Sinnesorgane, Berlin, L. Schumacher, 1881.
8. Frey, M. von: Beitrage zur Sinnesphysiologie der Haut, Leipsig, 1895.
9. Melzack, R., and Wall, P. D.: Pain mechanisms. A new theory, Science 150:971, 1965.
10. Casey, K. L., and Melzack, R.: Neural mechanisms of pain: a conceptual model, in Way, E. L. (ed.): New Concepts of Pain, F. A. Davis, 1967.
11. Melzack, R., and Wall, P. D.: Gate control theory of pain, in Soulairac, A., Cahn, J., and Charpentier, J. (eds.): Pain, New York, Academic Press, 1968.
12. Quillam, T. A.: Unit design and array patterns in receptor organs, in de Reuck, A. V. S., and Knight, J. (eds.): Touch, Heat, and Pain, Boston, Little, Brown & Co., 1966.
13. Cauna, N.: Fine structures of the receptor organs and its probable functional significance, in de Rueck, A. V. S., and Knight, J. (eds.): Touch, Heat, and Pain, Boston, Little, Brown & Co., 1966.
14. Iggo, A.: A single unit analysis of cutaneous receptors in C afferent fibers, in Wolstenholme, G. E. W., and O'Connor, M. (eds.): Pain and Itch. Nervous Mechanisms, Boston, Little, Brown & Co., 1960.
15. Keele, C. A., and Armstrong, D.: Substances Producing Pain and Itch, Baltimore, Williams & Wilkins, 1964.
16. Lim, R. K. S.: Pharmacologic viewpoint of pain and analgesia, in Way, E. L. (ed.): New Concepts in Pain, Philadelphia, Davis, 1967.
17. Bishop, G. H.: The relation between nerve fiber size and sensory modality. Phylogenetic implications of the afferent innervation of the cortex, J. Nerv. Ment. Dis., 128:89, 1959.
18. Winkelman, R. K.: Similarities in cutaneous nerve endings, in Montagna, W. (ed.): Cutaneous Innervations of the Skin, Advances in Biology of Skin, vol. 1, p. 48, London, Pergamon Press, 1960.
19. Weddell, G.: Studies related to the mechanism of common sensibility, in Montagna, W. (ed.): Cutaneous Innervation of the Skin, Advances in Biology of Skin, vol. 1, p. 112, London, Pergamon Press, 1960.
20. Lim, R. K. S., Liu, C. N., Guzman, F., and Braun, C.: Visceral receptors concerned in visceral pain and the pseudoaffective response to intra-arterial injection of bradykinin and other algesic agents, J. Comp. Neurol. 118:269, 1962.

21. White, J. C., and Sweet, W. H.: Pain, Springfield, Ill., Charles C Thomas, 1955.
22. Mountcastle, V. B.: Duality of function in the somatic afferent systems, *in* Brazier, M. A. B. (ed.): Brain and Behavior, vol. I, pp. 67-93, Washington, Amer. Inst. Biol. Sci., 1961.
23. Whitlock, D. G., and Perl, E. R.: Thalamic projections of spinothalamic pathways in monkey, Exp. Neurol. 3:240, 1961.
24. Perl, E. R., and Whitlock, D. G.: Somatic stimuli exciting spinothalamic projections to thalamic neurons in cat and monkey, Exp. Neurol. 3:256, 1961.
25. Mark, V. H., Ervin, F. R., and Yakovlev, P. L.: The treatment of pain by stereotaxic methods, Confin. Neurol. 22:238, 1962.
26. ———: Stereotaxic thalamotomy. III. The verification of anatomical lesion sites in the human thalamus, Arch. Neurol. 8:529, 1963.
27. Olds, M. E., and Olds, J.: Approach-avoidance analysis of rat diencephalon, J. Comp. Neurol. 120:259, 1963.
28. ———: Approach-escape interactions in the rat brain, Amer. J. Physiol. 203:803, 1962.
29. Cox, V. C., and Valenstein, E. S.: Attenuation of aversive properties of peripheral shock by hypothalamic stimulation, Science 149:323, 1965.
30. Pavlov, I. P.: Lectures on Conditioned Reflexes, New York, International Publishers, 1928.
31. Bell, C., Sierra, G., Buendia, N., and Segundo, I. P.: Sensory properties of neurons in the mesencephalic reticular formation, J. Neurophysiol. 27:961, 1964.
32. Engel, G. L.: Psychogenic pain and the pain prone patient, Amer. J. Med. 26:899, 1959.
33. Morgan, W. L., and Engel, G. L.: The clinical approach to the patient, Ch. 2, The Diagnostic Process, Philadelphia, W. B. Saunders, 1969.
34. Kellgren, J. H.: On the distribution of pain arising from deep somatic structures, with charts of segmental pain areas, Clin. Sci. 4:35, 1939.
35. Libman, E.: Observations on individual sensitiveness to pain, J.A.M.A. 102:335, 1934.
36. Blitz, B., and Lowenthal, M.: The role of sensory restriction in problems with chronic pain, J. Chronic Dis. 19:1119, 1966.
37. Melzack, R., Weisz, A. Z., and Sprague, L. T.: Stratagems for controlling pain: Contributions of auditory stimulation and suggestion, Exp. Neurol. 8:239, 1963.
38. Egbert, L. D., Battit, G. E., Welch, C. E., and Bartlett, M. K.: Reduction of post-operative pain by encouragement and instruction of patients, New Eng. J. Med. 270:825, 1964.
39. Beecher, H. K.: Generalization from pain of various types and diverse origin, Science 130:267, 1959.
40. Zborowski, M.: Cultural components in responses to pain, J. Social Issues 8:16, 1952.
41. Olin, H. S., and Hackett, T. P.: The denial of chest pain in 32 patients with acute myocardial infarction, J.A.M.A. 190:977, 1964.
42. Swanson, A. G., Buchan, G. C., and Alvord, E. C.: Anatomical changes in congenital insensitivity to pain, Arch. Neurol. 12:12, 1965.
43. Noordenbos, W.: Pain, Amsterdam, Elsevier Publ., 1959.
44. Sherman, E. D.: Sensitivity to pain, Canad. Med. Ass. J. 48:431, 1943.
45. Wolf, S., and Wolff, H. G.: Human Gastric Function, New York, Oxford University Press, 1943.
46. Klein, R. F., and Brown, W.: Pain descriptions in medical settings, J. Psychosom. Res. 10:367, 1967.
47. Denny-Brown, D.: The release of deep pain by nerve injury, Brain 88:725, 1965.
48. Head, H., and Sherren, J.: The consequences of injury to the peripheral nerves in man, Brain 28:99, 1905.
49. Wolff, H. G.: Headache, New York, Oxford University Press, 1963.
50. Macchia, B.: Position relief of pain. Important clue to clinical diagnosis of carcinoma of the pancreas, J.A.M.A. 182:6, 1962.
51. Tinling, D. C., and Klein, R. F.: Psychogenic pain and aggression. The syndrome of the solitary hunter, Psychosom. Med. 28:738, 1966.
52. Engel, G. L.: Fainting, ed. 2, Springfield, Ill., Charles C Thomas, 1962.
53. LeShan, L.: The world of the patient in severe pain of long duration, J. Chronic Dis. 17:119, 1964.

4

Headache*

HAROLD G. WOLFF
(May 26, 1898—February 21, 1962)

PATHOPHYSIOLOGY OF HEADACHE

Headaches fall into two major categories as regards their origin: (1) those that arise mainly as a result of stimulation of intracranial structures, and (2) those that occur upon stimulation of tissues that lie on the outside of and adjacent to the skull.

PAIN-SENSITIVE STRUCTURES OF THE HEAD

The pain sensitivity of the tissues covering the cranium, the cranium itself, and most of the intracranial structures has been ascertained from a series of patients during surgical procedures on the head by using a variety of stimuli. Some of the "pain pathways" and the mechanisms of headache are defined.

1. Of the tissues covering the cranium, all are more or less sensitive to pain, the arteries being especially so.

2. Of the intracranial structures, the great venous sinuses and their venous tributaries from the surface of the brain, parts of the

* Revised by Helen Goodell, Lawrence E. Hinkle, Jr., and E. Charles Kunkle.

dura at the base, the dural arteries, and the cerebral arteries at the base of the brain, the fifth, the ninth and the tenth cranial nerves and the upper three cervical nerves are sensitive to pain.

3. The cranium (including the diploic and the emissary veins), the parenchyma of the brain, most of the dura, most of the pia-arachnoid, the ependymal lining of the ventricles, and the choroid plexuses are not sensitive to pain.

Stimulation of the pain-sensitive intracranial structures on or above the superior surface of the tentorium cerebelli resulted in pain in various regions in front of a line drawn vertically from the ears across the top of the head. The pathways for this pain are contained in the fifth cranial nerve.

Stimulation of the pain-sensitive intracranial structures on or below the inferior surface of the tentorium cerebelli resulted in pain in various regions behind the line just described. The pathways for this pain are contained chiefly in the ninth and the tenth cranial nerves and the upper three cervical nerves.

Intracranial diseases commonly cause headache through more than one mechanism and by involvement of more than one pain-sensitive structure. From the data available, six basic mechanisms of headache from intracranial sources have been formulated: headache may result from (1) traction on the veins that pass to the venous sinuses from the surface of the brain and displacement of the great venous sinuses; (2) traction on the middle meningeal arteries; (3) traction on the large arteries at the base of the brain and their main branches; (4) distention and dilatation of intracranial arteries; (5) inflammation in or about any of the pain-sensitive structures of the head; and (6) direct pressure or traction by tumors on cranial and cervical nerves containing many pain-afferent fibers from the head.

Traction, displacement, and inflammation of pain-sensitive venous structures, arteries, cranial, and upper cervical nerves are chiefly responsible for headache arising from intracranial structures.

Headache from intracranial disease is usually referred pain. Local tenderness of the scalp may serve as an index to the structures responsible when a lesion produces

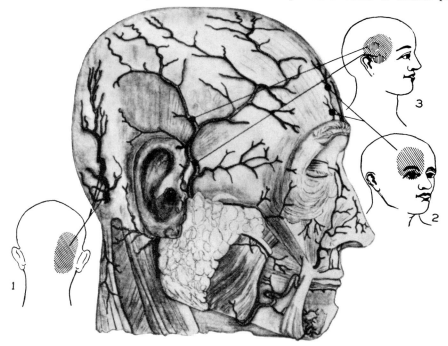

Fig. 4-1. The arteries of the scalp. Solid circles indicate the points of stimulation causing pain. The diagrams show the areas of pain following the stimulation of (1) the occipital arteries, (2) the supraorbital and frontal arteries, and (3) superficial temporal artery. (Ray and Wolff: Arch. Surg. 41:817)

direct irritation of pain-sensitive structures. However, disease of remotely separated pain-sensitive structures may cause pain and hyperalgesia in identical areas. Sepsis or fever of any origin may be associated with headache, but this is not referred pain. Pain referred to the head from disease of tissue elsewhere than the head does not occur, with the rare exception of pain in the jaw or the neck with angina pectoris. In paraplegics, headache may be associated with excessive distention of the urinary bladder or the rectum. Such headache results from dilatation of cranial vessels, secondary to a rise in systemic arterial pressure.

MECHANISM OF HEADACHE ASSOCIATED WITH CHANGES IN INTRACRANIAL PRESSURE

The headache so frequently associated with abnormally high or low cerebrospinal fluid pressure has long been the subject of con-

tradictory speculations. In a study of headache associated with changes in intracranial pressure, headache was regularly induced in normal erect human subjects by the free drainage of approximately 20 ml. of cerebrospinal fluid (about 10 per cent of the total CSF volume), the estimated vertex pressure falling to between minus 220 and minus 290 mm. from a normal of approximately minus 130 mm.

The headache that often follows lumbar puncture has predictable and unique features, all of which indicate its similarity to the drainage headache. It may appear a few hours to several days after lumbar puncture, lasting a variable period of days or, rarely, weeks. The pain is a dull, deep ache and may be throbbing. It is usually bifrontal and often also suboccipital. In the latter position it may be associated with moderate stiffness of the neck. Like drainage headache, post-

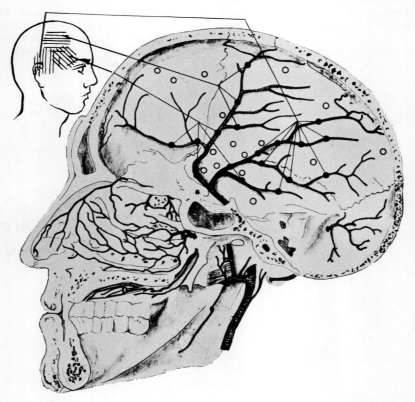

Fig. 4-2. Middle meningeal artery. Open circles indicate the point of stimulation of the dura without pain. Solid circles indicate the point of stimulation causing pain. The diagram shows three overlapping areas of pain in the parietotemporal region resulting from stimulation of different portions of the artery and its branches.

puncture headache was shown to be associated with a decrease in cerebrospinal fluid volume as evidenced by a fall in cerebrospinal fluid pressure. It was completely eliminated by the intrathecal injection of an amount of saline equal to that of spinal fluid removed. Its intensity was reduced by change from the erect to the horizontal position or by head flexion or extension. Its intensity was increased by bilateral jugular compression and by shaking the head (lowered "jolt threshold").

Therefore, the usual variety of postpuncture headache is similar in type and mechanism to the headache induced by drainage of cerebrospinal fluid. Its behavior suggests that it is caused chiefly by dilatation and traction upon pain-sensitive intracranial venous structures. It is probably secondary to the loss of cerebrospinal fluid removed for

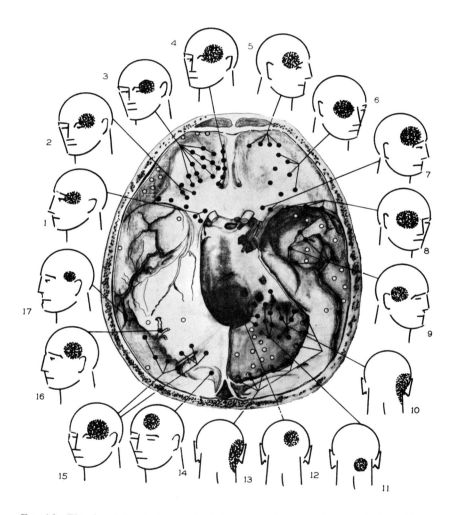

Fig. 4-3. The dural floor of the skull, the tentorium cerebelli and the adjacent venous sinuses and venous tributaries. Open circles indicate the points of stimulation without pain. Solid circles indicate the points of stimulation causing pain. The diagrams show the areas of pain following stimulation of: (1–8) the dura of the floor of the anterior fossa, (9–17) the middle meningeal artery, (10–12) the dura of the floor of the posterior fossa, (13) the inferior wall of the transverse sinus, (14) the superior wall of the torcular Herophili, (15) the superior wall of the transverse sinus and upper surface of the tentorium cerebelli and (16) the inferior cerebral veins. (Ray and Wolff: Arch. Surg. 41:825)

analysis, plus the prolonged leakage of fluid through the dural hole in the lumbar sac produced by the operator's needle. Prevention is facilitated by the use of a small bore lumbar puncture needle.

The headache so often associated with increased intracranial pressure has generally been assumed, but never proved, to be related to the increased pressure. Yet elevation of intracranial pressure in normal human subjects to abnormally high levels failed to cause headache. Headache homolateral to the lesion in a patient with a brain tumor was induced by lowering the intracranial pressure, but could not be induced by elevation of the pressure to a high level of 550 mm. That increased intracranial pressure is not the dominant factor in headache associated with brain tumor is suggested by an analysis of 72 patients in whom headache occurred almost as commonly (82 per cent) in 23 patients without increased intracranial pressure as it did (94 per cent) in 49 patients with increased pressure.

Hence, increased intracranial pressure is neither a prime nor an essential factor in the headache that may be associated with it.

From these data it is concluded that the headache associated with either decreased or increased intracranial pressure results from traction upon or displacement of pain-sensitive intracranial structures and is independent of generalized intracranial pressure changes per se.

BRAIN-TUMOR HEADACHE

The Quality and the Intensity of Brain-Tumor Headache. The headache associated with brain tumor is of a deep, aching, steady, dull nature. It is not rhythmic and seldom throbs. It is usually intermittent, but in one-tenth of the patients it is continuous. The headache is sometimes severe, but rarely is it as intense as that of migraine or of the headache associated with rupture of cerebral aneurysm, meningitis, or certain febrile illnesses, or of that induced by certain drugs. It is usually diminished in intensity by acetylsalicylic acid, or cold packs applied to the scalp, both indications of its moderate intensity. It rarely interferes with sleep. It may be aggravated by coughing, or straining at stool, and sometimes it is worse in the erect than in the recumbent position. It is commonly aggravated also by the onset of a minor infection. If there is any variation in intensity during the 24-hour cycle, it is worse in the early morning.

Even when the tumor directly compresses or extensively stretches cranial nerves containing pain afferents, the pain is not equal in intensity to that of tic douloureux, and indeed is often mild or absent.

One rare form of very intense headache may be encountered in patients in the terminal phase of brain tumor. This headache is generalized, paroxysmal, and agonizing and it may precede stupor or death. The pain may last for 30 seconds to half an hour, and may disappear suddenly.

Unless the pain is severe, nausea with tumor headache is slight. Vomiting occurs with displacement or compression of the medulla and is sometimes projectile (perhaps because it is unexpected when unaccompanied by nausea). The headache, when occipital or suboccipital, sometimes is associated with "stiffness" or aching of the muscles of the neck and tilting of the head toward the side of the tumor. The possibility of brain tumor should be appraised, (1) whenever severe and/or persistent headache begins in a patient who upon careful questioning reveals that he has not had headache previously; and (2) whenever a change occurs in the site, the quality, the intensity, and the temporal features of the head pain in those with a long history of headaches.

The Mechanism of Brain-Tumor Headache. Brain-tumor headache is produced by traction upon and displacement of intracranial pain-sensitive structures, chiefly the large arteries, veins and venous sinuses, and certain cranial nerves. There are two types of traction, which operate singly or in combination: local traction by the tumor upon adjacent structures; and distant traction by extensive displacement of the brain, either directly by the tumor, or indirectly by ventricular obstruction (internal hydrocephalus). Brain tumor may in addition press directly upon cranial nerves.

Headache as an aid in the localization of brain tumor is limited in its value by two facts: the headache may be remote from the site of its production, and the site of production of headache may be remote from the tumor.

In spite of these limitations, when it is interpreted in terms of known principles of intracranial pain production and pain reference, the headache of brain tumor may significantly aid in the diagnosis and the localization of the lesion. The following generalizations are useful:

1. Although the headache of brain tumor

is often referred from a distant intracranial source, it approximately overlies the tumor in about one-third of all patients.

2. Brain-tumor headache in the absence of papilledema is of great localizing value. In about two-thirds of such patients, the headache immediately overlies or is near the tumor; in all, when unilateral, it is on the same side as the tumor.

3. Headache is almost always present with posterior fossa tumor, but may be absent with any of the common types of supratentorial tumor.

4. Headache is usually the first symptom of posterior fossa tumor and is almost always over the back of the head, except in cerebellopontile angle tumors.

5. The headache of cerebellopontile angle tumors is frequently and sometimes solely postauricular on the side of the tumor.

6. Headache is the first symptom of one-third of supratentorial tumors and is rarely in the back of the head unless associated with papilledema.

7. When headache associated with brain tumor is both frontal and occipital it indicates extensive displacement of the brain and has little localizing value.

8. Brain-tumor headache is usually intermittent, but when it is continuous its value in localization is greatly enhanced. The history of the site and the distribution of headache, whether it was initially and predictably on the left or the right, frontal or occipital, may indicate the site of a lesion. In some instances, intracranial tumor is manifested by induced frontotemporal headache following sudden head rotation or jolting. If the induced headache is unilateral, the lesion is usually on the side of the head pain.

Experimental Evidence on Intracranial Vascular Mechanisms of Headache

The association of headache following intravenous histamine injection with increase in the amplitude of the intracranial arterial pulsations has been demonstrated photographically. Simultaneous records of systemic arterial blood pressure, cerebrospinal fluid pressure, temporal artery pulsations, and intracranial pulsations were made (Fig. 4-4). Such experimentally induced headaches were abolished by increasing the intracranial pressure, thereby giving extramural support to the cerebral arteries at the base of the brain. The demonstrated correlation is further evidence that headache can arise from dilatation and stretching of the pain-sensitive pial and dural arteries and their surrounding tissues.

Pressor Headache

Rapid and extreme increase in intravascular pressure in the arteries within the head will induce headache in most persons. Thus, upon bladder distention in paraplegics with lesions about T-6, a systemic pressor response is evoked which is associated with severe headache. This is abolished by increasing the intracranial pressure, demonstrating its intracranial origin. This phenomenon has been attributed by Whitteridge (1947) to a pressor reflex undamped by the usual compensatory alterations in peripheral resistance. It is most marked when the cord lesion is high thoracic or cervical.

Coincident with the pressor response facial flushing and a moderate to intense anterior headache are noted. The reaction subsides spontaneously after a few minutes. Preliminary studies by Thompson and Witham (1948) have shown that the pressor response and headache can be blocked by prior administration of a tetraethyl ammonium salt. Especially relevant is the observation by Schumacher and Guthrie (1949) that the headache can be eliminated by the artificial elevation of intracranial cerebrospinal fluid pressure by the intrathecal injection of saline. Therefore, it is probable that this variety of headache stems from distended intracranial arteries.

The massaging of a pheochromocytoma with subsequent sudden paroxysmal hypertension is associated with severe headache. Likewise, too rapid infusion of norepinephrine with sudden and extreme rise in systemic arterial blood pressure will cause headache.

No headache resulted from experimental bladder and large bowel distention in intact humans. It is inferred that, in normal persons with constipation or with urinary retention, the mechanism of any associated headache is not directly related to the viscus distention or to large bowel contraction.

Headache does not depend upon the integrity of sensation from the superficial tissues. The extracranial and the dural arteries play a minor role in contributing to the pain of headache experimentally induced by histamine. Cerebral arteries, principally the large arteries of the base of the brain, including the internal carotid, the vertebral and the basilar arteries, and the proximal segments of their main branches, are chiefly responsi-

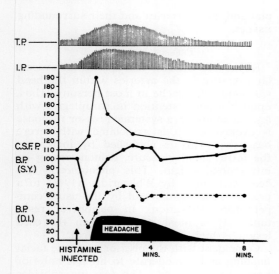

FIG. 4-4. Diagrammatic representation of the course of events during headache produced by histamine in subject G. The headache was most severe with rising blood pressure, and it should be noted that at this time the cerebrospinal fluid pressure is returning to its resting level from the high point reached after the injection of histamine. Increase in amplitude and rate of the temporal pulse (T.P.) and of the intracranial pulsation (I.P.) are indicated in the upper two shaded areas. The line C.S.F.P. indicates the cerebrospinal fluid pressure in millimeters of Ringer's solution. Systolic blood pressure is indicated by the heavy black line at B.P.S.Y., and the diastolic blood pressure is indicated by the broken line at DI.

ble for the quality and the intensity of such headache. Although there may be other less important afferent pathways for the conduction of impulses interpreted as headache following injection of histamine, (1) the fifth cranial nerve on each side is the principal afferent pathway for headache resulting from dilatation of the supratentorial cerebral arteries and felt in the frontotemporoparietal region of the head, and (2) the ninth and the tenth cranial and the upper three cervical nerves are the most important afferent pathways for headache resulting from dilatation of the arteries of the posterior fossa and felt in the occipital region of the head.

Kunkle has demonstrated that headache induced by intravenous histamine is also promptly eliminated by exposure to a posi-

tive acceleration of 3.0 to 3.6 "G" produced by the centrifugal force acting in a head-to-foot direction on a subject in the human centrifuge. The fall in intracranial arterial pressure produced by the centrifugal force reduces the pressure within the cranial arteries, and thus eliminates pain caused by average blood pressure thrusting on relaxed arterial walls.

These findings lend support to the previously stated formulation that headache experimentally produced by histamine results from the stretch of the walls of the intracranial vessels during the period in which they are hypotonic and unable adequately to absorb the shock of the systemic arterial pressure, since it returns to normal levels soon after the drug injection (see Fig. 4-4).

HEADACHE ASSOCIATED WITH FEVER

Observations of the amplitude of pulsations of the cranial arteries during headache associated with experimentally induced fever show that the spontaneous increase and decrease of intensity of the headache parallel the change in amplitude of pulsations in these arteries.

The observation was made moreover, that increasing the cerebrospinal fluid pressure in the subarachnoid space reduces the intensity of fever headache (Pickering). From fragmentary data it is likely that the headaches associated with acute infections, sepsis, bacteremia, nitrites, anoxia, hunger, hypoglycemia, caffeine-withdrawal, "hangover" and postconvulsive state are similarly due primarily to the distention of intracranial arteries.

HEADACHE RESULTING FROM TRACTION UPON INTRACRANIAL STRUCTURES

Head Jolting. In many normal subjects, sudden and vigorous head movement will elicit a fleeting headache in the frontal or temporal area on one or both sides.

For test purposes, a brisk rotary head movement to one side and back to the mid-position is carried out actively by the instructed subject. The maximum force of such a jolt can be recorded by means of a miniature accelerometer gripped between the teeth. In this way it is possible to measure in approximate terms the threshold force for induced jolt headache.

Kunkle has shown that the threshold to jolt headaches as here defined is usually very low in association with diffuse inflammation of intracranial meningeal and vascular structures, as in meningitis, and may be moderately low with distortion of intracranial anchoring vessels, as with brain tumor. Such evidence strongly suggests that jolt headache results from traction by the brain as it shifts in position within the skull case, exerted chiefly upon the major arteries, which anchor the brain at its base. With inflammation or sustained displacement of intracranial veins, particularly those tributory to the superior sagittal sinus, the pain from head jolting may arise in part from venous traction. The jolt threshold is greatly lowered during states in which intracranial arteries are known to be dilated, as after the injection of histamine. On the other hand, the threshold is not lowered in normal subjects during procedures that induce distention of intracranial veins, as with straining or bilateral jugular compression.

For these reasons, the rotary jolt maneuver is doubly useful: it produces an instructive experimental headache, and may be an aid in the detection of intracranial sources in clinical headaches (Fig. 4-5).

Other Features of Traction Headache. When headaches arise from sustained displacement of any or several of the structures anchoring the brain, the pain may be aggravated by coughing or straining, measures that produce sudden fluctuations in intracranial arterial, venous, and cerebrospinal fluid pressures.

The intensity of the headache is not reduced by compression of surface arteries of the head or by the administration of vasoconstrictor drugs.

The Headache Associated with Meningitis. The headache of meningitis is primarily related to the lowered pain threshold of inflamed tissues and structures within or adjacent to the coverings of the brain. Although generalized, the inflammatory changes are usually most marked in the basal dura and the pia and the adjacent blood vessels and nerves at the base of the brain. Under these circumstances, even slight jolting of the head and the usually painless arterial dilatation and distention during each cardiac systole become painful—thus, the characteristic throbbing headache.

Special Mechanical Stresses in Relation to Vascular Headache. When the human subject is turned to the inverted position, the adaptive response includes an increase in vasoconstrictor tone in the head, in which both the internal and external carotid branches share. Headache associated with arterial dilatation has in some instances been eliminated completely during this postural adaptation.

A vasomotor reaction of opposite type may occur following an abrupt fall in cranial arterial pressure. This is seen most dramatically in man in a unique circumstance:

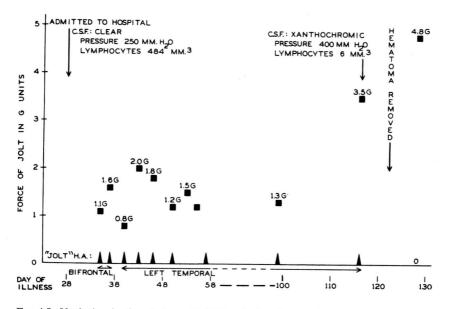

FIG. 4-5. Variation in threshold to "jolt" headache—in a patient with left temporo-parietal subdural hematoma.

during the phase of release from exposure to centrifugal force in the head-to-seat direction —increased positive G (Kunkle *et al.*, 1948). Presumably, in an attempt to maintain cranial circulation during such mechanical stress, there is a decrease in constrictor tone in head vessels, because, as the centrifugal force subsides and cranial arterial pressure rises to normal, flushing of the face is briefly observed. At this point in some subjects a transient headache develops. This symptom can conveniently be termed rebound vascular headache; whether the pain is principally intracranial or extracranial in origin has not been determined. A comparable reaction may explain the occasional occurrence of a trivial and fleeting headache in some individuals a few seconds after suddenly standing up from a recumbent position.

Migraine Headache

Definition. By "migraine headaches" we mean headaches of unknown cause which occur episodically and are produced by the painful dilatation of the arteries of the skull, scalp, and face.

The outstanding feature of the migraine syndrome is periodic headache, usually unilateral in onset, but which may become generalized. The headaches are associated with irritability and nausea, and often with photophobia, vomiting, constipation, or diarrhea. Not infrequently the attacks are ushered in by scotomata, hemianopia, unilateral paresthesia, and speech disorders. The pain is commonly limited to the head, but it may include the face and even the neck. Often other members of the patient's family have similar headaches.

Other accompaniments may be abdominal distention, cold extremities, vertigo, tremors, pallor, dryness of the mouth, excessive sweating, and "chilliness." Duration of attacks varies from a few hours to several days. They can be of any degree of severity. After an attack, patients often experience a period of buoyancy and well-being. In the interval between headaches gastrointestinal disturbances, notably constipation, may occur. Diarrhea is less frequent. Migraine may begin at any age, usually during adolescence. No age, social, intellectual, or economic group is immune. There are many variants of the migraine attack, and some phase of the syndrome other than headache may become the presenting complaint.

Classification. A useful classification of vascular headache of the migraine type has been made by a panel on Headache under the auspices of the United States Public Health Service:

A. Vascular headache with sharply defined, transient visual, other sensory and/or motor prodromes *(classic migraine)*. This headache is preceded by scintillating scotomata or visual field defects, which are transient, and sometimes by "numbness," "tingling," or paralysis of an extremity, or by periods of confusion, which also are transient. The headache appears as these phenomena subside. Typically, it is severe and is unilateral, frontal, and temporal at the time of its onset; but there are many variations in its severity and location. Type "A" headache is much less common than type "B" headache.

B. Vascular headache without striking prodromes *(common migraine)*. This headache is episodic, but it is much more variable in its characteristics than types "A" or "C." It is characterized by free intervals alternating with headaches, but there are no preceding visual prodromata; the intervals, the onset, and the severity are variable. The headaches are less often unilateral, and they may be occipital, parietal, periorbital, or generalized, as well as frontal or temporal in location.

Synonyms are "atypical migraine" or "sick headache." Calling attention to certain relationships of this type of headache to seasonal, environmental, occupational, menstrual, or other variables are such terms as: tropical, summer, Monday, weekend, relaxation, premenstrual, and menstrual headache.

C. Vascular headache, predominantly unilateral; associated on the same side with flushing, sweating, rhinorrhea, and increased lacrimation; brief in duration and occurring in closely packed groups separated by long remissions *(cluster headache)*.

This headache is almost always unilateral, of high intensity, brief, burning, and boring in character, and many attacks occur in quick succession, sometimes several in a 24-hour period for several days or weeks, followed by remissions lasting months or years; hence, the name, "cluster headache." The pain involves the region of the eye, the temple, the neck, and often one side of the face, and may spread into the teeth and extend into the shoulder on the involved side. Association manifestations are profuse watering and congestion of the conjunctiva, rhinorrhea, and nasal obstruction, increased perspiration, redness of the skin, and swelling of the temporal vessels. Kunkle, in a study of 90 patients, pointed to the unique tempo of the recurrence of cluster headaches as its most striking feature, although in a few patients the attacks occur sporadically instead of in groups. The thesis that endogenous histamine may be responsible for cluster-type headache is based on the facts that (1) unilateral headache in patients subject to these headaches can be experimentally induced by injection of a small amount of histamine and (2) "desensitization" to histamine is often followed by alleviation of headaches. However, similar therapeutic effects can be achieved by placebos. There is no conclusive evidence that histamine is involved in the headache mechanism in man.

Identical or closely allied conditions are: erythroprosopalgia (Bing); ciliary or migrainous neuralgia (Harris); erythromelalgia of the head or histaminic cephalgia (Horton); and petrosal neuralgia (Gardner et al).

D. Vascular headache, featured by sensory and motor phenomena that persist during and after the headache (hemiplegic migraine and ophthalmoplegic migraine).

E. Headache of possible vascular mechanism centered primarily in the lower face (lower-half headache). In this group are atypical facial neuralgia, sphenopalatine ganglion neuralgia (Sluder), and vidian neuralgia (Vail).

Incidence. It has been said that migraine headache is the most common complaint of civilized people, although few reliable data exist concerning its frequency. Grimes found that "of 15,000 individuals examined in general practice with reference to migraine, 1,200 or 8 per cent were afflicted." There are all gradients of migraine complaint from the most severe and disabling illness to trifling symptoms, and it is safe to say that less than half of the migraine victims ever consult a physician. It is a difficult syndrome to investigate because it usually disappears under conditions of intensive laboratory study; therefore, development of knowledge of the pathogenesis of migraine headache has been slow.

Hereditary Aspects. In the family pedigrees of 119 patients with the migraine type of vascular headache there were found to be 343 relatives with migraine, distributed in as many as five generations. Migraine occurred in the children of families having relatives with migraine with the following frequencies: 69.2 per cent when both parents had migraine; 44.2 per cent when one parent had migraine; and 28.6 per cent when neither parent had migraine. Applying genetic con-

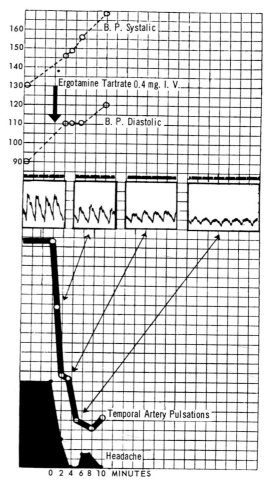

Fig. 4-6. Relation of amplitude of pulsations of temporal artery to intensity of headache after administration of ergotamine. The sharp decrease in amplitude of pulsations following injection closely paralleled rapid decrease in intensity of headache. Representative sections of photographic record are inserted. Average amplitude of pulsations before and after administration of ergotamine was ascertained by measuring individual pulsations from photographic record. Points on heavy black line represent these averages, as percentages. Initial or "control" amplitude was taken as 100 per cent. Interrupted line represents intervals of one second. (Wolff, H. G.: Headache and Other Head Pain, New York, Oxford)

cepts to these data, the hereditary character of migraine became highly significant; it appears that inheritance of the migraine headache trait is through a recessive gene with a penetrance of approximately 70 per cent.

The Pathophysiology of Migraine Headache

Vasodilatation. Changes in the intensity of these vascular headaches of the migraine type are related to changes in the amplitude of pulsations of the cranial arteries, chiefly the branches of the external carotid arteries. Reduction in amplitude of pulsations of the temporal artery by digital pressure on the carotid artery on the affected side is accompanied by reduction in intensity of the headache. Conversely, experimental distention of extracranial arteries by increasing the intravascular pressure results in pain. It has also been shown by means of observations and photographs, made both before and during action of *ergotamine tartrate* and of *norepinephrine*, that these agents *reduce the amplitude of pulsations* of the aforementioned arteries by about 50 per cent, and concurrently diminish the intensity of or terminate the migraine headache (Fig. 4-6).

There is considerable evidence against the view that classic migraine is chiefly due to dilatation of the dural and the cerebral arteries, since not even extremely severe attacks of migraine headache are reduced in intensity by raising the cerebrospinal fluid pressure as high as 800 mm. of water by means of a manometer system attached to a needle in the lumbar sac.

The internal and the external carotid arteries and the vertebral arteries have branches both in the subcutaneous tissue and in the meninges. The branches of the external carotid artery predominate numerically, both superficially and on the dura. On the other hand, the anterior meningeal artery arises from branches of the internal carotid artery, as do the superficial frontal and the supraorbital arteries. Since the area supplied by the latter structures commonly is involved in migraine headaches, branches of the internal carotid artery may contribute to the pain. Therefore, it is obvious that it would be arbitrary to contrast these arteries too sharply.

Although most attacks of migraine headache are limited to the temporal, the frontal, or the occipital region, some patients have pain elsewhere. In the face, below the eye, and behind and below the zygoma, severe throbbing pain, which seems to emanate from the back teeth of the upper jaw, occasionally occurs. Another variant is facial pain, which spreads behind the angle of the jaw, down the neck, and into the shoulder. The aching sensations in the shoulder sometimes are associated with the awareness of unusual throbbing in the neck.

The pains described can and probably do result from dilatation and distention of the extracranial portion of the middle meningeal artery, between its origin and the point of entrance into the skull, the internal maxillary artery, and the trunks of the external and the common carotid artery. It has been

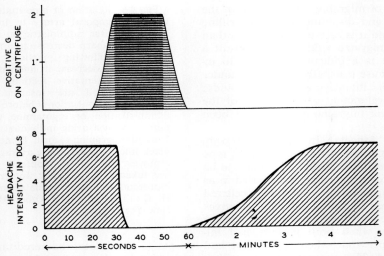

FIG. 4-7. Effect of centrifugation (positive G) on migraine headache in a woman, aged 22.

shown that the latter structures are sensitive to pain, and the sites in which pain is felt are the face, the neck, and the shoulder.

The effect upon migraine headache of reducing cranial intravascular pressure is demonstrated by a patient with migraine headache who was the subject of investigation on the human centrifuge. The headache in this 22-year-old female dental technician was either right frontal or generalized and had been recurring frequently for four weeks, in a setting of dissatisfaction with her work and increasing tension. The dominant stress centered about her inability, because of circumstances beyond her control, to maintain her usual high standards of performance. During exposure to centrifugal force of 2.0 G in the head-to-seat direction, the experimenter was able to eliminate the headache completely (Fig. 4-7).

It is likely, therefore, that, for the *fever* headache and that experimentally induced by *histamine,* the cerebral branches of the *internal carotid,* the *basilar,* and the *vertebral* arteries at the base of the brain are primarily responsible. To the migraine headache, however, the extracranial, and possibly the dural, branches of the *external carotid* artery are the chief contributors.

Muscle Spasm. An ancillary mechanism of pain during the migraine headache attack involves the sustained *contraction of the muscles* of the head and the neck. Pain in the head from any cause induces secondary contractions of these muscles, which, when maintained, become in themselves a source of pain. Although present in all, the amount of muscle spasm varies greatly from patient to patient.

Such painful contractions may persist for some time longer than the primary cause of the contraction, i.e., pain arising from cranial vasodilatation. This affords an explanation of the failure to obtain relatively prompt relief after ergotamine tartrate administration in some patients who have a major muscle component in their headaches.

Arteritis. There is still another factor in the failure to achieve prompt relief from migraine headache after the administration of ergotamine tartrate. After several hours of migraine headache, involving, for example, the temporal artery, this artery may appear prominent and distended and may become more easily palpable through the skin. Instead of being easily collapsible, it becomes rigid, pipelike, and less readily compressible by the palpating finger. Also, the artery may

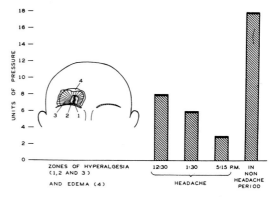

FIG. 4-8. Demonstration of the progressively lowered thresholds of deep pain during a vascular headache of the migraine type in the supraorbital region.

be tender when compressed. Patients so affected report that after the first hour or two of a migraine headache attack the quality of the headache changes in that the initial pulsating or throbbing is less conspicuous or even absent, and the pain becomes a steady ache. Under such conditions, ergotamine tartrate fails to eliminate headache promptly or even to reduce its intensity appreciably.

To account for such changes, it was postulated that following the sustained dilatation of a local artery of the head there occurs a transient change in the structure of the artery wall, namely, *thickening or edema of the muscular and the adventitial structures.* In order to lend validity to this concept, experiments were done in which the arteries of cats' ears were studied following prolonged vasodilatation by infusion for 2 hours of 10 ml. of mammalian Ringer's solution containing a vasodilator agent (0.05 mg. acetylcholine). The dilated artery walls were compared with the arterial walls of a control ear by means of serial sections. Measurements demonstrated thickening of the arterial walls of the infused ear. Also, the vasoconstrictor agent, ergotamine tartrate, was found to be less prompt and less effective in constricting arteries with such thickened or edematous walls, as compared with its action on vessel walls early in a headache.

Hyperalgesia. Contributing to the migraine headache attack is the heightened tenderness of tissues located in and about the painfully dilated large cranial arteries, associated with local edema. *Deep-pain-thresholds* of affected scalp tissues have been found to be *lowered greatly* during headache (Fig. 4-8), and the

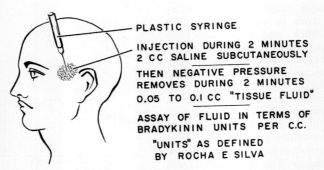

PLASTIC SYRINGE

INJECTION DURING 2 MINUTES
2 CC SALINE SUBCUTANEOUSLY

THEN NEGATIVE PRESSURE
REMOVES DURING 2 MINUTES
0.05 TO 0.1 CC "TISSUE FLUID"

ASSAY OF FLUID IN TERMS OF
BRADYKININ UNITS PER C.C.

"UNITS" AS DEFINED
BY ROCHA E SILVA

FIG. 4-9. Method of obtaining fluid from painful tissues for bioassay of "headache stuff."

lowered thresholds persisted for hours or days after spontaneous ending of the headache. Furthermore, it was demonstrated that the onset of certain migraine headaches is preceded by a lowering of the jolt threshold. In some instances this lowered threshold also persists for some hours after headache has subsided.

Humoral Factors. Sterile isotonic saline (2 ml.) was injected subcutaneously, and as much fluid as possible was withdrawn under gentle negative pressure during a two-minute

interval (1) from the tender regions of the heads of persons during headaches of a wide range of intensity, (2) from the tender region of the scalp following headache attacks, (3) from the nontender regions of the heads of persons subject to headache but during headache-free periods, and (4) from persons not subject to headache attacks (Fig. 4-9).

It was found that specimens of tissue fluid collected from the head during the headache attacks contain a substance that could be distinguished from serotonin, potassium,

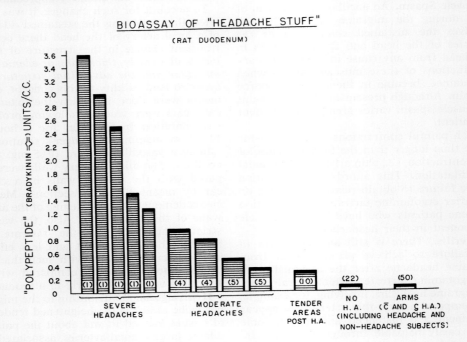

BIOASSAY OF "HEADACHE STUFF"
(RAT DUODENUM)

FIG. 4-10. Results of bioassay of tissue fluid from 23 subjects during vascular headaches of the migraine type.

ATP, substance P, acetylcholine, and histamine, although these and other substances also may have been present. The active substance relaxed the isolated rat duodenum, contracted the rat uterus, and depressed the blood pressure of the rat. A constant ratio of activity on these several assay preparations among several specimens of tissue fluid indicated that the observed activity of the specimens probably was due to a single substance.

The activity of the specimens could be stabilized by boiling. Incubation with chymotrypsin inactivated the stabilized specimens, indicating that the active substance remaining after stabilization is a polypeptide. The heat-stabilized substance had many of the properties of bradykinin, kallidin, or plasma kinin. However, when analyzed quantitatively using several assay procedures, including electrophoresis, it was evident that the substance is not identical to any of these, although it closely resembles them and is a polypeptide of the same general type. This polypeptide has been labeled *neurokinin* and has been found by Wolff and his associates to appear during neuronal excitation. It appears in tissue fluid of the skin of man during antidromic dorsal root stimulation and during axon reflex flare. It is not the result of vasodilatation alone since it is not released during reactive hyperemia. It also has been found in the cerebrospinal fluid of patients during vascular headache of the migraine type.

The neurokinin content of specimens collected during headache averages eight times as much and in rare instances may be 35 times as much as that of control specimens, and the amount is closely related to the intensity of the headache attack (Fig. 4-10). Following administration of ergotamine tartrate in subjects with headache, the intensity of headache, amplitude of cranial artery pulsations, local tenderness, and neurokinin activity all decrease concurrently. Lowered deep pain thresholds return to normal.

In addition to the polypeptide, headache fluid contains a *proteolytic enzyme*, capable of forming neurokinin (presumably by cleavage of a plasma globulin present in subsurface extracellular fluid).

The increased content of polypeptide (neurokinin) and protease found locally can account for many of the features of vascular headache of the migraine type. Neurokinin is an extremely powerful vasodilator. When injected intradermally, tissue fluids containing mixtures of neurokinin and protease induce pain and erythema, lower pain threshold, and increase capillary permeability.

Since the release or activation of neurokinin-forming enzyme and subsequent formation of neurokinin have been observed during neuronal excitation in man in a variety of circumstances, the potent hypotensive and

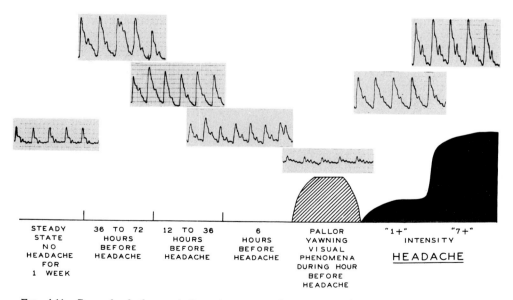

FIG. 4-11. Record of the variations in temporal artery pulsiations in a subject having recurrent vascular headaches of the migraine type.

vasodilator action of neurokinin and its formation during neuronal excitation suggest that it contributes to local vasomotor control in the central nervous system.

The Migraine Headache Attack as the Outcome of Central Nervous System Activity. Migraine headache attacks are linked to activity of the central nervous system since they often occur following a long period of alertness, striving, extraordinary effort or major frustration usually associated with feelings of anger and resentment. They may begin with vasoconstriction affecting the cerebral cortex and the retina. The painful local reaction in the extracranial vessels may thus be an epiphenomenon of the excessive operation of the normal mechanisms for functional vasodilatation within the central nervous system. A common innervation of the branches of the external and internal carotid arteries could lead to a simultaneous release of vasodilator substances both intracranially and extracranially. Thus, the pain of vascular headache of the migraine type can be seen as the outcome of the combined effects of *large artery dilatation* plus the action of *pain-threshold-lowering substances* accumulating in the blood vessel walls and perivascular tissue. These substances are implicated in local vasomotor control. Their accumulation, neurogenically induced, results in a *sterile inflammatory reaction.*

Craniovascular Instability and Vascular Headache. Repeated measurements over several days of the amplitude of pulsation of the cranial arteries by Marcussen and Kunkle, and later by Tunis, indicated that, in many subjects who have vascular headaches, the variation in tone of the artery walls during headache-free periods is far greater than in those who do not have recurrent headaches, and is greatest in the days preceding an attack (Fig. 4-11). These observations gave support to the concept that the cranial vasomotor apparatus of patients with vascular headaches is more labile than is that of persons who are not subject to headache.

Pharmacodynamic Properties of Methysergide Maleate Relevant to Vascular Headache of the Migraine Type. Methysergide, an ergot alkaloid, although lacking the capacity to terminate an existing headache, is often effective in reducing the number and severity of headache attacks when the agent is maintained at adequate blood levels. Although it does not by itself induce vasoconstriction, it does enhance the vasoconstrictor action of norepinephrine.

1. ANTI-INFLAMMATORY ACTION OF METHYSERGIDE. This agent is effective in diminishing edema formation induced by the injection of serotonin in the rat's paw. In order to show that this phenomenon was not specific to inflammation induced by serotonin, areas of

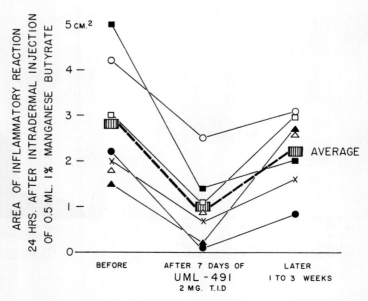

FIG. 4-12. The anti-inflammatory action of methysergide in seven human subjects.

sterile inflammatory response were produced through the subcutaneous administration of manganese butyrate to seven human subjects. The flare responses induced during methysergide therapy were significantly smaller than those induced either before or several weeks subsequent to its administration (Fig. 4-12). A verification of this study was made in animal experiments by Zileli in which the volume of inflammatory exudate in croton oil pouches was significantly less after pretreatment with methysergide.

2. INHIBITION OF VASOMOTOR REFLEXES. Dampening of the pressor reaction to carotid occlusion is a well-recognized property of many of the ergot alkaloids. In the anesthetized cat, this pressor response can be abolished by infusion of methysergide at a rate of 1.0 mg. per kg. per hour, suggesting a moderate depressing action on the vasomotor centers, thus dampening vasoconstrictor reflexes. Although the amounts of the agent required to *abolish* these reflexes in the cat are many times more than the amounts that are effective in the prevention of migraine attacks, it is possible that damping of vasoconstrictor reflexes also may be induced by methysergide in patients with migraine.

Evidence relevant to such a modifying effect on the sensitivity of vasomotor centers was afforded by a study of a series of persons subject to vascular headaches of the migraine type regarding the effect of this alkaloid on the carotid sinus reflex, the cold pressor reflex, and the breath-holding reflex. These were selected as samples of vasomotor reflexes that could be tested in man, although it is recognized that they represent different reactions than those implicated in vascular headache of the migraine type. The magnitude of these reflexes was studied before, during, and in some instances after the daily administration of 8 to 12 mg. amounts of methysergide in divided doses. It was observed that those subjects experiencing the most striking reduction or elimination of headache also exhibited the greatest inhibitory effect on their vascular reactions to noxious and painful stimulation.

3. INHIBITION OF CHANGES IN RESPONSIVITY OF CRANIAL VESSELS ASSOCIATED WITH SHIFTS OF BODY FLUID. The migraine attack is characterized by initial vasoconstriction followed by vasodilatation. When effective, methysergide prevents both the preheadache (visual loss) or vasoconstrictor phase and the headache or vasodilator phase. Of its two actions, inhibition of central vasoconstrictor reflex effects and augmentation of peripheral vasoconstriction produced by catecholamines, the former could be significant in inhibiting the initial vasoconstrictor phase of the attack, and the latter in minimizing the subsequent painful dilatation of the vasodilator phase.

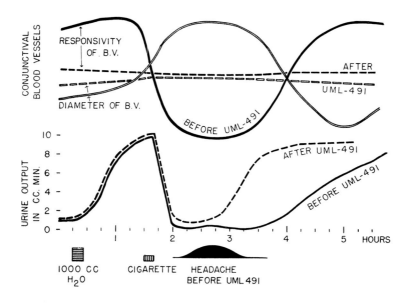

FIG. 4-13. Schema of damping effect of methysergide on blood-vessel responsivity.

On the other hand, it is conceivable that the prevention of the initial vasoconstriction makes the subsequent vasodilatation unlikely to occur.

Since initial fluid retention and subsequent diuresis are part of the migraine attack and changes in the reactivity of the bulbar conjunctival blood vessels occur during such periods of fluid shift, the effects of methysergide on these phenomena were studied. Fluid shifts were induced experimentally by evoking diencephalic reactions through nicotine. It was observed that concurrently with the oliguria the bulbar conjunctival vessels dilate and become less responsive to serial dilutions of norepinephrine. During the subsequent diuresis, all conjunctival vessels constricted and the response of these vessels to serial dilutions of norepinephrine returned to preoliguric levels. Headache was sometimes initiated during the vasodilator and oliguric phase and terminated shortly after, with the beginning of the vasoconstriction and diuresis. Prior administration of methysergide during 48 hours strikingly diminished the magnitude of both these vascular responses; no headache occurred (Fig. 4-13).

4. VASOMOTOR INSTABILITY AND VASCULAR HEADACHE. These data suggest that, in the prophylaxis of vascular headache of the migraine type, the peripheral actions of methysergide on cranial blood vessels are significantly supplemented by its effects on the nervous system. The magnitude of cranial vascular responsivity is reduced, thereby preventing crises of vasoconstriction and vasodilatation which characterize the migraine attack. These observations further support the thesis that *the migraine attack is the symptomatic manifestation of recurrent heightened reactivity of cranial blood vessels.* Moreover, the modification of vasomotor reflexes, concurrent with a period of reduction in the intensity and frequency of headache attacks, adds further support to the inference that *unstable cranial vasomotor functions* are a prime factor in the pathophysiology of this variety of headache.

Mechanism of Scotomata Associated with Migraine Headache. The preheadache phase of the migraine attack is sometimes featured by scintillating scotomata and areas of blindness. These result from vasoconstriction within the calcarine cortex, where vasoconstriction is indicated by changes in the electroencephalogram. It is no longer believed that retinal vasoconstriction causes scotomata, although sometimes within the retina constricted vessels can be seen and photographed by means of a slit lamp and microscope. In order to demonstrate further that dysfunction of the cerebral vasculature is responsible for the preheadache symptoms of scotomata, a vasodilator agent, amyl nitrite, known to affect cerebral vessels, was employed. It is justifiable to infer that cerebral vasodilatation induced without a fall in blood pressure increases cerebral blood flow, whereas a sharp drop in blood pressure, regardless of the state of the cerebral arteries, decreases the cerebral blood flow. Symptoms due to cerebral vasoconstriction should be overcome by cerebral vasodilatation in the presence of a sustained normal level of blood pressure, but they should be augmented by a fall in blood pressure with accompanying decrease in cerebral blood flow. Experiments based on these two potential actions of the vasodilator drug amyl nitrate were performed by a subject having preheadache scotomata who was skillful in observing his own visual fields.

It was apparent from such experiments that cerebral vasodilatation associated with a sustained normal level of blood pressure caused symptoms to disappear, whereas a procedure that decreased cerebral blood flow caused the symptoms to become worse. From this it may be deduced that cerebral vasoconstriction was responsible for the visual defect in this patient with migraine. It is also likely that the cause of the visual defect was not in the retina or the orbit, but within the cranial cavity.

The preheadache phenomena of migraine, i.e., visual disturbances, paresthesias, and dysarthria, associated with (and probably due to) cranial vasoconstriction, can be modified or abolished by certain agents that produce cranial vasodilatation. A series of patients was given a mixture of 10 per cent carbon dioxide and 90 per cent oxygen by face mask during the preheadache or early headache phase. This mixture abolished the preheadache phenomena and aborted the headache in most of the trials. Ten per cent carbon dioxide in air was less effective, having a shorter and more transient effect.

Pharamacodynamics of the Urine of Patients with Migraine. Water and electrolyte balance studies of persons with the migraine type of vascular headaches indicate that in about half of those having migraine headache there is retention of water, sodium, potassium, and steroids in the period just preceding the headache attack. During the retention phase, the creatinine output in the urine is reduced, suggesting that the renal vessels also participate in the vasoconstriction occurring about the head. With the onset of the headache and during the subsequent hours there is a diuresis of water, sodium, potassium, and steroids. The described changes are not related causally or mechanistically to the onset, the intensity, or the duration of the migraine attack. Instead, they are manifestations of the widespread bodily changes accompanying adaptive reactions during and after stressful periods. The migraine attack is a concurrent but independent feature.

Formulation of the Dynamics of the Migraine Attack. For a period of several hours to several days preceding the headache there is increased variability of the contractile state of the cranial arteries, indicated by facial flushing or pallor due to dilatation or constriction of extracranial vessels and by other transient cranial vasomotor phenomena, such as vertigo. In the hour preceding the headache, visual and other nonpainful sensory phenomena due to local constriction of cerebral arteries or, sometimes, retinal vessels occur in about 10 to 15 per cent of the instances. These may take the form of scintillating scotomata or visual field defects, such as unilateral or homonymous hemianopsia. As the vasoconstrictor preheadache phenomena recede, vasodilator headache manifestations commence, sometimes overlapping the last traces of preheadache phenomena, sometimes beginning after a short symptom-free interval. The pain is throbbing and aching in quality, is appreciably reduced by pressure on the common carotid and superficial arteries, and is characteristically modified by the action of vasoconstrictor agents.

The migraine attack is but one aspect of a diffuse disturbance in function occurring episodically during or shortly after periods of sustained purposeful activity or arousal, which may be accompanied by feelings of tension or anxiety. The headache itself may appear in a setting of fatigue or "letdown" after such a period. In certain circumstances, even during periods of sustained activity, the migraine headache or preheadache phenomena may diminish or actually fail to recur. However, other bodily or mood disturbances may be accentuated and become the basis of the dominant complaint. These other phenomena, referred to as *migraine equivalents*, include a variety of abdominal, thoracic, and extremity pains and nonpainful

attacks of vomiting, diarrhea, diffuse edema, transient mood disorder, and fever.

Individuals with migraine headache appear to be people who have a hereditary susceptibility to the development of episodes of painful dilatation of the arteries of skull, scalp, and face. These episodes are inclined to appear after a period of sustained purposeful activity, alertness, or arousal, during which there seems to be a relative constriction of the head vessels with a gradual increase in vasomotor instability in this region. The headache itself may be precipitated by any occurrence that leads to a general relaxation of body activities and accompanying vasodilatation. Deep sleep, warmth, alcoholic beverages, or the taking of nitroglycerine may bring on a headache. Often accumulated fatigue with a gradual slowing of activities suffices to initiate the episode. In many people who suffer with migraine the episodes occur only rarely and may be associated with such transient and demanding episodes as a trying business meeting, periods of scholastic examinations, a period of tense interpersonal relations, or an unusual period of hard work. Other people who are chronically prone to periods of anxiety or arousal because they are in periods of sustained interpersonal difficulty, because they are subject to depressive illness, or because of their own personality structures, may have headaches that are related to alertness, arousal, and tension, but are not immediately related to any obvious new situations or events in their daily lives.

Most people who have occasional vascular headaches do not appear to be outside of what might be called the "normal range of personality structure and behavior" for people in our society and our time. However, a significant number of migraine sufferers who come to the attention of the physician are rigid, ambitious, and perfectionistic people. If a person who has such a personality structure is also susceptible to migraine, his headaches may be unusually frequent and severe. Such people have found that doing "more than" and "better than" their fellows brings them many rewards. They strive continually to do an exceptional job at whatever they attempt, and often disregard their own bodily demands for rest. The outcome of this is usually a period of intense and unremitting activity which may be highly effective, but is nearly always followed by increasing tension, irritability, fatigue, and exhaustion. It is at this point that the headache often makes its appearance. This phenomenon is so frequently seen in migraine headaches that it has led to a belief that there is a "specific migraine personality." The present evidence suggests that there is no specific causal relationship between the personality and the headache, but that persons susceptible to migraine, who also exhibit this personality, are likely to have a peculiarly pernicious and disabling form of the illness.

Efforts to treat patients who have this syndrome by advising them about their characteristics and attempting to get them to behave in a different manner, not only encounter the underlying psychodynamic drives that tend to make the patients sustain this personality structure, but also encounter some very practical considerations. Many patients with migraine, although prostrated during and perhaps immediately after a headache, may thereafter have feelings of increased energy and effectiveness, which persist for several days to a week. This may be exhilarating to them, because they find themselves able to do a great deal and to accomplish many things in a short period of time. They are further urged to this behavior by the fact that they have fallen behind on their self-imposed schedule of work during their last period of headache. Furthermore, people who have migraine actually may accomplish a great deal. In our society people who do "more than" and "better than" others are those who are likely to rise to positions of responsibility within

their families, among their friends, and at their businesses. Any effort to get them to change their pattern of activity may be seen by them as posing a realistic threat to their positions.

Other carefully studied patients with migraine have been found to be involved in interpersonal situations of chronic conflict, characterized by periodic exacerbations. The following protocol is representative:

A 30-year-old Italian housewife had a history of almost daily unilateral headache of varying intensity and duration for about two months. Prior to this series of attacks she had had typical migraine headaches every few weeks since adolescence. The present series of headaches paralleled the development of a progressively severe feeding problem in her four-year-old daughter. The patient stated that her headaches followed meals with monotonous regularity. The child refused to eat, despite the patient's every effort to induce her to do so. At this persistent refusal, the mother would become angry and berate the child violently. Often she would attempt to force food between the child's clenched teeth. Failing this, the mother became so enraged several times that she assaulted her daughter so violently that the child was left stunned and bruised. Within an hour after such an encounter the patient would develop a high-intensity headache, usually unilateral, which required ergotamine tartrate or opiates for relief. Later this woman realized that she might seriously injure her daughter during one of these assaults and would therefore storm out of the

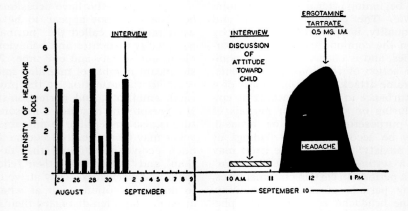

FIG. 4-14. Experimental precipitation of a migraine headache attack in a setting of mounting tension by the introduction of a topic arousing conflict, anger and guilt. Attack terminated by the intravascular administration of ergotamine tartrate. Initial interview on September 1, by dispelling guilt and conflict, reduced the frequency and intensity of attacks. The subsequent interview, intensifying these feelings, precipitated the headache.

room before she gave way to physical violence. Under such circumstances the subsequent headache would be more intense. The mother felt extremely guilty about her failure as a parent and was humiliated by the comments of neighbors who overheard her outbursts and observed the child's progressive loss of weight.

During her first clinic visit, the patient confessed her story to a friendly and sympathetic physician. She displayed considerable emotion during the interview and felt appreciably relieved at the end. She had no further headache during the following week, the first remission in months. At her next visit, the same physician adopted a stern and unsympathetic attitude. He scolded the patient for her behavior and criticized her for her failure to control herself in dealing with the child, pointing out the damage that she was doing to the child and to herself. All this the patient seemed to accept well, smiling and agreeing with the physician. The interview terminated after an hour and the patient left the clinic. Ten minutes later she developed a high intensity bitemporal and frontal throbbing headache accompanied by some blurring of vision and nausea. The headache was abolished within 30 minutes after the intramuscular injection of ergotamine tartrate (Fig. 4-14).

MECHANISM OF HEADACHE ASSOCIATED WITH ARTERIAL HYPERTENSION

Studies made of the headache associated with hypertension have revealed that essentially the same mechanism is operative in producing this pain as in producing the migraine headache. It is to be emphasized that this statement applies not to the so-called hypertensive encephalopathy of Fishberg, "hypertensive crisis," but rather to the frequent, severe and often incapacitating headaches suffered by hypertensive patients who may otherwise be free of symptoms. The term hypertensive headache is misleading, since it implies that the frequency and the severity of the headache are directly related to the level of the blood pressure.

Almost all of the patients with hypertension and associated headaches in this series had had headaches for many years. In numerous instances the headache was known to have preceded the onset of the hypertension and, in some patients, changed only in intensity with the rise in blood pressure.

The following data indicate that the pial and the cerebral arteries are not the prime contributors to the headache and that the headache associated with *hypertension*, like that of migraine, arises chiefly from the dilatation and distention of certain branches of the *external carotid artery:*

1. The headache was not relieved by increasing the cerebrospinal fluid pressure.

2. There was no increase in the amplitude of pulsations of the intracranial arteries during the headache, and the amplitude of pulsations of these arteries did not become less as the headache diminished in intensity.

3. Ergotamine tartrate, which in the head acts chiefly on the branches of the external carotid artery, reduced the intensity of the headache.

4. Manual pressure on the temporal, frontal, supraorbital, postauricular, or occipital artery decreased or abolished the headache.

5. Ligation of the middle meningeal or the temporal artery, especially the latter, decreased the intensity of the headache for some months.

It also has been observed that the headache in subjects with hypertension bears no direct relationship to the level of blood pressure or pulse pressure. The headache may be present when the blood pressure is relatively high, moderate, or low. By pressing the thumb upon the common carotid artery, the intensity of the headache is reduced with an accompanying decline in the amplitude of the pulsations. Decrease in the intensity of headache in the temporal region followed similar pressure upon the corresponding temporal artery. Furthermore, when ergotamine tartrate did succeed in decreasing the amplitude of pulsations of the cranial arteries appreciably for a shorter or longer period, the intensity of the hypertensive headache decreased, despite the fact that the ergotamine tartrate considerably increased the already elevated systolic and diastolic pressures. If little or no reduction of the amplitude of pulsation of the arteries occurred there was no reduction in the intensity of the headache.

The fact that the high level of blood pressure among hypertensive subjects is not a sufficient condition for headache does not justify the assumption that these phenomena are entirely unrelated. This would be contraindicated by the facts of common experience, since some persons with hypertension never had headache until the hypertension became established. It seems reasonable to postulate that a cranial artery, only slightly relaxed for whatever reason, would not distend as much, and possibly not to the point of producing pain, if the blood pressure were low. If, however, the sustained level were raised, distention would be greater and therefore pain might readily follow. In other

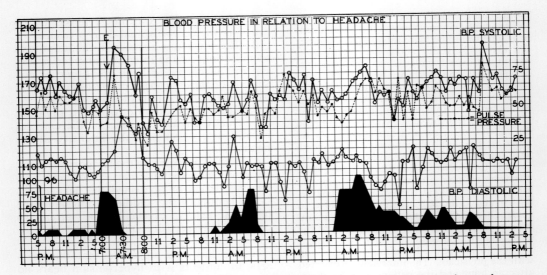

Fig. 4-15. Relation of blood pressure to headache in a patient with hypertension and associated headache. The fluctuations of the blood pressure and the incidence and severity of the headache vary independently. Thus, headache occurred with a B.P. of 140/75 on one occasion, whereas headache disappeared as the B.P. rose from 145/90 to 195/110 at another time. At E, to the left of the chart, is shown the record of a headache terminated by ergotamine tartrate.

words, a degree of change in the contractile state of the arterial wall, compatible with comfort when blood pressure is average, would be associated with pain when the blood pressure is elevated. During an average or normal contractile state of the arterial walls, distention does not occur and, correspondingly, there is no headache. Should this contractile state be impaired, as by stress, fatigue, or other conditions, distention and headache follow (Fig. 4-15). In brief, high blood pressure is a necessary, but not a sufficient condition for this type of headache. There is a significant relation between headache associated with hypertension and the contractile state of the cranial arteries.

This conception is supported by analogy with the experimental evidence described for histamine headache.

Headache with Temporal Arteritis

In the syndrome of arteritis of the temporal vessel, and sometimes of other cranial arteries, the associated headache is the main feature (Kilbourne and Wolff, 1946). Furthermore, when the inflammatory nature of the disorder is relatively inconspicuous, the localization of the headache and the associated tenderness of the temporal artery may lead to the erroneous diagnosis of atypical migraine. The headache is of high intensity, throbbing and persistent. It is felt as a deep ache and is also often burning in quality. Other features of the syndrome are not pertinent to this discussion.

Pain from Nasal and the Paranasal Structures

Quality and Intensity. The headache associated with frontal sinus disease is localized diffusely over the frontal region, and with antral disease over the maxillary region. The headache associated with sphenoid and ethmoid disease is experienced between and in back of the eyes and over the vertex. Commonly, when sinus disease is of sufficient duration, there is pain in the back of the head, the neck, and the shoulders, in addition to the headache experienced in the front and the top of the head.

Headaches are less frequent when the patient has been for some time in the recumbent position, or resting, and are less often present at night than during the day. Moreover, the pain associated with maxillary sinus disease gradually diminishes when the patient assumes the recumbent position with the diseased side uppermost. Relief in the recumbent position is not prompt, usually requiring about 30 minutes to be achieved.

The headache associated with frontal sinus disease commonly begins about 9 A.M., gradually becomes worse, and ends toward evening or on retiring. The pain associated with maxillary sinus disease often has its onset in the early afternoon.

In all instances the pain is of a deep, dull, aching, nonpulsatile quality. It is seldom, if ever, associated with vomiting or nausea. The headache that accompanies chronic sinus disease is of a low order of intensity. The headache associated with acute sinus disease is sometimes of greater intensity, but seldom very severe. Pain does not achieve the intensity noted in some instances of migraine, or of the headache associated with ruptured cerebral aneurysm, meningitis, or certain febrile illnesses, or of that induced by certain drugs.

The headache associated with disease of the nasal and the paranasal structures is commonly reduced in intensity or abolished by aspirin or codeine. The intensity of pain is increased by shaking the head or by the head-down position. The headache is intensified by procedures that increase the venous pressure, such as straining, coughing, or a tight collar. Also, it is intensified by states that increase the engorgement of the mucosa, such as anxiety and resentment, menstruation, cold air, sexual excitement, or the effects of alcohol.

Mechanism of Pain from the Nasal and the Paranasal Structures. The mucosa covering the approaches to the paranasal sinuses is found to be the most pain-sensitive of the nasal and the paranasal structures and cavities, whereas the mucosa lining the sinuses is of relatively low sensitivity.

On a 1 (minimum pain) to 10 (maximum pain) scale, a given faradic stimulus will produce pain of the indicated intensities at the following sites: tongue, 1; septum, 1 to 2; turbinates, 4 to 6; nasofrontal duct, 5 to 7; ostium of the maxillary sinus, 6 to 9; lining of frontal or maxillary sinus, 1 to 2 (see Fig. 4-16).

Most of the pain from faradic, mechanical, and chemical stimulation of the mucosa of the nasal and the paranasal cavities is re-

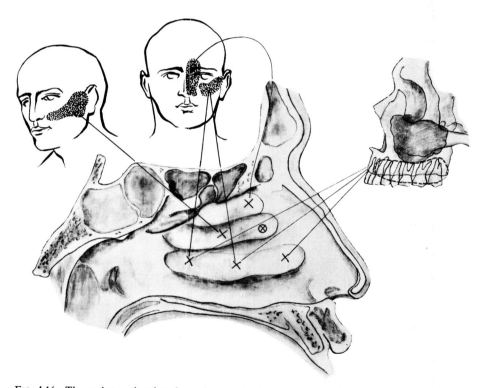

FIG. 4-16. The points stimulated on the turbinates are indicated by crosses, from which lines lead to the indicated areas in which pain of 4 plus to 6 plus intensity was felt. (Wolff, H. G.: Headache and Other Head Pain, New York, Oxford University Press, 1963)

ferred pain, i.e., it is felt at a site other than that stimulated. It is diffuse, sustained, of a deep, aching nature, and nonpulsatile. It is associated with lacrimation, photophobia, erythema, and hyperalgesia. The pain and its associated effects outlast the period of stimulation.

The pain thus produced experimentally is referred chiefly to those regions of the head supplied by the second division and, to a less extent, to those supplied by the first division of the fifth cranial nerve. When severe enough, or of sufficient duration, the pain spreads over most of the region supplied by that division of the fifth cranial nerve to which it is initially referred, and sometimes spreads from the region of the second to that of the first division.

The stimulation of several different sites results in pain referred to the same region. Thus, stimulation of the nasal structures near the mid-line results in the same area of referred pain as does stimulation of the ostium and the more lateral wall of the maxillary sinus.

A thin rubber balloon was inserted into the maxillary sinus of a subject through a fistulous opening, so that pressure could be applied to the walls of the sinus by inflating the balloon. When a pressure of 50 to 80 mm. Hg was maintained for two and one-half hours, pain of low intensity was experienced. It also was observed that sustained pressure within the sinus was accompanied by swell-ing and reddening of the turbinates and that the pain in the face could be abolished by procainization of the swollen, reddened turbinates, even while maintaining pressure.

Negative pressure within the sealed sinus resulting from applying suction of 100 to 150 mm. Hg for periods of a few minutes elicited a feeling of drawing in the face, which the patient described as the feeling that "her face would collapse." When the negative pressure was rapidly increased to 250 mm. Hg, however, an immediate intense pain was experienced on the side of the nose and in the teeth.

Pain in the back of the head or neck never results directly from stimulation of the mucosa of any of the nasal or paranasal structures. Such pain is due to the secondary effects of prolonged contraction of the cervical and head muscles.

Section of the fifth cranial sensory nerve foot in most instances causes the mucosa of the aforementioned areas to be insensitive, with the exception of the pharynx, the tonsils, the fossa of Rosenmuller, the eustachian tubes, the external auditory canal, and the ear drum.

Inflammation and engorgement of the turbinates, ostia, nasofrontal ducts, and superior nasal spaces are responsible for most of the pain emanating from the nasal and the paranasal structures. If a headache is not associated with turbinate engorgement and inflammation, it is in all probability not the

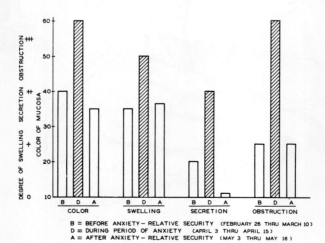

B = BEFORE ANXIETY — RELATIVE SECURITY (FEBRUARY 26 THRU MARCH 10)
D = DURING PERIOD OF ANXIETY (APRIL 3 THRU APRIL 15)
A = AFTER ANXIETY — RELATIVE SECURITY (MAY 3 THRU MAY 16)

FIG. 4-17. Sustained hyperemia, swelling, hypersecretion, and obstruction in the nose during 12 days of anxiety and resentment compared with control periods before and after.

result of disease of the nasal or the paranasal structures. Furthermore, if a zygomatic, frontal, temporal, or vertex headache is not greatly reduced in intensity or eliminated by shrinking or local anesthetization of the nasal structures, it also in all probability is not due to disease of the nasal or the paranasal structures.

Alterations in Nasal Function Occurring as Part of the Individual's Pattern of Adjustment to his Environment and Their Relevance to Headache. An example of this relationship is given in the following case history.

A young male subject who was a junior physician on a hospital staff made daily notes about his activities, his interpersonal relations and feeling states. In addition, his nasal function was observed each day, and records were made of the color of the nasal mucosa, the amount of secretion and of swelling of the nasal structures, and the degree of obstruction to inhaling air.

During a period in which the subject was exposed to serious threats to his independence, he was also subjected to threats to his career by an inefficient intern and to danger of losing the approval of his superiors.

He first tried to cope with the situation by suggesting a plan to maintain the ward's efficiency. When this failed, the subject began, in addition to his own work, to perform the neglected duties himself. At this time, be-

cause of his wife's pregnancy, it was necessary to give up his apartment and go to live in the home of a relative.

In this setting of threat to his career and the fear of loss of the approval of his senior colleagues, as well as the conflict arising from his being forced to sacrifice those symbols of independence that his own home represented, the subject developed an anxiety state with feelings of insecurity, guilt, resentment, and hostility.

Figure 4-17 demonstrates the increase in redness of the nasal mucosa associated with a significant increase in the amount of secretion, swelling, and obstruction sustained throughout this 12-day period.

DEVELOPMENT OF PAIN. During the entire period of conflict, the subject was aware of a constant "irritation" in both nostrils which, at times, developed the quality of a burning pain of low intensity. This was increased by forced inspiration, and associated with it there occurred a dull, aching pain, which spread from the bridge of the nose into the orbit and along the zygoma to the ear on each side of the swollen nasal structures. When the swelling shifted to the opposite nostril the pain correspondingly changed position. The pain, which also involved the teeth, especially those of the upper jaw, alternated with a "feeling of fullness," was worse during the working hours of the day,

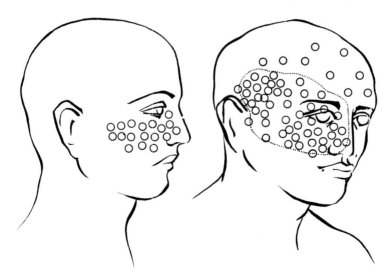

FIG. 4-18. Distribution of pain during nasal hyperfunction associated with emotional conflict: (*Left*) transitory reaction; (*Right*) sustained reaction during prolonged, intense conflict. This was associated with photophobia, lacrimation, congestion of the conjunctiva on the right, intense erythema, and "hyperalgesia" over the zygoma.

especially during periods of stress, and was minimal in the early morning and the late evening. When pain was relatively intense, local deep tenderness also was noted. Photophobia occurred, especially on the painful side, with injection of the sclerae and the skin of the cheek. Distribution of headache is shown schematically in Figure 4-18.

COMMENT. The data of this episode indicate that together with sustained conflict there may occur prolonged nasal hyperfunction accompanied by obstruction, facial pain, and tenderness. Such symptoms often are attributed to acute sinusitis. However, in this case no infection of the sinuses was demonstrated, and the disturbance with accompanying symptoms subsided completely when the subject's conflicts were resolved.

GENESIS OF PAIN FROM THE EYE

Headache associated with various ocular disorders has long been recognized as a clinical entity. Errors of refraction (hypermetropia, astigmatism), anomalies of accommodation, disturbances of muscular equilibrium, and glaucoma are universally described as causing headache. In addition, refractive errors are said to give rise to such other symptoms as aching of the eyes, sandy feeling in the eyes, pulling sensations in and about the orbit, and congestion of the conjunctivae.

Investigations have been made on the pain-sensitive structures, both superficial and deep, of the eye; on the headaches and the eyeaches associated with refractive errors and extraocular muscle imbalances; and on photophobia.

Using persons with normal eyes as experimental subjects, experimenters investigated the modalities of touch, pain, and temperature on both the conjunctiva and the cornea. Cotton wisps applied to the conjunctiva produced the sensation of touch without pain, and localization of the area touched was fairly accurate. Applicators cooled to below 30° C. were recognized as cool or cold, whereas above this temperature, up to 70° C., they were recognized only as touch. Sharp or pinching stimuli produced pain. Only pain and cold sensations were recognized on the cornea.

Patients with increased intraocular pressure described a sharp pain, which at first remained localized in the eyeball, then extended as a "bad ache" along the rim of the orbit, and finally throughout most of the area supplied by the ophthalmic division of the trigeminal nerve. Nausea and vomiting some-times accompanied such headaches. In patients having operations for strabismus under local anesthesia, pinching, sticking, or cutting the extraocular muscles caused no sensation, but traction produced prompt exclamations of pain. The pain was described as an aching sensation felt in the eye on the same side as the muscle stimulated and deep in the orbit. There was no consistent radiation of pain from traction on the extraocular muscles, and no pain was felt in the back of the head or the neck.

Traction on the iris tissue with a small toothed forceps or by chemical agents (mydriatics or miotics) caused varying degrees of pain in the eyeball, which in some instances was accompanied by radiation to the area supplied by the ophthalmic division of the trigeminal nerve on the same side.

It is recognized that hyperopia, astigmatism, and marked extraocular muscle imbalances can produce such symptoms as a sensation of ocular discomfort and aching, a feeling of heaviness in the head, and actual headache, which usually starts around and over the eyes subsequently radiates to the occiput and the back of the head.

The explanations of these symptoms are (1) that they are the result of the *sustained contraction of intraocular muscles* associated with excessive accommodative effort; and (2) that they are secondary to the unusually great and *sustained extraocular muscle contraction* resulting from the effort to produce distinct retinal images and single binocular vision with fusion.

Simple myopia, in contrast with the ocular defects just mentioned, usually does not produce headache. The reason for this is found in the fact that the myope, in attempting to improve his vision by the contraction of his eye muscles, actually makes his vision worse, and hence soon abandons the attempt.

Furthermore, it was found that experimentally induced hyperopia and astigmatism caused headaches, whereas induced myopia did not. Induced extraocular muscle imbalance caused tenseness and irritability, and, if prolonged, headache developed with abnormal electromyograms from the muscles of the head and the neck. Spontaneously occurring muscle imbalances produce the same symptoms and the same type of myograms.

Any severe headache may be accompanied by photophobia, which may be of two varieties. In the diseased eye in which inflammation of the iris and the ciliary body exists, light may cause intense pain felt in the eye and over the area supplied by the ophthalmic division of the fifth nerve, when the light stimulus is accompanied by movement of the inflamed iris. When the latter structure is immobilized, pain is allayed.

Another type of photophobia occurs in persons with healthy irides. It can be elicited by abnormally large amounts of light, or by normal amounts of light under certain conditions, such as surface irritation of the conjunctiva by chemical (2 per cent ethylmorphine hydrochloride) or by mechanical (a foreign body) means. Vascular congestion can be abolished without affecting such experimentally induced photophobia. On the other hand, the photophobia can be diminished by surface anesthesia, but not by mydriasis or cycloplegia. Surface anesthesia also reduces the normal winking responses to a bright light. This is probably due to abolition of the normal sensory impulses from air currents, lid pressure, etc. Photophobia may be absent in the presence of the Argyll Robertson pupil.

MUSCLES OF THE HEAD AND NECK AS SOURCES OF PAIN

Pain and tightness in the back of the head and the neck are frequent complaints. The sensations are variously described as a stiff cap, viselike, a weight, pressure, a tight band, a cramp, drawing, aching, or soreness. Tenderness throughout the trapezius muscles commonly is associated with these complaints and is most intense along the top of the shoulders and in the upper neck. Another common complaint is that of pain, pressure, or paresthesia over the vertex of the head. Here, tension in the neck is less obvious, but pain usually can be elicited by palpation of the trapezius muscles.

The effect of pain in the head upon the head and the neck muscles was studied in several series of observations. Muscle potentials were recorded on a two-channel ink writing oscillograph by means of solder electrodes applied over the frontal, the temporal, the occipital, and the neck muscles.

Headaches of short duration were induced by spinal drainage and by the intravenous injection of histamine. Contraction of the head and the neck muscles was observed in association with the pain, but no pain arose from the muscles themselves, probably because of the short duration of the induced head pain.

In another series, prolonged pain in the head was induced by means of repeated injections of 6 per cent saline into the right temporal muscle. This continuous pain in the head caused marked muscle contraction and secondary pain in the back of the head and the neck (Fig. 4-19).

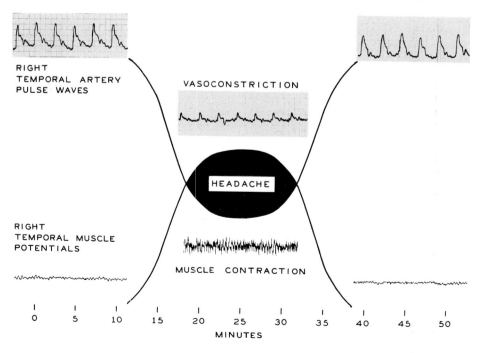

FIG. 4-19. Muscle contraction headache, right temporal region.

An irritant introduced into and left in the conjunctival sac sometimes reflexly caused contraction of the head and the neck muscles and gave rise to secondary pain and paresthesia in the scalp and the neck.

Abnormally sustained contraction of the external ocular muscles brought about by placing a +3D vertical prism in front of the dominant eye caused a sustained contraction in the neck muscles, followed by pain in the neck and the shoulder.

Observations made in patients with pain in the occiput and the neck associated with inflammation or other dysfunction about the head (pansinusitis, migraine headache, and caplike, vise, or pressure sensations), revealed sustained contraction of neck and head muscles. The intensity of the pain in the neck and over the back of the head could be modified by hot packs and massage.

These studies demonstrate that noxious stimulation in any part of the head, or emotional tension, lead to sustained contraction of the head and the neck muscles, secondarily giving rise to pain from the shoulders, the neck and the head.

Moreover, such muscles were tender upon palpation. Injection with physiologic saline solution of especially tender areas caused an increase in head sensations and pain, whereas injection of 1 per cent procaine solution into such areas relieved uncomfortable head sensations.

The exceedingly common "tension headache" found in tense, aggressive, and frustrated, anxious people also was associated with electromyographic evidence of prolonged contraction of the muscles of the head and the neck and with evidence from pulse wave records of constriction of the nutrient vessels to the muscles involved. Bilateral pulse waves recorded from the supraorbital, the temporal, and the occipital arteries during muscle-contraction headache intervals exhibited evidence of greater vasoconstriction than did records made in headache-free intervals. During such headaches subjects exhibited as much as a 10-fold increase in amplitude of action potentials from the involved muscles. Furthermore, reduction or elimination of tension through change in the subject's emotions and attitudes by modification of the life situation and by administration of phenobarbital for a few days reduced muscle contraction and vasoconstriction, and eliminated pressure, tight sensations, and headache.

TEETH AS A SOURCE OF HEADACHE

In a series of experiments in which electrical stimulation was applied to defective teeth it was demonstrated that, when an upper tooth was stimulated, pain was experienced at first locally, then diffusely in tissues supplied by the second division of the fifth cranial nerve. Noxious impulses arising from the lower teeth caused pain to be felt, at first locally and then diffusely, in tissues supplied by the third division of the fifth cranial nerve. If stimulation was sufficiently intense and prolonged, regardless of its site of origin, homolateral spread of the pain into all three divisions of the trigeminal nerve occurred. Homolateral hyperalgesia, both superficial and deep, and vasomotor reactions of tissues in the head remote from the site of the stimulated tooth were common.

Injections of procaine locally into the tissues involved in the area of headache associated with noxious impulses from a tooth, reduced in intensity but failed to eliminate pain and the sensation of fullness and tightness in areas adjacent to the region of anesthesia. However, blocking the noxious afferent impulses from stimulated teeth by peridontal infiltration with procaine completely and immediately relieved head pain.

Thus, it seems likely that the diffuse headache associated with disease of the teeth results from afferent impulses from the teeth, causing excitatory processes in the brain stem which spread to exert their effects on many other structures innervated by the fifth cranial nerve. Furthermore, when pain in the teeth is prolonged or severe, sustained contraction of the muscles of the head and the neck may occur, and in these patients pain and "tightness" may persist in the occiput and the neck for a short period, even after blocking the afferent impulses from diseased teeth.

CHRONIC OR RECURRENT POST-TRAUMATIC HEADACHE

A series of patients with headache following head injury was studied. The headaches were found to be of three varieties: (1) severe pain or circumscribed tenderness in a scar or site of impact; (2) a steady pressure sensation or aching pain in a circumscribed area or in a caplike distribution; (3) a throbbing and aching pain occurring in attacks usually unilateral and in the temporal or frontal region.

The first type was represented by those

patients who had tender areas in the scalp. These persisted sometimes for as long as 6 years after the trauma. Such tender spots often were related to visible scars and often were at or near the site of injury. Injection of the tender areas with isotonic saline accentuated the pain, whereas injection with procaine predictably eliminated it. It is inferred that the pain comes from stimulation of pain endings caught in the locally damaged tissue.

The second type resulted from sustained skeletal muscle contraction. It was demonstrated by means of electromyograms in these patients that pain in any part of the head induced a sustained contraction of the head or neck muscles sometimes remote from the original site of noxious stimulation, which in turn gave rise to steady pressure or aching pain in the head or the neck, the exact site depending upon the locus of the contracted muscles. However, such sustained and often painful contraction occurred even without tender scars or circumscribed areas of tenderness and was associated with tension and apprehension. In some instances these contractions represented unconscious protective immobilization of the head and the neck.

The third type of headache was caused by recurrent episodes of dilatation of cranial arteries. Such pain was reduced by compression of the painful arteries. Headache was eliminated by intramuscular injection of ergotamine tartrate. Such headaches also were associated with tension, anxiety, resentment, and fatigue.

Sometimes the same patient exhibited more than one mechanism of headache. Thus, in this series, post-traumatic headache and other sensations arose from structures on the outside of the head. Nearly all patients studied harbored resentment related to the circumstances of the accident, or fear that they had sustained permanent damage to their brains. Such emotional reactions and attitudes were intimately related to the aforementioned mechanisms of post-traumatic headache.

The mechanisms of the pain following head trauma (excepting epidural and subdural hematoma and subarachnoid hemorrhage) are therefore of three types: (1) pain due to local tissue damage; (2) pain due to sustained neck or head muscle contraction; (3) pain due to dilatation of the branches of the external carotid arteries.

DISCOVERY OF THE CAUSE: IMPORTANT CONSIDERATIONS IN DIAGNOSIS

INCIDENCE

The most commonly encountered headaches are vascular headaches of the migraine type and the headaches from sustained muscle contraction accompanying vasoconstriction and associated with anxiety and emotional tension. The headaches associated with fever and septicemia probably rank next in frequency, and then come those due to nasal and paranasal and eye disease. The headaches of meningitis, aneurysm, brain tumor, and brain abscess, although important and dramatic, are much less common.

INTENSITY

The most intense headaches are those due to ruptured intracranial aneurysm, meningitis, fever, migraine, and those associated with arterial hypertension. The subarachnoid hemorrhage resulting usually from ruptured intracranial aneurysm produces a headache that is sudden in onset, reaches great intensity in a very short time, and may be associated with feelings of faintness or with unconsciousness. The onset of pain is soon followed by the development of a stiff neck and the presence of blood in the lumbar spinal fluid. The very intense headache of meningitis is accompanied by a very stiff neck, which prevents passive flexion of the head on the chest. The spasm of the muscles of the neck associated with the intense headaches of migraine permits flexion of the neck.

The intensity of the headaches associated with brain tumors, brain abscesses, sinus disease, and eye disease is usually only moderate. Hemorrhage into the parenchyma of the brain seldom causes headaches unless the hemorrhage breaks through into the ventricular or subarachnoid spaces; then, intense headache may result. Also, hemorrhage into a brain tumor causing additional and serious displacement of the brain may result in a moderately severe headache.

Brain abscess may be a painless disorder unless associated with circumscribed meningitis or periostitis. However, when of long standing, brain abscess may produce headache because of generalized brain displacement and traction on pain-sensitive structures.

One rare form of very intense headache is encountered in patients in the terminal phase of brain tumor. This headache is generalized, paroxysmal, and agonizing and often ends in stupor. The pain may last for 30 seconds to 30 minutes and then disappear as quickly as it came, leaving the patient exhausted. With such headache the patient may pass into coma and die.

QUALITY OF HEADACHE

The headache of fever, migraine, hemangiomatous tumors, and those associated with arterial hypertension are characteristically throbbing or pulsating in quality. Headache from secondary muscle spasm associated with emotional tension or with eye or sinus disease has the quality of tightness or external pressure, and may be bandlike, caplike, or viselike. The headache of brain tumors and of meningitis, although occasionally pulsating, is usually of a steady aching quality.

SITE

Vascular headaches of the migraine type may occur anywhere in the head and the face and may involve the neck. The most common site is the temple, usually on the right side. The migraine headache at some time involves both the right and the left sides, although any one attack may be strictly unilateral. The headache of sinus or eye disease, shortly after its onset, is usually in the front of the head, roughly in the region near the site of stimulation; subsequently, the pain may be predominantly in the back of the head and the neck because of secondary muscle contraction. Headaches associated with pituitary adenomata and parasellar tumors are often bitemporal.

The headaches of posterior fossa tumors, early in the development of the tumor and before the beginning of general brain displacement, are usually over the occiput or behind the ear. Headaches from supratentorial tumors, before serious brain displacement occurs, are usually in the front or on the top of the head. Occasionally, if the tumor involves the dura and the bone, the headache may be near or over the site of the lesion. Early in the course of the tumor, or before general displacement of the brain has occurred, the headache is usually on the side of the tumor.

Subdural hematoma produces a headache of considerable intensity, usually localized over or near the site of the lesion, most commonly over the frontoparietal areas. The headache may be intermittent but is present, usually, some time each day, for weeks, months, or longer. A history of almost continuous headache from the date of injury is characteristic; there is no long "silent period" immediately after the injury.

The headaches associated with tumors of the cerebellopontile angle and acoustic neurinoma are often localized in the postauricular region. Like other brain-tumor headaches, they are intermittent, and of moderate intensity. They are associated with hyperalgesia of the postauricular region on the same side as the tumor. Headache is one of the earliest manifestations of acoustic neurinoma. Headache is a later manifestation of cerebellopontile angle tumors.

The muscle-contraction headaches or pressure sensations associated with emotional tension are usually first evident and most intense in the neck, the shoulders, and the occiput, but later spread to include the frontal region. They may be unilateral or bilateral.

Disease involving the dome of the diaphragm or the phrenic nerve causes pain high in the shoulder and the neck. Similarly, in rare instances, coronary occlusion and myocardial insufficiency cause pain in the lower jaw, high in the neck, and in the occiput. Disease and dysfunction of structures below the diaphragm do not ordinarily induce headache except indirectly through fever, sepsis, or bacteremia.

However, in special circumstances headache may occur with excessive distention of the urinary bladder or rectum. It has been demonstrated in paraplegics whose level of cord transection is T-6 or higher that excessive distention of the bladder or rectum results in a vascular pressor response in the segments below the level of the lesion. Prompt rise in blood pressure occurs, and cranial blood vessels not involved in the pressor response become dilated, causing headache.

TENDERNESS

During migraine headaches and often for some hours thereafter there is hyperalgesia or tenderness near the large arteries on the outside of the head in the affected region. As mentioned previously, it has been demonstrated that deep-pain thresholds are lowered. Also, there may be tenderness of the skin of the face as a result of inflammation of the nasal and the paranasal spaces. Muscle in a state of sustained contraction, secondary to pain anywhere in the head, may become tender on palpation. Thus, brushing and combing the hair may be a painful experience during or after muscle tension or migraine headache. With myositis and myalgia there may be tender areas in the muscles of the head and the neck. Because of the hyperalgesia, percussion of the head may cause pain over or near an underlying brain tumor.

Periostitis secondary to frontal, ethmoid, or sphenoid sinus disease or mastoiditis produces a pain of moderate to severe intensity associated with local tenderness at the site of disease. If the pain is sufficiently severe and continuous it may become generalized. If the mastoid or sinus disease is limited to the bone (osteomyelitis) it is usually completely painless. The tenderness or hyperalgesia associated with mastoid disease with periostitis is far greater than the hyperalgesia associated with posterior fossa brain tumor.

Tenderness at a site of head injury, and often associated with a scar, may persist for many years. Also, in post-traumatic headache there often occur tender muscles or nodules in parts of the head remote from the site of injury. Headache of the vascular type akin to migraine with tenderness over the arteries may be initiated by head injury.

Effect of Manual Pressure

Pressure upon the temporal, frontal, supraorbital, postauricular, occipital, and common carotid arteries often reduces the intensity of migraine headache and that associated with arterial hypertension. No other type is modified so definitely by manual pressure, although supporting the head makes any patient with headache feel more comfortable.

The headache or pressure sensations associated with emotional tension and resulting from sustained muscle contraction are intensified by firm pressure upon tender muscles or regions of tenderness.

Effect of Position of the Head

In many instances migraine headache is made worse by assuming a horizontal position and is relieved by an erect position. It is often made worse by ascending stairs, by moving about rapidly, or by lifting objects. Sitting quietly in an upright position often proves to be most comfortable. The recumbent position may at first make the headache associated with nasal and paranasal disease more intense, but subsequently the headache subsides. A sudden change in position, usually from the recumbent to the sitting and less frequently from the sitting to the recumbent, may make the headache of brain tumor

more intense. Unlike the migraine headache, the headache of brain tumor is often worse when the patient is in the upright position. The head-down position aggravates some headaches, except those due to spinal drainage and occasionally those associated with brain tumors. Shaking the head tends to augment the intensity of intracranial vascular headache and brain-tumor headache, but may reduce that due to muscle spasm from tension or that secondary to sinus and eye diseases. Muscle contraction headache is usually reduced in intensity by movements of the head and the neck which extend the contracted muscles. Straining at stool and coughing increase all but muscle headaches. Sharp flexion or over-extension of the head reduces the intensity of postpuncture headache.

Duration of Headache

Headache of the migraine variety may be as brief as 20 or 30 minutes, or it may last for days, or, rarely, for weeks. The usual headache is terminated within 24 hours. A striking feature of migraine is the complete freedom from headache between prostrating attacks. The headaches of brain tumor are intermittent, but usually occur during part of every day and vary in intensity from time to time. Headache associated with chronic sinus disease is intermittent but quite predictable; it may occur during the working hours of each day for weeks or even months.

Muscle contraction headache or pressure sensations associated with sustained tension and anxiety may persist for days, weeks, or even years.

Time of Day

Headaches associated with hypertension and migraine most commonly have their onset in the early hours of the morning, so that the patient awakens with the pain. Such migraine headaches characteristically diminish in intensity with the "setting of the sun" or in the evening. The headache of brain tumor, if it be connected in any way with the time of day, is more severe in the early part of the day, although not in the early hours of the morning. The headache associated with nasal and paranasal disease usually occurs in the morning and improves toward the late afternoon or when the patient retires. Headache associated with eye disease usually begins in the latter part of the day or evening.

Muscle contraction headache or pressure sensations are usually worse at the end of the working day.

DAY OF THE WEEK AND THE MONTH

Migraine headaches are common during week-ends, during the first period of vacation holidays, and immediately after vacation. They are very common just before the onset of menstruation. Patients with migraine often have fixed days of the week when their headaches occur.

SEASON OF THE YEAR

Headache associated with nasal and paranasal disease is usually more common during periods when the upper respiratory infections prevail, namely, the darker months of the year. Migraine headache occurs during periods of increased conflict, tension or stress for the individual; for example, during early fall for the school teacher, during "rush" or "holiday" seasons for the merchant, during very hot or humid weather for those who feel ineffective and prostrated during such climatic states.

MUSCLE SPASM

Contractions of the muscles of the head and the neck occur with all headaches. If the contractions are of sufficient duration, they themselves become a cause of headache. Headache and a very stiff neck accompanied by Kernig's sign are associated with widespread meningitis. The Kernig sign may be absent even late in the course of a carcinomatous invasion of the meninges at the base of the brain. Headache and stiff neck are common with tumors of the posterior fossa, but the stiff neck may be overcome by persuasion and passive movement of the head by the examining physician. Neck stiffness may sometimes occur with prolonged postpuncture headache.

Spasm of the muscles of the neck, the head and the back may become so great with meningitis that it cannot be relaxed and the patient assumes the position of opisthotonos. With posterior fossa tumors, muscle spasm may cause tilting of the head or lifting of the shoulder. The muscle spasm headache associated with prolonged anxiety and tension may cause backward tilting of the head and half closing of the eyes. Muscle spasm is always an accompaniment of migraine headache and is one explanation of the slow

relief afforded by ergotamine tartrate to some patients in whom this component is major.

PHOTOPHOBIA

Photophobia is associated with any headache experienced chiefly in the front or the top of the head. It is commonly noted in patients with meningitis, migraine, nasal and paranasal disease, eye disease, brain-tumor, and muscle-spasm headache. Congestion of the sclera and the conjunctiva may accompany such photophobia. If the intensity of the pain is very great, photophobia, lacrimation, and sweating of the homolateral forehead and side of the face also occur.

PERIODICITY

Headaches that begin in childhood or at puberty and occur especially with menstruation and at certain fixed intervals during many years are in all likelihood of the migraine variety. Migraine headaches often stop at menopause. On the other hand, they may occasionally begin at this time.

MUCOUS MEMBRANE INJECTION

Redness and swelling of the mucous membrane of the nose with or without nosebleeds may occur with migraine. Also, injection of the conjunctiva may be seen. Headache caused by disease of the nasal and the paranasal sinuses is always accompanied by obvious congestion of the turbinates and the nasal mucous membranes.

GASTROINTESTINAL AND VASOMOTOR DISTURBANCES

Anorexia, nausea, and vomiting, although most commonly associated with migraine headaches, may be associated with any headache, and the more intense the headache the more likely they are to occur. Vomiting without nausea may occur with brain tumors, especially those of the posterior fossa. Nausea and vomiting with little or no headache may occur in persons with migraine. The headache associated with sinus or eye disease is seldom associated with vomiting. Constipation often is associated with migraine, although diarrhea also occurs. Distention and flatulence are common in migraine and tension headaches, but are seldom associated with other headaches.

Excessive pallor and cold hands and feet are characteristic prodromal accompaniments of the migraine attack. Tachycardia and extrasystoles frequently are noted.

POLYURIA

Polyuria commonly is associated with migraine headache attacks and, with the exception of the headache associated with third ventricle tumors, seldom occurs with other headaches. Weight gain of several pounds preceding the migraine attack is common, but not invariable. It usually develops some hours before, but sometimes occurs well in advance of the headache (7 to 10 days). During subsidence of the headache, weight loss occurs, with increased rates of excretion of water, sodium, and potassium. However, these fluid and electrolyte changes are not related causally or mechanistically to the onset, the intensity, or the duration of the migraine attack. Instead, they are manifestations of the widespread bodily changes accompanying adaptive reactions during and after stressful periods. Thus the migraine attack is a concurrent but independent feature. Tension states with headaches may be linked with frequency of urination.

VISUAL DISTURBANCES

Both scintillating scotomata and visual field defects such as unilateral or homonymous hemianopsia may occur with migraine headaches. Such defects in vision may occur with brain-tumor headaches when the tumor is due to a lesion of the occipital lobes or is adjacent to the visual pathways. The visual disturbances of migraine, with the exception of blurred vision and diplopia, seldom occur with the headache but usually precede it. The visual disturbance is usually of short duration, persisting for less than an hour. Enlarged pupils and lacrimation may cause dimness of vision during a migraine headache, but when visual defects outlast the headache attack it is likely that one is dealing with cerebral vascular accident or a brain tumor. Defects in color vision and colored rings around lights may occur with the headache associated with glaucoma. Ptosis of the eyelid may be an accompaniment of the brain-tumor headache and occasionally that of migraine. It occurs with a rare variety of migraine called ophthalmoplegic migraine, in which case it is probably due to an aneurysm of the circle of Willis. Partial closure of the eyes due to muscle spasm may accompany any headache and give the impression of faulty vision.

VERTIGO AND OTHER SENSORY DISTURBANCES

Vertigo may be a forerunner of a migraine headache attack. Vertigo sometimes is associated with the headaches of brain tumors, although feelings of unsteadiness are more common. Fleeting vertigo with sudden movement or rotation of the head often accompanies the post-traumatic headache. Meniere's syndrome is frequently associated with headache. Other sensory disturbances, such as paresthesias of the hands and the face, may occur as a forerunner of the migraine headache. However, paresthesias that persist during or outlast the headache attack are more common in patients with brain tumors and in those with certain types of cerebral seizure.

MOOD

The wish to retire from people and responsibilities, a dejected, depressed, irritable, or negativistic mental state bordering on prostration or stupor is a dominant aspect of the migraine attack and in some instances may be more disturbing than the pain in the head. Apathy, listlessness, or even euphoria may be associated with brain-tumor headache. Depression is not a feature, although obviously a depressed person also may have brain tumor.

The headache associated with muscle contraction may occur in a tense, irritable person, but the patient is usually more willing to accept attention, massage, or medication in contrast with the patient with a migraine headache attack who commonly expresses the wish to be left alone. Exaltation or feelings of especial well-being are common sequels to the migraine headache attack. The suffering experienced with the headache of fever, meningitis, or ruptured aneurysm may be very great, and the mental state is that of reaction to intense pain.

SLEEP

Migraine headaches, even of the most severe type, do not disrupt sleep entirely, except for short periods. Those of brain tumor, sinus disease and muscle spasm permit sleep. Therefore, when an individual complains of long periods of sleep loss because of headache, it is well to consider anxiety or depression as the dominant aspect of the illness. The headache of meningitis usually interrupts sleep.

EYEGROUNDS

When headache is linked with papilledema, it is in most instances due to an expanding intracranial mass. However, in patients with brain tumor, headache often occurs without papilledema, and papilledema without headache. In the advanced phase of hypertensive encephalopathy, headache and papilledema are usual. Aneurysm and subdural hematoma may cause intense headache without papilledema. Meningitis does not affect the eyegrounds except possibly to induce slight suffusion. During migraine headache arterial and venous dilatation in eyegrounds is usual. Albuminuric retinitis may not be associated with headache; when headache is present, the two phenomena are not directly related.

FAMILY HISTORY

The headache of migraine and that associated with arterial hypertension are the only familial headaches. Evidence permits the assumption that inheritance of the migraine headache trait is through a recessive gene with a penetrance of approximately 70 per cent.

LEUKOCYTOSIS

The headaches of meningitis and subarachnoid hemorrhage are usually accompanied by leukocytosis; the headache of typhoid fever, by leukopenia. There may be leukopenia with the headache associated with influenza or grippe. Headache and stiff neck with slight, if any, leukocytosis is noted in leutic meningitis and sometimes in tuberculous meningitis.

The headache following severe convulsions or a series of convulsions may be associated with leukocytosis. The headache associated with brain tumor, particularly if it be in the frontal region, is sometimes accompanied by leukocytosis. Leukocytosis coupled with fever is most commonly associated with brain abscess.

CEREBROSPINAL FLUID

Headache and pleocytosis may be associated with meningitis, whereas the headache associated with the onset of acute infections outside the cranial cavity usually is accompanied by only a slight increase or no increase in the number of cells in the spinal fluid. Intracranial pressure may be increased with headache associated with brain tumor, but often no increase occurs.

The headache of brain abscess is commonly associated with a slight increase in the number of cells. The serologic test for syphilis of the spinal fluid is positive if luetic meningitis or gumma is responsible for the headache. The cerebrospinal fluid is normal during the headache of migraine, hypertensive vascular disease, or fever, and usually is normal in meningismus. When a headache results from a brain tumor in contact with the arachnoid space, there may be an increase in protein and cells in the spinal fluid.

Blood in the spinal fluid or xanthochromia not due to spinal cord injury or disease almost always is accompanied by headache. This combination commonly occurs with head injury, carcinomatosis (especially of the meninges), subarachnoid hemorrhage, and ruptured cerebral aneurysm. It less commonly occurs with subdural hematoma, meningioma, and glioma.

ELECTROENCEPHALOGRAMS

When electroencephalography is performed in a large series of patients with the complaint of headache, without reference to the type of headache, the number of abnormal records is not much different from that found in a similar group of headache-free individuals. However, the incidence of abnormal electroencephalographic records increases significantly when patients with vascular headache of the migraine type are studied. Patients having focal motor, sensory, or mental disturbances during one phase of a migraine attack are those most likely to have focal electroencepalographic abnormalities. These abnormalities may be separated into three broad categories:

1. Transient focal electroencephalographic changes that appear only very briefly along with a focal neurological sign, and then disappear almost simultaneously with the dwindling of the neurological defect (as with scotomata).

2. Transient focal abnormalities lasting hours or days. These are exemplified by the infrequent occurrence of hemiparesis accompanying and sometimes outlasting the migraine attack.

3. Persistent focal and/or generalized slow activity seen during headache-free intervals. This accounts for only a small percentage of the electroencephalographic changes.

ROENTGENOGRAMS

X-ray pictures of the head in patients with migraine or the headaches of hypertension, meningitis, ruptured aneurysm, and brain abscess, show nothing unusual. Aneurysm sometimes may be demonstrated by arteriograms. Moreover, x-ray examinations reveal nothing in at least half of the patients with brain tumor. Frontal hyperostosis is not in itself a cause of headache. Calcification of the falx, of the cerebral arteries, of the pineal body, or of the choroid plexus does not cause headache. A small sella turcica is in itself no cause of headache.

Chronic osteosclerosis of the mastoid region and increased density of the sinuses do not in themselves cause headache.

Disease of the nasal and paranasal sinuses can cause headache without enough change to be evident in x-ray plates. On the other hand, there may be serious disease of the sinuses with osteomyelitis without headache.

FACTORS THAT MODIFY HEADACHE

Decompression of the skull and removal of brain tumors very commonly afford relief of headache due to such tumors. This is not universally true, since headaches caused by pituitary adenomata often persist after the tumor has been removed.

Ligation or obliteration of the middle meningeal artery will sometimes relieve headache due to brain tumor even though the latter has become inoperable. Such procedures often fail, however, since traction upon other pain-sensitive structures may continue to cause pain.

Ligation of the superficial temporal artery or other superficial scalp arteries may reduce or eliminate migraine headaches in certain patients.

The evacuation of pus from beneath the periosteum and from the adjacent paranasal sinuses and mastoid cells often affords prompt relief of the headache associated with empyema of these regions. However, the persistence or development of frontal headache after simple sinusotomy is evidence of the presence of extradural infection, and possibly of subdural infection. Similarly, the persistence or development of postauricular or preauricular headache after simple mastoidectomy is good evidence for the existence of adjacent extradural, and possibly subdural infection.

CHEMICAL AGENTS THAT MODIFY AND THAT PREVENT HEADACHES

We are not concerned in this chapter with details of treatment; however, consideration of drug actions helps us to understand pathogenesis.

The effectiveness of analgesics is dependent entirely upon the intensity of pain and not at all on the site or origin or the particular mechanism inducing the pain. Thus, 60 mg. of codeine sulfate or 15 mg. of morphine sulfate may be necessary for the high-intensity headaches of meningitis, migraine, ruptured aneurysm, and of certain fevers such as typhus and typhoid fever, whereas agents such as acetylsalicylic acid, in 0.3-to-0.6-Gm. doses, are effective against other types of headache. Fortunately, the headache of brain tumor is seldom so intense as to require opiates.

Ergotamine tartrate if given parenterally in sufficient amounts and sufficiently early in the course of a headache will abolish or modify the headache of migraine. It is effective, through its vasoconstrictor action, on dilated cranial arteries. It does not affect other types, except those associated with arterial hypertension.

Norepinephrine, in a dilution of 4 ml. of an 0.2 per cent solution in a liter of 5 per cent dextrose and water, may be administered intravenously at an average rate of 4 drops per second, or at a rate sufficient to raise the systolic blood pressure 20 to 40 mm. Hg. It acts to relieve headache by vasoconstriction of cranial arteries. Mild headaches of the migraine type have been eliminated in 30 minutes with infusion of norepinephrine; severe headaches in 45 to 160 minutes.

Phenobarbital, if given over a period of days to weeks in amounts of 0.015 to 0.030 Gm. three times a day to people who have mild symptoms of anxiety and tension in association with their headaches, may help to reduce the frequency and severity of the headaches by reducing the degree of their arousal. Chlordiazepoxide ("Librium"®) in amounts of 5 to 10 mg. three times a day, and meprobamate in amounts of 400 mg. three times a day, may have a similar effect. In patients with a disturbed sleep cycle, the administration of phenobarbital 0.09 Gm. at bedtime, or amitriptyline ("Elavil"®) 50 to 100 mg. in the evening before bedtime, over a period of two weeks or more, may improve the sleep cycle and also help to ameliorate the headaches. None of these medications acts directly upon the cause of the headache itself.

Methysergide maleate ("Sansert"®) 2 mg. three to four times a day, given over a period of weeks, is often effective in diminishing the frequency and severity of vascular headaches and in preventing their occurrence. Methysergide, an ergot alkaloid, acts differently from ergotamine; it is effective in preventing both vasoconstrictor and vasodilator phases of the migraine attack. See discussion of its action earlier in this chapter. It is of no help in the treatment of headaches that are already established, but it is probably the most useful medication that is presently available for establishing a remission of a disabling cycle of frequent and severe migraine. This medication does have serious side effects in some patients, and must be used with caution. About 20 per cent of patients who are initially given this medication will develop an untoward reaction within the first few days or weeks of therapy. This is associated with aching pains in the calves or upper arms, nausea and abdominal discomfort, low abdominal pain, anxiety, fogginess or feelings of depersonalization, and very rarely chest pain. The medication should be stopped if any of these symptoms occur. In a small proportion of patients who receive this medication over a period of weeks or months, massive and generalized growth of fibrous tissue may appear. These most often occur in the retroperiotoneal region, but they have been reported to occur in the lung, in the pericardium, and in the subendocardial tissues involving the heart valves. Ureteral obstruction and developing uremia have lead to the discovery of some of these cases. Although the condition is said to remit spontaneously when the medication is discontinued and the number of cases observed has been few in relation to the number of those who have received methysergide, nevertheless, the following precautions should be used in the administration of this medication.

No patient who has a history of vascular disease or collagen disease should receive methysergide. Its use should be limited to those who are having a disabling vascular headache at least once a week. Each patient who receives the medication should be seen at intervals of at least every two weeks initially, and thereafter, at least every month. Every effort should be made to complete the course and discontinue the medication within six months. Those few patients who cannot avoid disabling headaches unless they are kept upon a small continuing dose of this medication should be observed at least every three months. Every patient who receives this medication should initially have an electrocardiogram, a chest x-ray, a urinalysis, and careful observations of his heart sounds and of the pulses in his radial, femoral, and dorsalis pedis arteries. The development of any of the symptoms just described, or any change in the physical or laboratory signs, should be a cause for discontinuing the medication.

LIFE SITUATIONS AND REACTIONS

Migraine headaches commonly occur when hereditarily susceptible persons become involved in patterns of activity or life situations which cause them to engage in sustained purposeful activity with arousal, anxiety, and tension accompanied by recurring fatigue and interpersonal conflict. No amount of therapeutic or preventive medication alone can take the place of helping the patient to understand himself, and to understand how his headaches are related to his pattern of activities and reactions to the life situations in which he is involved. Recognition of these, and alteration of them to some extent, will be more beneficial in producing a remission of the headaches than any other form of therapy.

BIBLIOGRAPHY

Camp, W. A., and Wolff, H. G.: Studies on headache. Electroencephalographic abnormalities in patients with vascular headache of the migraine type, A.M.A. Arch. Neurol. 4:475-485, 1961.

Chapman, L. F., Goodell, H., and Wolff, H. G.: Augmentation of the inflammatory reaction by activity of the central nervous system, A.M.A. Arch. Neurol. 1:557-582, 1959.

Chapman, L. F., Ramos, A. O., Goodell, H., Silverman, G., and Wolff, H. G.: A humoral agent implicated in vascular headache of the migraine type, A.M.A. Arch. Neurol. 3:223-229, 1960; Trans. Amer. Neurol. Ass., 85:42-45; 200-202, 1960.

———: Definition of a biochemical agent implicated in the mechanism of vascular headache of the migraine type, Trans. Ass. Amer. Physicians 73:259-271, 1960.

Clark, D., Hough, H. B., and Wolff, H. G.: Experimental studies on headache, observations on headache produced by histamine. A.M.A. Arch. Neurol. Psychiat. 35:1054, 1936.

Dalessio, D. J., Camp, W. A., Goodell, H., and Wolff, H. G.: Studies on headache. The mode of action of UML-491 and its relevance to the nature of vascular headache of the migraine type, A.M.A. Arch. Neurol. 4:235-240, 1961.

Dalessio, D. J. Champan, L. F., Zileli, T., Cattell, M., Ehrlich, R., Fortuin, F., Goodell, H., and Wolff, H. G.: Studies on headache. The responses of the bulbar conjunctival blood vessels during induced oliguria and diuresis, and their modification by UML-491, A.M.A. Arch. Neurol. 5:590-593, 1961.

Dalessio, D. J., Camp, W. A., Goodell, H., Chapman. L. F., Zileli, T., Ramos, A. O., Ehrlich, R., Fortuin, F., Cattell, M., and Wolff, H. G.: Studies on headache. The relevance of the prophylactic action of UML-491 in vascular headache of the migraine type to the pathophysiology of this syndrome, World Neurol. 3:66, 1962.

Eckardt, L. B., McLean, J. M., and Goodell, H.: Experimental studies on headache: the genesis of pain from the eye, Proc. Ass. Res. Nerv. Ment. Dis. 23:209, 1943.

Goodell, H. Lewontin, R. and Wolff, H. G.: Familial occurrence of migraine headache. A study of heredity, Arch. Neurol. Phychiat. 72:325, 1954.

Graham, J. R., and Wolff, H. G.: Mechanism of migraine headache and action of ergotamine tartrate, Proc. Ass. Res. Nerv. Ment. Dis. 18:638, 1937; Arch. Neurol. Psychiat. 39:737, 1938.

Grimes, E.: The migraine instability, Med. J. Research 134:417, 1931.

Holmes, T. H.: Goodell, H., Wolf, S. G., and Wolff, H. G.: The nose; an experimental study of reactions within the nose in human subjects during varying life experiences, Springfield, Ill., Thomas, 1950.

Kilbourne, E. D., and Wolff, H. G.: Cranial arteritis: a critical evaluation of the syndrome of "temporal arteritis" with report of a case, Ann. Intern. Med. 24:1, 1946.

Kunkle, E. C., Ray, B. S., and Wolff, H. G.: Studies on headache. The mechanism and significance of the headache associated with brain tumor, Bull. N. Y. Acad. Med. 18:400, 1942.

———: Studies on headache: An analysis of the headache associated with changes in intracranial pressure, Arch. Neurol. Psychiat. 49:323, 1943.

Kunkle, E. C., Lund, D. W., and Maher, P. J.: Analysis of vascular mechanisms in headache by use of the human centrifuge, with observations upon pain perception under increased positive G, Arch. Neurol. Psychiat. 60:253, 1948.

Kunkle, E. C., Pfeiffer, J. B., Wilhoit, W. M., and Hamrick, L. W.: Recurrent brief headache in "cluster" headache, Trans. Amer. Neurol. Ass: 77:240, 1952.

Kunkle, E. C., Hernandez, R. R., Johnson, W. T., and Baumann, J. A.: Adaptive responses of cranial vessels in the head-down position, Trans. Amer. Neurol. Ass. 87:151, 1962.

Marcussen, R. M., and Wolff, H. G.: A formulation of the dynamics of the migraine attack, Psychosom. Med. 11:251, 1949.

———: Studies on headache. 1. Effects of carbon dioxide-oxygen mixtures given during preheadache phase of the migraine attack; 2. Further analysis of the pain mechanisms in headache, Arch. Neurol. Psychiat. 63:42, 1950.

Ostfeld, A. M., Reis, D. J., Goodell, H., and Wolff, H. G.: Headache and hydration. The significance of two varieties of fluid accumulation in patients with vascular headache of the migraine type, A.M.A. Arch. Intern. Med. 96:142-152, 1955; Trans. Ass. Amer. Physicians 68:255, 1955.

Ostfeld, A. M., and Wolff, H. G.: Arterenol (norepinephrine) and vascular headache of the migraine type. Studies on headache, Arch. Neurol. Psychiat. 74:131-136, 1955; Trans. Amer. Neurol. Ass., p. 142, 1954.

———: Studies on headache: reactivity of bulbar conjunctival vessels during the migraine type of headache and muscle contraction headache (abstract), (Am. Fed. Clin. Res.) Clin. Res. 4:1956; Arch. Neurol. Psychiat. 77:113, 1957.

Ostfeld, A. M., Chapman, L. F., Goodell, H., and Wolff, H. G.: Studies in headache. Summary of evidence concerning a noxious agent active locally during migraine headache, Psychosom. Med. 19:199-208, 1957.

Ostfeld, A. M., and Wolff, H. G.: Studies on headache: participation of ocular structures in the migraine syndrome, Mod. Problems Ophthal. 1:634-647, 1957.

Pickering, G. W.: Experimental observations on headache, Brit. Med. J. 1:907, 1939.

Pichler, E., Ostfeld, A. M., Goodell, H., and Wolff, H. G.: Studies on headache. Central versus peripheral action of ergotamine tartrate and its relevance to the therapy of migraine headache, Arch. Neurol. Psychiat. 76:571-577, 1956.

Ray, B. S., and Wolff, H. G.: Experimental studies on headache, Pain-sensitive structures of the head and their significance in headache, A.M.A. Arch. Surg. 41:813, 1940.

Robertson, S., Goodell, H., and Wolff, H. G.: Headache; the teeth as a source of headache and other pain, Arch. Neurol. Psychiat. 57:277, 1947.

Robertson, S., and Wolff, H. G.: Studies on headache: distention of the rectum, sigmoid colon and bladder as a source of headache in intact humans, Arch. Neurol. Psychiat. 63:52, 1950.

Schottstadt, W. W., and Wolff, H. G.: Studies on headache. Variations in fluid and electrolyte excretion in association with vascular headache of the migraine type, Arch. Neurol. Phychiat. 73:158-164, 1955.

Schumacher, G. A., and Guthrie, T. C.: Mechanism of headache induced by distention of bladder and rectum in patients with spinal cord injuries, Trans. Amer. Neurol. Ass., 74:205, 1949.

Schumacher, G. A., Ray, B. S., and Wolff, H. G.: Experimental studies on headache. Further analysis of histamine headache and its pain pathways, Arch. Neurol. Psychiat. 44:701, 1940.

Schumacher, G. A., and Wolff, H. G.: Experimental studies on headache. (A) Contrast of histamine headache with the headache of migraine and that associated with hypertension. (B) Contrast of vascular mechanisms in preheadache and headache phenomena of migraine, Arch. Neurol. Psychiat. 45:119, 1941.

Simons, D. J., Day, E., Goodell, H., and Wolff, H. G.: Experimental studies on headache, muscles of the scalp and neck as sources of pain, Proc. Ass. Res. Nerv. Ment. Dis. 23:228, 1943.

Simons, D. J., and Wolff, H. G.: Experimental studies on headache: the mechanism of chronic or recurrent post-traumatic headache, Psychosom. Med. 8:293, 1946.

Sutherland, A. M., and Wolff, H. G.: Experimental studies on headache. Further analysis of the mechanism of headache in migraine, hypertension and fever, Arch. Neurol. Psychiat. 44:929, 1940.

Thompson, C. E., and Witham, A. C.: Paroxysmal hypertension in spinal cord injuries, New Eng. J. Med. 239:291, 1948.

Torda, C., and Wolff, H. G.: Experimental studies on headache. The pharmacodynamics of the urine of patients with migraine headache, Fed. Proc., Amer. Soc. Pharmacol. Exp. Therap. 2:44, March, 1943.

———: Experimental studies on headache: Transient thickening of walls and cranial arteries in relation to certain phenomena of migraine headache and action of ergotamine tartrate on thickened vessels, Arch. Neurol. Psychiat. 53:329, 1945.

Tunis, M. M., and Wolff, H. G.: Studies on headache. Cranial artery vasoconstriction and muscle contraction headache, Arch. Neurol. Psychiat. 71:425, 1954.

———: Studies on headache. Long-term observations of the cranial arteries in subjects with vascular headache of the migraine type, Arch. Neurol. Psychiat. 70:551, 1953.

Whitteridge, D., Gilliatt, R. W., and Guttmann, L.: Inspiratory vasoconstriction in patients after spinal cord injuries, J. Physiol. 107:67-75, 1948.

Wolff, H. G.: The cerebral circulation, Physiol. Rev. 16:545, 1936.

———: Personality features and reactions of subjects with migraine, Arch. Neurol. Psychiat. 37:895, 1937.

———: Stress and Disease, Springfield, Ill., Thomas, 1952.

———: Stress and adaptive patterns resulting in tissue damage in man, Med. Clin. N. Amer. 39:783, 1955.

———: Headache and Other Head Pain, ed. 2, New York, Oxford, 1963.

Wolff, H. G., and Tunis, M. M.: Analysis of cranial artery pressure pulse waves in patients with vascular headache of the migraine type, Trans. Ass. Amer. Physicians 65:240, 1952.

Wolff, H. G., Tunis, M. M., and Goodell, H.: Studies on headache. Evidence of tissue damage and changes in pain sensitivity in subjects with vascular headaches of the migraine type, A.M.A. Arch. Intern. Med. 92:478, 1953.

Zileli, T., Chapman, L. F., and Wolff, H. G.: Anti-inflammatory action of UML-491 demonstrated by granuloma pouch technique in rats, Arch. Intern. Pharmacodyn. 136:463, 1962.

Zileli, T., Goodell, H., Hinkle, L. E., and Wolff, H. G.: Studies on headache: the modifying effect of methysergide on the sensitivity of vasomotor centers and its relevance to vascular headache, Cornell Symposium on Headache, 1964.

5

Loss of Vision; Eye Pain

ROBERT D. REINECKE

Measurements of Visual Loss

Principal Locations of Pathologic Processes

Acute Visual Loss: Emergencies
WITHOUT PAIN OR FLASHES
Occlusion of Central Retinal Artery
PAINLESS LOSS OF VISION WITH A
FLASHING SENSATION
Retinal Detachment

Other Painless Sudden Loss of Vision
EYE HEMORRHAGES
Vitreous Hemorrhages
Pathologic Bleeding (Hematologic Disorders)
Rupture of Veins
Retinal Hemorrhages (Occlusion of Central Retinal Vein)
WITH DIABETES MELLITUS
Diabetic Retinopathy

With a Red, Painful Eye
ANGLE-CLOSURE GLAUCOMA

With Painful Eye Movements
RETROBULBAR NEURITIS

Painless Chronic Visual Loss
CATARACTS
Aging as a Factor

Metabolic Disorders
TUNNEL VISION
Glaucoma
Drug Toxicity
Retinitis Pigmentosa

Transient Visual Loss
HEMIANOPSIAS WITH FLASHES
Migraine
TRANSIENT MONOCULAR VISUAL LOSS
Carotid Insufficiency
Impending Occlusion of Central Retinal Artery

Hemianopsias

Distorted Vision with Blurring
CENTRAL SEROUS RETINOPATHY
SENILE MACULAR DEGENERATION
CHORIORETINITIS

Sudden Loss of Vision: Traumatic
HEAD TRAUMA
ELECTRIC SHOCK
DIRECT TRAUMA TO THE EYE
Physical Injury
Chemical Contact
Ultraviolet Exposure

MEASUREMENTS OF VISUAL LOSS

Visual loss may be of various degrees, from slight and subtle to profound. In this chapter most of the conditions discussed involve visual loss that is severe—the loss is sufficient that the patient is well aware that the vision has changed dramatically, often from excellent vision to no light perception. Neither the more subtle visual losses nor the poor vision associated with amblyopia will be discussed here; the latter can be considered a lack of development of vision rather than a loss of vision. In any instance of professed visual loss, careful evaluation and recording of the central vision and of visual fields is of paramount importance. Each eye is tested separately. By far the most satisfactory measurement of central acuity consists of determining the smallest line of a Snellen Chart which the patient can read accurately at twenty feet. Correction of refractive errors with lenses may be used if helpful. Vision is usually considered as within acceptable normal limits if it is 20/30 or better with or without glasses (correction by a lens). The second crucial measurement is that of the circumference of the visual field and detection within it of any areas of decreased or absent vision.

PRINCIPAL LOCATIONS OF PATHOLOGIC PROCESSES

Visual loss may be due to three principal types of pathologic processes. First, the optical properties of the eye may be impaired (cornea, aqueous, lens, or vitreous). Second, the retina may be damaged so that no signal can be converted from light energy to neural impulses (as with retinal detachment or retinitis pigmentosa). Third, the neural pathway may be impaired at the optic disc (as in glaucoma), the optic nerve (as in ischemic optic atrophy), the chiasm (as in pituitary tumors), or in the brain. The first two principal causes usually can be seen with the ophthalmoscope and the third can be studied with the visual field tests.

ACUTE VISUAL LOSS: EMERGENCIES

Sudden loss of vision requires emergency evaluation. Of the several conditions that can cause acute loss of vision, occlusion of the central retinal artery and angle-closure glaucoma must be treated immediately. Even though there are only two disorders that require prompt treatment, all cases must be studied immediately to determine the diagnosis and thus permit decision concerning which must receive emergency treatment. One of the conditions, occlusion of a central retinal artery, often produces irreversible blindness in the affected eye if the condition is not treated within one and one-half hours; some observers believe the condition to be hopeless if the patient is not seen within one-half hour after the occlusion.

WITHOUT PAIN: EMERGENCY

Occlusion of Central Retinal Artery

The central retinal artery is subject to the usual causes of occlusion—thrombosis, atherosclerosis, arteriolar sclerosis, and emboli. Often repeated showers of emboli are dramatic to watch but fortunately may spare the vision. There may be fat emboli after bone trauma, emboli from atheromatous plaques in the carotid (especially following arteriography), or off vegetations from diseased heart valves. Occasionally, emboli of carcinoma cells may be the cause. The site of the occlusion in the artery usually shows fibrosis and intimal proliferation. If inflammation such as that sometimes associated with temporal arteritis is the cause, the site is usually in the nutrient arteries of the optic nerve; there, giant cell proliferation can be seen in the wall of the artery.

After the retina has been permanently damaged by occlusion of the central retinal artery, the first pathological change is edema of the entire retina with accentuated swelling of the internal layers. As the edema disappears, the inner layers show irreparable damage to the bipolar and ganglion cells. Often the rods and cones are surprisingly intact if the retina is sectioned within a few weeks of the occlusion. Later sectioning of the retina, years after the occlusion, shows complete gliosis of the retina with few recognizable structures.

Experimental studies with cats and rats have indicated that the retina cannot tolerate ischemia for more than one and one-half hours. If circulation is restored prior to that time, recovery from the ischemia seems complete, although histologic changes such as endothelial proliferation in the arterial wall can be identified. Case histories of recovered vision after occlusion of central retinal arteries in humans are common, although the exact etiology and completeness of the occlusion are poorly if at all documented.

The patient with occlusion of a central retinal artery usually notes that vision is lost suddenly. He cannot distinguish light from dark. The symptom changes from blurring to complete loss of light perception in about 15 seconds, although in some patients there may be retention of light perception in the extreme temporal field. Others may report loss of the entire peripheral field and preservation of a small central field. In such patients a cilioretinal artery provides a separate flow of blood to the macular area; hence, the central field is maintained. Unfortunately, the cilioretinal artery is present in only a small percentage of persons. On the other hand, occasionally the cilioretinal artery only is occluded. These patients report the loss of central vision with preservation of the surrounding peripheral field. The rarity of the cilioretinal artery precludes the latter becoming a common occurrence.

Examination of an eye after recent occlusion of the central retinal artery reveals a fundus which is whiter than usual, with a cherry-red spot in the macula. This change is due to the retinal edema, which occurs soon after the occlusion. The fovea is the thinnest portion of the retina; hence it is less swollen, and shows the red choroid beneath it, giving the cherry-red spot. A more striking and dramatic feature is the visible stasis of blood in the retinal arterioles. The blood becomes separated into red clumps interspersed by areas of clear fluid. The degree of occlusion can be determined to some extent from this clumping: if the occlusion is complete, the blood clumps will not move. If, however, the occlusion is not complete, the blood will be seen to be moving slowly in the retinal arterioles. Even if the clumped blood is still moving to some extent, treatment should be employed, because the retina will suffer irreparable damage if the condition is allowed to persist. Occasionally, the blood will appear to be moving in the direction opposite to normal, and intermittently it will change direction of movement.

The diagnosis is relatively simple in the case of occlusion of a central retinal artery. The eye will appear as in Figure 5-1. As soon as the diagnosis is firmly made, is is well to try to raise the patient's blood pressure. Vasodilators may bring about a sudden lowering of the blood pressure, and thus have an untoward effect. The easiest means of temporarily raising the blood pressure is to have the patient exercise (perhaps run in place for a few seconds). The fundus then can be checked intermittently to see if the treatment has had any effect on the occlusion.

The principle behind this treatment is to raise the differential pressure of the artery proximal to the occlusion as compared with the pressure in the artery distal to the occlusion. Raising the systemic blood pressure is an obvious means of accomplishing this. Another means is to lower the intraocular pressure. Intermittent massage of the eye is the quickest and easiest means of lowering intraocular pressure. Massage of the eye has the added advantage of causing sharp changes in the differential pressure, so that the embolus may be dislodged or broken up and can move to the periphery of the retina. Diamox®, (acetazolamide) also may be administered intravenously in a dose of 500 mg. This drug will lower the intraocular pressure several more millimeters of mercury.

Increasing the concentration of carbon dioxide in the blood causes a moderate dilation of the central retinal artery and simultaneously raises the blood pressure. A 10 per cent CO_2 in 90 per cent O_2 mixture is used. If the CO_2 is to be effective, it must

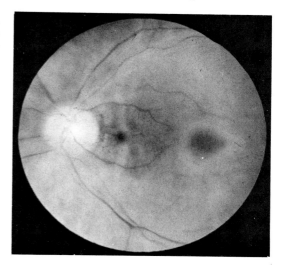

Fig. 5-1. The central retinal artery is occluded. Note the retinal edema. A small area has been spared temporal to the disc because a cilioretinal artery supplies the area. Note the dark (actually cherry-red) appearance of the macula.

be inhaled in about this concentration. If the mask fits so loosely that room air leaks in, or if the flow of gas is slower than the rate of inspiration, there will be no appreciable effect. One can easily test the effect of the arrangement by breathing the mixture oneself and noting if (as expected) a slight giddiness accompanied by moderate headache is produced within a few moments. An occasional patient will benefit from this technique and will report some return of vision as he uses the gas mixture. One can judge results by looking into the eye and observing the blood flow.

The direct pupillary reflex is extremely poor with occlusion of the central retinal artery and the resultant blind retina. Observation of the consensual reflex is valuable. It is elicited by shining a light into the fellow eye and observing that the reflex of the affected eye thus indirectly induced is normal. The poor direct pupillary reflex is of modest advantage to the doctor, because it allows a good view of the fundus through a relatively large pupil.

From time to time during treatment the intraocular pressure should be checked. If the preceding measures have failed to reduce the intraocular pressure substantively, one should lower the intraocular pressure by removing a small amount of fluid from the eye. It is to be emphasized that this should be done only by an ophthalmologist, because the potential complications of this maneuver can be severe and can result in as serious damage to the eye as the occlusion of the central retinal artery. Until recently, the aqueous was removed with a small cataract knife. A tiny incision was made in the cornea to allow a drop of aqueous to escape. With the availability in most emergency rooms of the very small caliber size 27 disposable needles, many ophthalmologists now prefer to use such a needle on a tuberculin syringe. The disposable needles are so sharp that they penetrate the cornea easily.

A question frequently asked is, "Should anticoagulants be given at once and perhaps continued indefinitely?" There is no evidence that anticoagulants dissolve a thrombus or embolus, and if the occlusion is alleviated by the means just described, there seems to be relatively little danger of the same artery occluding again.

While the preceding treatment is continued in an effort to establish blood flow to the retina, blood should be drawn from the patient and an erythrocyte sedimentation rate measured. If the rate is elevated, temporal and retinal arteritis is immediately suspected until proved otherwise. When the sedimentation rate report is available approximately two hours will have elapsed, and the success or failure of the emergency treatment of the occluded retinal vessel is usually already apparent. An elevated sedimentation rate is an indication for biopsy of the temporal artery. When arteritis is suspected, corticosteroid therapy in large doses may be given immediately (before biopsy and microscopic confirmation), and continued until one is assured that the patient does not have temporal plus retinal arteritis.

An occasional patient may have all of the symptoms of central retinal artery occlusion, yet on examination the blood flow may appear to be perfectly normal. There is nevertheless a sluggish pupillary reflex on direct stimulation and profound loss of vision. Upon comparison of the two discs, it is seen that the disc of the affected eye is ever so slightly boggy and is slightly paler than the other. The only vision in the eye may be some light perception in the lower temporal field. The other eye is completely normal. This situation usually occurs in patients over 55 years old. The presumed diagnosis is occlusion of the nutrient artery of the optic nerve. The blood supply of the retina is intact, but the supply to the optic nerve has been interrupted just behind the eye. Although the etiology may be atherosclerosis, the most likely diagnosis is the syndrome of "temporal arteritis." The sedimentation rate should be measured immediately and the patient should breathe the 10 per cent CO_2 in 90 per cent O_2 mixture. If the sedimentation rate is elevated, the diagnosis of temporal arteritis syndrome should be entertained. A biopsy of the temporal artery should be done, but it will be several days before the pathology report is returned. This situation is an emergency, and prompt use of systemic steroids may save the sight of the involved eye and certainly may save the sight of the other eye. If steroids are not started quickly, the other eye may well become involved with the same condition, and the patient may end up with total blindness in both eyes. This unfortunate train of circumstances may prevail even with steroid treatment.

The other possible serious effects of the temporal arteritis syndrome should be kept in mind when dealing with this disease. There may be a widespread polyarteritis. There may be arteritis of the coronary arteries with occlusion or similar effects on arteries elsewhere. General malaise and polymyalgia often occur, with daily spikes of fever to about 102° F.

PAINLESS LOSS OF VISION WITH A FLASHING
SENSATION: EMERGENCY

Retinal Detachment

Detachment of the retina causes mechanical stimulation of the rods and cones as it tears away from the pigment epithelium and floats free. This produces a noticeable visual sensation of flash and the patient usually will remember it as the signal immediately or shortly preceding loss of vision. He also may note that there appeared to be a "veil" over his eye either just before the flash or immediately after it. If the detachment involves only the peripheral portion of the retina, the patient will have only a partial visual field defect corresponding to the detachment. He will often comment on this as a "veil" over a portion of his vision. If the macula is detached, the vision is poor in that eye and the emergency nature of the condition is reduced; the prognosis is much poorer once the macula is off, no matter how successful or immediate the surgery may be in mechanically reattaching the retina. If the macula is still attached, the prognosis for visual improvement following surgery is much better. When the symptoms of a flash and veil are reported, the patient should be referred to an ophthalmologist.

Two types of retinal detachment are by far the most common. Among the two, the **rhegmatogenous** is more common. Rhegmatogenous indicates that the cause of the detachment is a hole in the retina. For reasons that are not known, if a retina develops a hole in it, fluid starts to collect beneath the retina from the site of the hole. If this is allowed to continue, the entire retina becomes detached. The treatment consists of mechanically closing the hole with a tamponade and producing scar tissue, which will permanently seal off the hole. Recent years have been fruitful in the development of new techniques, which cleverly accomplish that end.

The second most common form of retinal detachment occurs in the presence of an intact retina. In this condition the fluid collects under the retina as a result of **transudation;** e.g., when the blood is low in protein, as in advanced uremia. If the uremic condition is corrected, the retina reattaches itself. **Tumors** of the choroid, both primary and metastatic, also produce an exudation of fluid, which detaches the retina.

In retinal detachment, the fundus color is changed from bright red to dull pink. The blood vessels are not on one plane, but at various angles and at irregular distances; hence, they appear more tortuous than normal. If the detached retina has fluid under it, the raised blood vessels lie at various levels, and it is therefore hard to focus accurately; a high plus lens in the opthalmoscope is required. Careful examination with a special ophthalmoscope usually will reveal a hole in the retina. It is often difficult to determine whether the cause of the detachment is a hole or a tumor. Care is taken to be sure that no operation is undertaken on the retina that is detached by a tumor. Inflammatory conditions also may cause detachment of the retina, and such disorders must be considered in differential diagnosis.

When a retina becomes detached as a result of advanced **renal failure,** the retina repeatedly shifts position. The fluid that accumulates and causes the detachment is heavier than the surrounding fluid, and hence moves to the most inferior position possible in the eye. If the patient is sitting or standing, with the lower portion of the retina detached but the macula attached, the patient's vision is good. However, if the patient lies down for several hours, the fluid shifts to the most dependent part of the eye and the macula may detach. Such a patient will complain of poor vision for several hours each morning and find that his vision improves remarkably as the day progresses. If the renal problem can be corrected, the retinal detachment clears and the vision usually returns to normal. An occasional patient with no renal disorder or other known disease may have a retinal detachment that resembles the condition just described for the patient with renal failure. Such a **serous** detachment may continue for several years, may resolve, or may go on to blindness. Little is known as to the etiology of these serous detachments.

PAINLESS SUDDEN LOSS OF VISION

Eye Hemorrhages

Vitreous hemorrhages are a frequent cause for sudden painless loss of vision. Typically, the patient's vision was normal until he noted that a series of floaters began to drift in front of his eye, and that there appeared to be a red glow to everything. After a variable length of time, he notes that the vision gradually fades until all that remains is a vague awareness of light from darkness in that eye. Usually the history is noncontributory (see exception later under diabetes). The eye appears white, quiet, and painless. The pupillary reflex is good, although there may be a slight sluggishness on the affected side. Examination reveals only a black reflex. After dilation of the pupil, the reflex still may be black, or one may glimpse a red reflex above. Somewhere within the eye a retinal blood vessel has ruptured and allowed blood to flow into the vitreous. There is no immediate treatment for this except bed rest to allow the blood to settle out so that the retina can be examined carefully. The most common cause of retinal vessel bleeding is a tear in the retina which includes a blood vessel. If the tear in retina is across a good-sized blood vessel and can be seen to be under some tension from strands in the vitreous, surgical treatment is indicated. Research has led most authorities to implicate disturbances in the vitreous which cause traction bands, which in turn pull and tear the retina. The causes

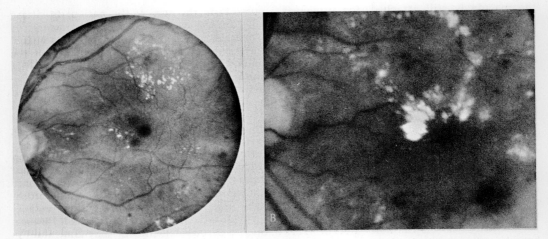

FIG. 5-2. Diabetic retinopathy. Note the scattered white "exudates" and the small dark spots which are small hemorrhages and microaneurysms.

and mechanisms involved in vitreous traction bands are not known. Occasionally blunt trauma will cause retinal tears. If a tear is not found and treated successfully, it can lead to retinal detachment, which may in turn lead to loss of vision. A black reflex means an intraocular hemorrhage until proved otherwise. During the time when the patient is at bed rest, studies should be done to detect possible **pathologic bleeding** from conditions such as hemophilia, sickle-cell anemia, or thalassemia. Hemophilia may produce hemorrhage from the retinal vessels. Sickle-cell anemia patients have tufts of new vessels growing out from the retina within the eye. These tufts are predisposed to hemorrhage and can be treated with light coagulation if found before severe hemorrhages occur. Thalassemia or cryoglobulinemia cause thrombosis of many veins, with resultant hemorrhages that can break out of the retina and produce vitreous hemorrhages.

Just as atherosclerosis may involve the arteries, so may it involve the central retinal vein and its branches. As the atherosclerosis proceeds, intimal proliferation continues until the stage is set for thrombosis at the exit of the vein from the eye. It is thought by some that the continued normal pulsation, with complete collapse and dilation of the vein, predisposes to thrombosis at this site. The immediate sequel to occlusion of either the central retinal vein or a branch is that the veins feeding the blocked vein become dilated and that any available collateral channels enlarge. If the central retinal vein is blocked there are no effective collateral channels, and the veins dilate to huge proportions with ensuing hemorrhages, which at first are in the nerve fiber layer, but may become deeper and sometimes break through into the vitreous.

RETINAL HEMORRHAGES

Occlusion of Central Retinal Vein

Localized hemorrhages within the retina may be extensive when there is occlusion of the central retinal vein. The patient complains that vision in the eye has gradually blurred over the past few days. The amount of visual loss is variable and is dependent upon whether or not the retinal hemorrhages are in the macula. The eye is normal in all external respects, including the pupillary reflex. The retinal picture however, is striking, with marked tortuosity of the retinal veins. There are hemorrhages about the entire retina in a random fashion if the occlusion involves the central retinal vein, or only over the distribution of the occluded retinal vein if a branch is involved. Many of the hemorrhages are flame-shaped, indicating that they are in the nerve fiber layer of the retina, but some of the hemorrhages are also found in the deeper layers of the retina. The hemorrhages are everywhere, and are especially prominent about the disc. The tortuosity of the veins exceeds that seen in papilledema.

If the patient is under 40 years of age, there is a reasonably good chance that he

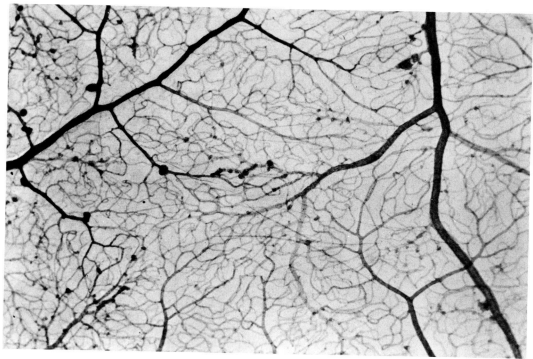

FIG. 5-3. Trypsin-digested retinal preparation from eye of a diabetic patient. Note the many aneurysms. A shunt has developed across the center of the figure. (From Cogan, D. G., and Kuwabara, T. K.: Capillary shunts in the pathogenesis of diabetic retinopathy, Diabetes 12:296, 1963)

will recover useful vision after occlusion of a central retinal vein. If he is well into his 60's, there is little likelihood that useful vision will be recovered. In fact, there is a fair chance in the older patient that within three months neovascularization of the iris may result in an intractable glaucoma, which may cause such pain that the eye must be removed. Little is known about the etiology of the neovascularization of the iris which sometimes follows occlusion of the central retinal vein. In such cases a delicate membrane of endothelial cells grows over the iris, and fine capillaries come with this membrane. The membrane covers the angle of the eye (that portion of the eye between the iris and cornea), where the aqueous normally drains. As the outflow channels are blocked, an irreversible glaucoma develops. Only a few eyes have survived such a chain of events, even with the most radical surgical treatment.

Even with early diagnosis of an occluded central retinal vein, there is little known effective therapy. Anticoagulants are ineffec-

tive. The main consideration is to detect possible causes that seem to favor the development of this condition. Raised intraocular pressure (glaucoma) or diabetes seem to predispose to the development of occlusion of the central retinal vein, but their mechanism is not known. If early open-angle glaucoma is detected and treated, there is less chance that the central retinal vein will become occluded in the other eye. If diabetes is present, it should be treated, but it is not known whether treatment of the diabetes helps to prevent occlusion of the other central retinal vein. Occasionally, especially in diabetes, the other eye becomes involved with the same dire outcome.

PAINLESS SUDDEN VISUAL LOSS WITH DIABETES MELLITUS

Young persons known to have diabetes for over eight years are prone to serious eye involvement, apparently as a specific result of this metabolic disorder. When the visual loss is first reported, it is often the result of progression of diabetic retinopathy, the de-

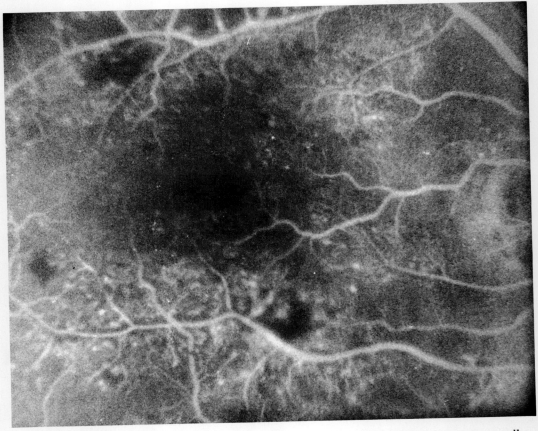

FIG. 5-4. Fluoroangiogram of the retinal vessels of a diabetic patient. Note the many small leaks of dye from the vessels and the many fine dots which represent aneurysms.

velopment of which has been observed as the diabetes has been treated, perhaps over a period of years. The first sign of diabetic retinopathy is slight engorgement of the retinal veins. At about this time, fine punctate hemorrhages can be observed. The fine dot hemorrhages are from small aneurysms, which are filled with blood. Serial photographs show that these small aneurysms are variable (Fig. 5-2). Such variation is due to many of them scarring, and becoming occluded and disappearing as the disease progresses. Concomitant with onset of aneurysms is enlargement of collateral fine venous channels. This is due to occlusion of other fine veins on the venous side of the capillary network. Many of these dilated collateral capillary channels can be seen ophthalmoscopically and are often termed neovascularization, although in fact they are just enlarged capillaries. Kuwabara and

Cogan have developed a technique that allows the retinal vessels to be studied on the flat after digesting away all other retinal tissue. This technique reveals that there are two types of retinal vessel cells, mural cells and endothelial cells (Fig. 5-3). Much of the damage in diabetic retinopathy seems to be due to damage to the mural cells. The reason for this susceptibility of the mural cells is not known. While there are changes going on in the vessel's wall, there are exudates being laid down in the deep layers of the retina. After a variable period of time, frank new vessel formation may begin and new vessels may break through the internal limiting membrane of the retina and appear as moving fronds, willowing in the vitreous. At any point the condition may suddenly become worse, often as a result of hemorrhage from the diseased vessels into the retina or into the vitreous.

Usually the sudden decrease in vision is due to a small hemorrhage in the macular area. This may be a small round hemorrhage similar to the many other small round hemorrhages which have been present elsewhere in varying degrees in the diabetic's eye (Fig. 5-4). Whether or not the hemorrhage hits the macular area seems to be a matter of chance. Macular involvement with consequent serious loss of vision may occur relatively early or late in the disease. If it is early, before there is a lot of scarring in the retina, the chances for absorption of the hemorrhage and the return of useful vision are much greater than if there is extensive scarring, and the region adjacent to the macula already is involved heavily with exudates, fibrous tissue, and other hemorrhages. The larger the hemorrhage, the poorer the prognosis for useful return of vision.

In a patient who has had the first decrease in vision due to diabetic retinopathy, the eye is white, quiet, and nonpainful. Upon examination of the fundus, the changes described previously probably will be seen with varying severity, the degree differing among patients. It is not infrequent that the retina at the time of the first complaint of visual loss already has been seriously and extensively damaged, with new vessels growing out of the disc into the vitreous, neovascularization of the retina and arteriovenous shunts in many places, exudates scattered about, many microeneurysms, and multiple hemorrhages. An eye in this condition has an extremely poor prognosis. Often a hemorrhage into the vitreous will further decrease the chances for any useful vision. In such an eye there may develop neovascularization of the iris with irreversible glaucoma. Occasionally there is bleeding from these new blood vessels, so that fresh blood can be seen in the anterior chamber. Once fresh blood is present in the anterior chamber the outlook is poor for salvaging vision in that eye.

In recent years, the retinopathy of some diabetic patients has responded favorably to ablation of the pituitary gland, although the pathophysiology involved is not known. Usually the teams who perform such an ablative procedure are strict in their criteria as to which patients may have the surgery. In general, one eye must be potentially salvable, with a macula that should be capable of good vision if the process of the diabetic retinopathy is reversed. Recently there have been some favorable reports on the use of lasers in the treatment of early stages of the vascular lesions of diabetic retinopathy.

Approximately eight years after the gradual onset and steady progression of severe diabetic changes, the patient will be blind in both eyes if there has been no treatment, and often in spite of the best treatment known. The same type of arteriolar disease causes renal failure to which the patient usually succumbs within approximately eight years after blindness occurs.

ACUTE VISUAL LOSS WITH A RED, PAINFUL EYE

Angle-Closure Glaucoma

The condition other than occlusion of the central retinal artery which requires immediate treatment (if the vision of that eye is to be saved) is angle-closure glaucoma. There is usually severe pain about and in the eye. The patient's systemic symptoms may be so severe that he will seek medical attention for nausea and vomiting rather than for the causal factor, the acute glaucoma with its eye pain and loss of vision. Finally, someone notes that the patient has a red eye, and an extremely high pressure is found in the eye. If only a complete history and review of systems had been taken, the patient would have related that his first symptom had been pain in the eye followed by blurring of vision. On occasion the patient with acute glaucoma will deny pain in or about the eye, yet will have severe systemic reactions with nausea and vomiting because of the high intraocular pressure.

The eye in acute glaucoma is red, and the pupil is fixed in mid-position, i.e., about 5 mm. in diameter. The anterior chamber is shallow. The depth of this chamber can be estimated by comparing the position of the iris (with respect to the cornea) of an assistant or nurse to that of the patient. In angle-closure glaucoma, the iris almost touches the cornea. The angle of the eye (the point where the iris joins the cornea, the site of fluid drainage from the eye) is actually closed. Since the eye continues to produce fluid in the usual amounts, the pressure goes to extremely high levels. The normal pressure within the eye is about 20 mm. Hg. When the angle closes, the pressure may go up to 60 mm. Hg or more. When the pressure reaches these levels, the cornea usually becomes steamy and loses its normal luster. The resulting loss of corneal transparency due to corneal edema causes some reduction in vision, but the pressure on the optic nerve head (i.e., the optic disc) seems to be the principal reason for this reduction. If the eye has been normal up until the time of the acute attack, it often can withstand high pressure for a few days. Some eyes, however, cannot endure such high pressure, and irreversible blindness ensues. As a rule, the patient seeks medical attention for the acute pain in his eye, and the pressure can be lowered so that vision returns to normal and the patient does not experience any permanent loss of vision. After lowering the pressure medically, the ophthalmologist performs a peripheral iridectomy, which usually cures this form of glaucoma.

The pathophysiology of angle-closure glaucoma is strictly mechanical. The lens grows as the patient ages. Since the iris rests loosely against the lens, it can be understood that if the iris is pressed firmly against the lens surface the normal flow of aqueous from behind the iris to the front of the iris via the pupil will be blocked. This differential in pressure will balloon the peripheral portion of the iris forward. As the peripheral portion of the iris comes forward it is thrust against the outflow channels of the eye in the angle, and the intraocular pressure starts to rise. As the iris is ballooned forward, the pupillary border of the iris is thrust ever closer against the lens surface, and a vicious cycle of events is set into motion which makes the pressure continue to rise until relief by either medical or surgical intervention. Usually miotics are successful in relieving the pupillary block and opening the angle. Surgery can create a small opening in the periphery of the iris, so that the same cycle of events will not recur. If adhesions have not formed during the acute attack, such an eye is usually cured for life with such surgery.

When the patient seeks assistance, either because of loss of vision, pain in the eye, or the systemic effects of pressure, such as nausea and vomiting, the eye appears as previously described: red, with a fixed pupil and shallow anterior chamber. If the cornea is clear enough to permit inspection of the fundus, one may find that the central retinal artery is pulsating. Pulsation of the central retinal vein is a normal occurrence; however, any time the central retinal artery pulsates, something is wrong. Either the eye pressure is extremely high, or the diastolic pressure in the artery is very low. Condi-

tions that can cause the diastolic pressure to be extremely low are marked aortic insufficiency or stenosis of the common or internal carotid on that side.

What other conditions could mimic the symptoms described: a red, painful eye, decreased vision, a steamy cornea, and an anterior chamber that is marginally shallow? Iritis certainly may; however, in that condition the pupil is small and the patient complains of light bothering the eye. Would open-angle glaucoma (simple glaucoma) mimic the condition? No. Open-angle glaucoma, even in the advanced state, is a painless loss of vision with a white and quiet eye.

ACUTE VISUAL LOSS AND PAINFUL EYE MOVEMENTS

Retrobulbar Neuritis

Retrobulbar neuritis causes the patient to complain of decreased central vision, that is, poor visual acuity, in the affected eye. Concomitant with the poor vision is the symptom of pain upon movement of the eye in any direction. Retrobulbar neuritis can strike at any age, but is more common in persons 20 to 35 years old. It is one of the common first symptoms of multiple sclerosis and one of the common occurrences during later stages of the disease. Often a retrobulbar neuritis attack is isolated, even if the patient may ultimately prove to have multiple sclerosis.

The location of the inflammatory site in the optic nerve determines whether the condition will be classed as **papillitis, neuroretinitis,** or **retrobulbar neuritis.** The etiologies of these three variants of optic neuritis are equally obscure. Optic neuritis may occur in any of the three various forms at different times in the same patient. The differential diagnosis between the three types is made by the ophthalmoscopic appearance. If there is some swelling of the retina adjacent to the disc and there are cells in the vitreous which produce a haze, the condition is usually called *neuroretinitis.* When the swelling and inflammation is confined to the disc, with some haze in front of the disc, the term *papillitis* is used. When the disc is normal in appearance or slightly pinkish and typical field defects are present, the condition is classed as *retrobulbar neuritis.* By far the most common cause of optic neuritis is multiple sclerosis. The demyelination in the optic nerve is similar to that occurring in this disease elsewhere in the central nervous system. As the acute inflammatory state passes, the function of the optic nerve usually returns to normal, although occasionally severe visual defects and even blindness may result. The macular fibers are peculiarly susceptible to any inflammation of the optic nerve, and hence the central vision drops precipitously with a resultant central scotoma, which can be documented with visual field studies. The surrounding visual field is normal. This is in direct contrast with papilledema, in which the central visual acuity is usually normal, the blind spot is slightly enlarged, and the peripheral field is slightly and irregularly constricted. Exceptions to involvement of the macular fibers with optic neuritis do occur, but are of sufficient rarity that a careful search for other causes should be made whenever optic neuritis seems to be present but central vision is good.

The typical patient with **retrobulbar neuritis** states that he suddenly noticed that he could not see from one eye. He may have awakened and promptly become aware of poor vision, or it may have come on, usually rather suddenly, during the course of the day. The visual acuity may be only moderately reduced or may be down to only light perception. More commonly, the vision is decreased to about 20/800. If a visual field is done, the field of the asymptomatic eye is found to be normal. The affected eye usually is found to have a central scotoma, the density of which is related to the visual loss. The pupil of that eye will be found to respond sluggishly to direct light stimulation, but quite briskly to consensual stimulation with light. Inspection of the fundus is not helpful, except to rule out other causes of decreased central vision. The optic nerve head may appear slightly flushed but is generally normal if the patient has not had prior attacks of retrobulbar neuritis. If there have been prior attacks, the nerve head appears to be slightly greyish on the nasal side of the disc. It is essential to be sure that the macula of the eye is normal, because some patients have central serous retinitis, which mimics the symptoms of retrobulbar neuritis with the exception of a lack of pain upon movement of the eye. Such patients have a slight serous accumulation in the macular area. They usually complain more of a distortion of vision than of the distinct visual loss, which is so typical of the patient with retrobulbar neuritis.

The pain on movement of the eye is thought to be the result either of the generalized inflammation of the posterior portion of the orbit or of inflammation of the optic nerve. The latter explanation depends on the optic nerve having some pain fibers that respond to the movement of the nerve as the eye is moved. Many persons have experienced a pain that is similar to the pain of retrobulbar neuritis after performance of some unusual task, which requires much more than usual eye movement for long periods of time. Driving a car for about eight hours is such an example for most of us. For many hours thereafter, up to 24 or more, any movement of the eyes is slightly painful.

There is no known effective treatment for retrobulbar neuritis at the present time, although some believe that steroid therapy helps. Controlled studies are in progress on the efficacy of steroids and ACTH treatment. Since most patients recover spontaneously, the study must be statistically secure to be convincing. The amount of initial visual loss does not seem to be related to the return of vision, from either a chronological or percentage point of view. In most correctly diagnosed patients, vision will return spontaneously. We must stress "if the diagnosis is correct," because retrobulbar neuritis is one of the most misdiagnosed conditions that the ophthalmologist sees. Conditions from detached retinas to hemianopsias caused by meningiomas are seen with disturbing frequency after initial diagnosis of retrobulbar neuritis has been made, and a month or so has passed, waiting for it to "clear up." Whenever retrobulbar neuritis is suspected, examination of the eye by an ophthalmologist is indicated.

PAINLESS CHRONIC VISUAL LOSS

CATARACTS

Cataracts are by far the most common cause of slowly progressive loss of vision. Typically the patient is well past middle age and has noted that his vision has become less acute. Oncoming headlights have become so bothersome that he has given up night driving. He has had some trouble with reading distant signs and near print unless the light is just right. All of these complaints have persisted, despite changing glasses several times. He may well have had his glasses prescribed by an optometrist rather than by an ophthalmologist, and hence has not had a medical evaluation of his eyes.

There is difficulty in discerning the details of the fundus. In fact, there is a great deal of difficulty in getting the position of the ophthalmoscope adjusted so that annoying reflexes do not preclude a view of the fundus. The physician's troubles in looking into the eye are exactly those of the patient in seeing out of it. Accordingly, viewing the eye with an ophthalmoscope should give some idea as to how well the patient is able to see. After the pupil is dilated, one may be able to see into the eye quite well, and if one rechecks visual acuity at that time, it will have increased as a result of the dilation.

Often it is helpful to measure the visual acuity in a lighted as well as in a darkened room. Many patients with slight or early cataracts will be able to see surprisingly well (with reflexly dilated pupil) in a darkened room, but in a lighted room (with constricted pupil), they may be able to read only 20/200.

When cataract first appears in the patient past age 55 medical studies seldom reveal a cause for the cataract. In the great majority of such patients the cataract is attributed to aging and is not associated with any systemic disease. In the patient under age 55, a thorough medical study is more often productive. Any evidence of diabetes, hyperparathyroidism, or drug toxicity should be sought. Past injury or inflammation of the eyes also may predispose to cataracts.

The pathophysiology of cataracts is not established insofar as etiology is concerned. About all that can be said is that most severe metabolic defects will have some effect on the metabolism of the crystalline lens. Even subtle changes in the biochemistry of the lens result in profound cataractous changes, because the equilibrium within the lens is a tenuous one. The slightest change will cause one or two lens cells or fibers to change their metabolism sufficiently that small amounts of extracellular fluid will result in tiny bubbles in the crystalline lens. As the changes within the lens fibers continue, the fibers themselves start to accumulate fluid and become opaque. Since the lens is constantly growing much the same as a tree trunk, events that affect the lens even subtly will leave their chronologic mark in it. Hypocalcemic tetanic episodes result in fine lens opacities, which can be related to the time the patient had the attacks, much as a wound in the trunk of a tree can be cata-logued in time by an imperfection in the symmetry of the rings of the trunk. Uncontrolled diabetes can produce swelling of the lens which is temporary, but most changes in the lens are permanent opacities, which often progress until the lens is opaque and must be removed if vision is to be restored.

TUNNEL VISION

Constriction of the visual fields produces few symptoms until the condition is far advanced. Since most of the conditions which produce tunnel vision do not produce sudden changes, the patient can gradually accommodate to the limitations in range and turn his eyes or head to compensate for the restriction of field. Not infrequently, the patient will have an increased incidence of auto accidents, or he will report frequently bumping into things that he should have easily seen. A patient whose visual fields are severely constricted typically enters a room very unsure of himself and searches about with head and eyes for the chair just offered him. Often, he stumbles over low tables or stools about the office.

The confirmation of tunnel vision is relatively easy through use of simple confrontation fields. When the diagnosis is thus proved, tangent screen fields should be done to quantitate the changes. Tunnel vision is not uncommon in hysteric persons and care should be taken not to talk or "suggest" an hysteric subject into a constricted field.

Glaucoma, retinitis pigmentosa, and **quinine toxicity** are the principal causes of tunnel vision. A careful drug history should be taken in such patients. Quinine, a now infrequently used drug, is one of the few which causes a constriction of the visual field.

Glaucoma

Glaucoma is relatively easy to diagnose as a causal factor of the restricted field since the optic disc of such a patient will have severe cupping which is responsible for the reduced visual field. The intraocular pressure is high, but is not necessarily found to be elevated at the particular moment of every examination. If glaucoma is suspected, the patient should be referred to an ophthalmologist for confirmation and treatment.

The degree of loss of the peripheral vision in glaucoma patients parallels the severity of the cupping of the optic disc. As the nerve fibers are stretched over the edge of the disc, they become irreversibly damaged. Since the fibers to the periphery of the retina penetrate the optic disc on the edges, they are the first to be damaged. The fibers that supply the macula usually are resistant to this damage, because they penetrate the disc in a more central fashion, and the cupping seems to advance less rapidly on the temporal side of the disc in which these fibers principally lie. The field loss is therefore greater on the nasal side. In a young child, the whole eye will enlarge if the intraocular pressure is allowed to remain high. In the adult, the eye is extremely tough and the weakest point is the optic disc; hence it is the point that yields to pressure, becomes cupped, and damages the optic fibers.

Drug Toxicity

The mechanisms by which quinine or other drugs cause constriction of the visual field are not known.

CHRONIC PAINLESS TUNNEL VISION AND NIGHT BLINDNESS

Retinitis Pigmentosa

Patients with retinitis pigmentosa usually complain of night blindness, which precedes the restriction of field. Diagnosis is usually easy because the retinal picture is typical in most patients. One of the most diagnostically reliable fundus changes is constriction of the retinal arterioles. In fact, if the arteries are not constricted, much doubt is cast upon the correctness of the diagnosis. The optic disc may have a slight yellowish appearance, but appears normal in most cases. In the periphery of the fundus, the typical picture of retinitis pigmentosa is present: the pigment clumps are scattered about in a largely random fashion, but with a moderate predilection for areas around the arterioles. The amount of pigment clumping seems to have little relation to the field changes in a patient.

The rods are selectively destroyed first, which accounts for the night blindness and the constriction of the visual field. The progression of the disease continues, until all of the vision is finally gone. The rate of progression varies from patient to patient. The general rule is that, the younger the age at which the disease first becomes symptomatic, the more rapid the progression. If the disease is manifested by age 12, the patient probably will lose useful vision by age 30. Despite this rule, there are enough exceptions to make exact prediction in individual cases highly uncertain.

There are variations from the classical retinitis pigmentosa pattern which are so subtle that special testing is necessary to determine the disease process with certainty. When the diagnosis is in doubt, the electroretinogram is used for confirmation. The electroretinogram utilizes the electrical response of the retina to the impingement of light. Absence of "a" and "b" waves is characteristic of retinitis pigmentosa. Subtleties of the electroretinogram may predict the mode of genetic transmission.[2] A picture indistinguishable from the classical case of retinitis pigmentosa often is seen in the disease a-beta-lipoproteinemia (Bassen-Kornzweig syndrome). There is no treatment for retinitis pigmentosa, but careful counseling should be given to these patients even before field loss is severe, especially about automobile driving, particularly at twilight.

TRANSIENT VISUAL LOSS

HEMIANOPSIAS WITH FLASHES

Migraine is a common problem, with headaches dating back to a fairly early age of the patient. However, the aura of migraine frequently does not start until the patient is in his 20's or later. The visual aura of migraine is so typical that it is almost diagnostic of the disease. The typical patient suddenly notes that he can see only one-half of objects. About that time he notes a flashing in his vision, just at the periphery of the scotoma. Often the scotoma will advance to the mid-line (in both eyes) and gradually recede, with the flashing continuing throughout the existence of the scotoma. The analogy of a prairie fire is helpful, in which the borders of the area are "burning," leaving behind the black remnants. The visual aura of scintillating scotomas usually lasts almost exactly 20 minutes. Within a few minutes after the aura, headache begins which may or may not be incapacitating. An occasional patient is almost incapacitated by scotomas, but bothered only slightly by headache. In fact, sometimes very careful history-taking is necessary to determine if there is any headache present in relation to the scotomas. In the typical migraine patient the scintillating scotomas are an almost complete hemianopsia. The loss of vision may be on the right in one attack, on the left in another. The hemianopsias are central in origin and hence are congruent; that is, if the visual fields of the two eyes are compared during the attack, they will be exact in their replication. They are *homonymous hemianopsias*, involving the same side (either left or right) of both eyes. The exact symmetry of the scotomata and the EEG changes during the aura of a migraine attack suggest strongly that the visual part, at least, of the pathology of the attack involves abnormal vasospasm of the occipital cortical arteries. For a further discussion of the pathophysiology of migraine, see the section on Migraine in the chapter on Headache.

Most patients will have an uncomfortable sensation during the aura, and some will develop nausea and vomiting. Typically there is nothing unusual noted when the fundus is examined during an attack. An occasional observer has noted some increased tortuosity of the retinal veins during the aura of an attack.

TRANSIENT MONOCULAR VISUAL LOSS

Carotid insufficiency and **impending occlusion of the central retinal artery** are the two most common causes of transient monocular blurring of vision. Typically, the attack lasts less than a minute. The diagnosis can usually be confirmed by measuring the diastolic blood pressure of the central retinal artery with an ophthalmodynamometer. The patient usually complains that the vision of the affected eye becomes greyer and greyer, until finally no vision is left. When the vision returns, the greyness appears first, and finally objects appear sharp again. A patient seldom takes the trouble to cover one eye and then the other to ascertain which eye is really bothering him. If the patient has not actually tested one eye at a time, the physician may be misled by accepting the patient's assumption that his condition is monocular, when in fact it is not. All too often patients will interpret an hemianopsia as a blurring of the eye on the side of the hemianopsia, rather than a defect in one side of *both* visual fields. As a result, the transient blurring reported in one eye is not that at all, but rather a transient hemianopsia, which might be caused by insufficiency of the basilar artery. In the latter case, the ophthalmodynamometer readings are normal.

Repeated transient monocular loss of vision should be studied by obtaining arteriograms of the carotids. Surgical removal of stenosis in a carotid artery frequently has been successful.[27,28]

HEMIANOPSIAS

Hemianopsias occurring in both eyes may be congruous, i.e., exact duplicates or not. The field defects may be mirror images of each other, or even monocular. The representation of the distribution of the visual pathways is so constant that the pattern of the hemianopsia will usually lead to the correct localization of the lesion. Often the doctor is misled into discounting the likelihood of an hemianopsia simply because the field defect is not dense. Many times the only way in which an hemianopsia can be established is to have the patient describe the relative brightness of objects on either side of his visual fields. Basically the hemianopsias are produced either by pressure on the optic nerve, tracts, radiations, or visual cortex, or by ischemia of any part of the visual pathway.

The differential diagnosis of hemianopsias of all kinds will not be given here, but it should be noted that most patients interpret hemianopsias as blurred vision rather than as field defects. When the patient has a left hemianopsia, he will have difficulty in finding the starting letter of a line of print, consistently missing the first two or three letters on the vision chart of each line. The patient with a right hemianopsia will be able to see each letter but will often have difficulty in following the line and will often skip the last letters of each line. Field defects may be severe, even if central visual acuity is still good. One patient who had most of her visual cortex ablated had a visual field of only two degrees to the left of fixation in each eye. Yet, with these two degrees, she was able to read slowly 20/15 letters.

DISTORTED VISION WITH BLURRING

Central serous retinopathy has been mentioned as a cause of sudden blurring of central vision. However, vision is distorted more than blurred by this condition. The loss of vision typically is not permanent, occurs in males who smoke too much tobacco, and runs a course of several weeks, usually returning to normal after that time and often recurring about the same time in each of several consecutive years. The retina appears normal in all areas except the macula. A small amount of fluid collects under the macula, and the macula itself is slightly edematous. The changes are subtle and require careful examination to be seen. Only a relative field defect can be plotted with such a patient, and that done with difficulty. The etiology of this condition is not known, and little is known about the pathology. Recently, fluorescein angiography of the retinal vessels has shown tiny leaks in the vasculature in the affected area. This finding has caused some ophthalmologists to treat such cases with the laser if there are signs of advancement rather than the usual regression. Most authorities are skeptical of such treatment because the treatment is considered as possibly more dangerous than the disease in regard to long-term visual prognosis.

A much more common condition, which strikes persons in older age groups, is **senile macular degeneration.** Typically there are some cystic changes in the retina followed by bleeding under the retina from the choroid. Unfortunately, the cause of this degeneration is not known and prognosis for sight is poor. The vision drops suddenly to about 20/200 or worse, and only minimal return of vision is expected. The eye is white and quiet with normal pupillary reflexes. The fundus is normal with the exception of the macular area, which shows varying amounts of blood under and in the retina, occasionally breaking through the retina to lie in front of it. The only consolation to the patient is that he will seldom lose peripheral vision. Even with severe loss of central vision, he can get about and continue to take care of himself. The other eye is commonly affected, but often several years intervene between the time the first is involved and the second is afflicted. There are no known systemic diseases associated with this condition.

Occasionally there is **localized chorioretinitis** of the macular area. The definitive causes of chorioretinitis are few and usually not found. However, *toxoplasmosis* may cause such a central lesion and should always be considered, particularly in the young. Occasionally a roundworm or other *parasite* may find its way into the eye and set up an inflammation about the macula. When some form of chorioretinopathy is discovered through the complaint of sudden visual loss, the eye specialist's opinion is valuable. Not uncommonly the patient may have had the condition for many years and only discovers the loss of vision when he accidentally covers one eye and finds that the vision in the other eye is poor. It is thus helpful to have an expert's opinion as to the age and acuteness of the condition.

SUDDEN LOSS OF VISION: TRAUMATIC

HEAD TRAUMA

Severe head trauma with skull fractures, but without direct damage to the eyeball, occasionally is associated with loss of vision, either immediately at the time of the trauma or so shortly thereafter that it is hard to decide upon the exact course of events which did take place. In such a case one eye is normal, but the other may have various amounts of vision—usually quite poor. The direct pupillary reflex of the involved eye is weak. The fundus is normal and the optic disc appears to be normal. Skull x rays show that there is a fracture extending into the sphenoid bone and directly into the optic foramen. The immediate question is, "Should the optic foramen be unroofed so that the optic nerve can be spared the compression implied by the fracture line and the possible hemorrhage?"

This line of reasoning seems appropriate until one examines the results of unroofing the optic foramina in such patients. The statistics do not bear out the contention that this is a useful procedure. Often the general condition of the patient is sufficiently precarious that a major operation at that time seems unwise, especially since the results for vision are so poor. Most clinicians believe that the optic nerve is damaged at the time of the acute trauma and the subsequent swelling does not add materially to the poor prognosis. Within two months such a patient, with or without surgery, usually develops optic atrophy on the affected side. The only exception to these conservative, nonoperative conclusions concerns the patient who has documented good vision in the affected eye after the accident and *subsequently* loses vision. Such a case does merit surgical exploration, since there may be severe retrobulbar hemorrhage. Care must be taken to see that such hemorrhage does not damage the eye from retrobulbar pressure on the eye and nerve. If progressive proptosis develops, insertion of a large needle into the retrobulbar space can be used to aspirate the hemorrhage. Placement of such a needle must be done with care, because the optic nerve can be damaged by the needle. If the proptosis develops without signs of hemorrhage in the lids or under the conjunctiva, thought must be given to the possibility of an arteriovenous communication in the cavernous sinus area. Arteriography will be indicated in such cases.

ELECTRIC SHOCK

Severe electric shock about the head may result in sudden loss of vision from which it may take hours to recover. Typically, the patient receives a shock on his forehead of sufficient intensity to knock him down and cause a short period of unconsciousness. When he regains consciousness, he cannot see. Such a patient is often hysterical by the time the doctor sees him. The eyes are white and quiet. The pupillary reflexes are absent or extremely sluggish. The fundi appear normal. The pupillary reflexes slowly come back to normal and objects begin to appear as grey forms; finally color perception and good vision return. The exact mechanism behind this series of events is not known, but some observers believe that the massive electric shock effectively depolarizes all cells in the retina and that time is needed for the resumption of normal electrical activity, and hence for the return of vision.

DIRECT TRAUMA TO THE EYE

Physical Injury

The eye after direct trauma, especially when it is severe enough to cause loss of vision, should receive the gentlest treatment possible. Little is gained by forcing the lids open for a complete examination. The trauma attendant upon any manipulation may cause further severe damage to the eye. In such cases it is best to examine the eyes as little as possible and to seek the consultation of an ophthalmologist. In all likelihood he will inspect the eye only briefly to determine if an open wound is present. If such a wound is present, the complete examination will be done after the patient is given general anesthesia. If the eye has no open wound, the patient will probably be put at bed rest to allow any blood that is present to clear, so that the ophthalmologist can see into the eye to determine the extent of damage. If he cannot be sure in a few days, it may be necessary to explore the eye surgically to see if there are any posterior ruptures. The prognosis for such eyes is poor.

Chemical Contact

A strong caustic such as lye splashed upon the eye will cause severe damage. The extent of injury depends upon how quickly the harmful agent can be washed away. If prompt irrigation is done, eye and vision may be saved. If no irrigation is performed until the patient reaches the care of an ophthalmologist, the eye may be lost. In all cases in which a foreign substance is splashed upon the eye, the immediate treatment is generous irrigation with plain water. The eyelids should be forced open and a gentle but continuous stream of water directed into the eye for a minimum of five minutes. If there is reason to believe that the foreign substance was an acid or an alkali, it is important to test the pH of the eye from time to time with pH paper. The irrigation should be continued until the pH is 7. Then a period of five minutes may be allowed to pass, and the pH of the eye is again tested. If the pH has risen or fallen, further irrigation should be carried out until the pH remains normal after irrigation. Following irrigation, antibacterial eye drops may be put in the conjunctival cul-de-sac. If the cornea is chalky white, prognosis for vision is poor. However, if the eye looks reasonably good, and the irrigation was thorough and done immediately after the accident, there is an excellent chance that vision will be saved without heroic measures, such as corneal transplantation.

Ultraviolet Exposure

The loss of vision following exposure of the eyes to ultraviolet radiation is more imagined than real. What actually happens, about six hours after exposure to rays from a sun lamp or welding arc without proper protection, is onset of *acute keratitis*. The corneal epithelial cells are damaged and many of them die. The roughening of the corneas is extremely painful; so painful that the patient cannot voluntarily open his eyes, and hence will maintain that he is blind. Application of a drop or two of ½ per cent proparacaine will relieve pain and allow examination. The patient can then open his eyes freely. The conjunctivae are moderately inflamed. The corneas are a bit hazy. A drop of fluorescein will show scattered staining of the cornea, indicating devitalization of many corneal epithelial cells. All other parts of the eye are normal. Within 24 hours the eyes usually have recovered fully. One must not succumb to the pleas of the patient for proparacaine to apply for similar relief at home. Such local anesthetics have an inhibitory effect on healing of the cornea and should not be used more than a few times within 24 hours. Too frequent use may interfere with healing and cause chronic ulceration.

SUMMARY

Of the many possible causes of loss of vision, occlusion of the central retinal artery is the most urgent and requires immediate treatment aimed at increasing the pressure differential in the artery on the two sides of the occlusion. Breathing of a 10 per cent CO_2 in 90 per cent O_2 mixture may be helpful. Another condition requiring immediate medical attention is acute angle-closure glaucoma. A real possibility exists that the systemic effects of the high intraocular pressure may divert attention away from the eye to the GI tract, resulting in unnecessary delay in the treatment of the acute glaucoma. Such a delay may cause the sight of the patient to be irreparably damaged. In most conditions that cause a reduction of vision or pain in an eye, the symptoms are so characteristic and the signs are so prominent that the exact diagnosis can be made if an accurate history can be obtained and if the eye is examined carefully. Usually definitive diagnosis and treatment can be deferred to an ophthalmologist in serious or problem cases. However, the observations of the first doctor seeing the patient are invaluable in determining the probable diagnosis, in deciding whether emergency treatment is necessary, and in judging whether the attentions of an ophthalmologist are required.

REFERENCES

1. Allen, J. H. (ed.): May's Manual of the Diseases of the Eye, 24th ed., Baltimore, Williams & Wilkins, 1968, also Arch. Ophthal. 79(6):663, 1968.
2. Berson, E., Gouras, P., Gunkel, R., and Myrianthopoulos, N.: Dominant retinitis pigmentosa with reduced penetrance, Arch. Ophthal. 81(2):266, 1969.
3. Campbell, F. P.: Retina and optic nerve, Arch. Ophthal. 79:789, 1968.
4. Cibis, P. A.: Vitreoretinal Pathology and Surgery in Retinal Detachment, St. Louis, Mosby, 1965.
5. Cogan, D. G.: Lesions of the eye from radiant energy, J.A.M.A. 142:145, 1950.
6. ————: Neurology of the Visual System, Springfield, Ill., Thomas, 1966.
7. Cogan, D. G., and Kuwabara, T. K.: Capillary shunts in the pathogenesis of diabetic retinopathy, Diabetes 12:293–300, 1963.
8. Cullen, J. F.: Occult temporal arteritis: A common cause of blindness in old age, Brit. J. Ophthal. 51:513, 1967.
9. Delthil, S., Sourdille, J., and Legras, M.: Horton's syndrome and its ocular manifestations, Bibl. Ophthal. 76:196, 1968.
10. Dufour, R., and Rumpf, J.: Vascular Diseases in Ophthalmology, Basel, S. Karger, 1968.
11. Fessel, W. J., and Pearson, C. M.: Polymyalgia rheumatica and blindness, New Eng. J. Med. 276:1403, 1967.
12. Francois, J.: Vascular pseudopapillitis, Bibl. Ophthal. 76:188, 1968.
13. Freeman, H. MacK.: Lens and vitreous, Arch. Ophthal. 80:132, 1968.
14. Gordon, D. M.: Visual impairment in the older patient, J. Amer. Geriat. Soc. 15:1025, 1967.
15. Grant, W.: Toxicology of the Eye, Springfield, Ill., Thomas, 1962.
16. Hoffman, D. H.: Eye burns caused by tear gas, Brit. J. Ophthal. 51(4):265, 1967.
17. Hollenhorst, R. W.: Effect of posture on retinal ischaemia from temporal arteritis, Arch. Ophthal. 78:569, 1967.
18. Industrial and traumatic ophthalmology, Symposium of the New Orleans Academy of Ophthalmology, St. Louis, Mosby, 1964.
19. Kearns, T. P.: Neuro-ophthalmology, Arch. Ophthal. 79:87, 1968.
20. Kimura, S. J., and Caygill, W. M. (eds.): Retinal Diseases: Symposium on Differential Diagnostic Problems of Posterior Uveitis, Philadelphia, Lea & Febiger, 1966.
21. Levene, R.: Glaucoma, Arch. Ophthal. 81(3):421, 1969.
22. MacFaul, P. A.: Ciliary artery involvement in giant cell arteritis, Brit. J. Ophthal. 51:505, 1967.
23. McLenachan, J., and Loran, D. F. C.: Angle-closure glaucoma and inverse astigmatism, Brit. J. Ophthal. 51:441, 1967.
24. Newell, F. W.: Ophthalmology, St. Louis, Mosby, 1965.
25. Norn, M. S.: Diabetes mellitus and cataracts senilis. The frequency and complications of cataract extraction in diabetics, Acta Ophthal. 45(3):322, 1967.
26. Paton, D., and Goldberg, M. F.: Injuries of the Eye, the Lids, and the Orbit, Philadelphia, Saunders, 1968.
27. Bauer, R. B., et al.: Joint study of extracranial arterial occlusion, J.A.M.A. 208:509, 1969.
28. Browne, T. R., and Poskanzer, D. C.: Treatment of strokes, New Eng. J. Med. 281:594, 1969.

6

Problems of Communication: Speech and Hearing Ear Pain

FRANCIS I. CATLIN

INTRODUCTION: HOW HUMAN BEINGS COMMUNICATE

Sound production by the voice and its reception through hearing are the most common means employed for interpersonal communication. Human beings transfer messages between each other chiefly vocally, but regularly employ many other modalities. Beyond early childhood the vocal expression is verbal; that is, the child learns to form sounds with accepted meanings—he employs language. Other sound-transmission of meaning can be conveyed by codes: through tapping of a Morse key in telegraphy, by drumbeats, or gunshots, or music, etc.

Language or code transmission can be sent by various means and perceived through sight: e.g. by written or printed symbols, by colors, light flashes, smoke signals, etc. Sight perception is regularly employed to receive messages conveyed by movements: motion of another person's eyes, through facial expressions, through conscious or unconscious movements of the head, hands, and body.

Meaning can be conveyed by touch—interpersonal touch: a handshake, a caress, or a blow; or touch of an object: such as Braille.

We have mentioned the three senses most commonly acting as receivers in human communication: *hearing, sight,* and *touch.* When a sense is impaired for reception, or a means of sending messages is incompetent, either temporarily or permanently, other techniques can be developed: the mute learn to speak with their hands, the blind learn to read by touch (Braille).

The other two senses regularly receive messages, sometimes purposefully intended, often involuntarily transmitted. Through *smell* we perceive numerous scents and odors, from delicate and pleasant to highly obnoxious. A perfume may say, "I want to be attractive to you." A detective entering a room may discover by sniffing the air that a shot has just been fired. Even *taste* can transmit information: a certain spice in a food, etc.; or that someone forgot to wash the castor-oil spoon.

Problems of communication between human beings usually involve one or more of these four modalities:

1. Voice production—the ability to produce vocal sounds.

2. Word and sentence formation—the ability to form accepted meaningful units or groups of sounds singly or in various inter-relationships; that is, the use of language.

3. Hearing—the ability to perceive sounds through the auditory apparatus.

4. The mental or intellectual ability to interpret the meaning of spoken sounds; that is, to understand the language used. The language involved may range from the most primitive to the most sophisticated and complex; the intellectual equipment required may therefore vary widely.

In this chapter, our purpose is to discuss primarily the pathologic physiology concerned in disorders of speech and hearing.

NORMAL DEVELOPMENTAL EXPECTANCIES IN HEARING AND SPEECH

The signs and symptoms of disorders of human communication must be evaluated in terms of chronological development of the patient. The general dictum: "a child talks as he hears, and in the manner in which he hears," presupposes a certain level of neurological and intellectual development. The normal or abnormal child acquires language through certain patterns of learning procedure; the impaired adult, however, recovers impaired communicative skills through a learning mechanism which is often quite different, since relearning of acquired skills plus the development of secondary skills are involved. The diagnostician, therefore, must be acquainted with the normal developmental expectancies of communicative skills, which, for the child, are given in Tables 6-1, 6-2, and 6-3[1].

Failure of any child to conform to these norms, within a time lag of six months, should lead to concern that a communicative problem may exist.

POSSIBLE PATHOPHYSIOLOGIC MECHANISMS

The child born with impairment of his ability to hear or to vocally or verbally communicate has defects which may be in his brain, in certain nerves, or in other organs; these defects may result (1) from a genetic aberration, which may or may not be familial or hereditary; or (2) from a disorder affecting the maternal organism; or (3) from a a disorder specifically affecting the individual fetus afflicted.

All infants are of course subject to genetic, maternal, fetal, and post-natal influences and possible hazards. Such hazards may produce many other possible difficulties beside auditory and speech problems.

We are in this chapter first concerned with reminding ourselves of the primary elements in the pathophysiology of impairments of hearing and speech which may affect infants and young children, and are not attributable to post-natal factors.

Next we must consider all of the possible post-natal factors which may cause hearing or speech defects, the mechanisms through which they operate, and the types of derangements that result.

HEARING

Hearing Assessment in Children

Auditory Responses

Hearing acuity in the very young child is judged by behavioral responses (Table 6-1). Not until about the age of 3 years does testing with pure tone audiometry become useful.

Current auditory screening procedures for the newborn and the infant up to eight months of age appear to be of less value than a direct comparison of performance of the child with developmental expectancies *plus* a review of maternal and pediatric factors which might predispose the child to a communicative impairment, i.e., the "high risk register." The use of such a register or questionnaire is highly recommended. The high risk factors are investigated and pursued as warranted by the information disclosed. For details of the use of such check lists and questionnaires, see the system used by Utah.[2]

The following classification, which groups most of the types of factors, cannot go into detail, and is not exhaustive.

Maternal High Risk Factors

1. History of previous handicapped infant.

2. History of prematurity, stillbirth, etc.

3. History of complications during pregnancy or at delivery.

4. Illness (endocrine, cardiovasculorenal, anemia, nutritional, Rh incompatibility, etc.).

5. Illness (infections: rubella, syphilis, toxoplasmosis, influenza, etc.).

TABLE 6-1. SPEECH, LANGUAGE, AND HEARING

Communication Chart (Newborn to Age Three Years)*

Normal Developmental Expectancies; Responses to Acoustic Stimuli; the Learning of Language; Vocal, Verbal, and Speech Output

AGE	ACTIVITIES RESPONSES	PARENTAL AND OBSERVATION	OFFICE PROCEDURES	INTERPRETATIONS AND MEANING
Newborn	1. Startle-reflex to sound; more often to sudden sounds of moderate-to-loud intensity. 2. Arousal responses. Investigators have demonstrated that relatively loud sound will arouse the new-born infant from accustomed sleep state.	Not pertinent.	Not pertinent.	Not ideal time to test auditory responses. Lack of expected responses bears little relationship to later communication problems. Conditions which apparently lead to auditory or other communicative problems may not become operative until several days after birth. In neurologic terms, clinical motor responses in the early months are relatively simple (gross). At this stage, more complex "apparatus"—neurological pathways (ultimately used for communicative purposes), may or may not be intact.
4 months	Typically turns eyes and head in direction of sound source. Awakens or quiets to mother's voice. May change facial expression or vocalize in response to sound. (During babbling several speech sounds are used.) May open eyes when sound is pre-sented, or, when eyes are open, palpebral fissure size may increase. May be cessation of typical movement. May frown, smile, or search for sound. May jerk head toward sound source.	What does he do when you talk to him? Does he react when he cannot see you? Do you see him turn toward sound of crib toys? How does he use his voice at home? After 4 to 6 months of age, if child actually has severely impaired hearing, previously noted babbling may cease or be diminished.	Tester should kneel or squat behind and to side of mother's chair. Baby is seated on mother's lap and held upright. Using quiet voice say baby's name; say s-s-s-s-s-s or k-k-k-k-k-k or use noisemaking toys. Keep sound source at ear level, but out of baby's peripheral vision. Be careful not to use a vowel (uh) after S or K.	With these procedures one is not measuring baby's hearing, but indexing babies whose responses seem abnormal. Lack of expected response to sound does not necessarily mean impaired hearing, but that baby's status and development need to be studied carefully. Premature or mentally retarded infants may be slow in developing expected responses to sound.

Age	Behavior	Test Method	Comments
8 months	1. Turns head and upper torso toward interesting sounds (at level of quiet conversational voice).	1. Have you seen this?	Response should be prompt. Delayed responses suggest possible hearing involvement. Persistent turning to one side or searching for sound, but not identifying appropriate direction of its source suggests hearing problem. Failure to turn quickly in presence of other evidence of hearing suggests developmental lag and need for careful follow-up.
	2. Vocalizes with variety of sounds and inflections. Done spontaneously when alone. Gives vocal responses when somebody talks to him; e.g., smiles, giggles, coos.	2. What have you heard him say? What noises does he make?	
	3. Usually responds to familiar sounds (his name, telephone bell, vacuum cleaner, barking dog, and quiets to mother's voice.	3. What does he do if he hears father's footsteps, the vacuum cleaner, the telephone?	Item 3 responses indicate baby's developing ability to "understand" everyday sounds around him (listening and discrimination).
	4. Usually awakens when mother talks to him.	4. Does he respond to "no-no"? Does he jiggle to music?	
		5. Has babbling decreased?	
		Test at ear level. Baby should seek and find sound source. It is important to test from both sides out of baby's vision range. When baby does respond, reinforcement must be used to hold baby's attention. This is done by immediately repeating stimulus at a louder level while expressing approval of baby.	
12 months	1. Responds to a number of different sounds, often with different reactions, and seems to recognize them as different; e.g., jabbers in response to human voice, may cry when there is thunder, quiets when hears mother nearby (vacuum cleaner), and may frown when scolded.	1. Direct query and observation. What kinds of sounds and noises does he make when you talk to him? What does he do when he hears a loud noise?	1. Average behavior is similar to 8-month period (Item 3), but responses should indicate more differentiation among speech sounds.
	2. Demonstrates understanding of some words by appropriate behavior, e.g., points or looks at familiar objects on request.	2. Try to test with appropriate objects, by saying the word quietly without general conversation or instruction.	2. This behavior indicates early differentiation of speech sounds as symbolic meanings.
	3. Uses sounds. "Talks" to toys. This is an enjoyable experience for baby.	3. Direct query and observation. Does he "talk" to himself or make sounds as he plays with his toys?	3. One can look for changes in baby's "talking" as his attention and patterns of play change.

* Adapted from unpublished report of Special Ad Hoc Committee of Children's Bureau; Chairman, William G. Hardy, Ph.D., 1965. Table constructed by Frances R. Tucker of the Maryland State Department of Health, in consultation with Francis I. Catlin, M.D., and William G. Hardy, Ph.D., of the Johns Hopkins Medical Institutions.

TABLE 6-1. SPEECH, LANGUAGE, AND HEARING (CONT.)

Communication Chart (Newborn to Age Three Years)*

Normal Developmental Expectancies; Responses to Acoustic Stimuli; the Learning of Language; Vocal, Verbal, and Speech Output

AGE	ACTIVITIES RESPONSES	PARENTAL OBSERVATION AND OFFICE PROCEDURES	INTERPRETATIONS AND MEANING
12 months Cont'd	4. Tries to imitate some simple words.	4. If possible, have mother demonstrate this; he is more used to her manner of speaking.	4. This is evidence of developmental maturation. Many children use a few words at this age. However, babies may *not* imitate words at 12 months. Absence of verbal utterance indicates a need to inquire about verbal stimulation at home, parental attitudes, and expectancies; e.g., "Do you have time to sit and talk with him and let him jabber back?" "Does his father?"
18 months	1. Expect some progressive increase in child's vocabulary (more definite words) from that observable at 12 months.	1. Query and demonstration. How many understandable words does he use? More or fewer than he used a few months ago?	1. Note any apparent loss of words that were previously used. With a child who has severely impaired hearing, one can expect cessation or regression of previously noted babbling.
	2. Begins to identify part of body; e.g., may point to nose on request.	2. Demonstration, if possible. The baby should be able to show you his nose or eyes.	2. This is clear evidence of verbal symbolic understanding.
	3. Beginning to pay attention to, and identify, various sounds from considerable distance.	3. Note detail of parental anecdotes. It is important that auditory responses are identified without the use of visual cues. What does he do when refrigerator door opens in another room? When ice cream man's bell rings? When there is a fire siren? When you open a box of candy that he cannot see? Does he seem to react to music? with rhythm? Does he like to look at books with you, and turn the page?	3. Whereas at 8 to 12 months baby's auditory attention is limited to close environment, by 18-months he is responding to wider environment of sound; e.g., from another room, or from outside the house. If hearing loss has been acquired, he probably will not do this, and may show symptoms of regression in speech attempts previously made.

24 months

1. Can follow verbal commands with two components without the aid of gestures; e.g., "Pick up the block and give it to mother."
2. Can identify familiar objects when named.
3. Can spontaneously name familiar objects.
4. Initiates "sentences" of two or more "words", which are meaningful to listener.
5. Learns new (simple) word with only one presentation.

1 to 5. Screening requires demonstration as well as parental reporting. Often it is easier and more economic to let mother do the demonstrating. The responses should be observed and not simply accepted from parental statements. Mother can tell him to "Close the door and sit down"; "Pick up the block and give it to me"; "Get my purse and put it on that chair." Inquire whether he shows interest in musical introductions to regular television shows. Does he listen to music from a record player?

5. This is only one item in a battery of achievements for this age. If it can be demonstrated, this accomplishment represents a significant landmark. It is perhaps best to direct mother to undertake this. Failure to accomplish it on the part of a just 2-year-old may be related to various developmental states of affairs, any of which warrant careful investigation.

36 months

1. Can identify objects or activities with the use of pictures; e.g., "Show me the one that is good to eat." "Show me the one that you wear."
2. Identifies his or her own sex.
3. Understands some verbs, adjectives, pronouns, and prepositions.
4. Repeats a four-word sentence.
5. Uses some verbs, adjectives, pronouns, and prepositions.
6. May respond to pure tones from audiometer, as well as to speech.
7. Names familiar objects.

1. Should be readily demonstrated.
2. "Are you a boy or a girl?" Put correct reference first.
3. Preferably, this should be demonstrated with the use of toys in a doll house or other appropriate objects; up, down, in, on, under, big, little, you, me, I. "Put the baby in the big bed." "Make the dog jump." "Push the car."
4. Actually, he should be able to repeat and use four-word sentences.
5. This requires observation, or acceptable reports, of the child's typical behavior.
6. To be determined in appropriate circumstances by qualified testers.
7. This should be readily demonstrated.

1 to 7. Child should be using speech socially. Deviations from normal development which may become apparent at this time, and which generally require extensive diagnostic evaluation, include "the retarded child," "delayed speech," "motor interference," "impaired hearing," and "emotional disturbance." If he does not quite readily demonstrate these verbal capacities, there is need for careful follow-up. If he uses jargon and gestures to try to control his environment, rather than words, hearing involvement may be suspected. There is always apt to be confusion between the dull child and the deaf child (frequently both conditions may be present). Further definitive measurement of hearing is readily available for the child of this age. Various kinds of audiometry can be done. These require special equipment and experience. (Routine pure-tone audiometry can be carried out with confidence with about 50 per cent of just 3-year-olds.

TABLE 6-2. VOCABULARY GROWTH*

AGE Years Months		NUMBER OF WORDS
0	10	1
1	0	3
1	6	22
2	0	272
2	6	446
3	0	896
3	6	1222
4	0	1540
4	6	1870
5	0	2072
5	6	2289
6	0	2562

TABLE 6-3. VERBAL OUTPUT*

AGE Years Months		AVERAGE LENGTH OF "SENTENCES" (Number of Words)
1	6	1.2
2	0	1.7 to 1.9
2	6	2.7 to 3.1
3	0	3.0 to 4.2
3	6	4.3 to 4.7
4	0	3.4 to 5.4
4	6	4.6 to 5.5
5	0	3.6 to 5.7
5	6	4.4 to 5.1
6	0	3.7 to 6.6
6	6	5.0 to 5.4
7	0	7.3
8	0	7.6

6. Other hazards (drugs, alcohol, radiation, etc.).

7. Age (under 16 or over 36 primigravida; or over 40, multigravida).

Infant High Risk Factors

1. Gestational age under 36 or over 42 weeks.

2. Birth weight under 4 or over 11 lbs.

3. Trauma at birth.

4. Apnea at birth.

5. Neonatal shock, jaundice, bleeding, or severe anemia, or severe hypoglycemia.

6. Evidence of a genetic defect (e.g., phenylketonuria, etc.).

TESTS OF HEARING AND OTOLOGIC EXAMINATION

A competent otologic examination to rule out disease of the ear is essential. When the otologic picture is normal, assessment of the neurologic and psychologic status of the child is most important.

Childhood auditory impairments may be genetic, congenital, or acquired. In small infants, this differentiation may be difficult because of the time-lag between the causative event and the period when impairment of performance is noticed. Some conditions may be recognized early: deformities of ear, lip and palate are readily apparent. However, palatal incompetence and choanal atresia occasionally escape early diagnosis. Gross deformities of the inner ear structures are fortunately rare and usually found in association with obvious external and middle ear malformations.

* These normative data can serve as a guide for checking status of vocabulary development and amount of expressive speech.

Hearing impairment may present in several ways. The age of onset, the character of the hearing impairment and the nature of the underlying disease all exert a direct bearing upon the symptomatology. The eight-month-old infant may fail to turn toward the source of sound; the two-year-old may be unable to identify familiar objects when named.

Mild hearing impairments may not be detected under average listening conditions. Under more difficult listening conditions, such as in the classroom, a child with a mild hearing impairment can be, and often is, classified mistakenly and unfairly as being uncooperative, unresponsive, erratic, or diffident, or as having a "behaviour problem." The more severe hearing impairments create a recognizable communicative dysfunction unless the hearing loss is unilateral, although an alert parent or teacher may recognize the latter condition.

Hearing impairment in the pre-school (4 to 6 year old) and school age child is most commonly the result of upper respiratory infection and its sequelae. For the most part, such predisposing conditions are self-limiting, and the hearing impairment is therefore transient. However, some of these conditions, although potentially reversible, can cause permanent damage to the auditory system unless treatment is prompt and adequate. One must not forget that prolonged auditory impairment in the preschool child may seriously delay and impair the normal acquistion of speech and language skills. Such delay may have long-term effects in many spheres upon the development of the person.

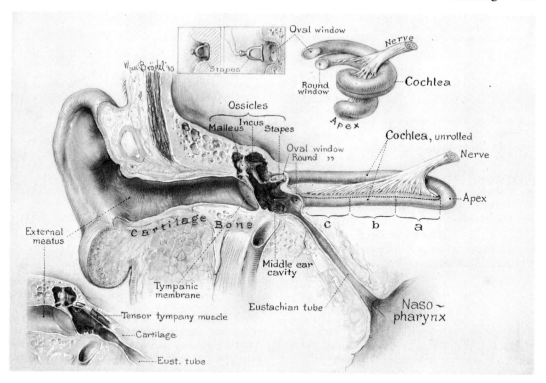

FIG. 6-1. Schematic drawing of the ear showing the relationships of the external, middle, and internal parts. The cochlea has been unrolled to show the relation of (a) the apical third, (b) the middle third, and (c) the basal third to the oval and round window niches of the middle ear space. (Department of Art as Applied to Medicine, Johns Hopkins University School of Medicine, an original drawing by Max Brödel)

ANATOMY AND PHYSIOLOGY OF AUDITORY APPARATUS

Some knowledge of the normal mechanisms of the auditory system is essential for an understanding of the symptomatology of hearing impairment. As the site of the underlying condition has a direct effect upon the symptomatology, these mechanisms will be described briefly (Fig. 6-1).

Sound-Conduction Mechanism of the Ear

The peripheral auditory system may be divided into three parts. Two of these, the external auditory canal terminating in the tympanic membrane, and the middle ear, containing the sound-conducting ossicles (malleus, incus, and stapes) that transmit vibrations from the tympanic membrane to the inner ear via the stapes footplate, constitute the conductive mechanism by which airborne sound is effectively transmitted to the fluid-encased structures of the inner ear. Without the "transformer action" of the tym-

panic membrane and ossicles, airborne sound would be reflected from the inner ear, with a resultant loss of auditory sensitivity.

Impairment of the transmission mechanisms of the external and middle ear produces a *conductive hearing impairment.* The loss of auditory sensitivity tends to be fairly uniform over the useful frequency range of the ear: that is, low-pitched sounds are attenuated to the same extent as are high-pitched sounds. Consequently, if the speaker raises the volume of his voice sufficiently, the listener with a conductive hearing impairment can usually understand the message. Tinnitus, or head noise, is occasionally noted with a conductive hearing impairment, especially when the underlying condition is otosclerosis with fixation of the stapes footplate.

Inspection of the external auditory canal and tympanic membrane may reveal an external auditory canal problem as the cause for the conductive hearing loss.

ETIOLOGY OF CONDUCTIVE HEARING
IMPAIRMENT IN THE EXTERNAL EAR

Causes of conductive hearing impairment in the external ear include:

Atresia of the external auditory canal

Narrowing, or collapse, of the external auditory meatus

Impacted cerumen

Impacted foreign body in the external canal

Polyp or tumor of the external auditory canal

Infection: furunculosis, external otitis, "swimmer's ear"

Edema from trauma or drug reaction

Exostoses, when such bony growths are large and obstruct the canal

Deformities of the tympanic membrane: congenital abnormalities, scarring, large perforations, etc.

Some of these deformities are visible to the naked eye. Most, however, can be readily detected by examination with the electric otoscope. In such instances, the pneumatic otoscope assists in the determination of mobility of the tympanic membrane, as with scarring and questionable perforations. One sign which is useful in the presence of external ear infection is tenderness of the auricle or tragus or both to pressure or to motion. Such tenderness is usually absent in a patient with a middle ear infection unless there is an associated necrotizing mastoiditis; in such circumstances, tenderness over the mastoid cortex may also be expected.

A congenital collapse of the external auditory meatus is frequently overlooked, especially when co-existing with an external otitis for which it may be a predisposing cause.

Impacted cerumen, foreign bodies or exudate are usually evident upon inspection. A pulsating discharge in the external auditory canal is usually evidence of a middle ear infection, although it is occasionally found in severe external otitis. Tympanic membrane perforations must be fairly large to cause significant hearing impairment. A small perforation with a significant hearing loss usually means that other middle ear factors are involved.

ETIOLOGY OF CONDUCTIVE HEARING
IMPAIRMENT IN THE MIDDLE EAR

Disorders of the middle ear which affect hearing include the following:

Acute inflammation

Chronic inflammation

Impairment of ossicular function (scarring, destruction, disruption from trauma)

Cholesteatoma

Serous exudate or hemorrhage

Tympanic membrane retraction secondary to Eustachian tubal obstruction

Tumors of the middle ear

Otosclerosis

Congenital malformations of the middle ear structures.

These conditions of the middle ear produce a conductive type of hearing impairment in three ways: (1) by "loading" the tympanic membrane with exudate, transudate, new growth, or cholesteatoma, or by alteration of normal middle ear pressure; (2) by decrease in mobility of the ossicles from scarring, exudate, transudate, otosclerosis or ossicular anomaly; or (3) by destruction of continuity of the ossicular chain from infection, trauma, new growth or cholesteatoma.

Acute Otitis Media. In children, acute otitis media is the most common condition encountered with symptoms of ear pain, hearing impairment, and often, associated upper respiratory infection with rhinorrhea, nasal obstruction, postnasal discharge, cough, sore throat and fever. Early acute otitis media may show retraction of the tympanic membrane, followed by evidence of fluid in the middle ear, a straw color or reddish tinge to the tympanic membrane and loss of the normal light reflex of the membrane, followed by bulging of the membrane, loss of normal landmarks and subsequent rupture of the membrane with release of a pulsating purulent discharge and corresponding decrease in otalgia. The presence and degree of ear pain constitute a useful index of the severity of the inflammatory process. Ear pain is apt to be severe in an acute fulminating process and mild or absent when the condition is mild.

The appearance of tympanic membrane in acute otitis media may be confused with that occurring in several other conditions. At times, a flecked, dull membrane is found in external otitis, which may resemble that of otitis media. In the middle ear condition, however, the auricle and tragus are not commonly tender and a conductive type of hearing impairment will be found, whereas the auricular appendage is usually very sensitive with external otitis, and there is frequently no hearing impairment if the external auditory canal is patent and free from debris. Occasionally, spread of an acute infection from the middle ear will distort the tympanic membrane into various shapes. Such distortions may be confused with blebs of the tympanic membrane found in some acute viral infections. In the latter condition, however, there is often an absence of hearing impairment, and the blebs collapse, with the release of clear fluid, to reveal an otherwise relatively normal tympanic membrane. Extension of the middle ear infection to the mastoid bone may be revealed by pain provoked upon palpation of the mastoid cortex. There is swelling of the cortex resulting in an anterior-inferior displacement of the auricle, which is usually painful to touch, or in tenderness and swelling below the apex of the mastoid process (Bezold's sign). Other sequelae to acute otitis media may be manifested by persistent perforation of the tympanic membrane, otorrhea, or the growth of polyps or cholesteatoma within the middle ear space or in the development of a scarred, thickened and often immobile tympanic membrane. Less severe infection may result in persistent fluid in the middle ear behind an intact membrane, plus an associated conductive hearing loss. In the presence of such signs of chronicity, one should look for signs and symptoms of malnutrition, poor hygiene, chronic tonsil and adenoid disease, sinusitis, or palatal abnormalities.

Serous Otitis Media. Another common affliction of the middle ear in children is serous otitis (media), manifest by tympanic membrane retraction (occasionally fullness or a normal position), a straw colored or reddish fluid in the middle ear and signs of a conductive hearing loss. The tympanic membrane is usually thin, glistening and intact, but altered in appearance by the fluid partially or completely filling the middle ear space. A fluid level, when present, will commonly shift in position with a change in attitude of the head. Occasionally an appearance of bubbles in the middle ear will be found. Pain and tenderness are characteristically absent. This condition is fairly common in adults also and results from impairment of the Eustachian tubal function. Infection, tubal obstruction by adenoids or new growths and allergy are the most common causes. A history of allergy may be associated with allergic changes in the nasal mucosa, particularly in the posterior part of the nose and nasopharynx: pallor and edema of the mucosa, occasionally hyperemia; polypoid degeneration of the posterior turbinate mucosa; nasal or nasopharyngeal polyps; edema of the Eustachian tubal orifice. Adenoid obstruction may produce nasal blockage, mouth breathing, snoring, evidence of ethmoid sinus infection (postnasal discharge) and the so-called "adenoid facies." In adults, a tumor of the nasopharynx must always be suspected particularly if the otologic condition is unilateral and accompanied by head pain or evidence of cranial nerve palsy (indicating an extension of the process to the middle cranial fossa). Metastasis to a cervical lymph node may also be an early presenting symptom.

Tympanosclerosis and Otosclerosis. When a conductive hearing impairment is found in the presence of a normal-appearing tympanic membrane and external auditory canal, the examiner should inquire about previous ear infections and investigate the family history regarding hearing impairment. In children, tympanosclerosis or scarring of the ossicular mechanism is a common cause. In young adults, the possibility of otosclerosis must be entertained. Examination of the ear may reveal a flushed or reddish color of the promontory, or medial wall of the middle ear, as seen through the tympanic membrane. This color results from an active otosclerotic process in the promontory region, but may be absent if this particular area is not involved. Anesthesia of the tympanic membrane in otosclerosis has also been described (Itard-Cholewa's sign). Tinnitus, or head noise is a frequently associated symptom found on the side of the involved ear.

Tumor of the Middle Ear. Tumors of the middle ear are relatively uncommon. Some rapidly progressive malignant tumors may be confused with the clinical picture of a severe necrotizing otitis media. Any situation in which a proliferation of tissue in the middle ear is found requires prompt biopsy. Congenital anomalies of the middle ear may

Resonance. The selective modification of laryngeal-produced sound by the anatomical and physiological characteristics of the speech mechanisms.

Articulation. Sound production and the selective modification of the voiced and unvoiced breath stream by the articulatory segments of the speech mechanisms (tongue, teeth and lips). A function interrelated with resonance.

Pronunciation. Arrangement of speech sounds in prescribed sequences of syllables with the application of proper syllable stress.

Language comprehension and use. The symbolization process involving the formulation and comprehension of language and other symbolic forms.

A communicative set. Enables the individual to have a willingness and readiness to speak, a confidence in one's communicative ability, plus the urge to communicate.

When an impairment of speech function is suspected, one must look for signs and symptoms of impairment of these basic functions, as well as of the speech-producing structures: the respiratory mechanism, larynx, tongue, teeth, hard and soft palate, lips, pharynx, and nasal cavities. In general, the respiratory or breathing mechanism will be adequate if the speaker can provide adequate sub-laryngeal pressures at appropriate times, accelerate or decelerate the volume of air flow at will, inspire and exhale at will and otherwise regulate his breathing patterns. The respiratory mechanism is seldom a factor in major communicative problems unless there is paresis of the respiratory structures or a severely impaired pulmonary reserve.

DISORDERS OF PHONATION

Phonation is the auditory experience of laryngeal voice production which is culturally appropriate for human communication. Certain parameters, such as pitch, show normal variations with respect to age, sex and socio-economic status. Abnormalities of phonation (voice) cannot always be easily distinguished from impairments of articulation or of resonance.

Certain characteristics are commonly used to describe phonation:

Pitch level. The central tendency of fundamental frequency of vocal cord vibration about which intonation variations habitually occur.

Loudness level. The average (characteristic) level of intensity of phonation.

Control. The ability to initiate, maintain, and discontinue phonation at will.

Intonation. The habitual variation of pitch, loudness and control of phonation appropriate to speech meaning and the circumstances of the communicative situation.

Quality. The overall characteristics of laryngeal produced sounds which are not the results of articulatory or of resonance effects.

Loss or absence of the ability to phonate. Voice disorders are frequently complex in nature. They are comparatively rare in incidence. Phonatory (voice) impairments may be classified as organic or non-organic (functional). *Every voice disorder should be studied for signs of organic impairment.*

Hoarseness, a combination of the acoustical features of breathiness and harshness, is rare as a non-organic disorder (as in "false-cord" phonation), but is relatively common as a sign of laryngeal pathology. Painless hoarseness is one of the early symptoms of cancer of the larynx. Associated symptoms include voice fatigue, frequent need to clear the throat, and, on occasion, chronic dryness or rawness of the throat. One should question for a history of excessive smoking or voice misuse (as in singers and public speakers), as well as for signs and symptoms of hiatus hernia and esophageal regurgitation.

Hoarseness, breathiness, and weak voice intensity in the adult should lead to suspicion of a growth on the vocal cord, vocal cord paralysis, or myasthenia gravis. Vocal cord paralysis is most commonly the result of trauma (especially surgical trauma). Bilateral vocal cord paralysis with the cords approximated (bilateral abductor paralysis) can produce frightening symptoms in some patients: apprehension, dyspnea, and labored respiration and speech.

Hoarseness and its first cousin, stridor (a harsh, high-pitched sound which is very audible), should lead the diagnostician to investigate the intrinsic as well as possible extra-laryngeal causes. Such study is especially urgent when these symptoms appear in small children. Intra-laryngeal causes include: inflammatory conditions, tumors, cysts, congenital anatomical abnormalities, neurological problems, trauma and intra-laryngeal foreign bodies. Among the extra-laryngeal causes are: congenital anatomical abnormalities, tumors, cysts, inflammatory conditions of the neck and mediastinum, and foreign bodies in the esophagus.

Ventricular phonation is characterized by hoarseness, low pitch, a moderate-to-weak intensity, reduced inflection and a raspy quality to the voice.

Diplophonia, the true production of two fundamental frequencies by the vocal cords, is rare.

Aphonia, or loss of voice, may result from organic causes, such as damage to the larynx, or from non-organic conditions, such as aphonia of psychogenic origin. With either organic or psychogenic aphonia, *whisper speech,* a sound produced by laryngeal air flow instead of by vocal cord vibration, may be employed.

Falsetto, a voice of higher pitch than appropriate for age and sex of the speaker, is most often the result of socio-cultural conditions, although it has been reported following laryngitis, trauma or shock. While use of falsetto may be appropriate for singing and under certain cultural conditions, it frequently dates from puberty and is more likely to occur if the true voice is bass. The falsetto voice does not necessarily have to be very high in pitch.

One should also consider other conditions which may affect phonation: hearing loss which impairs the individual's self-monitoring mechanisms; reduced auditory memory span; poor or inconstant pitch placement; and faulty discrimination and use of intensity and quality. All of these parameters of speech are affected by internal and external feedback systems. The functions of all of these systems must be evaluated just as carefully as the physical apparatus for the production of speech sounds, if the interpretation of signs and symptoms is to be of value.

Signs and Symptoms of Articulatory Disorders

Learning to articulate the standard sounds of a language is an experience of all communicating individuals. Since speech is a learned activity, the majority of speech disorders occur during the childhood or developmental period and, to a lesser degree, in the aging population in the form of aphasia and laryngeal disease.

Most childhood speech problems are articulatory disorders; that is, defective production of acceptable speech sounds. All physiological measurements show ranges of variation. Speech sounds are no exception. As Van Riper and Irwin[7] have noted, however, **certain criteria** can be employed to describe abnormalities of articulation. These include:

Intelligibility. The degree to which intelligibility is impaired.

Frequency and consistency of error. The number of errors heard by the listener and the consistency with which they occur.

Type of error. Some articulatory errors are more noticeable than others. Many errors are so close to the variations of normal utterance that they can scarcely be termed errors. Others deviate widely; for example, compare the effects of omissions, substitutions and distortions.

Conditions of communication. Society uses different tolerance levels for variations in pronunciation in terms of the type of communication used. More variation is tolerated in casual conversation than in formal platform speech. Articulation errors tend to be overlooked by the listener during stressful or emotional environmental situations.

Status within the culture. Judgment regarding the quality of articulation in speech is also based upon the listener's evaluation of the status of the speaker in his culture. Errors made by a child and accepted as normal would be considered abnormal for adult use. Two factors are apparent: the standards of language usage are frequently employed as signs of cultural status. Closely related to this factor of cultural status is the fact that the standards of acceptable pronunciation undergo continual change just as do other cultural activities.

Subjective criteria of abnormality. The prior criteria have been defined primarily in terms of listener reaction. In some instances, the speaker, because of anxiety, may attribute defects to his own speech which are nonexistent. Other persons may refuse to recognize articulatory errors which are real. A few refuse to believe that their speech is in any way defective. They are unable to isolate their errors sufficiently to perceive them.

Clearly, the identification and interpretation of articulatory disorders is not a task for the layman.

Other forms of defective speech include voice disorders which can **mimic articulation disorders** (and vice-versa). *Lalling* refers to slurred and defective articulation resulting from reduced tongue-tip activity. *Hyponasality,* as in muffling of the *m, n* and *ng*

TABLE 6-4. LANGUAGE DEVELOPMENT
AND APHASIA

STAGE	STATE OF DEVELOPMENT	TYPE OF APHASIA
I	Pre-language: characterized by speechlessness.	Global
II	Pre-language: characterized by meaningless autistic and echolalic phoneme use.	Jargon
III	Progressive acquisition of comprehension. Oral expression of words and neologisms, largely unrelated to meaning or below level of comprehension.	Pragmatic
IV	The beginning use of substantive language, progressing through nominal, verbal and adjectival words. Characterized by one or two-word groups as complete expression.	Semantic
V	The use of syntax or grammar in oral expression.	Syntactic

sounds, occurs with nasal or nasopharyngeal obstruction (as in acute coryza). While occasionally described as a voice disorder, Van Riper and Irwin consider hyponasality to be an articulation problem in which certain sounds are produced defectively.

Although cleft palate speakers are described as having characteristically *hypernasal* voices, their speech seems more nasal if it contains many consonant articulation errors than if it contains few. Apparently, hypernasality and misarticulation are closely related.

Misarticulations are also found in the speech of individuals with certain *dental conditions*, such as severe malocclusion. Misarticulation frequently occurs with *cerebral palsy* and as one of the speech defects of *aphasia*. Defective articulation, often accompanied by disorders of voice pitch and loudness, is frequently encountered in those whose learning mechanisms are hampered by severe *hearing impairments*, especially in young children.

Delayed speech is a common wastebasket diagnosis. Whereas the term properly refers to children with late onset of speech who nevertheless go through an orderly process of speech development, this diagnostic label is often applied to other conditions in which misarticulation and impairments of vocabulary, use of syntax, and general language awareness are intermixed in various proportions. Many of these children exhibit poor auditory memory (seldom better than the achievement of the normal two-year-old) and impaired language comprehension. Many also have difficulty in reading. One should look for related emotional, intellectual (maturational) or socio-economic factors.

Similarly, the person learning *a new language* needs to acquire new skills in articulation, vocabulary, syntax, intonation and language comprehension. Traces of the characteristics of the first language learned in childhood are apt to remain to modify another language learned later in life.

Cluttered speech is described by Weiss[8] as "hurried in rate, yet hesitant," with repetition of syllables and short words, slurring with speed, and with syntactic deformation of longer sentences. Many of these speakers demonstrate poor auditory memory and omissions.

Stuttering, on the contrary, is not an articulatory problem but an interruption of the ongoing process of expressive speech which is characterized by part-word (syllable) repetitions, intermittent sound prolongations and irregularity in the rate of verbal expression. Stuttering becomes eminent when the performance of speech occurs under stress. Even speakers classified as "normal" may stutter if environmental conditions are sufficiently stressful. The debate over the behavioral versus organic etiology of stuttering remains unresolved.

LANGUAGE

Language comprehension and use implies the willingness and ability to formulate and utilize meaningful symbols for the comprehension of speech stimuli (vision, etc.), and for the initiation of appropriate motor output (speech output, gesture, etc.). A simplistic division of impairments of language comprehension into acquired versus developmental conditions is appealing but often unsatisfactory. Several reasons exist: too little is known about the relationship of language comprehension to the neurophysiology of the central nervous system; current tools for evaluation of the language function are, at best, gross; and the ability of the individual to comprehend and use language changes continually.

Some authors have offered a diagrammatic outline in which the five stages of normal language development are compared with corresponding stages of aphasic disturbance found in impaired adults. See Table 6-4.

The average infant may be expected to reach stage III at a twelve to eighteen month level, stage IV at about the two year level and stage V by three years of age. Failure to achieve these levels may be related to factors other than the ability to develop language. The diagnostician should consider the psychological stimulation provided (or not provided) by the child's environment, the presence and nature of associated hearing and speech defects, and the non-verbal mental age of the child, when compared with his peer group. A recent survey of the problems of classification may be found in: "Human Communication and Its Disorders," prepared by the National Institute of Neurological Diseases and Stroke.[9]

PAIN IN THE EAR

The differentiating characteristics between ear pain caused by otitis externa and by otitis media have previously been discussed. An outline of some of the common causes of pain in the ear with the localizing signs and symptoms follows:

1. **Primary pain—arising from disorders of aural structures**

    A. Auricular pain
    Frostbite
    Trauma
    Infection (soft tissue or perichondritis)
    (The foregoing conditions are usually self-evident, with an inflammatory reaction locally, hemorrhage or abrasions in the case of trauma, and swelling of the soft tissue.)
    Tumors
    Cysts (especially if infected)

    B. External auditory canal
    Abrasion or laceration (as with a foreign body)
    Furunculosis
    External otitis (swimmer's ear)

    Herpes oticus (with otic eruption, other signs of facial involvement; facial paralysis, sensory-neural hearing loss)
    Tumors

    C. Tympanic membrane
    Trauma
    Laceration/perforation
    Bullous myringitis

    D. Middle ear
    Aerotitis media (generally retraction of tympanic membrane and inflammation of middle ear mucosa)
    Acute otitis media
    Chronic otitis media with acute superinfection
    Acute mastoiditis
    Tumors

2. **Referred pain—arising from adjacent structures**

    A. Nasopharynx
    Acute nasopharyngitis
    Tumors of the nasopharynx (usually invasive)

    B. Dental origin
    Pulpitis
    Impaction

    C. Sinusitis
    Acute, usually sphenoid or maxillary

    D. Pharynx, mouth
    Infection (tonsils, pharyngeal spaces, etc.)
    Tumors

    E. Neck
    Infection of the triangular spaces and their contents
    Tumors (uncommon unless invasive).

REFERENCES

1. Tucker, Frances R.: Speech and Hearing (adapted from unpublished report of Special Ad Hoc Committee of Children's Bureau, Chairman, William G. Hardy, Ph.D., 1965), Maryland State Department of Health, 1969.
2. Utah State Division of Health, Maternal and

Child Health Section: Maternal and Infant High Risk Check Lists, 1967.

3. Cushing, H.: Tumors of the Nervus Acusticus and the Syndrome of the Cerebellopontile Angle, Philadelphia, Saunders, 1917.

4. Erickson, L. S., Sorensen, G. D., and McGavran, M. H.: A review of 140 acoustic neurinomas (neurilemmoma), Laryngoscope 75: 601–627, April 1965.

5. Riley, E. C., Sterner, J. H., Fassett, D., and Ward Sutton, W. L.: Ten years with industrial audiometry, Journal of American Industrial Hygiene Association, 22:151–159, 1961.

6. Johnson, W., Darley, F. L., and Spriestersbach, D. C.: Diagnostic Methods in Speech Pathology, New York, Harper and Row, 1963.

7. Van Riper, C., and Irwin, J. V.: Voice and Articulation, Englewood Cliffs, N. J., Prentice-Hall, 1958.

8. Weiss, D. A., and Beebe, H. H.: The Chewing Approach in Speech and Voice Therapy, New York, S. Karger, 1955.

9. Human Communication and Its Disorders—An Overview, National Institute of Neurological Diseases and Stroke, National Institutes of Health, Bethesda, Maryland, 1969.

7

Sore Tongue and Sore Mouth

RICHARD W. VILTER

**Normal Morphology and Physiology
of Tongue and Mouth**

Medical History and Physical Examination

**Systemic Diseases That May Cause
Sore Tongue and Sore Mouth**
NUTRITIONAL DEFICIENCY DISEASES—
VITAMIN B COMPLEX, VITAMIN C,
AND RELATED DEFICIENCY STATES

Other Systemic Diseases

Local Oral Lesions

Since the earliest day of medicine, the tongue has been a barometer of health. Hippocrates[1] correlated the dry, heavily coated, fissured tongue with fever and dehydration, and he associated a poor prognosis with the red, ulcerated tongue and mouth of the patient with protracted dysentery.

With the medical renaissance of the eighteenth and the nineteenth centuries, observations on the state of the tongue and the mouth became as important as the taking of the pulse. Indeed, by 1844 glossology had become so important a part of the medical art that a Dr. Benjamin Ridge proposed the fantastic theory that the viscera were represented by definite areas on the tongue and that an abnormality in a viscus was reflected in this predetermined area. The physician was not alone in holding the tongue in high regard. The patient and his family often considered it the only sure indicator of health or disease and regarded that physician poorly who did not greet his patient with the request, "Stick out your tongue, please." Such aphorisms as "raw red tongue—raw red gut" or "coated tongue—constipation" stem from this period.

During the first half of the twentieth century, the science of medicine rapidly outstripped the art, and many reputable physicians, aware that the beliefs of previous centuries were frequently "old wives' tales,"

preferred to confine their observations to such newly developed instruments as the fluoroscope and the electrocardiograph. Observation of the tongue and the mouth was so simple that it was frequently neglected and, in fact, often considered as the mark of the "old-timer."

In recent years, however, observations of the condition of tongue and mouth have begun to assume new diagnostic importance. Interpretations have been based upon controlled clinical observations rather than upon empiricism. The change began about 1900 with William Hunter's description of the glossitis of pernicious anemia.[2] Later, hematologists such as Minot and Murphy[3] substantiated Hunter's observations and made use of them as diagnostic measures; but the present emphasis on the significance of oral lesions primarily is due to the work of nutritionists such as Spies,[4,5] Jolliffe,[6] Sydenstricker,[7,8] Sebrell,[9] and Kruse[10,11] who have stressed the importance of tongue and mouth lesions in the early diagnosis of nutritional deficiency diseases. The complicated mechanisms whereby the tongue and the mouth mirror the abnormalities of the body as a whole have only begun to be unraveled, but knowledge of metabolic diseases is increasing rapidly. Already, the importance of questioning the patient concerning soreness or burning of the tongue and of careful examination of the tongue have been re-established.

This chapter is concerned with the description, the interpretation, and the differential diagnosis of *painful* abnormalities of tongue and mouth which reflect metabolic disease. Wherever possible the altered physiology responsible for the abnormalities provides the background for the discussion.

NORMAL MORPHOLOGY AND PHYSIOLOGY OF TONGUE AND MOUTH

Under normal conditions the ventral surface of the tongue is covered by smooth, pink, mucous membrane and lymphoid follicles. On its dorsal surface the filiform, fungiform, and circumvallate papillae, containing the end organs of taste, produce a rough grayish-red appearance. The twelve large mushroomlike circumvallate papillae are arranged in an inverted V-shape at the base of the tongue. The hairlike filiform papillae, the most numerous type present, are fine projections of mucous membrane capped by tufts of squamous epithelial cells and usually are arranged in rows parallel to the row of circumvallate papillae. These inverted V-shaped rows gradually merge into parallel straight lines on the anterior surface of the tongue, and finally at the tip this regular arrangement is lost. The fungiform papillae are conical or mushroom-shaped and are covered by smooth, thin epithelium. They are larger than the filiform papillae among which they are scattered and usually occur in greatest abundance at the tip and the sides of the tongue. The thick epithelial tufts of the filiform papillae give the tongue its characteristic gray-white coating, whereas the globular, pale-red fungiform papillae give the tongue a speckled-pink appearance.

The tongue is usually not furrowed except for a mid-line groove. A common variant is the "scrotal" tongue, which appears more bulky than usual and many irregularly placed grooves and furrows transect it. However, the general arrangement and the appearance of the papillae are unaffected.

In health, the buccal mucous membrane has an even grayish-red color and may be crossed by fine grayish ridges where it settles between the rows of teeth when the mouth is closed. By close inspection, particularly if a small magnifying glass is used, one can distinguish a meshwork of tiny blood vessels just under the epithelium from which this color is derived. The mucous membrane covering the gums has a somewhat lighter red color. The gingival margins and the interdental papillae (the projections of gum between the teeth) have the same appearance as the rest of the gum.

The exposed portions of the lips are dry, vermilion in color, and usually are marked by slight superficial vertical wrinkling. Inside "the line of closure" the lips are moist and of the same even grayish-red color as the rest of the oral mucous membrane. The hard palate is usually a pale pink and shades gradually into the deeper pink and red color of the soft palate and the uvula.

This highly vascularized mucous membrane, like the skin, is constantly shedding its outermost layers. Metabolic changes, particularly those affecting capillaries and the formation of new cells, may easily alter this process and thereby alter its appearance. Like the skin, the mucous membrane has many highly differentiated appendages (papillae of the tongue, interdental papillae, and teeth), which react in predictable fashions under abnormal conditions. The oral cavity is dark, moistened by saliva and traumatized by the acts of chewing and smoking. Food, which collects in crevices and is attacked by bacterial saprophytes, ferments and forms the nidus for growth of pathogenic organisms. Such points of irritation have decreased tissue resistance and are frequently the first areas visibly affected by metabolic disturbances.

MEDICAL HISTORY AND PHYSICAL EXAMINATION

The physician may be approached by his patient primarily because of sore burning tongue and mouth "as though scalded by hot coffee," or this complaint may be uncovered only after careful history-taking in a patient who has some apparently unrelated difficulty, such as shortness of breath, weakness, or anxiety.

A careful investigation of the complaint of sore tongue and mouth is essential if the history is to be helpful. Such investigation should be directed toward establishing the onset, the duration, and the relationship of the sore tongue to seasons of the year, to types, quantity and quality of food, to smoking, alcohol ingestion, therapy with drugs, such as heavy metals, and to emotional disturbances. The relationship to other symptoms, especially those of the gastroenteric tract, is of great importance. Frequently an extremely accurate impression of the pathologic process responsible for the complaints can be gained by such a search. Even in the absence of a specific complaint referable to the oral cavity, this area deserves close scrutiny, because some patients with well-defined pathology either have no referable complaints or are so inured to them that they are ignored. Conversely, symptoms of sore tongue and mouth may be present and clinically significant even though no gross morphologic change is visible.

In most instances a careful gross examination of the oral cavity will give the internist as much useful information as he could gain from biomicroscopic examination and the use of other technical refinements. Occasionally, a small hand lens is helpful in studying detail of very early lesions.

In considering the *pathologic physiology* or *mechanisms* that may lead to *sore tongue* or *sore mouth,* a division into (1) systemic and (2) local conditions may be made. The systemic disorders include those of nutritional origin and a large and varied miscellaneous group.

SYSTEMIC DISEASES THAT MAY CAUSE SORE TONGUE AND SORE MOUTH

NUTRITIONAL DEFICIENCY DISEASES—VITAMIN B COMPLEX, VITAMIN C, AND RELATED DEFICIENCY STATES

Etiology. Nutritional deficiency diseases usually occur for one of the following reasons: (1) deficient intake of essential nutrients because of poverty, ignorance, anorexia, food fads, or diets prescribed or self-imposed; or because alcohol or vitamin-free carbohydrate is substituted for foods rich in essential nutrients; (2) deficient absorption of essential nutrients because of gastroenteric tract diseases, such as chronic ulcerative colitis and the malabsorption syndromes; (3) failure of utilization of essential nutrients as may happen when the liver is damaged; (4) requirements increased beyond the normal dietary intake as may occur in pregnancy, lactation, chronic febrile states, and hyperthyroidism; (5) increased elimination of essential nutrients in urine, feces, or vomitus as may occur in chronic diarrheal states; (6) decreased production of certain essential nutrients by colon organisms following prolonged oral administration of antibiotic drugs, especially sulfonamides; (7) blockade of chemical reactions by which essential nutrients are converted into biologically active compounds, competition of metabolically inactive analogues with their biologically active relatives for a locus on a protein apoenzyme, or destruction of the completed coenzyme. An example of blockade is the inhibiting effect of aminopterin (4-amino pteroyl glutamic acid) on folic acid reductase, preventing the conversion of folic acid to its active form, tetrahydrofolic acid. An example of competition can be found in the inhibitory effect that 4 desoxypyridoxine (a vitamin B_6 antagonist) has on enzymatic reactions, such as transamination, in which pyridoxal phosphate serves as a prosthetic group. Finally, irradiation may destroy coenzymes or apoenzyme-coenzyme complexes, or drugs like isonicotinic acid hydrazide may

conjugate with pyridoxal to form an inactive isonicotinic acid hydrazone. Should the history indicate that one of these situations may pertain, a close search should be made for symptoms and signs of nutritional deficiency disease.

Incidence of Nutritional Deficiency Diseases. Nutritional deficiency diseases tend to occur in the spring and to a lesser degree in the autumn. This seasonal variation holds true whether the deficiency is due to inadequate diet or is secondary to one of the other etiologic factors listed in the preceding paragraph.[12]

These diseases are most common in women during the childbearing period, in children during the period of rapid growth and development, and in men after their most productive years have passed. Bachelors and widowers who cook for themselves or eat in restaurants are prone to develop these diseases. Since wheat flour enriched with niacin, thiamin, riboflavin, and iron generally has been available throughout the United States of America, and with the improvement of the general standard of living of most American families, the incidence of full-blown nutritional deficiency disease has been reduced nearly to zero.

The diet still may be inadequate in very low income families, food faddists, chronic alcoholic addicts, or persons under the stresses of adolescence, pregnancy, lactation, chronic infections, hypermetabolic diseases, malabsorption, and old age. Less than 5 per cent of the robust people in the United States eat diets that are marginal in essential nutrients. Enough food is available so that no one need eat a deficient diet.[13] Only through continued elevation in the standard of living and repeated efforts at nutritional education for all people will nutritional deficiency disease be eliminated. Until this millenium is reached, the physician must be on the alert constantly for the symptoms and signs suggestive of the disordered metabolism resulting from insufficient essential nutrients.

Pathologic Physiology and Chemistry. A patient's sore tongue and mouth may be the only grossly visible sign that he has nutritional deficiency disease. Yet he is sick in every cell of his body and, indeed, has been biochemically sick for a variable period of time (the prodromal period of the deficiency state) prior to the appearance of the first gross or microscopic lesion. The vascularity, constant moisture, bacterial flora, foci of infection, and recurring slight traumatization, which are characteristics of the oral cavity, account for the frequency with which the earliest morphologic changes occur here. The deficiency diseases do not induce changes in resting tissues as quickly as in tissues undergoing constant regeneration and repair.

The abnormalities that occur in the mouth and tongue as a result of two different deficiency states may be identical. Conditions unrelated to deficiency disease also may produce the same changes in these organs. Although these observations have always puzzled students of nutrition, it is probable that the explanation lies in the rather restricted spectrum of changes possible in the tongue and mouth. One possible change is vasodilation, causing hyperemia and redness. Atrophy or hypertrophy of the epithelium, capillary rupture with submucous hemorrage and infarction, ulceration, and necrosis are still others. When one considers these limits on the possi-

bilities of reaction and the close chemical relationships of the nutritional deficiency diseases, it is not surprising that they frequently cause very similar changes in the tongue and the mouth. These oral lesions are the readily visible manifestations of gross or microscopic cellular damage, tissue inflammation, and hyperemia occurring in the esophagus, the stomach, and the intestine,[14] of lesions of the skin which may at this time be visible only under the microscope,[15] and of chemical changes in muscle, liver, and other viscera[16] which may be detected with the aid of highly specialized biochemical and bacteriologic technics.[17,18]

These chemical abnormalities of which we have some slight knowledge are the primary causes for the visible structural changes. Information gained from investigations in the respiration of yeast cells, bacteria, and various animal tissues indicate that many of

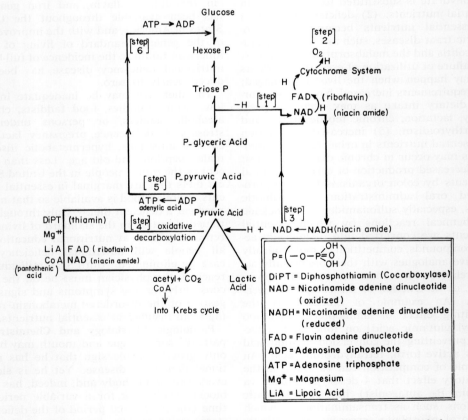

FIG. 7-1. A schematic representation of the Emden-Meyerhof pathway of carbohydrate oxidation illustrating the probable mechanism through which B-complex vitamins control and implement these reactions and the chemical interrelationships of these vitamins.

the vitamins, particularly the vitamins of the B complex and probably vitamin C, are integral parts of complex respiratory enzymes or catalysts.[19-22] These vitamins, after undergoing certain changes in the body, enter into and implement oxidation-reduction reactions, which allow the cell to breathe, perform work, and liberate energy. In the process, the catalyst is inactivated and then is regenerated, although the body is constantly incurring some loss of the catalyst or its progenitors through excretion. When these substances are absent, the cells lose their ability to utilize oxygen and die. When there is a deficiency of these substances, the body utilizes whatever stores of these essential substances may be available for such emergencies. Alternate and possibly less efficient reactions, which do not require the deficient substance also may be called into play. Only after these protective mechanisms break down does the essential respiration of the cell suffer and illness occur. Thus, the process of depletion is usually a long one, and all possible homeostatic mechanisms are utilized to protect vital cell functions.

Many of the B-complex vitamins are essential for certain biochemical chain reactions, each vitamin being responsible for the normal completion of one or more stages. The vitamins influence these processes after being chemically incorporated into coenzymes.

These coenzymes are organic compounds which, in the presence of specific protein enzymes, catalyze oxidation, reduction, transamination, decarboxylation, phosphorylation, and many other critical cellular reactions. Without either the coenzyme or the protein apoenzyme, the reaction stops. For instance, niacin, thiamin, riboflavin, and adenylic acid are essential for normal carbohydrate metabolism of yeast cells and probably of animal tissues also.

Figure 7-1 represents a simplification of the many reactions that may be involved in carbohydrate metabolism. It is included in this schematic form to facilitate visualization of the interrelated functions of many of the B-complex vitamins.

Niacin is an essential part of nicotinamide adenine dinucleotide (NAD), formerly called diphosphopyridine nucleotide (DPN). It is also an essential component of nicotinamide adenine dinucleotide phosphate (NADP), formerly called triphosphopyridine nucleotide (TPN). Thiamin is a component of cocarboxylase (diphospho thiamin) and transketolase. Riboflavin, also a precursor of several coenzymes, combines tightly with specific protein enzymes to form flavoproteins. It can fulfill its coenzyme role only when it is phosphorylated (riboflavin-5-phosphate) or when it is in the form of a nucleotide (flavin adenine dinucleotide). Adenylic acid may act as a means for carrying phosphate through reversible phosphorylation to adenosine diphosphate and adenosine triphosphate.

Nicotinamide adenine dinucleotide (NAD), in conjunction with its specific protein enzyme, catalyzes the conversion of a "triose phosphate" to phosphoglyceric acid (Fig. 7-1, step 1). In this oxidation reaction, it accepts a hydride ion (proton plus two electrons), (it acts as a dehydrogenase), and temporarily is reduced (to NADH), having oxidized the substrate, "triose phosphate." However, it may be regenerated by donating its excess hydride ion to flavin adenine dinucleotide, and in this manner it regains its original oxidized form (NAD). The flavin adenine dinucleotide is reduced when it receives this hydride ion, but is reoxidized when it transfers the hydride ion through the cytochrome system to oxygen (step 2). On the other hand, NADH may donate its hydride ion to pyruvic acid, thus implementing the reduction of pyruvic acid to lactic acid (step 3). In either case, NAD is made available again for the primary dehydrogenating reaction. Energy released in this NAD $\leftrightarrows$ NADH reaction is utilized for the phosphorylation of adenosine diphosphate to form the triphosphate (ATP).

Cocarboxylase, in conjunction with its specific protein enzyme, catalyzes the decarboxylation and oxidation of pyruvic acid through intermediate metabolites to carbon dioxide and water. It is regenerated when lipoic acid accepts the carbon remnant of pyruvic acid (acetate) from it. The acetate finally is shifted to coenzyme A and thence into the Krebs tricarboxylic acid cycle, while lipoic acid is regenerated through the action of nicotinamide adenine dinucleotide and flavin adenine dinucleotide (step 4). Adenylic acid after having been converted into adenosine diphosphate acts as a phosphate carrier by accepting phosphate ion from phosphopyruvic acid. It becomes adenosine triphosphate (ATP), and in turn transfers its energy-rich phosphate to hexose (step 6). Through this reaction, hexose phosphate and adenosine diphosphate are formed.

The B-complex vitamins are involved also in the direct oxidative pathway, which is fre-

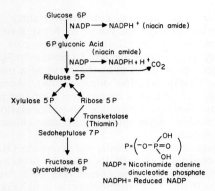

FIG. 7-2. Direct oxidative pathway for glucose or the hexose monophosphate shunt. The roles played by niacin and thiamin are indicated in this diagram.

quently called the hexose monophosphate shunt (see Fig. 7-2). Glucose-6-phosphate is oxidized to 6-phosphogluconic acid by the enzyme glucose-6-phosphate dehydrogenase, for which NADP (nicotinamide adenine dinucleotide phosphate) is the coenzyme. Further NADP-dependent oxidation occurs when phosphogluconic acid is converted to 3-ketogluconic acid 6-phosphate. Carbon dioxide is lost from the first position and ribulose-5-phosphate is formed. After some internal rearrangements, a 2-carbon ketone from xylulose-5-phosphate is transferred to ribose-5-phosphate to form sedoheptulose-7-phosphate. This transketolase reaction is catalyzed by thiamin diphosphate. Further rearrangements occur, leaving ultimately glyceraldehyde phosphate and fructose-6-phosphate.

It is probable that these and other vitamins of the B complex are essential for similar reactions in protein, fat, steroid, and nucleic acid metabolism. Pyridoxal phosphate, the coenzyme form of vitamin B_6, acts as a decarboxylase,[20] transaminase,[21] desulfurase,[22] and racemase[22] for certain amino acids. It is also essential for the conversion of tryptophane to nicotinamide derivatives (NAD),[23] and possibly for the interconversion of the essential fatty acids,[24] linoleic, and arachidonic acids. Pantothenic acid takes part in an enzyme system concerned with acetylation,[25] and folic acid and vitamin B_{12} are intimately connected with the formation of nucleotides and nucleic acid,[26,27] as well as phospholipid formation and the degradation of histidine through single carbon unit transfer.

The relationship of the B-complex vitamins to respiration and energy production has been stressed in the foregoing paragraphs. Emphasis also should be directed toward the role of these micronutrients in a much broader area of biochemistry. In many instances, the intermediates of these pathways as well as the level of reduction of the coenzymes exert a controlling influence on metabolic processes other than energy production. For instance, the level of NADH may be an important regulator for urate reabsorption by the renal tubule, for fat oxidation and mobilization, and for the direction of carbohydrate metabolism. The hexose monophosphate shunt pathway links with the glucuronic acid pathway through which uridine diphosphoglucuronic acid is formed, an important mechanism for mucopolysaccharide formation. Many drugs and bilirubin are excreted as glucuronides,[27b] and abnormal operation of the latter pathway may be important in producing the ground substance and basement membrane abnormalities found in patients with diabetes mellitus.[27a]

A strong reducing agent, vitamin C, is probably essential to many oxidation-reduction systems and phosphatase activity, although its exact chemical function has not yet been defined. It is essential to the normal metabolism of tyrosine and phenylalanine.[28] When vitamin C is deficient in animals, premature infants, or adult humans, intermediate phenolic products of the metabolism of these two amino acids appear in the urine in large amounts. A similar abnormality occurs when there is insufficient folic acid,[29] and it seems likely that a close biochemical relationship exists between ascorbic acid and folic acid. Ascorbic acid or other reducing agents are essential for the protection of the folic acid coenzymes (tetrahydrofolic acid and related compounds) from oxidative influences. This is another example of vitamin interdependency.

The biochemical abnormalities attendant upon vitamin C depletion probably lead to the basic pathologic changes of the scorbutic state, the failure of normal formation of collagen and intercellular cement substance. These fundamental abnormalities result in increased fragility of capillaries and decreased strength of fibrous tissue and other tissues of mesenchymal origin—the basic abnormalities of clinical scurvy.[30]

A discussion of all of the possible chemical aspects of nutrition and nutritional deficiency diseases is beyond the scope of this chapter.

PLATE 1

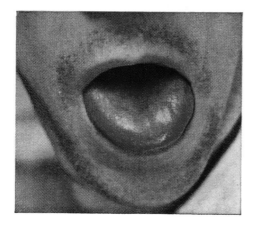
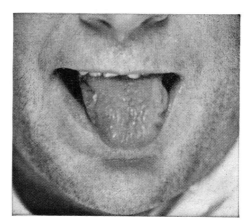
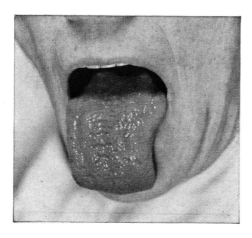
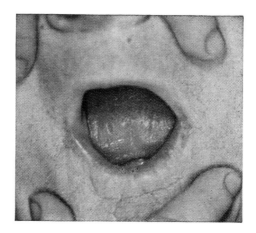

(*Upper left*) Acute pellagrous glossitis in a patient with pancreatic insufficiency and steatorrhea. The tongue is scarlet red, swollen and uncoated. Discrete hyperemic papillae are obscured by the swelling. Healing fissures are visible at the angles of the mouth. These are due to associated riboflavin deficiency.

(*Upper right*) Acute pellagrous glossitis superimposed on chronic pellagrous glossitis in a chronic alcoholic addict. The tongue is red, smooth, slick and deeply furrowed. No papillae are visible.

(*Lower left*) Magenta tongue of riboflavin deficiency in a patient with long-standing congestive heart failure and anorexia. The blue-red color is distinctive. There is moderate papillary atrophy which is probably the result of an associated chronic niacin deficiency.

(*Lower right*) Cheilosis of riboflavin deficiency in a patient with hepatic cirrhosis. These are superficial fissures and erosions at the mucocutaneous junctions of the angles of the mouth. The tongue is magenta.

PLATE 2

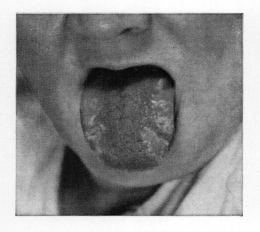
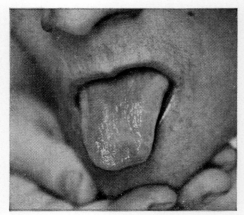

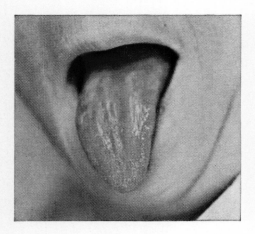
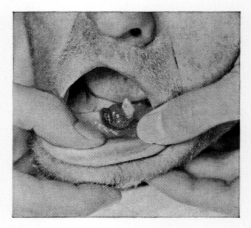

(*Upper left*) Geographiclike tongue in a patient with uncontrolled diabetes mellitus and neurotic vomiting. The bulbous papillae at the tip are of the "cobblestone" variety. This lesion cleared when diabetes mellitus was controlled and an adequate diet was supplemented with niacin and riboflavin.

(*Upper right*) Atrophic glossitis in a Negro patient with microcytic hypochromic anemia. The tongue is extremely smooth, pale and devoid of papillae.

(*Lower left*) Atrophic glossitis with leukoplakia. The posterior portion of the tongue is atrophic and streaked with thin whitish keratotic epithelium.

(*Lower right*) Acute scorbutic gingivitis. The gum surrounding the one remaining tooth snag is swollen and blue-red. The edentulous portion of the gum is normal.

Actually, biochemists only have scratched the surface of this very important subject. The chemical reactions cited, although they may be incomplete and possibly inaccurate in the light of future developments, illustrate most clearly the chemical relationships of the vitamins and in turn of the vitamin-deficiency diseases. These reactions show why nutrition must be adequate in all essential nutrients before health can be optimum.

Multiple Deficiency States. Deficiency diseases seldom occur as single clinical entities, although for didactic clarity they will be described as though they did. Under natural circumstances they almost always occur as multiple deficiency states. Deficient diets seldom if ever are lacking in only one essential nutrient. For instance, food deficient in one of the vitamins of the B complex is apt to be deficient in all of these vitamins and probably in minerals and protein also. In addition, many of the vitamins and minerals are essential for closely related biochemical reactions in the cells (Fig. 7-1), for the release of energy through the Krebs cycle and for the formation of the active coenzyme forms of other vitamins.

Niacin Deficiency (Pellagrous Stomatitis and Glossitis). As the niacin concentration in the tissues decreases, the deficient person may become aware of burning sensations in the tongue following the intake of hot or spicy foods. The continuous burning resembles the sensation commonly experienced following the ingestion of extremely hot coffee. This complaint may come and go; it is usually most intense during spring and fall seasons and is associated with mild anorexia, fatigue, nervousness, irritability, alternating periods of constipation and diarrhea, and burning sensations in the epigastrium. As the deficiency becomes severe, or a complicating disease develops which increases the body requirement for niacin, the mouth and the tongue may become so sore that it is impossible for the patient to ingest or swallow anything but liquid food. Concomitantly, other symptoms and signs may develop such as severe watery diarrhea, burning erythematous skin eruptions, cheilosis, angular stomatitis, seborrhea or dyssebacea in the nasolabial folds, mental confusion, delirium, and occasionally spastic paraplegia.

While the deficiency is mild, there may be no gross abnormalities visible in the tongue and the mouth, even though these structures may be hyperesthetic. If the deficiency continues or increases in severity, the fungiform papillae become increasingly vascular and prominent, imparting a distinctive redness to the tip and the sides of the tongue where these papillae are most numerous. At this stage these papillae stand out as swollen red globules on a background of apparently normal filiform papillae. However, the filiform papillae may be affected later. Those at the tip and the lateral margins are affected first, and from these areas the process usually spread backward toward the circumvallate papillae. The filiform papillae become swollen, denuded of epithelial tufts, hyperemic and fused in certain areas, giving the tongue an edematous, slick, fissured, fiery scarlet-red appearance. All coating is absent, and the teeth leave indentations along the margins of the swollen organ. Minute ulcerations may appear which enlarge and become infected with staphylococci, hemolytic streptococci, Vincent's organisms, or fungi. These ulcers frequently are covered with a white or gray membrane. Occasionally only one portion of the tongue, usually an area located at the tip or the side, is involved. This involved area may move from place to place on the tongue, leaving atrophic spots behind. This type of localized painful excoriation of the tongue has been called "Moeller's glossitis" in older literature.

The same fiery redness observed on the dorsal surface of the tongue occurs on the ventral surface and in the smooth mucous membrane of the cheeks, the gums, and the soft palate. The mucous membranes of the stomach, the rectum, the vagina, and the anterior urethra are affected similarly. The nasal mucous membrane frequently remains pallid in contrast with its boggy blue-red appearance in virus diseases such as influenza. Often superficial ulcerations may occur, particularly where the sharp edges of broken teeth irritate contiguous buccal mucous membrane. At this stage, the mouth and the tongue are extremely painful, and saliva may drool from the mouth and over the pillow and the bed clothes. All types of food are shunned by the patient because of the pain.

Remissions and exacerbations in this clinical picture may be anticipated even though the patient receives no crystalline vitamin or diet therapy. Morphologic changes that tend to be permanent occur as the deficiency state continues over months or years. In point of time this may be called a chronic deficiency state. The hyperemic, swollen vascular papillae, both fungiform and filiform, become flattened, atrophic, and gradually disappear, leaving a ridged or furrowed "bald" tongue. This bald tongue during periods of remission may be quite pallid, but during periods of exacerbation may again become fiery red. Frequently, even at this stage, the hyperemic rudiments of the papillae can be seen with the naked eye as small pinpoint red dots, especially along the tip and the sides of the tongue. The mucous membranes of the buccal cavity are affected by the same atrophic process, the interdental papillae of the gums recede, and secondary pyorrhea and other infections of the gums are common. Patients with chronic vitamin B complex deficiency diseases frequently lose their teeth at an early age because of these gum changes.[31]

The syndrome just described has been shown to be the result of niacin and tryptophane lack. Such a deficiency state has been induced in human beings by corn diets deficient in these substances but fortified with the other essential nutrients.[32] Glossitis occurred when the deficiency state was acute, whereas dermatitis was more likely when the deficiency state was induced more slowly. Whitish plaques and ulcerations developed under the tongue, cheilosis and angular stomatitis were observed as were diarrhea, irritability, restlessness, and weakness. This clinical picture developed when the niacin and tryptophane intakes were 4 and 180 mg., respectively, each day. Slightly more niacin and tryptophane provided by a "wheat diet" appeared to be protective.

With adequate therapy, acute pellagrous glossititis clears rapidly, frequently within 24 to 48 hours. In those patients with more chronic disease and glossal atrophy, regeneration of papillae may occur in time, usually after weeks of therapy. Much of the apparent regeneration observed early in the course of therapy is due to the disappearance of edema. The longer the period of deficiency, the slower and more incomplete the process of regeneration. Papillae may never regenerate on chronically scarred tongues, even after the most adequate therapy.

Riboflavin Deficiency (Ariboflavinosis). Riboflavin deficiency once was the most common deficiency disease in the southern part of the United States.[33] Symptoms related to the tongue and the mouth are usually mild. It is difficult to be sure that the usual burning sensations in the tongue experienced by the patient with riboflavin deficiency are caused by a lack of riboflavin or an associated deficiency of niacin. Tenderness and soreness at the corners of the mouth and along the lips usually are caused by cracking of the surface epithelium and secondary infection. In some patients moderate or severe morphologic changes in the tongue and the mouth due to riboflavin deficiency may produce no symptoms at all. The eyes, however, may burn, itch, or feel as though sand has found its way into them, and the patient usually is weak, irritable, and lacking in appetite.

As a rule, the first oral lesion is a painless grayish papule.[9] This lesion occurs at one or both of the angles of the mouth. The papule enlarges and gradually breaks down, resulting in a fissure, secondary infection, ulceration, and yellowish heaped-up crusts—angular stomatitis or perlèche (to lick).[34] The lips become red and fissured (cheilosis). Remissions are common, as in all deficiency diseases, but unless the diet is improved, relapse is almost certain. The process is extremely indolent, and remissions or relapses may persist for months. After several relapses the angles of the mouth may be scarred permanently.

The buccal mucosa of the cheeks is usually affected along with the angles of the mouth.[35] At first, the fine reticulated vascular pattern previously described as normal for this area is obliterated by engorgement, and the mucous membrane has a flat, dull-red color. With progression, the mucous membrane becomes edematous, grayish, and pebbly. It tends to exfoliate in sheets, causing a distinctive mottled or moth-eaten appearance; some areas are gray-pink and others dull red. Because of the swelling, the occlusal line becomes prominent, and individual tooth imprints may be visible. The lips are involved in the same process. That part of the lips within the line of closure has the same pebbly, moth-eaten, dusky-red appearance as the rest of the buccal mucous membranes. The vermilion borders of the lips exfoliate, dry, fissure, and crack (cheilosis). The line of closure is usually well-demarcated and exhibits a striking dusky-red color. The end stage of this stomatitis is an atrophic moth-eaten mucous membrane.

The tongue is affected less frequently in riboflavin deficiency. The fungiform papillae enlarge and become hyperemic, followed by a similar process affecting the filiform papillae. However, they do not lose their shape or surface epithelium as in niacin deficiency. In contrast, the epithelium thickens and becomes edematous, which produces the rows of bulbous hyperemic papillae of the so-called "cobblestone tongue." (This term has been applied to syphilitic glossitis with leukoplakia in the older literature.) Since thickened edematous mucous membrane covers the hyperemic vascular tuft of each papilla, the tongue is a diffuse dusky red or magenta color. This magenta tongue contrasts sharply with the brilliant scarlet red tongue of niacin deficiency.[7] The magenta color of the tongue may be deepened by the sluggish circulation in the dilated vessels of the papillae, essentially stagnation cyanosis.

Concomitantly, other grossly visible tissue changes due to riboflavin deficiency may occur. Conjunctival injection and diffuse superficial keratitis[36] are common findings. Erosions similar to cheilosis may occur at the ocular canthi, in the nasolabial folds, or at the mucocutaneous junction of the anus and of the vagina. Hypertrophy of the sebaceous glands over the bridge of the nose associated with plugging of the ducts of the glands may lead to a rough "sharkskin" effect. This process frequently affects the skin in the nasolabial fold as well as on the nose, and has been called dyssebacea. Seborrhealike dermatitis may occur in the nasolabial fold as well. Pure riboflavin deficiency induced in human beings by a diet containing 0.55 mg. of riboflavin daily caused angular stomatitis and cheilosis, and seborrhealike lesions of the scrotum and the external genitalia, but the magenta tongue, lesions of the oral mucosa, and of the eyes were not reported.[37]

After repeated episodes of acute riboflavin deficiency, scars may be found at the angles of the mouth and less commonly in the corneae. The mucous membrane of the mouth is thin and mottled. The tongue and the lips are fissured and dry. It is possible that some of the senile changes in conjunctivae, corneae, lenses, and skin, such as fatty and hyaline deposits, pingueculae, arcus senilis, cataracts, atrophy of the skin, senile hyperkeratoses, etc., are in part the result of chronic riboflavin and other long-standing vitamin-deficiency states.

Other B-Complex Deficiency States. No specific oral lesions in human beings can be related to a deficiency of thiamine, pantothenic acid, para-aminobenzoic acid, choline, or inositol. Rosenblum and Jolliffe[38] described a lesion characterized by irregular desquamation of the mucous membranes of tongue and buccal cavity leading to small whitish patches on a dull reddish-purple background suggestive of riboflavin deficiency. The lesion, however, responded to pyridoxine after niacin and riboflavin had failed to induce healing. Smith and Martin[39] reported cheilosis typical of riboflavin deficiency which responded to pyridoxine after riboflavin had failed. Vilter and his associates[40] have described oral lesions in 50 patients with vitamin-B_6 deficiency induced by desoxypyridoxine, a vitamin-B_6 antagonist.* The deficiency state could be induced most readily when the patient was on a diet poor in the vitamin B complex, but, with larger doses of the antagonist, it occurred in patients on a normal hospital diet. Erythema and atrophy of the tongue occurred in 14 patients, cheilosis and angular stomatitis in 3. The oral mucosa was involved, also, in either a diffuse or spotty erythematous process. A much more common lesion was seborrheic dermatitis, beginning in the nasolabial folds and spreading over the cheeks, the chin, the eyebrows, the forehead, down the neck, and over the shoulders. Peripheral neuritis occurred also. Patients with this deficiency state excreted abnormally large amounts of xanthurenic acid in the urine after a test dose of tryptophane, suggesting that the conversion of tryptophane to nicotinamide coenzymes was impaired. All of these lesions failed to respond to niacin, thiamin, and riboflavin, but improved within 48 hours after the administration of any of the vitamin-B_6 group (pyridoxine, pyridoxal, or pyridoxamine). Patients studied by Sydenstricker, Singal and Briggs[42] developed manifestations of biotin deficiency on a diet poor in B-complex vitamins but supplemented with the available crystalline members of this group, except biotin. The absorption of biotin from the gastroenteric tract was limited sharply by including desiccated egg white, containing the protein avidin (which combines with biotin and prevents its absorption), in an amount equivalent to 30 per cent of the total calories. The changes in the tongue varied from the geographic type to general atrophy of the lingual papillae or marginal atrophy. Cure resulted in

---

* A vitamin antagonist is usually a chemical analogue of the essential nutrient, so similar in structure that the cell cannot differentiate between the two. The antagonist, or "antimetabolite," as it is sometimes called, is biologically inactive and induces deficiency of the active metabolite by replacing the active substance in biologic reactions, bringing the reaction to an end.[41]

three to five days after the administration of from 150 to 300 μg. of biotin per day.

Acute folinic acid deficiency induced by aminopterin or amethopterin, antagonists of the reaction that converts folic acid to folinic acid, may cause very severe soreness and ulceration of the mouth and the tongue. These lesions usually begin as erythematous patches on the buccal mucosa or gums; the superficial epithelium sloughs and ulcers appear. These spread and may involve the entire oral cavity. Since the drugs mentioned above are among those used in persons with acute leukemia, the lesions frequently become purpuric, and infected with all varieties of organisms. If antibodies and cortisone have been administered also, fungal infections are frequent. The lesion cannot be differentiated with assurance on morphologic grounds from the purpuric secondarily infected ulcerating lesions of the acute leukemic process. However, lesions due to acute leukemia come and go irrespective of the drug being administered, and improve as a clinical remission is induced, whereas the lesions due to aminopterin toxicity usually respond rapidly when folinic acid is given.[41]

Such observations illustrate the morphologic counterpart of the biochemical interrelationships of the B-complex vitamins which have already been stressed. The fact that deficiences of different vitamins should induce similar morphologic changes in the tongue and mouth is not surprising when one recalls these chemical interrelationships, and the probability that the tongue and the mouth can respond only in a few ways to damage. These observations also illustrate the lack of specificity of a morphologic oral lesion for a deficiency of one member of the vitamin B complex. The lack of specificity of these lesions will be discussed in subsequent sections.

Atrophic Glossitis (Hunter's Glossitis; Beefy Tongue). As this chapter is written, atrophic glossitis cannot be considered as a disease entity. The acute glossal lesions of many systemic diseases (including those already described) may lead to atrophy of the glossal mucous membrane if adequate treatment is not given (see Fig. 7-3). We only can describe the lesion, catalogue the disorders that may be responsible, and speculate on their clinical similarities and probable metabolic interrelationships.[43-49]

The following are conditions with which

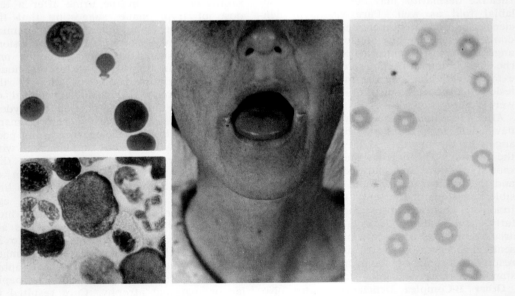

FIG. 7-3. (*Center*) Chronic atrophic glossitis and angular stomatitis in a patient with mixed vitamin B-complex deficiency disease. Similar lesions of tongue and mouth occur in patients with macrocytic megaloblastic anemia. (*Left, top*) Macrocytic erythrocytes. (*Left, bottom*) Bone marrow megaloblast. Patients with microcytic hypochromic anemia of chronic blood loss and iron deficiency also develop this lesion of tongue and mouth. (*Right*) Microcytic hypochromic erythrocytes.

TABLE 7-1. SYNDROMES CHARACTERIZED BY ACUTE GLOSSITIS OR GLOSSAL ATROPHY
AND MACROCYTIC ANEMIA CLASSIFIED ACCORDING TO PRESENT CONCEPTS
OF ETIOLOGY AND THERAPY

TYPE OF MACROCYTIC ANEMIA	CLINICAL CHARACTERISTICS					PROBABLE DEFICIENCY	INDICATED THERAPY
	FREE HYDRO-CHLORIC ACID	COM-BINED SYSTEM DISEASE	DIAR-RHEA	STEATOR-RHEA	RESPONSE TO PARENTERAL VITAMIN B_{12}		
Pernicious anemia	0	+	±	0	++++	Vitamin B_{12} due to intrinsic factor lack	Parenteral vitamin B_{12}
Nutritional macrocytic anemia	±	0	+	0	++++	Vitamin B_{12} and folic acid	Vitamin B_{12} Folic acid
Sprue	±	0	+	+	++	Folic acid and vitamin B_{12} due to malabsorption	Folic acid Parenteral vitamin B_{12}
Vitamin-B_{12} refactory megaloblastic anemia	±	0	±	0	±	Folic acid coen-zymes due to metabolic error	Folic acid
Megaloblastic anemia of pregnancy	±	0	±	0	±	Folic acid coen-zymes due to fetal demands, vomiting, and dietary lack	Folic acid
Megaloblastic anemia of infancy	±	0	±	0	±	Folic acid, ascorbic acid due to dietary lack	Folic acid Ascorbic acid

atrophic glossitis frequently is associated:

1. Vitamin-B_{12} deficiencies:

a. Addisonian pernicious anemia, due to a genetically conditioned lack of the mucoprotein substance called "the intrinsic factor," without which physiologic amounts of vitamin B_{12} cannot be absorbed from the intestinal tract[50,51] (see Table 7-1)

b. Postgastrectomy pernicious anemia, due to surgical removal of the stomach and elimination of intrinsic factor[52]

c. Fish tapeworm infestation, which interferes with the activity of the intrinsic factor[53]

d. Intestinal blind loop syndromes, and other mechanical gastrointestinal abnormalities, which allow proliferation of microorganisms that interfere with absorption of vitamin B_{12}[54]

e. The Vegans syndrome, or pure vegetarianism, which results in dietary deficiency of vitamin B_{12}[55]

2. Folic acid deficiencies:

a. Megaloblastic anemia of pregnancy, due to metabolic demands of the fetus for folic acid, maternal dietary inadequacy, and vomiting[56]

b. Vitamin-B_{12}-refractory megaloblastic anemia, due, it is thought, to failure of the metabolic processes responsible for the conversion of food folic acid to the coenzyme forms[57]

c. Megaloblastic anemia of cirrhosis, due to dietary lack of folic acid and to possible increased demands for folic acid as a result of liver failure[58]

3. Combined deficiencies of folic acid, vitamin B_{12}, and ascorbic acid

a. Nutritional macrocytic anemia[47]

b. Megaloblastic anemia of malabsorption syndromes, particularly sprue,[59-61] a disease of obscure etiology, which results in deficiencies of all the hematopoietic vitamins, but especially folic acid. Diseases of the small bowel, such as gluten enteropathy, regional ileitis, intestinal lipodystrophy, lymphoma, and tuberculosis are other examples[62]

c. Megaloblastic anemia of infancy,[63] a combined dietary deficiency of folic acid and ascorbic acid due to an unsupplemented milk diet. (Ascorbic acid deficiency in the adult may result in megaloblastic anemia when the dietary supply of folic acid is marginal or when alcohol ingestion increases the requirements.[70])

4. Iron-deficiency (microcytic hypochromic) anemia[64] due to blood loss

5. Idiopathic atrophic gastritis with achlorhydria

6. Chronic vitamin-B-complex deficiency disease

7. Glossal atrophy of unknown cause.

Symptomatically, the tongue and the mouth feel dry, and there are exacerbations and remissions of burning and tingling sensations and paresthesias of taste. Atrophy is the most prominent morphologic feature. In a quiescent phase the tongue is small, slick, and glistening. All vestiges of papillae except the circumvallate are absent, and the mucous membrane is thin. It is usually ridged and furrowed where the atrophic process has involved muscle underlying mucous membrane. If the patient is very anemic, the color of his atrophic tongue will usually be a faint pink. If he is moderately anemic, the color will be a dull red.

With exacerbations of the pathologic process which may occur at any time before adequate therapy is administered, the mouth is extremely sore so that only liquid foods can be tolerated. Diffuse swelling may occur, and the color may become the raw, bluish-red, shiny hue of rare beefsteak. Anemia must be severe (usually red blood cell count under 1.5 million or hemoglobin under 4 gm.) before the tongue remains pallid.

If the tongue is examined closely during these periods of pathologic activity, multiple small pinpoint red dots corresponding with the hyperemic capillaries of the atrophied papillae usually are visible. Small superficial ulcerations, erosions, and hemorrhages may occur in the mucous membrane. The ulcerations may become secondarily infected with any of a number of pathogenic or saprophytic bacteria or molds. In periods of remission and exacerbation the buccal mucous membranes have essentially the same appearance as does the tongue. Erosions at the angles of the mouth similar to those seen in riboflavin deficiency occur frequently, especially in association with chronic iron deficiency.

Periods of exacerbation usually correspond with or immediately precede periods of activity in the causative disease, e.g., a relapse in the anemia of pernicious anemia, although occasionally they occur while the anemia is under control or many years before anemia or other signs of the fundamental disease appear. Acute or atrophic glossitis also may appear as a manifestation of sprue before the appearance of steatorrhea.[65]

Each of the diseases with which atrophic glossitis is associated usually is characterized also by gastrointestinal disturbances, hypochlorhydria, achylorhydria or achylia gastrica, anemia that is macrocytic and megaloblastic (except in iron-deficiency states), and by multiple vitamin-deficiency diseases. Among the macrocytic anemias with glossitis, separation can be made on the basis of one or more distinctive clinical or laboratory manifestations or by demonstrating that a specific therapeutic agent will induce a remission of the glossal atrophy and the anemia (Table 7-1). The use of vitamin B_{12} labeled with radioactive cobalt has improved the accuracy with which some of the conditions resulting in glossal atrophy and megaloblastic anemia can be differentiated. When vitamin B_{12} is given orally to a patient with pernicious anemia, only a minute amount is absorbed. However, when the same dose is given with intrinsic factor, vitamin B_{12} is absorbed as effectively as in normal persons. Patients with sprue absorb vitamin B_{12} poorly whether or not intrinsic factor is given. Patients with dietary deficiencies of vitamin B_{12} or folic acid absorb vitamin B_{12} normally without added intrinsic factor. The physiologic defect of patients with intestinal lesions such as blind loops or pouches may be clarified by showing that tetracycline will frequently improve vitamin B_{12} absorption under these conditions.[86-88]

In addition to the data given in Table 7-1, iron will relieve the anemia, glossitis, and cheilosis of iron deficiency; niacin and riboflavin will relieve the glossitis and cheilosis of pellagra. Idiopathic atrophic gastritis and glossitis sometimes are benefited by folic acid, vitamin B_{12} or parenteral liver extract, or B-complex vitamins. Only too often no effective therapeutic agent can be found.

There is no explanation that is entirely

satisfactory for the morphologic similarity of the acute and the chronic glossal changes that occur in these apparently different deficiency states.

Deficiencies of the folic acid coenzymes and vitamin B_{12} interfere with the transfer of single carbon units, the former in a direct manner, the latter indirectly. Vitamin B_{12} seems to be necessary for certain reduction reactions of biological importance. Through these functions, both vitamins are involved in chemical chain reactions that culminate in the synthesis of nucleic acids. These reactions are blocked by a deficiency of either of these vitamin systems.[27] Studies of the growth requirements of certain microorganisms have suggested that the formation of thymine deoxyribotide is blocked by deficiencies of both vitamins. The formation of other purine and pyrimidine nucleotides may be blocked also, but such deficiencies are not so rate-limiting as is a deficiency of the thymine derivative. Since thymine,[66] uracil[67] and orotic acid[68] (a precursor of pyrimidines) given in large doses will induce remissions in persons with pernicious anemia, it is probable that the same relationship holds in human metabolism.

The megaloblast, which is characteristic of the bone marrow cytology in persons with pernicious anemia and related macrocytic anemias, may be a primitive erythroblast with abnormal or deficient nucleoprotein.[27] Cytologic changes similar to those seen in the megaloblast have been observed in the cells of the stomach and other mucosal surfaces, indicating the widespread involvement of tissues in these deficiency states,[69] the tongue no less than other parts of the gastroenteric tract. Since ribose nucleic acid (the cytoplasmic and nucleolar type) controls the formation of protein, and deoxyribose nucleic acid (the nuclear type) governs the processes of cell division and is the template for the formation of messenger RNA, one readily can see that fundamental aspects of cellular growth and multiplication are involved when folic acid or vitamin B_{12} are lacking.

The B-complex vitamins, niacin, riboflavin, vitamin B_6, and biotin (see preceding sections) have many different functions, most of which are concerned with the release of energy; iron is essential for the oxygen transport capacity of hemoglobin, and for the activity of the respiratory enzymes, catalase, and the cytochromes. A deficiency of any of these substances adversely affects the metabolism of all of the cells of the body, but certain areas, because of local conditions and demands, show the deficiency effects most strikingly. The tongue and the mouth are such areas and react to all these deficiency states in essentially the same way— with vasodilatation, inflammation, and edema, followed eventually by atrophy of the papillae and the surface mucosa. It is true that there are few other ways in which these tissues can react to injury, and this may be the real explanation for the similarity of appearance. On the other hand, all of these essential nutrients are chemically dependent upon each other and control fundamental reactions involved in the release of energy and the regeneration of cells. This, too, may be a common denominator.

Vitamin-C Deficiency (Scurvy). The principal complaints referable to the oral cavity in clinical scurvy are soreness, swelling, and bleeding of the gums. In advanced cases the distress may be so great that the patient is unable to chew food. Lesions usually occur late in the development of the clinical disease. Pyorrhea and other diseases of the gums seem to be predisposing factors favoring earlier occurrence. Gross lesions occur seldom, if ever, in edentulous scorbutic patients.

The first oral lesions of scurvy usually occur in the interdental papillae,[11] spread to the gingival margins and finally to the alveolar mucous membrane. They do not ordinarily extend beyond the alveolar-labial junction. Capillary dilatation and congestion are the earliest visible changes. The interdental papillae and then the gum itself become a deep blue-red color as blood extravasates into these tissues. Swelling occurs and the interdental papillae and the gingival margins may become so edematous that collars of swollen blue-red friable mucous membrane surround the teeth, and in advanced cases may almost cover them. Debris and microorganisms collect or are already present in pockets along the gingival margins. Infection and ulceration may spread from these areas to involve and destroy much of the gum. Infarction and gangrene of the interdental papillae may occur. Only in the most severely affected cases does one observe spontaneous oozing of blood or frank hemorrhages. Usually trauma is necessary to induce bleeding. When bleeding does occur, it is seldom excessive or exsanguinating. The breath is fetid, and salivation is increased.

As the process subsides, atrophy of the interdental papillae and retraction of the gums from about the teeth occur. With repeated exacerbations and remissions of the scorbutic process, there may be extreme recession of the gums from about the teeth. The net result may be the same as that following long-standing pyorrhea. The teeth loosen, rotate, or fall out in advanced cases because of rarefaction and reabsorption of alveolar bone. The gum becomes pale and scarred. Should an acute deficiency of vitamin C supervene, the gum may again become so blue-red and swollen that the atrophic phase is completely masked.

Other characteristic lesions of scurvy are: (1) follicular hyperkeratoses and perifollicular hemorrhages, especially on the extremities; (2) larger confluent ecchymoses, especially around the joints and the popliteal spaces or at sites of slight trauma; (3) painful, tender, sometimes swollen joints (hemarthroses); and (4) in children subperiosteal hemorrhages may occur before the gum changes are visible. In adults, normocytic or moderately macrocytic anemia usually occurs only after a prolonged period of severe vitamin-C depletion.[70] The anemia responds to the administration of vitamin C and seems to be due to interference with blood formation by the vitamin-C deficiency as well as by deficiencies of other essential nutrients, especially folic acid. Infants and children who have scurvy may develop more severe anemia, sometimes quite rapidly, because of loss of blood into the extensive subperiosteal hemorrhages.

OTHER SYSTEMIC DISEASES

Many systemic diseases or local irritative processes may produce lesions that at some stage are morphologically similar to those that occur in the vitamin-deficiency states. These various conditions must be recognized and understood in order to avoid mistakes in determining the mechanism producing the sore tongue or sore mouth.

Cirrhosis, Nutritional or Postnecrotic. Vitamin-deficiency diseases are common in patients with cirrhosis, particularly in those with the nutritional (alcoholic addict) type. Anorexia or vomiting may bring about deficiency states in persons with postnecrotic cirrhosis, too. When dietary-deficiency disease is responsible, dietary improvement or supplementation of the diet with B-complex vitamins will overcome the lesion. However, very frequently one finds a very red tongue, sometimes with papillary atrophy, sometimes with papillary hypertrophy, but always with dilated, engorged capillaries in the papillae or their remnants. Usually the oral mucosa is spotted with erythematous lesions also. These lesions usually do not cause pain, and they do not respond to any of the B-complex vitamins, to liver, or to yeast. As the liver disease improves, these glossal and stomal lesions improve also. The reverse is true when liver failure ensues. Soreness may then appear to be due to superimposed moniliasis, which can be recognized by the white patches that appear on lips, tongue, or soft palate.

Inability of the damaged liver to form coenzymes from the B-complex vitamins usually is considered to be the cause for this type of glossitis and stomatitis. However, this is an unproved hypothesis, and the glossitis may be due to a vascular reaction similar to palmar erythema and spider angiomata.

Leukemia, Hypoplastic Anemia, Idiopathic and Drug-Induced Neutropenia, and Idiopathic Thrombocytopenia. Sore, swollen gums from which blood constantly oozes may be found in patients with any type of acute or subacute leukemia, severe hypoplastic anemia, malignant neutropenia, or thrombocytopenia. Thrombocytopenia and capillary damage are responsible for the bleeding into the tissues, and the breakdown of the barriers against infection is responsible for the redness, ulceration, and swelling. Secondary infection and ulceration may make the mouth extremely sore and foul. Particularly in neutropenic states in which no polymorphonuclear neutrophils can be found in the blood, the mouth, the pharynx, and the tonsils may be severely inflamed, swollen, ulcerated, and necrotic (agranulocytic angina). So much tissue may be destroyed by the necrotic ulcers or noma that a sinus tract may form, and the lesion may present itself externally on the cheek. In acute monoblastic leukemia,[71] and occasionally in other types of acute leukemia, infiltration of the tissues of the gums with leukemic cells may account for some of the swelling and necrosis. Careful hematologic studies, with particular emphasis on the differential white blood cell count, platelet count, and bone marrow examination will establish the diagnosis in these cases.

The Erythemas and "Collagen" Diseases. Certain diseases of obscure eiology, such as erythema multiforme, disseminated lupus erythematosus, and periarteritis nodosa may produce painful oral lesions.

Erythema multiforme, when severe, may affect the mouth as well as the skin, eyes, genitalia, lungs, and joints (Stevens-Johnson syndrome).[72] The lesions may be of any type. In severe cases, bullae or purpuric vesicles may form. Secondary infection usually is superimposed and the mouth, the gums, and the tongue rapidly become extremely sore and foul. The oral lesions seldom occur in the absence of the skin eruption. One variant, called Behçet's syndrome, is characterized by arthritis, conjunctivitis, urethritis, keratodermia blennorrhagica, and erosive mucocutaneous vesicles. Reiter's syndrome is the eponym used when arthritis, urethritis, and conjunctivitis predominate. The oral and dermal bullae of these conditions must be differentiated from pemphigus and pemphigoid.

Disseminated lupus erythematosus may produce areas of purpura on the buccal mucosa which progress to infarction, secondary infection and necrotic sloughs, and shaggy, grayish ulcer.[73] The diagnosis will depend upon finding one or more of the other protean manifestations of the disease: (1) disseminated erythematous skin lesions, (2) serous pleural, pericardial, and peritoneal effusions, (3) arthralgia and arthritis, (4) nephritis, (5) myocardosis, (6) leukopenia, and (7) the lupus cell phenomenon.

A diffuse orange-red discoloration of the tongue associated with burning sensations in the organ has been noted in persons with fulminating periarteritis nodosa. None of the vitamins of the B complex or liver extract improves this glossitis. The etiology of the glossitis is as obscure as the primary disease.

Lichen Planus. This dermatologic condition is associated frequently with oral lesions, plaques scattered irregularly over the tongue of a whitish cast, and pearly lacelike or spider-weblike threads on the oral mucous membrane. Occasionally, these occur without typical skin lesions. The etiology is unknown, but one usually finds strong psychogenic factors in affected patients.

Systemic Infections, Scarlet Fever, Syphilis. In the early stages of scarlet fever the tongue is coated and dry. After two or three days, however, epithelial exfoliation begins. At first, only the swollen, red fungiform papillae can be seen which, on the gray background of the coated filiform papillae, give the tongue a "raspberry" appearance. The exfoliation continues until all papillae, filiform and fungiform alike, appear to be swollen red knobs. This is the so-called strawberry tongue. The oral mucous membranes and the lips may partake in the same process, and appear redder than normal. This enanthem is seldom painful; at least any soreness is obscured by the highly inflamed sore throat and cervical lymphadenitis so characteristic of the disease.

Secondary syphilis also produces oral lesions, the mucous patches, which are painless unless secondarily infected. These lesions may appear anywhere in the oral cavity. They are usually circumscribed, flat, superficial white or gray patches, which bleed easily when scraped. They are teeming with spirochetes. If they are widespread over the tongue and if secondary infection occurs, the tongue may become fiery red, painful, and flecked with white patches. Under these conditions, secondary syphilitic glossitis easily may be confused with acute pellagrous glossitis. At times differentiation will depend upon a careful history and search for other signs of primary and secondary syphilis or deficiency disease.

Tertiary syphilis usually does not produce painful lesions of the mouth. Solitary or multiple gummata may destroy large areas of tongue, palate, and gingiva without causing soreness or burning sensations. An obliterative endarteritis in the tongue during the secondary stage of syphilis may lead in the tertiary stage to atrophy of epithelium and muscle (glass tongue or sclerosing glossitis). This condition may be confused with atrophic glossitis, but in syphilitic glossal atrophy, the extensive replacement fibrosis can be determined by palpation. It is frequently the precursor of keratoses and leukoplakia. The rhagades or scars about the angles of the mouth and the lips in congenital syphilitics must be differentiated from scars in the same areas due to chronic riboflavin and iron deficiencies.

Exogenous Intoxications, Heavy Metals. Subacute or chronic poisoning with mercury or one of its salts may cause severe swelling, redness, erosion, and ulceration of the mouth, the tongue, and the gums. Mercuric sulfide, formed in the mouth from mercuric salts excreted by the salivary glands, acts as the tissue irritant. Salivation is excessive and the salivary glands may be tender and swollen.

Bismuth and lead poisoning usually lead

to deposition of bismuth or lead sulfide in a black line along the gingival margins when teeth are present—the bismuth or lead line. The pigment may be deposited in any part of the mouth, the pharynx, or the gastroenteric tract, in which infection or putrefaction of food and debris liberate hydrogen sulfide. Stomatitis of varying degrees of severity may occur in either case, but more commonly with bismuth poisoning, since bismuth sulfide is a more potent tissue irritant than is lead sulfide.

Dilantin Gingivitis. An occasional patient who is taking dilantin (diphenylhydantoin) for the control of epilepsy may develop hypertrophy of the gums, particularly when his oral hygiene is poor. The gums become sore, swollen, and bleed easily. As the condition progresses, the swollen gums may almost cover the teeth. Drug hypersensitivity is believed generally to be the cause.

Endogenous Intoxication, Uremia. Ulcerated, bleeding, and necrotic lesions of the gums and oral mucous membranes may occur in the terminal stages of renal insufficiency, but are only rarely the presenting symptoms. Usually these lesions occur only when nitrogen retention is profound and when there is a high degree of metabolic acidosis. The lesion may be single and located at a point where a broken tooth has irritated the oral mucosa or the tongue, or may be diffuse and involve large areas of the mouth. When the gums are principally involved and are swollen and oozing blood, a mistaken diagnosis of scurvy may be entertained. It is probable that these lesions are similar to the mucosal erosions that may occur throughout the gastroenteric tract in uremia, principally in the stomach, the duodenum, and the colon. The exact pathogenesis is unknown, but it probably is related to capillary damage and tissue infarction.

Allergy. Local contact, inhalation, or ingestion of various allergens may cause localized or diffuse erythema, swelling and ulceration of the buccal mucosa, the gums, and the tongue with sensations of itching and burning.[74] It is reported that allergy to amalgam tooth fillings or minute galvanic currents induced between several types of metal fillings in the moist oral cavity may produce localized areas of irritation, erythema, and burning sensations. Local contact testing with the suspected allergen or the therapeutic test of elimination of the suspected allergen will aid in differential diagnosis.

Antibiotics. Penicillin hypersensitivity has been implicated as a cause of the burning sensations of the tongue and the mouth which occur in many patients given this drug, particularly in the form of lozenges or troches.[75] More commonly, however, a different mechanism is responsible. Suppression of the normal bacterial flora of the oral cavity by the antibiotic allows uninhibited growth of other organisms, particularly fungi.[76,77] *Moniliasis* of the tongue, the mouth, the esophagus, and, in fact, any part of the gastroenteric, the tracheobronchial, or the genitourinary tracts has been found, particularly in debilated patients given penicillin for long periods. The tongue and the mouth may become sore and inflamed, ulcers may form, and usually the physician will see small white patches on the mucous membrane from which monilia can be obtained in smear or culture. Similar lesions occur in patients receiving aureomycin, terramycin, tetracycline, and chloramphenicol.[76] Usually in these cases the tongue is swollen, the papillae are edematous, and in some areas fused, producing a cobblestone, fissured appearance. The color most frequently is orange-red, but occasionally the scarlet red of niacin deficiency or the magenta color of riboflavin deficiency is so closely mimicked that it is impossible to differentiate the lesions by appearance alone. Diarrhea, itching and burning about the anus and the vagina, flatulence, and intestinal discomfort occur even more commonly than the oral symptoms and have the same cause.[76] There is no evidence that any of these lesions are due to interference by the antibiotics in the metabolism of any of the vitamins, although this suggestion has been made.

Persons taking penicillin, particularly by the oral route, occasionally have developed a painless, black hairy tongue.[77] The papillary tufts are much elongated, thickened, and fused, and pigment deposited on these unsloughed papillae gives the tongue a yellowish-brown or black appearance. This type of tongue lesion may occur and remit spontaneously in persons who have not had contact with antibiotics. In either case, the cause is usually overgrowth with a fungus, such as *Aspergillus niger*.

The lesions do not respond to any of the vitamins, but disappear within a few days or several weeks after the antibiotic is discontinued.

Menopause. Burning sensations in the tongue and mild glossal atrophy may occur as manifestations of decreased production of estrogens after the menopause. These changes are probably similar to those that occur in the vagina—senile vaginitis. Improvement is prompt when estrogens are administered.

Neurologic Lesions. Hypoglossal nuclear lesions occurring in amyotrophic lateral sclerosis, syringomyelia, and related conditions may lead to glossal atrophy. The atrophy of the muscle is much more striking than the atrophy of mucous membrane. The tongue is smooth, deeply furrowed, and paretic. Fibrillary twitchings may be present, and inadvertent trauma from the teeth may lead to soreness and pain. Supranuclear lesions involving sensory and motor tracts may lead to contralateral parasthesias, numbness, and tingling sensations, as well as slight paresis. Such lesions are seldom, if ever, the only cause for the patient's visit to the physician. Associated neurologic abnormalities will suggest the correct diagnosis and interpretations.

Psychoneuroses. Sensations of burning, dryness, stinging, itching, soreness, or taste disturbance (metallic) in the tongue and the mouth without any related objective evidence of inflammation or lack of salivation may occur as a manifestation of anxiety neurosis, which is said to be related to lack of sexual gratification and similar frustrations. Women in the postmenopausal period are affected most commonly. Men have this symptom only occasionally. Cancerophobia seems to be a commonly associated factor also.[78] Usually patients with neurotic glossodynia have had their symptoms for long periods of time with exacerbations and remissions related to emotional upsets rather than to seasons of the year, periods of dietary insufficiency, anemia, or local irritative factors. Frequently such patients date the onset of the symptom to the administration of an antibiotic. Occasionally tooth imprints may appear on the tongue of tense, anxious persons, who speak very infrequently, and who press the tongue forward against the teeth. This may occur in the absence of true glossal swelling. The underlying emotional factors must be clear before such a diagnosis is made. It must be remembered that in the prodromal period of niacin deficiency burning of the tongue is common without change in gross morphology. During this prodromal period, the patient is usually emotionally unstable, irritable, and anxious. In the absence of a history suggestive of a psychoneurosis, a therapeutic test with niacin may be necessary. The physician also must be aware that a patient with a psychoneurosis manifesting itself by faulty function of the gastroenteric tract may not eat an adequate diet and therefore may develop niacin deficiency as a secondary disorder. Only through careful interpretation of all available historical data can the physician hope to understand the true sequence of events.

LOCAL ORAL LESIONS

The following types of local lesions of the oral cavity must be considered in differential diagnosis: acute and chronic oral sepsis, pyorrhea, granulomas, lesions due to local trauma and irritation, certain conditions thought to be developmental abnormalities, and lesions of unknown etiology.[79-82]

Vincent's Stomatitis. Of the acute infections, Vincent's stomatitis (trench mouth) is probably most common. This disease, caused by Vincent's spirochetes and fusiform bacilli, is highly contagious and may reach epidemic proportions. The acute inflammation may involve any or all structures of the oral cavity and the throat. Painful ulcers form on the gingiva, the buccal mucosa, or the tongue. They are deep and may destroy considerable tissue. Fever and leukocytosis are common. There is considerable evidence that this disease usually attacks previously devitalized oral mucous membranes. The organisms are common secondary invaders of pellagrous lesions. Although the infection may be acquired by persons with no apparent underlying disease, the careful physician always searches for evidence of nutritional deficiency or other devitalizing processes when he is confronted by a patient with Vincent's stomatitis.

Herpetic Gingivostomatitis and Aphthous Stomatitis. Herpes zoster and herpes simplex may attack the tongue and the mouth and lead to very painful vesicular eruptions. Herpetic gingivostomatitis due to the herpes simplex virus (the common cold sore) tends to remain localized on the lips and around the nose in adults unless they are severely debilitated. Rather commonly in children and rarely in adults, these painful vesicles, which rapidly form shallow whitish ulcers with a red areola, involve the entire oral cavity and tongue. There may be fever and lymphadenopathy associated with this infection, and occasionally the virus attacks the skin over parts or all of the body. Children may have several attacks of this very painful disabling condition.

When similar ulcers occur singly or in groups of two or three, within the mouth, at the base of the tongue, or on the lips, the condition usually is called aphthous stomatitis or canker sores. They, too, are suspected of being due to viral infection. Frequently they may become secondarily infected with staphylococci and streptococci. They may last for a few days or a few weeks and are prone to recur. When they heal, they leave no scar because of the very superficial epithelial involvement. These ulcers occur commonly in adolescent youths, and in malnourished adults. They tend to occur also in persons with poor oral hygiene. No clear-cut etiology for the recurrence of these lesions has been discovered. Deficiency disease, allergy, local trauma, and psychoneurotic mechanisms have been suspected. Since etiologic mechanisms are unknown, a multiplicity of therapeutic agents has been recommended, none of which is of proven value. Improvement in oral hygiene and diet, elimination of such habits as thumb-sucking, repeated vaccination with vaccinia virus, hyposensitization to bacterial invaders, and psychotherapy are only a few of the therapeutic methods that have been proposed.[83]

Isolated simple papillitis of the tongue is extremely common—the single swollen exquisitely tender papilla on the tip or the sides of the tongue which appears suddenly, lasts a day or so, then disappears, leaving the tongue apparently normal. Occasionally under magnification, such an involved papilla appears as though it has burst and extruded a yellowish content. The cause of this phenomenon is unknown.

Enteritis. A virus type of enteritis in infants described by Dodd and Buddingh may cause painful vesicles on the tongue and in the mouth.[84] Infections with yeasts and molds, such as thrush, ordinarily do not cause pain.

Chronic Granulomas. Of the chronic granulomas, tuberculosis, actinomycosis, and blastomycosis may produce painful inflamed ulcerations of the tongue, the lips, and the mouth. Primary syphilitic chancre is usually nonpainful. Secondary syphilitic lesions, tertiary gummata, and sclerosing glossitis already have been described.

Hyperplasia of the deep epithelial layers of the mouth and tongue frequently may follow long-standing metabolic, infectious, or irritative glossitis. When such hyperplasia results in hyperkeratosis of the surface epithelium and the formation of white translucent plaques, we call the lesions *leukoplakia*.

Leukoplakia is usually asymptomatic. It frequently appears on a background of syphilitic or metabolic atrophic glossitis and commonly occurs in those who use tobacco excessively. Its chief importance lies in the fact that it is a precarcinomatous lesion.

Tumors. Benign and malignant tumors of the tongue and oral mucosa are rare. They are usually nonpainful unless secondarily infected.

Local trauma caused by poorly fitted dentures, sharp broken teeth, excessively hot coffee, or caustic and irritative medications may produce inflammatory changes and burning sensations lasting several days or as long as the trauma persists. Pipe smokers are acquainted with burning sensations in the tongue after excessive smoking.

An interesting lesion morphologically similar to the angular stomatitis of B-complex deficiency diseases may occur in edentulous patients or those whose dentures no longer are satisfactory because of shrinking of the alveolar ridge.[85] Because of malocclusion, the closed mouths of such patients often have deep crevices at the angles. Saliva and debris collect in these crevices, irritate and erode skin and the mucous membranes, and eventually cause deep, secondarily infected fissures. These perlèchelike lesions do not respond to vitamins of the B complex alone, but heal when the creases are eliminated by adequate dentures. It is probable that dietary deficiency in the beginning is often a contributory factor, but B-complex vitamins will not induce healing until the local traumatic factors of stagnant saliva and secondary infection are removed by mechanically opening the "bite."

Pain or burning sensations in the tongue and the mouth may occur in trifacial neuralgia, xerostomia (particularly in mouth breathers), and has been described in Costen's syndrome (auriculotemporal nerve disturbance due to temporomandibular joint displacement). The appearance of the mucous membranes is not altered in these conditions.

Certain other conditions of the tongue of developmental or unknown etiology also must be considered in differential diagnosis. Median rhomboid glossitis, a congenital anomaly possibly arising from remnants of the tuberculum impar, appears as a plaque on the dorsum of the tongue just anterior to the circumvallate papillae. The surface is smooth and glistening and covered with stratified squamous epithelium. It is painless and harmless.

Geographic tongue (glossitis areata exfoliativa—wandering rash of the tongue) usually appears at an early age. The surface of the tongue is divided into irregular zones by zigzag white lines, which are formed from thickened hypertrophic filiform papillae. Within these lines, the filiform papillae have atrophied, and isolated fungiform papillae appear larger and redder than normal. These "hills and valleys" give the tongue the appearance of a relief map—the geographic tongue. These areas of atrophy and hypertrophy may migrate or remain stationary. Usually the condition is painless, although at times the patient may experience sensations of burning. The etiology is not established. In some cases it may be a manifestation of vitamin-B-complex deficiency disease. In others it seems to be related to neurogenic disturbances; in still others it seems to be congenital.

SUMMARY

A burning sensation or soreness in the tongue and the mouth may be more commonly a manifestation of systemic disease than of local pathology. This chapter attempts to correlate these symptoms and the hyperemic, swollen, or atrophied mucous membrane of vitamin-B-complex deficiency diseases, scurvy, pernicious anemia, and related erythrocyte maturation factor deficiency states, iron-deficiency anemia, achlorhydria, and atrophic gastritis, and to explain these changes in light of deranged cellular biochemistry. Other systemic and local diseases are considered which may produce the same general complaints. A burning tongue and mouth, evaluated by careful history and physical examination, frequently provide the key leading to the solution of an otherwise obscure diagnostic problem.

REFERENCES

1. Adams, F.: The Genuine Works of Hippocrates, New York, William Wood & Co., 1886; 2 vol.
2. Hunter, W.: Further observations on pernicious anemia (seven cases): A chronic infective disease, Lancet 1:221-224, 296-299, 371-377, 1900.
3. Minot, G. R., and Murphy, W. P.: A diet rich in liver in the treatment of pernicious anemia; study of 105 cases, J.A.M.A. 89:759, 1927.
4. Spies, T. D., and Cooper, C.: The diagnosis of pellagra, Int. Clin. 4:1, 1937.
5. Spies, T. D., Vilter, R. W., and Ashe, W. F.: Pellagra, beriberi and riboflavin deficiency in human beings, diagnosis and treatment, J.A.M.A. 113:931, 1939.
6. Jolliffe, N., Fein, H. D., and Rosenblum, L. A.: Riboflavin deficiency in man, New Eng. J. Med. 221:921, 1939.
7. Sydenstricker, V. P.: The clinical manifestations of nicotinic acid and riboflavin deficiency (pellagra), Ann. Inter. Med. 14:1499, 1941.
8. ———: Clinical manifestations of ariboflavinosis, Amer. J. Public Health 31:344, 1941.
9. Sebrell, W. H., and Butler, R. E.: Riboflavin deficiency in man, preliminary note, Public Health Rep. 60:2282, 1938; 64:2121, 1939.
10. Kruse, H. D.: The lingual manifestations of aniacinosis with especial consideration of the detection of early changes by biomicroscopy, Milbank Mem. Fund Quart. 20:262, 1942.
11. ———: The gingival manifestations of avitaminosis C, with especial consideration of the detection of early changes by biomicroscopy, Milbank Mem. Fund Quart. 20:290, 1942.
12. Bean, W. B., Spies, T. D., and Blankenhorn, M. A.: Secondary pellagra, Medicine 23:1, 1944.
13. Wells, O. V.: Current food trends, Nutr. Rev. 17:161, 1959.
14. Spies, T. D., Bean, W. B., and Ashe, W. F.: Recent advances in the treatment of pellagra and associated deficiencies, Ann. Intern. Med. 12:1830, 1939.
15. Moore, R. A., Spies, T. D., and Cooper Z. K.: Histopathology of the skin in pellagra, Arch. Derm. Syph. 46:100, 1942.
16. Axelrod, A. E., Spies, T. D., and Elvehjem, C. A.: Effect of nicotinic acid deficiency upon coenzyme I content of human erythrocyte and muscle, J. Biol. Chem. 138:667, 1941.
17. Evans, E. A., Jr. (ed.): The Biological Action of the Vitamins, A Symposium, Chicago, Univ. of Chicago Press, 1942.
18. Baumann, C. A., and Stare, F. J.: Coenzymes, Physiol. Rev. 19:353, 1939.
19. Devlin, T. M.: The relation of diet to oxidative enzymes, in Wohl, M. G., and Goodhart, R. S. (eds.): Modern Nutrition in Health and Disease, ed. 2, p. 446, Philadelphia, Lea & Febiger, 1960.
20. Bellamy, W. D., Umbreit, W. W., and Gunselus, I. C.: Function of pyridoxine; conversion of members of vitamin B_6 group into codecarboxylase, J. Biol. Chem. 160:461, 1945.
21. Schlenk, F., and Snell, E. E.: Vitamin B_6 and transamination, J. Biol. Chem. 157:425, 1945.
22. Snell, E. E.: Summary of known metabolic functions of nicotinic acid, riboflavin and vitamin B_6, Physiol. Rev. 33:509, 1953.
23. Ling, C.-T., Hegsted, D. M., and Stare, F. J.: The effect of pyridoxine deficiency on the tryptophane-niacin transformation in rats, J. Biol. Chem. 174:803, 1948.

24. Witten, W., and Holman, R. T.: Polyethenoid fatty acid metabolism. VI. Effect of pyridoxine on essential fatty acid conversion, Arch. Biochem. 41:266, 1952.

25. Lipman, F., Kaplan, N. O., Novelli, G. D., Tuttle, L. C., and Guirard, B. M.: Coenzyme for acetylation, a pantothenic acid derivative, J. Biol. Chem. 167:869, 1947.

26. Stokes, J. L.: Substitution of thymine for "folic acid" in the nutrition of the lactic acid bacteria, J. Bact. 48:201, 1944.

27. Vilter, R. W., Will, J. J., Wright, T., and Rullman, D.: Interrelationships of vitamin B_{12}, folic acid, and ascorbic acid in the megaloblastic anemias, Amer. J. Clin. Nutr. 12:130, 1963.

27a. Winegrad, A. I., and Burden, C. L.: Hyperactivity of the glucuronic acid pathway in diabetes mellitus, Trans. Ass. Amer. Physicians 78–158, 1965.

27b. Touster, O.: Essential pentosuria and the glucuronate-xylulose pathway, Fed. Proc. 19:977, 1960.

28. Woodruff, C. W., Cherrington, M. E., Stockell, A. K., and Darby, W. J.: The effect of pteroylglutamic acid and related compounds on tyrosine metabolism in the scorbutic guinea pig, J. Biol. Chem. 178:861, 1949.

29. Govan, C. D., and Gordon, H. H.: The effect of pterolyglutamic acid on the aromatic amino acid metabolism of premature infants, Science 109:332, 1949.

30. Wolbach, S. B., and Bessey, O. A.: Tissue changes in vitamin deficiences, Physiol. Rev. 22:233, 1942.

31. Mann, A. W.: Nutrition as it affects the teeth, Med. Clin. N. Amer. 27:545, 1943.

32. Goldsmith, G. A., Sarett, H. P., Register, V. D., and Gibbens, J.: Studies of niacin requirements in man. I. Experimental pellagra in subjects on corn diets low in niacin and tryptophane, J. Clin. Invest. 31:533, 1952.

33. Spies, T. D., Bean, W. B., Vilter, R. W., and Huff, N. E.: Endemic riboflavin deficiency in infants and children, Amer. J. Med. Sci. 200:697-701, 1940.

34. Stannus, H. S.: Problems in riboflavin and allied deficiencies, Brit. Med. J. 2:103-105, 140-144, 1944.

35. Sandstead, H. R.: Deficiency stomatitis, U. S. Public Health Rep. (supp. 169), 1943.

36. Cleckley, H. M., and Kruse, H. D.: The ocular manifestations of ariboflavinosis; progress note, J.A.M.A. 114:2437, 1940.

37. Horwitt, M. K., Hills, O. W., Harvey, C. C., Liebert, E., and Steinberg, D. L.: Effects of dietary depletion of riboflavin, J. Nutr. 39:357, 1949.

38. Rosenblum, L. A., and Jolliffe, N.: The oral manifestations of vitamin deficiencies, J.A.M.A. 117:2245, 1941.

39. Smith, S. G., and Martin, D. W.: Cheilosis successfully treated with synthetic vitamin B_6, Proc. Soc. Exp. Biol. Med. 43:660, 1940.

40. Vilter, R. W., Mueller, J. F., Glazer, H. S., Jarrold, T., Abraham, J., Thompson, C., and Hawkins, V. R.: The effect of vitamin B_6 deficiency induced by desoxypyridoxine in human beings, J. Lab. Clin. Med. 42:335, 1953.

41. Schoenbach, E. B., Greenspan, E. M., and Colsky, J.: Reversal of aminopterin and amethopterin toxicity by citrovorum factor, J.A.M.A. 144:1558, 1950.

42. Sydenstricker, V. P., Singal, S. A., Briggs, A. P., DeVaughan, N. M., and Isbell, H.: Observations on "egg white injury" in man, J.A.M.A. 118:1199, 1942.

43. Oatway, W. H., Jr., and Middleton, W. S.: Correlation of lingual changes with other clinical data, A.M.A. Arch. Intern. Med. 49:860, 1932.

44. Manson-Bahr, P.: Glossitis and vitamin B_2 complex in pellagra, sprue and allied states, Lancet 2:317, 356, 1940.

45. Abels, J. C., Rekers, P. E., Martin, H. E., and Rhoads, C. P.: Relationship between dietary deficiency and occurrence of papillary atrophy of tongue and oral leukoplakia, Cancer Res. 2:381, 1942.

46. Harris, S., and Harris, S., Jr.: Pellagra, pernicious anemia, and sprue; allied nutritional diseases, Southern Med. J. 36:739, 1943.

47. Moore, C. V., Vilter, R. W., Minnich, V. M., and Spies, T. D.: Nutritional macrocytic anemia in patients with pellagra or deficiency of the vitamin B complex, J. Lab. Clin. Med. 29:1226, 1944.

48. Castle, W. B., and Townsend, W. C.: Observations on etiological relationship of achylia gastrica to pernicious anemia: the effect of the administration to patients with pernicious anemia of beef muscle after incubation with normal human gastric juice, Amer. J. Med. Sci. 178:764-777, 1929.

49. Schieve, J. F., and Rundles, R. W.: Response of lingual manifestations of pernicious anemia to pterolyglutamic acid and vitamin B_{12}, J. Lab. Clin. Med. 34:439, 1949.

50. West, R., and Reisner, E. H.: Treatment of pernicious anemia with crystalline vitamin B_{12}, Amer. J. Med. 6:643, 1949.

51. Herbert, V., Castro, Z., and Wasserman, L. R.: Stoichiometric relation between liver receptor, intrinsic factor and vitamin B_{12}, Proc. Soc. Exp. Biol. Med. 104:160, 1960.

52. MacLean, L. D., and Sundberg, R. D.: Incidence of megaloblastic anemia after total gastrectomy, New Eng. J. Med. 254:885, 1956.

53. Nyberg, W.: The influence of *Diphyllobothrium latum* on the vitamin B_{12}-intrinsic factor complex. I. In vivo studies with Schilling test technique, Acta. Med. Scand. 167:185, 1960.

54. Doscherholmen, A., and Hagen, P. S.: Absorption of CO^{60} labeled vitamin B_{12} in intestinal blind loop megaloblastic anemia, J. Lab. Clin. Med. 44:790, 1954.

55. Wokes, F., Badenock, J., and Sinclair, H. M.: Human dietary deficiency of vitamin B_{12}, Amer. J. Clin. Nutr. 3:375, 1955.

56. Gatenby, P. B., and Lillie, E. W.: Clinical analysis of 100 cases of severe megaloblastic anemia of pregnancy, Brit. Med. J. 2:1111, 1960.

57. Mueller, J. F., Hawkins, V. R., and Vilter, R. W.: Liver extract-refractory megaloblastic anemia, Blood 4:1117, 1949.

58. Jandl, J., and Lear, A. A.: The metabolism of folic acid in cirrhosis, Ann. Intern. Med. 45:1027, 1956.

59. Darby, W. J., and Jones, E.: Treatment of sprue with synthetic *L. casei factor* (folic acid, vitamin M), Proc. Soc. Exp. Biol. Med. 60:259, 1945.

60. Butterworth, C. E., Nadel, H., Perez-Santiago, E., Santini, R., and Gardner, F.: Folic acid absorption, excretion and leukocyte concentration in tropical sprue, J. Lab. Clin. Med. 50:673, 1957.

61. Althausen, T. L., DeMelendez, L. C., and Perez-Santiago, E.: Role of nutritional deficiencies in tropical sprue, Amer. J. Clin. Nutr. 10:3, 1962.

62. Vilter, R. W.: Treatment of macrocytic anemias, A.M.A. Arch. Intern. Med. 95:482, 1955.

63. May, C. D., Nelson, E. N., Lowe, C. V., and Salmon, R. J.: Patholgenesis of megaloblastic anemia in infancy; an interrelationship between pteroylglutamic acid and ascorbic acid, Amer. J. Dis. Child. 80:191, 1950.

64. Moore, C. V.: Iron deficiency, *in* Wohl, M. G., and Goodhart, R. S. (eds.): Modern Nutrition in Health and Disease, ed. 4, Philadelphia, Lea & Febiger, 1968.

65. Jolliffe, N., and Fein, H. D.: Some observations on acute and chronic glossitis, Rev. Gastroent. 15:132, 1948.

66. Spies, T. D., Frommeyer, W. B., Jr., Vilter, C. F., and English, A.: Thymine; antianemic properties, Blood 1:185, 1946.

67. Vilter, R. W., Horrigan, D., Mueller, J. F., Jarrold, T., Vilter, C. F., Hawkins, V., and Seaman, A.: Studies on the relationships of vitamin B_{12}, folic acid, thymine, uracil and methyl-group donors in persons with pernicious anemia and related megaloblastic anemia, Blood 5:695, 1950.

68. Rundles, R. W., and Brewer, S. S., Jr.: Hematologic responses in pernicious anemia to orotic acid, Blood 13:99, 1958.

69. Klayman, M. I., and Massey, B. W.: Further observations on gastric cytology of pernicious anemia, J. Lab. Clin. Med. 44:820, 1954.

70. Vilter, R. W.: Vitamin C (ascorbic acid), *in* Wohl, M. G., and Goodhart, R. S. (eds.): Modern Nutrition in Health and Disease, ed. 2, pp. 337-392, Philadelphia, Lea & Febiger, 1960.

71. Forkner, C. E.: Clinical and pathological differentiation of the acute leukemias, A.M.A. Arch. Intern. Med. 53:1, 1934.

72. Soll, S. N.: Eruptive fever with involvement of the respiratory tract, conjunctivitis, stomatitis and balanitis, etc., Arch Intern. Med. 79:475, 1947.

73. Harvey, A. McG.: Systemic lupus erythematosus, *in* Cecil and Loeb (eds.): Textbook of Medicine, ed. 10, p. 641, Philadelphia, Saunders, 1959.

74. Goldman, L., and Goldman, B.: Contact testing of buccal mucous membrane for stomatitis venenata, Arch. Derm. Syph. 50:79, 1944.

75. Goldman, L., and Farrington, J.: Contact testing of the buccal mucous membrane with special reference to penicillin, Ann. Allerg. 4:457, 1946.

76. Woods, J. W., Manning, I. H., Jr., and Patterson, C. N.: Monilial infections complicating the therapeutic use of antibiotics, J.A.M.A. 145:207, 1951.

77. Wolfron, S.: Black hairy tongue associated with penicillin therapy, J.A.M.A. 140:1206, 1949.

78. Karshan, M., Kutscher, A. H., Silvers, H. F., Stein, G., and Ziskin, D. E.: Studies in the etiology of idiopathic orolingual paresthesias, Amer. J. Dig. Dis. 19:341, 1952.

79. Rogers, A. M., Coriell, L. L., Blank, H., and Scott, T. F. McN.: Acute herpetic gingivostomatitis in the adult, New Eng. J. Med. 241:330, 1949.

80. Thoma, K. H.: Oral Pathology: A Histological, Roentgenological, and Clinical Study of the Diseases of the Teeth, Jaws, and Mouth, ed. 2, St. Louis, Mosby, 1954.

81. McCarthy, F. P.: A clinical and pathological study of oral disease based on 2,300 consecutive cases, J.A.M.A. 116:16, 1941.

82. Jeghers, H.: Medical progress; nutrition; the appearance of the tongue as an index of nutritional deficiency, New Eng. J. Med. 227:221, 1942.

83. Ship, I. I., Merritt, A. D., and Stanley, H. R.: Recurrent aphthous ulcers, Amer. J. Med. 32:32, 1962.

84. Buddingh, C. J., and Dodd, K.: Stomatitis and diarrhea of infants caused by a hitherto unrecognized virus, J. Pediat. 25:105, 1944.

85. Ellenberg, M., and Pollack, H.: Pseudoariboflavinosis, J.A.M.A. 119:790, 1942.

86. Schilling, R. F.: Intrinsic factor studies. II. The effect of gastric juice on the urinary excretion of radioactivity after the oral administration of radioactive vitamin B_{12}, J. Lab. Clin. Med. 42:860, 1953.

87. Halstead, J. A., Swendseid, M. E., Lewis, P. M., and Gasster, M.: Mechanisms involved in the development of vitamin B_{12} deficiency, Gastroenterology 30:21, 1956.

88. Jerzy-Glass, G. B.: Intestinal absorption and hepatic uptake of vitamin B_{12} in diseases of the gastrointestinal tract, Gastroenterology 30:37, 1956.

8

Thoracic Pain

JOHN R. SMITH and ROBERT PAINE

Pain arising in the chest, in common with pain originating elsewhere, may occur in the presence of local lesions of no seriousness, or may indicate important somatic or visceral disease. Thoracic pain may be difficult to evaluate, particularly when it is of visceral type. Chest pain may be the only presenting indication of disease.

Information regarding many types and mechanisms of thoracic pain is fragmentary. Other forms of chest pain, such as that from the heart and the pleura, have been investigated more extensively. In the short space of this chapter it will not be possible to include detailed descriptions of all the types of thoracic pain. The mechanisms of the common and important forms will be presented briefly.

ORIGIN OF PAINFUL STIMULI

There is now convincing evidence that there are nerve fibers specifically concerned with the transmission of pain impulses.[1,2] Further evidence indicates that tissue damage from trauma, bacterial invasion, or other disease stimulates pain nerve endings by tissue tension or by chemical factors present in the injured tissue, or by both these factors together.[1] It is clear that a wide variety of pathologic changes may lead to tension or chemical irritation to provoke pain; on the other hand, extensive tissue damage may be incurred, without pain, if these factors are absent.

Tissue Tension. That tissue tension will provoke pain is seen readily when a single hair is plucked. The pain is undoubtedly produced by direct tension exerted on the nerve endings.[3] Tension, applied to a wide area of normal skin, must be considerable before pain occurs; but tension (and chemical factors) in inflamed skin may produce exquisite pain. Inflammatory reactions are intensely painful when associated with much exudation ("as in the painful boil before pus issues from it")[3] or with edema. Throbbing pain occurs with the rise of tension from each pulse wave into inflamed areas. Distention of the adventitia of blood vessels is said to be painful,[62,89] perhaps reaching a peak of severity in dissecting aneurysms of the aorta. Some workers have considered the pain of angina pectoris and myocardial infarction to arise from tension on the sheaths of the coronary arteries, although this explanation is now not widely accepted. Abnormal dilatation of hollow viscera has been shown to be painful.[5] The role of tissue tension in pain stimulation is therefore important. The preceding examples are only a few.

Chemical Factors. The nature of the chemical excitants of pain in tissue injury is not known with certainty. It has been suggested that the liberation of potassium ions stimulates pain endings.[3] Moore *et al.*[4] demonstrated that pain nerve endings are sensitive to potassium ions in certain concentrations. Acid changes in certain tissue (i.e., ischemic muscle) may be adequate to produce pain.[4] Lewis[3] speaks of a "pain-producing substance" present in normal tissue, which is liberated when injury to the tissue is sustained. It is well-known that the contraction of muscle when the blood supply is impaired (ischemic) may give rise to intolerable discomfort. Such a condition may occur, for instance, following an arterial embolus after which a limb may become ischemic. It is seen to a lesser extent in the course of Raynaud's disease. Lewis and his co-workers[63] and others[64] suggested that the pain of muscle ischemia results from the accumulation of "metabolites" in the tissue with widespread irritation of pain nerve endings (cf. Cardiac Pain). It is further possible that such metabolites may accumulate in tissue, with infections or other diseases, in sufficient concentration to provoke pain.

Whatever such chemical factors may be, they operate, often together with tension within the tissue, to cause discomfort.

With these fundamental pain stimuli in mind, many painful symptoms find reasonable explanations when considered in relation to the known or to the suspected pathology in a given clinical problem.

Pathways of Pain. The impulses of all painful sensations below the level of the cranial nerves enter the spinal cord by fibers traversing the posterior ganglia and the dorsal roots and are transmitted to neurones in the posterior horns. The somatic and the visceral pain fibers share these pathways. Therefore, impulses from visceral nerve endings arrive at the same reception point among the posterior horn cells as do impulses of somatic origin. An appreciation of this merger into a common path is essential to the understanding of the distributions of pain in visceral disease. *Visceral pain will be noted in that somatic area with which it shares a final common path.*

The precise localization of somatic pain differs from the wider distribution of visceral pain because, in general, visceral pain is transmitted to several segmental levels, whereas somatic pain is transmitted to a single level. However, it is important to realize that the intensity and the duration of

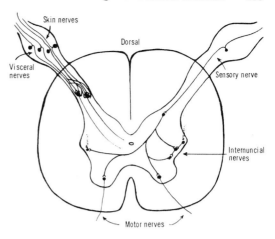

Fig. 8-1. Diagrammatic sketch of a cross section of the spinal cord illustrating certain nervous connections to explain the reference of pain. It is generally believed that visceral pain fibers may synapse in the spinal cord with certain neurones transmitting pain sensation from the skin. When these visceral pain fibers come under intense stimulation, the stimuli may affect the cutaneous neurones because of the crossed synapses, so that a sensation of cutaneous pain is simultaneously experienced. Referred pain may be due in part to reflex muscle spasm, also mediated through intraspinal nerve connections as shown at the right of the diagram.

painful stimuli also influence the extent of spread of pain to adjoining segments, whether the reception is visceral or somatic. For instance, a traumatic injury to one digit may, after a time, be followed by discomfort in the entire arm and shoulder.

Extension of pain to other levels demonstrates the existence of intermediate neurones connecting the posterior horn cells with other areas in the cord. These include the spinothalamic tract, the intermediolateral nuclei, and the anterior horn cells as well as internuncial cells connecting with the higher and lower segments of the cord. Impulses transmitted to the spinothalamic tract result in thalamic and cortical action in the awareness of pain. Impulses transmitted to the intermediolateral (sympathetic) nuclei may call forth the sympathetic discharges responsible for causalgic states, and impulses transmitted to the motor cells of the anterior horn produce the reflex muscular spasm associated with pain.

PAIN ARISING IN THE CHEST WALL

The integument and the muscles of the chest wall are subject to essentially the same diseases as similar tissues elsewhere. The pain-sensory innervation of these tissues is conveyed to the dorsal roots through the cutaneous and the intercostal nerves. Generally, pain arising from the thoracic integument and other superficial tissues is sharply localized. Furuncles and other infections, contusions, and abrasions of varying severity may produce superficial, well-localized pain. Owing to the anatomic peculiarities of the thorax, pain of distinctive nature may arise from involvement of muscles, nerves, and bone. These will be considered separately.

INTERCOSTAL NERVE PAIN

Irritation of the intercostal nerves may arise from a *neuritis* of those nerves, resulting from trauma, systemic or upper respiratory infections or other toxic cause, or pressure upon the nerve.[7] The neuritis often is aggravated by exposure to cold. The onset of the pain is usually sudden. The pain is localized in the intercostal space, the patient being readily able to identify the exact site of tenderness. The nature of the pain may be stabbing, lancinating, burning, and, in severe cases, occurring in paroxysms when the patient breathes deeply, coughs, or moves suddenly. We have been interested in the frequency with which intercostal neuritis is localized about the precordium, leading the patient to believe that he has heart disease. However, in intercostal nerve irritation, localized tenderness may be found along the course of the inflamed nerve, and slight pressure elicits paroxysms of pain. Pressure points where tenderness is maximum may be located near the vertebrae, in the axillary lines, or near the parasternal lines.

Herpes zoster is a distinctive form of dorsal root irritation producing an acute inflammatory dermatosis. The disease occurs more frequently in persons who are chronically ill, or in malnourished individuals.[7] The sensory root ganglia and corresponding peripheral nerves may be involved in any region, although the process is usually restricted to a few successive roots and nerves. The formation of herpetic lesions generally is heralded by intense burning, or knifelike pain along the nerve course. When the intercostal nerves are affected, the patient may be aware of pain extending from the spine along the lateral thoracic wall to the anterior midline. The movements of the trunk and of respiration may be restricted because of the pain. The pain is continuous and usually is punctuated by paroxysms of increased severity. Frequently the pain of herpes zoster is incapacitating and continues for many weeks, even after the herpetic lesions have healed. During the disease, hypesthesia of the skin occurs; hyperesthesia is rare. The nature of herpes zoster is imperfectly understood. It appears to arise from irritation and intense hemorrhagic inflammation of the sensory root ganglia; the peripheral nerves show degeneration of fibers and occasionally evidence of active inflammation. Stern[8] has obtained a virus from the lesions which is similar to that of varicella. Antibodies have been demonstrated in patients convalescing from herpes zoster which are capable of neutralizing the virus present in the lesions. Others, however, have suggested[9] that, although there is a specific viral etiologic agent in herpes zoster,[100,101] the lesions may be precipitated by bacteria, by neoplasms, by chemical agents, and by other noninfectious, irritating agents.

Holmes[10] has called attention to *slipping rib cartilages* as important causes of chest pain. He notes that the costal cartilages of the eighth, ninth, or tenth ribs, on either side, may loosen from their fibrous attachments; this is followed by deformity—a curling upward of the end of the cartilage on the inner aspect of the rib, in close relation to the intercostal nerve. The condition is of traumatic origin. The manifestations of pain are varied. Usually the pain is a dull ache, often tolerated for years. Occasionally the pain is acute, stabbing, paroxysmal in type, incapacitating in severity. Localized tenderness to pressure over the lesion is present. The usual chronicity of the disease, together with location of the pain and the tenderness, ordinarily makes the diagnosis clear.

MYALGIA

Irritation of muscles is a frequent cause of somatic pain. Apparently muscle is a tissue from which only one sort of pain is produced; the discomfort is aching in nature.[6] The intense aching pain occurring during exercise of ischemic muscle is well-known.[63] Muscle pain of the same nature was noted by Lewis[6] when isotonic acids or hypertonic solutions were injected directly into the tissue. Firm squeezing of a muscle will likewise produce the pain. Muscle pain, if sufficiently intense, may be referred to other dermatomes common to the muscle itself, although often the pain is well-localized at the site of muscle injury.

Inflammation of muscles and pain may occur in a great variety of pathologic processes.[12,13] These processes may be local (e.g., trauma, hematomas) or diffuse (e.g., systemic infections, trichinosis, myositis ossificans, etc.). Perhaps the most common conditions provoking muscular pain about the chest result from exercise of "untrained" muscles of the shoulder girdle. Incessant or paroxysmal severe cough may render the intercostal muscles painful. Fibromyositis involving the shoulder muscles may occur; it presents no particular problem of identification, because the shoulder and the arms may be tender on motion, and the muscles are readily palpated for tenderness. Myositis involving the intercostal muscles may give rise to marked discomfort, and nodules and induration in the muscles[12] may be present. Another form of myalgia has been emphasized by Mendlowitz.[14] He noted in a large group of soldiers that strain of the pectoralis minor muscle may cause marked discomfort in the anterior chest wall. The pain was aching in character and was confined, in general, to the area of the muscle, including the corresponding shoulder. The pain did not radiate to the arms. Involvement of the left pectoralis minor muscle produced symptoms superficially resembling cardiac pain. Curiously enough, Dixon[12] found that pain of muscular origin may be relieved partially by the use of nitrites. This fact should be borne in mind lest the condition be confused with smooth-muscle pain.

OSTALGIA

The sources of pain from bone are the numerous sensory nerve endings in the periosteum and, to a lesser extent, in the endosteum. Therefore, bone disease may be present without pain until these structures are involved. Affections of the periosteum give rise to intense pain, usually well-localized, whereas chronic disease, often affecting the bone marrow and endosteum, may result in poorly localized pain of varying severity. Reference of the pain to corresponding body segments may occur by the mechanism already described. Trauma (with or without fracture) resulting in periostitis and acute osteomyelitis may affect the bony thorax or the spine. Exquisite tenderness occurs over the affected point.[7] The pain is sharp and severe. In osteomyelitis the pain may be continuous for many hours.

Bone pain in syphilitic aortitis may be continuous and so severe as to be incapacitating. Recently we have observed a number of cases of aortitis and aneurysm with gradual erosion of the sternum and contiguous costal cartilage. In these cases there was unremitting, well-localized pain, boring or burning in type. The usual analgesics provided little or no relief.

Intense, aching, boring back pain may occur in malignant metastases to the thoracic vertebrae,[15] as it does from carcinoma of the prostate or hypernephroma; often it is referred to the corresponding dermatomes. The pain is constant and usually requires continuous narcotization. Frequently, in our experience, the metastatic vertebral lesions cannot be seen roentgenographically, but their presence may be suspected from the intense symptoms and the finding of carcinoma elsewhere. Mediastinal tumors, other than aortitis, may provoke chronic aching or dull chest pain (often substernal) by pressure against the spine or the ribs. Hodgkin's disease and lymphosarcoma are common examples. Leukemia has long been known to produce costal pain in its advanced stages, particularly producing areas of point tenderness in the sternum.[16] Multiple myeloma, osteitis deformans and sarcoma, involving the ribs or the thoracic spine, may likewise cause ostalgia.

POSTERIOR ROOT PAIN

The clinical and the pathologic features of dorsal root pain and its differentiation from underlying visceral pain have been emphasized repeatedly.[102] Dorsal root pain refers to irritation, mechanical or otherwise, of the dorsal radicles in the proximity of the spinal cord. As with the other forms of somatic pain described before, root pain may be felt at the point of irritation, but is frequently referred to points along the peripheral course of a nerve. Root irritation of the thoracic spinal segments is often referred to the lateral and anterior chest wall.[17]

The lesions producing dorsal root pain may be toxic or infectious (radiculitis), but the pain is more frequently the result of mechanical irritation of the root due to spinal disease or deformity. Bony spurs about the intervertebral foramina in hypertrophic osteoarthritis may irritate the nerves upon motion of the spine.[19] Narrowing of the intervertebral spaces by compression of the intervertebral disks may bring pressure on the nerve trunks. Cervical ribs and apposition of the anterior scalene muscle to the brachial plexus have been noted to produce root pain referred to the chest wall.[19]

Smith and Kountz[17] observed that dorsal root pain may be caused by *thoracic deformity* alone. They reasoned that, in early osteoarthritis, swelling and thickening of the intervertebral disks straightens and lengthens the spine so that the spinal cord is drawn cephalad. This exerts tension on the spinal nerves in their exit through the intervertebral foramina, and they are irritated upon motion. As the spinal arthritis progresses, the vertebral bodies are thinned anteriorly with final anterior collapse to produce kyphosis (the characteristic hump). In this way, the spinal canal is even more lengthened, the spinal nerves are constantly taut, and irritation of nerves occurs upon motion of the column.

The pain of dorsal root irritation is often stabbing, or there may be twinges of sharp aching pain localized in the spinal region. The pain is accentuated upon motion, such as bending, use of the arms, or torsion of the trunk. Patients with spinal osteoarthritis commonly awaken at night in pain, pre-

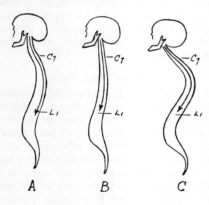

FIG. 8-2. Diagram showing position of the spinal cord with respect to abnormal degrees of vertebral flexion and extension. A illustrates normal spinal curvature. The end of the cord lies at the level of L-1 or L-2, indicated by arrow point. B and C show abnormal dorsal straightening and kyphosis occurring in spinal osteoarthritis. In both instances the neural canal is lengthened and the cord is relatively displaced cephalad. Tension is exerted on the spinal nerves.

sumably because relaxation in sleep allows the spine greater flexion and irritation of nerves by osteophytes or tension. Reference of the pain to the lateral and anterior chest wall is common; it may be sharp, but is often dull and aching in nature. Occasionally the discomfort is projected to one or both arms through branches of the brachial plexus. Referred pain occurring about the sternum and the shoulders, often paroxysmal, may resemble angina pectoris closely and sometimes is confused with it.[17,18] The confusion may be heightened by the partial relief obtained by the use of nitroglycerin.[18] Careful study of these patients will reveal a history of back pain; the pain is more superficial than heart pain (cf. Cardiac Pain), is only indifferently relieved by nitrites, and usually is associated with exertion involving the upper part of the body.

Upper anterior and posterior chest pain can result not only from dorsal root irritation but also from cervical disorders, because the distribution of nerves originating as high as C_3 and C_4 may extend as far caudally as the nipple line. The pectoral, the suprascapular, the dorsal scapular, and the long thoracic nerves originating in the lower cervical level can, upon irritation, cause pain in the chest, the midscapular, and the postscapular areas.

Although the anterior or ventral roots are motor in type, they can be productive of a dull deep boring type of discomfort when stimulated and can, therefore, produce a form of discomfort different from that attributed to posterior root disturbance. The anterior roots also play a role in the production of somatic echoes of visceral pain.

Breast Pain

With the accumulation of extensive data concerning disease of the mammary tissue, particularly carcinoma, increasing importance has been attached to the prompt investigation of the symptoms or signs of breast disease.

The sensory nerves of the breast are gathered into the second, third, fourth, fifth, and sixth intercostal nerves through the terminal brachial and medial antebrachial cutaneous twigs of the lower four of these nerves.[20] In addition, pain fibers in the second intercostal nerves have a common connection with the intercostobrachial nerve of the brachial plexus. A few pain fibers may ascend in the second and third cervical nerves from the region of the clavicles. Further more, sensory impulses from the medial brachial and medial antebrachial cutaneous nerves, as well as from the ulnar, may enter the spinal cord in the same segments as sensory impulses from the breast tissue innervated by the upper intercostal nerves. Diffusion of pain from the breasts passes around the chest and into the back, along the medial aspects of the arms and occasionally over the neck.[21]

The integument of the breasts, including the nipples and areolae, shows accurate localization of painful superficial stimuli in common with integumentary structures elsewhere. Pain from cutaneous incisions, furuncles, contusions of the surface, and similar lesions is superficial and is generally readily identified by the patient. Fissuring of the nipples and inflammation in the papillary ducts and areolae will often produce intense, well-localized pain. The breast parenchyma seems to be peculiarly insensitive to painful stimuli[20] except when the stimulus occurs as the result of distention of the stroma. Such stromal distention may be confined to a small segment of the parenchyma (e.g., in some cases of carcinoma), or may involve large portions of the glandular tissue. Furthermore, it is possible that invading, malignant tumor tissue may involve pain nerve endings, so that pain may be severe and even constant. Inflammatory lesions, in addition to distending the stromal tissue, irritate sensory nerve endings and may produce severe pain.[22]

Inflammatory breast disease is a common cause of breast pain. The citation of a case of acute puerperal mastitis will exemplify certain types of mammary pain. We observed a young woman with bilaterally fissured nipples, two weeks postpartum. Localized pain in the nipples was so intense that nursing became almost impossible. There was intense pain to palpation of all of the breast tissue, which was engorged and grossly nodular. The pain, sharp, cutting, and aching, was referred to the axillae and along the medial aspects of the arms to the little and the ring fingers. There was a fever of 104° F. With infections of lesser severity, the symptoms may be misleading. Veil[23] studied a case of cellulitis of the breast displaying intermittent precordial pain and radiation of the discomfort to the left arm. Angina pectoris was considered to be present; however, with clearing of the cellulitis, all symptoms disappeared.

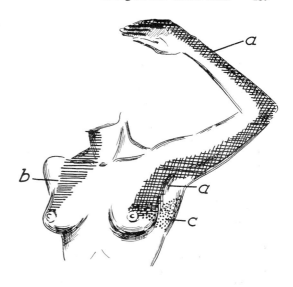

Fig. 8-3. Diagram illustrating diffusion of pain arising from the breasts. Cross-hatching (*a*) shows reference of mammary pain into axilla and along medial aspect of the arm. Pain (*b*) may be projected to supra-clavicular level and into the neck. Breast pain may diffuse around the thorax (*c*) through the intercostal nerves (see text). Pain may be referred to the back and to the posterior aspects of the shoulder girdle (not shown).

Benign and malignant tumors of the breasts are common causes of painful symptoms. It seems possible that a tumor that is situated so as to produce distention of the mammary parenchyma, or involves pain nerve endings, may account for the pain.[20] However, large tumors may be present without necessarily provoking the symptom. The position and the nature of the neoplastic tissue would therefore appear to be primarily concerned in determining the presence of pain.

Mastodynia is one of the most common conditions producing mammary pain. The onset of pain is gradual, during months or years; frequently it is intensified in the premenstruum. The discomfort is present particularly in the upper outer quadrant of the breast, which is firm, thick and tender to palpation. The pain, at first, may be intermittent, occurring only at the premenstrual period, but later may be persistent. Jarring or movement of the breasts may accentuate the pain. It may radiate to the inner aspects of the arms as a dull (or intense) ache and is aggravated by motion of the arms. These breasts show imperfect lobular development with increased periductal stroma, epithelial proliferation, and changes tending toward cyst formation and adenosis.[21]

Other tumors and chronic inflammatory disease cause mammary pain that resembles mastodynia. Or there may be an aching within the breast, a prickling sensation, or lancinating pain projected along the side of the breast and into the axillae and the arms.[22,24] Cheatle and Cutler[25] state that the pain of carcinoma may be lancinating or stabbing, radiating to the characteristic places. The breast may ache incessantly, and the patient attempts to support it to prevent jarring. Cheatle and Cutler[25] further state that localized nodularity, tumor, and stabbing pain (if present) occurring in the same place in the breast calls for immediate investigation as to the presence of carcinoma. Pain in neoplastic breast disease is not uniformly present.

PAIN ARISING FROM THE TRACHEA, THE PLEURA, AND THE DIAPHRAGM

TRACHEOBRONCHIAL PAIN

The symptom of substernal pain from acute tracheitis is familiar to most persons. The discomfort is usually felt under the upper portion of the sternum and it is frequently described as a burning sensation. Coughing accentuates the discomfort. This pain is often accompanied by similar pain lateral to the sternum at points corresponding to the positions of the major bronchi. Sharp foreign bodies, such as fishbones, in

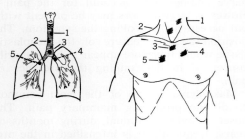

FIG. 8-4. When a bronchoscope is introduced into the tracheobronchial tree and when faradic stimulation is applied at points 1, 2, 3, 4 and 5, the patient may recall pain occurring at the corresponding points marked on the figure of the thorax. Note that the points of pain are homolateral to the areas of stimulation. Diagram based on the observations of Morton and his coworkers.[27]

the wall of the upper trachea may cause continuous pain in the anterior aspect of the neck.[26] Some patients with irritating foreign material, carcinoma,[28] or inflammatory lesions in the major bronchi will localize pain with accuracy in the right or left anterior chest, corresponding to the particular bronchus involved. Because of this, it is assumed generally that tracheobronchial pain is referred to sites in the neck or anterior chest at the same levels as the points of irritation in the air passages.

Although lower respiratory tract pain is common, the symptom has received scant attention. Investigation[27] indicates that stimuli applied directly to the tracheal or bronchial mucosa, in patients *under bronchoscopy,* are construed as painful sensations in the anterior cervical or anterior thoracic area. In addition, the pain is on the homolateral side of the neck or chest to the point of stimulation. The sites of pain are consistent and symmetrical. Morton *et al.*[27] further showed that section of the vagus nerves (below the recurrent laryngeal branches but superior to the pulmonary plexus) abolished the pain on the side of the vagus section. The cough reflex also was abolished. In a few instances, pain of tracheobronchial origin was referred to the contralateral side following vagotomy. These observations reaffirm the older suggestions that the pain-sensory innervation of the trachea and large bronchi is carried entirely in the vagus trunks. On the other hand, the finer bronchi and the lung parenchyma appear to be free of pain innervation.[26] Graham[26] frequently has cauterized the mucosa of small open bronchi through openings in the chest wall, the patient being unaware of the procedure except for cough from the smoke of searing tissue. Likewise, extensive disease may occur in the periphery of the lung without the occurrence of pain until the process extends to the parietal pleura. Pleural irritation then results in pain.

PLEURAL PAIN

It seems well-established that the parietal pleura is amply supplied with pain endings, and that the visceral pleura is insensitive. These facts were brought out in the interesting experiments of Capps and Coleman.[29] They introduced a large trochar and cannula into the pleural space in patients with pleural effusion, and stimulated various places on the pleural surfaces by means of a silver wire passed through the cannula.

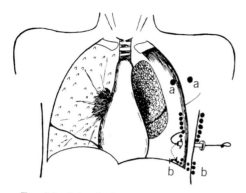

FIG. 8-5. Stimulation of the parietal pleural membrane by means of a silver wire produces sharp pain. Such stimuli to the parietal pleura of the anterior, lateral and posterior chest wall is referred to the superficial tissue at corresponding points in the wall (*a* and *b*) as shown in this sketch. Pain from pleural irritation is usually well localized.

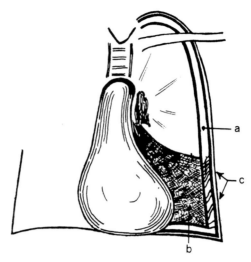

FIG. 8-6. Schematic diagram showing lobar consolidation and acute fibrinous pleurisy. The pleural space (*a*) is drawn in exaggeration, beneath which the consolidated lung lobe (*b*) is shown. Multiple fibrinous strands are represented by the small lines (*c*). Movement of the pleural surfaces in respiration will exert tension upon the fibrinous strands, pulling upon the parietal pleural membrane. Such tension upon the parietal pleura probably produces the exquisite pain which characterizes the disease, in addition to tension caused by widening of the interspaces on movement and friction of the inflamed surfaces. Actually, the fibrinous deposit is dense so that individual strands are not visible, and the pleural membranes show acute inflammation.

They found that the visceral pleura and the lung parenchyma were insensitive to such stimuli, but that stimulation of the parietal pleura gave rise to sharp pain. The pain could be well localized by the subject. It seemed clear, therefore, that pain arising from pleural irritation depends upon involvement of the parietal pleural membrane. Pain fibers, originating in the parietal pleura, are conveyed through the chest wall as fine twigs of the intercostal nerves. Irritation of these nerve fibers results in pain in the chest wall —usually construed as arising in the skin— which may be sharply localized, knifelike, and cutting in nature and accentuated on any respiratory movement. Arising in the most inferior portions of the pleura, the pain may be referred along the costal margins or into the upper abdominal quadrants. The discomfort often is relieved dramatically by anesthetization of the skin.[30]

The mechanism by which painful stimuli are initiated in an inflamed parietal membrane has been the subject of some discussion. It has been held generally that friction between the two pleural surfaces, when the membranes are irritated and covered with fibrinous exudate, produces the sharp pain. Other theories suggest that intercostal muscle spasm due to the pleurisy, or stretching of the parietal pleura, causes the characteristic pain. The latter theory is consistent with Bray's observation[31] that during inspiration the superior excursion of the ribs widens the intercostal spaces appreciably. The widening of the spaces, he reasoned, stretches the parietal pleural membrane; when the pleura is inflamed, such stretching irritates the pain fibrils, and sharp cutting inspiratory pain results. Although pleural stretching may be concerned in the production of pleural pain, other mechanisms have been suggested. There is evidence that pulling or tugging upon the membrane causes severe pain. Goldman[32] observed that patients with artificial pneumothorax often develop pain when adhesions between the pleural surfaces are present. He believed that if adhesions are present when a lung is forcibly collapsed in pneumothorax therapy, traction on the parietal pleura by the adhesions results in pain. This suggestion affords an interesting explanation for the pain of acute fibrinous pleurisy. The paroxysms of

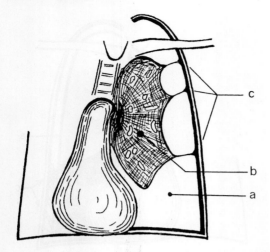

FIG. 8-7. Schematic diagram, showing partial collapse of the left lung by air in the pleural cavity (*a*) (pneumothorax). Complete collapse of the lung (*b*) is prevented by a number of "string" adhesions (*c*). It is readily understood how forcible collapse of a lung may produce tension upon the parietal pleural membrane when adhesions are present (as illustrated here); such tension explains the pain of pneumothorax when pleural adhesions are present.

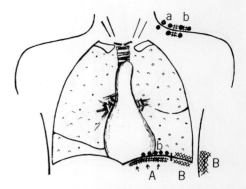

FIG. 8-8. Irritation of the pleura of the central area of the diaphragm (solid circles) causes pain along the superior ridge of the trapezius muscle and supraclavicular fossa (solid circles); stimulation of the marginal diaphragmatic pleura (xx) provokes pain at corresponding points in the thoracic wall (xx). Similarly, irritation of the central diaphragmatic peritoneal surface produces pain in the shoulder and neck of the same side and stimulation of the marginal peritoneal surface results in pain referred to the abdominal wall (xx).

pain may be due to many points of traction upon the irritated parietal pleura by countless fibrinous strands, as well as by stretching of the membrane upon costal movement. It also seems probable that irritation is further augmented by simple friction (clinically manifested by a friction rub) between the roughened surfaces of the pleural membranes.

Pleural pain is frequently encountered in acute fibrinous pleurisy complicating pulmonary inflammatory disease. Pneumonic processes reaching the extreme periphery of the lung cause a visceral pleuritis which quickly involves the contiguous parietal pleura. Pulmonary infarction may give rise to pleurisy if the infarcted tissue extends to the pleural surface. Krause and Chester[33] found that pain was one of the most common symptoms in their series of cases of pulmonary infarction. Tumor, especially bronchiogenic carcinoma,[34] may be attended by severe, continuous pain when the tumor tissue, extending to the pleurae through the lung, constantly irritates the pain nerve endings in the pleura. The occurrence of spontaneous pneumothorax is often signalized by severe pain, usually in the upper and lateral thoracic wall, and is aggravated exquisitely

by any movement and by the slight cough and dyspnea which accompany it.[35] It is probable that adhesions, brought under tension by rapid recession of the lung, cause such pain. Spontaneous pneumothorax may occur without pain.

As stated before, pleuritic pain is knifelike or "stabbing" in nature and its position is usually easily defined by the patient. Laughing, coughing, or even normal respiratory movement will produce paroxysms of exquisite pain. The notable exception is invasion of the parietal pleura by tumor, with which pain endings are constantly irritated.

DIAPHRAGMATIC PAIN

The diaphragmatic pleura receives a dual pain innervation through the phrenic and the intercostal nerves. Capps and Coleman,[29] using the technic described before, found that stimulation of the central portion of the diaphragmatic pleura with a wire resulted in sharp pain referred to the region of the superior ridge of the trapezius muscle (the somatic segmental area innervated by nerves of common origin to the phrenic). The peripheral rim, anteriorly and laterally, and the posterior third of the diaphragmatic pleura have pain fibers reaching the fifth and sixth intercostal nerves.[36] Stimulation of the peripheral portions of the diaphragmatic pleura

Fig. 8-9. Diagram of a transverse section through the thorax at a level immediately superior to the heart. The mediastinum and its contents are shown, together with the pleural and pericardial membranes. The pleuropericardial space is particularly exaggerated to accentuate its relationships clearly. (Based on an illustration in Gray's Anatomy of the Human Body, ed. 22, Philadelphia, Lea & Febiger.)

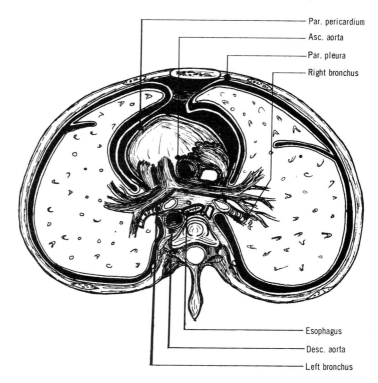

Par. pericardium
Asc. aorta
Par. pleura
Right bronchus

Esophagus
Desc. aorta
Left bronchus

results in sharp pain felt along the costal margins. The latter pain may be projected to the epigastrium, subchondral regions, or lumbar regions by the lower thoracic somatic nerves. The peritoneal surface of the diaphragm apparently is supplied by the same pain-sensory innervation, because stimulation of the central diaphragmatic peritoneum results in pain along the upper border of the trapezius.[29,37] Stimulation of the periphery of the diaphragmatic peritoneum causes pain reflected along the costal margins.

It is easy to understand, therefore, how affections of the diaphragm may be localized clinically by the position of the referred pain. *Diaphragmatic pleurisy*, secondary to pneumonia or pericarditis, is common, and sharp pain occurs along the trapezius or costal margins, accentuated upon the diaphragmatic motion in coughing or deep breathing. *Subphrenic abscess* may produce painful symptoms that are similar to diaphragmatic pleurisy. There may be tenderness to palpation about the costal margins with sharp pain occurring upon marked excursion of the diaphragm. Irritation of the central portion of the diaphragmatic peritoneum produces sharp pain in the shoulder on the affected side.

Herniation of abdominal viscera through a diaphragmatic hiatus may give rise to lower chest or upper abdominal pain.[38] It is often difficult to decide whether the pain originates in the diaphragm or from the anatomic distortion and disturbed function of the herniated viscus. Diaphragmatic hernias may provoke mild epigastric distress or pain simulating that of peptic ulcer. Reference of discomfort to the lower sternal area may resemble seizures of cardiac pain closely.[39] The overlapping of symptoms appears to depend on pain reference mechanisms of common distribution.

An interesting type of lower chest pain, attributed to the diaphragm, is "stitch"—a sharp pain occurring about the costal margin upon exertion. It was attributed by Moor[40] to interference with diaphragmatic motion. Capps[41] studied the sideache occurring on strenuous exertion at the right costal border in normal persons. He reasoned that diaphragmatic anoxemia might precipitate the pain. It seems reasonable that pain originating in the muscle of the diaphragm may be referred to the level of diaphragmatic attachment and the corresponding intercostal nerve.

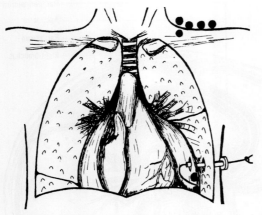

Fig. 8-10. Diagrammatic sketch of cannula and silver wire in the pericardial sac. Most of the pericardial surface is insensitive to pain, but stimulation of the sac at the level of intercostal spaces 5 to 6 produces pain referred to the superior border of the trapezius muscle and supraclavicular fossa.

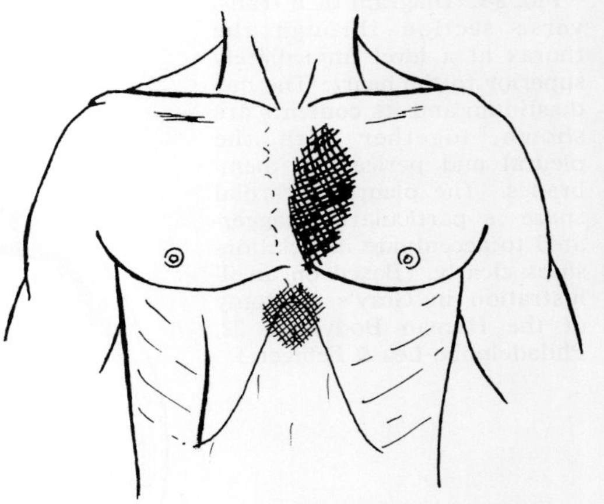

Fig. 8-11. Crosshatching illustrates the common sites of pain in pericardial disease. The pain may be substernal or to the left of the sternum and may be felt in the epigastrium. In some instances, pain may be more extensively referred (see text).

PAIN ARISING FROM ORGANS CONTAINED IN THE MEDIASTINUM; MEDIASTINAL PAIN

Pain arising from the mediastinum or its contained organs is frequently difficult to evaluate. Regardless of its origin, pain arising from various mediastinal structures has much in common and is frequently referred to identical peripheral sites. The subject is as difficult to present as such pain may be to interpret at the bedside. As an approach, it is well to recall that the mediastinum is a *space* bounded by structures that can give rise to pain in themselves. Disease of the thoracic spine, affections of the esophagus, the pericardium, the pleurae, and other structures produce pain that may be referable to the mediastinum. On the other hand, inflammatory lesions and tumors within the mediastinum may provoke pain if extensive or critically located. A few of the more common forms of pain arising from the mediastinum and mediastinal organs will be considered briefly.

Pericardial Pain

The mechanism of pain arising in pericardial disease is puzzling. One might think of the acute pain of pericarditis as occurring from the movement of opposed, inflamed pericardial membranes, or consider that pain may be produced by marked distention of the sac by fluid. However, the experiments of Capps and Coleman[29] indicate that there are very few pain fibers in the pericardium. Using their cannula and silver-wire technic, they stimulated the endothelial surfaces of the pericardium in patients with pericardial effusion. No pain resulted from scratching the visceral surface. With the same stimulus no pain occurred in the parietal layer except when the *parietal membrane* was stimulated opposite the *fifth and the sixth* intercostal spaces. Such stimulation resulted in sharp pain about the superior border of the trapezius as in central diaphragmatic stimulation (see Fig. 8-10). From these findings it seemed probable that a few pain fibers in the lower parietal pericardium, adjacent to the diaphragm, are carried in the phrenic nerves, but that elsewhere the pericardial membranes are devoid of pain sensation.

It remains to be explained why pain usually substernal or immediately to the left of the sternum, occurs in some cases of *acute pericarditis*. Since the pericardium is largely insensible to pain, it seems probable that irritation of contiguous structures must occur to cause the pain of pericarditis. The parietal pleura and the pericardium are in close apposition (see Fig. 8-9) in the mediastinal enclosure. Inflammation from an acute pericarditis then easily might spread to the neighboring pleura, producing pain,[29] or even to other mediastinal tissues. The situation of the pain (substernal or to the

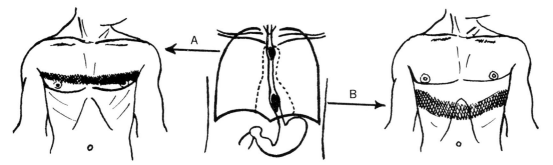

FIG. 8-12. Esophageal pain may be projected around the chest at the level of the spinal segment corresponding to the esophageal lesion. Schematically, pain from a lesion in the esophagus corresponding with the 4th thoracic spinal nerve (represented by arrow A in the central figure) may be referred as a band of pain about the thorax. An esophageal lesion at the level of the 7th or the 8th spinal nerves may manifest itself in pain about the chest following the course of those nerves (arrow B).

left of the sternum) is in keeping with the segment of pleura which may be involved. Barnes and Burchell,[42] studying pain in apparently benign pericarditis, noted that difficulty in swallowing, deep breathing, or torsion of the trunk frequently accentuated the pain, suggesting that an associated inflammation of the esophagus and other mediastinal structures was present.

As noted, acute pericarditis may be accompanied by pain that is substernal, along the left sternal border, or occasionally, epigastric. The pain is often sharp, lancinating, and paroxysmal; it may be continuous. The pain of pericarditis may be severe, closely resembling that of myocardial infarction[42] (cf. Cardiac Pain), although it is less agonizing and usually requires no narcosis for relief.

Pericardial effusion, often massive, is usually not accompanied by painful symptoms; however, in the series studied by Camp and White,[43] pain occurred not infrequently. Pericardial effusion may be manifested as a feeling of fullness within the chest, or as intermittent or continuous frank substernal pain, or ill-defined pain.[44] Distress of essentially the same nature may occur in tuberculous pericarditis.

ESOPHAGEAL PAIN

Esophageal pain, occurring as the only symptom, may be confusing because of its similarity to other visceral thoracic pain. Such pain presents itself as deep thoracic pain, or it is referred to corresponding somatic segments, conforming with visceral referred pain in general. However, other symptoms, such as progressive dysphagia, regurgitation of freshly eaten solid food, together with persistent pain or pain upon swallowing, suggest esophageal disease.

The esophageal mucosa appears to be more sensitive to pain in its upper portion than in the middle and the cardiac regions. Acid, regurgitated from the stomach, produces an unpleasant burning sensation in the upper thoracic, cervical, and nasopharyngeal regions, with no sensation referable to the lower esophagus.[47]

Pain arising from the muscular portion of the tube is clearly demonstrated in the experiments of Paine and Poulton.[45] They introduced tubes, to the ends of which balloons were affixed, into the esophagus. When the balloons were inflated in the lower esophagus, a burning pain was induced, becoming "gripping" in character when the subject swallowed. Paine and Poulton reasoned that distention of the organ is painful, and that muscle contraction, attempting to overcome distention, results in paroxysmal cramping pain. These observers further noted that pain from the distended esophagus may be substernal or epigastric or may be referable to the back, but that the level of the referred pain corresponds closely to the level of the distended portion of the esophagus through successive spinal segments. Thus, the higher the pain in the esophagus, the higher the level of pain felt about the sternum and the back.

Heartburn. Probably the most common symptom involving the esophagus is "heartburn." Heartburn is a vague term, and there is considerable difference of opinion as to the exact nature of the symptom. It may best be described as a "hot" or burning sensation occurring substernally or about the heart following a meal. It disappears within a short time. Heartburn has been attributed to regurgitation of acid gastric content into the esophagus, reversed esophageal peristalsis, or failure of the cardia to open promptly upon deglutition. Alvarez is of the opinion that, whatever the cause, it may be initiated by reversed gastric peristalsis.

Acute esophagitis may be caused by the swallowing of foreign bodies, such as bones or other sharp objects, spicy foods, and as a complication of acute infectious disease. The mucosa as well as the muscle may be involved. Paroxysmal pain upon deglutition is one of the most constant symptoms, the pain being substernal and radiating to the back. There is often no discomfort when the esophagus is quiescent, although dull discomfort frequently persists. Chronic esophagitis, often seen in chronic alcoholics and heavy smokers, or following acute disease, may produce essentially the same symptoms. In phlegmonous esophagitis, painful symptoms are accentuated markedly,[15] accompanied by fever, chills, nausea and vomiting and great fetor of the vomitus. There may be constant substernal and back pain, so accentuated upon swallowing that taking food is nearly impossible. Carcinoma of the esophagus, in itself, provokes no pain, although pain occurs with the esophagitis which frequently complicates it.

Cardiospasm (spasticity of the cardia) may not be accompanied by distress.[46] However, pain upon deglutition often occurs which is substernal, epigastric, or along the left border of the lower thoracic spine.

Esophageal pain, therefore, is referred to the sternum or back at the level of the lesion. Although the type and location of pain per se may be inconclusive, the occurrence of painful dysphagia and regurgitation of undigested food material, necessitating a liquid diet, and weight loss at once suggest esophageal disease.

MEDIASTINAL PAIN

Extensive mediastinal distortion from tumors or other disease may occur without producing painful symptoms. Indeed, enormous mediastinal tumors may be present with no discomfort to the patient other than cough, dyspnea, and moderate wheezing. Mediastinal lymph nodes involved by Hodgkin's disease,[53] neurofibromata, or other tumors may not give rise to pain unless nervous structures are involved. In explanation of such clinical phenomena it seems possible that the mobility of the mediastinum, together with the resiliency of the tissues that bound it, may allow for considerable distortion without necessarily irritating pain-sensitive structures. However, many mediastinal tumors do provoke pain, usually in association with dyspnea and cough.[51] The pain first may be manifest by a sensation of substernal weight or "oppression" which is ill-defined. Over a period of weeks or months the pain may become severe. The discomfort usually remains substernal, but varies greatly in intensity. Involvement of the esophagus by tumor in the posterior mediastinum may produce pain upon swallowing. Certain tumors, such as carcinoma of the lung apex (Pancoast),[54] may be accompanied by sharp axillary, shoulder, and subscapular pain radiating along the medial aspects of the arms. Large aneurysms of the aorta may produce symptoms, particularly when they exert pressure upon the chest wall, although vague discomfort appears to arise from the aneurysms themselves in some instances[55] (cf. Aortic Pain).

Spontaneous mediastinal emphysema is frequently accompanied by agonizing pain. The syndrome has been vividly described by Hamman,[50] who believes it to be more common than is generally thought. From his observations, it appears that rupture of the lung may occur through an attenuated alveolus; the air then dissects along fascial planes to the mediastinum. Pneumothorax occasionally complicates mediastinal emphysema, and it has been suggested that some cases of pneumothorax may result from unrecognized mediastinal emphysema. The condition often occurs when the individual is making no effort and is sitting or lying quietly. The accident is generally heralded by intense, agonizing substernal pain, radiating to the nape and to the shoulders. It seldom radiates to the arms. Such pain may persist for hours; indeed, a needle may have to be inserted into the mediastinum to permit the escape of air before relief is secured. In some instances the pain is milder, although it is "oppressive" and is substernal in location. Frequently a distinctive crepitus is heard, synchronous with the heartbeat, indicating the presence of air about the heart.

Mediastinal pain may be caused by acute inflammatory disease, or by traumatic rupture of the esophagus, or disintegration of the esophageal wall from carcinoma.[15,48] Occasionally inflammation may be caused by the passage of infection through lymphatics or by burrowing along the fascial planes of the neck.[48,49] Under such conditions the complaint of constant substernal pain is common, but the site of the pain is difficult to localize. The pain may seem to be present in the back, particularly if the vertebrae are involved, and percussion of the dorsal spine may elicit paroxysms of pain. Tenderness of the sternum occasionally has been noted. Pain may be accentuated upon swallowing if the esophagus is affected by the inflammatory process. Sudden motions of the trunk may be accompanied by severe discomfort. Painful symptoms of this nature should raise the question of mediastinitis, particularly if there are indications of infection in the neck, esophageal disease, or other lesions, such as retroperitoneal infection or pneumonia.

Chronic mediastinitis may arise as the result of tuberculosis, or following other chronic infections.[51] Occasionally, mediastinitis occurs for which no cause can be elicited, as described by Pick.[52] Chronic mediastinal inflammation may give rise to pain (together with dyspnea). The discomfort may be a severe, unremitting substernal oppression, or a burning and aching sensation substernally or in the precordium. Some cases may run their course with little or no pain. Frequently, striking physical signs occur which point to the underlying disease.

CARDIAC PAIN

ORIGIN OF CARDIAC PAIN

In 1768 William Heberden accurately described the symptomatology of angina pectoris.[56] As Osler aptly put it, Heberden said little about the cause of the disease and had the "good fortune to get very close to the truth in what he did say." Herrick's[57] classic description of acute coronary occlusion in 1912 gave impetus to the study of the recognition and cause of coronary insufficiency and cardiac pain. One consideration was almost immediately apparent, namely, that cardiac pain results from diminution or cessation of blood flow to the myocardium.[58,59,60] How such diminution of flow causes pain has remained a controversial question to date. Some authors have held that anoxemia of the myocardium provokes pain.[60] Others believe that important vasomotor reflexes or spasm of the vessels account for paroxysms of heart pain, the painful impulses arising from the vessels themselves. Others postulate that pain is provoked by distention of the walls of the coronary vessels. Wenckebach[61] suggested that sudden distention of the coronary arteries proximal to a point of occlusion or sudden distention of the aortic wall might provoke paroxysmal pain, a view that subsequently was amplified by Gorham and Martin.[62] However, these viewpoints have remained largely speculative for lack of conclusive support from animal experiments[60] and clinical observation.

At present, the conception most widely held in explanation of cardiac pain is that heart pain results from an *accumulation of metabolites* within an ischemic segment of the myocardium. The theory had its inception in the work of Lewis, Pickering, and Rothschild.[63] They applied pressure to an arm by blood-pressure cuff and noted the occurrence of intolerable pain a short time (70 seconds) after exercise of the arm was begun. Similar occlusion of the resting arm was not followed by pain despite the development of intense cyanosis. The conclusion was reached that during ischemic muscular contraction a substance is produced which causes pain, but that anoxemia alone does not produce such discomfort. Katz *et al.*[64] pursued this idea further and presented striking evidence that a substance, or substances, produced during muscular contraction, accumulates in the presence of ischemia and anoxia and provokes intolerable pain; angina pectoris and intermittent claudication were thought to be due to this mechanism. Thus, it seems possible that ischemia of the myocardium, whether it be transient (causing angina pectoris) or prolonged (producing the pain of myocardial infarction), may set off pain impulses by causing rapid accumulation of metabolites within the heart muscle.

Although coronary angiography has provided precise information regarding the coronary arteries of the intact human, other catheterization techniques have extended the knowledge of myocardial function from experimental animal preparations to the normal and diseased human heart.

These experimental and clinical investigations have demonstrated the predominantly aerobic nature of cardiac energy production. Oxidative processes within the heart muscle consume carbohydrate (glucose), fatty acids, lactate, and amino acids. The final combustion of each of these fuels is in the Krebs tricarboxylic acid cycle, which takes place within the mitochondria. Until the point of entry into this cycle, metabolic breakdown of glucose can proceed in the absence of oxygen and can produce small quantities of useful energy in the form of adenosine triphosphate. In the hypoxic state, pyruvate derived from glucose or amino acids is converted to lactate and is metabolized no further. The processes of the mitochondria are paralyzed in the absence of oxygen supply and the heart muscle, deprived of sufficient energy-rich ATP, rapidly loses the ability to contract.

In patients with coronary disease, areas of the myocardium deprived of normal arterial blood supply have been subjected to *venous* catheterization for analysis of the blood that drains the areas of ischemia. As anticipated, ischemic areas of myocardium have been distinguished by excessive quantities of lactate in their venous effluent. Other observations have demonstrated loss of contractility in these regions, a loss reflected in left ventricular failure during periods of coronary insufficiency.[110,111]

RESTRICTION OF CORONARY FLOW

From the foregoing discussion, it seems probable that the inception of cardiac pain results from *myocardial ischemia.* Furthermore, the evidence indicates that failure of myocardial nutrition occurs most frequently from insufficiency of the coronary circulation. The anatomic and physiologic factors governing the coronary blood flow have been investigated extensively and are of importance to the understanding of the genesis of ischemia of the heart muscle. These principles will be considered briefly.

The blood supply to the myocardium may be retarded or arrested by obstruction or distortion of the lumen of the arteries, and by changes in dynamics of flow from valvular disease, heart failure, or other mechanical disturbances. Another consideration is the reflex effect upon the coronary vessels which reduces the caliber of the arteries.

Obstructive lesions of the coronary vessels are encountered frequently at necropsy in the hearts of patients who have suffered attacks of cardiac pain.[65] The lesions are usually atherosclerotic. Less commonly, the coronary ostia may be narrowed critically in syphilitic aortitis, or the arteries may be occluded by emboli from endocardial disease within the left cardiac chambers. Atherosclerotic narrowing of the lumina may be so

marked that adequate coronary flow is maintained only at rest. Therefore, a rise in work load of the heart brought about by exertion or emotional stimulation may result in myocardial ischemia because of the failure of the vessels to provide the increased amounts of blood required. Under these conditions, the patient may suffer attacks of heart pain on effort. During rest, the coronary circulation again is adequate to meet the minimum requirements of the heart muscle; the attacks of pain cease.

Coronary Angiography. In recent years, coronary angiography has carried these studies from the postmortem table to the clinical radiology department, where with minimal risk the state of the major coronary vessels may be visualized in the living patient.[112]

By the insertion of an intra-arterial catheter in retrograde fashion through the aorta to the ostia of the coronary arteries, delineation of each coronary artery can be accomplished by injection of a radio-opaque dye.

In patients afflicted with coronary disease, angiography may reveal a variety of lesions. There may be a single isolated segment of narrowing or occlusion. Of the three major coronary arteries (the anterior descending, the left circumflex, and the right coronary arteries) the anterior descending is the most frequently diseased. It provides blood supply to the anterior and interventricular septal portions of the left ventricle and adjacent portions of the right ventricle. The right coronary artery is often the nutrient vessel for the conduction apparatus between the atria and ventricles and for the posterior, diaphragmatic portions of the ventricles. Because of their common blood supply, diaphragmatic or posterior myocardial lesions often are complicated by atrioventricular conduction defects, partial or complete heart block.

When isolated, lesions within the coronary tree most often lie within the proximal portions of the vessels near their ostia. However, the left coronary artery above its bifurcation into the anterior descending and left circumflex arteries is seldom found to be occluded by angiography, since interruption provokes ischemia of such wide extent as to be rarely compatible with survival.

Other patients present multiple lesions within the coronary tree, involving more than one of the three vessels with one or more points of narrowing or occlusion. In general, those patients in whom pain is most easily precipitated by exertion or for whom discomfort occurs during rest or upon the minimal stress of eating are found to have the more numerous angiography abnormalities. The specific referral of pain to arms, neck, or face does not appear to be related to the pattern of angiographic lesions.

Coronary angiography has clearly demonstrated the occurrence of coronary spasm manifest by minute-to-minute fluctuations of the vascular lumen, but, remarkably, change in vessel caliber has not been associated with pain regularly, and pain has occurred during angiography without spasm. The possibility that contraction of small vessels distal to those visualized by this technique is productive of myocardial ischemia cannot be excluded.

With relatively few exceptions, coronary angiography has revealed abnormalities in *all patients* who have been afflicted with angina pectoris or myocardial infarction. Consequently, the technique has been of great value in identifying the state of the coronary circulation in atypical cases.

The sudden obstruction of a major coronary vessel (usually by thrombosis) and the occurrence of frank myocardial infarction may be attended by violent pain. Fortunately, in many of these patients the remainder of the coronary circulation is sufficiently intact to assure cardiac function until the infarct heals.

It is interesting that some patients may have extensive coronary artery disease without infarction and without having suffered pain or impairment of cardiac function. Blumgart and his associates[65] have pointed out that gradual occlusion of the principal coronary vessels may be accompanied by the development of extensive anastomoses between the branches of the right and left coronary arteries. An effective collateral circulation then is established to enhance the circulation around points of obstruction (Fig. 8-13). Such enhancement of the circulation may sustain myocardial function for many years. The devious networks of vessels which bridge the occlusions of large arteries have been shown in various ways.[65,66] Smith and Henry[66] ligated major coronary vessels in the extirpated hearts of dogs. Subsequent perfusion of the vessels with an opaque material indicated that the twigs included in the obstructed area were filled readily by the rich anastomoses derived from neighboring

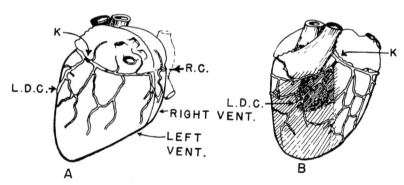

A   B

FIG. 8-13. (A) Diagrammatic sketch of a heart in which a theoretically *slow* occlusion has developed in the left circumflex coronary artery (at point K), and a second partial occlusion farther along the course of the vessel. Collateral channels from the left descending coronary artery (L.D.C.) and from the right coronary artery (R.C.) are shown in exaggeration, permitting circulation about the point of occlusion. Establishment of such collateral blood supply may be important in sustaining anatomic and functional integrity of the myocardium following obstruction of major vessels. (B) Sketch of a heart in which the left descending coronary artery is theoretically occluded *suddenly* at point K. Wide crosshatching indicates general area of ischemia distal to the obstruction. Although blood vessels near the point of occlusion may be filled, thorough irrigation of these vessels is lacking and an infarct forms in the area indicated by dense shading.

arteries (Figs. 8-14 and 8-15). Prinzmetal and his co-workers[67] were able to demonstrate that red blood cells labeled with radioactive phosphorus readily penetrated areas distal to the obstruction in the beating hearts of dogs and man, because of the rich collateral blood supply. They suggested that blood flow through collateral channels operates to limit the size of infarcts, thereby lessening the danger of cardiac rupture as well as promoting the process of healing. On the other hand, it is evident that further occlusions of arteries of the collateral system again may increase myocardial ischemia, or result in infarction of the muscle, possibly with attacks of cardiac pain.

Convincing experimental evidence also has been evolved to show that other mechanisms may operate to increase the coronary flow. Gregg et al.[68] observed marked increases in coronary arterial inflow when the right ventricle was placed under increased work by constriction of the pulmonary artery. The increased flow was evident even when the aortic blood pressure diminished. They considered the augmented flow to be due to dilatation of the coronary arteries by metabolites present in the working cardiac muscle. Similar observations were made by Smith and Jensen[69] in experimental acute heart failure. They demonstrated that, when the hearts of heart-lung preparations were made to fail by the administration of a toxic substance, there was a sharp increase in coronary inflow—even as the systemic blood pressure and cardiac output diminished. The phenomenon could be explained only by coronary dilatation. Therefore, it seems possible that any increase in work load for the heart muscle will result in greater blood flow from dilatation of the vessels. These experiments offer no clue as to the possible duration of coronary dilatation in hearts placed under chronic strain. Nevertheless, it is

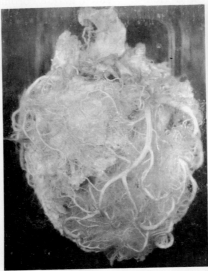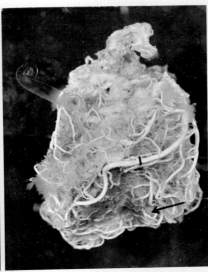

Fig. 8-14 (*Left*). Cast of the coronary arterial system of a dog heart filled with Neoprene latex. The heart muscle and blood vessels have been removed by digestion in concentrated hydrochloric acid. Delicate tracery of fine arteries and capillaries is preserved in the casting, which is suspended in water.

Fig. 8-15 (*Right*). Neoprene latex casting of the coronary arteries of a dog heart. The left descending coronary artery is prominently displayed on the surface of the cast. Previous to injection of the arteries with Neoprene, the left descending coronary vessel was ligated at the point shown by the small black line. After injection with latex, the left descending coronary artery distal to the ligation (black line) was filled from collateral vessels. The area below this artery (indicated by arrow) failed to fill with latex, leaving a depression in the casting. The specimen indicates that an abundance of anastomoses exists between the major coronary arteries and that the vessels which were not injected occupy a smaller area than would be expected from ligation of a large artery. (Smith and Henry: J. Lab. Clin. Med. 30:462) likely that the effects of coronary dilatation, and even of increased anastomotic circulation, may be neutralized largely by extensive narrowing and hardening of the vessel walls or by progressive occlusion of essential collateral channels. The flow may be insufficient to correct ischemia resulting from increased work, and exertional attacks of heart pain occur. Furthermore, it is observed often that drugs administered for the purpose of causing coronary dilatation appear to be ineffective, possibly because of previous continued dilatation of all of the vessels.

Interference with the dynamics of the coronary flow may be more difficult to understand. Passage of blood through the coronary vessels is dependent upon the head of pressure, the resistance to flow through the vascular bed, and the pressure existing at the venous end of the circuit. It must be assumed also that an optimum quantity of blood is available for irrigation of the system. The resistance of the vascular bed is modified further by the compression and relaxation of intramural vessels by myocardial motion. Certain alterations of any of these factors may be detrimental. Aortic valvular disease (stenosis or insufficiency) may modify pressures at the aortic openings of the arteries, reducing the net flow into the system. In addition, it is possible that *dilatation* of the chamber, with stretch of the myocardium, impedes the flow. When the inflow of blood is measured into an *atrial branch* of the coronary system, dilatation of the atrial chamber inhibits the inflow into the artery even when a high perfusion pressure is maintained.[70] Other evidence indicates that most of the blood which passes through the coronary arteries is returned to the right cardiac chambers through the coronary sinus, the anterior cardiac veins, and the thebesian system of veins. Therefore, the elevation of right intraventricular pressure and right atrial tension (increased venous pressure) of sufficient degree may reduce the effective pressure gradient between the pressure head (in the aorta) and the escaping venous blood, with consequent diminution of flow through the capillaries.[71] It is easy to visualize that in congestive heart failure, or in other conditions tending to *raise tensions in the right cardiac chambers*, the coronary flow may be impeded.

It has been postulated for many years that reflex coronary vasospasm may occur transiently, provoking myocardial ischemia and attacks of angina pectoris. However, coronary spasm has been difficult to produce in experimental animals, and the concept must be considered to be unproved.[60] It is notable that patients with attacks of angina pectoris frequently observe an increase in the severity and the frequency of the seizures when they are chilled and exercising. Riseman and his associates[72,73] exercised patients with angina pectoris in heated and cold rooms. These patients did not tolerate exertion in the cold room as well as in the warm air, and attacks of cardiac pain were definitely more frequent. In addition, a greater incidence of anginal attacks was noted by patients who were exercising in a warm environment when their hands were chilled by immersion in ice water or when they were holding ice cubes. These workers considered their findings as evidence that *reflex coronary constriction* may be an important factor in the precipitation of anginal seizures. This viewpoint and the alternate contention (that the angina of exertion occurs because of sudden increase in cardiac load and a disproportionately small coronary circulation) have not been reconciled completely. In light of the physiologic evidence now at hand, it is possible that both mechanisms of reducing coronary blood flow may operate to produce cardiac pain.

Occasionally, cardiac pain may be precipitated when the dynamics of the coronary circulation are normal. It is not uncommon for patients suffering from *pernicious anemia* to have attacks of angina upon exertion, presumably because of the primary lack of nutrition to the myocardium. Large doses of *epinephrine* may augment the work of the myocardium, beyond the existing coronary flow, and cause pain.[74,109]

In some instances the administration of digitalis in cardiac failure has been noted to produce angina pectoris or to intensify the frequency and severity of attacks[75]; fortunately, this is not the usual occurrence with the use of digitalis.[76]

With reference to any of these mechanisms, it appears to be basically important that *attacks of cardiac pain occur when critical myocardial ischemia is produced, either by an absolute diminution of the coronary blood flow or by increased demand on the heart out of proportion to the available blood supply.*

CHARACTERISTICS OF HEART PAIN

For convenience of discussion, cardiac pain will be considered as (1) paroxysmal (angina pectoris) and as (2) the pain of myocardial infarction.

Angina Pectoris. Typically, angina pectoris is characterized by the occurrence of substernal pain on exertion. Patients describe the pain as an "oppression," a tightness or crowding within the chest, or a heaviness substernally. Occasionally the sensation is said to be that of a viselike gripping of the sternum and the lateral chest, and less commonly it is described as burning. The pain is rarely severe; more often it is of moderate intensity. It is never stabbing, never precipitated by coughing or respiratory movements. As the pain radiates to the upper extremities and elsewhere, the sensation is characterized as an ache, a numbness, tingling, or other vague discomfort. The location of the pain is usually under the upper portion of the sternum, but it may be felt beneath the entire extent of the sternum. Anginal pain is usually, but not always, substernal. It may occur to the left of the sternum, in the precordium.[77] Under such conditions, the pain must be studied carefully, since pain in the precordium or in the region of the apical impulse is common to other disorders. Therefore, the occurrence of precordial pain must be interpreted with great care.[11]

The discomfort of angina pectoris commonly radiates from the substernal region. Frequently, the sensation is projected over the left pectoral region to the left shoulder and along the medial aspect of the left arm to the elbow.[77] The pain may be projected further through the forearm to the hand along the distribution of the ulnar nerve. Less commonly, the pain radiates to the right shoulder and arm with or without concomitant left-sided projection. Reference of the pain to the shoulders and to the inferior part of the neck has been described; these patients may have the sensation of a portmanteau clasped about the neck.[78] Occasionally, the pain is referred to the neck as a constriction, or as a pain in the left side of the neck and face. We observed a patient in whom substernal pain radiated through the neck and localized as a severe ache in the left temporomandibular joint; movement of the mandible intensified the pain. Radiation of the substernal discomfort to the epigastrium and the right costal margin also may occur, but such pain always has a thoracic component as well.[77]

Attacks of angina pectoris often are precipitated by excitement or exertion. They may occur at night as in aortic valve disease, or after meals. The paroxysms usually last a few minutes to a half hour and usually disappear quickly when the patient rests[77]; frequently the subject is forcibly halted by the severity of the attack. The administration of nitroglycerin or other powerful vasodilating drugs dispels the attack, and so many sufferers are taught to carry nitroglycerin or amyl nitrite with them to allay the seizures.

The pain of acute myocardial infarction is similar to that of angina, although gener-

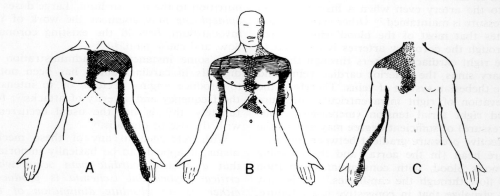

Fig. 8-16. Positions and common points of reference of cardiac pain. (A) Area of substernal discomfort projected to the left shoulder and arm over the distribution of the ulnar nerve. Reference of pain may be confined only to the left shoulder, or to the shoulder and along the arm only to the elbow. Less frequently pain may be referred to the right shoulder and arm (B) or to both shoulders, arms and hands simultaneously. Occasional radiation to the epigastrium and right upper abdominal quadrant may take place. Projection of anginal pain to the back is also encountered less frequently (C); reference is usually to the area of the left scapula or the interscapular region.

ally more severe and more prolonged. It is variously described. To some, it is an intolerable crushing or clutching, substernally or over the precordium; to others, it is a viselike gripping of the chest, or a pain the awfulness of which defies description.[79] The agony may be extreme. It often diffuses widely through the chest. Strong persons sometimes toss, pace the floor, and tear at the breast in anguish. In some patients the pain is moderate, or may be only slight. Unlike angina, the pain continues for hours and often is controlled only by large doses of morphine.

Radiation of the pain is similar to that of angina. When the pain is referred to the upper abdomen and is of explosive severity, the resulting upper abdominal symptoms may resemble acute hemorrhagic pancreatitis, perforation of a peptic ulcer, or other forms of acute abdominal conditions requiring surgery.[80,81] There may be muscle guard or even abdominal rigidity, which, together with fever and leukocytosis, frequently causes confusion. When the heart pain is referred to the right upper quadrant and back the condition is likely to be confused with cholecystitis.[81] In some patients the onset of myocardial infarction is signalized by a sensation of distention in the epigastrium, so that the patient believes himself to have "acute indigestion."

Myocardial infarction is followed not infrequently by a *painful disability of the shoulders and hands,* characterized initially by mild to severe pain in one or both shoulders.[103,104] Pain may arise immediately, or weeks or months after the infarction. There may be tenderness and limitation of motion of the shoulder, suggestive of periarthritis. Later the hand may become swollen, glossy, stiff, and painful upon motion.[82,83]

The etiology of the "shoulder-hand syndrome" is uncertain. It may be in part the result of persistent stimulation of the intermediolateral nuclei of the sympathetic nerves by internuncial transmission from the posterior horn cells. It is thought that chronic sympathetic stimulation can produce changes in blood flow to these somatic areas and contribute to musculoskeletal changes in the extremity.

Similarly, prolonged reflex stimulation of the anterior horn cells may provoke chronic spasms of somatic muscles, and subsequently inflammation of muscle and related cartilaginous structures. A mechanism seems evident which causes the tender spots on the chest wall and arm in the presence of myocardial disease. The basic similarity of this thoracic muscle spasm to the muscular rigidity in acute abdominal disease should be noted. It is also clear that the presence of similar tender, trigger areas does not necessarily relate *specifically* to a *visceral* disease, because it could result from any long-standing posterior horn cell stimulation, regardless of its origin. Once the tender area has developed, it is often self-perpetuating, supplying its own afferent pain sensation to maintain the reflex sensory motor arc. Not infrequently, one observes patients who, after myocardial infarction, complain of persistent anterior chest pain with the fear that the symptom results from continuing active myocardial ischemia. However, the myocardium may be healed and the pain stimuli may originate in the spastic muscles at the site of somatic referral; the somatic pain now may be both the cause and the result of the persisting muscle and joint irritation.

It is possible that operative procedures for the relief of "intolerable angina pectoris" often are effective because they do, in fact, involve incision of the sensory or motor nerves of this somatic-somatic sensory-motor cycle. Ligation of the internal mammary artery, a procedure formerly used in such cases, was effective occasionally, possibly because of interruption of the anterior intercostal nerves at the site of incision. Similarly, injection of procaine into the painful areas of the chest wall may result also in the interruption of the self-sustaining cycle and incur the permanent relief of pain.

After myocardial infarction and following operative procedures upon the heart, one or more episodes of chest pain, fever, and perhaps cough and dyspnea may occur.[105,106,107,108] There is often evidence of pericarditis, pleurisy, and pneumonitis in such instances. The pain is usually of a pleuritic or pericarditic type and can be distinguished from the pain of myocardial ischemia. The pathogenesis of these postinfarction and postcardiotomy syndromes may relate to the demonstrated presence of *antiheart antibodies* in the serum of these patients. It may be postulated that infarction, or incision, of the heart releases previously bound substances into the circulation to which the individual reacts with the production of antibodies. It has been postulated that the autoantibodies then attack the antigen in the pleura, pericardium, or myocardium, and incite an inflammatory reaction at these sites.

Precordial ache and tenderness. Functional precordial pain occasionally has been confused with cardiac pain.[11] Patients become alarmed at the occurrence of pain about the heart, and the physician should not be led into the pitfall of hasty or superficial consideration of these symptoms. White[11] has described carefully the "heart pains which are not angina."

Many persons complain of an aching about the heart when they are fatigued at the day's end. Others may notice sharp twinges of pain in the area of the apex beat, and the chest wall at that point is tender to pressure. Tense, hyperkinetic, easily fatigued persons frequently suffer from heartache. Such patients are often in good health and show no evidence of disease anywhere. In neurocirculatory asthenia and in some other types of neurosis, intense precordial aching

FIG. 8-17. (A) Course of cardiac sensory fibers along sympathetic nerves through the white rami and into the posterior spinal root. (B) Pathways of the fibers in the cervical and dorsal region. (C) Intraspinal pain tracts transmitting pain impulses from the heart to corticosensory areas. The ascending internuncials pass from the posterior horn cranially as far as the spinal nucleus of the trigeminal and provide the pathways of referral of cardiac pain to the arm, neck, and face.

or stabbing pain is often the principal complaint; a few of these patients are semi-invalids because of the pain and the belief that they are suffering from a fatal illness. On the other hand, precordial pain not infrequently occurs in the presence of marked cardiac enlargement. Although the discom-

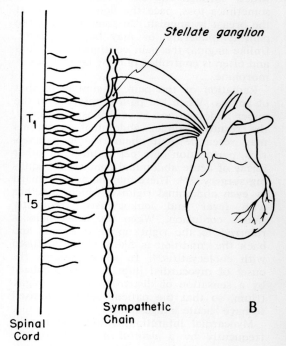

B

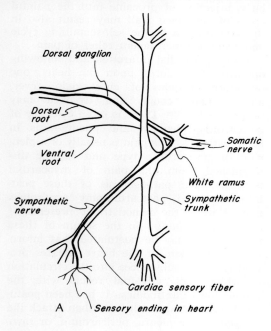

A

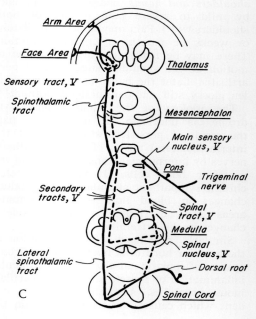

C

fort may be transient, it often persists for days and requires large doses of analgesic drugs. Because of its association with heart disease, the symptom may be confused with true cardiac pain. We observed a 19-year-old girl with acute rheumatic myocarditis and heart failure. The heart was greatly enlarged. She complained bitterly of sharp pain localized about the apex impulse, and palpation of the area revealed rather exquisite tenderness upon light pressure.

It is often difficult to find an explanation for precordial ache, particularly in persons of good mental and physical health. Possibly the constant impact of the heart against the chest wall irritates the intercostal muscles and nerves locally; fatigue then may translate the local irritation into symptoms of pain. This explanation would also seem to hold when such pain occurs with marked cardiac enlargement.

TRACTS AND REFERENCE OF CARDIAC PAIN

It seems well-established that pain fibers from the heart pass from the cardiac plexus, enter the upper five or six thoracic sympathetic ganglia (through which they pass without interruption), and thence on through the rami communicantes to the corresponding spinal (or dorsal root) ganglia. The cell bodies of these fibers lie in the spinal ganglia.[111] Afferent pain neurones also pass through the inferior, middle and superior cardiac nerves to the cervical sympathetic chains. They course downward to the inferior cervical and first dorsal (stellate) ganglion before passing across white rami into the dorsal roots. However, the majority of pain fibers from the heart course through the inferior cervical sympathetic and upper two or three thoracic ganglia. Elsewhere, they are much fewer in number. The pain neurones synapse with neurones of the second order in the posterior gray columns of the spinal cord (cf. Physiology of Pain). (See Fig. 8-17.)

Consideration of the anatomic transmission of cardiac pain immediately suggests the mechanism of reference of heart pain. It seems probable that the greater part of pain impulses reaching the upper dorsal ganglia are projected as pain in one or both pectoral regions; pain occurring along the inner aspects of the arms may result from common connections through the brachial plexus.

Within the central nervous system, as in the sympathetic chain, considerable longitudinal dispersal of fibers occurs. Internuncial fibers extending from the cervical posterior horns may run cranially as far as the spinal nucleus of the trigeminal nerve in the medulla. These are neurones, which provide the passageway for pain impulses arising in the heart to a final common path with facial sensation. Whatever the site of origin, referral of visceral pain depends upon merging of visceral and somatic afferents into a final common path. Although cardiac afferents in greatest numbers join with somatic sensory fibers in the upper thoracic and cervical area producing the commonplace pain referred to the arm, the sensory trigeminal plays a comparable somatic role. Referral is less frequent, apparently because of the relative scarcity of interneural connections between the upper cervical cord and the medullary nucleus of the trigeminal nerve. The more frequent occurrence of pain in the angle of the jaw than in the upper portions of the face appears to reflect the proximity of that portion of the facial sensory supply to greater numbers of cardiac internuncials.

Potential merging of cardiac and cranial afferents also is seen in the parallel courses of the spinothalamic and trigeminal tracts ascending through the medulla, pons, and mesencephalon. Their termination in adjacent areas of the thalamus may afford a third point of overflow of cardiac sensory impulses into the facial stream.

Immediately following coronary occlusion, collateral coronary flow has been found to be doubled. Subsequently, the enlargement of anastomotic vessels provides significant supply to areas of myocardial ischemia so that the area of damage or necrosis may be much smaller than would be expected from occlusion of the vessel. That the establishment of "adequate" collateral flow following occlusion generally requires several weeks is a major factor underlying the logic of the three- or four-week period of rest prescribed for patients after infarction.

It has been suggested that the common anginal symptom of substernal oppression may be reflex muscular contraction of the anterior intercostal muscles. If the pain barrage is severe, mass excitation of visceromotor reflexes such as sweating, lowered blood pressure, ashy cyanosis and other evidence of vasomotor disturbance, and nausea and vomiting may become prominent.

The relationship between cardiac pain and pain in the upper abdominal region is less readily explained. Miller[84] points out that difficulty in diagnosis arises when pain is referred to distant areas not directly related to the organ involved. In most persons, visceral afferent fibers converge upon a limited number of dorsal roots which come into relation with a restricted number of afferent somatic fibers. Therefore, in diseases of the heart, the gallbladder, the stomach, and other viscera, pain usually is referred to characteristic localities. With respect to the gallbladder, the visceral afferent pathways are numerous (extending from T_1 to T_{12}), and although the pain impulses are carried predominantly in the lower thoracic nerves, they may be included in many more segmental levels. In this way, gallbladder pain may be referred to segments commonly reserved for cardiac pain; acute heart pain may, in turn, be projected to the right upper quadrant and flank. Miller further notes that cardiac pain occasionally is transmitted over accessory afferent fibers. These are generally too few to carry impulses in any quantity, although in some individuals they may be in sufficient concentration to refer pain to divergent sites. Possibly such a mechanism accounts for the radiation of pain to the upper abdomen in cardiac infarctions and for the pain that resembles heart pain in acute abdominal accidents. In this connection, it is interesting that Wertheimer[85] and Leriche[86] observed the occurrence of severe anginal symptoms upon stimulation of the central end of the severed greater splanchnic nerves in patients at operation.

AORTIC PAIN

MECHANISM OF AORTIC PAIN

Clinical and experimental evidence indicates that the lesions of the aorta or of the smaller arteries in general may produce pain. The painful dilatations of the cranial arteries in migraine and the pain produced by arterial punctures for clinical studies are common examples. It is generally held that the adventitia of large blood vessels contain pain fibers.[89] Spiegel and Wassermann[90] found that acute stretching of the wall of the aortic arch produces pain. They demonstrated also that coating the aorta with irritating substances had profoundly painful effects. These authors concluded that aortic pain results from stimulation of the adventitia.

Afferent aortic pain fibers appear to run in close relation to those from the heart. White[88] has observed that the intractable pain of angina pectoris or aneurysm is abated by resection of the upper five thoracic ganglia, or the rami communicantes, or by interruption of the corresponding dorsal roots proximal to the root ganglia. Aortic pain neurones pass to the sympathetic chain ganglia from the aortic plexus, traverse the rami communicantes, and reach their cell bodies in the dorsal root ganglia (Fig. 8-17).

It has been suggested that the pain of dissecting aneurysm of the aorta occurs because of marked distention of the adventitial coat.[88] On the other hand, syphilitic aortitis may lead to aneurysms of great size without discomfort to the patient. Syphilitic aortitis may give rise to attacks of angina pectoris by reducing the coronary flow through involvement of the mouths of the coronary arteries. Occasionally aortitis may provoke substernal discomfort that is dull, burning, and continuous. Mills and Horton[55] have suggested that such pain in some cases of aortic aneurysm results from sudden distention of the aneurysmal sac. They observed that the pain was frequently aggravated by recumbency, by exercise, by cough, or upon deep breathing. In our experience aortitis and aneurysms due to syphilis have rarely been observed to produce painful symptoms, unless saccular dilatation had become so large as to impinge upon the chest wall or spine.

It is difficult to understand how the marked dilatation of syphilitic aortic aneurysm occurs with so little pain. Possibly in the slowly dilating aorta, adventitial distortion is gradual, and forceful stimuli to adventitial pain endings are not present. A further possibility is that afferent nerve endings may be destroyed largely by extensive syphilitic involvement of the vasa vasorum and the adventitia.

Quite in contrast to syphilitic aneurysms are the sudden disruptions of the aortic coats frequently accompanied by agonizing pain. *Dissecting aneurysms* apparently usually result from changes that first occur in the media. The pathologic changes in the medial coat lead to a rent in the intima, often just superior to the aortic valves. Blood enters under pressure from the lumen and splits apart the layers of the arterial wall. In the process of dissection, the muscle coats are torn apart, and the adventitia, in places, may be lifted from the underlying media. Intense distention of the portions of the wall outside of the burrowing column of blood occurs. We[91] have frequently observed dissecting aneurysms in open-chest experimental dog preparations. If the blood pressure is normal or high, and the aortic intima is then torn by a blunt instrument, blood burrows into the aortic wall so that the adventitia and a few strands of the medial coat are raised as a huge, bulbous purplish swelling which creeps distally along the aorta. The aneurysmal sac becomes thin and tenuous in places where there is subadventitial dissection; elsewhere the sac may be firmer from support of underlying dissected layers of the media. Seepage from the thinner parts of the sac usually occurs, terminating in rupture. Pathologic evidence indicates that a similar mechanical rending of the vessel may occur in patients.[92] The basic lesion leading to aortic dissection appears to be medial cystic necrosis[93] of the wall of the vessel.[94,95] The evidence offered by Bauersfeld[97] indicates that cystic disease of the media causes a rupture of the vasa vasorum with the formation of medial hematomas; the hematomas may split the aortic wall. Tension of the intima then tears the membrane and dissection is extended from pressure within the lumen. Most patients with dissecting aneurysms have had pre-existing arterial hypertension. Marked elevation of blood pressure may facilitate rapid disruption and final rupture of the aortic wall when a small tear in the intima has occurred.

CHARACTERISTICS OF AORTIC PAIN

Clinically, aortic pain is recognized most clearly when dissecting aneurysms occur. Such pain may be dramatic; it is sudden in onset and quickly becomes severe and agonizing. When the aneurysm is confined to the aortic arch, the pain is substernal or diffuses over the upper anterior chest. It may be projected to the shoulders.[92,96] Projection into the arms is infrequent. As dissection proceeds over the arch and into the descending aorta, extreme pain may be felt at the base of the neck and along the back —particularly in the interscapular area. The agony is continuous and requires heavy narcotization. Although grayish cyanosis and other signs of visceromotor reflex disturbances appear, the blood pressure usually is sustained. In the grip of such pain, some patients may be distraught: they may climb in and out of bed, roll about, assume grotesque postures, or press their chests against chairs or walls in an effort to obtain relief.[98] This behavior is in contrast with that of individuals with myocardial infarction, who may lie quietly, and often exhibit signs of collapse. Cases of dissecting aneurysm are described[92] in which symptoms have been transient or mild, suggesting angina pectoris. In some cases (usually found unexpectedly at necropsy) no pain has occurred, although the aorta may be extensively damaged.

Peery[99] has drawn attention to incomplete rupture of the aorta. This lesion is produced by an intimal tear without dissection of the vessel wall. It may provoke severe substernal pain of a "stabbing" or "tearing" quality, but it is not as severe as that of dissecting aneurysm. This pain may be confused with that of coronary occlusion. Incomplete rupture of the aorta can give way to dissection of the aortic wall at any time.

SUMMARY

The essential clinical features of thoracic pain have been presented briefly, and the painful symptoms interpreted in light of the underlying, known pathologic physiology. Pain arising from the chest wall, thoracic respiratory system, mediastinum, esophagus, and cardiovascular system is discussed.

REFERENCES

1. Heinbecker, P.: Heart pain, J. Thorac. Surg. 10:44, 1940.
2. Heinbecker, P., Bishop, G. H., and O'Leary, J.: Pain and touch fibres in peripheral nerves, Arch. Neurol. Psychiat. 29:771, 1933.
3. Lewis, T.: Pain, New York, Macmillan, 1942.
4. Moore, R. M.: Stimulation of peripheral nerve-elements subserving pain-sensibility by intra-arterial injections of neutral solutions, Amer. J. Physiol. 110:191, 1934.
   Dennis, J., and Moore, R. M.: Potassium changes in functioning heart under conditions of ischemia and of congestion, Amer. J. Physiol. 123:443, 1938.
5. Hamilton, J. B.: The pathways and production of pain, Yale J. Biol. Med. 9:215, 1936-37.
6. Lewis, T.: Suggestions relating to the study of somatic pain, Brit. Med. J. 1:321, 1938.
7. Behan, R. J.: Pain, New York, Appleton, 1920.
8. Stern, E. S.: Mechanism of herpes zoster and its relation to chicken-pox, Brit. J. Derm. 49:263, 1937.
9. Goeckerman, W. H., and Wilhelm, L. F. X.: Herpes zoster and herpes simplex, Arch. Derm. Syphilol. 35:868, 1937.
10. Holmes, J. F.: Slipping rib cartilage, with report of cases, Amer. J. Surg. 54:326, 1941.

11. White, P. D.: Diseases of the Coronary Arteries and Cardiac Pain, New York, Macmillan, 1936.

12. Dixon, R. H.: Cure or relief of cases misdiagnosed "angina of effort," Brit. Med. J. 2:891, 1938.

13. Schmidt, R.: Pain: Its Causation and Diagnostic Significance in Internal Diseases (Translation by Vogel and Zinsser), Philadelphia, Lippincott, 1911.

14. Mendlowitz, M.: Strain of the pectoralis minor muscle, an important cause of precordial pain in soldiers, Amer. Heart J. 30: 123, 1945.

15. Graham, E. A., Singer, J. J., and Ballon, H. C.: Surgical Diseases of the Chest, Philadelphia, Lea & Febiger, 1935.

16. Craver, L. F.: Tenderness of the sternum in leukemia, Amer. J. Med. Sci. 174:799, 1927.

17. Smith, J. R., and Kountz, W. B.: Deformities of the thoracic spine as a cause of anginoid pain, Ann. Intern. Med. 17:604, 1942.

18. Davis, D.: Spinal nerve root pain (radiculitis) simulating coronary occlusion; a common syndrome, Amer. Heart J. 35:70, 1948.

19. Reid, W. D.: Pressure on the brachial plexus causing simulation of coronary disease, J.A.M.A. 110:1724, 1938.

20. Fitzwilliams, D. C. L.: On the Breast, St. Louis, Mosby, 1924.

21. Geschickter, C. F.: Diseases of the Breast, Philadelphia, Lippincott, 1943.

22. Labbé, L., and Coyne, P.: Traité des Tumeurs Bénignes du Sein, Paris, Masson, 1876.

23. Veil, P.: Cellulite du sein et engine de poitrine, Arch. Mal. Cœur 25:703, 1932.

24. de Cholnoky, T.: Benign tumors of the breast, A.M.A. Arch. Surg. 38:79, 1939.

25. Cheatle, G., and Cutler, M.: Tumors of the Breast, Philadelphia, Lippincott, 1931.

26. Graham, E. A.: Personal communication.

27. Morton, D. R., Klassen, K. P., and Curtis, G. M.: The effect of high vagus section upon the clinical physiology of the bronchi, in 1949 Proc. Central Soc. Clin. Res., J. Lab. Clin. Med. 34:1730, 1949.

28. Bonner, L. M.: Primary lung tumor, J.A.M.A. 94:1044, 1930.

29. Capps, J. A., and Coleman, G. H.: An Experimental and Clinical Study of Pain in the Pleura, Pericardium and Peritoneum, New York, Macmillan, 1932.

30. Dybdahl, G. L.: The control of pleuritic pain by the use of cutaneous anesthesia, Permanente Fdn. Bull. 2:30, 1944.

31. Bray, H. A.: The tension theory of pleuritic pain, Amer. Rev. Tuberc. 13:14, 1926.

32. Goldman. A.: Personal communication.

33. Krause, G. R., and Chester, E. M.: Infarction of the lung; clinical and roentgenological study, A.M.A. Arch. Intern. Med. 67:1144, 1941.

34. Carlson, H. A., and Ballon, H. C.: The operability of carcinoma of the lung, J. Thorac. Surg. 2:323, 1933.

35. Ornstein, G. G., and Ulmar, D.: Clinical Tuberculosis, vol. II, G-21, Philadelphia, Davis, 1941.

36. Kiss, F., and Ballon, H. C.: Contribution to the nerve supply of the diaphragm, Anat. Rec. 41:285, 1928-29.

37. Hinsey, J. C., and Phillips, R. A.: Observations upon diaphragmatic sensation, J. Neurophysiol. 3:175, 1940.

38. Master, A. M., Dack, S., Stone, J., and Grishman, A.: Differential diagnosis of hiatus hernia and coronary artery disease, A.M.A. Arch. Surg. 58:428, 1949.

39. Jones, C. M., and Chapman, W. P.: Studies on the mechanism of the pain in angina pectoris with particular relation to hiatus hernia, Trans. Ass. Amer. Physicians 57:139, 1942.

40. Moor, F.: The cause of "stitch," Brit. Med. J. 2:282, 1923.

41. Capps, R.: Cause of the so-called side ache that occurs in normal persons, A.M.A. Arch. Intern. Med. 68:94, 1941.

42. Barnes, A. R., and Burchell, H. B.: Acute pericarditis simulating acute coronary occlusion, Amer. Heart J. 23:247, 1942.

43. Camp, P. D., and White, P. D.: Pericardial effusion; a clinical study, Amer. J. Med. Sci. 184:728, 1932.

44. Harvey, A. M., and Whitehill, M. R.: Tuberculous pericarditis, Medicine 16:45, 1937.

45. Paine, W. W., and Poulton, E. P.: Experiments on visceral sensation: I, The relation of pain to activity in the human esophagus, J. Physiol. 63:217, 1927.

———: Visceral pain in the upper alimentary tract, Quart. J. Med. 17:53, 1923-24.

46. Hurst, A. F., and Rake, G. W.: Achalasia of the cardia, Quart. J. Med. 23:491, 1929-30.

47. Alvarez, W. C.: An Introduction to Gastroenterology, New York, Hoeber, 1941.

48. Neuhof, H., and Rabin, C. B.: Acute mediastinitis; roentgenological, pathological and clinical features and principles of operative treatment, Amer. J. Roentgen. 44:684, 1940.

49. Furstenburg, A. C.: Acute mediastinal suppuration, Trans. Amer. Laryng., Rhinol. Otol. Soc., p. 210, 1929.

50. Hamman, L.: Spontaneous mediastinal emphysema, Bull. Hopkins Hosp. 64:1, 1939.

51. McLester, J. S.: Diseases of the Mediastinum, in Oxford Medicine, New York, Oxford Univ. Press.

52. Pick, F.: Ueber chronische unter dem Bilde der Lebercirrhose verlaufende Perikarditis (perikarditische Pseudolebercirrhose) nebst Bemerkungen ueber die Zuckergussleber (Curschmann), Z. Klin. Med. 29:385, 1896.

53. Middleton, W. S.: Some clinical caprices of Hodgkin's disease, Ann. Intern. Med. 11:448, 1937.

54. Pancoast, H. K.: Superior pulmonary sulcus tumor. Tumor characterized by pain, Horner's syndrome, destruction of bone and atrophy of hand muscles, J.A.M.A. 99:1391, 1932.

55. Mills, J. H., and Horton, B. T.: Clinical aspects of aneurysm, A.M.A. Arch. Intern. Med. 62:949, 1938.

56. Heberden, W.: Pectoris Dolor, *reprinted in* Classic Descriptions of Disease (Major), Baltimore, Thomas, 1932.

57. Herrick, J. B.: Clinical features of sudden obstruction of the coronary arteries, J.A.M.A. 59:2015, 1912.

58. Sutton, D. C., and Lueth, H. C.: Pain, A.M.A. Intern. Med. 45:827, 1930.

59. Pearcy, J. F., Priest, W. S., and Van Allen, C. M.: Pain due to the temporary occlusion of the coronary arteries in dogs, Amer. Heart J. 4:390, 1928-29.

60. Keefer, C. S., and Resnik, W. H.: Angina pectoris; A syndrome caused by anoxemia of the myocardium, A.M.A. Arch. Intern. Med. 41:769, 1928.

61. Wenckebach, K. F.: Angina pectoris and the possibilities of its surgical relief, Brit. Med. J. 1:809, 1924.

62. Gorham, L. W., and Martin, S. J.: Coronary occlusion with and without pain, A.M.A. Arch. Intern. Med. 62:821, 1938.

63. Lewis, T., Pickering, G. W., and Rothschild, P.: Observations upon muscular pain in intermittent claudication, Heart 15:359, 1931.

64. Katz, L. N., Lindner, E., and Landt, H.: On the nature of the substance(s) producing pain in contracting skeletal muscle; its bearing on the problems of angina pectoris and intermittent claudication, J. Clin. Invest. 14:807, 1935.

65. Blumgart, H. L., Schlesinger, M. J., and Davis, D.: Studies on the relation of the clinical manifestations of angina pectoris, coronary thrombosis, and myocardial infarction to the pathological findings, Amer. Heart J. 19:1, 1940.

66. Smith, J. R., and Henry, M. J.: Demonstration of the coronary arterial system with neoprene latex, J. Lab. Clin. Med. 30:462, 1945.

67. Prinzmetal, M., Bergman, H. C., *et al.*: Studies on the coronary circulation. III. Collateral circulation of beating human and dog hearts with coronary occlusion, Amer. Heart J. 35:689, 1948.

68. Gregg, D. E., Pritchard, W. H., Shipley, R. E., and Wearn, J. T.: Augmentation of blood flow in the coronary arteries with elevation of right ventricular pressure, Amer. J. Physiol. 139:726, 1943.

69. Smith, J. R., and Jensen, J.: Observations on the effect of theophylline amino-isobutanol in experimental heart failure, J. Lab. Clin. Med. 31:850, 1946.

70. Smith, J. R., and Layton, I. C.: The flow of blood supplying the cardiac atria, Proc. Soc. Exp. Biol. Med. 62:59, 1946.

71. Visscher, M. B.: The restriction of the coronary flow as a general factor in heart failure, J.A.M.A. 113:987, 1939.

72. Riseman, J. E. F., and Brown, M. G.: The duration of attacks of angina pectoris on exertion and the effect of nitroglycerine and amyl nitrite, New Eng. J. Med. 217:470, 1937.

73. Freedberg, A. S., Spiegel, E. D., and Riseman, J. E. F.: Effect of external heat and cold on patients with angina pectoris: Evidences for the existence of a reflex factor, Amer. Heart J. 27:611, 1944.

74. Herrick, J. B.: The coronary artery in health and disease, Amer. Heart J. 6:589, 1930-31.

75. Fenn, G. K., and Gilbert, N. C.: Anginal pain as a result of digitalis administration, J.A.M.A. 98:99, 1932.

76. Gold, H., Otto, H., Kwit, N. T., and Satchwell, H.: Does digitalis influence the course of cardiac pain? A study of 120 selected cases of angina pectoris, J.A.M.A. 110:895, 1938.

77. Harrison, T. R.: Clinical aspects of pain in the chest; I, Angina pectoris, Amer. J. Med. Sci. 207:561, 1944.

78. Gallavardin, L.: Syndromes angineux anormaux, Médecine 18:193, 1937.

79. Levine, S. A.: Coronary thrombosis, its various clinical features, Medicine 8:245, 1929.

80. Levine, S. A., and Tranter, C. L.: Infarction of the heart simulating acute surgical abdominal conditions, Amer. J. Med. Sci. 155:57, 1918.

81. Breyfogle, H. S.: The frequency of coexisting gallbladder and coronary artery disease, J.A.M.A. 114:1434, 1940.

82. Ernstene, A. C., and Rinell, J.: Pain in the shoulder as a sequel to myocardial infarction, A.M.A. Arch. Intern. Med. 66:800, 1940.

83. Askey, J. M.: The syndrome of painful disability of the shoulder and hand complicating coronary occlusion, Amer. Heart J. 22:1, 1941.

84. Miller, H. R.: Interrelationship of disease of the coronary arteries and gallbladder, Amer. Heart J. 24:579, 1942.

85. Wertheimer, P.: A propos des doleurs provoquées par l'excitation des grands splanchniques, Presse Méd. 45:1628, 1937.

86. Leriche, R.: Des doleurs provoquées par l'excitation des grands splanchniques, Presse Méd. 45:971, 1937.

87. White, J. C., Garrey, W. E., and Atkins, J. A.: Cardiac innervation; Experimental and clinical studies, A.M.A. Arch Surg. 26:765, 1933.

88. White, J. C.: The neurological mechanism of cardio-aortic pain, J. Nerv. Ment. Dis. 15:181, 1935.

89. Singer, R.: Experimentelle Studien über die Schmerzempfindlichkeit des Herzens und der grossen Gefässe und ihre Beziehung zur

Angina Pectoris, Wien. Arch. in. Med. 12:193, 1926.

90. Spiegel, E. A., and Wassermann, S.: Experimentelle Studien über die Entstehung des Aortenschmerzes und seine Leitung zum Zentralnervensystem, Z. Ges. Exp. Med. 52: 180, 1926.

91. Smith, J. R., and Paine, R.: Unpublished observations.

92. Flaxman, N.: Dissecting aneurysm of the aorta, Amer. Heart J. 24:654, 1942.

93. Erdheim, J.: Medionecrosis aortae idiopathica cystica, Virchow. Arch. Path. Anat. 276:187, 1930.

94. Sailer, S.: Dissecting aneurysm of the aorta, A.M.A., Arch. Path. 33:704, 1942.

95. Niehaus, F. W., and Wright, W. D.: Dissecting aneurysm of the aorta, J. Lab. Clin. Med. 26:1248, 1941.

96. Kountz, W. B., and Hempelmann, L.: Chromotrophic degeneration and rupture of the aorta following thyroidectomy in cases of hypertension, Amer. Heart J. 20:599, 1940.

97. Bauersfeld, S. R.: Dissecting aneurysm of the aorta: A presentation of fifteen cases and a review of the recent literature, Ann. Intern. Med. 26:873, 1947.

98. Tillman, Clifford: Personal communication.

99. Peery, T. M.: Incomplete rupture of the aorta; heretofore unrecognized stage of dissecting aneurysm and cause of cardiac pain and cardiac murmurs, A.M.A. Arch. Intern. Med. 70:689, 1942.

100. Weller, T. H., Whitton, H. M., and Bell, J. E.: The etiologic agents of varicella and herpes zoster: Isolation, propagation and cultural characteristics in vitro, J. Exp. Med. 108:843-868, 1958.

101. Wesselhoeft, C.: Chicken pox and herpes zoster, Rhode Island Med. J. 40:387-395, 1957.

102. Davis, D.: Radicular Syndromes with Emphasis on Chest Pain Simulating Coronary Disease, Chicago, Year Book Pub., 1957.

103. Steinbrocker, O.: Shoulder-hand syndrome, Amer. J. Med. 3:402, 1947.

104. Edeiken, J.: Shoulder-hand syndrome, Circulation 16:14, 1957.

105. Dressler, W., Yurkoksky, J., and McStarr, M.: Amer. Heart J. 54:42, 1957.

106. Dressler, W.: A post-myocardial infarction syndrome, J.A.M.A. 160:1379, 1956.

107. Weiser, N. J., Kantor, M., and Russell, H. K.: Posterior myocardial infarction syndrome, Circulation 20:371, 1959.

108. Gregg, D. E.: Physiology of the coronary circulation, Circulation 27:1128, 1963.

109. White, J. C.: Cardiac pain, anatomic pathways and physiologic mechanisms, Circulation 16:644, 1957.

110. Scheuer, J., and Brachfeld, N.: Coronary insufficiency: Relations between hemodynamic, electrical, and biochemical parameters, Circ. Res. 18:178, 1966.

111. Herman, M. V., Eliot, W. C., and Gorlin, R.: An electrocardiographic, anatomic, and metabolic study of zonal myocardial ischemia in coronary heart disease, Circulation 35:834, 1967.

112. Proudfit, W. L., Shirey, E. K., and Sones, F. M.: Selective cine coronary arteriography: Correlation with clinical findings in 1,000 patients, Circulation 33:901, 1966.

9

Abdominal Pain

RICHARD D. AACH

Despite the many recent advances in diagnostic and laboratory procedures, a carefully taken detailed history still plays an invaluable role in the diagnosis of intra-abdominal diseases. Of paramount importance in the history is the evaluation of pain. It is the rare patient with an abdominal disorder who does not complain of pain. Often it is the only or chief complaint. In contrast to pain in many other regions of the body, abdominal pain offers to the diagnostician a unique, and at times frustrating, challenge. Intense pain in any portion of the abdomen may be the result of a wide variety of conditions, some benign, others demanding immediate attention. Pain can be experienced in an area that is far removed from the actual site of the disorder, and various disorders involving different organs can produce pain of similar character. Nevertheless, important patterns exist which can lead directly to the correct diagnosis. The assessment of abdominal pain, therefore, demands critical judgment and a very careful search for all of its pertinent features.

HISTORY

Studies of the nature of abdominal pain date back more than 300 years. In 1760, the Swiss physiologist, von Haller, demonstrated that the visceral peritoneum, like the visceral pericardium and pleura, was insensible to mechanical stimuli, such as pinching and cutting. Despite the significance of these observations, little information was added until the turn of the last century. With the emergence of the fields of neuroanatomy and neurophysiology in the late 1800's, the problem of the sites of origin of abdominal pain became a subject of considerable interest. Soon there was controversy as to the existence of true visceral pain, and heated debate continued well into this century. Essentially, two schools of thought existed. One school, having Ross as an early champion, held that there were two distinct types of visceral pain: splanchnic, or true visceral pain, experienced in the region of the stimulated organ; and somatic, or referred pain, experienced in somatic structures served by the same neural segment. The second school, with Mackenzie as the main protagonist, believed that all visceral pain was referred pain. According to this concept, abdominal viscera lacked pain fibers. However, afferent pathways did exist which were capable of carrying nonpainful impulses from a visceral organ to the spinal cord via the sympathetics. These impulses could produce an "irritable focus" upon reaching the spinal cord, resulting in the stimulation of adjacent pathways, and thereby giving rise to the sensation of pain in somatic structures supplied by the same segment of the spinal cord. This view was supported by the studies of Lennander, who, like von Haller, demonstrated that abdominal viscera were insensible to the applications of heat and cold, clipping, cutting, and burning with caustics. On the other hand, pain was evoked when somatic nerves in the parietal peritoneum, mesentery, and

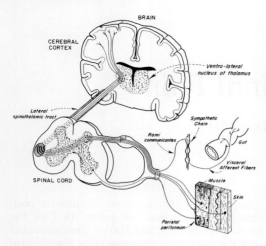

FIG. 9-1. Afferent pathways of abdominal pain. Afferent visceral fibers carried in the sympathetic chain pass via the rami communicantes to the spinal cord where their sensory impulses travel in the same pathways as do impulses of superficial and deep afferent somatic origins. After crossing to the opposite side the afferent impulses ascend in the laterospinothalamic tract to the ventrolateral nucleus of the thalamus and then to the postcentral gyrus of the cerebral cortex.

subserous connective tissue were stimulated by torsion or traction. The heat of this debate between the two schools has dissipated with time. Many of the hypotheses advanced during this early period of study have since been discarded. What remains, however, are many critical and careful observations. A notable example is the contribution of Head, who systematically mapped out the peripheral distribution of referred pain for each of the neural segments of the spinal cord. He also stressed that hyperalgesia was a common finding in an area of referred pain. To his credit, the term "Head zones of hyperalgesia" is still used to denote this important feature of referred pain.

It is now generally accepted that visceral structures do indeed have a sensory apparatus that can give rise to the sensation of pain when properly stimulated. Although it is less well-developed than the corresponding somatic sensory system with respect to size and number of nerve fibers, studies by Hertz, and later Ryle, demonstrate that pain can be elicited by stretching or distending visceral organs, or by their contraction if rapid and extreme in nature. The observations of Rene

Leriche added further evidence that true visceral pain could be produced by vigorous contraction of the intestinal tract. However, under certain conditions, even ordinary mechanical stimuli can evoke pain. The very thorough studies of Wolff and Wolf convincingly demonstrate that pinching or faradic stimulation gives rise to visceral pain when the mucosal surface of a visceral organ is inflamed, congested, or edematous. Further, ischemia due to vascular insufficiency also can lower the pain threshold, so that ordinarily nonnoxious stimuli can give rise to the sensation of pain. Pain of intra-abdominal origin, therefore, may originate from the parietal peritoneum, mesentery, splanchnic vessels, and visceral organs themselves under the appropriate circumstances.

PATHWAYS

Pain felt in the abdomen is either transmitted through spinal roots T-6 through T-12, or is referred to these segments through impulses traveling from neighboring structures in the chest, the extremities, or the pelvis. Some structures within the chest are innervated from segments as low as T-9; therefore, the location of the sensation of pain in the chest or abdomen does not necessarily establish the site of the disease with certainty.

Sensory impulses of somatic origin (integument and parietal peritoneum) travel via the cerebrospinal tract to the dorsal root ganglia, and then into the region of the posterior horn of the spinal cord (Fig. 9-1). In the gray matter, the impulses are transmitted to a second neuron, which crosses to the opposite side of the cord and ascends to the thalamus via the lateral spinothalamic tract. In the thalamus, impulses pass to a third neuron, whose axon ends in the cerebral cortex in the region of the postcentral gyrus.

Sensory impulses from visceral structures within the abdomen are carried by visceral afferent nerve fibers, which pass along the sympathetics to the dorsal root ganglia by way of the rami communicantes. From the dorsal root ganglia, these fibers enter the posterior horn of the spinal cord, along with somatic neurons. Once inside the central nervous system, sensory impulses of visceral origin travel along the same pathways as pain impulses arising in somatic structures.

The afferent visceral neurons are mainly of the small unmyelinated variety (Gasser's Class C). In contrast to the "quick," sharply circumscribed pain sensation derived from large myelinated somatic afferent neurons, impulses carried by afferent visceral fibers produce a "slow" aching pain, which is usually poorly localized.

TYPES OF DEEP PAIN

There are three general categories of deep abdominal pain:

1. **True Visceral.** True visceral pain is felt at the site of primary stimulation and may or may not be associated with referred pain. It is eliminated by infiltration of procaine into the site of noxious stimulation, or by blocking its afferent nerves. It is not altered by infiltration of procaine into other structures supplied by the same or adjacent neural segments. True visceral pain is characteristically dull and aching in character. It is diffuse and deep in location, often experienced in the midabdomen. The patient and physician may have a difficult time in trying to localize the site of the pain, which roughly corresponds to the segmental location of the visceral structure producing the sensory impulses. Examples of true visceral pain are the initial midabdominal pain of acute appendicitis, and the discomfort experienced early in intestinal obstruction or cholecystitis.

2. **Deep Somatic Pain.** Deep somatic pain arises from noxious stimulation of the parietal peritoneum and the root of the mesentery. Since pain impulses are transmitted via the cerebrospinal pathways, this form of pain is generally very intense and sharply circumscribed, and is appreciated in an area closely approximating that region being stimulated. Because the same pathways subserve the more superficial areas of the same neural segment, including the skin, deep somatic pain often is accompanied by referred pain. The sharply localized pain of acute appendicitis following the spread of inflammation to the parietal peritoneum or the intense pain of peritonitis are examples of deep somatic pain.

3. **Referred Pain.** Pain experienced at a site other than that stimulated, but in tissues supplied by the same or adjacent neural segments, is called "referred pain." Thus, painful stimulation of visceral or deep somatic structures gives rise to the sensation of pain in more superficial areas of the body (e.g., skin) supplied by the same, and occasionally neighboring, segments of the spinal cord. Spread of excitation occurs because impulses from visceral organs, and both superficial and deep somatic structures, share common pathways inside the central nervous system.

Referred pain may occur in addition to, or in the virtual absence of, true visceral and deep somatic pain. An entire dermatome or neural segment need not be involved. As a rule, however, referred pain usually is experienced only when the painful stimulus is sufficiently intense or when the pain threshold of a viscus or organ has been lowered by disease.

Characteristically, referred pain is sharp in character and relatively well-localized, often to the lateral aspects of the abdomen or back. The right subscapular pain of acute cholecystitis or biliary colic is an example of referred pain. A heightened degree of discomfort to other painful stimuli applied to the area of referred pain ("Head zones of hyperalgesia") and local tenderness frequently accompany and rarely may constitute the principal form of discomfort of an intra-abdominal disease. Alteration in effector or motor activity may also accompany referred pain. Skeletal muscle contraction, appreciated as "muscle guarding," often is demonstrable in the segment of referred pain. Muscular contraction, if prolonged, may itself be a new source of pain and local tenderness. In the same way, efferent impulses may stimulate other structures in the area of referred pain, including blood vessels and glands. This may be appreciated by observing a difference in the skin temperature and moisture in the region of referred pain. Hyperalgesia and muscle guarding are present to their fullest extent in association with the deep somatic pain of generalized peritonitis.

CLINICAL ANALYSIS

HISTORY

Because abdominal structures by and large have poorly developed sensory systems, and because afferent impulses travel over a limited number of nervous pathways, determining the source of abdominal pain can be very difficult. All too often, the findings on physical examinations are minimal or entirely absent. Therefore, the patient's history, past and present, is of extreme importance. Attention must be paid to details that are best obtained in a methodical fashion. If the patient is alert, the most accurate description is given when pain is being experienced or shortly thereafter. Questioning on more than one occasion may be required.

Patients vary widely in sensitivity to pain, in psychic and emotional reactions to pain, and in ability to describe their sensations of pain. Causes of variation among patients include such factors as age, education, and verbal ability. The patient may be able to describe his abdominal pain only in the most general terms. Words such as "gas pain," "cramps," or "indigestion" are heard frequently by the physician. The same terms may represent an entirely different pain experience to different individuals. Therefore, the physician, must not be content with such vague descriptions, but must characterize the patient's abdominal pain as to its (1) location, (2) quality, (3) temporal features, (4) intensity, (5) type of onset, and (6) reaction to circumstances, i.e., those that produce, intensify, or reduce it.

1. **Location.** The site of pain can be a very valuable clue to its origin. Pain of the upper gastrointestinal tract is usually experienced low in the anterior chest or high in the abdomen, often in the midline. For example, esophagitis is felt substernally or in the epigastrium, where the pain of a peptic ulcer also may be experienced. The pain of an active ulcer tends to be sharply localized; one finger can be pointed to the exact site of pain. On the other hand, the abdominal pain experienced in gastroenteritis, or in psychophysiologic gastrointestinal disease, usually is diffuse and poorly localized. Appendicitis and regional enteritis are examples of disorders that most often produce right-lower-quadrant pain, whereas diverticulitis usually gives rise to low abdominal pain, either in the midline or left lower quadrant. The pain of renal colic characteristically is felt in the flank, and radiates towards the groin, whereas the pain of cholecystitis usually is experienced in the right upper quadrant, where pain referred from basilar pneumonitis also may be felt.

2. **Quality.** Whether the pain sensation originates in the superficial or deep structures often can be determined by the quality of the pain. Pricking or itching pains come from superficial tissues such as the skin, whereas dull aching pain characteristically arises in deeper structures. The sensation of burning or "gnawing" is typical of peptic ulcer disease and peptic esophagitis.

3. **Temporal Features.** It is important to determine whether the pain is intermittent, continuous, pulsatile, or colicky in nature. The duration of a painful experience and its periodicity or frequency of occurrence in terms of minutes, days, or even season may provide valuable information. The pain of biliary tract origin is likely to be intermit-

tent, whereas the pain of pancreatic carcinoma often is agonizingly persistent and unchanging. An abdominal aneurysm may produce pulsatile pain. Intestinal obstruction or gastroenteritis is characterized by intermittent cramping pain ("griping") which comes and goes in a wave-like rhythm. In the female, intense but brief pain in the low abdomen or back, known as "mittelschmerz," may occur at mid-month between menstrual periods, at the time of ovulation. Exacerbations of peptic ulcer disease are most common in the spring and fall of the year, whereas the pain of psychophysiologic gastrointestinal disease often is related to periods of emotional stress which the patient may or may not recognize.

4. **Intensity.** In general, the intensity of pain is related to the severity of the abdominal disorder, especially if acute. Thus, the pain of biliary and renal colic, or of peritonitis usually is of high intensity, whereas the pain of psychophysiologic gastrointestinal disease and gastorenteritis is less severe. However, intensity is apt to be the most difficult feature of abdominal pain for the patient to describe accurately and for the physician to evaluate. This is because intensity of pain is largely a subjective quality and depends upon the patient's personality, his psychic and emotional state, as well as his previous pain experience and alertness. Further, age may also affect the degree to which a patient experiences pain; the pain of acute appendicitis may be much less intense in an elderly individual, to the point that this diagnosis may be overlooked. To evaluate the intensity of pain, the patient can be asked to compare it to a previous painful experience. "Is the pain as severe as the labor pains of childbirth?, of a previous gallbladder attack?, or appendicitis?" Also, the patient can be asked to grade the severity of the pain in terms of degree, from 1+ to 10+.

5. **Type of Onset.** The type of onset, whether gradual or sudden, may provide very useful information. The pain of cholecystitis often begins gradually and builds in intensity, whereas the pain of renal colic, rupture of a viscus with resultant peritonitis, or mesenteric artery occlusion usually begins suddenly, and is maximal from the very onset.

6. **The Circumstances which Produce, Intensify, or Reduce Pain.** Most abdominal pain may be produced or intensified under certain specific circumstances, and this characteristic often is very helpful in making the

correct diagnosis. The pain of vascular insufficiency of the small intestine ("abdominal angina") usually begins within an hour after eating (Bircher), whereas the pain of peptic ulcer disease is experienced later, one to two hours after a meal when the stomach is empty of food. The intestinal cramping pain, bloating, and diarrhea associated with deficiency of the small intestinal disaccharidase enzyme *lactase* occurs 30 minutes to 2 hours after the ingestion of milk. Coughing, straining, or sneezing is likely to accentuate the pain from lesions involving spinal roots. Pleuritic pain, whether felt in the chest wall or referred to the abdomen, is associated with breathing. Sudden movement may intensify the pain of peritonitis or give rise to pain in patients with hepatic metastases.

Equally important are the factors that reduce abdominal pain. The pain of peptic ulcer characteristically is relieved by antacids or the ingestion of food. Right-lower-quadrant pain of regional enteritis frequently disappears after defecation, usually urgent in nature. Locally applied heat often reduces the intensity of pain from muscle tension. A particular posture may minimize abdominal pain. For example, pain from a hernia often is modified by changes in the position of the body. The pain of pancreatitis may be reduced by sitting up and leaning forward. Intestinal colic may cause the patient to double up in a jack-knife position to seek relief. The patient with generalized peritonitis usually will lie on his back absolutely motionless because any movement increases pain.

PHYSICAL EXAMINATION

The same rules that apply to the general physical examination apply to examination of the abdomen. The examination must be systematic and thorough, beginning with inspection, then auscultation, and finally palpation and percussion. As the cardiac status is ascertained by evaluation of the patient in more than one position, so should the abdomen be examined. Abnormal masses may be felt only in certain positions, particularly if they are mobile. An enlarged spleen may be palpable only when the patient is lying on his right side. If at all possible, the patient should be examined during an attack of pain, because certain signs may be present only then. He should also be examined, if possible, when free of pain, when there is no muscle guard masking other symptoms, and when other reactions to pain are absent.

General inspection should include careful attention to the *position assumed* by the patient when he is experiencing pain. As mentioned earlier, strict immobility characterizes the patient with general peritonitis, whereas patients with biliary or renal colic writhe in agony. Lying with a flexed hip may indicate a psoas abscess, whether related to appendicitis or a perinephric abscess. An abnormally distended loop of bowel may be recognized simply by observing the anterior abdominal wall for visible peristalsis. Ascites can be suspected upon observing a protuberant abdomen, bulging flanks, or an adult with an umbilical hernia.

Although *auscultation* of the abdomen frequently does not yield meaningful information in a routine physical examination, it may be of extreme importance in the evaluation of abdominal pain. Complete absence of bowel sounds is found in advanced peritonitis or adynamic ileus of any cause. Pain coincidental with abnormally active, highly pitched bowel sounds is a feature of early mechanical bowel obstruction. The cessation of bowel sounds during an attack of pain of brief duration suggests biliary or renal colic with reflex ileus. Auscultation should not be limited to the characterization of bowel sounds. A bruit or a friction rub heard over the liver may be an important clue in the diagnosis of hepatic metastasis. Similarly, a friction rub heard over the spleen should suggest pain due to a splenic infarct.

Palpation of the abdomen may be of value in discovering enlarged organs or masses not normally present, such as neoplasm. Muscular rigidity or "guarding" is one of the most important early signs of inflammation and must be carefully looked for in patients with acute abdominal pain. The examination is done by gently palpating both sides of the abdomen simultaneously with both hands. Muscular guarding is unilateral in the presence of a fairly localized inflammatory mass, such as a walled-off abscess, and is bilateral in generalized peritonitis. Palpation also will elicit tenderness, which may be either superficial or deep. It is important to distinguish between superficial and deep tenderness, because deep tenderness implicates disease of visceral organs. However, it should be kept in mind that deep tenderness may be associated with overlying superficial tenderness through the mechanism of referred pain.

An attempt should be made to elicit *rebound* tenderness, a sign of peritoneal irritation. The physician should be aware that the subjective reaction of the patient to the sudden release of pressure on the abdomen may limit the value of this maneuver. Palpation of the abdomen is not completed until each of the sites of possible hernias (femoral and inguinal canals) has been examined.

Percussion of the abdomen usually does not play an important role in the assessment of abdominal pain. It may confirm the presence of an enlarged organ or abnormal mass found on palpation. Occasionally the liver can not be palpated but can be percussed. The percussion note over an abdominal mass (whether dull or tympanitic) will distinguish between a solid tissue mass or distended bowel. Free fluid in the peritoneal cavity usually is best recognized by demonstrating shifting dullness.

Finally, it should be remembered that abdominal pain can be a feature of extra-abdominal disease, not only of the chest or pelvis, but of the central or peripheral nervous system. For this reason, physical examination must not be limited to the abdomen.

LABORATORY TESTS AND DIAGNOSTIC PROCEDURES

Especially in recent years, the diagnostician has had available a wide array of laboratory tests and procedures, which often play an essential role in establishing the cause of abdominal pain. The scope of this chapter does not permit a detailed discussion or even a listing of all the useful tests, but mention should be made of some of the more recent diagnostic procedures now available in many medical centers and hospitals. These procedures do not supplant such time-tested studies as barium examination of the gastrointestinal tract, intravenous pyelograms, or the proctoscopic examination, but rather are useful when the more conventional, easier, and safer studies have failed to establish a diagnosis.

Within the past few years, *arteriography* has begun to play an increasingly important role in the diagnostic work-up. This radiologic procedure can be used to uncover a wide variety of intra-abdominal diseases. Neoplasm infiltrating the kidney, liver, or pancreas can be detected by the trained radiologist on the basis of alterations in the distribution and shape of blood vessels supplying these organs, or by "tumor staining." The arteriogram is the only method short of surgery which can demonstrate narrowing of the celiac axis or the superior mesenteric artery, and thus establish the diagnosis of "abdominal angina."

A second diagnostic approach of relatively recent vintage is the use of *radioisotopic scanning*. The demonstration of a "cold area" in the liver which has failed to take up an isotopically labeled substance, such as rose bengal or gold, is suggestive of a hepatic neoplasm, cyst, or abscess. Renal and pancreatic scanning also are coming of age, but, like the liver scan, present techniques do not visualize lesions less than 1 to 2 cm. in diameter, or enable the physician to distinguish between the various possible space-occupying lesions producing the abnormal scan.

In the past decade, peroral and percutaneous *biopsies* of intra-abdominal structures have become commonplace in many medical centers. These techniques have the advantage of not requiring surgery or general anesthesia. The percutaneous needle liver biopsy, when performed by a physician experienced in the technique, is an established method for making a definitive morphologic diagnosis of hepatic disease. Peroral biopsy of the small intestinal mucosa is being performed with increasing frequency. Microscopic examination of biopsy samples of intestinal mucosa can reveal the changes of celiac sprue, Whipple's disease, or intestinal lymphangiectasia. Further, analysis of the tissue for the activity of the enzymes that split the disaccharide sugars can confirm the diagnosis of lactase deficiency, causing milk intolerance with resultant abdominal cramping pain, flatulence, and diarrhea (Haemmerli).

Cytologic examination of aspirated fluid from the stomach, the esophagus, and the duodenum in patients suspected of having neoplasm of these organs or of the pancreas may reveal carcinoma cells.

Undoubtedly, present tests and diagnostic procedures will be improved or supplemented by new and better ones in the future.

ETIOLOGIC CLASSIFICATION OF ABDOMINAL PAIN

The common conditions and the diseases that can cause abdominal pain can be divided into (1) those involving structures within the abdominal cavity, and (2) those involving structures outside the abdominal cavity.

ETIOLOGIC CLASSIFICATION OF ABDOMINAL PAIN

1. Pain originating within the abdomen
    A. Disease of hollow organs
       Bowel, gallbladder, ducts, etc.
    B. Peritonitis
       Chemical or bacterial
    C. Vascular
       Mesenteric thrombosis, "abdominal angina," dissecting aneurysm
    D. Tension on supporting structures
       On mesenteries, distensions of capsules (liver, spleen, lymph nodes)

2. Pain originating outside the abdomen
    A. Referred pain
       From thorax, genitourinary tract, spine, spinal cord, pelvis, etc.
    B. Metabolic pain
       1. Endogenous
          Toxic: uremia, diabetic acidosis
          Allergic: food hypersensitivity?
       2. Exogenous
          Toxic: drugs, lead, etc.
          Biologic: bacterial toxins, insect and snake venoms, etc.
    C. Neurogenic Pain
       Spinal cord or root pain; tabes, causalgia, etc.
    D. Psychogenic Pain

Only those conditions seen most frequently are discussed below.

THE INTESTINAL TRACT

1. **Esophagus.** Pain impulses arising in the esophagus are carried by afferent nerve fibers, which course with the sympathetics and enter the spinal cord from the level of the lower cervical through the entire thoracic vertebrae. The fifth and sixth thoracic spinal segments are most heavily trafficked. In contrast to most of the other regions of the intestinal tract, esophageal pain corresponds relatively well to the site of the disease process. Thus lesions of the upper esophagus give rise to pain in the suprasternal notch or beneath the manubrium; those in the mid-esophagus produce pain deep to the mid-sternum; and pain due to disease of the distal esophagus usually is experienced beneath the xiphoid process or in the epigastrium.

The most common pain from the esophagus is "heartburn," a burning pain felt substernally and fairly well-localized over the site of stimulation. This pain has been shown by Jones to be due to spasm of the cardiac end of the esophagus. The spasm may be induced by mechanical, thermal, chemical, or electrical stimuli. The most common mechanism of heartburn in man is thought to include the regurgitation of highly acid gastric juice into the esophagus, which has already had its pain threshold lowered by the presence of engorgement or inflammation.

2. **Stomach.** The studies of Wolff and Wolf have shown convincingly that pain of considerable intensity is produced by either mechanical or chemical stimulation of the gastric mucosa, if it is inflamed, congested, or edematous. Deeper structures, either the muscular layer or serosa, can give rise to painful sensations when the stomach vigorously contracts, especially when the stomach wall is inflamed. Afferent impulses enter the cord at the level of the seventh to ninth dorsal roots. The pain of gastric origin is most often felt in the epigastrium, usually in the midline or in the left upper quadrant.

3. **Small and Large Intestines.** Noxious impulses from the small intestine travel in splanchnic pathways, but enter the cord slightly lower than do those from the stomach, from T9 to T11. The afferent innervation of the colon above the sigmoid is also carried in the sympathetic trunks. Below this level it is probably supplied mainly by afferent fibers through its mesentery from the lower thoracic and upper lumbar segmental nerves, without involvement of sympathetic or parasympathetic pathways. The rectum, however, does receive afferent nerves through the parasympathetic rami from S2 to S4.

Like the pain of a gastric ulcer, that due to a peptic ulcer of the duodenum is most often experienced in the epigastrium, usually in the midline or close by. It may not be possible to distinguish between the pain of a gastric ulcer and that of a duodenal ulcer. Both may be sharply localized, burning in character, beginning approximately one to two hours after meals and relieved by eating or antacids. A change of any kind in this pattern of pain of ulcer disease should suggest *penetration* into neighboring structures, such as the pancreas. Such pain is apt to be deeper, boring, less well-localized, persistent rather than intermittent, and not relieved by food or antacids.

There is poor localization of pain in disease affecting other regions of the intestine. As a general rule, pain from the small intestine is periumbilical, with some tendency for jejunal lesions to be felt in the upper left quadrant, and ileal pain to be felt in the right lower quadrant. Pain arising from colonic disorders generally is experienced in the lower half of the abdomen, and is relatively diffuse. Cecal and ascending colon pain usually is felt in the right lower quadrant. Pain of transverse and descending colon origin is located typically in the left lower abdomen. Disease of the sigmoid colon often produces suprapubic pain, or pain posteriorly in the region of the sacrum.

As described earlier, intestinal pain is typically colicky in nature. Each wave of pain is brief, usually lasting less than a minute. In between attacks of pain the patient may be entirely symptom-free. Audible bowel sounds can be heard at times synchronous with pain, and the patient may double-up or feel the urge to defecate. Indeed, in gastroenteritis, "irritable colon syndrome," and regional enteritis, pain may abate following the passage of stool. Intestinal obstruction, whether due to adhesions, strangulated hernia, intussusception, volvulus, or a constricting neoplasm, generally is characterized by colicky pain. Partial obstruction may give rise to repeated attacks of colicky pain, eventually ending in complete obstruction. If the site of obstruction is high in the intestine, vomiting is a prominent feature, the vomitus at times appearing "fecal" in character. If the obstructive lesion is low in the intestinal tract, distension and obstipation are more prominent early features than vomiting. In patients with acute mesenteric artery occlusion, abdominal pain may be continuous rather than colicky. Persistent pain also characterizes peritonitis; muscular rigidity, hyperalgesia, and tenderness to palpation are frequent accompanying features.

Enzyme deficiency may cause colicky abdominal pain, bloating, and diarrhea. The lactase deficiency of infants with intolerance to the lactose of milk is an example of this. Lactase deficiency is also frequent in adults, and is much more common among Negroes than among white persons. Evidence suggests that the enzyme deficiency may be genetically transmitted (Bayless). The enzyme lacking in adults may not be the same one that is deficient in infants; adults with the disturbance have not commonly had milk intolerance as infants. Ingested lactose is not digested, and remains in the intestinal lumen. A great deal of fluid enters the lumen to dilute this hypertonic load. The excess fluid causes distention, abdominal cramps, and increased peristalsis. In addition, the undigested lactose is fermented to lactic acid and this also acts as a cathartic. Carbon dioxide is also produced by this fermentation and contributes to the resultant bloating and frothy diarrhea.

Celiac disease of children or adults (nontropical sprue, idiopathic steatorrhea) is one of the hereditary *malabsorption syndromes*. Practically all patients suffering from this disease have abdominal discomfort; about 25 to 30 per cent have, at times, quite severe cramping pain. Large, pale, fatty, bulky stools are characteristic, often with diarrhea. There is a typical histologic alteration of the jejunal mucosa (blunt or absent villi, lengthened crypts, etc.). Diagnosis may be made by peroral suction biopsy. Present concepts of the pathophysiology involved are that the mucosa lacks one or more peptide-hydrolyzing *enzymes* that normally complete the digestion of gluten; the remaining peptides (in the gliadin fraction of the cereal protein, gluten) damage the epithelial absorbing surface of the small intestine; multiple manifestations of malabsorption result. Gluten-free diets have resulted in remission of the symptoms and improvement in the appearance of the mucosa; resumption of gluten intake causes a relapse. Generalized disaccharidase deficiency due to epithelial cell damage occurs, affecting lactase particularly. Milk or lactose ingestion may cause cramping abdominal pain and diarrhea.

One of the most serious and yet most frequent causes of severe abdominal pain is *acute appendicitis*. It is common to both sexes and all ages. Even laymen are familiar with it, as often the cause of right-lower-quadrant pain. However, in most instances, acute appendicitis begins not with right-sided pain, but with pain in the epigastrium or in the region of the umbilicus. Pain is soon followed by nausea and often by vomiting. Several hours after illness begins, pain classically shifts to the right lower quadrant, to an area frequently referred to as "McBurney's point," which is halfway between the umbilicus and the anterior superior spine of the ilium. In this region, deep tenderness, muscular rigidity, and cutaneous hyperalgesia usually can be demonstrated. Fever of 102° to 103°F and leukocytosis are characteristically present by this stage. If perforation of the appendix is to be avoided, surgery should not be delayed beyond this juncture. In patients with a retrocecal or pelvic appendix, pain may begin in the right lower quadrant. In such patients, and in elderly and debilitated persons, pain may be less intense and deep tenderness and muscle guarding are correspondingly less evident. Rectal examination may be of considerable value because it may elicit pain in the region of the appendix and a tender inflammatory mass may be palpated.

Acute gastorenteritis may produce pain, sometimes similar to that of acute appendicitis. Distinguishing features usually are: vomiting more common at the onset in the former, soon followed by diarrhea, which is rare with appendicitis; muscle guard and rebound tenderness and pain absent in the former, characteristic in the latter; often several associates or family members affected in the former.

Perforation of carcinoma of the colon may cause pain, tenderness, muscle spasm, vomiting, fever, and leukocytosis, and is difficult to distinguish from the clinical picture of acute appendicitis, especially in older persons.

Other conditions that may cause pain resembling that of acute appendicitis are discussed later in this chapter in the section on the acute abdomen. Still other conditions causing pain resembling that of acute appendicitis may originate in the organs located in the pelvis of the female and are discussed in the section on the genitourinary tract.

Diverticulitis of the colon is yet another important cause of serious abdominal pain of intestinal origin. In contrast to appendicitis, this condition is limited to adults, almost always of middle age and beyond. Because the sigmoid colon is the most frequent site of diverticula, the pain of acute diverticulitis is located in the lower abdomen, either in the midline or the left hypogastrium. When experienced in the latter region, the clinical picture has been likened to "left-sided appendicitis." Diverticula also may occur in the cecum and ascending colon, and diverticulitis in these locations can be confused with acute appendicitis. A previous history of similar attacks, and of derangements in bowel habits, and the absence of early epigastric or periumbilical pain do not assure, but favor, the diagnosis of diverticulitis.

PANCREAS, LIVER, AND BILIARY TRACT

Afferent impulses from the pancreas, biliary tract, and liver appear to travel in the same pathways as do those from the stomach and duodenum. The common pathways explain, in part, the difficulty that can be encountered in the differential diagnosis of epigastric pain. The more common painful disorders involving these structures include cholecystitis, biliary colic, acute pancreatitis, pancreatic carcinoma, and rapid hepatic enlargement.

The pain of *biliary tract origin* is usually experienced along the distribution of T8 or T9. In acute cholecystitis, right-upper-quadrant pain is most characteristic. Pain referred posteriorly to the angle of the scapula suggests a stone impacted in the cystic duct, and may occur alone or in association with pain in the right hypochondrium. Occasionally, pain may be referred to the right shoulder via the phrenic nerve. In acute cholecystitis, it is common to obtain a history of the onset of pain several hours after the ingestion of a large meal. During an attack, pain gradually builds in intensity, and although it may wax and wane, it does not entirely disappear until after the attack is over. Tenderness and muscular rigidity in the right upper quadrant are common findings, and occasionally an inflammatory mass or distended gallbladder may be palpable. The patient with acute cholecystitis is febrile and appears toxic. It should be remembered that the pain of cholecystitis can be atypically located in the chest, where it can be confused with the pain of coronary insufficiency or acute myocardial infarction. The passage of gallstones through extrahepatic bile ducts typically gives rise to biliary colic. The pain of biliary colic is sudden, intense, and paroxysmal. It is usually more localized than the pain of cholecystitis, but it can be felt either anteriorly in the right upper quadrant or posteriorly in the right subscapular area. Biliary colic is more frequently accompanied by vomiting and less often accompanied by muscular rigidity than is cholecystitis. In some instances, gallstones lodged in the common bile duct may be "silent", i.e., they may not produce pain; rather, recurrent episodes of fever and chills (Charcot's fever) may be the principal abnormality. An elevated serum bilirubin and alkaline phosphatase, a nonvisualizing gallbladder or one containing stones, or a dilated common bile duct on roentenographic studies of the biliary tract should lead to the correct diagnosis.

Diseases of the *pancreas* are among the most difficult intra-abdominal disorders to diagnose correctly. The pain of acute pancreatitis is usually sudden in onset, continuous in character, and epigastric in location; often it spreads to one or both flanks. It is almost always accompanied by vomiting. Shock may occur early in a severe attack; however, one or more of these features frequently is absent. A history of alcoholism or gallstones, or the presence of mild jaundice and a very high level of amylase in the serum or peritoneal fluid should help establish the correct diagnosis. The pain of pancreatic carcinoma may be either continuous and unrelenting or intermittent. Although it is usually located in the upper left abdomen or epigastrium, the patient may complain only of back pain, poorly localized. Carcinoma of the pancreas is one of the most difficult causes of abdominal pain to diagnose. Anorexia, severe weight loss, or depression, in association with upper abdominal pain should suggest this diagnosis. Later signs of far advanced disease include biliary tract obstruction, steatorrhea, and diabetes. All too frequently, the correct diagnosis is made very late in the course of the disease despite consultation with numerous physicians, including psychiatrists.

The hepatic parenchyma is insensitive to pain but *the liver's capsule*, when rapidly distended, can evoke right-upper-quadrant pain. Acute fatty infiltration of the liver in the alcoholic; the swollen edematous liver of cardiac decompensation; the inflamed swollen liver of viral or toxic hepatitis; and the enlarged liver with tumor or hepatic abscess are examples.

PERITONITIS

Peritonitis is most commonly due to rupture of a diseased viscus. Appendicitis or perforated peptic ulcer are the most common causes of peritonitis. Other causes include rupture of the gallbladder, perforation of a diverticulum, and pancreatic disease. Gastric fluid, bile, or pancreatic juice in the abdominal cavity initiates a violent and severe peritonitis manifested by immediate and intense pain (chemical peritonitis), whereas perforation of a viscus lower in the intestinal tract produces a more slowly developing picture of peritonitis (bacterial peritonitis).

In the acute state, beginning as chemical peritonitis, the role of enzyme action and of secondary anaerobic infection is frequently of importance in causing a rapid and enormous accumulation of peritoneal fluid. The amount of fluid in the peritoneal cavity may reach as much as one-third of the total plasma volume. Very sudden intense pain may, in itself, cause shock; massive fluid derangement is apt to cause shock; together, they account for the high mortality rates in such conditions.

Rupture of a liver abscess may be the cause of peritonitis (more frequently amebic, less often pyogenic). Perforation of an amebic ulcer of the colon will provoke peritonitis.

Free blood in contact with the peritoneum causes peritonitis, and may result from *trauma* to a viscus (spleen, liver, gallbladder, intestinal tract) or from a ruptured graafian follicle, ruptured tubal pregnancy, etc.

Pneumococcal peritonitis may occur from bacteremia or lymphatic spread of systemic infection. Diagnosis is made by examination of the purulent ascitic fluid. In children, especially young girls, pneumococcal peritonitis occurs occasionally. The vagina and fallopian tubes are presumably the portal of entry, and smears from the cervix may reveal the organism. In the nephrotic syndrome, particularly in children, peritonitis is a frequent complication; often there may be repeated episodes.

Streptococcal peritonitis is rare, but may occur from bacteremic spread from an upper respiratory infection, or in scarlet fever or erysipelas, or as a complication of an operative procedure or puerperal infection.

Gonococcal peritonitis may spread from salpingitis. The onset may be severe and sudden, but systemic symptoms tend to subside in a few days and the signs usually become those of a localized pelvic infection.

Tuberculous peritonitis may begin suddenly with severe abdominal pain, prostration, and high fever. Ascitic fluid may accumulate rapidly, causing distention and discomfort, and requiring tapping to afford relief. More characteristically, the onset is insidious, with moderate, poorly localized pain. The organism reaches the peritoneum by extension from lesions in the intestine, lymph nodes, or genital tract, or by hematogenous spread. The peritoneal infection may become chronic. It is the most common cause of ascites without leg edema in children. Adhesions may form, matting the intestines and omentum together. Often diarrhea occurs, and sometimes signs of partial intestinal obstruction due to bowel stenosis are present. The abdomen may be slightly or very tender, and is usually distended, with areas of tympanites and dullness, and with shifting fluid in the flanks. It is doughy to palpation, with tumor masses.

THE GENITOURINARY TRACT

Renal and urethral pain arise from afferent impulses that reach the spinal cord via the lower splanchnic trunks and the lower two thoracic and first lumbar segments. The pain of acute pyelonephritis is felt in the costovertebral angle posteriorly. Palpation or pressure over the area may elicit extreme discomfort. The passage of a renal stone or blood clot into the renal pelvis or ureter gives rise to "renal colic." An unforgettable experience for those unfortunate enough to be afflicted, the pain of renal colic is excruciating. It comes and goes in waves and typically is located in the flanks, radiating to the lower abdomen, often ending in the groin. Extreme restlessness characterizes the patient with renal colic, and frequency of urination and hematuria also may be present. Bladder pain, as in cystitis, is experienced suprapubicly, although pain due to lesions of the bladder trigone and urethra is felt at the distal tip of the urethra.

Prostatic pain is experienced in the perineum or lower lumbar region, where it may be confused with skeletal, muscular, nerve, rectal, or even renal pain. Pain arising from the testes or spermatic cord is largely felt in situ, although occasionally it may be referred to the hypogastrium.

Although far less common than dysmenorrhea or the pain of labor, the more serious causes of acute abdominal pain arising *in the female* are those related to ectopic pregnancy, torsion of an ovarian cyst, and pelvic inflammatory disease, usually due to gonococcal infection. Ectopic pregnancy, with its ever present danger of Fallopian tube rupture, must be seriously considered in any female of reproductive age with lower abdominal pain of colicky type who has not menstruated for one or more months. The recent onset of "morning sickness," tender enlarging breasts, and scant uterine bleeding are helpful clues when present. Pain due to torsion of an ovarian cyst usually is experienced laterally low in the abdomen. If located on the right side, it may be confused with the pain of acute appendicitis. The pain of acute pelvic inflammatory disease generally is continuous, and often is accompanied by signs of peritoneal irritation. An inflammatory mass that is exquisitely tender is found on pelvic examination, which may also reveal a purulent vaginal discharge containing intracellular gram-negative neisseria organisms.

OTHER CAUSES OF ABDOMINAL PAIN

Mention already has been made of the occurrence of abdominal pain due to *thoracic disease.* Thus, lower lobe pneumonia may produce severe upper quadrant abdominal pain, which may even be associated with muscular rigidity. However, the finding of pleuropulmonary abnormalities above the diaphragms in patients with abdominal pain does not insure a thoracic origin. Persons suffering from abdominal disorders frequently also have pathologic changes above the diaphragm. Pleural effusion may be seen in patients with pancreatitis, and atelectasis is not an uncommon finding in cholecystitis and various forms of liver disease.

Since *retroperitoneal and skeletomuscular structures* share the same afferent pathways as visceral organs, lesions involving these structures also may give rise to abdominal pain. Spinal cord and vertebral lesions also can produce abdominal pain, usually in a segmental or radicular distribution. A history of trauma, the characteristics of the pain (particularly with respect to posture), and definitive findings in the physical examination should permit separation of visceral from somatic origin of pain in most instances.

Abdominal pain may be seen in a variety of *systemic disorders.* The abdominal pain of acute intermittent porphyria, uremia, or diabetic ketoacidosis may simulate the pain of an "acute surgical abdomen." Lastly, sickle cell crises, lead intoxication, and snake and insect bites are very rare causes of abdominal pain.

THE ACUTE ABDOMEN

Use of the term "acute abdomen" usually is reserved for a situation in which the patient is suddenly incapacitated by very intense abdominal pain, which may or may not be associated with fever, nausea, vomiting, and shock. The special feature on examination is finding spasm of the abdominal muscles, sometimes amounting to a boardlike rigidity. In such circumstances, a surgical consultation is imperative, although operative intervention may not necessarily be required. Many of the causes of an acute abdomen have already been discussed. Appendicitis is the most common cause. Other causes include intestinal obstruction, perforation of a viscus with peritonitis, and vascular occlusion of mesenteric vessels with infarction of the bowel (Cope). The acute abdomen presents as an emergency problem, and yet more errors are made through failure to take time to question and examine the patient than from delay occasioned by a careful analysis of the problem. When the parietal peritoneum is an important source of the pain, an unusual or abnormal position of an organ such as a rotated sigmoid may cause confusion, as may the failure to take into account the complex peritoneal gutters through which pus may travel to a site distant from its origin. Thus, the corrosive fluid from a perforated ulcer may spread down the right pericolic gutter to produce intense pain and muscle spasm in the right lower quadrant. Conversely, fluid from a ruptured appendix may spread upward to the suprahepatic or infrahepatic spaces. The same principles apply to the diagnosis of the acute abdomen as to other less dramatic situations involving abdominal pain. Again, intrathoracic conditions must be considered: careful examination of the chest is indispensable.

Among the laboratory tests that are particularly helpful in the differential diagnosis of the acute abdomen are the white blood cell count and the serum amylase determination. In acute appendicitis, the white blood cell count usually is elevated, but rarely above 25,000 per cu. mm. Pneumonia, however, which may produce a confusing picture of abdominal pain, is often associated with a very high white blood cell count. On the other hand, acidosis associated with diabetes or renal disease may be accompanied by abdominal pain and a normal white blood cell count, by the presence of ketonemia and ketonuria in the case of diabetes, or an elevated blood urea nitrogen level in the case of renal failure. The serum amylase is most characteristically elevated in acute pancreatitis (with levels of higher than 600 mg. per cent usually achieved). In an acute exacerbation of chronic pancreatitis, however, the serum amylase may be normal. Perforation of a peptic ulcer near the pancreas may produce elevation of serum amylase reaching 400 mg. per cent. Other procedures that may be helpful in differential diagnosis include sickle cell preparations, examinations of the blood for hemoglobinopathies, and Ehrlich's test of urinary porphobilinogen. Roentgenologic examination of the abdomen is often helpful, particularly if there is free air in the abdominal cavity indicating an intestinal perforation, or air-fluid levels within the lumen of the gut indicating intestinal obstruction. Gallstones may, of course, be visualized, as may occasionally, calcification of the pancreas or blood vessels. The introduction of barium into either end of the intestinal tract may help in diagnosis, but use of barium is to be avoided if perforation is suspected. Arteriography may demonstrate occlusion of a major mesenteric artery. Another procedure that may be of substantial help is the "peritoneal tap." Fluid so obtained should be examined by immediate inspection: is it serous, hemorrhagic, purulent, or chylous? It should be studied microscopically by proper cytologic and staining techniques for red blood cells, leukocytes, bacteria, and neoplastic cells. It should be cultured for possible infectious organisms and tested for pancreatic enzymes.

In conditions requiring prompt or possible surgical intervention, the diagnosis must be made quickly. An hour or two delay in surgery may increase the likelihood of a serious, and possibly fatal, outcome.

BIBLIOGRAPHY

Bayless, T., and Rosensweig, N.: Incidence and implications of lactase deficiency and milk intolerance in white and Negro populations, Johns Hopkins Med. J. 121:54, 1967.

Bircher, J., Bartholomew, L. G., Cain, J. C., and Adson, M. A.: Syndrome of intestinal arterial insufficiency (abdominal angina), Arch. Intern. Med. 117:632, 1966.

Cope, Z.: The Early Diagnosis of the Acute Abdomen, ed. 13, London, Oxford Univ. Press, 1968.

Haemmerli, U. P., *et al.*: Acquired milk intolerance in the adult caused by lactose malabsorption due to a selective deficiency of intestinal lactase activity, Amer. J. Med. 38:7, 1965.

Head, H.: On disturbances of sensation with especial reference to the pain of visceral disease, Brain 16:1, 1893.

Hertz, A. F.: The Goulstonian lectures on the sensibility of the alimentary canal in health and disease, Lancet 1:1051, 119, 1187, 1215, 1911.

Jones, C.: Digestive Tract Pain, Diagnosis and Treatment. Experimental Observations, New York, Macmillan, 1938.

Lennander, K. G.: Uber die Sensibilitat der Bauchhohle und uber lokale und allgemeine Anasthesie bei Bruch-und Bauchoperationen, Zbl. Chir. 28: 209, 1901.

Leriche, R.: The Surgery of Pain, p. 434, Baltimore, Williams & Wilkins Co., 1939.

MacKenzie, J.: Some points bearing on the association of sensory disorders and visceral disease, Brain 16:321, 1893.

Ross, J.: On the segmental distribution of sensory disorders, Brain 10:333, 1888.

Ryle, J. A.: Visceral pain and referred pain, Lancet 1:895, 1926.

———: The clinical study of pain with special reference to pains of visceral disease, Brit. Med. J. 1:537, 1928.

von Haller, A.: Memoires sur la Nature Sensible et Irritable des Parties du corps Animal. Tome Quatrieme, contenant les Responses Faites a Differentes Objections, p. 232, Lausanne, S. D'Arnay, 1760.

Wolff, H. G., and Wolf, S.: Pain, Springfield, Ill., Charles C Thomas, 1948.

10

Urinary Tract Pain
Hematuria and Pyuria

ALAN D. PERLMUTTER and *ROBERT S. BLACKLOW*

URINARY TRACT PAIN

Anatomic and Physiologic Conditions

The urinary tract consists of organs and structures serving varied functions. The kidneys are involved in the formation and excretion of urine by the filtration of plasma and by the secretion and reabsorption of small molecules and ions. The ureters conduct the urine, by peristalsis, to empty into the bladder. The bladder serves the dual functions of storage and evacuation. The urethra is the pathway to the exterior, and its voluntary sphincter helps provide urinary control.

The kidneys are paired organs in the upper retroperitoneum, below the diaphragm, usually opposite the T2 to L2 vertebral bodies. The ureters extend from the upper retroperitoneum into the true pelvis. The bladder in the adult is extraperitoneal and within the bony pelvis, except for the dome, which when distended can be palpated in the hypogastrium.

Nerve Supply to the Urinary Tract

The kidneys and ureters are innervated by both the sympathetic and parasympathetic components of the autonomic nervous system (Fig. 10-1). Parasympathetic innervation to the kidney is derived from the vagus; the function is not known.[1] Sympathetic fibers are derived from the thoracolumbar trunk, T6 to L3 inclusive, mainly T10 to L1. These fibers travel in the superior, middle and inferior splanchnic nerves. Preganglionic fibers terminate in the semilunar (celiac) ganglion and, for the inferior splanchnic nerve, in the aorticorenal ganglion. Postganglionic fibers enter the renal plexus, a network of nerves intimately associated with the renal vascular pedicle. From this plexus, fibers supply the intrarenal arterial system and calyces. Branches extend to the renal capsule, upper ureter, and adrenal. A few fibers connect to the opposite renal plexus. The pathways of postganglionic nerves vary; the inferior splanchnic nerve is inconstant. Some nerve fibers pass directly to the renal plexus, together with branches of first and second ganglia of the lumbar sympathetic chain. Some of these direct connections may represent sensory (afferent) pathways traveling with sympathetic afferent fibers. Stimulation of efferent nerves to the kidney alters urine formation by changes in intrarenal arterial tone.[1,2,3]

Afferent nerves from the kidney are both myelinated and unmyelinated. Some of these nerves monitor changes in renal venous pressure[4] and distention of the renal pelvis

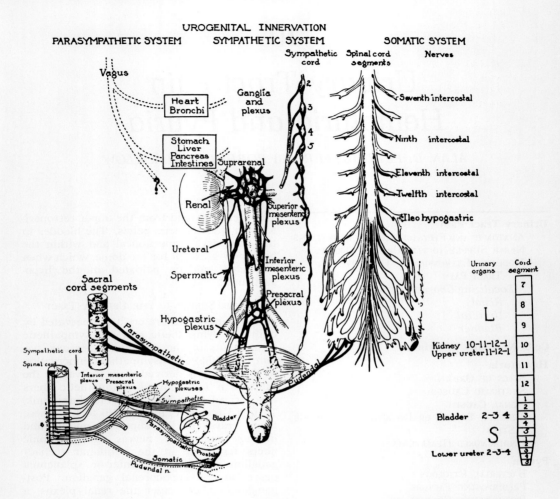

FIG. 10-1. Diagrammatic representation of urinary tract innervation. (Campbell, M. F., ed.: Urology, Philadelphia, Saunders, 1963, pp. 1-46)

and capsule. The anatomy and neurophysiology of the renal sensory pathways is poorly understood. Sensory fibers and receptors have not been demonstrated in the human kidney, and sensory endings have not been identified in the renal pelvis or upper ureter, although myelinated fibers are present.[5] In human subjects undergoing a unilateral sympathectomy under procaine block, pain responses were elicited by stretching or compressing the renal pelvis, pedicle, or ureter near the ureteropelvic junction. Unilateral sympathectomy from T7 to 11, and division of the greater and lesser splanchnic nerves at the celiac ganglion eliminated these pain responses. No contralateral pain was sensed. During the same studies, upper ureteral pain

was eliminated when the T12 and L1 ganglia were excised.[6]

Innervation of the ureter is by multiple fibers extending from a meshwork of retroperitoneal plexuses. These include renal, spermatic, aortic, inferior mesenteric, hypogastric, and inferior vesical plexuses, and fibers from the celiac and aorticorenal ganglia. The terminal ureter receives parasympathetic branches from S2, 3, and 4, which segments also supply the bladder.[3,7]

Ureteral afferents from the upper ureter are found in the 11th and 12th thoracic, the first, and possibly the second lumbar nerves. Distal ureteral afferents enter the second, third, and fourth sacral segments. Although the proximal ureter has a sensory innervation, sensory terminations have been identified only for the lower ureter, where sensory fibers pass through the muscularis into the mucous membrane. Connections have been demonstrated between nerve fibers to the ureter and the plexuses which supply the ovary, testis, and parietal peritoneum.[5,7,8]

The bladder has a triple innervation: sympathetic, parasympathetic, and somatic. The parasympathetic pathways of the bladder—S2, 3, and 4—provide motor function for coordinated voiding. Afferent parasympathetic fibers mediate the desire to void, proprioception, and pain. All of these sensory and motor pathways run together in the pelvic nerves (nervi erigentes).

The sympathetic supply to the bladder is found in the hypogastric plexus, also referred to as the hypogastric or presacral nerve. The sympathetic pathways to the bladder provide motor innervation to the trigone; sectioning of these nerves does not result in an altered voiding pattern. Sympathetic afferents provide additional subjective awareness of bladder distention, pain, and less specific abdominal discomfort from vesical distention.[9,10] This sensory input reaches the cord at T9 or even higher. From studies in patients with traumatic paraplegia, it has been observed that awareness of distention is decreased as the cord lesion becomes more proximal, and disappears completely at T6 to T4.[11]

Sensory receptors have been detected in the mucous membrane of the bladder, proving that pain stimuli can originate in the mucous membrane. Since the sensory fibers run through the muscularis, contraction of the bladder wall may also cause pain. The sensory fibers are more concentrated near the ureterovesical junction, the bladder neck, and the trigone in decreasing density, and are less well-developed in the remainder of the bladder.[5]

The urethra has a rich sensory innervation from S2, 3, and 4 via the pudendal nerve, a mixed somatic nerve, which also contains motor fibers to the external urethral sphincter. Some sensory receptors within the urethra respond to flow, others to urethral distention.[12] Thermal sensation is also present in the urethra, and plays a role in awareness of urination. As contrasted with desire to void, imminence of voiding is from urethral sensation and from traction on the bladder neck and trigone by the contracting bladder.[10]

Modes of Expression of Urinary Tract Pain

Because of the extensive and variable distribution of nerve fibers to the urinary tract, pain patterns are protean. The proximity of urinary organs to intraperitoneal structures and the extensive collateral nerve supply through the celiac and other plexuses are two reasons why localization of disease processes by site of pain may be difficult. As with other visceral pains, urinary tract pain is less well-localized than corresponding somatic pain involving the same dermatomes; one reason for this is the decreased density of innervation of the involved viscus as compared to skin. Visceral and skin afferents probably converge at different levels in the nervous system: impulses converge on the same secondary or tertiary neuron. Localization of visceral pain is also learned. Children localize urinary tract pathology less well than adults. Accuracy and body awareness tend to become greater with experience, growth, and development.[13]

Localizing Characteristics

Renal pain follows acute stretching of the capsule or distension of the collecting system. Pain of renal origin is classically felt in the posterior subcostal and costovertebral region, and is usually aching in nature, although severe, boring pain may be present. Hyperesthesia of associated dermatomes (usually T9-10) may occur. Radiation forward around the flank into the lower abdominal quadrant (T11-12), and ipsilateral or generalized abdominal pain, spasm of abdominal muscles, and even rebound tenderness occur with severe discomfort; often these latter symptoms exist alone, or exceed the posterior pain. Nausea, vomiting, and paralytic ileus accompany severe acute pain. Pain referred to the contralateral abdomen has been described,[14] but this is exceedingly rare.

Distention of the ureter is painful. The most common cause is an obstructing calculus, which has descended from the kidney, with sudden dilatation of both kidney and ureter. Unusual pain patterns may result, but typically, pain of ureteral origin starts in the costovertebral angle, and radiates to the lower abdomen, upper thigh, testis, or labium on the same side. The pain is usually excruciating, and the patient writhes about, unable to obtain relief. In contrast, with the pain of peritonitis, the patient lies quietly because motion increases the discomfort.[15]

If the calculus has reached the ureterovesical junction, urgency, frequency, and stinging referred to the urethra and glans of the phallus may be noted. Rectal tenesmus is sometimes another symptom of sudden low ureteral obstruction. As with renal pain, ileus with distention, nausea, and vomiting can occur. Acute urinary retention has also been noted.

Severe ureteral pain most often is felt as crescendo waves of colic. Once thought to be due to ureteral spasm or hyperperistalsis proximal to the acute obstruction, this pain has been shown to be caused by distention of and trauma to the ureter itself. Amplitudes of contraction pressure higher than normal have not been recorded in acutely obstructed ureters; rather the resting pressure rises and the amplitude of the contraction complexes falls as the ureter progressively dilates.[16] Upon physical examination, hyperesthesia of associated dermatomes (T12 and L1) and tenderness to palpation over the ureter and kidney, with or without rebound, may be present.

Chronic renal and ureteral pain tend to be vague, poorly localized, and atypical, and easily confused with that from other visceral or somatic lesions.[17] Complete examination, including urinalysis and urographic study, is required for a differential diagnosis. Other possible causes of acute or chronic pain of a similar nature include a perforated viscus, intestinal obstruction, cholecystitis, retrocecal appendicitis, acute seminal vesiculitis, pelvic inflammatory disease, tubo-ovarian abscess, ruptured ectopic pregnancy, twisted ovarian cyst, or any other cause of peritonitis or peritonismus.

When inflammatory lesions of the upper urinary tract extend beyond the collecting system, adjacent structures become involved. Perinephritis or perinephric abscess may irritate the diaphragm, resulting in shoulder pain; with periureteral disease, pain may occur on movement of the adjacent ileopsoas muscle. Rebound tenderness results when the adjacent peritoneum becomes inflamed.

Bladder pain is suprapubic or low abdominal, usually associated with great urgency, tenesmus, and dysuria. Inflammation of the urethra and bladder neck may result in a "hot" or burning sensation, because of stimulation of previously described thermal receptors in the urethra. Frequency and urgency result from stimulation of the proprioceptive and sensory receptors in the bladder wall and urethra. Upon examination, suprapubic and sometimes urethral tenderness may be observed, and if the infection arises in the prostate gland, a swollen, tender, hot gland is palpable.

The foregoing review of urinary tract pain has considered the pertinent anatomic and physiologic factors. The modes of presentation and expression have been described. The reasons for the variability of symptoms that are encountered have been discussed. Many of the disturbances resulting in urinary tract pain are inflammatory conditions of which hematuria or pyuria are important manifestations.

CELLS NORMALLY IN URINE

Both red blood cells and white blood cells (predominantly polymorphonuclear leukocytes) are found in normal urine in small numbers. Their route and their mode of entry into the urinary tract is unclear. That the ratio of red blood cells to white blood cells in blood is 1000:1 and in urine is 1:30 suggests that these cells do not come from minute hemorrhages along the urinary tract.[18] In the presence of urinary tract disease, increased numbers of red cells and white cells are found in the urine; it is only when these blood elements are seen in casts that one may be certain that they derive from the kidney,[19,20] unless red or white cells are collected by ureteral catheterization.

HEMATURIA

Hematuria is the presence of red blood cells in the urine. Bleeding from the urinary tract, whether gross or microscopic, is a serious sign. It should be looked upon with the same gravity as abnormal bleeding elsewhere in the body. Gross hematuria is not always red. The color of bloody urine depends upon the amount of blood present and the pH of the urine. In an acid urine, the color is often brown or smoky; in an alkaline urine, the color is red. Not all red urine is blood: cell-free hemoglobin or myoglobin stain the urine red. Drugs, food pigments, and metabolites may also color the urine red: azo dyes, phenolphthalein, indole alkaloids, beets, and porphyrins are among these substances.

Red blood cells may be found in the urine of healthy individuals. The classic studies of Addis,[21] Goldring,[22] and others[23,24] have established that the normal excretion of red blood cells per 12-hour period for healthy adults is up to 400,000 cells. In children aged 4 to 12 years, up to 600,000 red blood cells per 12 hours may be found.[25] An investigator from one insurance company diluted 600,000 red blood cells in 300 ml. of clear urine and found about 2 red blood cells per high-power microscopic field after handling the specimen in the usual manner.[23] In 6,000 consecutive male and female urine specimens examined by one observer, 78 per cent had no red blood cells per high-power field, and 94 per cent had one or less[26] (Fig. 10-2). These two studies suggest the normal limits of erythrocytes in urine as under 2 per high-power field.

Vigorous exercise, lordotic posture, acute febrile illness, dehydration, and unbalanced dietary intake may produce microscopic hematuria in the absence of serious disease of the urinary tract.[22,24,27]

Site of Origin. Hematuria may be classified on an anatomic or an etiologic basis. Noting whether hematuria is initial, total, or terminal may help in the localization. *Initial*

hematuria suggests the urethra as the source; *terminal hematuria* suggests the posterior urethra, trigone, or bladder base. *Total hematuria* means that red blood cells are dispersed throughout the urinary stream and suggests origins from the kidney, ureter, or bladder. Hematuria accompanied by red blood cell *casts* indicates a renal origin, such as acute or subacute inflammatory lesions of the glomeruli and renal parenchyma.

Systemic causes of bleeding may present with hematuria. A complete listing is beyond the scope of this chapter, but some of the more common causes are the following: hemophilia, anticoagulant therapy with either heparin or vitamin K antagonists, thrombocytopenia, polycythemia vera, hyperglobulinemic syndromes with generalized vascular bleeding, scurvy, and sickle-cell disease. Extra-urinary-tract pathology, such as endometrial, cervical, and rectal neoplasms, may

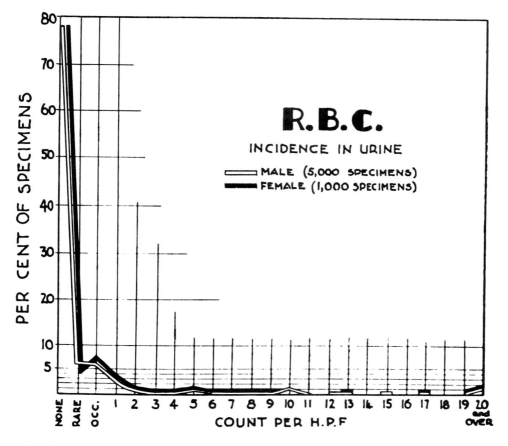

FIG. 10-2. Red blood cell counts in the sediment of 5,000 consecutive male and 1,000 consecutive female urine specimens received at the John Hancock Mutual Life Insurance Company. (Adapted from Wright, W. T.: Arch. Intern. Med., 103:76, 1959)

invade the urinary tract and produce hematuria. Endometriosis involving the urinary tract produces cyclical bleeding with the menses.

Renal. Polycystic renal disease, renal artery embolism, renal vein thrombosis, cortical necrosis, renal infarction, acute tubular necrosis, angiitis, periarteritis nodosa, systemic lupus erythematosus, allergic purpura, acute and chronic glomerulonephritis, focal glomerulonephritis, acute pyelonephritis, malignant nephrosclerosis, postradiation nephritis, hereditary nephritis, sponge kidney, Wegner's granulomatosis, nephrocalcinosis, and nephrotoxins are all examples of renal parenchymal lesions that bleed. Since many of these are associated with glomerulitis, red blood cell casts will also be present. Proper history, physical examination, and laboratory studies, including (if necessary) renal biopsy, will help in the differential diagnosis.

Discussion. Tumors, urinary tract obstruction, calculi, and infection account for over 60 per cent of hematuria in adults. Painless total hematuria is suggestive of a tumor in the urinary tract, and at least 20 per cent of the people with this presenting symptom will prove to have a urinary tract neoplasm. Tumors of the renal parenchyma produce hematuria when the kidney pelvis has been invaded. The bleeding may be variable in volume and amount, often with clots.[28] Tumors of the upper collecting system and ureter (those parts of the urinary tract lined with transitional cell epithelium) also present with bleeding in over 74 per cent of the cases;[29] the bleeding is painless and has no distinctive characteristics as to amount and timing. Gross hematuria occurs in 60 to 90 per cent of bladder tumors.[30]

Depending upon the anatomical location of a urinary tract neoplasm, the bleeding may be initial, terminal, or total. It is apparent that complete urologic visualization of both the upper and lower urinary tract is required to diagnose hematuria. Techniques used to localize the source of bleeding include intravenous urography, cytoscopy, retrograde ureteropyelography and aortography with selective injection of contrast material into the renal artery to outline the abnormal vascular supply of the tumor. Assays of certain enzymatic activities in urine have also proved helpful in the differential diagnosis of urinary tract neoplasms. Wacker and his co-workers[31] have found the urinary activities of lactic dehydrogenase and alkaline phosphatase to be reliable indicators of neoplastic cellular growth in the absence of bacterial contamination of urine or lysis of cellular elements.

Renal, ureteral, and bladder calculi, acute, chronic, and interstitial cystitis, vascular malformations of the bladder, prostatic venous congestion secondary to benign prostatic hyperplasia, and radiation cystitis are all common lower urinary tract causes of hematuria.

Hematuria may also occur in association with pyuria when there is urinary tract infection. In acute pyelonephritis, renal tuberculosis, and leptospirosis, the damaged blood vessels are probably in the kidney. Painless hematuria, "sterile" pyuria, and an acid urinary pH should suggest renal tuberculosis. The bladder is often the source of the hematuria in leishmaniasis and genitourinary schistosomiasis. Once again, history, physical examination, and appropriate laboratory studies will aid in the diagnosis.

Trauma must not be neglected as a significant cause of bleeding from the kidneys and bladder. Whether or not trauma is associated with pain depends upon the extent of renal capsule distention or tear and upon the extent of blood and urine extravasation into the retroperitoneum. A study on boxers by Kleiman[32] demonstrated a correlation between injuries from boxing, hematuria, and morphologic and physiologic changes in the upper urinary tract.

Undiagnosed hematuria, referred to in the past as "idiopathic hematuria" or "renal epistaxis," may require vigorous and repeated studies in an attempt to find the cause. When the etiology has not been discovered, the listing should be: *"hematuria, cause to be determined."* It is hoped that newer techniques of study, including renal angiography and biopsy, will reduce undiagnosed cases to a minimum, and reduce the temptation either to operate upon or to neglect patients with hematuria of unknown cause.

PYURIA

Pyuria means leukocytes in the urine. A few white blood cells normally occur in the urine. Up to 2,000,000 leukocytes and nonsquamous epithelial cells per 12-hour period may be excreted by a normal male adult, with a mean of from 600,000 to 1,000,000.[21,24,33] Children from 4 to 12 years of age have a similar excretion rate, with the mean for girls slightly higher than that for boys.[25] This amount may also (as in red blood cells) be increased by fever, exercise, and diet.[22,24,27] A life insurance study demonstrated that 90 per cent of males had less than 2 white blood cells (or nonsquamous epithelial cells) per high-power microscopic field, and 76 per cent of noncatheterized females had less than 5 white blood cells per high-power field[26] (Fig. 10-3).

Pyuria, especially with clumping of white blood cells, denotes the presence of an inflammatory process in the urinary tract and indicates the need for (1) complete bacteriologic studies, and (2) studies to localize the site of the infection, and (3) its type. White blood cell **casts** localize the infection to the renal parenchyma. However, the number of leukocytes in the urine may be little indication of the severity of the lesion in the urinary tract, since pyuria may be intermittent or absent when associated with chronic pyelonephritis, perinephric abscess, renal cortical abscess, or total obstruction of a kidney or ureter.

Bacteriuria may be present without pyuria. It has been emphasized recently that chronic pyelonephritis with sight to even severe bacteriuria may be associated with little or no significant pyuria.[34] This observation has been noted for many years by pathologists. Several British workers have proposed that the white blood cell excretion rate[33] in response to an intravenous injection of bacterial lipopolysaccharide or prednisolone may be used as a diagnostic measure to detect the inflammation of chronic pyelonephritis. A rise in white blood cell excretion rate to over 400,000 cells per hour in response to the aforementioned stress was found in all but two of 67 patients with chronic pyelonephritis.[35] Other workers have found that the white blood cell excretion rate on the side of the lesion in unilateral chronic pyelonephritis is elevated.[36] It is known that some bacterial pyrogens are lipopolysaccharides; perhaps transitory pyuria during an acute febrile illness also may be mediated in this manner. The finding of "glitter cells" in the urine (leukocytes with characteristic supravital staining and granular motility) had been thought to be indicative of renal infection. However, studies have shown this phenomenon to be nonspecific, and one must urge caution against overinterpretation of the glitter-cell phenomenon as pathognomonic for renal infection.[37-39] These cells have also been found in prostatic fluid, vaginal secretions, oxalated blood, and joint fluids; the glitter cell may represent a damaged white blood cell.

Pyuria with a urine culture negative for the more commonly implicated bacteria is

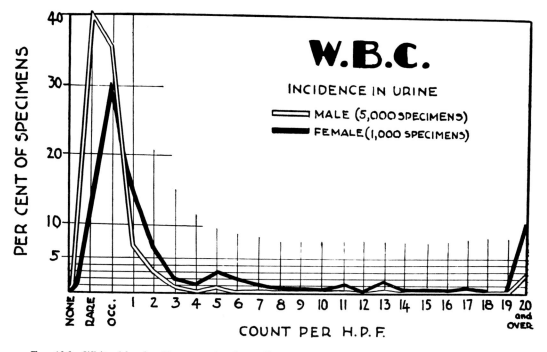

Fig. 10-3. White blood cell counts in the sediment of 5,000 consecutive male and 1,000 consecutive female urine specimens received at the John Hancock Mutual Life Insurance Company. (Adapted from Wright, W. T.: Arch. Intern. Med., 103:76, 1959)

called *sterile pyuria*. In this instance, cultures for tubercle bacilli and special studies for uncommon infections such as atypical bacteria (especially *mycoplasma* strains), parasites, and schistosomes should be undertaken.

Pyuria and an alkaline urine suggest a urea-splitting ammonia-producing organism, such as *Proteus vulgaris*. If pyuria persists after the infecting agent itself appears to have been eradicated, this is suggestive of obstruction, stasis (hydronephrosis, megaureter, or bladder hypotonia with persistent post-voiding residual), or abscess. Urgency, frequency, and suprapubic pain associated with a purulent urine are indicative of lower urinary tract infection.

In females, vaginal contamination, especially leukorrhea, may give an impression of pyuria. Adequate cleansing procedures before voiding and proper technique of collection will eliminate this error.

Pyuria may be initial, terminal, or total; and this is the basis of the three-glass test. Most of the white cells are found in the first glass with urethritis or urethral diverticulum, and in the first or third glass with prostatitis. White blood cells equally distributed in all three glasses define the source as the bladder or above. The three-glass test is, at best, qualitative: it indicates the possible rather than probable anatomic location of pyuria.

BACTERIAL ETIOLOGY

Pyuria indicates bacterial infection at one or more sites in the urinary tract. Bacterial infection may ascend upward or progress downward. Bacteria occasionally reach the urinary tract through the blood or lymph vessels during systemic infections, or metastatically from a locus elsewhere (abscess, empyema, etc.). The usual route, however, is from the anus through the urethra, with ascending infection. The bacteria involved most commonly are coliform bacilli, which are normal saprophytic inhabitants of the intestinal tract, particularly *Escherichia coli* (the colon bacillus) and *Aerobacter (Klebsiella) aerogenes*. Although harmless in the intestine, such bacteria may cause severe infection if introduced into tissues. Over 95 per cent of cases of acute pyelitis are caused by gram-negative enteric bacilli. A small percentage of cases of acute pyelonephritis results from infections with gram-positive cocci, enterococcus, and staphylococcus. Frequently, two or more kinds of bacteria may be active simultaneously in causing urinary

tract infection. Other microorganisms, which may be pathogens, are proteus, pseudomonas, chromobacteria, and fungi. In most instances, infection by microorganisms other than those of the coli-aerogenes group are related to previous instrumentation of the urinary tract (by catheter or cystoscope, etc.).

Normally, the urinary tract is free of bacteria except near the urethral meatus. Some bacteria, usually those commonly on the skin, such as staphylococci and diphtheroids, are normally present in the lower urethra. Cleansing of the urethral meatus and collection of a midstream urine sample when getting a specimen for culture or microscopic study will help to avoid these contaminants.

Urine specimens examined for cells, bacteria, or culture should be fresh; urine is a good medium for growth of bacteria. Measurement of the approximate number of bacteria present per milliliter in a freshly voided specimen will help to indicate whether infection is present and the severity of the infection. A drop of fresh uncentrifuged urine is placed upon a slide and stained with methylene blue or Gram's stain. If bacteria are found, the number exceeds that which may occur from urethral contamination, and probably is in the range of 100,000 per ml.; quantitative cultures should be done. If the yield indicates more than 100,000 bacteria per ml. of fresh urine, active infection is present; if 10,000 or less are found, they are probably not significant; if between 10,000 and 100,000 are found, they are indeterminate.

PREDISPOSING FACTORS

Factors predisposing to urinary tract infection include *trauma* and *stasis*. The epithelial membranes lining the tract may be damaged by a stone, by instrumentation, etc. Stasis may occur in hydronephrosis, with obstructing stones or prostatic hypertrophy, etc. Bacteria grow well in urine; a slowed flow provides time for greater multiplication, and a heavy inoculum results, increasing the possibilities of invasion of tissues along the tract.

CONDITIONS PREDISPOSING TO URINARY TRACT INFECTIONS

1. **Age and Sex. Infants** during the diaper period (early months to 2 years) have a high incidence of urinary tract infections because of fecal soiling of the urethral meatus. Because of the greater anatomical ease of contamination, females are affected much more often than males.

Women at any age, presumably because of

the short female urethra and its location, have urinary tract infections several times as commonly as men, except for *men in older age groups* who have prostatic obstruction.

2. **Pregnancy.** Acute urinary tract infections occur in 2 or 3 per cent of pregnant women, appearing usually in the last half of the pregnancy, or early in the puerperium. At this time, ureters and kidney pelves are somewhat dilated.

3. **Obstructive Disorders.** A stone, a stricture, a tumor, prostatic hypertrophy, or any condition impeding the free flow of urine causes stasis and favors urinary tract infection. Persistent obstruction results in hydronephrosis, increasing the incidence of pyelonephritis some 10 or 12 times.

4. **Neurogenic Bladder Dysfunction.** Neuropathies interfering with emptying of the bladder, especially if repeated catheterization has been done, are highly apt to result in urinary tract infection. This may occur in diabetic patients, those with spinal-cord injuries, multiple sclerosis, tabes dorsalis, etc.

5. **Diabetes Mellitus.** Among persons with diabetes mellitus significant bacteriuria is about 3 times as common, and pyelonephritis is about 4 times as common as among the nondiabetic population. Factors believed to cause this include: poorer tissue resistance, poorer circulatory supply, and possible neurogenic bladder dysfunction.

Cystitis is very common in diabetes. Pyelonephritis of all forms (acute, chronic interstitial, intrarenal abscesses, and necrotizing papillitis) are several times as common in the diabetic as in the nondiabetic population.

Necrotizing papillitis (medullary necrosis) occurs as a very severe and destructive form of pyelonephritis, occurring at times among persons with obstructive uropathy, in neurogenic bladder dysfunction, and especially if repeated instrumentation has been done. Those with diabetes mellitus are particularly susceptible to this often violent renal complication, developing it from 3 to 7 times as often as do nondiabetic persons. It is obvious that instrumentation should be avoided, especially in diabetics, whenever possible; catheterization should never be done, for example, simply to obtain a urine specimen for bacterial culture.

PYURIA—MOST COMMON CLINICAL PICTURES

Acute Pyelonephritis. The onset may be gradual, with frequency, dysuria, and fever; after a few days, sudden severe symptoms appear. Often there is no preliminary phase, but an abrupt onset with unilateral or bi-lateral flank pain, fever of 103° to 105°, frequently with one or more chills, sometimes nausea, and vomiting. There is leukocytosis, usually of 15,000 to 25,000. The urine reveals bacteria, usually on uncentrifuged direct stain; a culture usually shows growth in 24 hours, indicating a quantitative bacterial count above 100,000 per ml. However, diagnosis is not based upon the number of organisms—pyelonephritis may be present with any bacterial count. The centrifuged urine shows many leukocytes, often in clumps; frequently in uncentrifuged specimens, several white blood cells or masses may be seen per high-power microscopic field.

Acute pyelonephritis may subside with or without treatment. It may recur with symptoms almost unnoticed, or with manifestations of various severity. Frequently a chronic pyelitis develops which may be asymptomatic over long periods, even years. Gradual destruction of kidney tissue may take place; probably under such conditions repeated study of the urine would reveal pyuria and bacteria, although it is evidently often intermittent.

Chronic Pyelonephritis. Often progressive pyelonephritis or recurrent mild attacks of pyelonephritis may produce no signs or symptoms over periods of months or years. Sometimes manifestations are general and nonspecific, such as fatigue and normochromic anemia. Usually there is no fever or leukocytosis, and no flank pain (unless there is a calculus, or obstructive neuropathy, or exacerbation of acute pyelonephritis). If any of the predisposing circumstances just listed are present, repeated examination of the urinary tract and urine are indicated. The urine may be relatively free of leukocytes or microorganisms for long periods. Intravenous pyelograms may be informative.

When pyelonephritis is persistent and chronically progressive or if acute pyelonephritis recurs repeatedly, enough renal tissue may be destroyed so that evidence of renal failure may appear, such as elevation of the blood urea nitrogen, deficient concentrating ability, etc., often with elevated blood pressure.

Cystitis. Inflammation of the urinary bladder usually causes quite characteristic evidence. Often it is preceded by urethritis. Micturition is frequent, and urgent, and is accompanied by burning pain. There is discomfort and tenderness over the bladder and pyuria. Usually there is no leukocytosis and little or no fever.

If systemic symptoms appear, such as

prostration, nausea, or vomiting, or a fever over 101° F, concomitant infection should be suspected elsewhere, particularly in the prostate or kidney.

REFERENCES

1. Last, R. J.: Anatomy, Regional and Applied, ed. 3, p. 473, London, J. and A. Churchill, Ltd., 1966.
2. Lich, R., Jr., and Howerton, L. W.: Anatomy and surgical approach to the urogenital tract in the male, *in* Campbell, M. F. (ed.): Urology, pp. 1–46, Philadelphia, Saunders, 1963.
3. Colby, F. H.: Essential Urology, pp. 18–21, Baltimore, Williams and Wilkins, 1961.
4. Aström, A., and Crafoord, J.: Afferent activity recorded in the kidney nerves of rats, Acta Physiol. Scand. 70:10–15, 1967.
5. Hachiro-Seto: Studies on the Sensory Innervation (Human Sensibility), ed. 2, pp. 250–323, Tokyo, Igaku Shoin, Ltd., 1963.
6. Ray, B. S., and Neill, C. L.: Abdominal visceral sensation in man, Ann. Surg. 126:709–724, 1947.
7. Wharton, L. R.: The innervation of the ureter, with respect to denervation, J. Urol. 28:639–673, 1932.
8. Kiil, F.: The Function of the Ureter and Renal Pelvis, pp. 108–131, Philadelphia, Saunders, 1957.
9. Learmonth, J. R.: A contribution to the neurophysiology of the urinary bladder in man, Brain 54:147–176, 1931.
10. Nathan, P. W.: Sensations associated with micturition, Brit. J. Urol. 28:126–131, 1956.
11. Bors, E.: Segmental and peripheral innervation of the urinary bladder, J. Nerv. Ment. Dis. 116:572–578, 1952.
12. Todd, J. K.: Afferent impulses in the pudendal nerves of the cat, Quart. J. Exp. Physiol. 49:258–267, 1964.
13. Sinclair, D.: Cutaneous Sensation, pp. 185–189, London, Oxford Univ. Press, 1967.
14. Campbell, M. F.: Clinical Pediatric Urology, p. 4, Philadelphia, Saunders, 1951.
15. Cope, V. Z.: The Early Diagnosis of the Acute Abdomen, 13th ed., p. 24, London, Oxford Univ. Press, 1968.
16. Kiil, F.: Physiology of the renal pelvis and ureter, *in* Campbell, M. F. (ed.): Urology, pp. 81–117, Philadelphia, Saunders, 1963.
17. Goodwin, W. E.: Retroperitoneal causes of abdominal pain, *in* Mellinkoff, S. M. (ed.): Differential Diagnosis of Abdominal Pain, pp. 255–312, New York, McGraw-Hill, 1959.
18. Rofe, P.: The cells of normal human urine, J. Clin. Path. 8:25–31, 1955.
19. Page, L. B., DuToit, C. H., Ackerman, I. P., and Wang, Y.: Examination of the urine, *in* Page, L. B., and Culver, P. J. (eds.): A Syllabus of Laboratory Examinations in Clinical Diagnosis, pp. 292–341, Cambridge, Mass., Harvard, 1961.
20. Relman, A. S., and Levinsky, N. G.: Clinical examination of renal function, *in* Strauss, M. B., and Welt, L. B. (eds.): Diseases of the Kidney, pp. 80–122, Boston, Little, Brown, 1963.
21. Addis, T.: The number of formed elements in the urinary sediment of normal individuals, J. Clin. Invest. 2:409–421, 1926.
22. Goldring, W.: Studies of the kidney in acute infection, III. Observations with the urine sediment count (Addis) and the urea clearance test in lobar pneumonia, J. Clin. Invest. 10:355–367, 1931.
23. Larcom, R. J., Jr., and Carter, G. H.: Erythrocytes in urinary sediment; identification and normal limits, J. Lab. Clin. Med. 33:875–880, 1948.
24. Roberts, A. M.: Some effects of exercise on the urinary sediment, J. Clin. Invest. 14:31–33, 1935.
25. Lyttle, J. D.: The Addis sediment count in normal children, J. Clin. Invest. 12:87–93, 1933.
26. Wright, W. T.: Cell counts in urine, Arch Intern. Med. 103:76–78, 1959.
27. Sargent, F., and Johnson, R. E.: Effects of diet on renal function in healthy men, Amer. J. Clin. Nutr. 4:446–481, 1956.
28. Deming, C. L.: Tumors of the kidney, *in* Campbell, M. F. (ed.): Urology, pp. 895–989, Philadelpha, Saunders, 1963.
29. Scott, W. W.: Tumors of the ureter, *in* Campbell, M. F. (ed.): Urology, pp. 999–1026, Philadelphia, Saunders, 1963.
30. Jewett, H. J.: Tumors of the bladder, *in* Campbell, M. F. (ed.): Urology, pp. 1027–1100, Philadelphia, Saunders, 1963.
31. Amador, E., and Wacker, W. E. C.: Enzymatic methods used for diagnosis, *in* Glick, D. (ed.): Methods of Biochemical Analysis, vol. XIII, pp. 265–326, New York, Interscience, 1965.
32. Kleiman, A. H.: Hematuria in boxers, J.A.M.A. 168:1633–1640, 1958.
33. Houghton, B. J., and Pears, M. A.: Cell excretion in normal urine, Brit. Med. J. 1:622–625, 1957.
34. Kass, E. H. (ed.): Progress in Pyelonephritis, Philadelphia, F. A. Davis, 1965.
35. Little, P. J.: Diagnostic criteria of pyelonephritis, J. Clin. Path. 18:556–568, 1965.
36. Brumfit, W.: Urinary cell counts and their value, J. Clin. Path. 18:550–555, 1965.
37. Berman, L. B., Schreiner, G. E., and Feys, J. C.: Observations on the glitter cell phenomenon, New Eng. J. Med. 255:989–991, 1956.
38. Lippman, R. W.: Urine and the Urinary Sediment, ed. 2, Springfield, Ill., Thomas, 1957.
39. Porier, K. P., and Jackson, G. G.: Characteristics of leukocytes in the urine sediment in pyelonephritis, Amer. J. Med. 23:579–586, 1957.

11

Back Pain

RICHARD H. FREYBERG

Anatomic and Physiologic Considerations

Nerve Supply

Back Pain Arising From:

LESIONS OF THE SPINE

ABNORMALITIES OF ARTICULATIONS OF THE
SPINAL COLUMN

LESIONS OF LIGAMENTS AND MUSCLES

LESIONS OF THE SPINAL CORD AND MENINGES

FAULTY BODY MECHANICS

DISORDERS OF THORACIC, ABDOMINAL, AND
PELVIC VISCERA

MISCELLANEOUS CAUSES

ANATOMIC AND PHYSIOLOGIC CONSIDERATIONS

Pain in the back—"backache"—is one of the most common complaints encountered in the practice of medicine. The pathogenesis and the multiple causes of back pain may be appreciated readily if one understands the anatomy and physiology of the human back.

The major structures in the back are: the vertebral column with its stabilizing ligaments, the muscles with their tendinous attachments and fasciae, the spinal cord with its coverings and segmental spinal nerves, and the nutrient blood vessels. The spinal cord is enclosed within a column of vertebrae, each possessing an anterior weight-bearing body and a posterior arch that surrounds the spinal canal. The bodies of the vertebrae are separated one from the other by intervertebral disks, which act as cushioning devices for the spine, and the delicate spinal cord. Each disk is composed of a central expansile portion (the nucleus pulposus) surrounded by strong fibrous connective tissue (the annulus fibrosus). Each intervertebral disk, by force of the expansile center, tends to be spherical in shape, but the compression of the vertebrae between which the disk is sandwiched forces it into a flat ovoid mass. The body weight is balanced on the nuclei of these intervertebral disks (Fig. 11-1).

Movement of the vertebral segments of the spine is accomplished through diarthrodial joints located in pairs between the posterior arches of the vertebrae. The stability of the spine is provided by strong ligaments, which span the spinal column from segment to segment. Some ligaments extend longitudinally, connecting vertebrae throughout the length of the spinal column; others cross obliquely between two or three segments.

The spine articulates with the pelvis through the sacro-iliac joints, composed of cartilage-covered edges of the upper three sacral segments and the cartilage-covered surfaces of the iliac bones that oppose them. Strong fibrous tissue binds together the nonarticulating opposing surfaces of the spine and pelvis. Ribs, which enclose the thoracic organs, articulate with the dorsal spine.

An important part of the back is its mus-

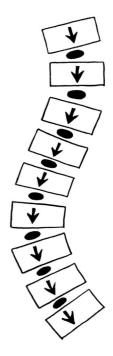

FIG. 11-1. This sketch illustrates the way in which the weight of the trunk of the body is balanced on the nuclei of the intervertebral disks.

culature, composed of three layers of muscles which help to stabilize the trunk of the body and produce many of its movements (Fig. 11-2). The muscles of the dorsal and lumbar back are surrounded by fascia; some muscles attach directly into this strong fascia.

In the canal of the spinal column, the spinal cord extends from the brain distally and terminates in the lowermost nerves and the ligaments, which anchor it caudally to the coccyx. From the spinal cord, pairs of nerves emerge at each vertebral segment. These innervate the trunk and extremities (described in a subsequent section of this chapter).

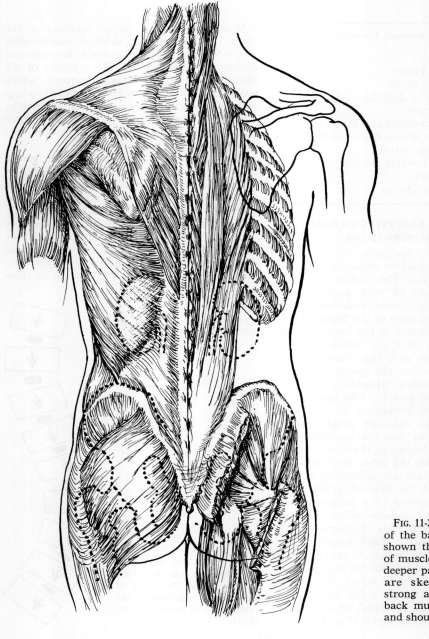

FIG. 11-2. The musculature of the back. On the left is shown the superficial layer of muscles; on the right the deeper paraspinous muscles are sketched. Note the strong attachments of the back muscles to the pelvic and shoulder girdles.

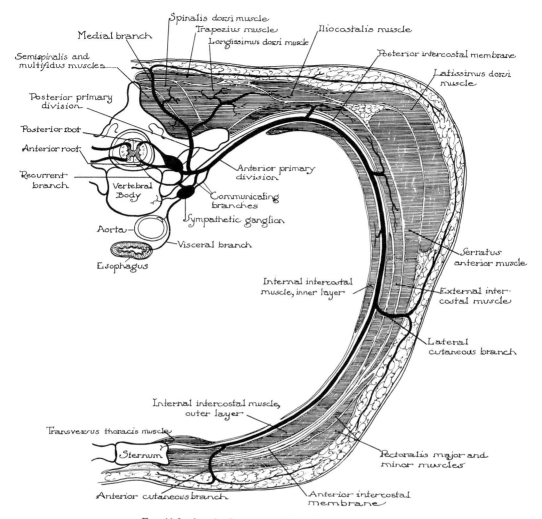

Fig. 11-3. A spinal nerve at the midthoracic level.

The back serves several important functions. It provides the principal support and stability for the body, and also provides for mobility of the trunk in all planes of motion. Many movements of the head and the extremities in relation to the trunk are accomplished by muscles located in the back. All movements of locomotion, standing, and sitting are effected by the back muscles producing movement at some joints of the spine and extremities while other joints are stabilized. The curves in the column strengthen it and add to its flexibility and to the protection that it provides against jarring the brain and stretching the spinal cord. Dorsal kyphosis favors proper lodgement of the thoracic organs. The springy intervertebral cartilaginous disks buffer the jolts of locomotion.

The two important functions of the spinal muscles are to supply postural tone and to provide movement to the trunk and to the structures attached to it. Postural tone, which is controlled by the autonomic nervous system, is normally maintained without effort or fatigue. In the erect position, the strong flexor and extensor muscles are kept in a balanced state of contraction by a static, postural, autonomic reflex mechanism. Should this function of the muscles fail, voluntary contraction of the muscles is required to supplement the autonomic function. This quickly leads to fatigue, faulty posture, and backache. Maintenance of a normal function of the back depends upon physiologic integrity of bones, joints, tendons, muscles, and nerves.

Abdominal and pelvic organs are secured in their respective positions largely by suspending ligaments attached to the back. Sensory, motor, and autonomic nerves leading to supporting structures of the torso and the extremities, and many nerves leading to viscera, pass through the back.

NERVE SUPPLY

It is important to understand the innervation of the structures in the back. Pairs of nerves emerge from the spinal cord through foramina in the column at each vertebral segment (Fig. 11-3). These nerves derive from the cord through two roots: the anterior root is composed solely of motor fibers, the posterior root contains only sensory fibers. Just distal to the foramen the two roots unite into one nerve, which divides near the spinal column into an anterior and a posterior branch. Near the point of division, a recurrent branch is given off which innervates the meninges covering the cord. Motor and sensory fibers are supplied to most structures of the back through the posterior branch. The upper spinal nerves group themselves to form a plexus innervating the upper extremity; the lower spinal nerves form a plexus which supplies important nerves to the lower extremity.

Smaller branches of regional nerves follow closely along blood vessels to reach their termination. The vertebrae are innervated much as are other bones: the cortex and the marrow cavity are poorly supplied, whereas the periosteum has rich sensory innervation. The numerous spinous ligaments also contain abundant pain fibers.[1] Muscles, fasciae, and tendons in the back are innervated as they are elsewhere. At their bony attachments the regional periosteum shares the nerve distribution to the tendons. The posterior articulations of the spine have a nerve supply comparable to that of joints in the extremities (see Chapter 12).

The parietal pleura, parietal peritoneum, and ligaments of the abdomen and pelvis which attach to the back are abundantly supplied with sensory nerves. In these structures, the mechanism of initiating painful stimuli depends chiefly upon stretching, distending, tearing, or severing the membranes containing terminal nerve fibers and end organs and upon chemical irritation (ex-plained in Chapter 12). Lesions affecting cartilage and bone without distorting the periosteal covering or irritating the soft structures attached thereto are relatively indolent; pain is produced chiefly when the periosteum, the ligaments, the fascia, and the other richly innervated soft structures are affected.

Within the spinal canal, painful stimuli may arise from irritation of sensory nerves, which are abundant in the meninges, from stretching or pressure upon the sensory roots of spinal nerves, or from stimulation of pain fibers in the spinal cord.

CAUSES OF BACK PAIN

It is clear from the foregoing discussion that many different types of lesions affecting one or another tissue in the back may cause pain. Accurate knowledge of anatomic and biomechanical features of the back is required to understand its disorders. The analysis of backache depends upon recognition of the nature and the location of the underlying illness; this requires complete, systematic examination of the entire body and shrewd evaluation of all of the findings in relation to the patient's complaints.

In the discussion that follows, no effort will be made to describe all of the disorders that may cause pain in the back, nor will the method of examination be discussed. Attention will be focused on the reasons for, and the mechanism of production of, back pain that results from various illnesses. Differential diagnosis of specific disorders will not be outlined; rather, the mechanism of production of the back pain by various causes will be emphasized—knowledge of which provides the logical basis for accurate diagnosis and proper therapy.

BACK PAIN ARISING FROM DISORDERS OF THE SPINAL COLUMN

Most diseases of the spine cause pain. The spine is frequently injured. If trauma is sufficient to *fracture* the spine, the resulting irritation of the periosteum, the stretch of ligaments, pressure from edema and hemorrhage, and spasm of muscles produce pain in the back. Spasm of the numerous large back muscles may add to the discomfort greatly. Displacement of bone fragments may be sufficient to cause pressure on the meninges, on the pain tracts in the spinal cord, or on the spinal nerve roots and so produce pain. *Dislocation* or *fracture-dislocation* of the spine causes pain in a manner similar to that of a simple fracture. Traumatic lesions are more apt to occur in the cervical and lumbar portions of the spine, in which there is normally more motion and less protection.

Spondylolisthesis (displacement of a portion of the spine on the remainder) occurs most often in the lumbar spine. This lesion develops at the site of a congenital spinal anomaly, at which point weakness or instability of the supporting structures allows displacement at times of physical strain to the low back. The bony displacement causes strain on adjacent ligaments and articulations, protective muscle spasm develops, and all of these changes contribute to the associated pain. Diagnosis is usually accurately made, based upon a history of lumbar back strain, physical abnormalities including a palpable "shelf" at the site of the malposition, painful flexion and extension of the low back, with limitation of these motions and characteristic findings in roentgenograms of the spine.

Various metabolic disorders may cause *osteoporosis* of the spine. Decalcification alone is usually asymptomatic. However, the degree of pain and disability cannot always be correlated with the severity of the bone rarefaction shown in the radiogram. Some patients with extensive radiographic decalcification may have little or no pain.[2,23] If vertebrae become markedly osteoporotic, they may mold under the expansile pressure of the intervertebral disks and produce strain on regional tissues, which causes backache. Minor injuries to the osteoporotic spine may cause compression fracture of one or more vertebrae, usually in the lumbar or dorsal spine.[3] When this happens there is usually sudden, severe, regional back pain and, if there is pressure on nerve roots, radicular pain is added to the pain complex.

The most common *infections* that cause back pain are acute hematogenous osteomyelitis (staphylococcal) and tuberculosis of the spine (Pott's disease). Osteomyelitis in vertebrae has characteristics of osteomyelitis elsewhere: suppuration, abscess formation, bone destruction, sequestration, involucrum formation, periosteal elevation, penetration and dissection along muscle or fascial planes, soft tissue abscesses, and sinus formation. The type and the intensity of the pain depend upon the degree of stretching of the periosteum, the amount of irritation from the products of inflammation, and the stimulation of nerve endings or compression of fibers caused by edema and muscle spasm.

Tuberculosis of the spine is always a metastatic process resulting from hematogenous dissemination of tubercle bacilli. It may begin in a vertebra or in an intervertebral disk, whence it involves adjacent structures. In the early stages, pain and tenderness may be confined to a relatively small portion of the back in the region of the infection. As the tuberculous process advances, one or more vertebral bodies may collapse, causing an angular kyphosis (gibbus), which produces altered weight-bearing and strain of ligaments, muscles, and fascia. Muscle spasm may become extensive and cause more severe and widespread back pain. If a paraspinous tuberculous abscess develops it may press upon nerve roots or fibers, causing pain in the distribution of the nerve. An abscess may dissect between fascial planes to produce pain quite remote from the original lesion, or it may point into the spinal canal and cause irritation of the meninges. Purulent meningitis may develop if infection is liberated within the spinal canal; cord compression may cause transverse myelitis. A diagnosis of Pott's disease is usually readily proved by characteristic roentgenograms and the demonstration of tuberculous infection.[4]

Malignant neoplasm may occur in the spine —primarily *sarcoma*, more often *metastatic carcinoma* or *multiple myeloma*. Whatever the nature of the neoplasm, if tumor formation is small and does not irritate the periosteum there may be no discomfort. When the tumor enlarges so that it erodes the cortex and stretches or tears the periosteum, or weakens the support in the back so that strain of ligaments or joint capsules and muscle spasm result, or when there is direct pressure on nerves, back pain may be agonizing. It is often described as "expansile" or "boring" pain. It is usually present constantly, but it is intensified by weight-bearing and movement. Vertebral fractures may result from neoplastic destruction of the bone. Roentgenograms usually clarify the diagnosis.

PAIN ARISING FROM LESIONS OF THE
JOINTS AND INTERVERTEBRAL DISKS

The apophyseal joints, which are true joints with articular cartilage, joint capsule, and synovial membrane, may become inflamed, just as do extremity joints. The most common form of joint inflammation to affect the apophyseal joints is *ankylosing spondylitis* (formerly diagnosed as rheumatoid spondylitis, Marie-Strumpell disease, von Bechterew's disease, spondylitis adolescens). Much doubt has arisen regarding classification of this form of spinal arthritis; most investigators now consider this not to be rheumatoid arthritis of the spine because of many dissimilarities between this and classical rheumatoid arthritis affecting extremity joints, including absence of the rheumatoid factor in the serum in this form of spondylitis. However, the histopathologic features in the spinal joints in this disease are comparable to those of classical rheumatoid arthritis. Spasm of regional back muscles and the paraspinous calcification underneath spinal ligaments contribute to stiffness, immobility, and pain, and irritation of spinal nerve roots may produce radicular pain. Consequently, this disease is usually characterized by severe back pain and stiffness.

The disease usually begins with arthritis in both sacro-iliac joints and slowly spreads to involve apophyseal joints in an ascending manner. Over the course of years, the sacro-iliac joints usually become ankylosed, and the posterior articulations that have been affected may become fused. Permanent stiffness of the spine may result from intra-articular ankylosis or from subligamentous calcification, or a combination of both of these pathologic processes. In the preankylosing stages, pain is the major disabling problem. The mechanism of production of pain in this type of spondylitis is the same as that for extremity joint rheumatoid arthritis (discussed in Chapter 12).

The pain that occurs characteristically in the early stages of this disease usually results from irritation of the fascia, the ligaments, and the tendons that attach to the low back. The back pain spreads upward as the inflammation ascends in the spine, and the parts affected earlier become less painful as stiffness and ankylosis develop. When spondylitis affects the dorsal spine, costovertebral articulations usually are involved in the inflammatory process, so that chest expansion becomes painful and restricted. Radiculitis may result from spinal nerve root irritation. Sneezing, coughing, and other movements that suddenly jar the back or increase the intraspinal pressure produce severe neuralgia in the back or along the thoracic or the abdominal segmental nerves.

Whenever a teen-age or young adult male complains of pain in the low back or thighs, ankylosing spondylitis should be suspected, and a roentgenogram of the pelvis and lumbar spine should be made.[5] Although sacro-iliac arthritis may exist without the development of spondylitis, it is wise to consider roentgenographic evidence of bilateral sacro-iliac arthritis indicative of early ankylosing spondylitis because of the frequency with which rheumatoid spondylitis begins in these joints. Errors in diagnosis may be made by following this policy; more often the correct diagnosis will be made sufficiently early to allow more effective treatment of this painful crippling disease.[6]

Tuberculosis may affect one sacro-iliac joint; it is very seldom bilateral. Disease of one sacro-iliac joint causes unilateral, regional back pain with or without muscle spasm. Tenderness is usually present only over the affected joint. Roentgenograms usually identify the lesion.

Low back pain that occurs after lifting or after vigorous physical activity that strains the low back often is considered by patients to be due to a *sacro-iliac disorder*. The once popular terms "sacro-iliac strain" or "throwing the sacro-iliac out" are based on fallacious reasoning.[7] Mechanical lesions of the sacro-iliac joints are rare.

The junctions between the vertebral bodies are not true articulations; motion is not accomplished by gliding or hingelike movement at these junctions. However, the segmental bony make-up of the spine, having fibro-cartilaginous disks between vertebrae, allows flexibility of the spine. Because it shares so extensively in almost all physical activities, the spine commonly undergoes changes because of wear and tear, which after several years results in degeneration of intervertebral disks and hypertrophic lipping and spurring at the edges of adjacent vertebrae.. Complete bony bridging between vertebral bodies may result from osteophytic growths. These changes characterize *osteoarthritis* of the spine, more correctly labeled osteoarthrosis or degenerative changes of the spine.[8] Irritation of ligaments, fascia, and other fibrous tissue about the spinal column accounts for the back pain, which is aggravated by standing and by movement of the spine. Osteophyte pressure on nerve roots commonly causes radicular pain. This type of degenerative disease commonly occurs in those parts of the spine where there is greater motion, i.e., the lumbar and cervical portions. Sacro-iliac joints are affected infrequently. Intra-articular ankylosis does not occur. Pain of an aching character (backache) is more common, but sharp pain may occur with motion in the spine. Diagnosis is not difficult, because roentgenograms show the characteristic osteophytes and degenerative changes in the disks.

At the lumbosacral junction, a flexible portion of the spine joins with the rigid pelvis at a place where there is considerable weight-bearing and where motion is important for lifting, stooping, and the like; consequently, *traumatic lesions* occur frequently at this site. With increased lordosis of the lumbar spine or excessive forward tilt to the pelvis, widening of the lumbosacral angle may be sufficient to cause strain of the longitudinal ligaments, and regional tendons and fascia, and in this way cause backache. This can be relieved by correcting the abnormal position. Often, the fifth lumbar disk is traumatized and degenerates, leaving a thin lumbosacral space that may also cause strain or pressure on regional tissues sufficient to cause backache.

If the anatomy of the back is understood, it should be expected that some lesions of the lower back may irritate the sciatic nerve roots. Low back pain and *sciatica* frequently occur simultaneously; sometimes sciatica is the only symptom of a lower back disorder.

Usually sciatic neuralgia is caused by a disorder arising in the spine.

Intervertebral disk disease is the most common cause of sciatic pain.[9,10] General features of the disk syndrome, its diagnosis, and treatment, will not be reviewed here—attention will be focused upon the pain characterizing this syndrome. Quite often severe pain begins suddenly with a "slipping" or "snapping" which the patient experiences in the act of stooping, lifting, or arising from a sitting or lying position. This pain is usually in the midline; the patient often cannot straighten his back because of pain and muscle spasm. Sneezing and coughing aggravate the pain. These attacks are believed by some investigators[11] to represent the beginning of degenerative changes in the disk with softening and loosening of the nucleus pulposus and its posterior displacement within the disk, which then produces pain by stretching the posterior spinous ligament (Fig. 11-4). The symptoms of the disk lesion in this stage (without actual hernia-

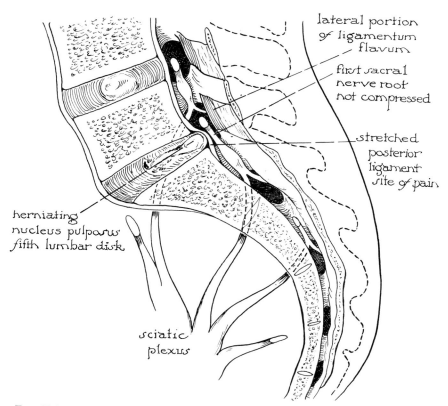

FIG. 11-4. Posterior displacement of the nucleus pulposus without herniation may stretch the posterior spinous ligament and may not protrude sufficiently to compress nerve roots. (Keegan, J. J.: J.A.M.A. 126:868)

tion) may be relieved by maneuvers that will straighten the spine and readjust pressure so that the nucleus is returned to its normal central position, thereby relieving the pressure on adjacent ligaments and eliminating the irritation set up by the displacement.

True herniation of the nucleus pulposus occurs when there is a tear of the annulus and a sufficient amount of the nucleus escapes underneath the posterior longitudinal ligament. There is then a tumor within the spinal canal that usually causes pressure on a nerve root (Fig. 11-5). Such a rupture may be sudden or gradual. Symptoms indicating unilateral nerve-root compression are the distinguishing characteristics. The patient usually complains of aching pain in the superior midgluteal region, with sharper, more variable pain radiating down the posterior thigh and calf (sciatica).

Several factors are involved in the compression of a nerve root by herniation of an intervertebral disk fragment.[12,13] Usually the herniation is located to one side of the midline directly beneath an emerging nerve root. If the spinal canal is large, the herniated fragment may displace the root and may not compress it. In such instances there may be several episodes of back pain without definite root symptoms. In most persons there is considerable flattening or narrowing of the spinal canal at the lumbosacral junction, so that herniation at this level usually compresses the nerve root against the ligamentum flavum and lamina. The nerve root is fixed laterally, and herniation of the disk usually occurs medial to it, so that compression develops in the narrow lateral angle of the spinal canal beneath a portion of the ligamentum flavum.

The earliest and most common complaint of nerve root irritation from herniation of a disk in the lumbar region is superior midgluteal pain. This is best explained as resulting from compression of the posterior primary division of the nerve against the

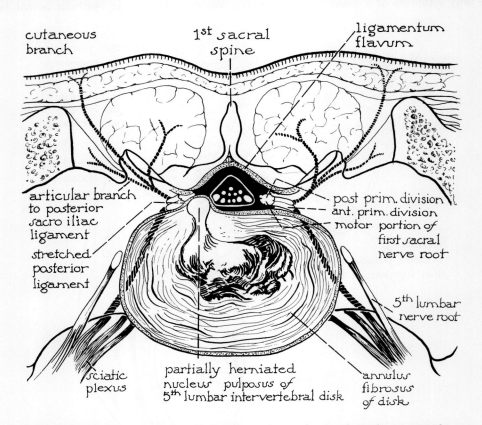

Fig. 11-5. Showing how herniation of the nucleus pulposus through torn annular tissue may produce an intraspinal tumor that will compress a nerve root and cause sciatica. (Keegan, J. J.: J.A.M.A. 126:868)

ligamentum flavum (Fig. 11-5). In this division are the fibers that supply sensation to the gluteal region. The central portion of the medial half of the root contains the sensory fibers that form the anterior primary division of the nerve to the leg. Greater compression may involve the anterior primary division of the root which joins with other roots to form the great sciatic nerve, which innervates most of the lower extremity below the knee.

Each of the roots forming the sciatic nerve has a segmental distribution, both motor and sensory (Fig. 11-6). The areas of the limb usually reported to be the sites of pain and paresthesia from disk lesions are the posterior thigh and the calf, the lateral portion of the ankle, and the foot. These segments are supplied by the first sacral root. The portion of the limb innervated by L-5 is more lateral on the thigh and the leg, the front of the ankle, the top of the foot, and the second, third, and fourth toes. Since all nerve roots have different dermatomes, determining the location of pain by careful history taking and the demonstration of sensory changes in the limbs will indicate the nerve root involved and will locate the level of the disk lesion. If the roots supplying the heel or patellar areas are compressed, these deep tendon reflexes will be diminished, or absent, thus contributing important diagnostic localizing information.

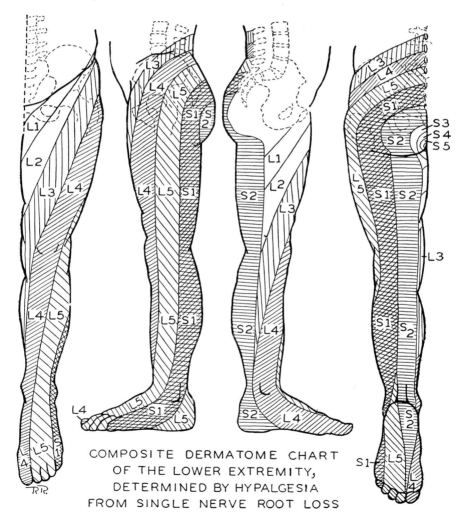

COMPOSITE DERMATOME CHART
OF THE LOWER EXTREMITY,
DETERMINED BY HYPALGESIA
FROM SINGLE NERVE ROOT LOSS

FIG. 11-6. Dermatome charts of the lower extremity. (Keegan, J. J.: J.A.M.A. 126:868)

The majority of disk lesions occur in the lumbar region at L-5 or L-4, accounting for the high incidence of lower back pain and sciatica. The nerve root commonly compressed by protrusion of disk L-5 is S-1; by disk L-4 the compressed nerve is L-5, etc. When unilateral nerve root pain, loss of reflex, and dermatome hypalgesia exist as the chief characteristics of a patient's illness, the pathologic condition must be related directly to involvement of a nerve root on that side. The recognition of the first sacral root syndrome strongly suggests herniation or protrusion of the L-5 disk and eliminates most other causes of back pain. If there is complete herniation of the nucleus pulposus through a tear of the annulus, tension on the annulus and longitudinal spinous ligament ceases, and there is no longer pain in the back (an early symptom); there may be only nerve root irritation, causing pain and sensory changes in the limb.[14]

Lesions of disks in the cervical portion of the spine will produce the same type of pain in the back and pain and altered sensation from nerve root pressure as described for the lumbar disk syndrome. The only difference is in the location of the back pain and the involvement of the upper extremities instead of the lower.[15] Movements of the head and neck aggravate the discomforts. "Whip-lash" injuries may cause the *cervical discogenic syndrome*.[16]

Lesions of the Ligaments, the Fascia, and the Muscles

Although involvement of the ligaments, the fascia, and the muscles contributes much to the discomfort of disease primarily affecting the spinal column and its articulations, these structures are subject to relatively few primary pathologic processes causing backache. All or any of these soft tissues may be injured in performing heavy work, especially lifting, pushing, or pulling in a stooped position. In sports or accidental injuries, these structures alone may be traumatized. When there is no true joint dislocation, so-called *back strain* or *sprain* is the result of incomplete tears or stretching of the tendons at the site of their attachments or unusual use of muscles so that soreness and muscle spasm occur. The erector spinae, quadratus lumborum, latissimus dorsi, and trapezius are the muscles commonly injured in these ways. Diagnosis of such injuries depends chiefly upon knowledge of the circumstances of the injury and

upon elimination of dislocation-fractures, disk lesions, etc., by careful studies, *including roentgenograms*.

Pain in the back frequently results from *spasm of the muscles*, which occurs as part of a protective mechanism for a lesion in the spinal column. Myalgia, muscle tenderness, and stiffness are commonly experienced following unusual exercise or exposure to dampness and cold. Suppurative myositis in the back is very rare. *Myositis* usually exists as part of a generalized disease, such as trichinosis. Muscle biopsy may be required to establish the diagnosis.

One of the diffuse connective tissue ("collagen-vascular") diseases—*polymyositis* may cause back pain.[31] It usually involves the muscles in the interscapular and posterior shoulder girdle groups, and less often the lower back muscles. Weakness of the inflamed muscles, and later atrophy commonly accompany the pain. Tenderness varies considerably. Muscle biopsy showing inflammation, fibrinoid degeneration, and atrophy is diagnostically characteristic.

A common clinical entity affecting the muscles and the fascia causing backache is that form of nonarticular rheumatism called *fibrositis, myofibrositis*, or *"muscular rheumatism."* This condition is often incorrectly diagnosed as spinal arthritis, from which it needs to be differentiated. In fibrositis the posterior neck, the shoulders, the interscapular region, and the lumbar region are the most frequently affected. The onset may be abrupt so that it causes an acute painful stiff neck or sore stiff lower back (lumbago). Severe muscle spasm prevents motion of the involved part and produces the pain characterizing this condition. The neck becomes rigid in a position of partial rotation or tilt to one side when the cervical area is affected; a list or a stoop develops when the trouble is in the lumbar back. The jarring of walking may cause so much pain that the patient prefers to remain in bed. When the onset is acute its termination also usually is rapid and complete.

When this disorder has a more insidious onset the pain is usually a dull ache, worse after a night's rest or prolonged inactivity when a "jelling effect" is noted. With activity, pain and stiffness lessen; consequently, through the middle of the day the patient is relatively comfortable, but toward evening, with fatigue, stiffness and aching become worse. The affected tissues usually are tender to pressure and squeezing. Pressure over "trigger points" may produce more widespread discomfort. Differentiation from spinal arthritis is established by normal roentgenograms and the absence of features of a systemic disease.

In this form of nonarticular rheumatism, no characteristic histopathologic changes exist. It is likely that the clinical features result from chemical or physiochemical alterations in the fibrous tissue. Studies of stiffness exhibited in many connective tissue diseases indicate that stiffness is accounted for by changes in the elasticity and the viscosity of the tendons more than by changes in the muscles or the joint capsules.[17]

Unless the adjacent soft tissues are irritated, osteoarthritis of the spine causes little or no discomfort; indeed, it is common to find degenerative changes when roentgenograms of the spine are made when no pain has been experienced in the region of the abnormalities. However, degenerative changes in the spine may produce pain, stiffness, and limited motion through the mechanism of irritation of the fibrous tissue structures adjacent to the affected spine. This is a syndrome often referred to as *secondary fibritis* (a fibrositis secondary to spinal osteoarthritis).

Degenerative changes in cervical disks and vertebrae frequently cause *irritation of roots of spinal nerves* entering the brachial plexus, producing shoulder or arm pain. In such instances there is usually neckache, along with more severe pain in the dermatomes of the cervical nerves affected. Movement of the head and the neck increases the pain in the neck and intensifies the component of arm discomfort. Roentgenograms differentiate this from other conditions with which it might be confused.

Lesions of the Spinal Cord and the Meninges

Trauma of sufficient violence to injure the spinal cord or the meninges almost invariably causes extensive injury to the supporting tissues of the back, which is the chief cause of the resultant back pain. *Infection* of the spinal cord and its coverings sometimes is the cause of back pain. Anterior poliomyelitis, for example, usually is characterized in the early stages by posterior headache and stiff neck. In the invasive stage of the disease these symptoms appear to result from reflex phenomena caused by the inflammation, edema, and irritation of the invaded nervous tissues. If there is localization of the virus in motor cells supplying spinal muscles, pain and tenderness of the corresponding muscles result.

Diseases that irritate the meninges cause back pain *via* the recurrent branch of the spinal nerve, which carries sensory fibers from the meninges (Fig. 11-3). The discomfort results chiefly from *reflex spasm* of back muscles causing stiff neck (meningismus) and leg signs (Kernig's, Lasegue's, and others) characteristic of meningitis. However, back pain is not a prominent symptom of meningitis. Study of the spinal fluid establishes the diagnosis.

Neoplasms that originate in the spinal cord or its coverings may produce regional back pain by stretch of, or pressure on the meninges, or by invasion of supporting structures of the back. Pain from spinal cord tumors is referred to the sites of distribution of the peripheral nerves affected more often than it occurs in the back. When spinal cord tumors cause back pain or referred pain, there are usually characteristic sensory and/or motor changes. Clinical examination, study of the dynamics and the characteristics of the spinal fluid, and roentgenograms of the spine usually indicate the nature of the trouble.

Back Pain from Faulty Body Mechanics

Many people who have dull back pain do not have a disease localized in any structure of the back; rather, they have a postural defect that strains the back as a whole. In order to understand backache that results from faulty body mechanics it is necessary only to stand for several hours in an unnatural stooped position. Strain of the muscles, the tendon attachments, the fascia, the ligaments, and the joints causes aching that may persist for days. In a like manner, defective posture may strain tissues that tend to compensate for a postural defect, and thus produce continuous and prolonged pain.[18]

Inequality of leg length, arthritis of the hip, scoliosis, and other lesions that cause imbalance of the paired structures of the back or alter the line of weight-bearing may cause back pain. The disturbance in the line of weight-bearing may be in the anteroposterior plane. Examples are dorsal kyphosis, increased lumbar lordosis and "sway-back" from disproportionate abdominal obesity or gravidity. Any abnormal pos-

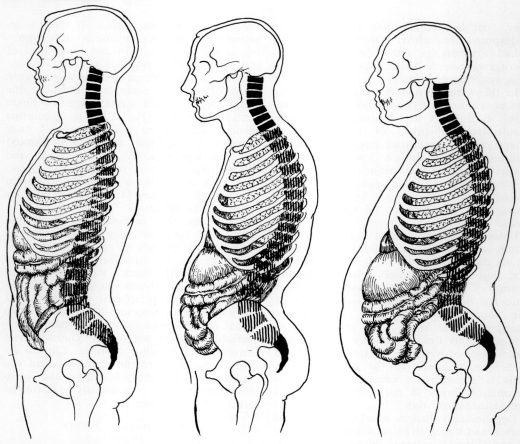

FIG. 11-7. The postural disorder of "slouch back" (center) and this abnormal posture combined with obesity (right) contrast sharply with normal posture (left).

ture causes strain on some of the vertebral joint capsules, on the intervertebral ligaments, the tendon attachments, and the muscles of the back. Postural tone of the back muscles, normally maintained without effort or fatigue by the autonomic nervous system, is then partly maintained by voluntary contraction of muscles in the back. This leads to fatigue and back pain. The discomfort is added to by the strain on the joint capsules and the ligaments in the spine at points where the increased curvature exists.[19]

The disturbed relationships of many parts affected by the "slouch" position of the back (with increased dorsal kyphosis, increased lumbar lordosis, and a more horizontal position of the pelvis) are illustrated in Figure 11-7. Obesity with a protuberant abdomen produces added backache. Forward displacement and ptosis of the abdominal viscera

causes strain on the suspensory ligaments that attach to the back, thus producing aching pain in the back.

Proper supports for pes planus, exercises to correct postural defects caused by weak torso muscles, restoration of good standing, sitting, and sleeping postures, and correction of accentuated spinal curvatures are beneficial remedial procedures. The relief obtained from proper correction attests to the importance of faulty body mechanics as a cause for backache.[20]

BACK PAIN SECONDARY TO LESIONS OF THORACIC, ABDOMINAL, OR PELVIC ORGANS

In other chapters, the mechanism of reflex pain originating in somatic structures and referred to viscera is explained. The converse of this, *viscerosomatic referred pain*, is another cause for aching or severe pain in the back. *Lesions in the peripheral portion of the lungs* which may irritate the posterior parietal pleura may cause back pain in the thoracic region. With this type of back pain there are usually important respiratory symptoms that do not accompany primary back pain. Mediastinal tumors (neoplasm and aortic aneurysm) may cause back pain. Saccular aneurysms may erode vertebrae or ribs, causing severe boring pain or radicular pain from irritation of spinal nerve roots. Dissecting aortic aneurysms commonly cause agonizing pain in the back.

Pain in the back is more apt to result from visceral disease in the abdomen and pelvis than from intrathoracic illness. The mechanism whereby *gallbladder disease, liver abscess,* or *right subdiaphragmatic abscess* cause pain referred to the right shoulder is well-known. Backache or sharp pain in the back frequently results from *lesions of the gastrointestinal tract.* In most instances, visceral dysfunction causes prominent gastrointestinal symptoms, and backache is a lesser complaint, but many investigators have reported instances of duodenal ulcer in which back pain was the only symptom.[21,22,24] In most instances, back pain from peptic ulcer is a dull ache in the midline (or slightly to either side) between D-5 and D-10. Frequently, these patients have been studied by an orthopedist, neurologist, neurosurgeon, gynecologist, and internist without finding cause for the pain until massive hemorrhage or roentgenograms indicate the existence of the gastrointestinal lesion.

Low back pain may be caused by disease of the colon or the rectum, especially when constipation exists. The classic balloon experiments of Jones[21] indicate a mechanical basis for the backache due to disorders of the intestine. A distended balloon in the duodenal cap sometimes caused pain in the back or pain that radiated from the xyphoid process through the abdomen to the back. When a balloon was distended in the second portion of the duodenum, pain often occurred in the back or around the margin of the thoracic cage. Distention of the colon frequently caused low backache; sometimes this was the *only* symptom. These studies show that most, if not all, symptoms caused by these disturbances are fundamentally associated with local distention of the gut either above an area of spasm or above an area of organic disease which causes constriction of the bowel. The splanchnic nerves enter the cord from D-5 to D-12. Nerves to the stomach

and the duodenum probably originate in the upper portion of this section of the cord. It has been shown that evulsion of the splanchnic nerves performed under local anesthesia causes severe pain. Often low backache is caused by spasm or dilatation of the colon, and promptly disappears when the bowel disorder is relieved. Lumbosacral pain due to distention of the sigmoid colon is promptly relieved by an enema, indicating that the pain is on a mechanical basis.

Perforation of a peptic ulcer may cause pain referred to the back. An ulcer in the posterior wall of the stomach or the duodenum and *penetrating into the pancreas,* or a carcinoma of the pancreas, sometimes causes low back pain. Agonizing lumbar back pain may be produced by *acute pancreatitis* or *dissecting aneurysm* of the abdominal aorta.[25]

There are records of a number of instances in which low back pain in the midline or slightly to the right side was caused by an inflamed and distended *retrocecal appendix.* Sudden onset of pain in this region should always make one suspicious of this lesion.

Painful disorders of the kidney parenchyma or capsule usually produce flank pain. Experimental studies of Ockerblad[26] indicate that *obstructive uropathies,* which produce stretching of the capsule of the kidney, cause pain in the flank. The average area of pain was found to be small (8 to 10 cm. in diameter). If pain and tenderness exist in one or both costovertebral angles the urinary tract should be investigated for a causative lesion.

Inflammation in the *prostate* and the *seminal vesicles* may cause low lumbar or sacral pain. Many references have been made to the frequency with which chronic lower back pain is caused by infection or other diseases of the pelvic organs. Chronic lower back pain due to pelvic disease rarely occurs in patients who do not have other more prominent symptoms that would lead to consultation with a urologist or a gynecologist.

It should be emphasized that low back pain in females is usually *not* due to pelvic disorders. Congestion at the onset of menses, the mechanical burden of the late stage of pregnancy, and some pelvic tumors may cause backache for obvious reasons. Sometimes severe infection in the female pelvic organs may cause reflex pain in the low back. However, uterine displacement and low-grade pelvic infection seldom cause backache.

Miscellaneous Causes of Pain in the Back

In the prodromal stages of various febrile illnesses, backache may exist along with generalized aching in the extremities. Sometimes septicemia may be ushered in by severe back pain, but soon malaise, fever, and other symptoms indicate the nature of the disease.

It is important to realize that some persons who complain of backache have no organic disease anywhere to cause it. Some of these persons are maliciously feigning pain that does not exist. Experiences in the armed forces have revealed a high frequency of "psychogenic rheumatism" occurring as a somatic manifestation of psychoneurosis. Boland and Corr[27] reported that the lower back is the most frequent site of this manifestation and that, in the group of soldiers studied, back pain was much more often due to psychoneurosis than to intrinsic disease of the spine or to organic rheumatic disease. *Psychogenic backache* is very difficult to diagnose because there are few reliable characteristics. Careful study often reveals unusual localization of pain or bizzare radiation, which does not conform to any anatomic pattern.[28] Usually it is uninfluenced by factors that intensify or relieve the pain of organic diseases. Other psychoneurotic manifestations are frequently present. Most difficult is the problem of proper evaluation of the psychogenic back pain coexisting with organic disease capable of producing backache.[29,30]

SUMMARY

Back pain may be caused by disease in any of the many structures in the back. Causes of back pain are explained on the basis of underlying pathologic physiology. The responsible disease sometimes is evident immediately; in the majority of cases, it can be determined through a thorough, systematic study. The complex structure of the back and the multiplicity of ailments to which the component tissues are subject make it imperative to approach the problem in each patient with an unprejudiced viewpoint and to evaluate carefully all of the evidence in an orderly fashion. Many mistaken diagnoses originate in the narrow viewpoint of specialists who fail to realize that the cause for back pain may lie outside their specialty. The orthopedist must realize that back pain may not be due to structural disease of the back, the gynecologist cannot account for all cases of low backache on the basis of pelvic disease, the neurologist can explain only some of the instances of back pain on lesions of the spinal cord or peripheral nerves, and the internist must realize that the different forms of arthritis or nonarticular rheumatism do not always account for pain in the back. Perhaps in no other medical problem is it so important to consider all of the possibilities and to pursue a systematic study to a logical conclusion.

A carefully elicited and complete history of the manner of onset, the location, the radiation and the nature of the pain, the factors that aggravate it, and those that relieve it, should be obtained. Thorough physical examination should include special back and leg maneuvers to allow recognition of disturbance of structure and function if they exist. Examination of the thorax should be made whenever pain is located in the upper part of the back. When there is lower back pain, examination of the abdomen, the pelvis, and the rectum, including direct visualization of as many of these parts as can be seen, may be required. Roentgenographic examination of the spine and the pelvis is an invaluable aid, and in some instances special x-ray procedures (such as myelography) may be helpful. Studies of blood cytology and chemistry, erythrocyte sedimentation, and urinalysis are usually indicated. A systematic investigation, supplemented by specialists' examinations seasoned by experience, should solve most problems of disease producing pain in the back correctly. There are usually anatomic or physiologic disturbances to indicate a structural basis for back pain. Disturbances of posture usually can be recognized as a basis for faulty body mechanics. If back pain is referred from visceral disease, symptoms and signs of such disease will usually be found, if sought.

Pain in the back ranks among the most common problems of medical diagnosis. Knowledge of the structure and the function of the back and the lesions that produce pain, thorough study, and intelligent interpretation of all findings, usually will yield the solution.

REFERENCES

1. Kellgren, J. H.: On distribution of pain arising from deep somatic structures with charts of segmental pain areas, Clin. Sci. 4:35–46, 1939.

2. Moldawer, M.: Senile osteoporosis. The physiologic basis of treatment, A.M.A. Arch. Intern. Med. 96:202, 1955.

3. Freyberg, R. H., and Gascon, J.: The problem of pathologic fractures in patients with rheumatoid arthritis receiving prolonged corticosteroid therapy, Proc. X International Congress on Rheumatic Diseases, ed. Minerva Medica, vol. 1, pp. 378–382, Turin, Italy, 1961.

4. Harrold, A. J.: Tuberculosis of the spine, a reassessment of the problem and the results of conservative treatment, Postgrad. Med. J. 31:495, Oct. 1955.

5. Polley, H. F.: Symposium on rheumatic diseases; diagnosis and treatment of rheumatoid spondylitis, Med. Clin. N. Amer. 39:509, Mar. 1955.

6. Hollander, J. H., et al.: Arthritis, ed. 7, Philadelphia, Lea & Febiger, 1966.

7. Cleveland, M., Aldridge, A. H., Bosworth, D. M., Ray, B. S., and Thomas, S. F.: Management of low back pain, Proc. New York Acad. Med. 35:778–800, 1959.

8. Wilson, J. C., Jr.: Degenerative arthritis of the lumbosacral joint, the end-space lesion, J.A.M.A. 169:1437, 1959.

9. Rose, G. K.: Backache and the disc, Lancet 1:1143, 1954.

10. Gill, G. G., and White, H. L.: Mechanisms of nerve-root compression and irritation in backache, Clin. Orthop. 5:66, 1955.

11. Keegan, J. J.: Diagnosis of herniation of lumbar intervertebral disk by neurologic signs, J.A.M.A. 126:868–873, 1944.

12. Jacobs, J. E.: Neuralgia and backache, Western J. Surg. 64:202, 1956.

13. Bradford, F. K.: Low back and sciatic pain, J. Indiana Med. Ass. 50:559, 1957.

14. Morrell, R. M.: Herniated lumbar intervertebral disc—cutaneous hyperalgesia as an early sign, Milit. Med. 124:257, 1959.

15. Jackson, R.: The cervical syndrome, Clin. Orthop. 5:138, 1955.

16. Hackett, G. S.: Whiplash injury, Amer. Pract. 10:1333, 1959.

17. Wright, V., and Johns, R. J.: Physical factors concerned with the stiffness of normal and diseased joints, Bull. Hopkins Hosp. 106:215, Apr. 1960.

18. Denny-Brown, D.: Clinical problems in neuromuscular physiology, Amer. J. Med. 15:368–390, 1953.

19. Gaston, S. R., and Schlesinger, E. B.: Symposium on orthopedic surgery; low back syndrome, Surg. Clin. N. Amer. 31:329, 1951.

20. Wilson, P. D., Jr.: in Hollander, J. H., et al. (eds.): Arthritis, ed. 7, pp. 1282–1326, Philadelphia, Lea & Febiger, 1966.

21. Jones, C. M.: Back pain in gastro-intestinal disease, Med. Clin. N. Amer. 22:749–760, 1938.

22. Gilson, S. B.: Back pain in peptic ulcer, New York J. Med. 61:625–627, 1961.

23. Howell, D. S.: in Hollander, J. H., et al. (eds.): Arthritis, ed. 7, pp. 973–991, Philadelphia, Lea & Febiger, 1966.

24. Compere, E. L.: Symptom-complex of visceral spinal pain, Illinois Med. J. 74:434–442, 1938.

25. Burt, H. A., Fletcher, W. D., and Mattingly, S.: Pitfalls in the diagnosis of backache, Ann. Phys. Med. 2:1, Jan. 1954.

26. Ockerblad, N. F.: Urological backaches, Kansas City Med. J. 21:22–24, 1945.

27. Boland, E. W., and Corr, W. D.: Psychogenic rheumatism, J.A.M.A. 123:805–809, 1943.

28. Levy, R. L.: Psychogenic musculoskeletal reactions, Med. Bull. U.S. Army Europe 12:175, 1955.

29. Wolff, H. G.: Stress and Disease, Springfield, Ill., Thomas, 1953.

30. Sundt, P. E.: Psychogenic rheumatism, Proc. Roy. Soc. Med. 48:66, 1955.

31. Pearson, C. M.: Polymyositis, Arthritis Rheum. 2:127, 1959.

12

Joint and Periarticular Pain

RICHARD H. FREYBERG

Anatomic Considerations

Physiologic Considerations

Pathogenesis of Articular and
  Periarticular Pain

Diagnostic Considerations

Monarticular Pain

Polyarticular Pain

Nonarticular Pain

Pain in and about the joints is one of the most common complaints with which the physician is confronted. The first symptom, and usually the chief complaint of most rheumatic diseases is pain in the region of the affected joints; it usually persists throughout the active disease. Arthralgia and periarticular pain also are prominent symptoms of many nonrheumatic systemic diseases. In addition to joint pain, there may be pain in the ligaments, tendons, muscles, fascia, and the periosteum. All of these tissues are importantly involved in many rheumatic diseases. Knowledge of the mechanisms of production of articular and periarticular pain is an important basis for accurate diagnosis and for proper therapy.

ANATOMIC CONSIDERATIONS

Early studies of the innervation of the joints and the periarticular connective tissues have been summarized by Gerneck.[1] Using more modern investigative procedures, this subject has been restudied by several investigators. Much of the following anatomic discussion is based upon studies made by Dr. Charley J. Smyth and the author while collaborating in the Rackham Arthritic Research Unit at the University of Michigan.

Joints receive their nerve supply from mixed nerves, which also innervate the muscles, the bones, and the skin of the sur-rounding area. Following along the blood vessels to the joints, the articular nerve branches supply the joint capsule, and terminal branches of unmyelinated and some finely myelinated fibers are distributed through the synovium and the subsynovial tissue, adjacent ligaments, and the regional periosteum. In the outer portion of the joint capsule, larger branches of the articular nerves divide to form a rich plexus from which finer branches course (usually along the arterioles into the subsynovial tissue, in which a secondary plexus may form close to the synovial surface), or they may terminate separately in synovial and subsynovial cells.

Nerves terminate in the joint capsule and in the synovium in one of three ways:

1. In a fine network, which often surrounds an arteriole close to the inner lining of the capsule (Fig. 12-1, Parts 1, 2 and 5, and Fig. 12-2 top, right)

2. As free nerve endings, close to or actually in the surface of synovial cells (Fig. 12-1, Parts 3 and 4, and Fig. 12-2 top, left)

3. In a special end organ (infrequently), which is an oval, laminated structure (Fig. 12-2, bottom, left and right) usually found deep in the fibrous portion of the capsule. This end organ appears to be a form of pacinian corpuscle, and very likely functions as a pressure sense end-organ, as this type of corpuscle is known to function when located in the fascia, the tendons, and the muscles.

No nerves are found in articular cartilage or in compact bone. Usually, nerves travel to articular structures alongside blood vessels; since joint cartilage is avascular, it is to be expected that this tissue should contain no nerves. This is important in connection with affections primarily involving the articular cartilage, such as degenerative disease of joints (osteoarthritis).

Periarticular tissues are abundantly innervated, and in all of these structures, the nerve endings are like those found in the joint capsule.[2,3] The smaller fibers from these various tissues form larger bundles, which become parts of the dorsal spinal nerve root of that segment. The constituent parts of these nerves synapse in similar spinal cord segments. Therefore, it is clear why stimuli originating in structures *about* the joints may give rise to a type of painful sensation considered by some patients as originating *in* the joint tissue.

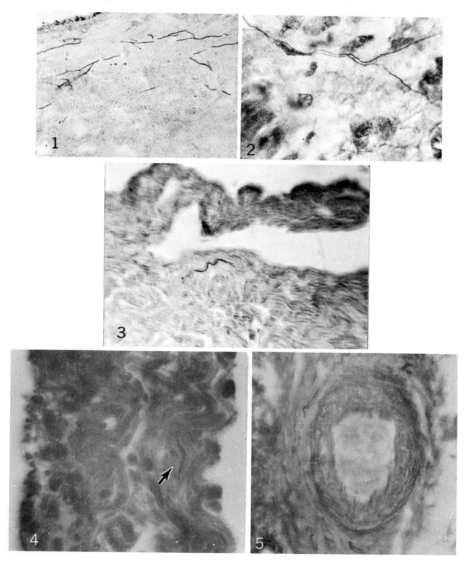

Fig. 12-1. Sections of human joint capsule, showing silver-impregnated nerve fibers. (1) Very near the synovial surfaces at the top of the section there is a rich plexus of small unmyelinated nerves. (2) A higher magnification of subsynovial tissue shows fine unmyelinated fibrils dividing, joining in a knotlike mesh, and separating again. (3) A single unmyelinated nerve very close to the synovial surface near the base of a villus. (4) High-power magnification of a villus cut in longitudinal section, showing a single nerve fiber just beneath the surface. (5) High-power magnification of a synovial blood vessel, showing numerous unmyelinated nerve fibers in or near the adventitia.

PHYSIOLOGIC CONSIDERATIONS

Lennander[4] found all of the articular and the periarticular structures (articular capsule, the synovium, the muscle, the tendon, the fascia, the ligament, the cancellous bone, and the periosteum) to be sensitive to pain; the articular cartilage and the cortical bone were insensitive. These results were found to be consistent in patients under different conditions including varying degrees and types of anesthesia and without anesthesia. These findings have been confirmed by others.[5-7] The only structures about which there is doubt concerning sensitivity to pain are the fibrocartilaginous menisci of the knee joints. It has been reported[2] that direct stimulation of the menisci causes no pain, that displacement is painful, and that electrical stimulation causes pain. In these studies, the possibility that the impulses might have originated in surrounding tissue to

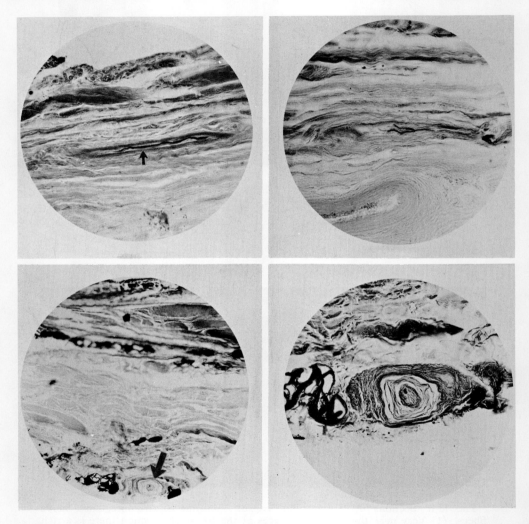

FIG. 12-2. Sections of human joint capsule stained with osmic acid. (*Top, left*) A subsynovial nerve containing myelinated fibers. Note its proximity to the surface synovial cells at the top of the section. (*Top, right*) Higher magnification of subsynovial tissue, showing a branching myelinated nerve alongside an arteriole. (*Bottom, left*) Deep in a joint capsule (synovium at top) is a laminated nerve end-organ, a pacinian corpuscle. (*Bottom, right*) Higher magnification of a pacinian corpuscle located deep in the fibrous tissue of the joint capsule.

which the stimuli spread cannot be excluded.[8]

The type, the localization, and the distribution of pain arising from structures in and about the joints have been studied extensively by Lewis and Kellgren; their fundamental research will be reviewed here in some detail. Kellgren[9] injected muscles in various locations with hypertonic saline solution and observed that pain was always felt diffusely and was referred in a spinal-segmental pattern. Ligaments irritated in a like manner gave rise to pain similar to that produced in muscle: a continuous ache felt *deep* in the structures involved. This pain was associated with tenderness of the deep structures in a distribution corresponding to the location of the pain; tenderness enabled the persons studied to localize the discomfort accurately to the areas stimulated. Experiments repeated in the same subjects gave remarkably constant results, even though weeks elapsed between observations. Charts of the distribution of pain produced by injection of intraspinous ligaments showed segmental areas of pain which did not correspond exactly with the dermatomes of skin tenderness; this variation suggests that distribution of *deep* pain and tenderness corresponds with the segmental innervation of the *deep* structures rather than of the integument. Pain that arose from the periosteum covering the tibia, the sternum, the vertebral spines, the acromion and the olecranon processes, or the phalanges (bone structures all of which are close to the surface) was confined to the neighborhood of the point stimulated, whereas pain that arose from the deeply situated periosteum was felt more diffusely. Stimulation of nerve endings in the deep fascia in the trunk and the limbs, in the subcutaneous ligaments and the tendon sheaths such as those in the wrists and ankles, and in superficially placed tendons (the patellar and the Achilles tendon), also caused more localized pain like that from superficial periosteum. Deeply situated intermuscular fascia and ligaments, when stimulated, gave rise to pain over a larger area, such as that arising from deeply located periosteum. Whether pain arising from a given structure is felt as localized or more diffuse pain depends upon the location of that structure (superficial or deep) more than upon the nature of the tissue (periosteum, ligament, tendon, or fascia).

Pain arising from muscles of the extremities usually is localized in the neighborhood of the joints that are moved by those muscles, if those joints are in the segmental pain areas corresponding with the nerve supplying those muscles. Pain from smaller joints, such as those in the hands and the feet, tends to be more localized, whereas pain arising in larger joints (the hips and the shoulders) usually is more segmental in distribution. Thus, pain arising from disease in the hip joint and the quadriceps femoris muscle often is felt in the knee, and pain arising in the tibialis anticus muscle may be localized in the ankle joint.

The extensive investigations of Gardner[10–13] indicate without doubt that the joint capsules and the ligaments are sensitive to painful stimuli. There is less clear evidence that the nerves shown in histologic specimens to terminate in the synovial lining of the joint capsules are pain receptors. Various methods used experimentally to stimulate nerve endings in the synovial lining may also have stimulated pain receptors in the deeper layers of the joint capsule. However, the studies of Kellgren and Samuel,[7] conducted in the human knee joint, indicate that, although the synovial membrane is relatively insensitive, some areas of the synovia are definitely pain-sensitive. The majority of the nerves in the synovial membrane are autonomic in origin and are contained in the blood-vessel walls, whereas the fibrous joint capsule and articular ligaments are supplied with somatic nerves, with a variety of specialized and unspecialized nerve endings.[7,13]

Lewis and Kellgren[14] studied referred somatic pain in relation to referred pain originating in a viscus. It was found that, at its height, somatic pain experimentally produced in the trunk was accompanied by muscle rigidity and deep tenderness. With induced pain in the extremities, muscle spasm and tenderness were less evident. These features of somatic pain are similar to corresponding abnormalities associated with visceral pain. The nature of somatic pain was found to be exactly like that known to have visceral origin: it was constant, of unvarying intensity, and the quality differed from the burning pain originating from the skin or the mucous membranes. Induced somatic pain frequently was accompanied by paresthesia and subsequent hyperalgesia similar in type and location to such symptoms occurring with visceral pain. Lewis[15] demonstrated that pain of deep somatic origin cannot be distinguished from that of visceral origin, and that deep somatic and visceral structures are supplied by a common set of afferent nerves, stimulation of which produces similar pain and reflex phenomena. It is not surprising, therefore, that pains associated with various rheumatic disorders of the spine, thorax, shoulders, and arms may simulate the syndrome of angina pectoris caused by heart disease.[16]

Until recently it was thought that pain fibers were carried only in the somatic nerves entering the spinal cord through the posterior roots. The reports of Herfort[17,18] indicate that at least a portion of the pain fibers from the lower extremities arrive at the cord centers through the autonomic pathways. Herfort has reported substantial relief of pain due to arthritis in the hip and knee joints by performing "extended lumbar sympathectomy." Severing the lumbar sympathetic chain along the retroaortic plexus and sectioning the decussating fibers in the prevertebral plexus relieved joint pain in the lower extremities in the majority of arthritic patients upon whom operations were performed. Herfort believes this surgical procedure accomplishes the benefit by "the ablation of afferent pain pathways running from the articular surfaces of the lower extremities and traversing the lumbar paravertebral sympathetic trunks and the retroaortic plexus."[17] These observations appear to support the thesis that important sensory innervation of the articular structures of the hip, the knee, and the ankle joints is derived from the lumbar *sympathic* ganglia. Support for this thesis is also provided by the report[19] that transient diminution of pain resulted from the administration of tetraethylammonium bromide to patients with rheumatoid arthritis. Furthermore, neuropathic joint changes did not occur in any of the sympathectomized patients; this would indicate that the *peri*articular and *extra*capsular tissues are not denervated by section of the lumbar sympathetic trunks, and that there is preservation of the extracapsular protopathic sensation providing the sense of joint position.

PATHOGENESIS OF ARTICULAR PAIN

The mechanism of excitation of pain-conducting nerve fibers in rheumatic disorders differs in various diseases. The experiments of Lennander[4] have shown that, when tissues about joints are stimulated by pinching, tearing, cauterizing by acid or heat, cutting, sticking, or use of electric currents, the same type of pain results. Lewis[15] confirmed these observations and also has consistently initiated pain by injection of chemical irritants. Knowing that pain can be induced by such different types of stimuli, one readily understands why most abnormalities of the joints and the periarticular tissues are accompanied by pain.

The nature of the stimuli differs in various types of disease. *Postural abnormalities* and *traumatic joint lesions* produce pain by stretching, pinching, or tearing supportive tissues (the ligaments, the joint capsule, the tendons, the fascia, and the periosteum). *Neoplastic diseases*, by reason of growth of the tumor and the resultant destructive changes, interrupt continuity, stretch, pinch, or otherwise irritate pain nerve fibers and their endings. *Inflammation*, which characterizes so many rheumatic diseases (infectious arthritis, rheumatic fever, rheumatoid arthritis, gouty arthritis, bursitis, and tenosynovitis), excites pain by chemical irritation, stretching, tension, and, if there are destructive changes of supporting tissues, by pressure upon nerve endings that are normally protected. *Swelling of the joint capsule* and periarticular tissue or *hydrops* of joints produces pain by stretching the joint capsule, as shown by the relief resulting from aspiration. Absence of discomfort when joint tissues are loosely distended by noninflammatory edema indicates that pain accompanying inflammation of articular structures must be produced by some stimulus other than mechanical irritation. *Chemical irritants* formed by the inflammatory process appear to act as important excitants of pain in nerve endings.

Traumatic or inflammatory joint disease often is accompanied by *spasm* of adjacent muscles; this contributes to the pain by adding the discomfort of muscle pain or by stimulation of nerve endings in the periosteum through fascial and tendinous attachments. Faulty body mechanics also may add traction and strain.

DIAGNOSTIC CONSIDERATIONS

The diagnostic significance of joint pain will be considered from two aspects:

1. The evaluation of differences in articu-

lar and periarticular pain and the relation of these variations to definite causes.

2. The consideration of characteristics of rheumatic pain occurring in the more common forms of rheumatic diseases, and the correlation of this symptom with associated abnormalities. It must be appreciated that joint pain may be influenced by many things other than the nature of the pain stimulus. Some persons complain bitterly of discomfort that others may consider trivial; there are wide variations in the threshold and the tolerance for pain.

A detailed description of the pain is fundamental to the correct interpretation of the symptom. For correct analysis of pain as a symptom it is necessary to know the *nature* of the pain, its *localization* or *distribution,* its *constancy* or *variability,* and the *factors that accentuate and relieve it.* Different patients may describe pain quite differently; common adjectives used are dull, aching, sharp, burning, tearing, pulling, boring, and the like. Even though the patient's intelligence, vocabulary, and impressionability may influence his description, the nature of the pathology is a very important factor in accounting for true basic differences in type and severity of pain in and about joints.

MONARTICULAR PAIN

Pain in only one joint may result from a number of different local disorders.

Trauma frequently affects only one articulation. When trauma results from a single injury, it usually is of sufficient severity that the etiologic diagnosis is evident from the history. Such trauma commonly originates from sports injuries, occupational injuries, violence, or accidental injuries. Trauma to a joint usually results in one of the following types of pathology: strain, sprain, synovitis, fracture of bone extending into the joint, tear of ligaments, tendons or capsule (often resulting in internal joint derangements, which thereafter cause recurrent joint pain following relatively minor injury), or joint dislocations. The pain resulting from traumatic joint lesions varies in character depending upon the extent of the injury, the joint involved, the tissue reaction to the trauma, and other factors.

Sometimes traumatic joint lesions heal in such a way as to disturb the patient's posture or to produce abnormal weight-bearing. During ensuing years, degenerative lesions may develop in the damaged joint and thus

account for monarticular pain. The hip, knee, ankle, and foot are more apt to exhibit such lesions; they occur more commonly in older individuals, who have led very active lives. This group of disorders overlaps the field of osteoarthritis and will be considered in more detail in the discussion of that disease.

Neoplastic disease affecting only one joint is rare and usually is a primary tumor (fibroma, fibrosarcoma, or synovioma). A bone tumor adjacent to a joint may cause pain in the articulation, or pain is referred to it, especially during motion of the joint. Neoplasms are likely to cause severe pain frequently described as "expansile" or "boring." Irregular joint swelling, and characteristic roentgenograms, usually indicate the nature of the pathology.

Degenerative joint changes frequently cause joint pain in older adults (osteoarthritis, osteoarthrosis). Although several joints usually are affected, it may involve a single weight-bearing joint (hip or knee).

Septic Joint. This form of joint disease has decreased in frequency greatly since the advent of effective antimicrobial therapy. Infection of articular structures may result in the accumulation of pus within the joint cavity—a "septic joint." This disorder is usually characterized by severe throbbing pain, which increases as the joint capsule becomes more distended with pus. The patient keeps the affected part in the position of greatest comfort; this characteristic attitude is helpful in the diagnosis. Movement of the affected joint increases the pain because of the increased tension and stretching of the inflamed joint capsule. Unless prompt and adequate treatment is instituted, there may be extensive destruction of articular cartilage and subchondral bone. Study of aspirated synovial fluid and characteristic roentgenograms usually leads to the correct diagnosis. Culture of the pus reveals the nature of the infecting organism and indicates the proper antimicrobial therapy.

Tuberculosis commonly affects a single joint. Tuberculous infection may extend into a joint from a focus in an adjacent bone, or tuberculous joint synovitis may be a metastatic lesion. Characteristically, the disease progresses slowly and the pain is mild at first; however, the pain usually is aggravated by weight-bearing and movement of the joint. Destruction of cartilage and bone usually causes greater pain and more joint dysfunction. After destructive changes occur, the roentgenographic appearance may be diagnostic.[20] The mild character of the inflammation accounts for the "cold" or "cool" joint. Since bone and joint tuberculosis is secondary to tuberculous infection elsewhere in the body, identification of the primary infection is helpful in the diagnosis. Tuberculin tests should be made in suspected cases. Often the true nature of the infection is not learned until joint aspiration or biopsy is performed. The possibility of tuberculous arthritis always should be considered when a patient has painful monarticular joint inflammation; however, this type of infectious arthritis is much less common since dependable treatment for tuberculosis has been available.

Neuropathic joint disease often is painless. However, mild or moderate discomfort occurring at a joint that may exhibit much swelling and hypermobility should make one suspect a Charcot's joint. Special diagnostic studies usually clarify the diagnosis.

The sudden onset of severe monarticular pain associated with severe joint synovitis, especially if it is located at the "bunion-joint" in an adult male, always should suggest an attack of *gouty arthritis* (to be described later).

Rheumatoid arthritis commonly affects many joints, but in some instances, especially in children, it may begin and persist for many months in only one joint. This possibility must be considered in evaluating monarticular pain.

Nonarticular Rheumatism. Frequently a bursa located near a joint becomes inflamed as a result of trauma, infection, or in association with systemic rheumatic diseases. The swelling or distention of the sac with fluid may stimulate the pain nerve endings, which are numerous in and about all bursae. Because movement of the adjacent joint adds to the irritation, the increased pain caused by moving the joint may erroneously be ascribed to disease in the articulation itself. However, bursal pain is elicited only by those motions that disturb the relationship of the bursa, whereas with joint inflammation usually all motions of the affected joint cause pain. The tendons, the tendon sheaths, the muscles, and the fascia near a joint may be affected in a similar manner and give rise to "joint pain." When a periarticular disorder exists alone, the location of the swelling and the tenderness, and the fact that pain is produced or accentuated only by certain motions of the adjacent joint, serve to differentiate such a lesion from joint disease. It is important to distinguish nonarticular from articular rheumatism, because the treatment and the prognosis differ depending upon which tissues are affected.

SINGLE JOINTS INVOLVED

The diagnostic significance of monarticular pain arising in various anatomic locations will now be considered.

Finger Joint. Pain in a single finger joint usually is due to trauma. The nature and the severity of the pain vary according to the nature of the injury. Diagnosis is based on the history of recent injury, physical findings, and roentgenographic findings. A typical example of such a lesion is the "baseball finger," which is traumatic arthritis produced by the extension of a fracture of a phalanx into the adjacent joint, frequently the terminal interphalangeal joint.

Wrist. Sprains, strains and fractures of the wrist are common. One lesion characteristically located at the wrist is "ganglion," a localized swelling of one or more of the tendon sheaths which becomes filled with gelatinous fluid. This swelling may be painless but usually there is dull, aching pain. If the ganglion enlarges rapidly, pain may be severe. Diagnosis is made readily by recognition of the cystic nature of the swelling, accompanied by local signs of inflammation.

Elbow. Pain at this joint frequently results from trauma, because this articulation is vulnerable to injury. At the tip of the elbow, the olecranon bursa is frequently traumatized. The pain usually is sharply localized to the inflamed bursa and there may be marked tenderness, crepitant fluctuation, and palpable increase in local heat. Swelling of the distended bursa may be considerable. The pain from acute bursitis usually subsides quickly with proper treatment. Chronic olecranon bursitis is common in patients with rheumatoid arthritis and gout.

Another common cause of elbow pain is "tennis elbow," or *epicondylitis*, which results from severe and repeated pulling of the forearm muscle tendons at their insertion into the humeral epicondyle.[21] Foregoing physiologic and pathologic considerations of joint pain readily explain why pain produced by such a lesion would be considered by the patient to be caused by arthritis in the elbow joint. Tenderness sharply localized to the epicondyle, pain accentuated by forceful contraction of the muscles of the forearm, and absence of signs of inflammation at the elbow joint capsule serve to distinguish this lesion.

Shoulder. Most shoulder pain is not due to arthritis! Besides *fractures* and *dislocations* (concerning which there is usually no problem of diagnosis), there are several forms of periarthritis that cause pain about this joint.

One or another form of periarticular (nonarticular) connective tissue disease commonly causes the painful stiff shoulder.[22,23] The most common cause of the painful shoulder is *calcific tendonitis.*[24] What was usually labeled "bursitis" of the shoulder has been shown to be, in fact, an inflammation of one of the tendons inserting into the greater trochanter of the humerus, usually the tendon of the supraspinatous muscle.[25] This condition has an acute onset, characterized by severe pain localized in the subacromial region of the shoulder, where there is sharply localized tenderness. Restricted motion in abduction and in abduction combined with rotation makes it difficult or impossible to get the hand behind the back at the level of the waist or the neck. These features of the syndrome aid in the diagnosis. Because of the proximity of the involved tendons to the deltoid muscle, pain may be referred to the humeral attachment of the deltoid muscle. Frequently, calcium salts are deposited in the inflamed portion of the tendon and this condition is then referred to as *calcific* or *calcareous tendonitis*. If the calcium deposit ruptures through the peritendinous tissues, it may localize in the subacromial bursa, which lies over the supraspinatus tendon. Then the condition is complicated by *calcific bursitis*. Frequently calcific tendonitis and subacromial bursitis coexist. Infrequently bursitis exists alone, producing similar shoulder pain. From the character and localization of the pain it is impossible to know whether the lesion is in the tendon, the bursa, or both.

Pain is produced, in part, by distention of the tendon, or the bursa, or both, and is frequently promptly relieved by puncturing the surface of the distended structure, or aspirating the distended bursal space.

When tendonitis or bursitis exists, there is pain upon abduction and rotation of the shoulder, and upon movement that stretches the inflamed tendon or bursal walls, but flexion and extension do not cause pain. Arthritis of the shoulder produces pain upon motion in all planes.

Tendonitis may develop insidiously; in such cases pain and tenderness are similar in location to those of bursitis, but less severe. Calcium salts may be deposited in the tendon; more often they are not. The character of the pain is the same, unless a firm calcium deposit develops that may in itself cause or aggravate the pain started by the tendonitis.

Persistence of tendonitis and/or bursitis at the shoulder may cause irritation of other fibrous structures around the shoulder joint capsule and a chronic condition of *adhesive capsulitis* may develop, producing dull aching pain and diffuse minor tenderness, which causes progressive limitation of all motions of the shoulder until the motion becomes almost nil. This is the so-called "frozen shoulder," a poor, but descriptive term for the almost motionless, painful, stiff shoulder.

If trauma causes a tear in the tendons attaching to the humeral trochanter, or if there is a tear in the musculotendinous cuff, abduction of the shoulder cannot be initiated, a helpful diagnostic characteristic of this lesion. Tears of the musculotendinous cuff of the glenohumeral joint capsule account for a large percentage of cases of shoulder pain. In this condition, pain is sharply localized to the site of the pathology.

Another form of periarthritis of the shoulder is *bicipital tenosynovitis*. This lesion is characterized by pain and tenderness over the bicipital groove and around the tendon of the long head of the biceps muscle. The pain can be initiated by movement of the arm requiring contraction of the biceps muscle, and there is persistent tenderness over the lesser tuberosity of the humerus.

Brachial neuritis characteristically causes a more severe and sharp pain that radiates through the distribution of the involved nerves, and in this way it can be differentiated from shoulder joint or periarticular disease. Associated abnormalities in these conditions also aid in diagnosis.[26]

Shoulder pain may be the principal or the only symptom of *osteoarthritis* involving the joints and interspaces between cervical vertebrae 4 and 5, or 5 and 6, resulting in osteophytic lesions causing pressure on the spinal nerves that innervate the shoulder. Production or accentuation of the pain by movement of the neck are characteristic of this condition; roentgenograms confirm the diagnosis.

Since the nature of pain from visceral disease has been found by Lewis and Kellgren to be indistinguishable from that caused by somatic disease, it is not surprising that the shoulder *(left or right)*, innervated by nerves from the same segment that supplies the heart, should be the site of pain after myocardial infarction.[27,28] Absence of aggravation by shoulder motion and detection of signs of cardiac or coronary artery disease help to establish the diagnosis.

Disease of the gallbladder, the liver, or the right basilar pleura may stimulate nerves in the right diaphragm and cause pain felt in the *right* shoulder. This pain may be sharp, stabbing and severe and may be followed by a dull ache. It usually can be differentiated from the discomfort of shoulder disease by its characteristic location in the scapular region and the absence of signs of shoulder joint abnormality.

Hip. This large, important weight-bearing joint, because of its deep location, cannot be examined as satisfactorily as can most other joints. To learn the cause of hip pain, it is often necessary to conduct extensive studies, employing indirect observations. During childhood, *osteochondritis* of the femoral head,[29] *separation* and displacement of the capital femoral epiphysis, and *tuberculosis* frequently cause hip pain. Recalling the discussion concerning the reference of pain originating in deep structures to more superficial areas supplied by nerves from the same spinal segment, it is understood readily that persons with disease of the hip may complain of pain along the anterior aspect of the thigh or at the knee. Similarly, associated with hip pain from any cause, pain along the distribution of the femoral nerve is the rule. Such pain should suggest lesions at the hip rather than in the lower back, disorders of which are most frequently associated with leg pain of sciatic or obturator nerve distribution.

Sometimes hip pain and associated anterior thigh discomfort is caused by strain or tension of the hip-joint capsule. Degenerative changes in cartilage or bone may result from trauma sustained years before the pain begins. With these types of post-traumatic disorders, pain may occur only at a certain point in a particular motion of the joint. No other abnormalities exist. The lesions are important only because of the discomfort.

Septic arthritis of the hip joint is usually very painful, chiefly because the capsule of this large articulation is so firm that it is relatively nonexpansile; consequently, a small amount of purulent intracapsular fluid causes great tension of the capsule, resulting in severe pain. The position of the lower extremity in flexion, abduction, and external rotation gives greatest relaxation of the capsule and explains the characteristic attitude of the patient afflicted with this lesion.

Osteoarthritis (malum coxae senilis) is a very common cause of hip-joint pain in adults past middle age. The pain of this disorder is usually of the dull aching type, felt chiefly when bearing weight, and is accentuated by walking. It gradually grows more severe, and sometimes incapacitates the patient. The mechanism of production of this pain is discussed in the section on degenerative joint changes. Good general health, absence of clinical and laboratory signs of inflammation, limitation of motion at the affected joint, and characteristic roentgenograms help to establish this diagnosis.

Pain located at the greater trochanter may be due to underlying bone disease; more often it is caused by *trochanteric tendonitis* or *bursitis*. Although less common than similar lesions about the shoulder, tendonitis or bursitis should be considered when tenderness is localized in the region of the femoral trochanter and when the hip joint is normal. The pain of this lesion is often described as being felt "in the hip."

Knee. Pain occurs at the knee more often than at any other joint. The knee joint is a large joint, important in locomotion and weight-bearing; it is a complex joint, the structures of which can readily be injured or inflamed; and it is situated in a vulnerable location in the body.

Trauma is frequently responsible for knee pain. The numerous traumatic lesions common to other joints will not be considered in this connection, but the lesions peculiar to the knee deserve special mention.

Numerous intra-articular structures may be strained, torn, or otherwise injured so as to cause internal derangement of the joint, which usually produces severe pain.

The manner of production of the injury and the localization of the pain may indicate the nature of the lesion. When the injured structure is rather superficial, sharp localization of tenderness may be diagnostic of the traumatized structure. For example, tenderness localized bilaterally adjacent to the patella at or below the level of the tibio-femoral joint line indicates injury of the infrapatellar fat pad; tenderness at a point midway between the patella and the internal collateral ligament is characteristic of tear of the anterior portion of the internal semilunar cartilage; and tenderness localized to the medial aspect of the knee at the joint line usually results from injury of the internal collateral ligament. Painful locking of the joint is usually the result of a movable fragment attached to an internal structure, such as a semilunar cartilage, or to the pressure of a loose body in the joint. All of the lesions are painful because of stretching, pinching, or tearing of joint structures richly innervated by sensory nerves.

Pain localized at the site of attachment of the patellar tendon, and produced by extension of the leg at the knee in an adolescent child, is characteristic of partial separation of the tibial tubercle (Osgood-Schlatter disease). The pain is due to tension on the sensitive, traumatized tissues of the epiphysis by contraction of the quadriceps muscle. Tenderness sharply localized at the tubercle and characteristic roentgenograms establish the diagnosis.

Massive hemorrhage into the knee joint cavity (frequent in hemophiliacs) causes diffuse, severe pain, accentuated by standing or by movement of the joint. History of injury, tender diffuse swelling of "doughy" consistency, and discoloration from superficial hemorrhage suggest the nature of the lesion; aspiration proves the cause of the swelling and pain.

The knee is frequently painful because of *osteoarthritic changes*. Pain from this disease is dull or aching in nature and is usually felt only with weight-bearing movement of the knee during climbing or descending stairs or hills, walking on uneven ground, or arising from a sitting position. In large measure it is produced by irregularities of weight-bearing surfaces or osteophytic projections straining the sensitive tissues around the articular surfaces (the synovium,

the fibrous capsule, the ligaments, the periosteum, etc.).

The knee is frequently the site of *neuropathic joint disease*, diagnostic features of which have been described.

Pain in the posterior aspect of the knee may be caused by *cystic swelling* of the joint capsule or one of the tendon sheaths, usually that of the semimembranosis tendon. The cyst results from distention of the inflamed synovial membrane or from the escape of synovial fluid in the knee joint into bursae or tendon sheaths. Swelling, producing tension or traction, accounts for the localized pain, which is relieved by aspiration or surgical removal of the sac.

It is appropriate to caution again that dull, aching pain felt anteriorly at the knee may be caused by a hip-joint disorder, and if the knee and the surrounding structures are normal, disease of the hip should be suspected and searched for.

Ankle. This joint is particularly subject to sprain, which causes pain in the lateral or medial aspect of the joint, depending upon whether the injury caused forced inversion or eversion of the foot. Other traumatic lesions common to many joints need no special mention here. Monarticular arthritis of the ankle is uncommon.

Foot. Injury or inflammation of the Achilles tendon or the Achilles bursa causes pain and tenderness localized at the sites of these structures. Foot strain frequently results from relaxation of the anatomic arches. The postural disturbance resulting from *pes planus* may be sufficient to cause posterior leg pain, or even backache. Diffuse pain felt on the plantar aspect of the foot may be caused by strain or inflammation of the plantar fascia. Metatarsal pain may be due to pinching of the nerve between the fourth and fifth metatarsal bones (Morton's metatarsalgia), to stretching of the capsule of a metatarsophalangeal joint or the adjacent periosteum (Freiberg-Kohler's disease), or to periosteal irritation from fracture of a metatarsal shaft (march fracture). The history of metatarsal pain existing months before other joints become affected with *rheumatoid arthritis* has been sufficiently frequent that one should suspect this disease whenever an adult complains of foot strain or metatarsal pain and tenderness. Clavus, callus, or bunion formation usually can be readily identified as causes of local pain at the toes. Severely painful inflammation localized at the medial aspect of the bunion joint in male adults is characteristic of *acute gouty arthritis* of the first metatarsophalangeal articulation (podagra).[30]

POLYARTICULAR PAIN

Systemic Disorders. Aching in and about many joints is usually part of the symptomatology of a constitutional disease. Many acute systemic infections, during their prodromal or early clinical stages, cause diffuse aching, including multiple arthralgias. The mechanism of production of arthralgia in such diseases is not known. The nature of the disease causing such somatic pain usually becomes evident by the early development of characteristic features.[31] The rheumatic symptoms lessen or disappear early in the illness. Severe joint pain may be a prominent symptom of a generalized nonrheumatic disease such as acute leukemia.

Infectious Arthritis. Gonococcal arthritis, once a common form of specific infectious arthritis, now is less common because antimicrobial therapy is so effective for the initial infection. Between 10 and 20 days after the onset of gonorrhea, if there is systemic invasion of gonococci, the patient experiences marked malaise with aching throughout the body. A few days later, the general aching and arthralgia subside, and signs of inflammation appear in a few joints, in which pain becomes intensified. The pain of gonococcal arthritis is due to the effects of inflammation of the joint capsule. If purulent arthritis develops, the characteristics of septic joint disease appear. The possibility of gonococcal joint disease always should be kept in mind, because adequate therapy is very effective in accomplishing prompt cure, and unrecognized or inadequately treated gonococcal infection in a joint may rapidly cause irreparable destruction of the articular cartilage and consequent crippling.

Other infections, such as meningococcal and pneumococcal diseases, may be complicated by infectious arthritis involving multiple joints with clinical features similar to those described for gonococcal arthritis. All forms of specific infectious arthritis are relatively rare now that antimicrobial therapy is so effective. Culture of joint fluid, aspirated from an infected joint, usually establishes the etiology of the joint disease.

Rheumatic Fever. This febrile disease occurs primarily in children and young adults. The joint pain of rheumatic fever is usually so characteristic that it is very helpful in diagnosis. The onset of the arthritis of rheumatic fever usually begins shortly after a hemolytic streptococcal infection in the tonsils or the pharynx. Several joints, usually paired joints, become inflamed; the synovitis worsens rapidly, so that within 24 hours the joints are markedly swollen, red, hot, and exquisitely tender. Intense pain may be so severe that the slightest jarring of the bed or the weight of bed clothes on the affected joints causes excruciating pain. After several days, inflammation subsides in the affected joints and moves to others; thus the disease is characterized by "migratory" arthritis. No anatomic or functional residua remain after the joint inflammation subsides.

If one recognizes these typical features, the diagnosis usually can be made correctly. The joint pain is entirely due to the inflammation, is quantitatively related to its severity, and leaves as the synovitis subsides. Salicylates more quickly and completely relieve the joint pain and inflammation of acute rheumatic fever than that of any other disease. The existence of carditis or chorea, and normal appearance of the joint structures in roentgenograms, are valuable diagnostic aids.

Gouty Arthritis. No discomfort produced by rheumatic disease is more characteristic than the pain of an acute attack of gouty synovitis. The disease occurs almost exclusively in adult males. The sudden onset of severe pain of increasing intensity in one or more joints, often the bunion joint of the foot (podagra), is typical. After only a few hours the affected joints may be intensely inflamed and severely painful. There is exquisite tenderness at the inflamed joint. Without treatment the inflammation and the discomfort usually subside after several days, leaving no residual abnormality. The patient resumes normal activity and continues to feel entirely well for months or years until another similar painful bout of gouty arthritis may be experienced in joints previously affected, or in other articulations.

Provocative factors include overeating, irregular meals, purine-rich foods, alcoholic debauches, fatigue, exposure to severe cold or dampness, ill-fitting shoes, excessive physical activity, and many other irregularities of life. The attacks tend to increase in frequency and severity; joint destruction may develop in the repeatedly affected joints because of urate deposits in articular cartilage and subchondral bone or adjacent soft tissues. Gout should be suspected from the history of a typical attack in an adult male. The clinical impression is strengthened by finding hyperuricemia; the diagnosis can be proved only by the demonstration of urate crystals in tophi or joint fluids.[32]

It is not known whether local concentration of urates in joint structures is a factor in production of the attack of gouty arthritis, but it has been shown by Seegmiller[33] that injection of urate *crystals* can produce synovitis simulating gouty arthritis. The discomfort of acute gouty arthritis is entirely due to the synovitis. In chronic tophaceous gout, the structural changes in the joints add to the pain when the joints are moved or support weight.

In doubtful cases the diagnosis is aided by observing dramatic relief of inflammation and pain by the proper administration of colchicine. The fact that it is so dependably effective in gout and usually valueless in other rheumatic disorders makes the use of colchicine a helpful diagnostic therapeutic test.[34]

Similar attacks of acute joint synovitis may occur because of the precipitation of calcium pyrophosphate microcrystals in joint structures which cause "crystal-induced synovitis" identical to that of gouty synovitis. Identification of the calcium crystals in aspirated joint fluid and the observance of a fine "calcium line" deposited in articular cartilages clarify the diagnosis and differentiate this "pseudogout" from true (urate) gout.[35]

Rheumatoid Arthritis. A very common cause of polyarticular pain is rheumatoid arthritis. The joint abnormalities of this diffuse connective tissue disease begin with inflammation of the synovium and the joint capsule. The joint inflammation becomes chronic, but because the inflammation is commonly not severe, the pain is usually described as "dull" or "aching" in character. The joint discomfort is intensified by movement of the joint and by weight-bearing, which adds strain and tension on the joint capsule and the periarticular structures. When joint fluid accumulates, distention of the inflamed capsule adds to the joint pain and restricts motion.

As the disease progresses the synovitis causes cartilage destruction, resulting in ir-regularities in the surface of the articular cartilages. There may be a grating type of discomfort when the joint is moved. Additional pain may be caused by muscle spasm. After crippling results, the joint deformities are additional causes of pain. The paresthesia and the neuralgic and the myalgic pains which frequently occur in this disease are, at least in part, due to inflammatory infiltrations in the perineurium of peripheral nerves and in muscles,[36,37] or to the neuropathy caused by vasculitis.[38]

Much discomfort from this disease is due to nonarticular abnormalities, especially irritation of the muscles and the periarticular connective tissue, as shown by the early beneficial response to corticotropin and corticosteroids. Benefit from these hormones in the rheumatoid patient usually begins with relief of stiffness, allowing greater and easier motion, *followed* by significant decrease in the joint inflammation.

In the very early stage of the disease there may be nothing to differentiate rheumatoid arthritis from other diseases with polyarticular nonpurulent inflammation. As the disease progresses, the chronicity with remissions and relapses, the evidence of systemic illness with slight fever, leukocytosis, elevated erythrocyte sedimentation rate, anemia, malnutrition, skin and muscle atrophy, development of joint deformity and ankylosis and the characteristic roentgenographic changes make diagnosis easy. Demonstration of the rheumatoid factor in serologic tests is a helpful confirmatory diagnostic aid, but is usually not possible in early stages of the disease when help in diagnosis is most needed. Rheumatoid arthritis affects individuals of any age, but is much more frequent in young and middle-aged adults. Juvenile rheumatoid arthritis (Still's disease) usually has characteristics similar to the adult disease.[39] Chronicity, greater constitutional changes, muscle, skin and bone atrophy, joint deformities, and the absence of carditis help to differentiate the disease from rheumatic fever, with which it is frequently confused.

Features clinically indistinguishable from classical rheumatoid disease frequently characterize the syndrome of systemic lupus erythematosus. Visceral inflammation and the demonstration of the lupus factor (L. E. cell, antinuclear antibodies, etc.) help to identify this syndrome.[40]

Degenerative Joint Changes. Osteoarthritis

(degenerative disease of joints) is about as common a cause of joint pain as rheumatoid arthritis. This disorder begins as a degenerative change of articular cartilage which slowly progresses to cause thinning of the cartilage, irregular joint surfaces, and irritation of the periosteum covering the adjacent bone, with resultant osteophytic and hypertrophic changes. Since articular cartilage contains no nerves, as long as the disease is confined to that structure, the degeneration may progress subtly and indolently. After articular cartilage becomes eroded and osteophytes develop, movement of the joint and weight-bearing produce pain as a result of strain and tension on the sensitive supporting periarticular fibrous tissues. Joint pain in osteoarthritis largely is due to ligamentous or muscular strains or to mild synovitis.[41] When the affected joints are not being subjected to weight-bearing or movement, the patient usually is comfortable.

The sharply contrasting pathology of these two common forms of chronic arthritis—rheumatoid and osteoarthritis—fully explains the differences in the joint discomfort accompanying these disorders. Osteoarthritis is a disease of older adults who usually are constitutionally healthy; it is a local joint disorder chiefly affecting the weight-bearing articulations. These characteristics, together with the absence of physical or laboratory signs of inflammation, usually clarify the diagnosis.

Because of the frequency of degenerative joint changes in older persons, it is not unusual for persons beyond middle age who develop joint inflammation due to rheumatoid arthritis to exhibit characteristics of both diseases. Gouty synovitis or specific infectious arthritis may also occur with osteoarthritis.

Nonarticular Rheumatism—Fibrositis. A painful rheumatic disease that should be differentiated from common forms of chronic arthritis is nonarticular rheumatism, frequently called "primary fibrositis," "muscular rheumatism," or "periarthritis." This occurs frequently in adults of middle or older age. Joints are not affected, but the adjacent fascia, muscles, tendons, and ligaments are involved. There is no characteristic histopathology in the affected nonarticular connective tissue. The abnormality appears to be due to chemical or physicochemical changes of undefined nature.

This disease may be quite widespread or may be localized to certain parts such as the neck, the lumbar spine, shoulders, or hands. The discomfort usually is described as "not a pain but an aching soreness" associated with stiffness of the affected parts. Symptoms usually are worse in the morning after a night's rest, as though the muscles had congealed; with activity through the day, the pain and stiffness lessen and may disappear. Toward evening, along with fatigue, the discomfort tends to increase. Diagnosis is based on the *pattern* of symptoms and physical findings, and the exclusion of other diseases. In differentiation, the absence of physical and roentgenographic signs of abnormality of joint structures, the absence of fever, leukocytosis, anemia, and undernutrition, and the presence of a normal erythrocyte sedimentation rate all are helpful.[42,43]

Polymyalgia Rheumatica. During the past decade, a syndrome has been described consisting of severe pain and stiffness in the neck, shoulders, arms, and sometimes the hips and thighs, occurring usually in elderly persons. Joints are not inflamed. The discomfort is localized in muscles; hence, the name "polymyalgia." Fever and high erythrocyte sedimentation rate commonly are found with this rheumatic disorder. In many, but not all patients with this syndrome, giant cell arteritis has been found in biopsy studies. When arterial biopsy is negative, diagnosis depends upon elimination of other rheumatic disorders and the dramatic and prompt response to salicylates or corticosteroids. Prognosis is comparatively good.[44,45]

Unexplained Arthralgia. Sometimes patients complain of constant or oft-recurring pain involving many joints, when repeated physical examination and laboratory studies fail to reveal any evidence of joint disease. The pain usually is described as a "soreness" or "aching"; it may be constant or intermittent. Etiologic possibilities include psychogenic, allergic, or "toxic" factors. Present knowledge of the pathogenesis of such joint pain is lacking. Often it is necessary to diagnose "arthralgia, cause unknown." It is wise to observe these patients for a long time to learn whether such pain is a prodromal manifestation of slowly developing chronic arthritis.

SUMMARY

Joint pain and periarticular discomfort are very common symptoms of a variety of different diseases. For full understanding of joint and periarticular pain, and in order to interpret these symptoms profitably in diagnosis, it is necessary to understand the anatomic and physiologic bases for articular pain. It then is necessary to analyze the mechanism of production of the pain by different pathologic processes. This information, together with an understanding of the pathologic and clinical characteristics of the various diseases, provides a basis for the utilization of the joint pain to maximum advantage in diagnosis.

The nature of the discomfort of a few diseases of joints and periarticular structures is so characteristic that correct diagnosis can be suspected and even made from the analysis of the pain alone. In most instances, however, pain calls attention to the fact that a disorder affecting the joints or periarticular structures exists, and its nature suggests the cause, but diagnosis can be made with confidence only after correlating all of the clinical and laboratory data with the symptoms.

REFERENCES

1. Gerneck, I.: Ueber die Nerven den Synovialmembran (Vorlansige Mitteilung), Arch. Orthop. Unfallchir. 28:599-604, 1930.
2. Stilwell, D. L., Jr.: The innervation of tendons and aponeuroses, Amer. J. Anat. 100: 289, 1957.
3. ———: Regional variations in the innervation of deep fasciae and aponeuroses, Anat. Rec. 127:635, 1957.
4. Lennander, K. G.: Mitt. Grenzgeb. Med. Clin. 15:465, 1906.
5. Lewis, T.: Suggestions relating to study of somatic pain, Brit. Med. J. 1:321-325, 1938.
6. Kellgren, J. H.: On distribution of pain arising from deep somatic structures with charts of segmental pain areas, Clin. Sci. 4: 35-46, 1939.
7. Kellgren, J. H., and Samuel, E. P.: The sensitivity and innervation of the articular capsule, J. Bone Joint Surg. [Brit.] 32S:84, 1950.
8. Raszeja, F., and Billewicz-Stankiewicz, J.: Sur l'innervation de la capsule articulaire du genou chez le lapin, Compt. Rend. Soc. Biol. 115:1267-1268, 1934.
9. Kellgren, J. H.: Observations on referred pain arising from muscle, Clin. Sci. 3:175-190, 1938.

10. Gardner, E.: Nerve supply of muscles, joints and other deep structures, Bull. Hosp. Joint Dis. 21:153, 1960.
11. ———: The innervation of the knee joint, Anat. Rec. 101:109-130, 1948.
12. ———: The nerve supply of diarthrodial joints, Stanford Med. Bull. 6:367-373, 1948.
13. ———: Physiology of movable joints, Physiol. Rev. 30:127-176, 1950.
14. Lewis, T., and Kellgren, J. H.: Observations relating to referred pain, viscero-motor reflexes and other associated phenomena, Clin. Sci. 4:47-71, 1939.
15. Lewis, T.: Pain, New York, Macmillan, 1942.
16. Ernstene, A. C., and Kinell, J.: Pain in shoulder as sequel to myocardial infarction, A.M.A. Arch. Intern. Med. 66:800-806, 1940.
17. Herfort, R. A.: Extended sympathectomy in treatment of chronic arthritis, J. Amer. Geriat. Soc. 5:904, 1957.
18. Herfort, R. A., and Nickerson, S. H.: Relief of arthritic pain and rehabilitation of chronic arthritic patient by extended sympathetic denervation, Arch. Phys. Med. 40: 133-140, 1959.
19. Howell, T. H.: Relief of pain in rheumatoid arthritis with tetraethylammonium bromide, Lancet 1:204, 1950.
20. Rose, G. K.: Tuberculosis of the knee joint, Brit. J. Clin. Pract. 13:241, 1959.
21. Tegner, W. S.: Tennis elbow, Postgrad. Med. J. 35:390, 1959.
22. Steinbrocker, O., Neustadt, D., and Bosch, S. J.: Painful shoulder syndromes, their diagnosis and treatment, Med. Clin. N. Amer. 39:563, 1955.
23. Albert, S. M., and Rechtman, A. M.: The painful shoulder, Amer. Pract. 7:72, 1956.
24. Mosley, H. F.: Disorders of the shoulder, Clin. Sympos. 11:75, 1959.
25. Smyth, C. J., et al.: Rheumatism and arthritis (Twelfth Rheumatism Review), Ann. Intern. Med. 50:366-494, 634-801, 1959.
26. Bucy, P. C., and Oberhill, H. R.: Pain in the shoulder and arm from neurological involvement, J.A.M.A. 169:798, 1959.
27. Steinbrocker, O.: The painful shoulder, in Hollander, J. L., et al. (eds.): Arthritis, ed. 7, pp. 1233-1274, Philadelphia, Lea & Febiger, 1966.
28. Morgan, E. H.: Pain in the shoulder and upper extremity: visceral causes considered by the internist, J.A.M.A. 169:804, 1959.
29. Monnet, J. C.: Osteochondritis deformans, J. Okla. Med. Ass. 52:376, 1959.
30. Smyth, C. J.: Diagnosis and Treatment of Gout, in Hollander, J. L., et al. (eds.): Arthritis, ed. 7, pp. 923-946, Philadelphia, Lea & Febiger, 1966.
31. Freyberg, R. H., et al.: Rheumatic manifestations of systemic diseases, Clin. Orthop. Related Res. 57:3-101, March-April 1968.

32. McCarty, D. J., and Hollander, J. L.: Identification of urate crystals in gouty synovial fluid, Ann. Intern. Med. 54:452, 1961.

33. Seegmiller, J. E., Howell, R. R., and Malawista, S. E.: Inflammatory reaction to sodium urate; its possible relationship to genesis of acute gouty arthritis, J.A.M.A. 180:469, 1962.

34. Freyberg, R. H.: Gout, Arthritis Rheum. 5:624, 1962.

35. McCarty, D. J., Jr., Gatter, R. A., and Brill, J. M.: Crystal deposition diseases: sodium urate (gout) and calcium pyrophosphate (chondrocalcinosis, pseudo-gout), J.A.M.A. 193:129-132, 1965.

36. Freund, H. A., Steiner, G., Leichtentritt, B., and Price, A. E.: Peripheral nerves in chronic atrophic arthritis, J. Lab. Clin. Med. 27:1256-1258, 1942.

37. ———: Nodular polymyositis in rheumatoid arthritis, Science 101:202-203, 1945.

38. Johnson, R. L., Smyth, C. J., Holt, G. W., Lubchenco, A., and Valentine, E.: Steroid therapy and vascular lesions in rheumatoid arthritis, Arthritis Rheum. 2:224, 1959.

39. Grokoest, A. W., Snyder, A. I., and Schlaeger, R.: Juvenile Rheumatoid Arthritis, Boston, Little, Brown, 1962.

40. Talbott, J. H., and Ferrandis, R. M.: Collagen Diseases, New York, Grune & Stratton, 1956.

41. Kellgren, J. H.: Some painful joint conditions and their relation to osteoarthritis, Clin. Sci. 4:193-205, 1945.

42. Rosenberg, E. F., Classification and management of fibrositis, Med. Clin. N. Amer. 42:1613-1627, 1958.

43. Graham, W.: Fibrositis and nonarticular rheumatism, Phys. Ther. Rev. 35:128, 1955.

44. Gordon, I., Rennie, A. M., and Branwood, A. W.: Polymyalgia rheumatica: biopsy studies, Ann. Rheum. Dis. 23:447-455, Nov. 1964.

45. Davison, S., and Spiera, H.: Polymyalgia rheumatica, Clin. Orthop. 57:95-99, March-April 1968.

13

Pain in the Extremities

WILLIAM F. COLLINS and *JOSEPH H. GALICICH*

INTRODUCTION

Establishing the cause of pain in an extremity can be difficult because of the many elements that must be considered as possible pathophysiologic factors. Some of these are the numerous and various conditions that can affect the several different tissues of the extremity, the reactions of the tissues involved, and the secondary reactions that can occur in adjacent tissues. They include the possibility of pain radiating into the extremity from lesions of the spinal roots and peripheral nerve plexuses, referred pain from lesions of organs such as the heart or kidney, and pain from central nervous system lesions. They also include the problem of pain radiating to more proximal areas of the extremity from lesions of the foot or the hand, and into more distal portions of the extremity from lesions of the proximal joints or muscles. There is also the consideration of systemic disease that may appear first as pain in an extremity. Probably the most difficult problem, however, is the differentiation between pain and suffering, (which includes the emotional and psychological responses to the pain) or even more commonly, a determination of what portion of the complaints that the patient has is actually pain caused by an organic lesion and what is arising from his total experience of suffering. The exposed position of the extremities and the necessity of their constant use in the activities of daily living contributes not only to their susceptibility to injury, but also to the marked disability the patient suffers with the painful extremity. Disability appears to contribute frequently to conscious or subconscious fear that the pain signifies a more serious disease than is actually true. Suffering caused by this fear contributes to the complaints and to the physician's difficulty in determining the cause of pain.

In considering any complaint, the etiology is most easily determined from the history. If the information contained in the history is to be effectively used, the history must often contain not only the type, onset and duration of the complaint, as well as factors that alter the symptoms, but also the past history, family history and a review of systems. A history that is inaccurate or too brief is a common cause for error in discovery of the pathophysiology of pain in an extremity. The physician also must do a complete physical examination, as well as examination of the extremity involved. Too often a complaint of pain in an extremity is investigated as though the extremity were isolated from the body, so that if the examination of the extremity reveals no positive findings, the physician concludes that the patient has no physical disease process as a basis for the complaint and diagnoses the cause as psychosomatic. The presence of possible contributory evidence such as contingent compensation for accident or injury may only strengthen the physician's confidence in his judgment instead of being simply another aspect of the history. On the other hand,

and perhaps even worse, is precipitous resort to unwarranted diagnostic tests or surgical approaches on finding an isolated positive physical sign such as a loss of reflex or change in muscle size in an extremity. This can be not only incorrect, but also dangerous for the patient.

This section is organized about anatomical divisions of the tissues of the extremities. This organization may give the reader the impression that the approach to understanding pathophysiologic processes which may produce pain is through an etiological listing of causes of aberration of function as they relate to anatomical structures of the extremity. While this may be a secondary process in the determination of the cause of such a complaint, it should be superimposed upon the total evaluation of the patient. Failure to realize the importance of total evaluation of the patient will allow this chapter to become a source of error rather than the source of aid the authors intended it to be.

PAIN ORIGINATING IN THE SKIN

Types of lesions of the skin that can cause pain are numerous. They include trauma, tumors, allergic reactions, infection, as well as many pathological changes of unknown etiology and various reactions of the skin that reflect systemic disease. There are, however, distinct characteristics of pain from lesions of the skin that extend throughout this wide variety of conditions. These distinctive attributes include accurate location and a special quality. The feeling is sharply localized and is described as similar to a previously experienced sensation from a burn, cut or scrape of the skin. Typically and nearly always, there is alteration in the appearance of the skin or subcutaneous tissue in the area involved. If these criteria are not met, it is best to look elsewhere for the cause of pain which the patient feels on the surface or in the subcutaneous tissue of an extremity.

The reason that the characteristics of pain are so constant in primary skin lesions is that the lesion involves sensory endings of the peripheral nerves. The deformation or injury of these primary endings conveys impulses that are similar to, if not the same as, impulses that are recognized through experience as coming from noxious stimuli on the surface of the body. The nervous system accurately localizes stimuli that arise on the surface of the body. The peripheral nerve ending must have an altered environment which either through stretching, pressure or alteration in metabolic function causes it to propagate impulses such that the subject feels pain. Changes in the skin detected by visual and tactile examination complete the reasons for these characteristics of painful skin lesions.

Pain perceived as being on the surface of the body but not well localized or accompanied by no alteration in the skin, or that is described in an unusual fashion, should make the examiner consider alteration in the function of the nerves or blood supply to the area rather than a primary lesion of the skin. There may be secondary reactions of the skin and subcutaneous tissue from lesions of the blood vessels or nerves resulting in visible and palpable skin lesions (e.g., as in herpes). It is the description of poorly localized discomfort and sensations which are difficult for the patient to describe in relation to previous experience that gives the clue that the pathology is not primarily in the skin. This group of afflictions in which peripheral nerve and/or blood vessel pathology is present causes the greatest difficulty in diagnosis of pain referred to the surface of an extremity. The distribution of the pain in the area of a dermatome, or a peripheral nerve, or over the specific area of the blood supply can be the clue that leads to the diagnosis of a more systemic or proximal disease process.

PAIN ORIGINATING IN BONE

Pain from bone lesions is caused by irritation of, or tension on the peritosteum; alteration in the function of joints proximal or distal to the bone involved; or changes in the function of overlying tissues, such as nerves, ligaments, tendons or bursae. With the exception of mild discomfort from distention of the marrow cavity or compression of cancellous bone, bone itself appears to have little, if any, pain sensitivity. Pain caused by lesions of bone is less well localized than that from lesions of more superficial tissue and often is described as an ache or a deep pain in the general area of the diseased tissue. When a peripheral nerve is also involved, the pain radiates to the peripheral distribution of the nerve, thus sometimes causing difficulty in differentiating the lesion from a primary peripheral nerve lesion.

Common disorders of bone causing pain are *trauma, neoplasms, infection, metabolic disorders including scurvy, rickets,* and *hyperparathyroidism,* and *Paget's disease.*

The pain from fractures comes from stretch, tearing and irritation of the periosteum and surrounding tissue. The site of the fracture, beside showing anatomical deformity, also shows swelling and evidence of hemorrhage. There is tenderness locally and focal pain when stress is placed on the fracture site by proximal or distal manipulation of the bone. Pain of infections and tumors may simulate each other with aching discomfort, often made worse by dependency of the extremity. The severity of the pain reflects, in general, the rapidity with which the lesion is enlarging and the amount of irritation such enlargement causes. Infections such as syphilis (periostitis) or osteomyelitis from bacteria of low virulence may become very extensive before much discomfort is felt. Tumors that are slowly growing may act in the same fashion and, therefore, benign tumors are at times huge before any discomfort is felt. On the other hand, highly malignant, rapidly growing neoplasms or infections from highly virulent organisms may cause pain when the lesion is very small, even before detectable by x-ray examination. When either infection or tumor breaks through the periosteum, there is often a dramatic decrease in pain. Such events illustrate and emphasize the part which the innervation of and stresses upon the periosteum have in the pain of these conditions. Pain from metabolic disorders and from Paget's disease relate to a combination of factors including deformities of bone, irritation and stretching of periosteum, and stress on joints. The discomfort may vary markedly from patient to patient depending upon severity, location, and nature of the disease process.

X rays of bones and joints taken by proper techniques and studied by experts yield highly significant information concerning pathophysiologic processes causing bone pain. The characteristic appearance of certain tumors may be noted. Hypertropic osteoarthropathy may be detected. Gouty, rheumatoid, and osteoarthritis have distinctive roentgenologic features. Osteomalacia and vitamin D deficiency cause typical changes. Hyperparathyroidism causes certain bone peculiarities, with cysts and demineralization. Paget's disease has special features. The history, physical, and laboratory findings help the roentgenologist in his contribution toward elucidating the pathophysiologic process.

Fractures or deformities of bone usually reveal in x rays characteristics of their causes: perhaps trauma acting on normal bone, perhaps trauma, stress or weight-bearing acting upon poorly developed or weakened or diseased bone.

When history and physical examination suggest possible bone involvement as a cause of pain, x-ray study is necessary. Because pain with bone disease is often poorly localized, and since there is the possibility of soft tissue and joint involvement at a distance from the lesion, x rays should be made of the entire extremity. For comparison, x rays of the opposite matching extremity are frequently of great help.

PAIN ORIGINATING IN MUSCLE

In contrast to bone, muscle is generously supplied with free nerve endings considered to be pain endings. Distribution of nerve endings is not as dense as in skin; therefore needle puncture or incision of muscle is much less painful than of skin. Inflammation, compression, or alteration in the blood supply of muscle, however, results in severe agonizing pain in part localized to the area of the muscle involved, but also referred to overlying soft tissue and, at times, to the entire extremity. When a muscle is traumatized or is involved in a painful disease process it usually responds with increased tone, which may result in spastic contraction or cramping. Increased tone from injury or from spasticity of neurological disease can in itself cause pain in muscle, related joints, fascia or bursa by altering their normal function. Diffuse pain of an entire extremity sometimes arising from conditions affecting a single muscle or a group of muscles can, at times, be difficult to diagnose as being related to the muscle. Helpful findings in such conditions are tenderness of the muscle involved, increase in pain in the whole extremity when that muscle is compressed, and increase in the pain of the extremity when that muscle is used.

Conditions of muscle causing pain can be considered under the following categories: *trauma, systemic infection, alteration in blood supply, inflammation* and *neoplasms.*

Trauma. A traumatized muscle usually is painful, has increased tone, and is tender. The subject experiences increased pain when it is used and some relief of pain with rest. The mildest type of muscle trauma causing pain is that encountered after strenuous exercise by an unconditioned subject. The cause of the pain is not understood, but may relate to retained metabolic products. The pain usually begins at four to six hours after use and reaches its maximum intensity in forty-eight to seventy-two hours. Mild exercise, heat and massage relieve the pain. The pain of muscle contusion is caused by hemorrhage within the muscle and begins within minutes after the injury and may continue for days or weeks. Rupture of a muscle may consist of rupture of just a few fibers, rupture of the fascial envelope of the muscle, rupture of the main muscle mass, or rupture of the tendon of the muscle. Examination will reveal marked tenderness over the area of partial rupture. There is tenderness with rupture of the fascia but the prominent finding is protrusion of the muscle mass through the fascia. With a major rupture of the body of the muscle or a rupture of the tendon, there is loss of function of the muscle, tenderness at the point of rupture, and contraction of the muscle mass proximal to the rupture. The pain of traumatic lesions of muscle may be localized or referred to the entire extremity. History of trauma and local findings clarify the diagnosis.

Myalgia of Systemic Infection. The cause of the diffuse myalgia with high fever or with viral infections with or without high fever is not known. The discomfort is usually a relatively mild pain that parallels the course of the fever or the illness, and while it may involve proximal extremity muscles more than other muscle groups, it is generalized. A diagnostic problem is the occasional patient with residual focal areas of tenderness and pain in the area of the scapula or shoulder. This condition is usually diagnosed as focal myositis or fascitis and is particularly common after viral infections. Such disorders usually seem to start with the illness but persist when the remainder of the muscle aches are gone. They frequently cause more difficulty and more pain with radiation into an extremity than when the entire myalgic syndrome was present. They usually respond to heat and analgesics, particularly salicylates, but at times require physiotherapy or local injections of corticosteroids.

Altered Blood Supply. One of the most severe pains known is that secondary to inadequate blood flow to a working muscle. A common cause of altered blood flow to an extremity is arteriosclerosis of either the major vessel of the limb or the more proximal *arterial trunks*. "Intermittent claudication", by which is meant cramping pain in the muscle with use, is a common presenting symptom of arterial insufficiency. Although most common in the lower extremities, it occurs in any extremity where there is significant arterial insufficiency and the muscles are used. Diagnosis can be made from the history of recurrent pain with activity and confirmed by palpation of the peripheral pulses, comparison of blood pressure in the opposite limb and oscillometry in the extremity. A similar pattern of complaints from impaired blood supply can also occur with Buerger's disease or altered blood supply secondary to *small vessel occlusion* rather than major vessel occlusion. Acute arterial occlusion by *emboli* will be discussed under arteries in this chapter, but if collateral blood supply is established after the acute embolic episode, the patient can present with a picture similar to that of arteriolar disease. At times, arteriography is necessary to separate the three conditions, i.e.: arteriosclerosis, arteriolar occlusion, and embolization.

Acute venous thrombosis may also cause evidence of vascular insufficiency to a muscle in part by altered blood flow through the vessels secondary to increased venous pressure, and in part from secondary arterial spasm. Sympathetic block will often partially relieve the pain. In summary, muscle pain from arterial insufficiency has as the basic pattern of complaint, pain and cramping in the distribution of muscles being used and relief of such pain when either the muscles are put at rest, the circulation improved, or both. Venous obstruction causes some of the same complaints, but the discomfort is usually milder in degree and more frequently relates to dependency of the extremity and edema of the tissues as much as to activity of the muscle.

Inflammation. Myositis or inflammation of muscle may be present as an acute or chronic process, either general or focal, usually with pain, tenderness, and weakness of the muscles involved. With involvement of muscles of the extremities, particularly and more commonly of the proximal muscles, pain may be referred into the extremity involved. The term used to describe generalized myositis is polymyositis. However, this is not a single clinical entity but rather a description of the pathological changes seen in muscles secondary to a few known infective agents such as Coxsackie virus, or parasites (for example, trichinella spiralis or tinea soleus), and more commonly as a response to collagen disorders, carcinoma, or with no known cause. The onset of polymyositis can be very acute or slowly progressive, and the severity of the pain relates to the acuteness and severity of the reaction. In general, the acute onset of polymyositis is more common in the young, while the chronic course is more common in the adult, but either may occur at any age. Polymyositis secondary to parasitic infestation is rare and, in general, unless repeated infestation of the parasite occurs the inflammatory reaction is brief and not severe, usually lasting five to ten days. Viral infections of muscles also are usually relatively brief, with moderate inflammatory response. Inflammatory reaction of a single muscle or muscle group secondary to bacterial infection is very rare, except under conditions of marked debilitation or altered blood supply in a muscle. It is most commonly seen following open trauma with inadequate wound débridement or poor control of adjacent hemorrhage. Following such a wound, clostridia infections must be considered when swelling and pain extends along a muscle or a fascial plane of a muscle within or adjacent to the penetrating wound.

Much more common is the idiopathic polymyositis or the polymyositis associated with **collagen disorders** or **carcinoma.** As mentioned, the onset may be acute, particularly in children, with severe inflammatory reaction in the muscle and in subcutaneous and dermal tissue above the muscle. Myositis with involvement of the skin has been termed dermato-myositis. The onset may be accompanied by fever and polymorphonuclear leukocytosis. The proximal muscles of the extremities are more commonly involved than the distal. They become tender and weak. Chronic myositis is more common in older persons. With weakness and tenderness of muscle, there may be alteration in function of joints of the extremity so that pain results secondarily from joint derangement. Examination may reveal fasciculations as well as tenderness and atrophy of muscles. The diagnosis is best made by electromyographic studies and surgical biopsy. Occurrence of chronic polymyositis with carcinoma, particularly of the stomach, breast and lung, has been known for many years and, at times, is the first indication of the presence of the neoplasm. However, it is most commonly seen with the dissemination of the neoplasm. In summary, aside from the bacterial infection of a single muscle which has been damaged by trauma or secondary to a penetrating wound of a muscle, infection of a muscle is relatively rare. Inflammatory response in muscles secondary to viral or parasitic infection usually shows tenderness of the muscle and pain on use of the muscle. The acute or chronic development of weakness, tenderness and pain in the muscles of the extremities more marked in proximal than distal extremities, should suggest the presence of polymyositis and a search for possible related diseases as collagen disorders and carcinoma should be undertaken.

Tumors. Tumors of muscle are extremely rare and usually are diagnosed by the presence of tenderness, weakness, and a mass in the area of the pain and tenderness. The pain of such tumors is related to the rate of growth and the alteration of the function of the muscle. Primary tumors such as rhabdomyosarcoma or desmoids are extremely rare. Rhabdomyosarcomas are malignant, rapidly growing, often painful and present an enlarging mass within the muscle. Pains from such lesions constitute a very minor portion of the complaints of pain in an extremity.

PAIN ORIGINATING IN JOINTS

The causes and mechanisms that produce joint pain are discussed in other chapters. Analysis of joint pathophysiology will not be repeated here. A few aspects of joint pain are, however, relevant to a discussion of pain in the extremities. Pain in joints is usually localized to the area of the joint involved, although more accurately in distal than in proximal joints. The pain is increased by movement of the joint and by pressure on the joint. There is often tenderness of the tissues around the joint. Therefore, increased pain with movement of a joint and tenderness of the periarticular tissues are significant localizing signs. Pain from a joint, in addition, may be referred to the muscles acting on the joint, probably secondary to both altered tone in the muscle and altered mechanisms of action. Joint pain, as with other deep pain in an extremity, can be referred to the entire extremity, to a distal portion of the extremity (as in the shoulder-hand syndrome), or may be a basis for reflex sympathetic dystrophy. The *shoulder-hand* syndrome almost always contains elements of reflex sympathetic dystrophy and consists of an aching, burning stiffness with altered vasomotor tone in the hand distal to the painful shoulder. When the reflex dystrophy in the extremity is the major part of the syndrome (most frequent in the upper extremity), sympathetic block with a local anesthetic is indicated. When the pain is primarily in the joint with mild referral to the distal part of the extremity, injection of tender areas around the joint with local anesthetic alone or in combination with corticosteroids will often relieve both the joint and the extremity pain. Both sympathetic block and local injection have therapeutic, as well as diagnostic merits, since their effects often long outlast the duration of action of the local anesthetic. Chronic conditions of joints that produce great limitation of joint function and severe alteration in anatomical configuration, particularly in rheumatoid conditions, will not respond to such injection unless local disease processes can be arrested and joint mobility restored. Therefore, injections in such conditions have little diagnostic value. Pain in a joint is usually localized, but may be referred both distally and proximally in the extremity, is usually increased by movement of the joint, and is accompanied by tenderness of the periarticular tissues.

PAIN ORIGINATING IN ARTERIES AND VEINS

Although arteries and veins contain pain-sensitive nerve endings, pain due to disease of blood vessels in the extremities is almost always the result of altered vascular perfusion within other tissues of the limb, chiefly muscle, peripheral nerve and skin. The character and extent of the resulting signs and symptoms of the vascular disease, including pain, depend upon whether the arterial or venous side of the circulation is primarily involved, upon the character of the disease process itself, its anatomical site, and usually the rate of its progression. Sudden occlusion of the major artery to a limb, resulting for example from a large embolus, almost always produces prompt pain and paresthesias throughout the limb secondary to ischemia of nerve trunks and muscles and is usually followed by paralysis. Arterial insufficiency, as mentioned under the section on muscles, classically produces distal pain with exercise if larger trunks are involved: e.g., of the thigh with aortic bi-furcation disease and of the calf with occlusive disease of the femoral artery. With more severe restriction of arterial blood supply there may be aching pain in the extremity even at rest, usually relieved somewhat by placing the limb in a dependent position. Aneurysms of the peripheral arteries are usually painless; diagnosis is most often made by finding a pulsating mass. However, because of their frequent approximation to major peripheral nerves, pressure produced by an aneurysm may result in paresthesias and pain in the distribution of one or more involved nerves.

Raynaud's phenomenon or intermittent vasospasm in the upper extremities precipitated by cold or emotion may exist as a primary disease, usually in young women, or may be associated with Buerger's disease, atherosclerosis or collagen diseases such as scleroderma, rheumatoid arthritis, or lupus erythematosus. Patients with this affliction complain of intermittent pain and paresthesias in the digits on exposure to cold and concomitantly note sudden pallor of the fingers resulting from vasospasm of the dermal arterioles, cyanosis, and then reactive hyperemia. Trophic changes of the skin of the digits and even gangrene may ensue. When this phenomenon is suspected, one should consider also the possibility of other peripheral arterial disease. A careful evaluation of all peripheral pulses should be made as well as a search for disorders predisposing to arterial occlusive disease such as diabetes, hypercholesterolemia, atherosclerosis, and the collagen diseases.

Venous disease may or may not give rise to pain. Superficial venous thrombosis often presents as local, painful swelling and the tender thrombosed vein can usually be palpated. Thrombosis of deeper veins, most common in the lower extremities of bedridden patients, should be suspected if pain occurs in the lower extremities or if swelling of one or both legs is present. Examination for changes in girth of the calf, calf tenderness and tenderness along the course of the major veins of the lower extremities should be part of the routine care of all postoperative and bedridden patients. Chronic venous insufficiency, usually with varicose veins, often gives rise to the complaint of aching and a feeling of heaviness, particularly after prolonged standing. There may be edema of the legs, and cyanosis. Often there is spotty brown pigmentation. Pain and pruritus secondary to induration and ulceration of the skin is not uncommon in these patients.

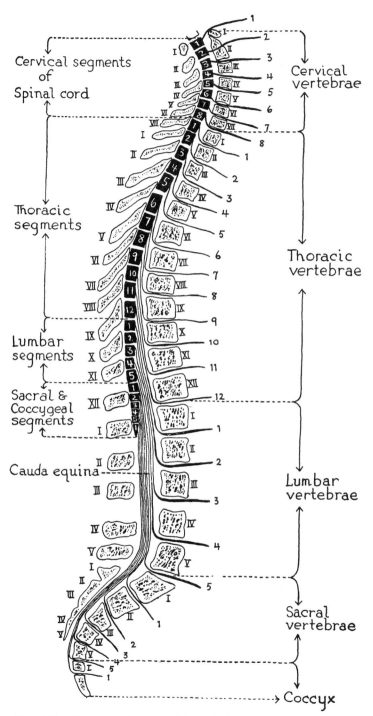

Fig. 13-1. Diagram of the position of the spinal cord segments with reference to the bodies and spinous processes of the vertebrae. Note also the place of origin of the nerve roots from the spinal cord and their emergence from the corresponding intervertebral foramina. (Modified from Tandler and Ranzi. Strong and Elwyn: Human Neuroanatomy, Baltimore, Williams & Wilkins)

PAIN FROM LESIONS OF THE NERVOUS SYSTEM

CENTRAL NERVOUS SYSTEM LESIONS

Although occasionally tumors of the spinal cord will so alter vasomotor responses as to cause a syndrome similar to Raynaud's phenomenon or reflex sympathetic dystrophy, the major central lesions that can cause pain in an extremity are of two types. The first is the *thalamic pain syndrome* in which thrombosis (usually of a branch of the posterior cerebral artery perfusing the thalamus) causes transient paralysis, marked loss of position, vibratory and touch sensation on half of the body, and moderate loss of pin prick perception. This is followed shortly by severe painful dysesthesias (pain from usually non-painful stimuli such as light touch). This syndrome (described by Dejerine and Roussy) results from conditions most difficult to treat, but fortunately is usually self-limiting. The second central lesion which causes pain in an extremity is secondary to the paralysis caused either by *loss of spinal cord or cortical-spinal tract function.* This is almost always related to immobilization of a joint or spasticity. It can be differentiated from the thalamic pain syndrome in that there is no dysesthesia and, therefore, light touch does not exacerbate it, while movement of an extremity, particularly of the proximal joints does increase the pain. Its treatment is by mobilization of the joints involved and, at times, by rhizotomy or other methods to decrease the spasticity.

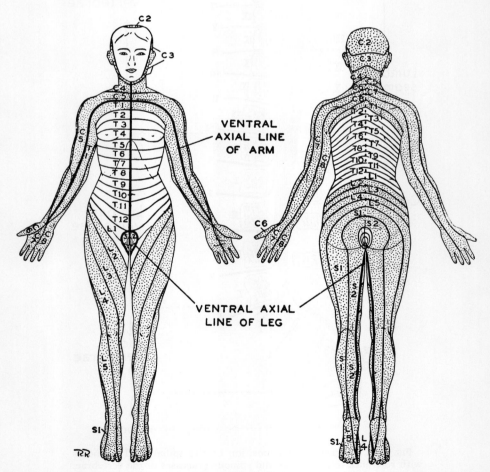

FIG. 13-2. Dermatome chart, with new patterns in the extremities based on single nerve-root syndromes. (Keegan, J. J. and Garrett, F. D.: Anat. Rec. 102:411)

SPINAL ROOT AND PLEXUS LESIONS

The upper extremity is innervated by the anterior rami of the fifth cervical through the first thoracic spinal nerves; the lower extremity by anterior rami of the second lumbar through the second sacral spinal nerves. The spinal nerves are formed in, or just beyond, the spinal foramina by the junction of the dorsal and ventral spinal roots peripheral to the dorsal root ganglia which lie outside the dura, usually in the spinal foramina. The central processes of the dorsal root ganglion cells enter the spinal cord in small bundles in an almost unbroken line along the dorsolateral sulcus. Similarly, the axons of the spinal motor

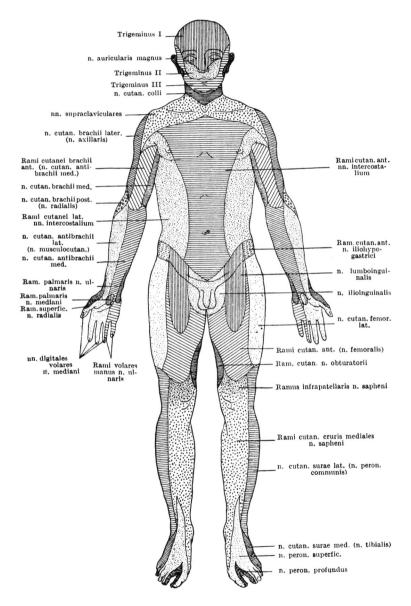

FIG. 13-3. Diagram of superficial skin innervation on the ventral surface of the body. (After Flatau.) (Grinker, Roy R.: Neurology, ed. 3, Springfield, Thomas)

neurons emerge from the ventrolateral sulcus as groups of small filaments which coalesce to form the ventral roots. The roots cross the spinal subarachnoid space and pierce the dura separately. The lower cervical and upper thoracic roots take a relatively short course obliquely downward through the subarachnoid space. The lumbar and sacral roots, collectively called the cauda equina, have a long course in the spinal canal

since the end of the spinal cord, the conus medullaris, lies at the level of the first lumbar vertebra. This discrepancy between the vertebral level and the underlying spinal cord segments and nerve roots, illustrated in Fig. 13-1, is important in the anatomical localization of lesions of the spinal cord and nerve roots. Soon after formation, the spinal nerves divide into a smaller posterior ramus and a larger anterior ramus. The posterior

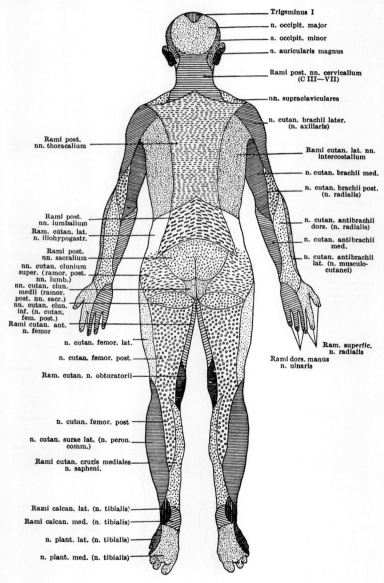

Fig. 13-4. Diagram of the superficial skin innervation on the dorsal surface of the body. (After Flatau.) (Grinker, Roy R.: Neurology, ed. 3, Springfield, Thomas)

TABLE 13-1. COMMON MONORADICULAR SYNDROMES

	PAIN	TENDERNESS	PARESTHESIAS & SENSORY DEFICIT	WEAKNESS, FASCICULATION & ATROPHY	REFLEX CHANGES
SIXTH CERVICAL	Radiation from neck into lateral arm & forearm; interscapular pain	Lower cervical spine, brachial plexus, median nerve	Dorsal & lateral aspect of thumb	Biceps	Diminished biceps reflex
SEVENTH CERVICAL	Same as Sixth Cervical	Lower cervical spine, brachial plexus	Index finger & usually middle finger	Triceps	Depressed or absent triceps reflex
EIGHTH CERVICAL	Radiation from neck into medial arm and forearm; interscapular pain	Lower cervical spine, brachial plexus, ulnar nerve	5th & ulnar half of 4th finger ulnar side of hand	Intrinsic hand muscles	None
FOURTH LUMBAR	Back pain radiation into anterior thigh	Mid-lumbar spine Femoral nerve	Anterior thigh just above knee	Quadriceps	Depressed or absent knee reflex
FIFTH LUMBAR	Back pain radiating into buttocks & posterior aspect of thigh	Low lumbar spine Sciatic & occasionally superficial peroneal nerves	Dorsum of foot and great toe	Dorsiflexors of foot and great toe	None
FIRST SACRAL	Same as Fifth Lumbar	Lumbosacral junction Sciatic nerve	Lateral aspect foot & small toe	Plantar flexors of foot (calf)	Depressed or absent ankle reflex

rami supply the paravertebral musculature and skin about the dorsal midline. The motor and sensory components of the anterior rami innervating the extremities undergo a somewhat complex re-arrangement into the peripheral nerves within the brachial and the lumbosacral plexuses.

The peripheral processes of a given dorsal root ganglion may be carried by more than one peripheral nerve, but the integrity of the area of skin supplied by that ganglion, the dermatome, is maintained, i.e. unbroken. However, contrary to the impression that might be gained from dermatomal maps (Fig. 13-2) a given area of skin is not solely supplied by fibers of one dorsal root ganglion. The dermatomes overlap in such a manner that the area of skin supplied by one dorsal root ganglion is also usually supplied by adjacent ganglia. Thus, to surgically denervate a dermatome, at least three posterior roots, not one, must be sectioned. Overlapping of sensory innervation to the skin (Figs. 13-3, 13-4) by adjacent peripheral nerves occurs as well, but not to such an extent since the peripheral nerves usually carry fibers from more than one dorsal root. Section of a major peripheral nerve almost invariably renders some area of skin anes-

thetic. The concept of the dermatome versus innervation by the peripheral nerves is important in that it often aids in localization of a lesion and sometimes in the exclusion of disease in the malingerer or hysterical individual.

Nerve Root Lesions

A common cause of extremity pain is a lesion affecting one or more dorsal nerve roots. Because of their close proximity, the ventral as well as the dorsal roots are usually involved in the pathological process with the consequence that weakness and reflex changes result as well as pain and sensory deficit. Exceptions to this rule may be found for example in herpes zoster infection which may be confined to the dorsal root ganglion. The initial and usually the most prominent feature of the radicular syndrome is intermittent lancinating pain which radiates from one side of the midline of the body into the distribution of the involved root. Radicular pain is usually associated with actions that produce traction on the roots such as coughing or sneezing, movement of the adjacent spine or, in the case of lumbar root involvement, maneuvers such as straight leg raising which stretch the peripheral nerve trunks and by contiguity, the nerve roots. By the same token, positions that reduce the tension on irritated nerve roots such as holding the arm above the head when a lower cervical root is involved, may relieve the pain. Reflex spasm of the local paravertebral musculature is often present and may account for aching pain in the neck or back. With irritation of the lower cervical nerve roots, interscapular pain is often present, perhaps due to the distribution of the posterior primary rami.

The distribution of the radiating pain may be of some help in localizing the involved root, especially in the upper extremities, but of more aid is the distribution of associated paresthesias often described as a "pins and needles feeling" or "numbness" which often can be recognized as conforming to a dermatomal pattern. Examination of the patient with a radicular lesion usually reveals limitation of motion of the associated portion of the spine, tenderness over the spinous processes adjacent to the lesion or along the course of the peripheral nerves which convey the radicular fibers and sensory loss conforming to a dermatomal pattern. Concomitant involvement of the corresponding anterior root produces a specific pattern of muscle weakness while the combined lesion of both roots may produce loss of a specific stretch reflex. The patterns of sensory, motor, and reflex changes produced by lesions of the most commonly affected nerve roots innervating the extremities are illustrated in Table 13-1.

It should be stressed that any patient suspected of having a nerve root lesion should have a complete neurological examination and x rays of the spine. The proximity of the nerve roots to the spinal cord in the cervical and thoracic region makes it highly possible that the same lesion producing a radicular syndrome may also impinge on the spinal cord and, therefore, necessitate an entirely different course of action than if only the nerve root is involved.

Trauma, Herniated Discs, Hypertrophic Changes in Vertebrae. The most frequent cause of radicular pain is acute or chronic nerve root compression. Most commonly, this compression is secondary to structural changes of the spine adjacent to and in the foramen through which the nerve roots exit. These changes usually are secondary to degeneration of the intervertebral disc with either extrusion of the nucleus pulposus beneath the root and/or hypertrophic bony changes about the interspace consequent to loss of joint function. Under such circumstances, relatively minor trauma may produce root injury.

Although herniation of intervertebral discs can be bilateral and thus occasionally can produce bilateral nerve root compression, the most common symptomatic herniation is in a posterolateral position and gives rise to a monoradicular syndrome. Clinically significant intervertebral disc herniation occurs most often at the last two lumbar interspaces i.e. between L4-5 or L5-S1 with most of the remainder at the L3-4 interspace. Less common, but not infrequent, are cervical disc herniations, the majority of which involve the C5-6 or the C6-7 interspace. Without objective evidence of nerve root compression, the diagnosis of a herniated intervertebral disc should rarely be made. In the lumbar region, the disposition of nerve roots is such that posterolateral herniation does not compress the nerve exiting at the corresponding intervertebral foramen but rather impinges on the set of anterior and posterior nerve roots which cross the disc in their course to the foramen immediately caudad. Thus, disc herniation at the interspace between the 4th and 5th lumbar vertebral bodies usually compresses the 5th lumbar nerve and herniation at the lumbosacral junction produces signs and symptoms referable to the first sacral nerve. In addition to low back pain, the patient will have the appropriate monoradicular syndrome listed in Table 13-1. In the cervical region, posterolateral disc herniation impinges on the nerve roots exiting at the corresponding foramen, but because the first cervical nerve exits between the first cervical vertebra and the skull, the nerve roots involved likewise do not correspond to the interspace by number. Herniation at the C5-6 interspace produces a radicular syndrome of the 6th cervical nerve and herniation at the C6-7 interspace produces a radicular syndrome of the seventh cervical nerve.

Nerve root compression with consequent pain, usually bilateral, is frequently seen in fracture-dislocation of the spine and in compression fractures of vertebral bodies weakened by osteoporosis or invasion by neoplasm or infection. Nerve root trauma without evidence of vertebral fracture may result from high velocity accidents in which there is stretching of nerve roots consequent to forced bending of the spine alone or in association with transmitted traction produced by forceful movement of the extremities.

Neoplasms that originate within or invade the spinal canal or spinal foramina may produce root compression and pain. Such neoplasms may be either extradural or intradural. Extradural neoplasms are usually of metastatic origin. They can arise from many sites, but the lung, breast, kidney, prostate, and those of the lymphogenous series are the most common. These tumors often invade the spinal canal after having metastasized to the vertebrae or, if in a paravertebral location, may grow into the canal through the intervertebral foramina. The radicular syndrome in any patient known to have had a primary tumor with a predilection for bony metastasis is presumptive evidence for invasion of the spinal canal even if plain x rays of the spine appear normal. This fact is of importance since, if the disease process is unchecked, the spinal cord eventually will be compressed either by the tumor alone or, more commonly, in association with a pathological compression fracture of one or more vertebral bodies.

The common intradural extramedullary tumors are the Schwannoma, the meningioma and the ependymoma of the filum terminale. Schwannomas (neurofibromas) almost constantly originate on a posterior root. They may have an extradural component as well, growing through the foramen to produce a dumbbell-shaped mass. The hallmark of this type of tumor, an enlarged foramen, may often be seen on the plain x ray. Meningiomas occur with about the same frequency as Schwannomas, but are more prevalent in the female and have a predilection for the thoracic region. Meningiomas usually occur in the ventrolateral portion of the spinal canal and, therefore, when in the cervical or thoracic region are apt to produce unilateral radicular pain. In contrast, intradural tumors of the lumbar spine since they are in contact with the multiple roots making up the cauda equina often produce severe bilateral pain in the lower extremities. Ependymomas originating in the filum terminale, Schwannomas, dermoid and epidermoid tumors are the most common intradural neoplasms in this area.

Primary spinal cord tumors rarely give rise to radicular pain. Patients with such intramedullary tumors may, however, have paresthesias in the extremities variously described as numbness, tingling, or a feeling of coldness. Children especially complain of persistent spine pain and often have spinal deformities such as torticollis and scoliosis. The correct diagnosis is rarely made until there is definite evidence of loss of spinal cord function. This is unfortunate since intramedullary tumors, usually slowly growing (astrocytomas, ependymomas), often produce widening of the spinal canal easily seen on plain x rays.

Inflammation of nerve roots, although often invoked as a cause of the radicular syndrome (radiculitis) is much less common than nerve root compression. Pyogenic infection in a paravertebral position or in the epidural space may produce root inflammation and pain, but the former more commonly produces pain by compression and inflammation of the adjacent spinal nerves and plexuses and evidence of rapid spinal cord compression is a more prominent feature of the latter. Bacterial, viral, and chemical meningitis often produce multiple bilateral nerve root inflammation which is the basis for Kernig and Brudzinski signs. Arachnoiditis following pyogenic and chemical meningitis may cause chronic root pain presumably by constriction of roots or interference with their blood supply. This is seen most frequently in the lumbar region in patients who have had multiple myelograms.

Isolated infection of the roots themselves is rare except for herpes zoster. Patients whose ganglia are infected with the causative virus often complain of pain and dermatomal sensory disturbances, usually hyperalgesia, before the eruption occurs. The classical skin eruption may not appear for one to two weeks after the onset of pain. Sometimes there is post-herpetic chronic pain in the distribution of the involved nerve root—again, usually a burning hyperalgesia —presumably due to a selective loss of the larger sensory fibers with preservation of at least some of the smaller nerve fibers conveying pain. This same mechanism may be operative in tabes to produce the "lightning" pains.

Some of the so-called post-infecitous neuritides such as the Guillain-Barré syndrome may be associated with root pain, but this is not usually a prominent feature. The painful syndromes following viral infection are more apt to be due to inflammation of the plexuses and peripheral nerves. Similarly, diabetes, while occasionally the cause of radicular pain, usually affects the distal nerves.

Lesions of the Brachial or
Lumbosacral Plexuses

Anatomical differences in the plexuses supplying the upper and lower extremities make each subject to several unique disease processes; therefore the two will first be discussed separately. The brachial plexus, formed by the anterior rami of the lower four cervical nerves and a large portion of the first thoracic nerve, extends from the neck to the axilla. It emerges between the medial and anterior scalene muscles, passes over the cupula of the lung, then beneath the clavicle, over the first rib into the axilla, where it surrounds the axillary artery. Its relatively long exposed course makes the brachial plexus subject to direct trauma and, because of the mobility of the shoulder girdle, to stretch injury. Its relation to the major arteries of the limb makes the brachial plexus liable to injury from aneurysms of the subclavian and axillary arteries as well as to several syndromes that may involve the arteries as well as the plexus. Finally, proximity to the lung makes possible involvement of the plexus by lung neoplasms and infection.

Pain caused by lesions of the brachial plexus is usually extremely severe and is precipitated or exacerbated by any movement of the plexus in relation to the surrounding structures: e.g., movement of the neck, deep inspiration, or movement of the shoulder. Distribution of pain and associated neurological deficit is highly variable—depending, of course, on the portion of the plexus affected. Tumors involving the plexus are usually either metastatic or arise in the adjacent lung. In the case of such malignant tumors, the pain is often unremitting and rapidly involves the entire upper extremity as does the neurological deficit. With superior sulcus tumors (Pancoast's syndrome), a Horner's syndrome is often present. Benign tumors of the brachial plexus, usually neurofibromas, either isolated or in association with von Recklinghausen's disease, usually have as symptoms less pain and slowly progressive neurological deficit. With any neoplasm involving the plexus, there may be tenderness over the plexus and a mass may be apparent on palpation.

Of especial note in regard to lesions of the brachial plexus which cause extremity pain is a symptom complex variously termed the *scalenus anticus syndrome, the cervical rib syndrome,* or *the thoracic outlet syndrome.*

This entity most often occurs in women of asthenic build and consists of pain in the medial arm and forearm often accompanied by feeling of coldness in the affected hand and sometimes associated with paresthesias involving the same distribution of the pain and in the fourth and fifth digits as well. The pain and dysesthesias may be made worse by turning the head to the opposite side and abducting the shoulder. On examination, the same maneuvers may reproduce the pain and at the same time cause obliteration of the peripheral pulse. However, pulse obliteration occurs in a high percentage of normal subjects under these conditions and the presence of this sign, therefore, does not necessarily make the diagnosis. Radiographic demonstration of a cervical rib is of much more aid in the diagnosis although its presence is not necessary for the syndrome to exist. The cause of this condition is the result of chronic pressure on the lower portion of the brachial plexus with or without associated compression of the subclavian artery. If a cervical rib, an unusually large transverse process of the seventh cervical vertebra, or a fibrous band from the transverse process to the first rib is present, the lower portion of the brachial plexus as well as the subclavian artery may be draped over it. Essentially the same anatomical abnormality may result from an unusually narrow thoracic outlet with compression resulting from the abnormally narrow confines between the first rib and the scalenus anticus muscle and clavicle.

The protected position of the lumbosacral plexus largely prevents it from being subjected to direct trauma. It is, however, subjected to disease processes occurring in the area, including invasion by carcinoma of the cervix, rectosigmoid or prostate. Psoas abscess, now uncommon, may affect the lumbar plexus. A lumbosacral neuritis resulting from x-ray treatment of the above mentioned neoplasms is occasionally seen. Diagnosis of pain of lumbosacral plexus origin is made on the basis of the distribution of the pain and neurological deficit. A thorough physical examination with special attention to rectum and pelvis, plain x rays of the lumbosacral spine and pelvis and diagnostic procedures such as proctoscopy, barium enema, and intravenous pyelograms are indicated in patients suspected of having a lesion of the lumbosacral plexus.

In addition to the disease processes mentioned above, it should be remembered that both the brachial and lumbosacral plexuses are subject to many of the inflammatory and metabolic processes to be discussed under the subject of peripheral nerves. The brachial plexus especially may be the site of an extremely painful neuritis following generalized viral infection, post vaccination, or injection with horse serum. Diagnosis of the etiology of such pain, in the case of post-infectious neuritis, must be made mainly on the basis of exclusion of the more common conditions.

PERIPHERAL NERVE DISEASE

Trauma. A common cause of pain in the extremities is trauma to a peripheral nerve. The trauma may be acute or recurrent. The latter, while it may be the result of external forces, usually relates to anatomical variations in the tissues around the nerve, occupational hazards necessitating unusual positioning of extremities, or preexisting disease causing increased sensitivity of the nerves to minor trauma. Acute injuries of nerves can be caused by compression, stretch, contusion or laceration. In such injuries the history relates onset of pain or difficulty to injury and diagnosis is usually quite clear. Degree and duration of pain, however, is variable and in some instances appears almost inverse to the severity of the injury, that is, the patient with relatively minor injury may have prolonged and severe complaints, while the more severely injured may have only brief discomfort. The problem is to recognize which painful syndromes of nerve injury are self-limiting and which require therapy for relief.

It is important first to recognize that although all nerve injuries are painful, only a small portion of the pain, and this usually over a brief period of time, comes from the trauma itself. The major portion of the pain complaint is related to other factors, such as altered sensation in the distribution of the nerve, altered function in the extremity, particularly as it affects joints, the paresthesias of regenerating nerve fibers, and the altered blood flow in a denervated area related to increased or decreased vascular tone. Since, with the exception of the pain of tissue damage all these causes for pain may take many months to subside, narcotics should not be given, except, if necessary, at the most early stage when the wound is the cause of the pain. The long-term use of narcotics may in itself be a cause of pain since the patient's addiction, recognized or unrec-

ognized, may be the factor prolonging the complaint. The pain of altered or lost sensation is difficult to recognize, but it is usually described as either a thick, heavy feeling, a tight, pressing, boring sensation, or it is described in terms of such graphic nature as, "in a vise", "twisted and pinched" or some other comparison that the patient can barely characterize. The use of such descriptions or the statement that the numbness is unbearable should alert the doctor to the fact that the patient is anxious, depressed, fearful, or some combination of these, or is the type of person who finds altered sensation in any portion of his body unbearable. Occasionally, and this is quite rare, some of the descriptions are used to describe the pain of reflex sympathetic dystrophy. This entity will be discussed later in this chapter. The pain of altered sensation also has a characteristic of being worse when the patient is unoccupied, particularly when he attempts to sleep and is least severe when he is occupied by a demanding task or a pleasurable sensation. These attributes suggest the best treatment, namely, reassurance by the physician, use of mood-altering drugs, and a return of the patient to his occupation or at least some occupation as rapidly as possible. Analgesics, nerve blocks, and extensive physiotherapy will usually increase the patient's fixation on the area of nerve loss and make him dependent, rather than independent, and delay his return to his normal activities. A goal for the physician and the patient is for both to determine the best possible means of using the damaged area so that the patient can return as rapidly as possible to active and effective life, for altered function in extremities cannot only be frustrating in attempting to perform daily activities of living, but both disuse and mal-use of joints can increase the pain in the extremity. Appropriate bracing so that a hand or a leg can be used, brief physiotherapy that the patient can do himself with weekly or bi-weekly supervision, often can alleviate a major portion of this type of pain. The parasthesias of regenerating nerve are best handled by assuring the patient that they are not only temporary, but are evidence of recovery and not a sign of difficulty. The discomfort of a swollen, engorged extremity can be treated by elevation, appropriate compressing with elastic stockings or arm and hand garments, and by total immersion of the affected part for periods in warm water. Relief obtained by these maneuvers can be diagnostic as well as therapeutic. The syndrome of reflex vaso-constriction will be discussed under reflex sympathetic dystrophy.

The incidence of prolonged, painful syndromes from nerve injury is difficult to determine. While they relate to all types of acute nerve injury, there is a higher incidence of vasomotor difficulties of the vasoconstriction type from partial injuries due to compression, stretch and contusion, and a higher incidence of altered sensation, discomfort and joint discomfort with lacerations of nerves. The problems encountered with incomplete laceration of nerves or with neuromas in continuity are too complex to discuss in this chapter, but the presence of partial loss of motor and sensory function distal to the nerve injury and the high incidence of parathesias in stretch injury coupled with the usual inability to afford significant relief by surgery is well recognized. At times, the only recourse is to convert the partial lesion to a complete lesion by surgically destroying the nerve, even at the price of loss of some motor function, since it appears that the presence of a neuroma in continuity in the nerve or the partial loss of function that may occur following neuropathy is less well tolerated than total loss of function.

Entrapment Neuropathies. Recurrent peripheral nerve injuries are usually less severe, but they may produce marked disability, usually from pain. They are most easily considered by placing them within the category of peripheral entrapment neuropathies. The entrapment neuropathies require a combination of restriction of nerve movements, often as they pass through a fibrous or osseous-fibrous canal, adjacent to an area of movement of an extremity. They are, therefore, found most commonly at or adjacent to joints. Almost all entrapments are painful, some mildly, some severely. In those that involve nerves to the skin, as in entrapment of a digital nerve, the acute pain is localized to the area of involvement of the nerve and to the area of its peripheral innervation. Entrapment of a nerve which is mainly motor and contains few superficial or skin sensory fibers may produce pain referred to the muscle supplied or joints moved by the muscle. There may be accompanying tenderness of the involved muscle, but rarely is the tenderness as great as with primary disease of muscle. Entrapment of a nerve supplying both skin and

muscle gives a combination of these symptoms.

Entrapment syndromes have in common a pattern of presenting symptoms relating to the recurrent injury of a peripheral nerve. The injury usually first causes mild loss of function in the larger fibers of the nerve and irritation of the small fibers and may progress to total loss of function in all the fibers of a peripheral nerve. The first symptom is usually pain and paresthesias in the distribution of the nerve with some subjective numbness. This is followed by increasing pain and weakness of the muscles supplied by the nerve and progressive numbness. The pain at first may be of an aching type which is poorly localized to the deeper structures, while the loss of sensation and the paresthesias are referred to the specific superficial areas of innervation. Total loss of function in the peripheral nerve is rare, for usually the symptoms cause the patient to decrease the activity of the extremity, allowing time for partial recovery. Knowledge of the anatomy and function of the nerve is necessary to recognize the syndrome, for some of the symptoms may mimic other diseases such as bursitis, arthritis and neuralgia.

In the upper extremity, probably the most common entrapment syndrome of peripheral nerve is that of the **median nerve at the wrist,** the "carpal tunnel syndrome". It occurs most often in persons with occupations necessitating considerable flexion, extension and rotation of the wrist, or in those who have marked alteration of the soft tissues around the wrist joints, as seen in rheumatoid arthritis, acromegaly or after wrist fractures. Loss of sensation in the palm over the distribution of the median nerve, atrophy of the thenar eminence, tenderness over the carpal ligament at the wrist, and Tinel's sign at the same area indicate the point of entrapment. Complaints of numbness, paresthesia and weakness of the hand with the above findings and evidence of a decrease of nerve conduction across the wrist measured by electroneurography confirm the diagnosis. Resting of the wrist, particularly in a neutral or slightly flexed position is not only therapeutic, but often diagnostic. Injection of steroids to reduce inflammatory reaction in the area may be either temporarily or permanently curative. Surgical decompression, however, is often required. A less common entrapment of the median nerve may occur *just below the antecubital fossa* where the nerve is crossed by the pronator teres. The syndrome can be quite similar to entrapment at the wrist except that the Tinel sign is over the pronator teres and there is usually weakness of the flexors of the first four digits.

The second most common entrapment syndrome in the upper extremity is of the **ulnar nerve at the elbow.** This has often been termed "tardy ulnar paralysis," the description relating to the frequency with which it is seen following fractures at the elbow. It is more often seen as a result of recurrent minor injuries to the ulnar nerve as it passes below the medial epicondyle of the humerus where the nerve is covered only by fascia and skin. Such injury may occur from repetitive blows to the "funny bone" or by constant pressure exerted when leaning on the elbow while reading or writing. The presenting symptom is usually aching pain in the forearm, paresthesias in the ring and little finger, and progressive weakness of the ulnar musculature. Palpation of the ulnar nerve as it crosses the medial epicondyle may reveal tenderness and thickening as compared with the opposite arm. Diagnosis is confirmed by demonstrating loss of motor and sensory function within the distribution of the ulnar nerve, and the slowing of conduction by electroneurography as it passes the epicondyle. The most effective therapy for ulnar entrapment is transplantation of the nerve to the antecubital fossa. Less common entrapments are of the radial nerve as it passes through the supinator muscle, causing weakness of extensor of the fingers and pain in the mid-forearm, and entrapment of the suprascapular nerve as it winds around the lateral edge of the spine of the scapula. In this latter condition, the distribution of the pain is poorly localized to the area of the posterior and lateral aspects of the shoulder and usually can be diagnosed by pain on palpation of the nerve at the scapular spine, weakness of the actions of the supraspinatus and infraspinatus muscles and increase in pain with movement of the partially abducted arm to the opposite shoulder.

In the lower extremity entrapment syndromes are less frequent, and usually more difficult to diagnose. The most common is the entrapment of a digital nerve between the metacarpal heads with the production of a neuroma, sometimes called Morton's neuroma. The digital nerve most often involved is that between the third and fourth metacarpal heads. The pain radiates to the ad-jacent sides of the toes. There also hypesthesia and hypalgesia can be demonstrated. Increase in pain with pressure over the metacarpal heads or between the web of the toes can be diagnostic. The next most common peripheral nerve involved is the peroneal nerve. Loss of function is caused by repeated trauma or prolonged pressure on the nerve as it crosses the fibular head or from a severe blow to the same area. It is most commonly seen in patients with some mild peripheral neuropathy, who have a habit of crossing their legs. Loss of motor function in the distribution of the nerve and mild hypesthesia with aching, usually referred to the dorsum of the foot or the arch of the foot, is a common complaint.

A common entrapment syndrome that presents as thigh pain is seen in obese patients who wear tight clothes or in whom sagging of the abdominal subcutaneous fat has become very prominent. The entrapment causes paresthesia and loss of sensation in the lateral aspect of the thigh. The syndrome is commonly known as meralgia paresthetica and relates to entrapment of the lateral femoral cutaneous nerve as it passes just anterior to the anterior superior iliac spine beneath Poupart's ligament. It is common in pregnancy, in obese persons, and in many persons who attempt to contain protuberant abdomens with firm undergarments. It is usually best treated by making the diagnosis and reassuring the patient that it is not a serious condition. The pain is often self-limiting or can be decreased with exercises and strengthening of the abdominal muscles and decrease in weight. A nerve entrapment of the lower extremities that can be quite confusing in relation to other causes of sciatica is the entrapment of the sciatic nerve at the sciatic notch. This may give symptoms indistinguishable from lumbar disc disease, but usually the patient has tenderness which is referred to the area of the sciatic notch with a Tinel sign at this point. Injection of the piriformis muscle and the placement of local steroids in the area can be both diagnostic and therapeutic.

Reflex Sympathetic Dystrophy

Reflex sympathetic dystrophy has been known for over one hundred years, but is still poorly understood. An early description of the symptoms was published by Weir Mitchell, based on his experience with wounds of the extremities during the Civil War, but it has been described since then by many clinicians and is known under different names depending on the presenting or primary symptoms. A few examples of these syndromes which fall under this general category are *causalgia*, the name used by Mitchell to describe the burning pain of partial nerve injury; *Sudeck's atrophy*, the name used to describe the muscle atrophy and decalcification of bone that occurs following soft tissue and bone injuries of the extremities; and the *shoulder-hand syndrome*, a term used to describe the pain and vasomotor changes in the hand that can occur with lesions of the shoulder joint. Although the most severe syndromes are seen with partial lesions of peripheral nerves, all these syndromes have similar changes apparently related to altered control of sympathetic innervation, and all respond in varying degrees to blocking the function of the sympathetic nervous system with local anesthetics or by surgical means.

In peripheral nerve lesions, the syndrome is seen most commonly with incomplete lesions of the median, ulnar and sciatic nerves, with preservation of pain function, but decrease in touch and pressure sensation distal to the lesion. The patient usually complains that any stimulus, particularly light touch, causes a burning over the distribution of the area of injury, which gradually spreads to involve the whole extremity. The pain often is so intense that the patient will spend hours keeping the hand or other involved part moist and protected from any contact or stimulus. On examination, the major changes are increased sweating, vasoconstriction, smoothness (atrophy) of the skin, and marked limitation of all joint movement. With lesions of joints or soft tissue, such as bursitis of the shoulder, fractures of the wrist, or fractures of the small bones of the hand, the same syndrome may appear with less severity. In all instances, if the syndrome continues long enough, x ray shows decalcification and physical examination reveals swelling, smoothness of skin, vasomotor constriction, increased sweating, limitation of movement of joints, and eventually atrophy of muscles. Diagnosis is confirmed and therapy best commenced by sympathetic block with a local anesthetic. The marked improvement that occurs following block is diagnostic as well as therapeutic. The syndrome is most often confused with the pain of regenerating nerve, of anesthesia dolorosa or of painful scars,

none of which respond to sympathetic blocking.

The pain of regenerating nerve has been discussed previously, as has the pain from loss of sensation. This latter is usually exacerbated by any procedure that increases loss of sensation. Short-term blocks of the peripheral nerve involved may be temporarily successful in relieving pain, but with repetition, the effect is lost and with sectioning of the nerve, the pain becomes more severe. The pain of painful scars is also difficult to treat and to understand. At times, the syndrome is caused by entrapment of a nerve in scar, but most often there appears to be nothing wrong with the scar and no entrapment. The pain can be quite striking, particularly in that it radiates both distally and proximally, is exacerbated by any touch or movement of the scar, and is usually unremittingly present unless the patient's attention is diverted from the area. The possibility of neuroma formation in the scar is always a consideration, but re-excision of the scar, attempted approximation of any nerves, or injection of the area usually is ineffective. Cutting nerves proximal to the painful scar or altering the sympathetic function of the area does not give any permanent relief.

In summary, reflex sympathetic dystrophy is a condition of altered vasomotor function, usually secondary to an injury to an extremity. The most severe symptoms are observed following partial injury of a peripheral nerve. The symptoms usually are burning pain, increased sweating, coldness, swelling and altered joint function in the extremity. Decrease in sympathetic innervation to the extremity either by blocking with local anesthetic or by surgical excision controls the syndrome in a majority of cases.

Neuropathy and Neuritis

One of the causes of pain in an extremity can be neuropathy or neuritis of peripheral nerve. These degenerative or inflammatory processes can be difficult problems not only because of the many possible etiologies, but also because the disorders are, in general, poorly defined, are not well understood, and can simulate many other conditions. Some diagnoses, such as sciatic neuritis or cervical radiculitis, have almost disappeared because compression of the spinal roots by herniated lumbar or cervical intervertebral discs has been recognized as the most common cause, rather than inflammatory or degeneratve reaction. There are, however, many neuropathies and neuritides of peripheral nerves that present with pain in an extremity or extremities. It is these conditions that will be discussed in this section.

The terms neuropathy and neuritis in themselves can be confusing because many authors use them interchangeably and some include the term neuralgia as a synonym for neuritis. Neuralgia is a general term that describes pain from involvement of a peripheral nerve without any implication of the etiology. The term neuritis is often used to describe painful dysfunctions of peripheral nerve, while the term neuropathy is sometimes confined to non-painful dysfunction of peripheral nerve. It is, however, more logical to use the classification proposed by Wechsler in which lesions characterized by parenchymal degenerative changes are called *neuropathies* and those characterized by inflammation are termed *neuritis*. Although inflammatory responses to degenerative processes do occur in the peripheral nerve, the classification proposed by Wechsler is, in general, a consistent and valid one. In defense, however, of defining the terms by the presence or absence of pain, it should be recognized that acute inflammation of peripheral nerve, which is a rare affliction, is very frequently painful, whereas degenerative change, which is more common, is frequently non-painful.

The etiological classification of neuropathies includes those that are secondary to toxic substances, to deficiency states or metabolic disorders, to collagen and allied disease, to familial diseases, or to unknown causes. Neuritides fall under the headings of infectious, allergic, toxic and idiopathic.

Neuropathy

Nutritional disorders may cause polyneuropathy from lack of intake of certain nutrients (starvation, malnutrition, alcoholism), or abnormal loss of nutrients (vomiting, diarrhea, etc.), or accelerated metabolism, especially as it affects nerve tissue (febrile illness, hyperthyroidism, alcohol). The nutrients especially implicated are thiamine (the lack of which causes beri-beri), niacin (the lack of which causes pellagra), pyridoxine, and pantothenic acid.

Polyneuropathy is a nonspecific result in the main trophic nerve cell and axon of any condition unfavorable to the metabolic activity of the cell.

When body tissues must supply most or all nutritional needs (as in partial or complete starvation), extreme weight loss may ensue, but evidences of vitamin deficiency such as neuropathy may not develop. The explanation seems to be that the tissues of the body, at least for a limited period, can provide a fairly complete and well-balanced array of all requirements.

Nutrition of nerve cells depends very largely upon adequate utilization of glucose. In diabetes neuropathy may occur as a consequence of repeated hypoglycemia from over-treatment with insulin, or it may occur with chronic hyperglycemia and under-treatment with insulin. In both instances the cell suffers from impaired glucose metabolism. Smoother control of the blood sugar does relieve numbness, pain and tingling in the extremities in some patients, especially younger, insulin-sensitive patients.

Generous therapy with thiamine occasionally relieves symptoms of neuropathy even when diabetes is under optimal control. Perhaps glucose utilization is accelerated and thiamine requirements are greater in these instances.

Symptoms of neuropathy develop most often in older diabetic persons in whom vascular disease has impaired the blood supply to the peripheral nerves, and often to the spinal cord as well. Neurological symptoms may be mild, but sometimes constitute the full picture of tabes. Optimal control of glucose metabolism and treatment with thiamine seldom afford relief.

The two most common peripheral neuropathies that are painful are *diabetic neuropathy* and *alcoholic neuropathy*. Diabetic neuropathy occurs as one of two basic types, mononeuropathy or symmetrical distal polyneuropathy.

Mononeuropathy in the extremities most often affects the femoral or sciatic nerve and may be caused by occlusion of vasa nervorum. It presents with sudden onset of pain over the peripheral distribution of the nerve and partial loss of both motor and sensory function. It can gradually resolve over a period of three to six weeks and may occur in mild or even undiagnosed diabetes. The sudden loss of function of the femoral nerve or the sciatic nerve in one extremity with considerable pain over the distribution of the nerve should always be considered as possibly related to diabetes.

The **polyneuropathy of diabetes** which appears with symmetrical distal involvement is more common. It usually has a rather insidious onset with sensory loss, particularly with impairment of detection of position and vibration. Decreased reflexes become apparent, followed by periods of painful paresthesias and vasomotor disturbances. In many patients these painful episodes seem to have little reference to the activity or severity of the diabetes and the neuropathy itself appears to progress regardless of the manner in which the diabetes is treated, or what nutrients (thiamine, niacin, etc.) are supplied. This lack of relationship to either treatment or severity of the diabetes indicates that the neuropathy in many cases is probably secondary to a metabolic or vascular defect of the diabetic which is not directly related to any known nutrient need, or glucose metabolism or its control by insulin.

Ischemic mononeuropathy involving femoral or sciatic nerves can also appear as mononeuropathy multiplex; that is, it affects many peripheral nerves simultaneously. A common presentation is the onset of acute or sub-acute pain in the proximal areas of the extremity, particularly the hip, with asymmetrical muscle wasting and weakness of the legs, but with very little sensory loss. As with other mononeuropathies, the process is usually self-limiting; but because of the extent of its involvement it can be quite disabling. There may be persistence of weakness and pain secondary to the altered function in the extremity after the neuropathy subsides.

Alcoholic neuropathies are clinically similar to the symmetrical distal polyneuropathies of diabetes and appear to relate to deficiencies in diet, particularly lack of thiamine, rather than to direct toxic reaction to alcohol. As with diabetic neuropathy, insidious onset is common with, at times, exacerbation following a particularly prolonged episode of poor nutrition and heavy alcohol intake. At the outset there may be vasomotor disturbances, paresthesias and pain in the stocking or glove distribution. These symptoms usually respond to massive doses of thiamine and other vitamins. Without such treatment they can progress to a disabling combined sensory and motor neuropathy.

Another deficiency neuropathy is that seen with *pernicious anemia* that relates to a lack of vitamin B-12. This often presents as paresthesias and dysesthesias in the lower extremities and may progress to an increasingly painful and disabling neuropathy as the central nervous system disease progresses. The presence of a peripheral neuropathy in a patient with combined system disease is an indication for massive doses of vitamin B-12. The dosage and blood levels of vitamin B-12 necessary to reverse both the central nervous system and peripheral nervous system disease are often out of proportion to those required to reestablish normal peripheral blood indices.

Another metabolic neuropathy that may present as acute abdominal and/or extremity pain is the neuropathy associated with *porphyria*. This usually presents with more motor than sensory loss. The motor loss can be so severe that the findings suggest the Guillain-Barré syndrome. The demonstration of abnormal porphyrins in the blood and urine are necessary for the diagnosis.

A rare, painful neuropathy that probably falls into the metabolic group is the neuropathy of *amyloidosis*. It is difficult to diagnose for it usually appears as a distal, symmetrical, sensory-motor neuropathy, similar to other distal neuropathies. It can, however, present as an asymmetrical neuropathy, particularly in the lower extremities. The presence of abnormal physical signs related to the systemic aspects of amyloid disease, particularly hepatomegaly, myocardial impairment and renal disease is helpful in differentiating the condition from other neuropathies.

The neuropathies associated with *collagen diseases* often resemble the neuropathies of diabetes, particularly mononeuropathy multiplex, but they can appear as a distal polyneuropathy. Often the neuropathy appears as severe intractable pain with a marked vasomotor component causing altered vasomotor reflexes with vasodilatory and vasoconstrictive aspects as demonstrated by a bluish or red mottling of the skin of the extremity. The involvement appears to be mainly an inflammatory process in blood vessels of the peripheral nerve with involvement of the adventitia and thickening of the intima.

Isolated painful neuropathies with sensory loss, particularly of position and vibration, may accompany *carcinoma*. It is more common, however, for the painful neuropathies associated with carcinoma to be seen in conjunction with polymyositis in which proximal weakness of the extremity as well as dysfunction in the peripheral nerve is present. The weakness secondary to polymyositis may cause considerable pain due to the altered function of the proximal joints. The picture can be confusing and present mainly as pain in the extremity with proximal weakness, loss of reflexes, and decrease in position and vibratory sensation.

Toxic neuropathies have been related to ingestion of heavy metals, exposure to organic solvents and ingestion of or exposure to insecticides. A painful polyneuropathy of heavy metal ingestion is arsenical polyneuropathy. This may present in the chronic phases as a neuropathy quite similar to alcoholic neuropathy, that is, with conspicuous sensory findings, vasomotor changes, and burning pain in a glove-like or stocking distribution. In such conditions, the differential diagnosis between alcoholic neuropathy and arsenical poisoning may depend on the demonstration of abnormal levels of the heavy metal. The organic solvents that have been implicated in peripheral neuropathy include carbon disulphide and carbon tetrachloride. Both these solvents usually present with paresthesias and motor weakness with little or no sensory loss. On the other hand, benzene or trichloroethylene can produce rapid onset of polyneuropathy with marked weakness and sensory changes in the limbs. At times, both may present as neuropathies with severe pain and paralysis.

There are so many organic compounds used in insecticides which can cause sensory or motor neuropathies that it is difficult to list them. Compounds containing ortho and para dichlorobenzene or pentachlorophenol have been most frequently implicated. Neuropathy following oral ingestion, inhalation or surface absorption has been reported. The possibility of polyneuropathy being caused by one of the insecticides must always be considered when the subject has been exposed to them.

Two of the **familial neuropathies** that should be considered since they may present as pain are the neuropathy of Dejerine-Sottas disease or interstitial hypertrophic neuropathy, and that of progressive peroneal muscular atrophy or Charcot-Marie-Tooth syndrome. Hypertrophic interstitial neuropathy may appear with shooting and cramping pains in the extremities and progressive peroneal weakness, but it is usually associated with nystagmus, scanning speech, tremor and ataxia. These findings as well as the presence of increased thickness of the nerves identify this condition. Progressive peroneal muscular atrophy most often presents as a painless neuropathy that involves the peroneal nerve initially, but involves other nerves as it progresses. The progressive loss of both sensory and motor function in a peroneal nerve, evidence of peripheral neuropathy elsewhere in the body and a familial incidence identify this condition. Rarely it may present as pain in the back and thighs secondary to the muscle weakness of the lower extremities.

Peripheral Neuritis

Peripheral neuritis is less common than peripheral neuropathy and falls into one of three categories: infectious, allergic or idiopathic. Polyneuritis has been described following practically every acute infectious disease and although in some, particularly viral infections, there appears to be evidence for direct involvement of the nerves, usually the pathophysiologic process in the nerves appears to be a relatively non-specific reaction to an infectious disease. The onset is usually signalled by paresthesia with muscle and nerve tenderness followed by weakness and areflexia. The sensory phenomena consisting of paresthesias, hyperesthesias and dysesthesias in the hands and feet in a stocking and glove distribution may precede or be replaced by pain. The severity of the pain can be quite variable. Patients often complain that light touch, pressure or movement of a joint increases the pain greatly. The resemblance between polyneuritis and polyradiculitis (the Guillain-Barré syndrome) has been noted. While in the former the sensory component is quite marked and the motor loss is distal, in the latter, the sensory component is often minimal, mainly subjective, and there is striking weakness of the proximal musculature. The course of postinfectious polyneuritis may be acute or sub-acute, lasting days or weeks. It may progress so that the roots are involved and it is indistinguishable from the Guillain-Barré syndrome or it may clear rapidly despite major loss of peripheral nerve function. Postinfectious polyradiculitis or Guillain-Barré syndrome is more common than postinfectious polyneuritis but rarely presents with complaint of pain in the extremities. At the onset, paresthesias, which some patients describe as painful, may occur, but the rapidly progressive areflexia, weakness and paralysis are the main problems.

Another infectious neuritis that should be considered, *herpes zoster*, is basically a viral infection of the dorsal root ganglion, but may also involve the peripheral nerve. The dermatome skin distribution, tenderness along the peripheral nerve, and altered sensation in the area of involvement make it pertinent to this discussion. *Syphilis* must always be considered and the shooting pains of tabes dorsalis should be easily recognized by the paroxysmal onset, the loss of deep tendon reflexes, impaired posterior column function and pupillary changes. The peripheral neuritis of *diphtheria* rarely begins in an extremity unless a diphtheritic infection occurs in an ulcer of the extremity. Direct involvement of the peripheral nerve by a local infection occurs in such disorders as abscess following trauma or in devitalized areas of an extremity.

Allergic polyneuritis sometimes occurs following serotherapy. It has been observed after the administration of tetanus and diphtheria antitoxins and usually involves the nerves proximal to the area of injection. Since injections are often given in the upper extremity, paralysis of the proximal muscles of that extremity with pain over the distribution of the upper brachial plexus is a common presentation with onset two to three days after injection. Allergic neuritis may follow injection of various sera and particularly occurs as a part of or sequel to serum sickness. Recovery is usually slow with sensory symptoms disappearing first and motor symptoms last.

SUMMARY

Pain in the limbs may be caused by disorders involving any of the structures or tissues of the extremities, or by disturbance elsewhere with the sensory phenomena referred to the limbs. Pain originating in the various sites tends to reveal the point from which it arises by certain qualities and by its location. The nature of the pathologic process resulting in pain may be mechanical, chemical, thermal, toxic, nutritional, metabolic, circulatory, or may involve combinations of these categories. The type of pain, its distribution, and the associated clinical phenomena yield important clues as to its cause.

BIBLIOGRAPHY

1. Adair, F. E., and McLean, J.: Tumors of peripheral nerve system with report of 2782 cases, A. Res. Nerv. and Ment. Dis., Proc. 16:440, 1937.
2. Baile, A. A., Sayre, G. P., and Clark, E. C.: Neuritis associated with systemic lupus erythematosus: A report of five cases, with necropsy in two, Arch. Neurol. and Psychiat. 75:251, 1956.
3. Bennett, A. E.: Horse serum neuritis: with report of five cases, J.A.M.A. 112:590, 1939.
4. Billig, D. M., Hallman, G. L., and Cooley, D. A.: Arterial embolism, Arch. Surg. 95:1, 1967.
5. Brain, R., and Henson, R. A.: Neurological syndromes associated with carcinoma; the carcinomatous neuromyopathies, Lancet 2:971, 1958.
6. Chambers, R. A., Medd, W. E., and Spencer, H.: Primary amyloidosis with special reference to involvement of the nervous system, Quart. J. Med. n. s. 27:207, 1958.
7. Croft, P. B., and Wadia, N. H.: Familial hypertrophic polyneuritis: Review of a previously reported family, Neurology 7:356, 1957.
8. Echlin, F., Owens, F. M., and Wells, W. L.: Observations on major and minor causalgia, Arch. Neurol. and Psychiat. 62:183, 1949.
9. Fischer, C. M., and Adams, R. D.: Diphtheritic polyneuritis—a pathologic study, J. Neuropath. Exp. Neurol. 15:243, 1956.
10. Fleming, R.: Refsum's syndrome; an unusual hereditary neuropathy, Neurology 7:476, 1957.
11. Gifford, R. W., Jr., Hines, E. A., Jr., and Craig, W. McK.: Sympathectomy for Raynaud's phenomenon: Follow-up study of 70 women with Raynaud's disease and 54 women with secondary Raynaud's phenomenon, Circulation 17:5, 1958.
12. Gilpin, S. F., Moersch, F. P., and Kernohan, J. W.: Polyneuritis; a clinical and pathologic study of a special group of cases frequently referred to as instances of neuronitis, Arch. Neurol. and Psychiat. 35:937, 1936.
13. Greenburg, L.: Diagnosis and treatment of occupational metal poisoning, J.A.M.A. 139:815, 1949.
14. Guillain, G., de Sèze, S., and Blondin-Walter, M.: Etude clinique et pathogénique de certaines paralysies professionelles du nerf sciatique poplité externe, Bull. Acad. Nat. Med., Paris, 111:633, 1934.
15. Keegan, J. J., and Garrett, F. D.: The segmental distribution of the cutaneous nerves in the limbs of man, Anat. Rec. 102:409–438, 1948.
16. Kirtley, J. A., Riddell, D. H., Stoney, W. S., and Wright, J. K.: Cervicothoracic sympathectomy in neurovascular abnormalities of the upper extremities: Experiences in 76 patients with 104 sympathectomies. Ann. Surg. 165:869, 1967.
17. Kopell, H. P., and Thompson, W. A. L.: Peripheral Entrapment Neuropathies, Baltimore, Williams & Wilkins, 1963.
18. Lewis, T.: Pain, New York, Macmillan, 1942.
19. Love, J. A.: The surgical management of the scalenus anticus syndrome with and without cervical rib, *in* E. V. Allen, N. W. Barker, and E. A. Hines, Jr., eds., Peripheral Vascular Diseases, ed. 3, Philadelphia, W. B. Saunders Company, 1962.

20. Martin, M. M.: Diabetic neuropathy; a clinical study of 150 cases, Brain 76:594, 1953.

21. Roos, D. B.: Transaxillary approach for first rib resection to relieve thoracic outlet syndrome, Ann. Surg. 163:354, 1966.

22. Semmes, R. E.: Ruptures of the Lumbar Intervertebral Disc, Springfield, Ill., Charles C Thomas, 1964.

23. Spencer, F. C.: Peripheral arterial disease, *in* Schwartz, S. I., ed., Principles of Surgery, New York, McGraw-Hill, 1969.

24. Spurling, R. G.: Lesions of the Cervical Intervertebral Disc, Springfield, Ill., Charles C Thomas, 1956.

25. Spurling, R. G.: Lesions of the Lumbar Intervertebral Disc, Springfield, Ill., Charles C Thomas, 1953.

26. Wechsler, I. S.: Multiple peripheral neuropathy versus multiple neuritis, J.A.M.A. 110:1910, 1938.

27. Woltman, H. W., and Wilder, R. M.: Diabetes mellitus; pathologic changes in the spinal cord and peripheral nerves, Arch. Int. Med. 44:576, 1929.

14

Clubbed Fingers and Hypertrophic Osteoarthropathy

BERNARD S. LIPMAN and EDWARD MASSIE

Terminology

Relationship of Clubbing to Hypertrophic Osteoarthropathy

Recognition
  CLINICAL FEATURES
  LABORATORY TESTS
  X-RAY FINDINGS

Medical Importance

Pathology

Pathogenesis

Clubbing is a physical sign characterized by bulbous changes and diffuse enlargement of the terminal phalanges of the fingers and toes.

Hypertrophic osteoarthropathy generally is considered to be a further extension of the clubbing process. A chronic proliferative subperiosteal osteitis involves the distal ends of the extremities and is manifested by the digital clubbing and in addition by swelling, pain, and tenderness over the larger involved bones and over the accompanying joints. However, some authors still believe that real differences in clinical significance exist between clubbing and osteoarthropathy and that the etiology and the pathogenesis of these two conditions are different. It is important to define the terms separately.

Many different names have been proposed for what we now know as clubbing and hypertrophic osteoarthropathy. The phenomenon of clubbing has been called *Hippocratic fingers, drumstick fingers, parrot-beak nails, watch-glass nails,* and *serpent's head fingers.*

Hypertrophic osteoarthropathy has been called *pulmonary hypertrophic osteo-arthropathy* (originally by Marie[1]), *secondary hypertrophic osteo-arthropathy, hyperplastic*

osteo-arthropathy, toxigenic ossifying osteoperiostitis, Marie-Bamberger syndrome, and numerous other names. As information accumulated, it became apparent that the bone lesions were characterized by the deposition of new-formed periosteal bone and that sometimes there were also joint manifestations; moreover, it became apparent that such changes were not limited strictly to an association with diseases of the lung.

The terms now generally accepted are *hypertrophic osteoarthropathy* for the changes in the larger bones and joints and *clubbing* for the distal extremity changes in toes and fingers.

RELATIONSHIP OF CLUBBING TO HYPERTROPHIC OSTEOARTHROPATHY

At first there was thought to be no relationship between clubbing and hypertrophic osteoarthropathy. They were described separately and considered to be independent entities. Under the unified theory, they have been considered as variations of the same process: hypertrophic osteoarthropathy being the more advanced stage with manifestations not only in the fingers but also in the more proximal parts of the extremities. This relationship is supported by the following facts: (1) The two conditions, either separately or together, occur in association with the same diseases. (2) Clubbing of the fingers is a constant characteristic finding in hypertrophic osteoarthropathy, although varying in degree. (3) The osseous changes in simple clubbing resemble those of hypertrophic osteoarthropathy.

As would be expected of the milder, earlier manifestation, clubbing is seen much more frequently than the more advanced state called hypertrophic osteoarthropathy.

As early as the fifth century B.C., Hippocrates[2] described curving of the fingernails in a case of empyema. In the latter part of the nineteenth century, von Bamberger[3] and Marie[1] drew attention to distinctive changes in the extremities associated with certain diseases of the lungs and heart. Since these early reports, numerous publications have appeared dealing with the intriguing physical evidences in the extremities of more serious internal disease and with the problem of how they are related. Mendlowitz[4] in his review (1942) gave 337 references. Much remains obscure, particularly concerning the pathologic physiology. As Samuel West[5] stated in 1897, "clubbing is one of those phenomena with which we are so familiar that we appear to know more about it than we really do."

RECOGNITION

CLINICAL FEATURES

The symptoms of clubbing are almost entirely objective, particularly in cases that are developing slowly; usually the patient is not aware of the deformity until it is brought to his attention. Recognition is not difficult if one keeps the possibility in mind and observes the extremities carefully. Occasionally, especially in cases secondary to lung tumors, the more rapid onset of changes in the pulp and nail bed attract the patient's or his manicurist's attention and should alert the physician to the necessity of a chest roentgenogram. In cases of acute clubbing, a feeling of warmth, a burning sensation, sweating, and rarely pain in the fingertips may occur. It is important to detect early clubbing.

Because of its diagnostic implications the condition in its early stages may at times be confused with other abnormalities of the fingers. Early clubbing should be differen-

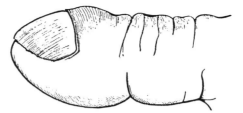

FIG. 14-1. Drawing of a clubbed finger from Marie's classic report. (Marie, P.: Rev. de méd. 10:1)

tiated from: (1) simple curving of the nail, which is seen normally—especially in the Negro; (2) chronic paronychia, in which the soft tissues at the base of the nail are swollen and no change occurs in the nail bed itself; (3) Heberden's nodes, which lie more proximally and rarely cause diagnostic difficulty; (4) chronic infectious arthritis, in which the swelling is periarticular and no change is apparent in the nail bed; (5) epidermoid cysts of the bony phalanges; and (6) felons, where there is associated pain and absence of changes in the other fingers. Early in the process of clubbing, thickening of the fibroelastic tissue of the nail bed produces a definite firm transverse ridge at the root of the nail, best observed on the dorsal aspect of the finger. Lovibond[6] noted this "profile sign." When one views a normal finger from the side, one sees an obtuse angle of about 160° between the base of the nail and the adjacent dorsal surface of the terminal phalanx. This angle is referred to as the "base angle" and is clearly demonstrated in the normal thumb. In early clubbing the base angle is obliterated and it becomes 180° or greater.[99] This "profile sign" is one of the best means of detecting the beginning stage of true clubbing.

Figure 14-2A illustrates the normal base angle of approximately 160°; Figure 14-2B

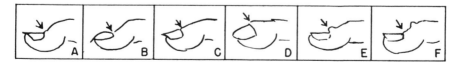

FIG. 14-2. Characteristic profile configurations of the finger. (A) Normal finger, illustrating the base angle of the nail (usually about 160°). (B) "Curving" of the nail, a variation of the normal. The base angle is undisturbed. (C) Early clubbing, with the base angle obliterated—positive "profile sign." (Club fingernails may also be curved.) (D) Advanced clubbing, with base angle greater than 180°. Base of nail projects upward. Over-all area of nail is increased. (E) Chronic paronychia, with fundamental base angle unaltered. (F) Heberden's node, with normal base angle. (Lovibond: Lancet 1:363)

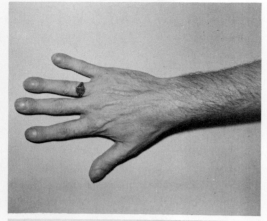

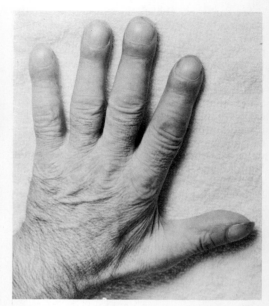

FIG. 14-4. Clubbed fingers in a 59-year-old man with carcinoma of the lung.

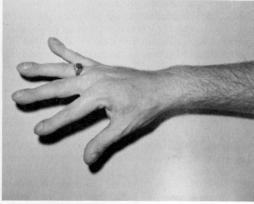

FIG. 14-3. Eleven-year-old girl with cyanosis from congenital heart disease (tetralogy of Fallot).

shows curving, an alteration that may be present in many normal finger nails. Notice that the base angle is not interfered with, in spite of the fact that the distal nail is considerably curved downward. If the original nail is curved, the clubbing will accordingly be accompanied by curving. Figure 14-2C illustrates the characteristic base angle obliteration in early clubbing; Figure 14-2D shows advanced clubbing (the base angle is greater than 180° and projects dorsally). In Figures 14-2E and 14-2F, illustrating chronic paronychia and Heberden's nodes, respectively, the base angle persists undisturbed.

Clubbing usually occurs first in the thumb and index finger, spreading to the other digits later. In the advanced stage there is an increase in all tissues of the finger tips, the soft tissues as well as the nails, so that

the ends of the fingers assume a bulbous appearance. In Figure 14-3, note the typical clubbed fingers in a girl with congenital heart disease. The overlying skin as well as the volar pads are smooth, shiny and bright pink in color. The vascular bed gives a lilac or cyanotic hue to the nails. Witherspoon[7] pointed out that the return of color following slight pressure on the finger nail is characteristically slower than normal. The base of the nail may be elevated so that its outline is seen beneath the skin's surface. Furthermore the nail can be rocked back and forth as if it were floating on a soft edematous pad. Patients may complain of *excessive sweating,* a feeling of *warmth,* or a *burning sensation* in the fingertips; pain is rare but may occur in cases of very acute clubbing. Abnormally frequent filing or clipping of the fingernails is often necessary because of the *accelerated* rate of growth, and longitudinal striations in the nail may appear. Hangnails form readily, due to the rapid growth of the cuticle, resulting often in acute and chronic paronychia. In long-standing cases, particularly in congenital heart disease, dorsiflexion with hyperextensibility of the distal phalangeal joints may be present. Figure 14-4 illustrates the appearance of clubbed fingers in a man with carcinoma of the lung.

Various forms of clubbing ("drum-stick," "watch-glass" "parrot-beak," and "serpent's head") have been described, and these variations now are known to be attributable to the duration and the degree of the process as well as to differences in the initial anatomy of the digits. Clubbing of the toes nearly always develops in association with clubbing of the fingers but is more difficult to recognize because of the wide range in the shape of normal toes. The early stage may be recognized best in the large toe. Successive measurements of the nail surface are at times necessary to confirm the diagnosis. Several authors, Mendlowitz,[4] Angel,[78] and Buchman and Hrowat,[79] report the presence of clubbing (swelling, thickening, and furrowing of the skin) over the nose, the molar region, the eyelids, and the ears.

Berry[102] has divided clubbing into two general types, depending upon the difference in their appearances. One type is associated with congenital, cyanotic heart disease with terminal phalanges that are dusky, richly vascular, and frequently accompanied by a reddish-brown pigmentation of the skin proximal to the lunule. This type of clubbing histologically is associated with increased vascularity, vasodilation, and increased flow of blood to the fingertips. There appears to be a relationship between the amount of clubbing and the degree of polycythemia. The other type of clubbing frequently is associated with chronic pulmonary disease and the fingertips have a less engorged, drier, and more pallid appearance. Histologically the enlargement of the distal phalanx is composed mainly of connective tissue overgrowth between the nail plate and the bone.

Hypertrophic osteoarthropathy should always be sought for in the presence of clubbing. Locke[8] stated that "Every case of hypertrophic osteoarthropathy so far recorded has shown well-developed clubbing of the fingers and toes, and it is regarded as an absolutely constant sign of the disease." On the other hand, review of the literature[69,75,77] reveals that clubbing occasionally may be absent in an otherwise typical case of pulmonary osteoarthropathy or that clubbing manifests itself later than the bone changes. Locke reported 39 cases of "simple" clubbing in which 12 (30 per cent) showed roentgen evidence of periosteal proliferation of the long bones indicative of hypertrophic osteoarthropathy. Such findings bear out the close association of these two conditions. Hypertrophic osteoarthropathy in its early stages may be asymptomatic and detectable only on roentgenograms; on the other hand, the onset may be heralded by *aching pains* in the joints and *tenderness* along the shafts of the involved bones. The pain may be severe, aggravated by movement, and may precede detectable roentgenographic changes. It may vary in intensity from a slight discomfort to a deep, dull aching pain, which is transient. The skin over the involved areas may be warm, reddened, and thickened by a brawny nonpitting edema. In some series, pain in the bones has been the only presenting complaint in as high as 40 per cent of the cases, the underlying more serious disease having caused less evident symptoms or none at all. Such bone and joint symptoms warrant careful search for evidence of clubbing and osteoarthropathy and search for the underlying cause (chest roentgenograms, etc.). Craig[9] and others have implicated *arthralgia* as one of the earliest clinical manifestations of intrathoracic lesions, the hypertrophic osteo-

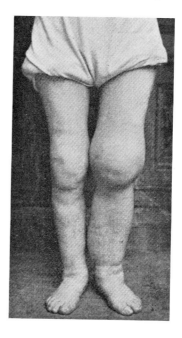

Fig. 14-5. Enlargement of both legs, particularly the left, in a case of hypertrophic osteoarthropathy. Note the large effusion in the left knee joint. (Norris and Landis: Diseases of the Chest, ed. 6, Philadelphia, Saunders)

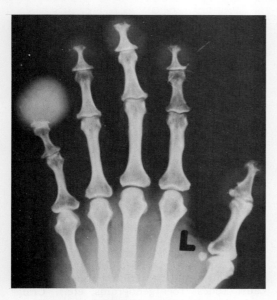

FIG. 14-6. Roentgenographic appearance of hand in patient also exhibiting changes in many other bones. Note resorption of terminal phalanx of the fifth digit, also narrowing of shafts and osteoporosis of other phalanges of this digit. In some of the phalanges of the other fingers osteoporosis predominates, in others there is thickening of the cortical bone. (D. C. Weir, St. Louis)

arthropathy in such cases being an early complication. Symptoms of pulmonary osteoarthropathy may precede by 1 to 18 months the detection of localized lung lesions, particularly neoplastic disease of the chest, in contrast with suppurative lung processes in which the onset of symptoms of osteoarthropathy tends to lag behind respiratory and systemic manifestations.[70,71,72,76] Early diagnosis of cancer of the lung may be hastened by early detection of hypertrophic osteoarthropathy. The pains in the extremities are occasionally mistaken for rheumatoid arthritis or hypertrophic osteoarthritis. A moderate degree of joint *effusion* may be seen along with some limitation of motion. Partial or complete ankylosis has been reported in advanced cases. *Edema and hypertrophy of the subcutaneous tissue* of the limbs are observed (Fig. 14-5).

Osteoarthropathy may occur at any age. Gottlieb *et al.*[80] reported clubbing and osteoarthropathy in a two-year-old infant with chronic pyopneumothorax. Kennedy re-

ported similar findings in a 7½-month-old infant with multiple lung abscesses from birth.

Hypertrophic osteoarthropathy was at one time confused with acromegaly, in which enlargement of the hands and feet is characteristic. There may be awkwardness of gait and clumsiness of movement in the hands and fingers due to the increased size and weight of the limbs in advanced stages of hypertrophic osteoarthropathy. The diagnosis also may be confused with thrombophlebitis, venous stasis, congestive heart failure, nutritional edema, or peripheral neuropathy. Several reports mention the presence, in association with osteoarthropathy, of muscular weakness; bone pain, which is deep-seated, burning in character and aggravated by lowering of the extremities; dusky discoloration of the fingertips; stiffness of the fingers; increased sweating; skin lesions, characterized by redness, glistening appearance, and warmth over the affected areas; increased hair growth; and broadened or cylindrical appearance of the distal thirds of the extremities produced by thickened skin and a firm, hard, pitting edema.[69,74] Spontaneous fractures may occur, apparently due to extreme osteoporosis.

The changes associated with clubbing are *usually gradual* in onset, taking place over a period of many weeks, months, or years. However, they have been noted to appear *within one week* of the onset of the underlying disease.[11] Similarly, hypertrophic osteoarthropathy may be evident in a few weeks or not until a period of as much as 20 years after the onset of the associated malady. Clubbing and hypertrophic osteoarthropathy may disappear and reappear synchronously with remissions and exacerbations of the underlying disorder. Changes in the degree of clubbing have been used as a gauge of the activity of the concomitant disease. Disappearance of the phenomena in the extremities has been reported following successful medical or surgical treatment of chronic pulmonary infections, subacute bacterial endocarditis, mediastinal and pulmonary tumors, cyanotic congenital heart disease, ulcerative colitis, regional ileitis, amebic dysentery, and sprue. Improvement, and even disappearance, have occurred also after collapse therapy in pulmonary tuberculosis, following antiluetic therapy in syphilis of the lung, and in subjects with chronic mountain sickness after descent to sea

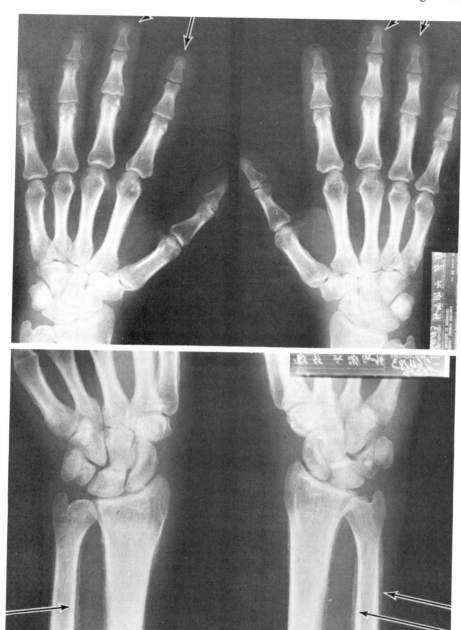

FIG. 14-7. Roentgenogram of hands and distal forearms in a case of clubbing and hypertrophic osteoarthropathy. Note the periosteal proliferation (noted by arrows) along the shaft of the radius, the ulna, the metacarpals and the phalanges. Burrlike proliferation of the distal phalanges is also present as indicated by arrows.

level.[4,12] In fact, failure of improvement in the osteoarticular manifestations following successful management of chronic lung infections should arouse suspicion of an underlying malignant process.[73] Vogl *et al.*[69] reported a case in which the general downhill course and the intractability of the pulmonary infection and of the symptoms of osteoarthropathy led to surgical exploration and detection of an underlying lung cancer.

A remarkable occurrence confirmed by many observers is the very rapid disappearance of pain in the bone which may occur following removal of a pulmonary tumor or other etiologic factor. Pain may disappear in 24 to 48 hours, thus suggesting the importance of circulatory or toxic (perhaps chemical) factors in the causation of the pain rather than the bone changes themselves being directly responsible. Flavell,[81] believing that the manifestations of osteoarthropathy were caused by a neural reflex from the lung, reported five inoperable cases of carcinoma of the lung in which vagotomy on the affected side provided immediate relief of symptoms. Steroid therapy and phlebotomies also have been suggested as therapy for symptomatic relief in inoperable cases[82]; the value of these measures is unproven.

LABORATORY TESTS

The most common abnormal laboratory finding is an elevated sedimentation rate. In addition, various other altered laboratory tests may occur as a result of the underlying disease processes. Since the concentrations of phosphorus and of alkaline phosphatase in the blood may be elevated during destruction and repair of bone, these values also may be changed in hypertrophic osteoarthropathy. This aspect bears further study.

X-RAY FINDINGS

The roentgenologic changes are variable and depend upon the intensity and the duration of the pathologic process. In early clubbing there is usually no radiologic evidence of alteration. Somewhat later, a burr-like proliferation of the tuft of one or more of the terminal phalanges may appear. In long-standing cases of clubbing, atrophic changes occur ranging from simple osteoporosis to complete resorption (see terminal phalanx, fifth digit, Fig. 14-6). Erosion of the terminal tufts is rare; not infrequently, however, there is atrophy and spindling

(narrowing of the shafts) of the terminal, and sometimes of the other phalanges and of the metacarpals and metatarsals (Fig. 14-6). The phalanges may show considerable elongation and prominent tufts when the clubbing occurs in childhood prior to cessation of growth. The development of newly formed periosteal bone in the terminal phalanges has been reported only rarely.

Fully developed hypertrophic osteoarthropathy produces distinctive roentgenographic alterations. These are generally extensive and involve earliest and most frequently the tibia, the fibula, the radius, the ulna, the femur, the humerus, the metacarpal, and the metatarsal bones. Later the phalanges, the clavicles, and the pelvis may be implicated and, very rarely, the tarsals, the carpals, the vertebrae, the ribs, the scapulae, and the skull.[4,14,15] Some authors state that the skull and the mandible are never involved. Characteristically roughened, uneven, linear densities, which represent the newly formed periosteal calcium deposits, are observed along the shafts of the involved bones; the appearance suggests that of chronic periostitis (Fig. 14-7). The periosteal reaction is usually most evident along the distal half of the long bones. The densities are thickest in the region of the peripheral epiphyses and at the points of muscular insertions. With remissions and exacerbations of the underlying disease, the repeated layered calcification in the periosteum may give a laminated x-ray appearance. The periosteal new bone may vary from the simple, smooth, parallel type of normal new bone to the rough, irregular, lacelike appearance of abnormal periosteal proliferation. In advanced cases, osteoporosis of the cancellous portion and thinning of the cortex of the original bone are found. Pathologic fractures may occur. Occasionally osteoporosis of the newly formed periosteal bone is seen. It should be pointed out that the roentgenographic diagnosis of hypertrophic osteoarthropathy is doubtful in the absence of definite periosteal proliferation. The new bone may be from 1 to 10 mm. in thickness. Gall *et al.*[73] noted that, in the early stage of development, the periosteum showed signs of inflammation, thickening, and early division into two layers. The outer layer showed an accumulation of inflammatory cells. The inner layer consisted of a fibrillary intercellular substance that was soon replaced by an osteoid matrix. The new subperiosteal bone layer fused with the original cortex, and numerous osteoclasts appeared and caused focal areas of bone resorption. A thickened spongy shaft with a rarefying osteitis of the older bone resulted.

The new subperiosteal bone is formed chiefly near the epiphyses and at the points of musculotendinous insertions. It tends to progress to the proximal ends of the bones, but these changes seldom are seen in areas covered by the articular capsule. If the new subperiosteal bone displaces the thickened periosteum rapidly, pain and tenderness may occur, but if the process progresses slowly there may be no discomfort. Various parts of the skeleton may show different stages of the disease, which may advance rapidly in one area while regressing in another.

MEDICAL IMPORTANCE

Clubbing and hypertrophic osteoarthropathy, although often relatively innocuous in themselves, owe their importance to the fact that usually they are associated with significant underlying diseases. However, these conditions may be absent even in the severe forms of the diseases with which they are often associated. Furthermore, clubbing may occur as an isolated condition, unassociated with any known systemic disorder, an example being hereditary clubbing.

The frequent association of these pathological changes in bones with chronic pulmonary diseases is well-recognized. Of the 144 cases of hypertrophic osteoarthropathy reported by Locke,[8] 113 (78 per cent) were associated with diseases of the respiratory tract. Review of more recently published reports indicates that between 75 and 80 per cent of cases with clubbing and hypertrophic osteoarthropathy are associated with diseases of the pulmonary system; 10 to 15 per cent occur with diseases of the cardiovascular system; 5 to 10 per cent are associated with lesions of the gastrointestinal tract, including the liver; and another 5 to 10 per cent fall into a miscellaneous group. Of the associated pulmonary diseases reported by Locke,[8] tuberculosis (20 per cent), bronchiectasis (19 per cent), malignancy (7 per cent), and empyema (5 per cent) occurred most frequently. However, the great recent progress of thoracic surgery has brought the realization that the percentage of persons who develop clubbing and hypertrophic osteoarthropathy which is secondary to bronchiectasis or pulmonary malignancy is higher than was thought. Poppe[16] reviewed 129 cases in which lobectomy was done at Barnes Hospital for bronchiectasis or chronic lung abscess. Of these, 103 patients (79 per cent) had clubbing in varying degrees. Of 276 tuberculous patients at Koch Hospital in St. Louis surveyed by Poppe,[16] 71 (25 per cent) revealed evidence of clubbing.

Skorneck and Ginsburg[83] emphasize a distinction between clubbing and osteoarthropathy. In a three-year roentgenologic study of 390 patients with pulmonary tuberculosis they found no cases of osteoarthropathy; in three patients who were misdiagnosed as tuberculous and in whom osteoarthropathy was found, the final correct diagnoses were lung cancer in two and pyogenic abscess in one. The authors went so far as to state that the finding of osteoarthropathy, but not clubbing, militates against a diagnosis of tuberculosis. In the presence of hypertrophic osteoarthropathy, intrathoracic neoplasm is the most important condition to be excluded. In the cardiovascular group of diseases, clubbed fingers were present in association with cyanotic congenital heart disease in 132 (13 per cent) of Abbott's[17] 1,000 cases. Friedberg[18] noted clubbing in about 66 per cent of fatal cases of subacute bacterial endocarditis, whereas Blumer[19] reported the incidence of clubbed fingers in subacute bacterial endocarditis to be 18 of 48 cases (36 per cent). Trever[95] described two cases of congenital cyanotic heart disease with long-standing clubbing and hypertrophic osteoarthropathy, emphasizing the distinction between simple clubbing and osteoarthropathy. In congenital cyanotic heart disease the literature shows a high incidence of clubbing but a low incidence of osteoarthropathy, and no case of osteoarthropathy occurred earlier than the age of 11. In the acyanotic child with clubbed fingers, a congenital heart malformation is unlikely, and an extracardiac cause should be sought. Moreover, when one congenital defect is discovered it is well to look for others, since multiple embryological defects are the rule. Polydactyly, syndactyly, hypoplastic or absent thumb, simian creases, brachydactyly with index finger overlapping third finger and the fifth finger over the fourth, with a tightly clenched fist, shortened fifth finger, arachnodactyly with lax joints, and telangiectasia of fingertips are some additional abnormalities of the hand, other than clubbed fingers, which are associated with congenital major cardiovascular defects.[99]

The various diseases that should be suspected in the presence of clubbing or hypertrophic osteoarthropathy are as follows:

Pulmonary Group. Bronchiectasis[20]; primary and secondary tumors of the lung,[21,22] bronchus,[9,23] mediastinum,[4] thymus,[24] and chest wall[25]; chronic empyema[1,26,27]; lung abscess[28,29]; fibroid pulmonary tuberculosis with excavation[30,31]; chronic pneumonitis[2,8]; emphysema associated with chronic suppurative conditions[32]; pneumoconiosis[2]; neurogenic tumor of the diaphragm[98]; atelectasis[10]; cystic disease of the lung[33]; chest deformities[26]; syphilis of the lung[34]; actinomycosis[35]; Hodgkin's disease involving the lung or mediastinum[36]; pulmonary hemangioma[37,38]; and aortic aneurysm with compression of the lung.[39]

Levine[106] recently has proposed a new physical sign: the *yellow rounded digit*. It combines tobacco-stained and clubbed fingers of cigarette smokers. The staining involves the terminal phalanges and nails of the index and middle fingers of either hand. Among 13 patients having the sign who were followed for a year, ten, or 77 per cent, proved to have bronchogenic carcinoma.

Cardiac Group. Cyanotic congenital heart disease with a venous-arterial shunt (right to left flow)[6,16,40,41,42]; subacute bacterial endocarditis[17,18,48] (rare in bacteria-free stage)[4]; chronic congestive heart failure[44]; and cardiac tumors.[4]

Hepatic Group. Cholangiolytic or Hanot's type of cirrhosis; obstructive biliary cirrhosis secondary to bile duct obstruction; cirrhosis associated with chronic malaria; hepatomegaly with amebic abscess; and, rarely, in portal cirrhosis.[45]

Gastrointestinal Group. Chronic ulcerative colitis; regional enteritis; intestinal tuberculosis; chronic bacillary and amebic dysentery; sprue; ascaris infestation; multiple polyposis of the colon; abdominal Hodgkin's disease; pyloric obstruction and gastrectasia associated with carcinoma of the pylorus or duodenal ulcer; and, rarely, in carcinoma of the colon.[4,46,47,48] Hollis[103] reported a patient with severe hypertrophic osteoarthropathy secondary to a myxoma of the lower esophagus without local invasion or metastases and with regression of the osteoarthropathy following removal of the myxoma.

Mixed Group. Idiopathic; hereditary; postthyroidectomy; nasopharyngeal tumors; pituitary gland abnormality; myxedema due to I[131]; generalized lymphosarcomatosis; chronic mountain sickness (Monge's disease); chronic osteomyelitis with amyloidosis; and pseudohypertrophic muscular dystrophy.[4,10,49,50]

Miscellaneous Group. *Unilateral clubbing* may be present in aneurysm of the subclavian artery, the innominate artery, or the arch of the aorta; lymphangitis; brachial arteriovenous aneurysm; and superior sulcus tumor (Pancoast tumor).[51,52,53]

PATHOLOGY

The pathology of clubbing and hypertrophic osteoarthropathy has received comparatively little consideration because of the difficulty in securing postmortem finger specimens for study, the inability to obtain suitable preparations for examination, and our inadequate knowledge of the normal histology of the finger tips. However, on the basis of various reports in the literature, the pathologic changes appear to consist chiefly of hypertrophy and hyperplasia.[2,8,12,54,55,56,57,58] There is increased proliferation of all tissues of the finger tip, especially in the fibrous elastic portion of the nail bed and in the fatty connective tissue of the ball of the finger. Corresponding with an increase in the underlying substance, there is an increase in the cross-sectional area of the nail. Newly formed capillaries have been observed, as well as dilatation and increased thickness of the walls of the small blood vessels in the end of the finger. The terminal phalanx may show increased thickness of its periosteum and of the ungual process itself or, in advanced cases, complete resorption of the bone. Bigler[84] stated that the shape of the clubbed digit is the result of the increased thickness of the nail bed. He stated that the nail bed is loosely textured, with large fibroblasts in a reticular network. The glomera are increased, as are extravascular lymphocytes and eosinophils. In chronic clubbing the increased thickness is due to increased collagen deposition in the nail bed with no evidence of edema.

In hypertrophic osteoarthropathy there is calcification of the periosteum, and islands of newly formed periosteal bone may be found along the shaft of the long bones, thickest in the region of the peripheral epiphysis and at the points of musculotendinous insertions. There is thinning of the cortex of the original bone and osteoporosis of the cancellous portion. Bone resorption may extend to the new periosteal bone, leaving a thin trabeculated space between the cortex and the periosteum. In patients with exacerbations and remissions, one sees multiple laminations suggestive of tree-trunk layers. Pathologic fractures may occur if thinning and osteoporosis exceed the capacities of the reparative processes. With joint involvement (which occurs in approximately one-third of the cases), the joint capsule and the synovial membrane occasionally are thickened, and there may be fluid collection within the joint capsule. Proliferation of the subsynovial granulation tissue associated with lymphocytosis and fibrinoid degeneration of the synovial membrane has been reported, resulting in pannus formation. Pressure from the pannus can produce degeneration of the cartilage with erosion; if this occurs, the process may terminate in ankylosis.

PATHOGENESIS

The pathogenesis of clubbing and hypertrophic osteoarthropathy has been in dispute since the time when these conditions first were recognized. Because of their diagnostic significance, they have engaged the interest of many clinicians, and numerous theories have been proposed—none of which has, to this date, been proved. In the eighteenth century it was thought that clubbing was due to emaciation, as described in the works of Laennec.[59] Pigeaux[59] in 1832 advanced the theory that circulatory alterations caused edema and increased cellularity of the connective tissue of the finger tip, resulting in clubbing. In the latter part of the nineteenth century, following the classic papers of Marie[1] and von Bamberger,[3] the theory that chronic infection might be responsible was widely accepted. The popularity of this theory soon was shared by the toxic hypothesis. (Circulating toxins were believed to act on susceptible peripheral capillaries and thus produce the characteristic changes.) However, the association of clubbing and hypertrophic osteoarthropathy with pulmonary neoplasms and congenital heart disorders provided evidence that these theories were inadequate. Verrusio[60] and others later postulated the mechanical theory, which proposed that clubbing was due to capillary stasis resulting from back pressure. The fact that clubbing was rarely seen in patients with heart failure and the fact that actual pressure measurements[61] failed to substantiate the presence of stasis were cited as evidence against this hypothesis. Numerous addi-

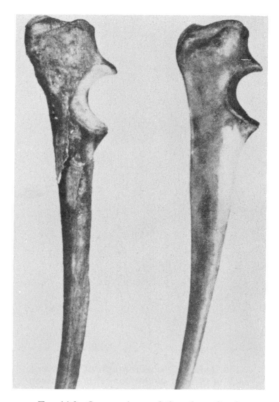

FIG. 14-8. Comparison of the ulna of a dog with experimentally induced hypertrophic osteoarthropathy (*left*) with ulna of a normal dog (*right*). Note the roughened, irregular, elevated areas of the new-formed periosteum on the left. (Mendlowitz, M. and Leslie, A.: Amer. Heart J. 24:141)

tional theories have been suggested, such as vitamin deficiency,[57] malfunction of the endocrine glands (pituitary,[62] thyroid,[60] parathyroid,[60] and gonads[60]), nerve injury,[32] lymph stasis,[63] change in blood volume,[64] increased intracranial pressure,[60] and reflex nerve impulses from peripheral pulmonic nerve fibers influencing the formation of arteriovenous anastomoses in the limbs.

Many attempts have been made to study clubbing and hypertrophic osteoarthropathy in animals. A number of unsuccessful methods were tried to reproduce these conditions in rabbits, guinea pigs, dogs, cats, and monkeys.[2,28,65,66] It was not until 1940 that Mendlowitz and Leslie[67] successfully induced hypertrophic osteoarthropathy experimentally in one of three dogs by anastomosing the left and adjacent main pulmonary artery to the left auricle, resulting

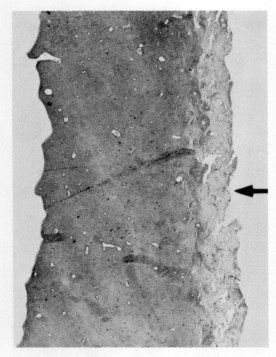

FIG. 14-9. Photomicrograph of transverse section of tibia of the dog with experimentally induced hypertrophic osteoarthropathy showing new-formed periosteum. (Mendlowitz, M. and Leslie, J.: Amer. Heart J. 24:141)

in a right-to-left heart shunt, simulating congenital heart disease with cyanosis. By this method they were able to produce the gross and microscopic evidences of periosteal proliferation seen in hypertrophic osteoarthropathy (Figs. 14-8 and 14-9). Careful studies revealed no change in the venous pressure, ether circulation time, or oxygen consumption. The main experimental finding was an increase in the cardiac output; the blood flow through the lungs remained relatively unchanged. Mendlowitz[61] also demonstrated the presence of increased peripheral blood flow in patients with acquired clubbed fingers by means of calorimetric and brachiodigital arterial blood pressure gradient methods. Furthermore, he was able to show that the accelerated fingertip blood flow waxed and waned with exacerbations and remissions of clubbing and the underlying disease. In 1959, Wilson confirmed Mendlowitz's findings of increased blood flow in clubbed fingers. He concluded that the increased flow passed largely through numerous arteriovenous anastomoses and was in excess of physiologic requirements, resulting in accelerated growth due to "forced feeding." Wilson noted that clubbing on the left hand regressed after ligation of the left subclavian artery in patients with tetralogy of Fallot who underwent surgical correction by the Blalock technique.

Blood flow and temperature regulation of the distal phalanges is a function of the glomus, as observed by Wilkins,[86] Grant and Bland,[87] Popoff,[88] and others. The glomus is a highly specialized arteriovenous anastomosis present in the digital nail beds and pads. It consists of an afferent artery joining the so-called Sucquet-Hoyer canal, from which two to five arterioles arise which subdivide into capillaries supplying the canal and related structures. The venous portion consists of a large receptacle forming a cape around the glomus and emptying into the subcapillary and deep veins of the digit. Reports concerning the influence of age on the number of glomera and the distribution of glomera vary according to the different counting techniques utilized. The fact that the glomus is a chief regulator of blood flow in the distal phalanx is established; its role therefore is inferred, but not proved, to be of major importance in the genesis of clubbing.[89]

Hall[90] in 1959 postulated that clubbing may be caused by a substance that is normally inactivated by the lungs and dilates the digital glomera. He suggested that this substance might be ferritin. Shorr[91] described a vasodepressor material (VDM) produced by ischemic skeletal muscle, spleen, and liver, which caused dilatation of the arteriovenous anastomosis in the mesentery and intestines of animals. The VDM material produced by the liver was identified as ferritin. Ferritin, in its *oxidized* form, was inert against epinephrine; but in its *reduced* form blocked the vasoconstrictive action of epinephrine. Crismon[92] reported that *rutin*, a flavonoid, blocked the vasodepressor effect of ferritin. Utilizing the reported findings on ferritin and rutin, Hall[90] performed a study on subjects with and without clubbing. The capillary blood flow through the fingertips was evaluated by a radiosodium (Na^{24}) clearance technique before and after the intravenous injection of rutin. Hall concluded from his findings that one of the possible causes of clubbing was the long-term result of dilatation of the glomera in the nail beds by the reduced ferritin, which had evaded oxidation. In view of the fact that there is controversial evidence in the literature on rutin and its effect on vaso-depressor materials (VDM) such as ferri-tin,[93] Hall's concept is stimulating but needs confirmation, particularly in regard to deter-mination of the amount of reduced ferritin as opposed to oxidized ferritin in subjects with clubbing.

Mauer[68] again raised the hypothesis that local tissue anoxia is the predisposing factor leading to clubbing. His thesis is based upon the fact that, in patients who have a disease associated with clubbing, the erythro-cytes are altered physically as evidenced by the elevated sedimentation rate. The deliv-ery and uptake of oxygen by the tissues are thus hindered by the altered physical state of the red blood cells and local anoxia re-sults. It is known, however, that tissue anoxia alone does not cause clubbing, since clubbing does not occur with the slow rate of flow and cold fingertips of Raynaud's syndrome. Mauer postulates that the in-creased blood flow present in clubbing is secondary to the anoxia and that the rapid flow, the associated tissue warmth, and the rouleaux formation are all factors in the pathogenesis of clubbing.

More recently it has been considered that the derangement of peripheral circulation may be dependent upon some pathologic intrathoracic reflex, which is promptly abol-ished by surgical removal of the primary lesion.[69] Flavell[81] reported prompt relief of pain due to osteoarthropathy by vagotomy on the side of the affected lung cancer in five cases. Trever reported a similar re-sponse of joint pains to atropinization. Further evidence in favor of the neural re-flex mechanism was furnished by Holling and associates,[104] who observed eight canine and six human subjects with osteoarthrop-athy secondary to pulmonary neoplasm. Division of the branches of the vagus in the hilus caused prompt regression of the osteo-dystrophy in all subjects. The validity of this neural concept could be investigated by preoperative and prompt postoperative capillary bed studies. Such studies may greatly contribute to solving the problem of hypertrophic osteoarthropathy.

Barnes et al.[94] showed that widespread vascular hypoplasia existed in arteriovenous aneurysm of the lung. Cudkowicz[96] and Armstrong[97] believed that a similar vascu-lar abnormality might be present in hyper-trophic osteoarthropathy. They examined the lungs of 15 cases with clubbing due to intrathoracic pathology. When they injected a radiopaque medium into the diseased lungs, they found occlusion of the major branches of the pulmonary artery in almost all cases. They demonstrated precapillary bronchopulmonary anastomoses, which di-verted bronchial blood into the low-pressure pulmonary artery bed distal to the occlusion. Since these anastomoses did not occur in normal, healthy lungs, and resembled the anastomoses found in clubbed fingers, the authors postulated that the resulting ische-mia of the lung set up antidromic impulses in the peripheral pulmonic nerve fibers which reflexly influenced the formation of the arteriovenous anastomoses in the limbs.

Gerbode et al.[105] produced hypertrophic osteoarthropathy experimentally in dogs, which had been rendered cyanotic by anas-tomosis of the inferior vena cava to the left atrium. They concluded that the patho-genesis of the osteoarthropathy that occurs in such a wide variety of apparently un-related clinical conditions is a common stimulus that appears to interfere with the gaseous exchange between the blood and the tissues of the extremities. In their ex-perimental cases, the significant factors appeared to be arterial anoxemia and in-creased peripheral blood flow, but the rela-tive part played by each of these factors is not clear. The arterial oxygen saturation in their animals varied between 54 and 81 per cent at rest. Mendlowitz, however, stressed that, in his experimental animals, no value below 92 per cent saturation was present and arterial anoxemia probably was not the most important factor. Mendlowitz based his argument mainly upon the fact that the oxygen consumption did not change. It is unlikely, however, that studies either of blood oxygen levels or of oxygen consump-tion give much information as to the actual degree of anoxia that is present in the tissue bed itself. Thus, one of the principal factors involved in the pathogenesis appears to be an increase in blood flow to the extremities, out of proportion to the requirements of the tissues. Tissue anoxia is also a factor. There are several possible mechanisms by which high flow rates might contribute to tissue anoxia. As stated previously, Mauer postu-lated that rouleaux formation not only re-duced the available diffusion surface of the red cells, but the relatively stable rouleaux formations are too large to traverse the capillaries and tend to be diverted through dilated arteriovenous anastomoses. Moreover, rouleaux embolism in the vessels may occur. Another mechanism whereby high flow rate may contribute to tissue anoxia is the fact that the blood may remain within the peripheral capillaries for a time that is insufficient for adequate gaseous exchange to occur. Another factor may be "axial streaming," which becomes very marked at high velocities; with this, the red cells become separated from the capillary endothelium by a wide zone of clear plasma.

The fact that hypertrophy and hyperplasia may result from circulatory changes often has been observed clinically. Arteriovenous fistulas, for example, are known to lead to myocardial hypertrophy as well as to abnormal increases in growth of single limbs. The increased growth of limbs has been stated to be common if the fistula is acquired before the closure of epiphyses. Sir Thomas Lewis indicated that the accelerated growth results from the more rapid flow of blood distal to the arteriovenous shunt, although the details of how the rapid blood flow produces increased growth in the face of diminished oxygen tension are lacking. Lovell postulated that increased blood flow in excess of tissue requirements produced accelerated growth due to "forced feeding." In the light of this theory, one may speculate that neurogenic, toxic, anoxic, endocrine, and other factors may be associated with the pathogenesis of clubbing and osteoarthropathy. The exact mechanism by which circulatory changes produce the definite hypertrophy and hyperplasia seen pathologically is still unexplained. Thus, in spite of extensive study and voluminous literature, the pathogenesis of clubbing and hypertrophic osteoarthropathy remains conjectural.

SUMMARY

Clubbing is characterized by bulbous deformity of the fingers and toes. As a diagnostic sign it is of great significance, since it suggests the presence of underlying diseases affecting certain organs and systems—particularly the lungs and the heart, and less often the liver and the gastrointestinal tract.

Hypertrophic osteoarthropathy represents a more advanced stage of the same process and is associated with the same disease conditions. Its presence should be considered particularly in those patients with clubbing who develop pain, tenderness, and swelling about the joints and along the shafts of the bones. The roentgenographic finding of periosteal proliferation and other characteristic bone changes confirms the diagnosis.

Recognition of these conditions is not difficult if one keeps the possibilities in mind and if one observes the extremities carefully. *Early* recognition can be a clue to the *early* diagnosis of intrathoracic malignancy.

REFERENCES

1. Marie, P.: De l' osteo-arthropathie hypertrophiante pneumique, Rev. Méd. 10:1, 1890.
2. Hippocrates, with English Translation by Jones, W. H. S., London, Heinemann, Loeb Classical Library, Prognostic Number 17, 2:35, 1923.
3. von Bamberger, E.: Ueber Knochenveranderungen bei chronischen Lungen- und Herzkrankheiten, Zr. Klin. Med. 18:193, 1890.
4. Mendlowitz, M.: Clubbing and hypertrophic osteoarthropathy, Medicine 21:269, 1942.
5. West, S.: Two cases of clubbing of the fingers developing within a fortnight and four weeks respectively, Trans. Clin. Soc. London 30:60, 1897.
6. Lovibond, J. L.: The diagnosis of clubbed fingers, Lancet 1:363, 1938.
7. Witherspoon, J. T.: Congenital and familial clubbing of the fingers and toes, with a possibly inherited tendency, Arch. Intern. Med. 57:18, 1936.
8. Locke, E. A.: Secondary hypertrophic osteoarthropathy and its relation to simple clubfingers, Arch. Intern. Med. 15:659, 1915.
9. Craig, J. W.: Hypertrophic pulmonary osteoarthropathy as the first symptom of pulmonary neoplasm, Brit. Med. J. 1:750, 1937.
10. Locke, E. A.: Clubbing and Hypertrophic Osteoarthropathy (Revised by A. Grollman), Oxford Medicine, vol. 4, p. 447, New York, Oxford, 1943.
11. Lipman, B.: Personal observations.
12. Blalock, A., and Taussig, H. V.: The surgical treatment of malformations of the heart in which there is pulmonary stenosis or pulmonary atresia, J.A.M.A. 128:189, 1945.
13. Weens, H. S., and Brown, C. E.: Atrophy of terminal phalanges in clubbing and hypertrophic osteoarthropathy, Radiology 45:27, 1945.
14. Temple, H. L., and Jaspin, G.: Hypertrophic osteoarthropathy, Amer. J. Roentgen. 60:232, 1948.
15. Holt, J. F., and Hodges, F. J.: Significant skeletal irregularities of the hands, Radiology 44:23, 1945.
16. Poppe, J. K.: Diagnostic significance of clubbed fingers, Dis. Chest 13:658, 1947.

17. Abbot, M. E.: Atlas of Congenital Heart Disease, New York, Amer. Heart Ass., 1936.
18. Friedberg, C. K.: Diseases of the Heart, Philadelphia, Saunders, 1949.
19. Blumer, G.: Subacute bacterial endocarditis, Medicine 2:105, 1923.
20. Whiteside, L. C.: A case of bronchiectasis with hypertrophic pulmonary osteoarthropathy, U.S. Nav. Med. Bull. 8:658, 1914.
21. Pulmonary hypertrophic osteoarthropathy in adenocarcinoma of the lung (Mass. Gen. Case 31281), New Eng. J. Med. 233:44, 1945.
22. Pulmonary hypertrophic osteoarthropathy in fibrosarcoma of the lung (Mass. Gen. Case 31271), New Eng. J. Med. 233:18, 1945.
23. Paterson, R. S.: Pulmonary osteoarthropathy, Brit. J. Radiol. 32:435, 1927.
24. Miller, F. R.: Carcinoma of thymus, with marked pulmonary osteoarthropathy, Radiology 32:651, 1939.
25. Konschegg, T.: Uber die Bamberger-Mariesche Krankheit, Virchow Arch. Path. Anat. 271:164, 1929.
26. Symes-Thompson, H. E.: Two cases of hypertrophic pulmonary osteo-arthropathy, Lancet 1:385, 1909.
27. Springthorpe, J. W.: Case of hypertrophic pulmonary osteo-arthropathy, Brit. Med. J. 1:1257, 1895.
28. Phemister, D. B.: Chronic lung abscess with osteo-arthropathy, Surg. Clin. Chicago 1:381, 1917.
29. Kerr, J.: Pulmonary hypertrophic osteoarthropathy, Brit. Med. J. 2:1215, 1893.
30. Zesas, D. G.: An den Osteoarthropathien bei Lungentuberculose, Med. Klin. 5:1480, 1909.
31. Kaplan, R. H., and Munson, L.: Clubbed fingers in pulmonary tuberculosis, Amer. Rev. Tuberc. 44:439, 1941.
32. Shaw, H. B., and Cooper, R. H.: "Pulmonary hypertrophic osteo-arthropathy" occurring in a case of congenital heart disease, Lancet 1:880, 1907.
33. Montuschi, E.: Clubbing associated with congenital lung cyst, Brit. Med. J. 1:1310, 1938.
34. Munro, W. T.: Syphilis of the lung, Lancet 1:1376, 1922.
35. Wynn, W. H.: Case of actinomycosis (streptothrichosis) of lung and liver successfully treated with a vaccine, Brit. Med. J. 1:554, 1908.
36. Parkes Weber, F., and Ladinghaus, J. C. G.: Uber einen Fall von Lymphadenoma (Hodgkinsche Krankheit) des Mediastinums verbunden mit einer hochgradigen hypertrophischen Pulmonalosteoarthropathie, Deutsch. Arch. Klin. Med. 96:217, 1909.
37. Rodes, C. B.: Cavernous hemangiomas of the lung with secondary polycythemia, J.A.M.A. 110:1915, 1938.
38. Plaut, A.: Hemangioendothelioma of the lung, Arch. Path. 29:517, 1940.
39. Lang, H. B., and Bower, G. C.: A report of a case of hypertrophic osteoarthropathy, Psychiat. Quart. 4:277, 1930.
40. Means, M. G., and Brown, N. W.: Secondary osteoarthropathy in congenital heart disease, Amer. Heart J. 34:262, 1947.
41. White, P. D., and Sprague, H. B.: The tetralogy of Fallot, J.A.M.A. 92:787, 1929.
42. Wahl, H. R., and Gard, R. L.: Aneurism of the pulmonary artery, Surg. Gynec. Obstet. 52:1129, 1931.
43. Cotton, T. F.: Clubbed fingers as a sign of subacute infective endocarditis, Heart 9:347, 1922.
44. Thorburn, W.: Three cases of "hypertrophic pulmonary osteo-arthropathy" with remarks, Brit. Med. J. 1:1155, 1893.
45. Rolleston, H. D., and McNee, J. W.: Diseases of the Liver, Gall-bladder, and Bile-ducts, London, Macmillan, 1929.
46. Schlicke, C. P., and Bargen, J. A.: "Clubbed fingers" and ulcerative colitis, Amer. J. Dig. Dis. 7:17, 1940.
47. Bennett, I., Hunter, D., and Vaughan, J. M.: Idiopathic steatorrhoea (Gee's disease); nutritional disturbance associated with tetany, osteomalatia, and anaemia, Quart. J. Med., N. S. 1:603, 1932.
48. Preble, R. B.: Gastrectasis with tetany and the so-called pulmonary hypertrophic osteoarthritis of Marie, Medicine 4:1, 1898.
49. Camp, L. J. D., and Scanlon, R. L.: Chronic idiopathic hypertrophic osteoarthropathy, Radiology 50:581, 1948.
50. Rynearson, E. H., and Sacasa, C. F.: Hypertrophic pulmonary osteoarthropathy (acropachy) afflicting a patient who had postoperative myxedema and progressive exophthalmos, Proc. Mayo Clin. 16:353, 1941.
51. Smith, T.: A case of aneurysm of the right axillary artery. Ligature of the subclavian; pyemia. Death on the twenty-second day. With remarks on clubbing of the fingers and toes, Trans. Path. Soc. London 23:74, 78, 1872.
52. Baur, J.: De l' hippocratisme dans les affections cardiovasculaires, Rev. Méd. 30:993, 1910.
53. Poland, A.: Statistics of subclavian aneurism, Guy. Hosp. Rep. 15:47, 1870.
54. Campbell, D.: The Hippocratic fingers, Brit. Med. J. 1:145, 1924.
55. Charr, R., and Swenson, P. C.: Clubbed fingers, Amer. J. Roentgen. 55:325, 1946.
56. Parkes Weber, F.: The histology of the new bone-formation in a case of pulmonary hypertrophic osteoarthropathy, Proc. Roy. Soc. Med. 2:187, 1908.
57. Crump, C.: Histologie der allgemeinen Osteophytose (osteoarthropathie hypertrophiante pneumique), Virchow Arch. Path. Anat. 271:467, 1929.

58. Thorburn, W., and Westamacott, F. H.: The pathology of hypertrophic pulmonary osteoarthropathy, Trans. Path. Soc. London 47: 177, 1896.

59. Laennec, R. T. H., and Pigeaux, D. M., *cited by* Mendlowitz, Medicine 21:269, 1942.

60. Verrusio, M., Massalongo, R., Danuco, I., and Sirshew, P., *cited in* discussion by Charr and Swenson: Amer. J. Roentgen. 55:325, 1946.

61. Mendlowitz, M.: Measurements of blood flow and blood pressure in clubbed fingers, J. Clin. Invest. 20:113, 1941.

62. Fried, B. M.: Chronic pulmonary osteoarthropathy; dyspituitarism as a probable cause, Arch. Intern. Med. 72:565, 1943.

63. Bryan, L.: Secondary hypertrophic osteoarthropathy following metastatic sarcoma of the lung, Calif. West. Med. 23:449, 1925.

64. Pritchard, E.: Familial clubbing of fingers and toes, Brit. Med. J. 1:752, 1938.

65. Compere, E. L., Adams, W. E., and Compere, C. L.: Possible etiologic factors in the production of pulmonary osteoarthropathy, Proc. Soc. Exp. Biol. Med. 28:1083, 1931.

66. van Hazel, W.: Joint manifestations associated with intrathoracic tumors, J. Thorac. Surg. 9:495, 1940.

67. Mendlowitz, M., and Leslie, A.: The experimental simulation in the dog of the cyanosis in hypertrophic osteoarthropathy associated with congenital heart disease, Amer. Heart J. 24:141, 1942.

68. Mauer, E. F.: Etiology of clubbed fingers, Amer. Heart J. 34:852, 1947.

69. Vogl, A., Blumenfeld, S., and Gutner, L. B.: Diagnostic significance of pulmonary hypertrophic osteoarthropathy, Amer. J. Med. 18: 51, 1955.

70. Berg, R., Jr.: Arthralgia as a first symptom of pulmonary lesions, Dis. Chest 16:483, 1949.

71. Deutschberger, O., Maglione, A. A., and Gill, J. J.: An unusual case of intrathoracic fibroma associated with pulmonary hypertrophic osteoarthropathy, Amer. J. Roentgen. 59:738, 1953.

72. Fischl, J. R.: Severe hypertrophic pulmonary osteoarthropathy. Report of a case due to carcinoma of the lung with operation and recovery, Amer. J. Roentgen. 64: 42, 1950.

73. Gall, E. A., Bennett, G. A., and Bauer, W.: Generalized hypertrophic osteoarthropathy, Amer. J. Path. 27:349, 1951.

74. Holmes, H. H., Bauman, E., and Ragan, C.: Symptomatic arthritis due to hypertrophic osteoarthropathy in pulmonary neoplastic disease, Ann. Rheum. Dis. 9:169, 1950.

75. Pattison, J. D., Beck, E., and Miller, W. B.: Hypertrophic osteoarthropathy in carcinoma of the lung, J.A.M.A. 146:783, 1951.

76. Robinson, W. D., *et al.*: Rheumatism and arthritis. Review of American and English literature of recent years, part II, Ann. Intern. Med. 39:498, 1953.

77. Shapiro, L.: Ossifying periostitis of Bamberger-Marie, Bull. Hosp. Joint Dis. 2:77, 1941.

78. Angel, J. H.: Pachydermo-periostosis (idiopathic osteoarthropathy), Brit. Med. J. 2:789, 1957.

79. Buchman, D., and Hrowat, E. A.: Idiopathic clubbing and hypertrophic osteoarthropathy, Arch. Intern. Med. 97:355, 1956.

80. Gottlieb, C., Sharlin, H. S., and Feld, H.: Hypertrophic pulmonary osteoarthropathy, J. Pediat. 30:462, 1947.

81. Flavell, G.: Reversal of pulmonary hypertrophic osteoarthropathy by vagotomy, Lancet 1:260, 1956.

82. Shapiro, M.: Hypertrophic osteoarthropathy, A.M.A. Arch. Intern. Med. 98:700, 1956.

83. Skorneck, A. B., and Ginsburg, L. B.: Pulmonary hypertrophic osteoarthropathy (periostitis): its absence in pulmonary tuberculosis, New Eng. J. Med. 258:1079, 1958.

84. Bigler, F. C.: The morphology of clubbing, Amer. J. Path. 34:237, 1958.

85. Wilson, G. M.: Local circulatory changes associated with clubbing of the fingers and toes, Quart. J. Med. 21:201, 1959.

86. Wilkins, R. W., Doupe, J., and Newman, H. W.: The rate of blood flow in normal fingers, Clin. Sci. 3:403, 1938.

87. Grant, R. T., and Bland, E. F.: Observations on arteriovenous anastomosis in human skin and in the bird's foot with special reference to reaction to cold, Heart 15:385, 1931.

88. Popoff, N. W.: Digital vascular system, with reference to the state of glomus in inflammation, arteriosclerotic gangrene, diabetic gangrene, thrombo-angiitis and supernumerary digits in man, A.M.A. Arch. Path. 18: 295, 1934.

89. Ribot, S.: Unilateral clubbing following traumatic obstruction of the axillary vein, A.M.A. Arch. Intern. Med. 98:482, 1956.

90. Hall, G. H.: The cause of digital clubbing, Lancet 1:750, 1959.

91. Shorr, E.: Intermediary and biological activities of ferritin, Harvey Lect. 50:112, 1954.

92. Crismon, J. M.: Rutin and other flavonoids as potentiators of terminal vascular responses to epinephrine and as antagonists of vasodepressor materials, Amer. J. Physiol. 164:391, 1951.

93. Williams, J.: The etiology of digital clubbing, Amer. Heart J. 63:139, 1962.

94. Barnes, C. G., Fatti, L., and Pryce, D. M.: Arteriovenous aneursym of the lung, Thorax 3:148, 1948.

95. Trever, R. W.: Hypertrophic osteoarthropathy in association with congenital cyanotic heart disease, Ann. Intern. Med. 48:660, 1958.

96. Cudkowicz, L., and Wraith, D. G.: A

method of study of the pulmonary circulation in finger clubbing, Thorax 12:313, 1957.

97. Cudkowicz, L., and Armstrong, J. B.: Finger clubbing and changes in the bronchial circulation, Brit. J. Tuberc. 47:227, 1953.

98. Trivedi, S. A.: Neurilemmoma of the diaphragm causing severe hypertrophic pulmonary osteoarthropathy, Brit. J. Tuberc. 52:214, 1958.

99. Silverman, M. E., and Hurst, J. W.: The hand and the heart, Amer. J. Cardiol. 21:116, 1968.

100. Regan, G. M., Tagg, B., and Thomson, M. L.: Subjective assessment and objective measurement of finger clubbing, Lancet 1:530, 1967.

101. Buchan, D. J., and Mitchell, D. M.: Hyper-

trophic osteoarthropathy in portal cirrhosis, Ann. Intern. Med. 66:130, 1967.

102. Berry, T. J.: The Hand as a Mirror of Systemic Disease, p. 104, Philadelphia, F. A. Davis, 1963.

103. Hollis, W. C.: Hypertrophic osteoarthropathy secondary to upper gastrointestinal-tract neoplasm, Ann. Intern. Med. 66:125, 1967.

104. Holling, H. E., Danielson, G. K., Hamilton, R. W., Blakemore, W. S., and Brodey, R. S.: Hypertrophic pulmonary osteoarthropathy, J. Thorac. Cardiov. Surg. 46:310, 1963.

105. Gerbode, F., Birnstingl, M., and Braimbridge, M.: Experimental hypertrophic osteoarthropathy, Surgery 60:1030, 1966.

106. Levine, H.: The yellow rounded digit, New Eng. J. Med. 279:660, 1968.

15

Arterial Hypertension*

ROBERT PAINE and WILLIAM SHERMAN

DEFINITIONS

The **blood pressure** is the force exerted from within against the walls of the blood vessels.

Normal Blood Pressure. No exact limits

* The authors express gratitude to Dr. Henry A. Schroeder for parts of this chapter based upon his treatment of this subject in the previous edition.

can be set because there are many fluctuating physiologic factors which normally exert effects upon the blood pressure. Arterial blood pressure should be thought of as responsive, variable, and in a dynamic, not a static, fixed state. Neverthless, we must have for practical purposes some norms in mind. In the newborn child arterial blood pressures are about 75 systolic and 40 diastolic. With increasing age there is a gradual rise to the average normal range for adults of 90/60 to 140/90. Up to age 14, upper normal limits are about 100/65; from age 15 to age 25 upper normal limits are about 120/80.

Systolic, Diastolic, and Mean Pressures. For standard purposes blood pressure is measured over the brachial artery in the upper arm while the patient is in a supine position. This is supposed to represent the pressure at the level of the heart. During ejection of blood from the heart with ventricular contraction, the arterial pressure rises rapidly to its peak, (the systolic value); during relaxation and filling of the ventricles, the pressure falls to its lowest point, (the diastolic value).

In an average adult with pressure measured at 120 mm. Hg systolic, 80 diastolic, the mean pressure is 100, and the pulse pressure is 40 (120 minus 80).

Arterial hypertension is elevation of the arterial blood pressure above ranges found normally in persons who are awake and at rest. In adults, persistent systolic pressures above 140 mm. Hg and diastolic pressures above 90 mm. should usually be considered abnormal.

Hypertension is not a disease; it is a physical sign of a cardiovascular disorder.

Malignant hypertension is severe, rapidly progressive diastolic arterial hypertension occurring with vasoconstriction from any cause; most often of unknown cause.

Systolic hypertension or **diastolic hypertension** may occur separately or they may occur together. Systolic hypertension is most closely related to cardiac output or arterial rigidity. Diastolic hypertension is particularly related to increased peripheral resistance, usually from arteriolar vasoconstriction.

PHYSIOLOGIC VARIATIONS

NORMAL PRESSURE GRADIENTS

The mean arterial pressure falls as the blood escapes from the aorta into the branching arterial tree. In the supine position the intravascular pressures are approximately as shown in Fig. 15-1.

PRESSURE LEVELS AND POSTURE

In the supine position the mean arterial pressure is normally about 100 mm. Hg throughout the arterial tree. In the erect posture, gravity and vasoconstrictive controls determine the pressures at various points in the vascular system. When standing, a normal adult has mean arterial pressures of about 100 mm. Hg at heart level, 60 in cerebral vessels and 170 in the dorsalis pedis artery. Veins, too, are subject to vasoconstrictive control by the sympathetic nervous system and intravascular pressure changes due to posture and gravity. In the veins of the foot pressure may be 90 mm. or above in the erect posture instead of the approximate 5 mm. normal in recumbency. The pressure at any point in the venous system below the level of the heart must be sufficient to balance the hydrostatic pressure of the column of blood intervening plus enough pressure to impart a linear velocity to the returning blood.

In normal persons there is usually a momentary fall followed by a sustained rise in arterial blood pressure when shifting from a recumbent position to a standing posture. The rise is from 5 to 15 mm. Hg and is apparent at both systolic and diastolic levels. It is caused by a reflex mechanism of the sympathetic nervous system which slightly overcompensates for the fall in pressure caused by gravity. Since the reflex takes about 30 seconds to operate, many persons experience slight faintness upon sudden standing.

If the reflex is not operating normally, or if it is depressed by ganglionic blocking agents, the pressure will remain lower in the erect posture. Much can be learned by first measuring the blood pressure while the patient lies horizontally and then while he is erect.

REGIONAL DIFFERENCES

The effective arterial pressures for the optimal operation of the greatly different parts of the body and the special needs of the various organs and tissues, vary widely from the fasting, resting state (see Fig. 15-1) to the state of accelerated activity of the organ or tissue. Pulmonary pressure and flow change with pulmonary activity. These parameters increase in the muscle tissues during exercise; gastrointestinal and renal pressure and flow rate increase with in-

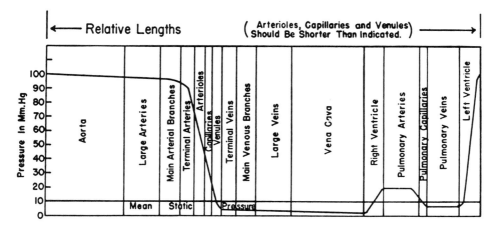

FIG. 15-1. The fall of pressure in the circulation through various anatomic divisions of the vascular system (after Green[2]). The relative length of each segment is indicated. Notice that most of the fall in pressure occurs in the smaller arteries and the arterioles. The static pressure is that which would be present during circulatory arrest.

creased activity of these tissues and so on throughout the body. Pressure and flow increase to skin and subcutaneous tissues when heat and fluid are being dissipated; they are restricted when heat and fluid are being conserved.

Thus the systolic and diastolic "blood pressure" readings which we may determine over the brachial artery in a person's arm are not the pressures in the left ventricle, or in the aorta, in the renal arteries, or in the arteries in the lower extremities, even when the whole arterial system is anatomically normal and is operating in a normal physiologic manner. Normal physiologic conditions may bring about variations in blood pressure levels between various areas; pressures are different from time to time in each area. Abnormal conditions or disease may cause reflections in the whole arterial system, in only one part, or in several parts of it.

Fluctuations in Blood Pressure. Blood pressure is not static; in any normal person it may vary considerably over a period of minutes to hours in response to various physiologic controls. The usual factors which may lead to minor or moderate **rises in pressure** are exercise, mental or physical stress, distraught emotional states and pain. Activity of sympathetic nerves and catecholamine secretion results in increased cardiac output and arteriolar vasoconstriction. The process may operate as a reflex, or the chain of stimuli may originate in high cerebral centers.

Decreases in pressure may occur if there is sudden loss of blood volume, in response to vasodilation or if there is a decrease in cardiac output. Mild or moderate pain usually elicits a rise, but severe pain may cause a great fall in blood pressure, shock and loss of consciousness. Sudden severe emotional stress also can cause fall of blood pressure and shock. Any cardiac disturbance leading to a fall in cardiac output may cause a fall in blood pressure: myocardial infarction, left ventricular failure, etc.

CIRCULATION, BLOOD FLOW, AND BLOOD PRESSURE

Blood ejected from the left ventricle by its contraction is propelled into the aorta, flows through the systemic circulation, and is returned to the right atrium. Fig. 15-1 shows the mean pressures and pressure gradients throughout the vascular system in a normal adult in the supine position. The circulation depends upon forceful projection from the heart into the arterial system and maintenance of a *vis a tergo* (force from behind), that keeps the blood moving forward through the vessels. Part of this energy is exerted by the blood against the walls of the blood vessels and may be measured as the **blood pressure.**

The blood pressure in the aorta and proximal great arteries, particularly the systolic value, depends primarily upon the force of ventricular contraction, the stroke volume, and the rate of ventricular contraction. The volume of blood in the circulatory system of an average adult is about 6 liters. A volume only slightly less than this, about 5 liters, is ejected from the left ventricle every minute (**cardiac output**). Since normal stroke volume at rest is about 70 ml., and normal heart rate is about 70 per minute 4,900 ml. of blood are ejected every minute. (Output is the product of stroke volume times rate.)

The cardiac output may be expressed in proportion to body size by using the **cardiac index**—the cardiac output per square meter of body surface. Average is about 3 L., normal range is from 2.2 to 4 L.

With maximally vigorous exercise, cardiac output may be increased to 4 or 5 times the normal, with cardiac indices of 12 to 15 L. This is accomplished chiefly through acceleration of the rate of ventricular contraction. Heart rate may increase by 250 per cent (70 to 175), but the stroke volume increase is only about 50 to 60 per cent. The increase in stroke volume is even less proportionately with less strenuous exercise. With vigorous muscular exertion there is increased force of cardiac contraction, and increased cardiac output (through high rate especially, as well as raised stroke volume). Both the impact of and the volume of blood per unit time ejected into the aorta and large arteries is considerably augmented. There is a consequent higher systolic blood pressure; from a resting value of 120 mm. Hg in a normal young adult it may reach 160 to 180 mm. or more.

FACTORS CONTROLLING BLOOD PRESSURE

Measurement of the arterial blood pressure is the assessment of the resultant of five chief factors: cardiac output, volume, viscosity, elasticity, and arteriolar and small artery cross-sectional area (peripheral resistance).

1. **Cardiac output** may be increased in exercise, fever, thyrotoxicosis, etc., with consequent elevation of blood pressure, chiefly of systolic values, but sometimes of diastolic levels also.

When cardiac output is low (myocardial disease, etc.), systolic hypotension results. If peripheral vasoconstriction is normally maintained or is increased, the diastolic pressure will be normal or high; the pulse pressure will therefore be narrow and small.

2. **The elasticity of the arterial walls** permits them to yield somewhat during systole and to retract during diastole. Expansion as the blood is received makes the systolic pressure lower than it would be in rigid vessels. The rebound retraction helps to maintain the propelling force in the interval between systolic contractions. The elastic return of the arteries to their original caliber after being stretched and the peripheral resistance of the arteriolar bed are the two chief factors that operate to maintain diastolic blood pressure.

When arteriosclerosis has limited the distensibility of the aorta and large arteries, systolic blood pressure is elevated. Just as there is lack of expansion of the vessels, there is lack of rebound retraction, with resultant rapid fall in pressure in diastole. Failure of the important elastic retractive support of the resting blood pressure may cause low diastolic pressure.

3. **Blood volume** affects blood pressure; high volume tends to raise it, low volume to lower it. With acute blood loss or dehydration there is apt to be hypotension, but increase in cardiac output or vasoconstriction may serve to prevent low blood pressure.

Severe polycythemia causes hypertension through two mechanisms: high blood volume, and high blood viscosity.

4. **Viscosity of the blood** is an important element in peripheral resistance to forward flow of the blood and thus directly affects blood pressure. "Blood is thicker than water," its greater viscosity being due to the small distortable particles (red blood cells) which constitute almost half its volume, and to the plasma protein content. About 60 per cent of the greater viscosity of blood is due to red blood cells, about 40 per cent to proteins.

The viscosity of blood in tubes is about 4 to 5 times that of water, but in the circulation (with normal hematocrit of 45 per cent) the factor is only about 2.2 times. In anemia with hematocrit of 25 per cent the relative viscosity is reduced to about 1.7; at 35 per cent, to 1.9, and the blood pressure would be quite low, were there no compensatory physiologic responses. As a result of severe anemia the cardiac output may be increased to 2, 3, or 4 times normal and there may be a high degree of vasoconstriction. These reactions to anemia can sometimes prevent severe hypotension and the resultant blood pressure may be only moderately low or even normal.

In polycythemia the relative viscosity, instead of the normal 2.2, is at hematocrit 55 per cent about 2.6, and at 65 per cent, about 3.0. The mean blood pressure may be 160 or more. Restoration of the erythrocyte count from 7 or 10 million to normal can restore normal blood pressure.

The onward propelling force falls greatly as the blood passes through the arterial tree into the smaller arteries. In these small vessels there is a greater proportionate contact of cells with vessel walls, therefore greater peripheral resistance and thus a greater *proportionate* effect of viscosity upon the blood pressure. In the smallest capillaries viscosity is especially high, as the cells are more in contact with each other and with the walls and are temporarily deformed as they pass through.

In the common forms of hypertension blood viscosity seems to be normal. In polycythemia and anemia, viscosity is abnormal and is an important determinant of blood pressure aberrations.

5. **Arteriolar and small artery caliber** is the chief determinant of peripheral resistance. The size of the lumina of these vessels depends upon their relative degree of contraction (vasomotor tone). The arterioles and small arteries are normally maintained in a state of partial constriction (normal tone). Further vasoconstriction raises resistance to blood flow and increases blood pressure. Vasodilation decreases resistance and lowers blood pressure.

The concept of peripheral resistance is often confusing to the student, depending as it does on the ratio of two measurable functions: pressure, and flow. Actually, this relationship is the analogue of Ohm's law: $E = IR$, where E is voltage or pressure, I is amperage, current or flow, and R is resistance (ohms). Thus, resistance is a ratio and can be expressed in arbitrary units.

The Poiseuille equation for flow of

homogeneous viscous fluids flowing through pipes states:

$$\text{fluid flow} = \frac{(\text{pressure difference})\,(\text{radius})^4}{(\text{vessel length})\,(\text{fluid viscosity})}\left(\frac{\pi}{8}\right)$$

Substituting this equation to indicate resistance:

$$\text{resistance} = \frac{\text{pressure}}{\text{flow}} = \frac{(\text{length})\,(\text{viscosity})}{(\text{vessel radius})^4}\left(\frac{8}{\pi}\right)$$

Blood is not, of course, a homogeneous fluid, but in general this formula is roughly valid for our purposes.

Resistance (if all other factors are unchanged) varies inversely as the fourth power of the radius of the lumen. If the radii of all vessels were reduced by 16 per cent, blood pressure would double. It thus is evident that small changes in caliber produce great changes in resistance and in

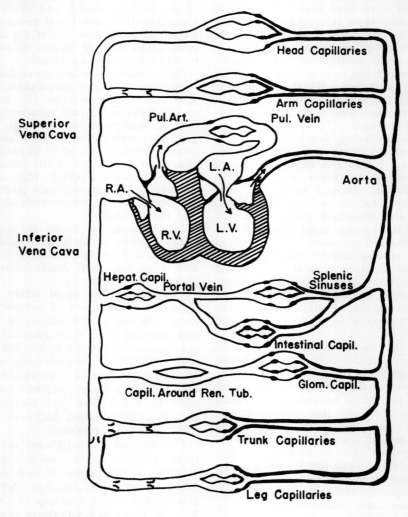

Fig. 15-2. Schematic diagram of the major parallel circuits in the body (from Green[2]). Each circuit contains a number of resistances in series, being the resistances offered by arteries and their branches, arterioles, capillaries, and veins; and a number in parallel, being collateral circuits. The kidney represents a special case with two in series; the portal circulation has two major ones in series and one in parallel (the spleen).

blood pressure. The diastolic pressure is the resultant of several factors, not vasomotor tone alone. The degree of vasoconstriction, however, profoundly affects the diastolic pressure and is its chief determinant when the other factors remain relatively constant. Persistent diastolic hypertension is the most common and most serious blood pressure disturbance in man and it usually results from chronic generalized vasospasm.

Adequate blood flow at optimal capillary pressure can be maintained at a wide range of central arterial pressures as long as cardiac output is normal. The determining factor is not the level of blood pressure nor wholly the cardiac output; it is the fall of pressure from major artery or aorta to capillary (Fig. 15-1).* Thus, a widely dilated vascular bed with a low blood pressure and adequate flow may provide plenty of capillary blood at normal intracapillary pressure and flow, with filtration and reabsorption of blood fluids and solutes proceeding normally. Likewise, adequate capillary pressure and flow may be maintained at very high pressures with intense vasoconstriction, the fall of pressure from aorta to capillary being great. The capillaries probably cannot distinguish between blood forced at high pressure through small pipes and the same amount of blood flowing at low pressures through large pipes. If a greater than normal part of the arterial pressure were transmitted to the capillary, its increased pressure would cause congestion, increased filtration of fluids and eventually rupture at a point where venous limbs could not carry the increased load. If a less than normal part of the arterial pressure were passed on to capillaries, lessened filtration, greater reabsorption of fluids and finally ischemic stasis and dehydration would result. Therefore, an intrinsic local mechanism for controlling pressure and flow probably exists. The purpose of the circulation, the heart, the lungs and the blood vessels is to provide capillaries with adequate blood at an optimal pressure for filtration and reabsorption. It is in this light that we must view the question of vasospasm.

Because the circulation is composed of a

series of shunts or resistances in parallel (Fig. 15-2), it is relatively easy to diminish the blood flow to one organ and increase that to another. Such large shifts occur constantly, during exercise when muscular flow is increased; during digestion when splanchnic flow is increased; during sleep when muscular flow may be low. These shifts are brought about by changes in the caliber of the arteries supplying the parts. Controlling factors are not well understood. Somehow the intrinsic needs of tissues for oxygen and food or for getting rid of metabolites determine the caliber of these vessels. Therefore we can postulate the presence of local regulatory mechanisms which in some way have general manifestations and affect other organs. These may be concerned with chemical agents produced at the site of need, although little is known about them.

FACTORS CONTROLLING VASOMOTOR TONE

The smooth muscle fibers in the walls encircling the arterioles normally are moderately contracted, so the lumina of the vessels are moderately constricted. A number of agents may act to relax and lengthen the muscle fibers, increase vessel cross-sectional area and lower blood pressure. Other agents stimulate the fibers to contract and thus reduce vessel caliber, increase peripheral resistance and raise blood pressure.

A knowledge of the anatomy and physiology of vascular smooth muscle aids in understanding some of the various factors which can influence the caliber of the arterial and arteriolar bed—for smooth muscle fibers can be affected directly by certain chemical substances applied to them from the blood, by other substances acting on nerves supplying the muscle fibers, by the nerves themselves through the formation and release of chemical substances at their end organs, and indirectly from sensitization or desensitization of their structures by outside influences. These various factors are considered separately.

Included in the influences determining vasomotor tone are:

Neurogenic Factors

The sympathetic portion of the autonomic nervous system has its origin in the posterior hypothalamus, where it receives connections from the cerebral cortex. Fibers pass through the spinal cord and out through the sympathetic ganglia. There is a center in the

---

* Green[2] has calculated the average pressure fall in various segments of the circulation of the dog as follows (mm. Hg): Aorta and large arteries, 2.8; main branches, 4.6; secondary branches, 4.8; tertiary branches, 13.4; terminal arteries, 4.5; terminal branches, 4.0; arterioles, 8.6. The greatest drop therefore occurs in arteries, not in arterioles.

medulla that supplies a part of the sympathetic vasoconstrictor outflow and acts as a synaptic junction for afferent fibers from the aortic arch and the carotid sinus. There are also medullary centers that regulate vasodilator effects and cardiac rate. Afferent impulses are transmitted from the carotid sinus and aorta (through glossopharyngeal and vagus nerves)—the "buffer nerve" mechanism. A rise in blood pressure inhibits outflow of sympathetic vasoconstrictor impulses; a fall in blood pressure augments sympathetic vasoconstrictor activity. Similar reflexes modify cardiac output.

The adrenal medulla may be considered a large sympathetic nerve ganglion; stimuli reaching it cause release into the blood stream of the chemical mediators epinephrine and norepinephrine for sympathetic nervous action. At the sympathetic nerve endings in the vessel walls the postganglionic fibers release norepinephrine, which stimulates the vascular smooth muscle to constrict. The amine is stored in granules within the nerve terminals until released by nerve impulses, much as epinephrine and norepinephrine are stored in chromaffin cells in the adrenal medulla.

The noradrenaline released at sympathetic nerve endings normally exerts most of its effects locally, at the site of liberation. Some "leaks" normally and constantly into the general circulation. The greatest increases in the venous concentration of norepinephrine occur during intense and frequently repeated sympathetic nerve stimulation. After release catecholamines have a short half-life, rarely exceeding two or three circuits of the circulation. Systemic effects of catecholamines are maintained by a low rate of basal secretion from the adrenal medulla. In response to stimuli, secretion is increased temporarily. Some persons have excessive secretory responses to stimuli, both central (anger, fear, etc.) and reflex (hemorrhage, hypoglycemia, hypoxia, etc.). There are some states of chronic adrenomedullary hypofunction, for example in children with spontaneous hypoglycemia. Whether there are disorders with sustained adrenomedullary hyperfunction in the absence of pheochromocytoma is controversial.

In the biosynthesis of the catecholamines, norepinephrine immediately precedes epinephrine. The latter is derived from norepinephrine by replacing one hydrogen on the tertiary nitrogen by a methyl group. This minor replacement alters the action of the hormone drastically. Its potency as a vasoconstrictor is reduced to about five-eights that of norepinephrine. Instead of acting as a general vasoconstrictor like norepinephrine, epinephrine in small amounts predominantly dilates (in muscle, especially), although it constricts the vessels of the skin. The net result is a rise of cardiac output (rate is increased by direct action on the accelerator), an increased systolic and a lowered diastolic blood pressure, and shunting of blood away from constricted areas into dilated areas. With physiologic amounts diastolic pressure is lower; with larger amounts, vasoconstrictor effects predominate and diastolic pressure is raised.

Epinephrine constitutes 80 per cent of the amines stored in the human adrenal medulla and accounts for most of circulating catecholamine effects; norepinephrine is the neurohormone released at sympathetic nerve terminals.

Central Nervous System. Impulses arising in the brain accompanying thought content or emotion may stimulate the vasomotor center in the hypothalamus. Impulses from the center are propagated through the sympathetic nervous system, cause vasoconstriction and elevate blood pressure. Part of the effect of sympathetic nerve stimulation is exerted through action on the adrenal medulla with release of circulating catecholamines.

Emotional shock or physical pain sometimes results in inhibition of the vasomotor center, stimulation of nervous system vasodilator mechanisms, fall in blood pressure, sometimes with loss of consciousness, and even death. See Fig. 33-1, p. 715.

Increase in intracranial pressure from a tumor or from any agent that heightens cerebrospinal fluid pressure may cause elevated blood pressure by reducing oxygen supply to the hypothalamic vasomotor center. When it is stimulated sympathetic nervous system response produces general vasoconstriction.

Carbon dioxide and oxygen supply to the vasomotor center greatly influence its function. Excess CO_2 stimulates the center, causes peripheral vasoconstriction and raises blood pressure. Deficient pCO_2 has an opposite effect and lowers blood pressure.

Excess oxygen inhibits the center and lowers blood pressure. Deficient pO_2 has an opposite effect and raises blood pressure.

A striking difference should be noted between the central effects of CO_2 and O_2 and their peripheral effects directly upon muscle fibers of the arteriolar wall. Peripherally the actions are opposite in effects upon blood pressure; excess pO_2 causes vasoconstriction and elevates blood pressure, excess pCO_2 causes vasodilation and lowers blood pressure.

In man these peripheral and central effects of contrary types tend to neutralize one another to a considerable extent. For example, hyperventilation lowers pCO_2, but usually has little effect upon blood pressure. The central vasodilator effect is counterbalanced by the peripheral vasoconstrictor effect (with cold, pale skin, etc.) which sustains the blood pressure that otherwise might have greatly fallen.

NEPHROGENIC FACTORS

Renal Ischemia and Vasoconstriction. Neurogenic vasospasm involves the renal vascular bed, which apparently is unique in that renal ischemia invokes the formation and release of humoral vasoconstrictor substances. The specialized circulation of the nephron, which has two arterioles, responds both to nervous stimulation and to the injection of catecholic amines by a relative decrease in caliber of the efferent arteriole, although both efferent and afferent arterioles can be affected. The net result is an increase in glomerular capillary pressure, an increased rate of filtration of blood, and a decreased total renal blood flow.

Just how and why this change calls forth "renal pressor mechanisms" is not understood. It depends upon reduction of renal blood flow by any means and is associated, perhaps, with diminished oxygen supply or with acidity of the cortex. At any rate, a proteolytic enzyme, *renin*, acts upon an α_2-globulin substrate, *hypertensinogen*, to produce a vasoconstrictor polypeptide, *hypertensin, angiotonin* or *angiotensin*. Why this happens can only be answered teleologically; the renin pressor system is one, and perhaps a major, protective mechanism against loss of blood flow through vital organs. Interestingly enough, angiotensin also appears to be antidiuretic. Other possible renal mechanisms set in motion by ischemia will be considered later.

Partial constriction of the renal artery of dogs is followed by a slow return of flow at a reduced pulse pressure, indicating "autonomous" control of the renal circulation. Renin may be released by diminution of the pulse pressure in the face of normal flow. A renal baroceptor which releases renin from the cortex has been suggested as a normal mechanism for controlling arterial pressure.

Vasodilator of renal origin. Many studies have indicated that renal tissue produces a circulating agent which causes vasodilation and combats renoprival hypertension. Evidence also suggests that the kidney makes a "natriuretic hormone" that promotes excretion of sodium. Whether there is but one such substance which may act both as vasodilator and natriuretic, or whether these responses are separate results from two or more agents is not known.

There is no agreement at present on the chemical nature of such an agent, but the **prostaglandin** designated PGA seems a likely candidate.[56] It is extracted from renal medullary tissue and is a potent vasodilator and natriuretic. Intravenous infusion of PGA into patients with essential hypertension has reduced blood pressure to normal. The prostaglandins are a group of cyclical fatty acids with diverse potent biological activities. Vasodepressor action of such a substance extracted from seminal fluid was reported in 1933.

Since PGA was found in 1965 in renal medulla (and called medullin) sufficient evidence has accumulated to permit speculation that it may normally exert an antihypertensive renal endocrine function and circulate as a natriuretic hormone. Such results support the concept that essential hypertension is not solely caused by hyperactive renal pressor mechanisms, but may be caused by deficiency of renal vasodepressor agents.

LOCAL INFLUENCES ON VASOMOTOR TONE

These may be grouped into various categories:

Altered sensitivity of vascular smooth muscle to catecholamines or other vasoconstrictors. Increased sensitivity may occur with sodium and adrenocortical hormones. In persons so affected, vasoconstriction and hypertension results. Decreased sensitivity is present with metabolic or respiratory acidosis, in myxedema, or adrenocortical deficiency. Vasodilation, with low blood pressure, results.

Relative supply of vasomotor stimulants or depressants. Locally high pO_2 causes vasoconstriction, low pO_2 elicits vasodilation. High CO_2 causes vasodilation. High H ion concentration evokes vasodilation.

Some of the above products of tissue metabolism and probably some others (particularly certain amines, e.g.: histamine, and serotonin, which is 5-hydroxytryptamine, etc.) are vasoactive and are believed to control directly and locally the caliber of arterioles and capillaries. The actual nature of many of these metabolites is not known. It is known, however, that muscular exercise causes great arteriolar and capillary vasodilation in the active muscles from effects of local products, with increase in the local blood flow that may reach 10 to 20 times the baseline. There is evidence suggesting that not only in muscle, but in other tissues and organs, a similar process operates whereby accelerated activity causes vasodilation. Thus, local controls may provide greater blood supply when needed.

Despite an increase of five-fold or more in cardiac output during exercise, there is little increase in mean blood pressure because of the great arteriolar and capillary dilation in the muscles.

A similar mechanism may operate in hyperthyroidism in which there is often extreme peripheral vasodilation. It seems likely that some metabolic derangement or by-product of excess thyroid hormone causes this vascular response and the low diastolic pressure. Systolic blood pressure is elevated because of high cardiac output (accelerated rate and raised stroke volume). Thyroid hormone directly increases myocardial contractility. The cardio-accelerator (sympathetic) center is hypersensitive to epinephrine in thyrotoxicosis. The heart itself normally responds to epinephrine and norepinephrine with increases in rate and force of cardiac contraction. These responses are augmented in hyperthyroidism.

Normal capillary tone is important in maintaining blood pressure. Most of the capillaries in muscle, for example, are normally closed. If all body capillaries are made to relax (e.g.: by a large dose of histamine) they will contain so much blood that venous return may be severely curtailed and circulatory failure will ensue.

Histamine causes arteriolar as well as capillary dilation. Histamine is liberated in antigen-antibody reactions, in response to various tissue injuries from physical trauma, and in response to other stimuli, such as heat and cold. It is also present in snake, wasp, and bee venoms.

Tissue damage not only releases histamine but also other substances: polypeptides of the pain-producing vasodilator "kinin" type from plasma; and serotonin (from plate-lets), also a pain-producer, in small amounts a vasoconstrictor, but in high concentration a vasodilator.

HORMONAL INFLUENCES

Circulating humoral substances from recognized endocrine glands affect vasomotor tone. They are discussed elsewhere in this chapter at appropriate junctures, and include the thyroid hormone, the adrenal medullary hormones, and the adrenocortical hormones.

Other circulating chemical mediators, sometimes called hormones, influence vasomotor tone of arterioles and capillaries. They also are discussed elsewhere and include renin, angiotensin, histamine, serotonin, prostoglandins and kinins.

OTHER CHEMICAL INFLUENCES

Of these, the most striking chemical influence is that of *sodium*. Sodium appears to act with certain steroids (cortisol, desoxycorticosterone acetate, aldosterone, etc.) to sensitize vascular smooth muscle to normally occurring vasoconstrictor substances (catecholamines, etc.).

When sodium is retained water retention also occurs, blood volume may increase, and hypertension may result. This mechanism sometimes seems to operate separately and at other times in addition to that proposed above.

PRIMARY AND SECONDARY HYPERTENSION

When the cause of hypertension is known it may be called **secondary,** when unknown, **primary,** or **essential.**

Systolic hypertension alone—not accompanied by diastolic elevation—always has a potentially ascertainable cause. These causes include *high cardiac output,* due to severe anemia, aortic insufficiency, arteriovenous fistula, thyrotoxicosis, beri-beri, heart block, and patent ductus arteriosus, and *rigidity of the aorta and main arteries* (arteriosclerosis).

Diastolic hypertension may or may not have a discoverable cause. When a cause is found, the hypertension is called **secondary.** In the great majority of instances the hypertension is from arteriolar vasoconstriction of unknown origin and is called **primary** or **essential.**

DIASTOLIC ARTERIAL HYPERTENSION

Persistent elevation of diastolic blood pressure may afflict as many as 10% of the adult population and is a major cause of illness and death. The primary concerns of this chapter are its etiology, its manifestations, and its consequences.

SYSTOLIC HYPERTENSION

Much less attention is given here to systolic hypertension since increased systolic pressure in the presence of normal diastolic tension is a common but much less ominous disorder. It is most frequently noted in elderly persons whose aortic elasticity has been so reduced by arteriosclerosis that the impact of blood ejected from the left ventricle is not buffered by systolic aortic expansion.

Persistent elevated systolic pressure with normal diastolic pressure, *especially in younger persons*, is more serious than previously thought. Findings of the Heart Disease Epidemiology Study at Framingham, Massachusetts, indicate that systolic pressure over 160 mm. Hg. for ages 39-59 is associated with a four-fold increased risk of coronary artery disease.

Insurance actuarial statistics have shown, moreover, that the *degree* of systolic hypertension is significant, particularly in patients with some elevation of diastolic pressure. In persons with diastolic pressures of 95, prognosis is progressively poorer with each gradation upward in systolic pressure.

The augmented stroke volume of aortic regurgitation or severe bradycardia may exceed the elastic capacity of even the normal aorta. Sharply accelerated cardiac output in anemia, arterio-venous fistula, thyrotoxicosis, beri-beri, or during exercise or excitement may similarly provoke abnormal systolic pressure.

DIASTOLIC HYPERTENSION

The great majority, perhaps 90 per cent, of the cases of diastolic hypertension are "essential" or of unknown etiology. Among them evidence of a *genetic factor* is impressive: forty per cent of the siblings of hypertensives are similarly afflicted; only five per cent of the offspring of normotensive parents develop high blood pressure while twenty-five per cent of children of a single hypertensive parent statistically become hypertensive. If both parents have essential hypertension, approximately one-half of the children develop hypertension at some time.[1]

Hemodynamic Abnormalities of Essential Hypertension

In most persons with uncomplicated primary (or "essential") hypertension there is no appreciable abnormality in cardiac output, pulse rate, volume or viscosity of blood, or in venous pressure. Peripheral arteriolar resistance is increased fairly uniformly throughout the body. Blood flow is unaffected throughout arteries and arterioles and capillaries because the arterial blood pressure is high. The high pressure provides a greater driving force that maintains adequate flow despite vasoconstriction.

The cardinal hemodynamic abnormality found in most instances of significant diastolic hypertension is an *augmented peripheral resistance*. A sizable minority, perhaps twenty-five per cent of early cases, are hypertensive because of *accelerated cardiac output* without altered resistance. These people may have a different disease; indeed they appear to have less impressive family incidence and to follow a more benign course, but even they, in later stages, develop increased peripheral vascular tone.

Following pressor stimuli, hypertensive patients fall again into two general categories. The majority have an exaggerated and prolonged peripheral arteriolar response; the minority react with augmented cardiac stroke volume and heart rate. The myocardial role in hypertensive pressor response has been documented in animals studied before and after cardiac denervation. When the heart has been thus excluded, the reaction to a variety of hypertensive procedures has been blunted and pressure has risen minimally. Participation of cardiac sympathetic apparatus in hypertensive states may be only a secondary adaptive factor in most cases, but may play the major role in the early hypertensive with markedly increased cardiac output.

No *convincing* evidence of an abnormality of *regional* blood flow has been offered in early hypertension although some observers have reported a reduction in dermal flow and an increase in muscle flow and have emphasized the similarity of this circulatory pattern to that of normal exercise. The earliest established disturbance of visceral circulation in essential hypertension is a restriction of renal blood flow. Just how early this derangement occurs and its significance in the pathogenesis of the hypertensive state will be discussed below.

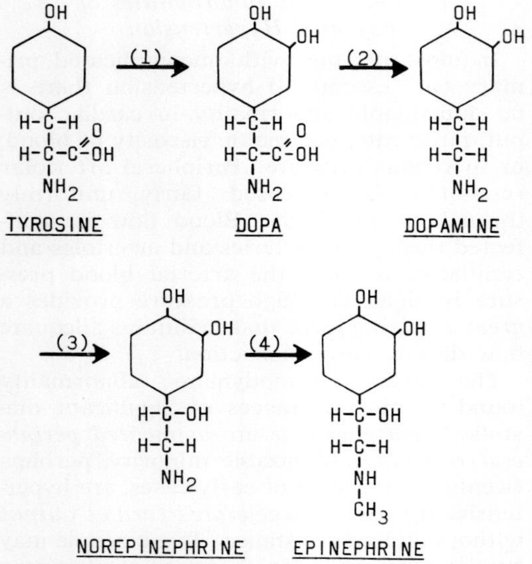

FIG. 15-3. Biosynthesis of catecholamines: (1) Tyrosine hydroxylase (mitochondrial), (2) Aromatic L-amino decarboxylase (cytoplasmic), (3) Dopamine β-oxidase (cytoplasmic granules), (4) Phenylethanolamine N-methyl transferase (cytoplasmic).

HYPERTENSION OF KNOWN CAUSE: RARE TYPES

In approximately ten per cent of patients studied, diastolic hypertension arises from a demonstrable cause. These "secondary" hypertensions are most commonly of renal or adrenal origin.

Pheochromocytoma. Perhaps the best understood is the syndrome due to pheochromocytomas. They occur in only about 0.25 per cent of hypertensive persons, but their pathophysiology is highly illuminating. These chromaffin tumors are usually found in the adrenal medulla but may arise in sympathetic ganglia or plexuses and occasionally lie in the organ of Zuckerkandl, the para-aortic area, urinary bladder, rectum, chest, or neck. In 10 to 20 per cent of cases pheochromocytomas are multiple. Within the cells of these tumors tyrosine absorbed from circulating blood is converted by mitochondrial and cytoplasmic enzymes to norepinephrine and epinephrine. (Fig. 15-3). Norepinephrine and epinephrine may remain physiologically inert within cytoplasmic granules or they may be released into cytoplasm and thence into intercellular fluid and circulating blood. The physiologic effects of these chromaffin tumors are not proportional to the size of the lesions or their catecholamine content, since a large tumor, rich in neurohormone, may release less active amine than a small one which stores little of its product. Some tumors resist the normal "feed-back" suppression of catechol production by epinephrine and norepinephrine. Rates of metabolic degradation of norepinephrine and epinephrine may vary also. Upon release from storage granules, the catecholamines may fall prey to cytoplasmic mono-amine-oxidase and be converted into inactive dihydroxymandelic acid or dihydroxyphenylglycol.

Epinephrine and norepinephrine secreted by the cell may interact with its receptor site or it may be o-methylated by catechol-o-methyl transferase found in parenchymal cells or it may be excreted unchanged in the urine or re-absorbed by sympathetic nerve endings and re-stored in cytoplasmic granules (Fig. 15-4).[2]

Various tumors produce epinephrine and norepinephrine in different proportions, some produce norepinephrine exclusively.

Norepinephrine and epinephrine are among the most potent vasoactive substances. They differ in their physiologic activities. Norepinephrine provokes intense systemic arteriolar constriction; only the coronary circulation responds with vasodilation. Epinephrine elicits a vigorous increase in cardiac con-

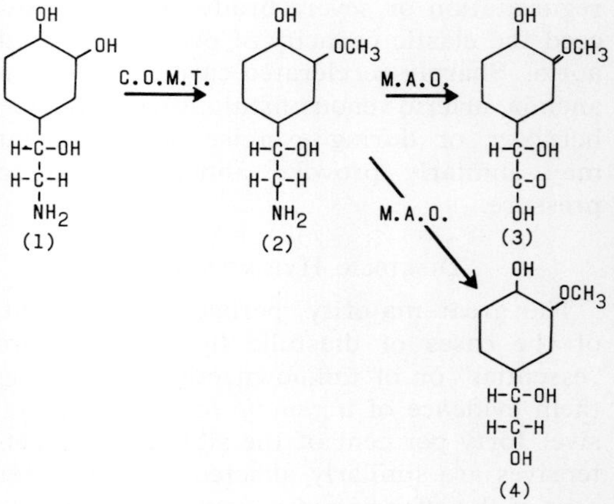

FIG. 15-4. Metabolism of circulating catecholamine. (1) Norepinephrine, (2) Normetanephrine, (3) Vanillyl mandelic acid (VMA), (4) Methoxy-hydroxyl phenyl glycol (MHP6).

Urine contains (1) (2) (3) and (4) and the comparable derivatives of epinephrine metabolism.

tractility, force and rate; it causes dilatation of arterioles in skeletal and cardiac muscle, but constriction of skin vessels. The sharp rise in arterial pressure after norepinephrine is due to augmented peripheral constriction, while the epinephrine response is predominantly the result of accelerated cardiac output.

The clinical manifestations of pheochromocytoma are those of excessive norepinephrine, epinephrine, or both. Usually, but not always, the release of these vasoactive hormones is paroxysmal rather than continuous. Almost three-fourths of patients with pheochromocytoma have paroxysmal symptoms of one sort or another. Spells of excessive sweating, weakness, abdominal pain, chest pain, palpitation, vasomotor phenomena, headache, and anxiety are characteristic. Hypertension may be paroxysmal, and patients may have symptoms long before elevated blood pressure is discovered.

However, persistent diastolic hypertension may be present.[3] In about 50 per cent of patients the classical syndrome with paroxysmal hypertension occurs; in the other half, there is persistent hypertension, and about a third of these have superimposed paroxysmal attacks.

Symptoms may be precipitated by a variety of situations which elicit catechol release: change of posture, exertion, pain, emotional stress, local heat, general anesthesia, meals, alcohol, smoking. Provocation of an acute rise in blood pressure by drugs is one of the means of clinical diagnosis of pheochromocytoma. Histamine, tyramine, or glucagon may provoke an abrupt rise in diastolic pressure, probably by stimulating release of catecholamine from the tumor. Blockade of catechol action with drugs blocking alpha-adrenergic activity, and resultant prevention or relief of hypertension is of diagnostic value. Phentolamine, in particular, has proved to be useful.

Quantitative determination of urinary catecholamines and their metabolites is of greatest reliability in recognition of pheochromocytoma. Twenty-four hour urinary excretion of catecholamines in excess of 100 mg. is highly suggestive. Values above 300 mg. are virtually diagnostic. Urinary VMA determinations are of value (Fig. 15-4). When pheocytoma is present urinary catechols or metabolites are found abnormally increased in 90 to 95 per cent of twenty-four hour specimens.

The metabolic effects of catecholamines

(chiefly from epinephrine) are often manifest. These include fasting hyperglycemia, glycosuria, accelerated glycogenolysis, and suppressed insulin release (alpha effect). Norepinephrine has little metabolic action. Despite these carbohydrate phenomena, ketoacidosis is remarkably absent even though free fatty acid release from lipoid tissue is often stimulated.[4]

Metabolic stimulation is seen in an elevated basal metabolic rate in one-third of these patients and loss of weight occurs in approximately one-fourth of persons with such tumors.

These neuro-tumors are sometimes familial and may occur in multiple sites. They may occur in association with neurofibromatosis and with thyroid tumors of neural crest origin (medullary thyroid carcinoma) which produce thyrocalcitonin. A syndrome of thyroid tumor, parathyroid adenoma, mucosal neuromas and pheochromocytoma has been described. Here the parathyroid hyperfunction may be in response to thyrocalcitonin. Another rare pluriglandular syndrome includes adrenal cortical hyperplasia in the presence of pheochromocytoma and appears to reflect catechol stimulation of ACTH release.

Although the therapy of pheochromocytoma is surgical removal, pre-operative management relies upon pharmacologic means of suppressing the alpha and beta adrenergic actions of epinephrine and norepinephrine. Phentolamine phenoxybenzamine effectively counters the vasoconstrictor (alpha) and propranolol combats the inotropic, chromotropic and vasodilator (beta) consequences of the catecholamines released before and during surgery. A surprising complication may result from the low blood volume found in these patients. Despite the hypertensive disorder, there may be postural hypotension. In fact, this may be a diagnostic clue. Especially during and after extirpation of the tumor, hypovolemia may induce hypotension and shock, and infusion of blood or plasma-expanding substances may be more important features of management than pressor agents.

Neurofibromatosis occurs in about 5% of pheochromocytoma cases. It may, even in the absence of chromaffin tumor, cause hypertensive disease if its associated vascular lesions involve the aorta or renal arteries sufficiently to disturb renal blood flow. Extensive vascular lesions can be a surprising feature of this uncommon disorder. Intimal hypertrophy, fragmentation of media and elastic lamina and adventitial fibrosis may compromise the blood supply of heart, gastrointestinal tract, endocrine organs and kidneys in particular.[5]

Adrenal Cortical Hypertension. An adrenal cortical role in blood pressure regulation is evident in the hypotension of Addison's disease, in the hypertension of many cases of adrenocortical hyperplasia or tumor, and in the pressor effect of corticosteroid hormone therapy. When massive, nonphysiologic quantities of glucocorticoids are administered in the treatment of shock, cardiac output is accelerated toward normal while peripheral arteriolar dilation occurs and systemic arterial pressure is bolstered. Chronic states of hypercorticism are often hypertensive whether they are iatrogenic or are the result of adrenocortical hyperfunction. Iatrogenic hypercorticism is usually the result of almost pure glucocorticoid therapy. Cushing's disease and Cushing's syndrome are often produced by combined mineralocorticoid and cortisol excess. Hypertension and cardiomegaly are almost always present, and are often accompanied by arteriolar nephrosclerosis identical with the lesions of essential hypertension.[6]

The mechanism of the hypertensive state in Cushingoid patients is controversial. Their polycythemia with augmented red cell volume and viscosity increases peripheral resistance while the expanded blood volume facilitates venous return and cardiac filling and output. A renal ischemic factor may be added when nephrosclerosis is present. Determinations of cardiovascular parameters in Cushing's syndrome, while scarce, seem to relate the arterial pressure primarily to the heightened peripheral resistance which cannot be accounted for by hyperviscosity alone.

Primary aldosteronism is a disorder of mineralocorticoid metabolism of far greater interest than its relative infrequency would suggest.[7] In this syndrome, exaggerated sodium retention and potassium excretion by the renal tubules causes hypokalemia, hypernatremia and benign hypertension. The patients complain most frequently of weakness, thirst, polyuria, and headache. Malignant hypertension is exceedingly rare, possibly because the sodium and water retention insures copious renal blood flow and delivery of sodium to the macula densa and juxtaglomerular apparatus. Two potent signals for renin release therefore are silenced. As expected, plasma renin concentration is less than normal, and this may militate against the onset of accelerated hypertension. Strikingly, edema does not appear in primary hyperaldosteronism. Sodium and water retention do engender an expanded blood and extracellular fluid volume, but several factors combine to make the process self-limiting. As noted, the distal nephron is presented with superabundant sodium and water. Once established, hypokalemic alkalosis curtails the potassium and hydrogen available for sodium exchange in the distal convolutions and persistent sodium retention is averted. Indeed, patients with advanced aldosteronism do not conserve salt normally. Hypokalemic tubular damage may accentuate salt and water loss and provoke polydipsia and isosthenuria.

In this disorder, hypertension develops in a setting without polycythemia and without participation of the renin-angiotensin mechanism. What then is its etiology? The expanded plasma volume alone can hardly be sufficient cause since even greater hypervolemia does not incite arterial pressure rise in other situations. Nor can hypokalemia be implicated since this electrolyte deficit is, if anything, hypotensive.

Serious consideration must be given to the relationship of *sodium retention* to the pathogenesis of this form of hypertension. A quantitative correlation exists between total body sodium and blood pressure. These patients consistently respond to negative sodium balance with a fall in pressure and suffer exacerbation of hypertension during supplemental salt intake. Experimental animals made hypertensive by mineralocorticoid (DOCA or aldosterone) administration respond similarly to fluctuations of salt intake with parallel changes in blood pressure, and become normotensive while being deprived of dietary sodium. Some evidence indicates that cortisol, DOCA, or aldosterone sensitize arteriolar vasomotor musculature to normally occurring vasoconstrictors.[1] Strains of rats have been bred which are consistently hypertensive while receiving abundant salt but are normotensive when given a low-sodium intake. The high blood pressure after Goldblatt clamping of the renal artery can be reduced but not made normal by natriuresis induced by diuretics.

Licorice. A unique cause of hypertension has been recorded in patients who have ingested enormous quantities of licorice. Their hypertension is the result of sharply increased cardiac output in the presence of normal peripheral resistance. The hypertension induced by licorice results from its steroid-like component glycyrrhetinic acid, which in chemical structure resembles deoxycorticosterone (DOCA) and aldosterone. There is sodium and water retention and potassium depletion similar to that in primary aldosteronism. Upon cessation of their strange habit, licorice eaters have promptly become normotensive.[10]

Myxedema. One-quarter to one-half of all hypothyroid patients are hypertensive. A causal relation between the two disorders is suggested by the fact that thyroid therapy has been followed by subsidence of blood pressure to normal in eight to fifty per cent of these cases. Elevation of pressure is especially remarkable in view of the slow, feeble heart action found in myxedema. Increased peripheral resistance is clearly responsible since cardiac output is consistently diminished. Cutaneous vasoconstriction may be a factor but narrowing of the visceral and muscular arterioles plays a more significant role.

In the coronary vessels, at least, arteriosclerotic changes may occur with normal frequency and severity in hypothyroidism so long as blood pressure is normal. When myxedema is complicated by hypertension, coronary narrowing is especially marked.[8]

Coarctation of Aorta. Elevation of pressure above the point of narrowing of the aorta might be the simple mechanical effect of the coarctation. The existence of additional factors becomes apparent after surgical repair of the aorta because blood pressure more often than not remains elevated for some days. In fact, only one-third of the patients in one series had reached normotensive limits upon discharge from the hospital, although most of the rest of the patients eventually did so after discharge. Carotid-aortic baroreceptors have been chronically adjusted to high pressure in the cranial half of these patients. It is reasonable to attribute very gradual post-operative easing of pressure to re-setting of these buffers. The discovery of hyperreninemia in coarctation indicates a renal ischemic element. Conceivably, the gradual subsidence of pressure after surgical repair parallels the improvement in renal blood supply. Paradoxically, the improved visceral blood supply sometimes causes severe abdominal pain associated with lesions in the small arteries and arterioles ascribed to the onslaught of higher

pressure upon vessels accustomed to chronic hypotension.[9]

HYPERTENSION OF KNOWN CAUSE: COMMONER TYPES

Renal Disease

To this point, we have considered hypertensive disorders of uncommon occurrence. Some in fact are "collector's items." All of the frequently seen varieties of secondary hypertension are caused by various forms of kidney disease. The association of **pyelonephritis** with hypertension has been well documented, although the mechanisms involved are controversial.[11] Hypertension has been present in as many as three-fourths of autopsy-proved cases of pyelonephritis. One of four malignant hypertensive patients have this form of kidney disease. Renal biopsies during sympathectomy revealed pyelonephritis in 15 per cent of patients.[12] Impressive cures of hypertension have followed the removal of the diseased kidney in unilateral pyelonephritis. There appears to be little doubt about the pathogenesis of the hypertension in these exceptional cases. However, one may legitimately ask which is cause and which is effect in the usual hypertensive pyelonephritic patient. The possibility that hypertension may facilitate pyelonephritis has been demonstrated in experimental animals in which hypertension induced by salt and mineralocorticoid administration and by angiotensin injection has increased the vulnerability of the kidneys to infection.

Evidence of infection may be difficult to detect in chronic pyelonephritis. Absence of bacilluria and pyuria is frequent. Indeed, even the pathologist may be unable to recognize pyelonephritis in advanced cases because these late lesions may be sterile and present non-specific end-stage architecture. Thus the hypertensive patient may conceal a related pyelonephritis despite the most careful scrutiny.[13] Clinically, radiographic discovery of diminished *renal size* may be the first clue to the presence of pyelonephritis, especially if the loss of renal mass is unequal. The pathogenesis of hypertension in pyelonephritis has been ascribed to *renal ischemia* induced by intrarenal endarteritis. Whatever the relationship between these two diseases, there is not an invariable association, for one-third or more of patients with chronic atrophic pyelonephritis never experience hypertensive disease.

In **glomerulonephritis,** modest blood pres-

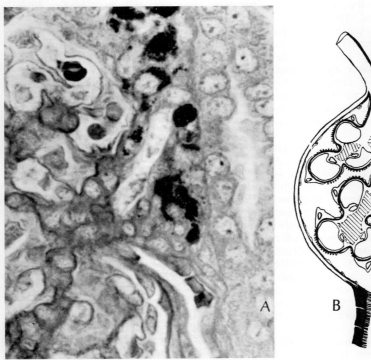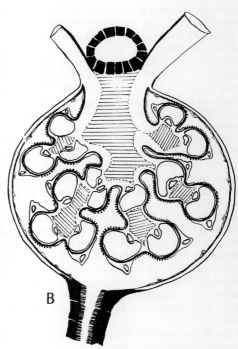

FIG. 15-5. (A) Vascular pole of the glomerulus showing both efferent (*left*) and afferent (*right*) arterioles. Juxtaglomerular cells with dark granules are in the wall of the afferent arteriole, but extend close to where the efferent arteriole leaves the glomerulus.

(B) Diagram of the glomerulus showing the relation of various parts of the J-G apparatus. Granulated cells of the afferent arteriole and specialized cells in the macula densa are seen in close apposition.

sure increase is, in frequency, second only to edema among signs developed in the acute stage. Although blood pressure levels have been related to fluid and sodium retention by their generally parallel behavior, the cause of the hypertension is unknown, although increased cardiac output and normal peripheral resistance have been documented. Excretory insufficiency usually appears in chronic glomerulonephritis before arterial blood pressure increases. Here too, its pathogenesis has not been determined although renoprival and ischemic mechanisms may be at work.[14]

Possible Pathophysiology

At least three different mechanisms may be considered as possibly operating to produce hypertension resulting from renal parenchymal diseases such as pyelonephritis and glomerulonephritis:

(1) **Loss of a renal anti-hypertensive fac-** tor that may be a normally occurring vasodilator and possibly also a natriuretic agent. Evidence that such a naturally occurring "hormone" produced in renal medullary tissue ("medullin") may be related to renoprival states is suggestive but needs further proof.[56,57]

(2) **Excess of renin production** with augmentation of renin-angiotensin activity and resultant vasoconstriction. However, except during malignant hypertension, peripheral renin activity is usually normal in renal parenchymal disease.[57]

(3) **Hypervolemia with sodium and water retention** has been demonstrated to be an important factor in the hypertension of many patients with renal parenchymal disease.[57]

Conclusions. It is probable that one or more of the three pathophysiologic processes cited, and possibly others, may operate to produce hypertension occurring with renal parenchymal disease. They may operate singly, or together, at varying degrees and at different times in the same patient. Among different patients, there is differing proportionate importance of the various mechanisms, permitting occasional instances of relatively "pure" single causes. More often there are combinations of two or more causes.

Renal Ischemia

While the hypertensive processes that are involved in parenchymal kidney diseases are still conjectural, one form of renal disorder is of special interest since it may offer an insight into the basic mechanisms underlying renal and perhaps essential hypertension. Obstruction of the main renal artery is often followed by the abrupt onset of hypertension or by the sudden aggravation of mild high blood pressure.[15] The patient may experience severe flank pain and thus call attention to the site of the trouble. More often, he is unaware of a renal problem. Upon examination, a high pitched murmur may be heard over the upper abdomen, flanks or costo-vertebral angle. Most often, the obstructive lesion is atherosclerotic, but, particularly in young women, a fibromuscular obstruction may be present distally in one or both renal arteries.

The renal venous blood of these patients, like that of Goldblatt's animals, contains abnormal amounts of vasopressor material which has been identified as *renin*. Renin has been characterized as an enzyme which acts upon a circulating globulin substrate formed in the liver to yield a decapeptide, angiotensin I. Angiotensin I is converted to the vasopressor octapeptide *angiotensin II*. Renin has been found in the renal cortex and has been identified in the granules of the specialized cells of the afferent renal arterioles which with adjacent cells in the distal renal tubule comprise the *juxtaglomerular apparatus* (Fig. 15-5).

Renin is released into the blood that is flowing through the renal arterioles when the distension of the afferent arteriole is diminished. Experimentally, the reduction of *renal blood pressure* by placement of a clamp on the aorta above the renal arteries is followed in a few minutes by detectable quantities of renin in the renal venous blood.[16,17] Secretion occurs even when the degree of aortic constriction is so slight that renal blood *flow* does not change. Neither flow nor variation in pulsation (pulse pressure) signals renin release.

Renin secretion responds also to variation

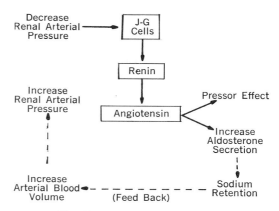

Fig. 15-6. See discussion in text.

in the *quantity of sodium* presented to the macula densa. Under experimental conditions, reduction in distal tubular sodium provokes release of renin while provision of increased sodium to the macular region forestalls renin release even in the presence of intra-renal hypotension. The anatomical proximity of the macula densa to the afferent arteriole is notable in view of these observations.

Sympathetic nerve fibers parallel the renal arterioles to the afferent entry into the glomerulus but go no farther. Of great interest is the observation that *sympathetic nerve stimulation* elicits renin secretion. The significance of this relation will be considered below.

Angiotensin II is not only the most potent pressor found in man; it is an equally important stimulant to adrenal cortical function. In the presence of angiotensin the zona glomerulosa of the cortex hypertrophies and *aldosterone secretion increases*. Consequently, resorption of sodium in exchange for excreted potassium and hydrogen is accelerated in the distal portion of the nephron and if this action is extreme and prolonged hypokalemic alkalosis ensues.[18]

A negative feed-back effect of aldosterone upon renin secretion results from the retention of sodium and water. The hypervolemic state probably supresses renin secretion by distending the afferent renal arteriole or by presenting increased quantities of sodium to the macula densa (Fig. 15-6). In all forms of hypertension, this inverse relation between serum sodium concentration and renin secretion exists, but these controls which are present normally may become deranged in the hypertensive state.

TABLE 15-1. RENAL ARTERIAL LESIONS

	AGE	SEX	ANGIOGRAPHIC APPEARANCE	PATHOLOGY
Atherosclerosis	Older	—	Asymmetric narrowing, Post-stenotic dilation, Occasional total occlusion.	Atherosclerotic with plaques.
Intimal fibroplasia	Young	—	Segmental circumferential narrowing, Post-stenotic dilation and aneurysm.	Collagen deposit and elastic duplication.
Medial fibroplasia with aneurysms	Middle age	Female predominance	String-of-beads.	Destruction of media and intima with fibrosis.
Fibromuscular hyperplasia	Young and middle age	Rare	Concentric narrowing with post-stenotic dilation.	Fibro-muscular hyperplasia.
Subadventitial fibroplasia	—	Female predominance	No aneurysm Severe stenosis often.	Fibrosis of adventitia.

Angiotensin per se also supresses renin release even when the angiotensin concentration is too small to elevate arterial pressure. This constitutes another feed-back control.

The circulating concentrations of renin and angiotensin gradually fall while the hypertension persists after renal arterial constriction. The chronically hypertensive animal soon appears to have no abnormality of renin or angiotensin. Animals chronically infused with angiotensin behave similarly. They require less and less angiotensin to maintain the hypertensive state until finally the infusion is so slow that circulatory levels are "normal" and no further sodium retention occurs. The possible relevance of this hypertensive state to essential hypertension (in which renin-angiotensin-aldosterone levels are normal) is impressive.

Hypertension in these chronically infused subjects may be abolished by sympathetic blockade and can be reduced by sodium depletion. The potentiation of angiotensin pressor activity by sodium suggests a vicious cycle of events, unlike the effect of sodium upon renin release.

A role of the sympathetic nervous system in renovascular hypertension has been noted in the demonstration of renin stimulation by sympathetic activity. The *potentiation of angiotensin effect by catecholamines* is a second point of synergistic action between the renin and sympathetic pressor mechanisms. Observations of renovascular hypertensive subjects provide other evidence of this synergism. Cardiac output is usually greater in these patients than in normal or essential hypertensive persons. Responses to tilt, Valsalva procedure and to beta adrenergic blockade are compatible with the participation of adrenergic activity in renovascular hypertension.

Angiotensin provokes increased permeability of vascular walls, and arterial vessels in renal hypertensive animals contain excessive water and sodium. This edema may play a part in the constriction of arteriolar lumina.

Tests for Renal Ischemia

The excretory function of the kidney following renal arterial constrictions is marked by diminished excretion of water and sodium. "Split function tests" (testing the two kidneys separately) have employed this phenomenon to identify patients with renal artery stenosis. The ability to dilute is embarrassed in the constricted kidney, a change which has been attributed to diminished delivery of sodium to the more distal portion of the nephron where sodium resorption generates "free" water.

Other clinical procedures employed to demonstrate renal artery stenosis include the *intravenous pyelogram*. The affected kidney may be smaller than its normal mate. When the lumen of the renal artery was less than 50 per cent constricted, 26 per cent of patients have been found to have reduced kidney size; 50 to 80 per cent arterial constriction produced renal atrophy in 60 per cent of cases, while over 80 per cent narrowing provoked this change in 75 per cent of cases with at least 1 to 1.5 cm. disparity in length of the two kidneys.

The injected dye may appear more slowly on the affected side because the slower glomerular filtration rate propels the dye more slowly into the tubular mass. Pictures recorded one, two and three minutes after injection are especially useful. The concentration of opaque dye in the renal pelvis may also reflect the inequality in water resorption. Final fading or wash-out of dye is also delayed as a result of the diminished renal blood flow and glomerular filtration rate.

The *radioactive renogram*, using radioactive mercury provides another means of displaying the impairment of perfusion through the affected kidney.

Of paramount value is the *renal arteriogram*.[19] Dye injected into the aorta or renal arterial orifices provides precise anatomical information about the renal obstruction. A variety of lesions of atherosclerotic and fibromuscular types can be recognized. (Table 15-1). It is not sufficient, however, merely to see an obstruction because many "normal" normotensive persons have constrictions. It is essential to demonstrate renal misbehavior as well. The most reliable evidence in confirming the presence of renal ischemic origin of hypertension is the finding of *increased concentrations of renin* in renal venous or peripheral venous blood. Indeed, the proof of elevated plasma renin content is the most reliable prognostic sign of possible successful surgical cure of hypertension.

Peripheral renin activity (PRA) in human hypertensive patients is high when the hypertension is malignant (with grade IV optic fundi), whether the hypertension is (1) essential, or associated with (2) renal artery stenosis, or with (3) chronic glomerulonephritis. If the hypertension is benign, the PRA may be elevated in half or more of patients with renal artery stenosis. In benign hypertension of essential type, or occurring with chronic glomerulonephritis, the PRA is normal.[57]

Such data and many other studies suggest that the renin-angiotensin cycle is responsible for hypertension only in consequence of renal arterial disease.

Restoration of normal blood pressure by nephrectomy or by renal arterial repair depends upon the health of the opposite organ; if the hypertensive state has produced vascular changes (nephrosclerosis) in the "good" kidney, hypertension will very likely persist. The remarkable situation has occurred in which repair of the obstructed artery has not been effective until the nephrosclerotic opposite kidney has been removed.

ESSENTIAL HYPERTENSION

The possibility that *essential hypertension* is in fact a form of *renal ischemic disease* has been championed since the classic work of Goldblatt. If obstruction of the main renal artery is not present, ischemia has been attributed to the sum effect of sclerotic lesions in multiple renal arterioles (arteriolar nephrosclerosis). Whether arteriolar nephrosclerosis *precedes* or *follows* hypertension remains the controversial key question. Renal concentrations in essential hypertension are not increased in the benign, common form, but they are high in malignant hypertension of any form (essential, ischemic, or with renal parenchymal disease[57]). This does not exclude the ischemic-renin-angiotensin cycle as a possible cause of benign essential hypertension.

Some credence is due the possibility that **loss of renal parenchyma** deprives the organism of a normally-functioning vasodepressor system.[20] The implantation of normal kidney into animals with malignant hypertension induces a fall in blood pressure; extracts of renal tissue contain depressor material. Normal blood pressure has been produced in patients with essential hypertension during intravenous infusions containing a vasodilator agent (prostaglandin A, medullin) made from an extract of renal medullary tissue.[56] Salt-fed rats become severely hypertensive after bilateral nephrectomy, but develop only slight hypertension if both ureters are implanted in the vena cava, as effectively eliminating excretory function as a nephrectomy yet leaving renal parenchyma intact.

These suggestions of a reno-prival cause of hypertension are countered, however, by the observations upon anephric men maintained in water and electrolyte balance by dialysis. These patients have not become hypertensive unless fluid plus sodium retention inadvertently occurred. At present, therefore, the role of renal parenchymal loss in essential or in secondary renal hypertension is controversial.

POSSIBLE PATHOPHYSIOLOGY OF ESSENTIAL HYPERTENSION*

It is to be hoped that in the future we will have less necessity to conceal our ignorance with such empty terms as idiopathic, primary, or essential. We are learning much more about causes of chronic hypertension.

The vast literature on clinical and experimental studies of hypertension furnishes at least minimal support for many different pathologic disturbances of physiology which could cause essential hypertension. But, as yet there are many unanswered questions.

1. Essential hypertension has, in part at least, some *hereditary basis*. But, just what is the transmitted genetic trait? Is it excessive production of vasoconstrictor amines? Is it a psychological hypersensitivity? Is it lack of a vasodilator mechanism?—etc.

2. *Psychological origins* of many cases seem probable. The fanatic persons, the hard drivers, seem to succumb especially. Those most prone to, or fortuitously involved in, emotionally charged situations seem especially susceptible. Do psychological causes operate directly through the sympathetic vasoconstrictor system?

3. Persons apparently not hypersensitive, when subjected to unusually frequent or *constant stress*, seem especially prone.

4. Some persons have hypersensitivity of the carotid sinus, responding to even slight pressure with inhibition of the sympathetic vasoconstrictor system. Do other persons have *insensitivity* of such *vasodepressor* reflexes that might permit persistent vasoconstriction and the development of hypertension?

5. Peripheral *hypersensitivity* of the *sympathetic vasoconstrictor system* has often been demonstrated in essential hypertension. This suggests that in such instances even normal stimuli could produce chronic vasoconstriction.

6. Could there be an hereditary overproduction of *catecholamines* and other sympathomimetic amines?

7. Are persons apt to develop essential hypertension more sensitive to activation of the ischemia-*renin*-angiotensin-vasoconstriction system?

8. Is the zona glomerulosa of the adrenal cortex *over-responsive*, with production of excess *aldosterone* to ordinary stimuli?

9. Why does blood pressure fall in essential hypertension with *sodium restriction* even

when there is no hypervolemia? Low sodium in the distal renal tubules provokes release of renin. Supply of increased sodium to the renal macula densa forestalls renin release even with intrarenal hypotension. Does sodium itself sensitize the arteriolar smooth muscle?

10. Renal vascular malfunction may be causative. Renal tubular disorder may be a factor. Renal impairment tends to cause hypertension. Nephrosclerosis results from hypertension and tends to establish a vicious cycle. Is *renal susceptibility* to vascular or other disorder an hereditary trait predisposing to "essential" hypertension?

There is some support for many of the possibilities discussed. Further evidence is needed, to eliminate some possible pathological processes or to vindicate others.

Probably it will be found that not all essential hypertension has the same cause, and that in any one case several mechanisms may be involved in its production.

Possible Various Sequences in Pathophysiology

As proposed above, starting points and patterns of development may possibly be multiple in the development of "idiopathic" hypertension (it causes itself) or "essential" or "primary" hypertension (it's just there).

A few possibilities:

1. Persistent environmental stress causes *cerebral* connections with vasomotor centers to be chronically hyperactive in sending impulses down the sympathetic pathway. General sustained vasoconstriction results, with hypertension. Renal arterioles are especially affected, causing further vasoconstriction through activation of the renin-angiotensin system. Peripheral renin activity is found normal, as it is in animals with chronic ischemic renal hypertension. The condition persists for years. Nephrosclerosis develops, a consequence of chronic hypertension. The patient succumbs to renal failure.

2. The *carotid sinus is abnormally insensitive* and perhaps other centers in brain and arteries for perception of blood pressure and volume also fail to respond. Vasomotor activity therefore is excessive, being under no limiting control. There is extreme vasoconstriction. Hypertension develops which soon becomes malignant.

3. Excessive *sodium retention* is the chief problem, due to a possible hereditary overproduction of *aldosterone*, or perhaps to a genetic renal defect with excess sodium retention. Hypertension develops with resultant great cardiac hypertrophy. Accelerated coronary atherosclerosis is a consequence of the extreme hypertension. Death may occur either from myocardial failure or coronary occlusion with infarction.

---

* The editor, Cyril M. MacBryde, is the author of this section. He does not want the authors of this chapter held responsible for his speculations.

4. There is a *genetic hypersensitivity* of the arteriolar muscle fibers to vasoconstrictor stimuli, or perhaps an hereditary overproduction at each stimulus of norepinephrine at nerve endings. Generalized vasoconstriction results with hypertension. Ischemia of the juxtaglomerular apparatus sets into operation augmentation of the hypertension because of excess chronic activity of the renin-angiotensin response. Fatal effects might be from cerebral accident, cardiac effects or renal failure.

The above four theoretical sequences are given just as examples of conceivable clinical courses in the condition we call essential hypertension, to emphasize that it has many possible causes and a group of highly likely consequences.

COURSE AND CONSEQUENCES OF HYPERTENSION

LABILE HYPERTENSION

Hypertensive disease is usually preceded by a period of intermittent blood pressure elevation. Indeed, patients found to have occasional increased blood pressure on routine examination later develop diastolic hypertension three to four times as often as those whose early records are within normal limits. In one study, 5% of 20 to 24 year old patients whose first examinations revealed diastolic pressures below 90 mm. Hg subsequently became hypertensive, while 30 per cent of those whose initial diastolic pressures were 90 to 94 mm. Hg later were afflicted. Hypertension has appeared in later years among 46 per cent of young people whose original diastolic recordings were above 95 mm. Hg.

ASYMPTOMATIC STAGE

Following the early labile period, most patients enter a stage of uncomplicated and often "silent" (asymptomatic) hypertension which on the average lasts fifteen years and terminates in a five to ten year interval of organic complications.

ORGANIC CONSEQUENCES

The most frequent difficulties during this phase are cardiac, renal, retinal, and neurological (cerebral). Untreated, the average duration of hypertensive disease is approximately twenty years. Death, if due to the hypertensive state, is most frequently cardiac (over 50%), cerebral vascular (10 to 15%), or renal (10%). Fatal accelerated or malignant hypertension occurs in five per cent. In general, mortality appears to parallel the level of diastolic pressure.

Vascular Lesions in Hypertension. The arterioles and small arteries are immediate participants in the hypertensive process.[21] These vessels generate the pathologic peripheral resistance responsible for diastolic hypertension while at the same time they face the onslaught of elevated intraluminal pressure. On the one hand, changes are seen which reasonably can be related to their hypertonic state, and considered perhaps as *causes* of generalized arterial hypertension. Arteriolar muscle cells are more numerous and consume oxygen and metabolic substrate more rapidly than normal. The ongoing nature of muscular growth is reflected in accelerated incorporation of protein precursors into the media.

On the other hand, other changes occur which are more likely to be the *effects* of hypertensive stress than the cause. Hyaline degeneration of arterioles and small arteries is a characteristic lesion in "benign" hypertension. The amorphous deposits in the intima and media are of uncertain origin. They may, as suggested by electron microscopic studies, be accumulations of debris from endothelial and muscle cell membranes, or they may be collections of plasma constituents impounded in the arteriolar wall by high intraluminal pressure. Hyaline degeneration is more prominent in afferent renal arterioles and in the splenic, pancreatic, adrenal, and hepatic arterioles, but strikingly not in the coronary and cerebral vessels. The elastic lamina is split and strands of elastica permeate the media.

In the intima of hypertensive arteries layered between high intraluminal pressure and hypertonic muscular media, atherosclerotic lesions are far more numerous than normal, notably in the aorta, larger proximal arteries and the coronary and carotid cerebral vessels.

In toto, the hypertensive arterioles show luminal narrowing and wall thickening with histologic evidence of muscular hypertrophy and structural wear and tear. The resultant constriction of luminal diameter is so forceful that experimental perfusion of vessels under high pressure fails to dilate them open to normal size.[22]

It is necessary to point out the fact that these changes may not be present in every instance. Indeed, in Smithwick's large series of renal biopsies performed at the time of sympathectomy, one-third of the patients had no renal vascular lesion. Goldblatt, on the other hand, declares arteriolar nephro-

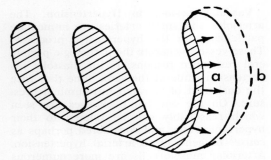

FIG. 15-7. Electrocardiogram in left ventricular hypertrophy. (a) The increased thickness of ventricular wall may prolong ventricular depolarization and thereby widen the QRS complex. (b) Increased surface area of depolarization wave front may increase voltage of the R wave.

sclerosis has been found in *every* hypertensive case he has examined.

As noted above, the severity, and not the cause, of hypertension influences the arterial and arteriolar pathology. When malignant hypertension with extreme elevation of pressure and renal failure occurs, a number of additional signs of vascular damage appear. "Onion skin" deposition of mucopolysaccharides, hyperplasia of muscle cells and duplication of elastic lamina are virtually always present. Necrotic and hemorrhagic areas are scattered in the wall. Cellular intimal hyperplasia further encroaches upon the narrowed lumen. Fibrinoid deposits, probably composed of fibrin and other plasma proteins, are most frequent in the arterioles of the gastrointestinal tract, pancreas and spleen but most characteristically in the kidney.[23]

At the opposite extreme, in early hypertension the arteriolar abnormality is most likely purely functional. In cases hypertensive because of high cardiac output, even the functional arteriolar lesion seems limited to a failure to relax normal arteriolar tone.

Renal Disease. Kidney disease, usually nephrosclerosis, is a common accompaniment of hypertension. So are pyelonephritis and other forms of infectious and vascular renal disease. Symptoms and course may be primarily from renal failure.

The Heart in Hypertension. When acute severe hypertension is induced in an experimental animal, the heart dilates because it fails to empty normally in systole. Myocardial fibers swell and fibrils loosen. The metabolic strain depletes myocardial stores of glycogen and creatine phosphate to ten or twenty per cent of normal, and lactate accumulates as the aerobic tricarboxylic acid cycle falls behind anaerobic glycogenolysis and fatty acid metabolism. As left ventricular diastolic pressure climbs, left auricular and pulmonary hypertension follow and pulmonary edema ensues. An astonishing myocardial hypertrophy begins. Myocardial weight increases *ten per cent per day*, protein synthesis is doubled, RNA content increases by one-third, and ATP slightly.[24]

This compensatory growth soon generates a balanced state of load and capacity, and all hemodynamic and myocardial metabolic parameters return to normal except for lactate excess and DNA deficit. In the hypertrophied myocardium, myocardial fiber enlargement apparently is not accompanied by capillary hyperplasia; thus a state of relative ischemia exists and is responsible for the accumulation of lactate.

Subsequently, compensated hypertrophy evolves into a final stage of myocardial degeneration with accumulation of fat, diminished protein synthesis, and depleted DNA, ATP, norepinephrine, and epinephrine.[25]

The clinical counterparts of this experimental model are seen in acute hypertensive states in which acute pulmonary edema may be the life-threatening event. More commonly, however, hypertensive disease generates a more gradual cardiac change. Left ventricular hypertrophy is detected on physical examination by displacement of the left cardiac border and apical impulse to the left. The aortic second sound is accentuated and often has a ringing tambour note. Roentgenograms of the chest reveal a rounded symmetrical enlargement of the left ventricle, or the heart may appear normal as the concentric hypertrophy forestalls dilation. Electrocardiographic tracings may also be normal, but more often present ST and T deviations of a characteristic form (Fig. 15-7).

Less often, voltage and/or duration of the ventricular complex (QRS) are increased. ST and T abnormalities may be attributed in part at least to the prolongation of conduction through the thickened left ventricular wall. As seen in Figure 15-7, normal depolarization moves outward from the Purkinje-endocardial inner layer generating the QRS complex. When depolarization reaches the epicardium, all layers of the wall are equally depolarized and an iso-electric segment (ST) results. Repolarization is initiated in the outer wall—the resulting positivity rolls inward, creating the T-wave.

When the ventricular wall is sufficiently

thickened, repolarization begins simultaneously in the subendocardial and subepicardial regions. There is no trans-wall difference in potential and the T-wave is flat. Still greater thickening causes the subendocardial layer to re-accumulate its positivity before the outer layers and the period of repolarization is marked by T-wave inversion and terminal ST depression. ST and T abnormalities probably reflect other factors as well (Fig. 15-8). Alterations in myocardial membranes by stretch, intramural pressure and cellular ischemia engendered by hypertrophy or by complicating coronary disease may play important roles. QRS voltage and duration seem to be more straight-forward indicators of myocardial thickness and surface area. While the numbers of myocardial capillaries probably do not increase in hypertensive hypertrophy, the proximal main coronary arteries may be slightly enlarged. Of greater significance, however, is the sharply accelerated development of **coronary atherosclerosis** seen in hypertension. The three coronary arteries may be involved in diffuse or spotty fashion especially in their proximal portions, the anterior descending artery somewhat more often than the circumflex or right vessels. Remarkably, atheromata are virtually absent from vessels penetrating the ventricular walls.

Hypertension and the Ocular Fundus. In the study of hypertension and the evaluation of the hypertensive patient, examination of the ocular fundi is of special importance for thus a direct assessment can be made of the presence of hypertension and its vascular effect. With this information, important inferences can be drawn about the state of the general circulation. New methods have helped to correlate the ophthalmoscopic picture with pathological findings. Serial photography of the retina during life combined with post-mortem injection studies of isolated retinal vessels have provided new basic information. An angiographic technique has recently been utilized to study the dynamic state of the retinal circulation.

The antomy of the retinal vascular tree has certain unique features.[26] Within the confines of the optic nerve, the central retinal artery and vein share a common adventitia. At arterio-venous (A-V) crossings on the retina, the adventitia is again shared. The wall of the central retinal artery abruptly thins as it passes the cribriform plate so that the wall to lumen ratio is only one to ten. After the first arterial branching on the retina, the wall thins again and the

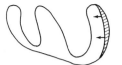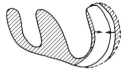

FIG. 15-8. Repolarization in left ventricular hypertrophy. Normally subepicardial myocardium repolarizes first, generating positive charge on the surface. Delay in repolarization of superficial myocardium creates altered sequence in recovery of charge. Subendocardial positivity may cancel or exceed surface charge and flatten or invert ST and T waves in surface leads over the free wall of the left ventricle.

muscular coat becomes discontinuous after the second major branching. It is essentially then an arteriole. The thinness of the arterial wall accounts for the nearly perfect optic transparency so that what is seen ophthalmoscopically is the column of blood in the vessel. The veins are also thin-walled, and at A-V crossings the lumina of the artery and veins are in intimate juxtaposition.

The retina itself is perfused by a dense capillary network arising abruptly from medium-sized vessels with only a precapillary arteriole intervening. The capillaries do not directly perfuse the outermost retinal layers that include the rods and cones. The macula also is devoid of direct blood supply.

Of importance is the total lack of anastomoses between individual retinal arterioles and also between the retinal and the choroidal systems.[27]

The retina, especially the macula, utilizes oxygen rapidly and requires abundant blood flow. The pressure in the central retinal artery is estimated by opthalmo-dynamometry to be about one-half that of the brachial artery; an unusually high tension is said to be transmitted to the capillary bed.

Control of the retinal circulation is primarily by autoregulation.[28] Elevation of mean arterial pressure provokes vasoconstriction, and a decrease produces vasodilation. Adrenergic nerve supply has not been demonstrated. In contrast to the vessels of the intracerebral circulation, the retinal vessels are more reactive to oxygen tension than they are to variation in carbon dioxide. Breathing one hundred per cent oxygen causes vasoconstriction. With a reduced oxygen supply the vessels dilate.

The vascular changes and retinopathies induced by sustained arterial hypertension are dependent on the pre-morbid state of the retinal vessels, the severity of the hypertension, and its duration. Other systemic diseases can modify and in fact may simulate the funduscopic lesions of hypertension. Usually in essential hypertension, vascular changes develop first and become gradually more advanced through years of sustained hypertension. If the integrity of the retinal vascular system is disrupted, **hypertensive retinopathy** appears. This term indicates the presence of any or all of the following:

Flame-shaped or deep hemorrhages
Exudates either of the "hard" or "soft," "cotton-wool" type
Retinal edema
Papilledema.

Severe hypertension arising in a young person may present with only retinal edema and relatively normal vessels.

The presence of sclerosis in the retina before hypertension becomes established modifies to a great extent both the type of vascular response and the degree of retinopathy.[29,30]

The arteriosclerosis of advanced age is known primarily to affect, in a patchy distribution, the larger arteries. However, the smooth muscle and elastic tissue of smaller arteries and arterioles are gradually replaced by acellular fibrosis. This "involutional sclerosis" is recognizable in the fundus. The arterioles are straightened and diffusely narrowed, with branching occurring at acute angles.

Development of diastolic hypertension in the person with retinal arteriosclerosis produces complex retinal arterial changes. Where the arterial segment is uninvolved with sclerosis and the contractile elements are intact, these portions constrict. The blood column appears pale, straight and narrow, especially in the arteriolar branches of the main vessels. On the other hand, in those portions of the artery (usually in the proximal vessels near the disc) where replacement of the media has occurred, the wall is passively dilated by the high intraluminal pressure. The latter segments will, therefore, appear wide, deeply colored and somewhat tortuous. A segment of arterial narrowing fortuitously located between two segments that have been passively dilated will simulate focal spasm.

The stress placed on the arterial wall due to sustained hypertension will hasten fibrous replacement in the hypertonic portions so that these areas eventually dilate, and the

entire length of the main retinal arteries appears wide, deeply colored and tortuous. The arteriolar branches of the main vessels are more resistant to fibrous replacement and tend to maintain their reactivity to the elevated arterial pressure. The narrowed straight arteriolar branches are sharply contrasted to the wide proximal vessels.

Histology of these vessels has been correlated with fundal photographs. The arterial walls of dilated segments are thinned and contain excessive collagen with hyaline degeneration.[30] Where the walls are relatively normal, the lumen tends to be narrow.

From a clinical aspect, the presence of sclerotic changes in the vessels implies less reactivity to excessive intraluminal pressure. This is consistent with the rarity of malignant retinopathy in the hypertensive patient past age sixty-five.

When severe hypertension occurs in a young person with normal vessels, the retinal arterioles respond with a generalized narrowing with or without focal spasm. The arteries tend to be straightened and shortened, pale in color and branch at acute angles. If the blood pressure elevation is transient, the vessels may return completely to normal.

In cases where the blood pressure elevation stabilizes at a high level, the retinal arterial tree undergoes a diffuse, reactive, compensatory sclerosis.[30] The arteries, originally narrowed due to "functional" hypertonus, gradually develop organic changes in their walls. This process involves a proliferation and hypertrophy of the media and subendothelial tissues that proceeds at variable rates in different segments of the retinal vascular tree. It eventually terminates in replacement fibrosis and severe narrowing of the lumen. The fundus shows narrowing of the arterial blood column that is often irregular and focally constricted. The smaller arteriolar branches are again relatively spared, and tend to maintain a diffuse hypertonus with straightening. Chronic narrowing, whether generalized or focal, is secondary to organic changes and will often remain unaltered for years despite normalization of the blood pressure with drugs or surgery.

Byrom has recorded the retinal arterial changes with serial photographs in rats with accelerated hypertension due to clamping of the renal artery.[31] Individual arteries became either focally or diffusely narrowed. Occasionally, segments of intense focal constriction alternated with dilated segments.

In the early stages, the narrowing could be transiently abolished by deep levels of anesthesia that measurably reduced the carotid blood pressure. After more prolonged hypertension, arterial constriction would no longer respond to anesthesia. Removal of the renal artery clamp and subsequent subsidence of hypertension resulted in disappearance of the vasoconstriction in a matter of days.

It should be evident that arterial narrowing is an important sign in hypertension. Comparison with adjacent veins and expression in terms of an arterio-venous ratio has been used to quantitate arterial diameter but there is a substantial overlap between normotensive and hypertensive patients.[32]

There are other important signs of advanced retinal arteriosclerosis. The most apparent is depression (nicking) of the vein at the arterio-venous crossing. More subtle is deflection in the course of the vein so that it crosses the artery at an angle approaching ninety degrees.

As A-V nicking becomes more pronounced, the vein is noted to taper on either side of the artery, and may be totally invisible under the artery. Occasionally on the upstream side of the crossing, the vein appears dilated as though its blood flow were impeded. Retinal arteriograms have shown that the venous blood flow is altered and turbulent at the point of severe A-V nicking. Venous thrombosis tends to occur at these points. Generally, the cause of A-V nicking is thought to be sclerotic thickening of both the adventitia between the vessels, but nicking has been noted in acute hypertensive states such as eclampsia when the taut hypertensive artery compresses the vein.

Other signs of diffuse retinal arteriosclerosis are based on the loss of transparency through the arterial walls. An early sign is the inability to see the veins as they cross under the arteries. The light reflex becomes broadened and more brilliant because the sclerotic media reflect more light. With progression of the arteriosclerotic process, the arteries develop a metallic color resembling a copper wire. And, in the most advanced stages, the vessel reflects light as a homogenous "silver wire." The blood column is invisible. Changes in the light reflex may be segmental, and different stages may be present in the same vessel. Pathologically, the portions of the vessels showing copper and silver "wiring" have advanced hyalin degeneration of the media.

Arteriosclerotic changes in the vessels and

TABLE 15-2. CLASSIFICATION OF RETINAL VASCULAR LESIONS

Grade I	Widening and increased brightness of light reflex from arteries, with slight depression of veins at A-V crossings with reduced visibility of underlying veins.
Grade II:	Copper color of arteries, definite depression and almost complete invisibility of vein at A-V crossing, deflection in course of vein at A-V crossing.
Grade III:	Silver color of arteries, depression and distal dilation of veins at A-V crossing, right angle A-V crossing, complete invisibility of vein on either side of artery.
Grade IV:	Arteries visible as white fibrous cords without blood column.

in the perivascular tissue may cause the appearance of white lines bordering the arteries. This sheathing may be evident earliest at the A-V crossings.

"Corkscrew" tortuosity of the smaller arterioles and venules in the macular region is also associated with retinal arteriosclerosis.

What conclusions can be drawn from arteriosclerotic changes in the retina? Wendland graded the arteriosclerosis (Table 15-2) in the fundi of a large series of non-diabetic patients with and without essential hypertension.[33] The fundi were categorized according to age group (below age 30, 30-45, 45-60, above 60) and diastolic pressures (less than 70 mm. Hg, 70-85, 85-100, 100-110, greater than 110). Patients over sixty years of age with a diastolic blood pressure less than 85 mm. Hg had less than a one per cent incidence of more than grade I retinal arteriosclerosis. In the same age group with a diastolic pressure below 70 mm. Hg, only five per cent showed *any* degree of sclerosis.

The above constitutes a significant negative correlation. With advanced retinal arteriosclerotic changes present in a non-diabetic patient, one can reasonably assume that hypertension is or has been present. The latter may be relevant in the hypertensive patient whose blood pressure has permanently fallen following a myocardial infarction.

On the other hand, what per cent of hypertensive patients with diastolic hypertension have signs of retinal arteriosclerosis? In Wendland's study, only forty-five per cent of patients less than forty-five years of age with diastolic pressure greater than 100 mm. Hg had more than grade I sclerosis. Duke-Elder quotes a number of studies in which as many as one-third of hypertensive patients have no changes in the ocular fundi. In one study where a large group of hypertensive patients were followed from four to eleven years, only about one-third developed A-V nicking. Shelburne has found advanced A-V nicking in a high percentage of patients with cardiomegaly as an indication of hypertension.[34]

Several large studies have shown a significant correlation between arteriosclerotic changes *in the fundi* and the degree of arteriosclerosis present *in renal biopsies* taken at the time of sympathectomy. Wendland found a close correlation, with eighty-seven per cent of renal and retinal arterioles not differing by more than one grade. (The renal arteriosclerosis was graded according to Bell's classification.)

Atherosclerosis in the larger vessels and particularly in the central retinal artery is accelerated in the hypertensive. Thrombosis in either the central retinal artery or vein is a major complication and is more frequent in the hypertensive.

When hypertensive retinopathy becomes manifest in the form of hemorrhages and "cotton-wool" spots, it may be assumed that the patient's eye changes are in the incipient stage. With resolution, the color becomes duller and granular and the exudate breaks up into smaller islands. When it has completely cleared, the retina usually appears normal.

Histologically, a "cotton-wool" spot appears to represent an area of anoxic edema and degenerated axons.[36] Injection studies reveal a capillary bed which is devoid of circulation. The capillary walls are intact but are without endothelial cells. The area stains heavily for fat which is thought to be a result of fatty degeneration of the endothelial cells. Partially or totally obstructed arterioles can often be identified. At the margin of the avascular area one sees capillary dilatation and often numerous capillary microaneurysms. As the exudate resolves, the circulation becomes re-established in the *same* capillary network.

It is important to emphasize that the presence of "cotton-wool" spots causes no subjective changes in vision. However, extensive edema of the retina with retinal detachment may cause major visual disturbances.

Capillary microaneurysms are well known in diabetes. They are also frequently present in advanced hypertension. In hypertensive retinopathy they are found at the margins of "cotton-wool" spots and in close relationship to retinal hemorrhages. With resolution of these lesions following treatment, the microaneurysms diminish in number. The capillary aneurysms are also seen in association with retinal venous occlusion, chronic uveitis, macroglobulinemia and sickle-cell anemia (see Chapter 5 on Loss of Vision).

Fluorescent retinal photography has greatly aided our understanding of the pathophysiology of hypertensive retinopathy. Sodium fluorescein is injected by either the intravenous or intra-arterial route. With injection of the contrast material into the brachiocephalic artery, a clear separation of the retinal arterial, capillary and venous phases is obtainable. The transit time is less than five seconds, and there is little or no parenchymal fluorescence in the retina until about ten minutes later when a rim of staining may appear at the edge of the optic disc. This technique has been extensively employed in serial studies of "cotton-wool" spots.[37,38]

Abnormal fluorescence may be seen up to two days before a visible "cotton-wool" exudate appears, indicating a local area of increased vascular permeability. When the exudate becomes visible, it can be seen from the capillary phase of the dye that there is no perfusion of the capillary bed in the involved area. A delayed collection of dye is seen in a rim of dilated capillaries and microaneurysms at the margin of the exudate. The latter show leakage of dye into the exudates. The involved areas show heavy fluorescence as long as thirty minutes after injection and the fluorescence spreads beyond the area of visible exudation.

It has been proposed on the basis of angiographic findings that damage to arterioles by spasm or temporary obstruction produces increased permeability of the arteriolar wall. Edema raises tissue pressure and closes the capillary bed, causing anoxia and swelling of the underlying nerve fibers.[39]

It should again be emphasized that "cotton-wool" exudates can be observed in a wide variety of disease states. They have been noted in diabetes mellitus, collagen diseases, fat embolism, dysproteinemias, Hodgkin's disease, leukemia and after severe blood loss.

"Hard" exudates are characteristic of the *chronic* stage of advanced hypertension. They are easily distinguished from "cotton-wool" spots. Following the onset of hypertensive retinopathy, the hard exudate appears a few weeks after the "cotton-wool" spot. Most commonly their location is in the macular area, where a so-called star figure may be visible. They are very slow in resolution. With arteriography there is no evidence of fluorescence in these lesions. Histologically, the exudate is situated in the deeper retina, and represents degeneration and phagocytosis of the outer plexiform layer. It stains heavily for lipids.

The onset of **papilledema** heralds the *malignant* hypertensive state. In the great majority its presence is accompanied by other manifestations of retinopathy. Occasionally, it has been found as the only funduscopic sign of accelerated hypertension. Absence of papilledema during malignant hypertensive encephalopathy has been described.

The etiology of the papilledema occurring with malignant arterial hypertension is controversial. Cerebrospinal fluid pressure is often elevated and capable of transmitting pressure back through the sheath of the optic nerve. However, grade IV fundi are not infrequently associated with normal and sometimes low cerebrospinal fluid pressure.

Papilledema is noticed in its earliest stages by detection of blurring of the nasal margins of the optic disc. Subsequently, the temporal margins also are obscured, and edema fills in the physiologic cup before spreading out from the disc. Clinically, there is enlargement of the blind spot. With more widespread edema, large segments of the retina may become detached with subsequent visual loss.

Fluorescent angiography in the patient with papilledema has revealed vascular abnormalities of the nerve head.[40] One sees a dense network of dilated capillaries and microaneurysms which extends beyond the disc margins. Leakage of dye is noted and intense delayed fluorescence occurs over the optic disc area extending beyond the disc margins. It has been proposed that this finding represents new vessel formation akin to diabetic neovascularization which also shows increased permeability for fluorescein dye. Papilledema is a dynamic hypertensive change and like arterial spasm, "cotton-wool" spots and hemorrhage, is responsive to therapy and is reversible.

Hypertensive Cerebrovascular Disease. The relationship between hypertension and cerebrovascular disease has for many years been known but poorly defined.

It is generally agreed that a majority of patients with primary intracerebral hemorrhage have antecedent arterial hypertension.[41] In a recent cooperative study involving nearly 5,000 patients investigated for signs and symptoms of ischemic cerebrovascular disease, almost forty per cent had hypertension. Prospective studies (Framingham) have implicated elevated blood pressure in the pathogenesis of ischemic brain infarction.[42] The incidence correlates directly with the magnitude of the pressure elevation regardless of age. Furthermore, autopsy series show heart weights greater than 400 grams in the absence of valvular disease in the majority of patients with either cerebral infarction or primary intracerebral hemorrhage.

Hypertension accelerates atherosclerosis of the cerebral circulation at the usual sites of predilection and a surprising number of these lesions have been found in the extracranial circulation. Of perhaps greater importance is the arteriosclerotic involvement of smaller arteries, especially the so-called penetrating branches supplying the internal capsule, basal ganglia, thalamus, pons, and cerebellum. These vessels are usually less than 300μ in diameter and are not visible in arteriogram. In patients with both cerebral infarction and diastolic hypertension (greater than 110 mm. Hg) approximately fifty per cent show no visible occlusive or significant stenotic lesions with four vessel angiography.[43] This is presumably a manifestation of small artery disease. In contrast, patients with only elevated systolic pressure and "stroke" (cerebral vascular accident) almost invariably have visible arteriographic lesions which are frequently in the neck.

The anatomy of the penetrating arteries makes them particularly vulnerable to chronic diastolic hypertension. They arise directly from large arteries such as the basilar and middle cerebral and are subjected to the full undampened pressure in the circle of Willis. These vessels have a strikingly high incidence of aneurysmal dilatation.

Fisher has described small (0.6-15 mm. in diameter) cystic lesions which are often multiple and located primarily in the territory supplied by the penetrating arteries.[44] These so-called "lacunes" he considered to be ischemic infarcts. Of 114 brains with these lesions taken from a large autopsy series, 111 had documented hypertension and nearly two-thirds had severe cerebral atherosclerosis. Although only a small number of vessels supplying the lacunes were studied in detail, the great majority showed total occlusion.

The small size of lacunes and their distribution favor minor neurological deficits with a tendency for recovery. Marshall and others described a series of patients with cerebral infarction occurring before age fifty-five.[45] Those with sustained diastolic pressure greater than 110 mm. Hg had small deeply situated lesions (not seen with arteriography) and were left with little residual disability. The normotensive group had a high incidence of large cortical lesions secondary to occlusion or stenosis of major arteries and had a poor recovery.

The territories of the brain supplied by the penetrating arteries are the principal sites of hypertensive intracerebral hemorrhage. Rupture of arteriosclerotic vessels subjected to high intraluminal pressure is a logical explanation, although the site of rupture is rarely found in autopsy material. Russell injected fresh brains with contrast material and using a dissecting microscope, found multiple microaneurysms of small arteries.[46] They were strikingly more frequent in the brains of persons known to have had hypertension and when present were very numerous. Their location was primarily in the penetrating arteries of the mid and hind brain. Histologically, they appeared to be true aneurysms.

Cole and Yates have confirmed the presence of microaneurysms using a similar technique in an autopsy series of 100 hypertensive patients matched for age and sex with normotensive groups.[47] A total of 53 brains contained numerous microaneurysms of which 48 were in the hypertensive group. Vessels of the same size and location again were involved. The presence of aneurysms correlated closely with the occurrence of small and large hemorrhages but not with infarctions. The lesions were rarely found before the fifth decade of life and were closely associated with extensive sclerotic changes in the parent vessels. The authors implied a pathophysiological relationship to hypertensive hemorrhages.

Before turning to hemodynamic considerations in hypertensive cerebrovascular disease, it is necessary to review briefly the control of cerebral blood flow (CBF). Much of our understanding comes from the work of Kety and Schmidt who introduced the nitrous oxide technique for measuring CBF and cerebrovascular resistance (CVR). A significant shortcoming of this method is that it fails to account for areas of brain that are devoid of blood supply and essentially removed from the circulation. Direct visualization of the surface vessels in experimental animals and in man has provided important information.

Man under normal physiological conditions maintains a CBF of 50 to 60 ml. per 100 grams of brain per minute (700-800 ml. per min. total) as calculated by the nitrous oxide method. These values correlate well with measurements using electromagnetic flow meters. The cerebral circulation is capable of highly efficient *autoregulation*. A normal CBF can be maintained with variations in the systemic mean arterial pressure (MAP) from 50 to 150 mm. Hg. This is accomplished by both intrinsic and extrinsic mechanisms.

The intrinsic regulation is sensitive, reacts within seconds, and is independent of the autonomic nervous system. It appears to be operative primarily at the small artery and arteriolar levels in the intracerebral circulation and is not present in the external carotid system. This response by the arterial wall to change in the intraluminal pressure is known as the Bayliss effect. With elevated pressures there is vasoconstriction; conversely, with decreased pressure, vasodilation ensues. CBF remains normal by a compensatory increase in CVR that rises linearly with the MAP and is not influenced by stellate ganglion blockade.

Changes in the chemical milieu are vital in the intrinsic regulation of CBF. The pial arterioles show a marked reactivity to tissue and arterial levels of pCO_2. Slight elevations cause vasodilation with increase in blood flow. The opposite occurs with reduction of pCO_2. The pO_2 in cerebral tissue is also a potent local stimulus. A decrease in pO_2 provokes vasodilation and an increase in blood flow, while an elevation in pO_2 causes the opposite effect. The hydrogen ion also independently influences CBF. A more acidic medium promotes vasodilation while alkalosis is a vasoconstrictor.

The major arteries of the monkey brain, the carotid and vertebral vessels, constrict in response to cervical sympathetic stimulation and decrease their blood flow from twenty to thirty per cent. Transient elevation of MAP following epinephrine injection is buffered by the major cerebral arteries so that the pressure in the circle of Willis is nearly normal.

In the uncomplicated phase of arterial hypertension, the CBF has been found to be normal.[47] The increased CVR is thought to be due to a generalized vasoconstriction that is capable of relaxation with pressure reduction. However, when evidence of cerebrovascular disease is present with more advanced hypertension, the CBF is significantly diminished. It has also been shown that persons with chronic hypertension have decreased ability to change CBF following carbon dioxide inhalation or hyperventilation. This is thought to be a manifestation of cerebral arteriosclerosis. In addition, the critical MAP level below which normal CBF cannot be maintained by autoregulation is higher in the chronic hypertensive patient.[48]

The widespread involvement of the small arteries and arterioles in sustained hypertension has important effects upon the ability of the brain to establish effective collateral circulation. An extensive arteriolar network exists in the pia mater which provides direct inter-connections with no intervening capillaries between medium-sized arteries. Thus, occlusion of a major cerebral artery distal to the circle of Willis causes a rapid dilatation of the pial vessels at the margin of the ischemic area and influx of collateral blood flow. Blood flows into the ischemic area because, (1) an arterial pressure gradient is established from the normally perfused areas to the ischemic tissue where decreased arterial pressure exists, and (2) the hypoxia and carbon dioxide accumulation promote vasodilatation of the bordering pial vessels. Occlusion of the middle cerebral artery in a healthy monkey has very little effect on the area of brain supplied by this vessel.[49] Large collaterals from the ramifications of the anterior and posterior cerebral arteries prevent tissue destruction.

The patient with chronic hypertension may be more vulnerable to infarction with occlusive cerebrovascular disease because the pial arterioles are subject to widespread arteriosclerosis and their ability to dilate widely is impaired, and thus, collateral blood flow is diminished. Denny-Brown and others have monitored patients with cerebrovascular insufficiency using electroencephalography before and after tilting on a tiltboard. Those with hypertension showed slowing of cortical activity in the involved area of brain with smaller reductions in systolic blood pressure than did normotensives.

Brain ischemia, itself, may produce a reflex pressor response if there is insufficient blood flow to the vasomotor center. There are well-documented reports of hypertension accompanying a transient cerebrovascular ischemic attack involving the vertebro-basilar system.[50]

The significance of cerebral vasospasm in the hypertensive patient remains controversial. Byrom has performed classical studies in rats with chronic renovascular hypertension in which he directly observed and photographed arterial vasospasm in the living animal through a permanent cranial window.[42] In the group of rats with benign hypertension, cerebral arterial spasm was rarely seen. At the times when the arterial pressure was exceptionally high, slight diffuse narrowing was noted. In the rats with malignant hypertension, the arteries and arterioles showed both focal and diffuse spasm. This was accompanied by pallor of the cortical surface. Focal spasms tended to remain in the same position. The signs in the animals with malignant hypertension were usually cerebral and consisted of generalized epileptiform convulsions, myoclonic contractions, local muscle weakness, and apathy progressing to coma. In animals surviving removal of the renal artery clip, dramatic relief of symptoms ensued. Approximately two weeks later, the cerebral arteries appeared normal.

Because the signs of encephalopathy cleared rapidly in certain animals with a reduction in blood pressure, Byrom suspected a functional abnormality that was not severe enough to produce tissue destruction. He therefore injected a dye (trypan blue) intravenously into rats with encephalopathy shortly before they were sacrificed. Multiple areas of blue staining were found in the cerebral hemispheres. The water content of the stained tissue was significantly higher than in the unstained areas. In only twenty-five per cent of these areas could evidence of structural damage be found with light microscopy. In rats with benign hypertension and in those serving as normal controls, no dye staining was found.

Apparently, a critically high intraluminal pressure produced diffuse arteriolar narrowing, focal spasm, and ischemic endothelial damage initially manifest by increased permeability of the vascular wall with focal edema. If the pressure continued to rise, the vasospasm became more intense with subsequent infarction, hemorrhage and diffuse edema.

Others have made observations on the cerebral arterioles of monkeys during acute hypertension produced by clamping the descending aorta. Generalized vasoconstriction occurred and was accompanied by severe brain swelling. The vasoconstriction sometimes produced perivascular hemorrhages and often outlasted the rise in pressure.

Other investigators induced segmental vasoconstriction (spasm) of the cerebral arterioles in chronic hypertensive anesthetized monkeys.[51] The spasm intensified with swings of blood pressure to higher levels. When systemic blood pressure was reduced by tilting the operating platform, a diffuse arterial and arteriolar dilatation occurred, but some focal constriction persisted. With restoration of systemic pressure, the segmental vasoconstriction returned exactly to its previous pattern. Even when a major artery was occluded, the anastomotic pial arterioles maintained some focal constriction. Segmental constriction impaired rapid readjustments of the cerebral circulation when threatened by ischemia. Segmental constriction could not be attributed to permanent changes in the vascular wall because topical papaverine caused rapid vasodilatation in the constricted areas.

When cerebral infarction occurs, the risk of hemorrhage is markedly increased in the presence of hypertension. Stimuli producing arteriolar reactivity in opposite directions are operating in this situation. Ischemia promotes vasodilation of anastomotic vessels, while the excessive intraluminal arterial pressure would elicit vasoconstriction. The net effect is vasodilatation with delivery of blood to the ischemic area under high pressure.

The brain edema that complicates accelerating hypertension may further compromise the cerebral circulation because the arterioles collapse when their intraluminal pressure falls below a critical closing pressure.

The hypertensive patient can present with a variety of neurologic signs and symptoms which range from minor to catastrophic. The frequency and pathophysiology of the headache associated with arterial hypertension is described in Chapter 4 (Headache). The small central cerebral infarct previously discussed may produce only minimal symptoms. Such infarcts are often not clearly discernible to either patient or physician.

Minor symptoms could conceivably follow leakage from a cerebral microaneurysm. Russell found suggestive histological evidence of hemorrhage into the areas immediately adjacent to aneurysms. Slit-like hemorrhages are also seen frequently in hypertensive brains without a history of stroke. Their origin is thought to be from rupture of a small vessel, but leakage from a microaneurysm has not been excluded.

Typical infarction is more frequent and tends to occur at an earlier age in the hypertensive patient. The classical picture of massive intracerebral hemorrhage is that of a sudden catastrophic event with rapid onset of coma. In such instances, large clinical studies show hypertension to be present in eighty to ninety-five per cent. Left ventricular hypertrophy is present in a similar frequency. Usually, normal activities have immediately preceded the hemorrhage. This is in contrast to ischemic cerebral infarction which typically occurs during the sleeping hours.

As the malignant phase of hypertension becomes established, cerebrovascular disturbances are more frequent, and the symptomatology more varied. Clarke and Murphy studied the neurological manifestations in a large series of patients with histological evidence of malignant hypertension.[52] Almost forty per cent had one or more of the following:

Acute brain damage in the form of hemorrhage or ischemia
Mental disturbance
Generalized or focal convulsions
Cranial nerve palsies
Dizziness or giddy feeling
Failing vision.

A true encephalopathy was rare. The neurological signs were frequently accompanied by elevated cerebrospinal fluid pressures and increased cerebrospinal fluid protein. Headaches, though of increasing severity in the malignant phase, did not correlate with the presence of other neurological symptoms. In a significant number, a neurological complaint announced the presence of the malignant phase. Jefferson noted frequent disturbances of gait and abnormalities of the pupils or ocular movements in patients with hypertensive cerebrovascular disease.[53] Many of his patients were originally suspected of having intracranial tumor before the correct etiology became apparent.

Focal areas of brain softening appear to be the underlying cause in the majority of cases with focal convulsions, mental deterioration, and cranial nerve palsies. The threshold for convulsive activity is said to be lowered by concomitant renal failure, which is often present. The visual impairment is attributable in almost all cases to papilledema or retinal pathology.

Hypertensive encephalopathy is a most dramatic acute or sub-acute disorder precipitated by a rise in arterial pressure that usually, but not always, reaches extremely high levels. The CBF is measurably decreased, and CVR reaches some of the highest recorded values.

The clinical manifestations include the following signs:

Severe headaches often accompanied by nausea and vomiting

Convulsions

Transient periods of mental confusion

Stupor sometimes progressing to coma

Impairment of vision.

Other evanescent focal neurological signs including cranial nerve palsies and even aphasias may be present.

These signs and symptoms cannot be ascribed to a lesion of a single cerebral artery. It is generally agreed that the clinical picture is induced by both focal and generalized ischemia caused by varying amounts of cerebral edema, necrotizing arteriolitis, small infarcts, and petechial hemorrhages. Though not proved in the human, it is thought that exaggerated arteriolar spasm plays a prominent role in the pathogenesis. Thus, symptoms and signs can rapidly abate with effective hypotensive therapy.

A clinical picture simulating encephalopathy can be produced in a hypertensive patient with injudicious hypotensive therapy.[54] Symptoms may be abolished by restoration of the cerebral blood flow when blood pressure is allowed to rise.

Cerebrovascular *consequences* of arterial hypertension have been discussed in some detail. However, there exists a diverse group of central nervous system disturbances in which hypertension appears as a *result* of direct or secondary stimulation of the vasomotor apparatus.[55]

Cortical (frontal lobes, especially), subcortical and hypothalamic stimulation can induce transient hypertension through a hypothalamic outflow to the medullary vasomotor center.

If pressure is applied to the dura mater of the intact brain so as to increase intracranial pressure, a rapid increase in systemic arterial pressure ensues. Arterial hypertension sometimes accompanies brain tumor, meningitis, encephalitis, head trauma, brain abscess, or obstructing hydrocephalus. Ar-

terial hypertension occasionally complicates polyneuritis (Guillain-Barré) or poliomyelitis, especially the bulbar type. Here, the pressor response is generally thought to be a manifestation of hypoxia due to involvement of the respiratory musculature, because the blood pressure returns to normal with mechanical pulmonary ventilation.

Some investigators have studied extensively the relationship between essential arterial hypertension and blood flow in the vertebral arteries determined at autopsy. They claim that an inverse relationship exists and speculate that brainstem ischemia precipitates the hypertension.

REFERENCES

1. Christy, N. P. (ed.): Recent advances in hypertension, Amer. J. Med. 39:616–645, 1965.
2. Green, H. D.: Circulatory system, physical principles, *in* Glasser, O. (ed.): Medical Physics, vol. 2, Chicago, Yr. Bk. Pub., 1950.
2a. Wurtman, R.: Catecholamines, New Eng. J. Med. 273:637, 693, 746, 1965.
3. Moorehead, E. L., Caldwell, J. R., Kelly, A. R., and Moracps, A. R.: Diagnosis of pheochromocytoma, J.A.M.A. 196:1107, 1966.
4. Spengel, G., Bleicher, S. J., and Ertel, N. H.: Carbohydrate and fat metabolism in patients with pheochromocytoma, New Eng. J. Med. 278:803, 1968.
5. Halpem, M., and Currarino, G.: Vascular lesions causing hypertension in neurofibromatosis, New Eng. J. Med. 273:248, 1965.
6. Scholz, D. A., Sprague, R. G., and Kernohan, J. W.: Cardiovascular and renal complications of Cushing's syndrome, New Eng. J. Med. 256:833, 1957.
7. Conn, J. W.: Aldosteronism and hypertension, Arch. Int. Med. 107:813, 1961.
8. Steinberg, A. D.: Myxedema and coronary artery disease, Ann. Int. Med. 68:338, 1968.
9. March, H. W., Hultgren, H. N., and Gerbode, F.: Immediate and remote effects of resection on the hypertension in coarctation of the aorta, Brit. Heart J. 22:361, 1960.
10. Koster, M., and David, G. K.: Reversible severe hypertension due to licorice, New Eng. J. Med. 278:1381, 1968.
11. Weiss, S., and Parker, F.: Pyelonephritis, its relationship to vascular lesions and to arterial hypertension, Medicine (Balt.) 18:222, 1939.
12. Merriam, J. C., Sommers, S. C., and Smithwick, R. H.: Clinico-pathologic correlation of renal biopsies in hypertension with pyelonephritis, Circulation 17:243, 1958.
13. Heptinsall, R. H.: Pathology of the Kidney, Boston, Little, Brown & Co., 1966.
14. DeFazio, V., Christensen, R. C., Regan, T. S., Baer, L. S., Morita, V., and Hellenis, H. K.: Circulatory changes in acute glomerulonephritis, Circulation 20:190, 1959.

15. Starney, T. A.: Renovascular hypertension, Amer. J. Med. 38:829, 1965.
16. DeChamplain, J., Genest, J., Veyratt, R., and Boucher, R.: Factors controlling renin in man, Arch. Intern. Med. 117:355, 1967.
17. Fitz, A.: Renal venous renin determinations in the diagnosis of surgically correctable hypertension, Circulation 361:942, 1967.
18. Slaton, P., and Biglieri, E.: Hypertension and hyperaldosteronism of renal and adrenal origin, Amer. J. Med. 38:324, 1965.
19. McCormack, L. S., Poutasse, E. F., Meaney, T. F., Note, T. J., and Dustan, H. I.: A pathologic arteriographic correlation of renal arterial disease, Amer. Heart J. 72:188, 1966.
20. Muirhead, E. F., Brooks, B., Kosinski, M., Daurets, E. G., and Heirman, J. W.: Renomedullary antihypertensive principle in renal hypertension, J. Lab. and Clin. Med. 67:778, 1966.
21. Page, I. H., and McCubbin, J. W.: Renal Hypertension, Chicago, Year Book Publishers, 1968.
22. Short, D.: Morphology of the intestinal arterioles in chronic human hypertension, Brit. Heart J. 28:184, 1966.
23. McCormack, L. J.: Vascular changes in hypertension, Med. Clin. N. Amer. 45:247, 1961.
24. Meerson, F. Z.: Compensatory hyperfunction of the heart and cardiac insufficiency, Circ. Res. 10:250, 1962.
25. Griggs, D. M.: Pathophysiology and biochemistry of end stage hypertensive heart disease, Amer. J. Cardiol. 17:621, 1966.
26. Becker, B., and Ley, A.: Retinal arteriosclerosis, Blumenthal, H. T. (ed.): Cowdry's Atherosclerosis, Springfield, Charles C Thomas, 1967.
27. Dollery, C. T., Henkind, P., Paterson, J. W., Ramalho, P. S., and Hill, D. W.: Ophthalmoscopic and circulatory changes in focal retinal ischemia, Brit. J. Ophthal. 50:285, 1966.
28. Ramalho, P. S., and Dollery, C. T.: Hypertensive retinopathy—caliber changes in retinal blood vessels following blood pressure reduction and inhalation of oxygen, Circulation 37:580, 1968.
29. Duke-Elder, S., and Dobree, J. H.: System of Ophthalmology, Vol. 10, Diseases of the Retina, St. Louis, Mosby, 1967.
30. Leishman, R.: The eye in general vascular disease: Hypertension and arteriosclerosis, Brit. J. Ophthal. 41:641, 1957.
31. Byrom, F. B.: The nature of malignancy in hypertensive disease—evidence from the retina of the rat, Lancet 1:516, 1963.
32. Nicholls, J.: The fundus oculi in hypertension an arteriosclerosis, Canad. M.A.J. 90:581, 1964.
33. Wendland, J. P.: Retinal arteriolosclerosis in age, essential hypertension, and diabetes mellitus, Trans. Amer. Ophthal. Soc. 64:735, 1966.
34. Shelburne, S. A.: Hypertensive Retinal Disease, New York, Grune & Stratton, 1965.
35. Moore, R. F.: The retinitis of arteriosclerosis, and its relations to renal retinitis and to cerebral vascular disease, Quart. J. Med. 10:29, 1917.
36. Ashton, N., and Harry, J.: The pathology of cotton-wool spots and cytoid bodies in hypertensive retinopathy and other diseases, Trans. Ophthal. Soc. U. K. 83:91, 1963.
37. Dollery, C. T.: Fluorescence retinal photography in Sorsby, A. (ed.): Modern Trends in Ophthalmology, 4th series, New York, Appleton-Century-Crofts, 1967.
38. Hodge, J. V., and Dollery, C. T.: Retinal soft exudates—A clinical study by colour and fluorescence photography, Quart. J. Med. 33:117, 1964.
39. Harry, J., and Ashton, N.: The pathology of hypertensive retinopathy, Trans. Ophthal. Soc. U. K. 83:71, 1963.
40. Dollery, C. T., Mailer, C. M., and Hodge, J. V.: Studies by fluorescence photography of papilledema in malignant hypertension, J. Neurol. Neurosurg. Psychiat. 28:241, 1965.
41. Bauer, R. B.: Evaluation of the stroke patient with respect to associated diseases, in Fields, W., and Spencer, W. (eds.), Stroke Rehabilitation; Basic Concepts and Research Trends, St. Louis, Warren H. Green, Inc., 1967.
42. Byrom, F. B.: The pathogenesis of hypertensive encephalopathy and its relation to the malignant phase of hypertension, Lancet 2:201, 1954.
43. Fields, W., and Spencer, W. (eds.): Stroke Rehabilitation; Basic Concepts and Research Trends, St. Louis, Warren H. Green, Inc., 1967.
44. Fisher, C. M.: Lacunes: Small, deep cerebral infarcts, Neurology 15:774, 1965.
45. Prineas, J., and Marshall, J.: Hypertension and cerebral infarction, Brit. Med. J. 1:14, 1966.
46. Russell, R.: Observations on intracranial aneurysms, Brain 86:425, 1963.
47. Cole, F. M., and Yates, P.: Intracerebral microaneurysms and small cerebrovascular lesions, Brain 90:759, 1967.
48. McHenry, L. C.: Cerebral blood flow studies in cerebrovascular disease, Arch. Intern. Med. 117:546, 1966.
49. Meyer, J. S., and Gilroy, J.: Regulation and adjustment of the cerebral circulation, Dis. Chest 53:30, 1968.
50. Montgomery, B. M.: The basilar artery hypertensive syndrome, Arch. Intern. Med. 108:559, 1961.
50a. Jellinck, E. H., Painter, M., Prineas, J., and Russell, R.: Hypertensive encephalopathy with cortical disorders of vision, Quart. J. Med. 33:239, 1964.
51. Mchedlishvili, G. I.: Vascular mechanisms pertaining to the intrinsic regulation of the cerebral circulation, Circulation 30:597, 1964.
51a. Rodda, R., and Denny-Brown, D.: The cerebral arterioles in experimental hypertension, Amer. J. Path. 49:53, 365, 1966.

52. Clarke, E., and Murphy, E.: Neurological manifestations of malignant hypertension, Brit. Med. J. 2:1319, 1956.

53. Jefferson, A.: Hypertensive cerebral vascular disease and intracranial tumor, Quart. J. Med. 24:245, 1955.

54. Ziegler, D. K., Zosa, A., and Zileli, T.: Hypertensive encephalopathy, A.M.A., Arch. Neurol. 12:472, 1965.

55. Tyler, H. R., and Dawson, D.: Hypertension and its relation to the nervous system, Ann. Int. Med. 55:681, 1961.

56. Lee, J. B.: Hypertension, natriuresis, and the renal prostaglandins, Ann. Int. Med. 70:1033, 1969.

57. Shapiro, A. P.: Hypertension in renal parenchymal disease, Disease-a-Month monograph, Chicago, Yr. Bk. Pub., Sept., 1969.

16

Palpitation and Tachycardia

EDWARD MASSIE

PALPITATION

The word palpitation is a derivative of the Latin *palpitare*, which means to throb. Palpitation is usually a less direful heart symptom than pain and dyspnea and is extremely common. It consists of an unpleasant sensation of the heart's action, whether slow or fast, regular or irregular. It is more frequently the result of the less important disturbances of cardiac rhythm, namely, premature beats and atrial paroxysmal tachycardia, or of forceful regular heart action, either rapid or slow, resulting from effort, excitement, toxins (as from tobacco, caffeine, or alcohol), or infection. Minor degrees of disturbance more easily produce palpitation if the subject is a nervously sensitive person. Less frequently it may be caused by a more important disorder of heart rhythm such as atrial fibrillation, atrial flutter, or venticular paroxysmal tachycardia.

It should be emphasized that palpitation and tachycardia often do not indicate a primary physical disorder but rather a psychic disturbance. They are the most important symptoms of cardiac neurosis. If such symptoms are analyzed critically it is seen that subjectively they result in what is termed heart consciousness and that they may be only manifestations of enhanced normal function. Various associated symptoms sometimes occur which are largely the result of more appreciative sensibilities. It is well-known that when a person becomes nervously exhausted or hyperirritable his sense of values and judgment are often somewhat distorted, especially in matters concerned with his physical and psychic well-being. If at such a time the patient has occasion to lift some object or walk up an incline, he may instantly notice rapid and forceful beating of his heart. This symptom usually disappears rapidly, but if similar experiences are repeated, he may become convinced that something serious has happened to his heart. The patient's nervous condition has brought about sufficient introspection, anxiety, and uncertainty to produce an increase of cardiac irritability and a decrease of the threshold at which palpitation, tachycardia, and the associated symptoms of cardiac neurosis become evident. Often the threshold of consciousness of the heart's action is so lowered that palpitation may be complained of when the rate and the rhythm are perfectly normal.

Palpitation is one of the most characteristic symptoms of neurocirculatory asthenia. In this condition it results, along with other symptoms of the disease, probably from an imbalance of the autonomic nervous system. Such an imbalance may be more or less constant in certain nervously hypersensitive individuals, but may also be precipitated in relatively normal persons by emotional or physical upsets acting reflexly on the autonomic nervous system.

The functional aspect of the symptom complex of palpitation was beautifully described in 1836 by John C. Williams* of Edinburgh who wrote a book on "Practical Observations on Nervous and Sympathetic Palpitation of the Heart, Particularly As Dis-

* Quoted in the third edition of "Heart Disease" by Dr. Paul D. White.

tinguished from Palpitation the Result of Organic Disease." He criticized the practice, usually followed up to that time, of attributing functional derangement of the heart to true heart disease. He taught that palpitation was

> frequently, by a careless observer, regarded as symptomatic of some serious organic or structural change being established either in the covering of the heart, its muscular texture, or in some of its natural valvular appurtenances. A careful and deliberate inquiry, however, will, in the generality of cases, enable us to strip them of their apparent obscurity and danger and reduce them to their place in nosological arrangement. Latterly there has been too great a rage for tracing diseases almost exclusively to vascular derangement. I deprecate this, because I am convinced of the increasing influence of the nervous system, both in health and in disease. A deservedly popular writer on medicine of the present day says, "The longer we live, the more we see; and the deeper we study, so much the more we shall become convinced, that not only are the primary impressions of morbific causes sustained by the sentient system of the human fabric, but it is here the primary morbid movements first begin, and are thence propagated to the vascular apparatus, which from that movement reacts upon, and is again influenced by the nervous system. No man, I am satisfied, can ever be a sound Pathologist, or a judicious practitioner, who devotes his attention to one of these systems in preference or to the exclusion of the other; through life they are perpetually acting, and inseparably linked together."

Williams goes on to quote a Dr. Baille as follows:

> There are in truth few phenomena which puzzle, perplex, and lead to error the inexperienced (and sometimes the experienced) practitioner, so much as inordinate action of the heart. He sees, or thinks he sees, some terrible cause for this tumult in the central organ of the circulation and frames his portentous diagnosis and prognosis accordingly. In the pride of his penetration he renders miserable for the time the friends and by his direful countenance damps the spirits of his patient. But ultimate recovery not seldom disappoints his fears and the Physician is mortified at his own success.

Neurocirculatory Asthenia. Palpitation is one of the most characteristic symptoms of neurocirculatory asthenia. This condition, first described during our Civil War, was very prevalent in World War I and again in World War II; therefore, it certainly merits detailed discussion. Among the current synonyms for this disease are "effort syndrome," "cardiac neurosis," "disorderly action of the heart," "soldier's heart," and "Da Costa's syndrome." The last term is derived from Da Costa's classical article on the irritable heart, published in 1871 and based upon his experiences as surgeon in the Northern armies in the Civil War. The incidence of this disease has since been found to increase sharply in wartime and to vary greatly from only a few cases among soldiers in military training to a considerable number under the strain and the hardship of combat. Although this condition came into prominence in World War I, it appears to have been even more of a problem in World War II.

Neurocirculatory asthenia of a pronounced degree is not too common in civilian life, primarily because those likely to develop the condition are usually able to avoid the factors of effort and nervous strain that help precipitate the undesirable symptoms. There is, however, no way to determine its frequency, because in the slight, and much more commonly unrecognized form, it is not likely to be recorded as a specific diagnosis. As a matter of fact, White and his associates were able to study a group of patients who had what was diagnosed in Army hospitals as neurocirculatory asthenia, and listed their various symptoms. Then, when a similar survey was made of the symptoms of patients on whom the diagnosis of *anxiety neurosis* had been made in the psychiatric wards, the similarity in symptoms was striking. Thus, it would seem that two patients with the same complaints and symptoms might have different diagnoses, depending entirely upon whether they were seen by a psychiatrist or an internist.

CLINICALLY neurocirculatory asthenia is characterized by such prominent symptoms as palpitation, chest pain, weakness, dyspnea, sighing respiration, sweating, tremulousness, dizziness, nervousness, headache and faintness, all of which are aggravated by excitement or effort and accompany or follow periods of anxiety, nervousness, or physical strain and infection. This symptom complex may occur as the only manifestation of illness or it may be a complication of many diseases, including structural disease of the heart or of other organ systems. The disease appears to be a result of fundamental imbalance of the autonomic nervous system. Such imbalance may be more or less constant in certain nervously hypersensitive or constitutionally inferior individuals, but may also occur in relatively normal persons after psychic or physical upsets which act reflexly on the autonomic nervous system. The patient may be acutely aware of the most minor variations in the heart rhythm or rate. Palpitation may be so severe as a result of an occasional extrasystole or even mild exertion that the patient becomes more or less incapacitated. In contrast with the characteristic symptoms listed above, there are no prominent physical signs in neurocirculatory asthenia. Tachycardia is often present, although the cardiac rate may be normal when mental and physical rest are established— only to increase again with slight exertion or with a disturbing thought. Such physical findings as cold, moist hands, excessive perspiration, tremor of the fingers, dermatographism and variable and slightly elevated blood pressure are frequently encountered. The heart itself, in the great majority of cases, is structurally normal and shows no significant murmurs. In addition, no characteristic laboratory findings have been identified in neurocirculatory asthenia.

Relationship of Palpitation to Organic Heart Disease. Persons with normal hearts may complain of palpitation whenever the force or the rate of the cardiac beat is increased to more than a moderate degree. On the other hand, patients with actual cardiac disorders as a rule are fortunately somewhat less sensitive than normal individuals to the force and the rate of the cardiac beat. Perhaps this is a result in part of habituation, so that even in the presence of irregular rhythms or of undue increases in rate, the abnormal stimuli do not penetrate the patient's consciousness and the reflex phenomena at the basis of palpitation are not produced. Atrial fibrillation often is present when the patient has no sensation of any heart disorder. Occasionally such patients temporarily have palpitation after restoration to normal rhythm, although none was experienced when atrial fibrillation was present. In cardiac decompensation with profound disturbances of rate and rhythm, palpitation is not infrequently absent even when dyspnea and orthopnea are severe.

Quite frequently extrasystoles are discovered of which the patient has no knowledge. Consciousness of an extrasystole is apt to be the awareness of a sudden premature forceful beat followed by a longer than usual pause, or, sometimes, there is chiefly perception of the hard post-extrasystolic contraction. In contrast, patients with aortic valve disease including the lesions of stenosis or insufficiency, in which the cardiac beat may be extremely forceful and heaving, usually experience no palpitation. Sometimes the sensations that develop from benign extrasystoles can be very disturbing, as well as peculiar and distinctive, and it is well to be familiar with them since the description of the symptoms given by the patient may establish the diagnosis without further examination. The sensations are described in such varied ways as "a flop of the heart," "twisting or skipping of the heart," "sinking or fading away of the heart," "a sudden lump or choking feeling in the throat," "the heart turns a somersault" and "like the sensation of a fish turning in water." There may be fleeting lightheadedness or transient pain in the precordial or substernal area. These disturbances usually appear when the patient is relaxing or about ready to fall asleep, since at this time he is apt to become more conscious of any sensation occurring inside his body and since at rest the heart rate is slower and the opportunity is greater during the longer diastolic pauses for premature beats to arise. The sensations are generally absent while the patient is active, walking or busily engaged in his affairs.

Although it has been said repeatedly that extrasystoles are usually of no serious significance and that normal people may have them, it was the animal experiments by Beattie and Brow which have made it possible to ascribe a definite neurogenic origin to them. They showed that, if certain nerve tracts coming from the hypothalamic region were cut in the animals with experimentally produced extrasystoles, the irregularity disappeared. They also found that, if these tracts were cut beforehand, the extrasystoles could not be produced by the same technic that always produced them in animals not subjected to this treatment. Thus it appears that there is a center in the brain that can initiate, or that is ultimately connected with, the formation of premature heart beats. This demonstration points to a structural neurogenic basis for conditions that have long been regarded as functional.

Relationship of Palpitation to Tachycardia. Palpitation, as previously stated, is a normal sensation when the force of the heart beat and its rate are considerably elevated, and the subject may not only say he "feels his heart pounding" but that it is beating "too hard," "too fast," or both. Slight exertion in normal persons may cause only a little shortness of breath. When the activity is a little more strenuous, one is apt to become aware of the thumping of the heart against the chest wall. After rest the thumping sensation may persist for a while after the rate has returned to normal, showing that one may be aware of a "harder beat" (greater systolic contraction and cardiac output) when the rate is not increased. Persistence of tachycardia with greater cardiac activity beyond a normal or physiologic range of time suggests impaired cardiac reserve. Many of the physical fitness tests employed by the armed services are based upon accurate, graded observations of these phenomena in response to standard amounts of muscular effort.

Fortunately, persistent tachycardia is usually not accompanied by continual palpitation, or at least not to the degree one might expect. Patients with cardiac decompensation with pulse rates of over 100 per minute even at rest may have little or no palpitation. Although palpitation is a common symptom in thyrotoxicosis there is often comparatively little consciousness of heart action. Persons with chronic infections resulting in long-standing fever and tachycardia often have no palpitation in spite of pulse rates that may be very rapid. It seems that in many of these instances physiologic readjustment takes place so that the subject becomes accustomed to the greater rate and often the greater force of the cardiac contraction. A *sudden* alteration in rate or rhythm or in the force of the beat is apt to be perceived promptly whether the heart is normal or diseased. This is true whether the change is toward a slower, more orderly beat or toward rapid, irregular contraction. Static conditions, even though quite abnormal, may not be accompanied by palpitation.

TACHYCARDIA

The term tachycardia is derived from the Greek words meaning quick and heart. Rapid action of the heart is the most common and obvious cardiac manifestation; accordingly, it is often the first to be discovered by the patient himself and by the physician. The rate of the heart beat is the expression of the property of rhythmicity (automaticity) inherent in all parts of the heart muscle, but most highly developed in the specialized muscle cells that constitute the normal pacemaker. This pacemaker in the right atrium can keep the heart beating rhythmically independently of all extracardiac factors, as, for example, in the excised heart. However, in the body this inherent rhythm is always being modified. A great number of physiologic control mechanisms are capable of influencing the rate of the heartbeat. Practically all of these can be included under two headings, *chemical control* and *nervous control*.

Chemical control of the heart is effected by certain ions and also by the more complex substances, hormones, secreted by the endocrine glands. The integrity of the living cell is dependent on a constant osmotic pressure of the surrounding extracellular fluid which the body guards by various homeostatic mechanisms. The concentration of the *sodium* ion in extracellular fluid is responsible for almost all of the osmotic pressure due to cations, and its constancy may be regarded as a measure of the constancy of the osmotic pressure. When the concentration of sodium in the blood increases, the posterior pituitary gland is stimulated to secrete the antidiuretic hormone, water is retained by the kidney, and the normal concentration of sodium and the normal osmotic pressure are restored. It is assumed that this is the general manner in which the primary abnormal retention of sodium leads also to abnormal retention of water in congestive failure. Other mechanisms probably also are concerned in the regulation of water balance in congestive failure, because water may be retained even when the sodium ion is below normal and the extracellular fluid is hypotonic.

Potassium is the predominant intracellular electrolyte. A normal concentration of intracellular and extracellular potassium is essential for normal myocardial contraction. In the isolated heart, potassium antagonizes the tendency of calcium to cause systolic standstill (calcium rigor). When present in excess, potassium prolongs diastole and may cause complete inhibition with arrest of the heart. Various observations have suggested an intimate relationship between the action of the potassium ion and the action of acetyl choline, the humoral effector agent produced by vagal stimulation. Potassium may participate in nerve stimulation and muscular contraction by altering cell permeability. Changes in the concentration of potassium may produce clinical symptoms because of impairment of muscular activity and/or

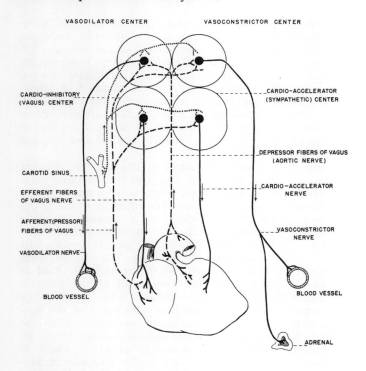

VASODILATOR CENTER   VASOCONSTRICTOR CENTER

CARDIO-INHIBITORY
(VAGUS) CENTER

CARDIO-ACCELERATOR
(SYMPATHETIC) CENTER

DEPRESSOR FIBERS OF VAGUS
(AORTIC NERVE)

CAROTID SINUS

CARDIO-ACCELERATOR
NERVE

EFFERENT FIBERS
OF VAGUS NERVE

AFFERENT(PRESSOR)
FIBERS OF VAGUS

VASOCONSTRICTOR
NERVE

VASODILATOR NERVE

BLOOD VESSEL

BLOOD VESSEL

ADRENAL

FIG. 16-1. Diagrammatic representation of the cardiovascular reflex mechanisms. Afferent vagal fibers are shown by broken lines; sinus nerve fibers, by a dotted line; efferent fibers to the heart and to the blood vessels, by a continuous line. The afferent fibers are represented as causing reciprocal effects upon the medullary centers. (Best, C. H., and Taylor, N. B.: The Physiologic Basis of Medical Practice, ed. 8, Baltimore, Williams & Wilkins, 1968)

changes in the cardiac mechanism and in the electrocardiogram. *Calcium* ions (with sodium and potassium) are essential to proper cardiac contraction. The perfused isolated heart will stop in diastole if there is no calcium; an excess of calcium causes systolic arrest (calcium rigor). Like digitalis, calcium increases systolic contraction. Fear of a dangerous potentiating effect is a basis for the purported contraindication to the injection of calcium in digitalized patients. Injected *parathormone* produces effects that are somewhat similar to those of calcium: an early increase in heart rate, followed by slowing and by cardiac arrhythmia characterized by premature beats and shifting of the pacemaker. The *adrenal* gland, when stimulated by its sympathetic nerve supply, secretes a mixture containing 80 per cent *l*-epinephrine and 20 per cent norepinephrine. The direct effect of *l*-epinephrine on strips of myocardium is to increase the speed, vigor, and power of myocardial contraction and to produce acceleration of the heart by acting on the pacemaker. In men, norepinephrine introduced into the bloodstream is reported to have a powerful vasoconstrictor effect on the peripheral vascular system but less effect on myocardial contraction. Increased con-

tractile properties of the myocardium are noted, but the heart rate slows.

The circulatory response to *hyperthyroidism* resembles that of a normal person to strenuous exercise. The cardiac impulse is diffuse and forceful. The heart is accelerated. There is good evidence that the tachycardia from excess thyroid hormone (*thyroxin*) represents a direct effect on the pacemaker activity of the myocardium. Hyperthyroidism imposes a heavy load on the myocardium, which must put out more useful work to supply the augmented metabolic requirement of the body while the efficiency of its contraction is diminished by tachycardia and by direct action of thyroid hormone on the myocardial fibers. When a patient with hyperthyroidism undertakes physical exertion, the circulatory reaction is exaggerated when compared to that of normal individuals performing the same task. In young persons the heart may compensate for this excessive load, but in older individuals cardiovascular reserves may become exhausted and heart failure supervenes. If coronary sclerosis is present, angina pectoris may become evident. Atrial fibrillation also is likely to occur because of increased myocardial irritability. *Hypothryoidism* with its decrease in thyroxin may result from spontaneous thyroid atrophy, surgical excision of thyroid tissue or as the result of thyroid irradiation. It principal cardiac effect is the development of a slow heart rate. The thyroid hormones act primarily and directly upon the heart itself and may also affect it through the mediation of its autonomic nerve supply. The hormone control of the heart comes into play slowly, after a significant latent period following the original stimulus initiating the cardiac response. In contrast, cardiac responses evoked by nervous influences usually occur promptly, the latent period between the stimulus and the effect being short. Furthermore, the response by way of the nervous system is of relatively short duration, the effect disappearing promptly when the stimulus ceases, whereas effects produced by hormones tend to persist, outlasting the stimulus for some time.

Nervous control of the heart is effected through the vagus and the sympathetic nerves. Figure 16-1 is a diagrammatic representation of the cardiovascular reflex mechanisms. The vagus may be considered to be the more important of the two nerves. It is tonically active at all times and exerts a continuous restraining influence upon the heart, keeping it beating at a slower rate than that which it would have if its intrinsic pacemaker, the sino-atrial node, were unchecked. This normal vagus tone is quite strong, and its removal leads to a marked and prompt increase in heart rate. Such removal or inhibition of the normal vagus tone is largely responsible for the tachycardia in nearly all of the clinical conditions associated with acceleration of the heart. Viewing the vagus nerve as the efferent limb of a reflex arc and the vagus center in the medulla as the center of the arc, the question arises as to what are the paths of the afferent impulses that reach the center and, by stimulating it, cause the heart to beat slower or, by inhibiting it, cause the heart to beat faster. Generally speaking, the potential afferent pathways capable of affecting the vagus center include all the afferent nerve fibers in the body. This concept means that all types of sensation from all parts of the body can affect the heart rate via the vagus center, although they may or may not do so according to circumstances. All afferent nerve impulses are conducted into some part of the central nervous system (spinal cord or brain), and, once within it, there is at least the possibility of

a pathway to every center within the central nervous system. The actual flow of impulses from afferent to efferent paths is regulated by the very complex functional organization of the central nervous system. Thus, sudden distraction by a loud noise (8th cranial nerve) or immersion in hot water (cutaneous nerves) may precipitate a change in pulse rate (vagus nerve) by this reflex mechanism. Obviously not every type or intensity of sensation is uniformly potent in this respect, and the cardiac rate is not continuously interfered with by the usual sensations. Afferent impulses from certain regions are especially predominant in influencing the heart rate.

It is not surprising that the more important afferent impulses for controlling the heart arise in portions of the circulatory system itself, especially those regions from which the heart receives and into which it discharges the blood. On the venous or receiving end, the Bainbridge reflex causes acceleration of the heart when the venous return is so excessive that it overdistends the *right atrium*. The sensory endings of this reflex arc are in the right atrium and the adjacent portions of the venae cavae and are stimulated by increased tension. The resultant nerve impulses course along the afferent fibers in the vagus and *inhibit the vagus center* so that the heart beats faster, thus tending to raise the heart output to balance the inflow.

On the arterial side is the *depressor reflex*, whose afferent fibers arise from the root and the arch of the aorta and run to the medulla within the vagus nerve. The initiating stimulus for these fibers is *tension* within the aorta; the higher the tension, the greater the stimulus. With elevation in the aortic pressure, afferent impulses ascend to and *stimulate the vagus center* so that the heart beats more slowly, and this action tends to reduce the blood pressure to its proper level. The reverse occurs also, in that lowered aortic pressure gives rise to afferent nerve impulses that inhibit the vagus center and so accelerate the heart by diminishing the vagus tone. A similar depressor reflex, dependent primarily upon the pressure within the carotid artery for its activity, has its afferent nerve endings in the *carotid sinus*, which is a specially innervated part of the arteries and the adjacent tissues located at the bifurcation of the common carotid artery. The afferent fibers from the carotid sinus reach the medulla by way of the glossopharyngeal and the vagus nerves and the sympathetic trunk. The initiating stimulus is either increased or decreased intracarotid pressure, tending to slow or accelerate the heart by affecting the vagus center in a similar fashion to the aortic depressor fibers already described. The highly developed nerve endings located in the *carotid body*, which is situated at the bifurcation of the common carotid artery, are *chemoreceptors* and are sensitive to oxygen lack and carbon dioxide excess. When either of these conditions is present, impulses from the carotid body aid in accelerating the heart.

The higher centers of the brain itself also may be considered to be one of the special regions for initiating afferent impulses for cardiac control, since *emotion* may cause nerve impulses to descend to the medulla where they may affect the vagus center sufficiently to cause a change in heart rate. *Increased intracranial pressure* usually is associated with slowing of the heart, brought about by overstimulation of the vagus center. The stimulation may be both due to direct mechanical effect on the vagus center cells in the medulla and to ischemia of the center from the adverse effect of the pressure upon its blood supply. Furthermore, *ischemia*, when not too severe, stimulates practically all of the medullary centers, including the vasomotor centers; therefore, increased intracranial pressure causes peripheral constriction and consequent elevation of blood pressure. The vascular hypertension thus produced in turn acts upon the aorta and the carotid sinus so as to stimulate the depressor reflexes already described and is therefore a secondary reason for cardiac slowing in increased intracranial tension.

The sympathetic and the vagus centers in the medulla together form a functional unit referred to as the *cardiac center*. The quantity and the quality of the blood reaching this center affect the heart rate. Slight hypoxia of the cardiac center causes increased cardiac rate, as does also a small excess of carbon dioxide; a high degree of oxygen lack causes slowing of the heart, and a large excess of carbon dioxide may lead to heart block. These effects occur by means of efferent impulses coursing along the vagus, or the sympathetic nerves, or both. Increased temperature of the blood going to the center increases cardiac rate. Increased intracranial tension from any local cause tends to decrease the blood flow to the cardiac center and results in heart acceleration.

The sympathetic nerve control of the heart is subordinate to the vagus control because under normal resting conditions it is quite inactive and upon stimulation the acceleration of the heart begins only after a definite latent period and develops gradually. If the normal sympathetic accelerating influence is entirely removed, the resultant cardiac slowing is usually negligible. In addition, the latency of the response upon stimulation of the sympathetic trunk renders it relatively ineffective when there is need of prompt increase in the activity of the heart. However, since its effect manifests itself later than that wrought by the vagus, it persists longer and so maintains the responses initiated via the vagus. Usually increased sympathetic tone simultaneously induces secretion of adrenalin, which further prolongs the acceleration of the heart. The sympathetic efferent nerve center is in the medulla. The afferent paths by which impulses may reach and affect it are identical with those already mentioned in connection with the vagus cardiac center. Similarly, the cardiovascular sensory areas of the right atrium, the root of the aorta, and the carotid sinus, which are related to vagus control, have an *analogously intimate relationship* with sympathetic control. Consequently, cardiac acceleration from an over-distended atrium, although predominantly brought about by inhibition of the vagus center, is partially produced by sympathetic nerve stimulation, and slowing of the heart by the vagus in the depressor reflex is enhanced by concomitant decrease in sympathetic tone. In most instances, however, the chief portion of the total response is effected through the vagus, and to a much lesser extent through the sympathetic.

Types of Tachycardia

The varieties and the causes of tachycardia are so numerous that a classification is necessary. The most common type of tachycardia is that originating in the sino-atrial node. This is called sino-atrial tachycardia or simply sinus tachycardia. Next in frequency is paroxysmal atrial tachycardia, followed by rapid heart action associated with atrial fibrillation and atrial flutter. A relatively rare, but more serious, form of tachycardia is that arising from the ventricles called ventricular tachycardia; this

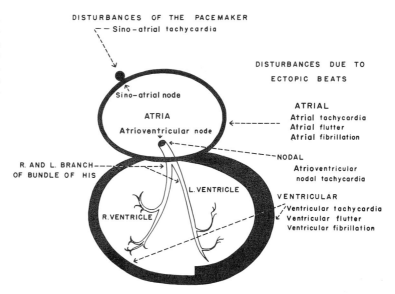

Fig. 16-2. Schematic diagram of arrhythmias associated with tachycardia. (Levine, S. A.: Clinical Electrocardiography, Oxford Loose-Leaf Medicine, vol. 2, New York, Oxford Univ. Press)

DISTURBANCES OF THE PACEMAKER
— Sino-atrial tachycardia

Sino-atrial node

ATRIA
Atrioventricular node

R. AND L. BRANCH
OF BUNDLE OF HIS

L. VENTRICLE

R. VENTRICLE

DISTURBANCES DUE TO
ECTOPIC BEATS

ATRIAL
Atrial tachycardia
Atrial flutter
Atrial fibrillation

NODAL
Atrioventricular
nodal tachycardia

VENTRICULAR
Ventricular tachycardia
Ventricular flutter
Ventricular fibrillation

may in turn predispose the heart to ventricular flutter and fibrillation. An infrequent form of paroxysmal tachycardia is that originating from the atrioventricular node. Figure 16-2 illustrates schematically the arrhythmias associated with tachycardia.

SINUS TACHYCARDIA

Sino-atrial tachycardia, sinus tachycardia, or simple tachycardia, as it is otherwise known, is defined by Herrman as a "sustained increase in the heart rate beyond the normal limits of the individual." Usually a rate of 100 beats or more per minute in a person over the age of 18 years is evidence enough to justify a diagnosis of sinus tachycardia. Although there is a wide range of the normal pulse rate at rest, a rate of over 100 beats per minute in the heart of a normal resting adult is infrequent. In contrast, the upper range of normal in children is about 120, whereas in infants it is 150.

Etiology. Sino-atrial tachycardia occurs in persistent form in many healthy individuals and is found normally as a trait in certain families. Transient sinus tachycardia is of daily occurrence in all individuals as a physiologic response to physical exertion, ingestion of food, emotion, pain, and the application of heat to the body. It is particularly apt to appear when alcohol, tobacco, coffee, or the like are used to excess. Caffeine, for example, acts by direct stimulation of the myocardium. Rarely, an individual will be found who can accelerate his pulse at will, and then usually because he has learned how to arouse an intense emotion. This ability has been used by malingerers to simulate heart disease. The effect is mediated through the sympathoadrenal system. Pathologic causes of sino-atrial tachycardia include especially *infections* and *fever;* the pulse rate in general rises about 9 beats per minute for each degree Fahrenheit of temperature elevation. This increase probably is partly due to the direct effect of the high temperature on the heart, because the beat of the excised heart has been shown to be accelerated by warming.

Another abnormal cause of tachycardia includes a group of noninfectious noxious disturbances, prominent among which is *thyrotoxicosis.* Thyroxin accelerates the heart beat by direct action on the heart muscle fibers and also, indirectly, by increasing the metabolic rate.

Another pathologic cause of tachycardia is *infarction* of some part of the body in a sufficiently large area to give rise to reactions with fever and often leukocytosis. *Shock* and *hemorrhage* usually produce tachycardia as a compensatory reflex reaction to the lowered blood pressure.

Certain *drugs*, particularly epinephrine (by direct effect on the myocardium and the conduction tissue), atropine (by blocking of vagal effects on the sino-atrial pacemaker), and the nitrites (through a carotid sinus reflex resulting in sympathoadrenal discharge), cause sinus tachycardia.

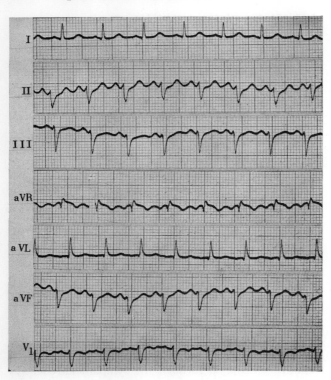

Fig. 16-3. Sinus tachycardia with a rate of 125 per minute. (Lipman and Massie: Clinical Scalar Electrocardiography, ed. 5, Chicago, Year Book Pub., 1965)

Episodes of *neurocirculatory asthenia* and *mental shock* often are associated with a rapid pulse. Sometimes the cause of the tachycardia cannot be definitely discovered.

The heart in *congestive failure* accelerates to a greater or less degree in an effort to maintain the volume of blood flow. Acceleration of beat, however, is not an intrinsic adaptation of the heart to increased work load, since, in the heart-lung preparation, accommodation to increased arterial resistance or greater venous return is accomplished without any change in the rate of the heart. It is not that the heart in such a preparation is unable to accelerate, because elevation in temperature is followed promptly by increase in rate. These observations on the isolated heart indicate that extrinsic mechanisms, nervous or chemical, are involved in the production of compensatory tachycardia in heart failure. Among the mechanisms that appear to be concerned are the Bainbridge and carotid sinus and aortic reflexes which have been discussed previously. It appears quite likely that, in the state of heart failure in which diminished cardiac output and elevated venous pressure are generally combined, these various reflexes are primarily responsible for for the production of tachycardia.

Symptoms. The symptoms displayed by an individual with sino-atrial tachycardia vary from little more than the objective sign of an increased pulse rate to a syndrome that may inhibit the normal activity of the patient. Palpitation is the most common of the symptoms encountered, although restlessness, agitation, apprehension, anxiety, and chest discomfort or pain also may be present, depending upon the symptom threshold and the nervous reactivity of the individual patient.

Diagnosis. As a rule, the diagnosis of sino-atrial tachycardia is obvious and clearly related to the exciting factor. The cardiac rhythm is usually regular, but shows fluctuations in rate in response to forced respiration and other physiologic stimuli, such as emotion and effort. In differentiating it from other forms of tachycardia, it should be remembered that sinus tachycardia has a gradual onset and a slight variation of the beat as compared with the abruptness and the marked regularity characterizing paroxysmal atrial or nodal tachycardia. Cases in which the increased pulse rate is due to psychogenic factors or an emotional imbalance generally exhibit a marked reduction in the pulse rate during sleep. Instances due to drug administration are easily singled out by a careful history. It would appear that many of the attacks called paroxysmal atrial tachycardia are really attacks of sinus tachycardia. Especially is this true when the heart rate is not above 150 to 160. The electrocardiographic findings in sinus tachycardia are illustrated in Figure 16-3.

Prognosis. The prognosis of sino-atrial tachycardia per se is good. In any given case it depends primarily on the fundamental cause of the tachycardia. In those instances where serious heart disease already is present, the myocardial or coronary reserve may be so limited that the tachycardia itself could precipitate heart failure.

PAROXYSMAL ATRIAL TACHYCARDIA

In this arrhythmia a rapid series of impulses originates in an ectopic focus in either atrium. This is the most frequent of the abnormal or ectopic tachycardias. Its incidence is impossible to determine with any degree of accuracy because many persons may have short paroxysms of this type of tachycardia lasting seconds or minutes that are not interpreted as such, either because they are not sufficiently troublesome to excite concern on the part of the person affected, or because there is no opportunity to obtain an electrocardiogram at the time of the paroxysms.

Mechanism. The mechanism of atrial tachycardia consists of a rapid and regular sequence of abnormal heart beats originating in the atrium either from a given point outside the normal pacemaker or as a type of movement re-entering the atrial muscle which in turn is recovering rapidly from its refractory stage. The site of origin of a paroxysm of atrial tachycardia may be in any part of the atrial musculature. The electrocardiographic picture resembles a series of premature atrial contractions occurring in quick succession. Electrocardiographically, the atrial complex differs from the normal P wave inasmuch as the origin of the impulse is abnormal and the course it takes through the atrium is likewise abnormal. The QRS complexes are similar in configuration to the QRS complexes of the basic mechanism unless aberration occurs. In such cases slurring, notching, or widening of the QRS associated with defective conduction is present.

Atrial tachycardia may be confused with nodal tachycardia, particularly when the P waves are not identifiable. The two conditions, in such instances, are frequently grouped together under the term supraventricular tachycardia. Difficulty at times may be encountered in differentiating slow paroxysmal atrial tachycardia from rapid sinus tachycardia. Paroxysmal atrial tachycardia has a rate which varies from 150 to 250 beats per minute.

Etiology. Paroxysmal atrial tachycardia may occur at any age, but it is rare in infancy. It is found more often in the absence of heart disease than in its presence; yet if we compare the relative incidence in normal persons and in cardiac patients we find a higher incidence in the cardiac patients. It is frequently associated with indigestion, overexertion, fatigue, excess use of tobacco, alcohol, or coffee. It may be psychogenic in origin and may start with a specific emotional reaction. It may be associated with various infections. Thyrotoxicosis should be suspected in every case until eliminated. Among the various forms of organic heart disease accompanied by paroxysmal atrial tachycardia, mitral stenosis probably has the highest incidence.

Symptoms. In most cases the patient is conscious of the disturbance of rhythm. The attack itself is instantaneous in onset and offset, and the patient is usually aware of this, describing it as coming on suddenly and stopping with a "thump." The patient complains of palpitation or fluttering of the heart, pounding in the chest, fulness in the neck; he becomes uneasy, nervous, dizzy, and apprehensive and desires to lie down. Occasionally there is pain over the heart, and there may be typical anginal distress even with radiation to the arms. Sometimes nausea and vomiting occur and then attacks often cease. This experience suggests to the patient that it is all produced by indigestion or some recently eaten food. After a length of time, varying from minutes to hours and even days, the attack ends and the patient quickly recovers either in good condition or in a sufficiently weak state to remain inactive for a day or two. The distress experienced depends primarily on the duration of the attack, the cardiac rate, and the condition of the heart before the attack occurred.

Diagnosis. The diagnosis of paroxysmal atrial tachycardia is simple in most cases. It is important to elicit evidence of an abrupt change in rhythm with an approxi-

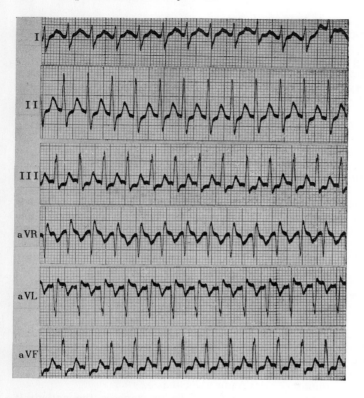

FIG. 16-4. Paroxysmal atrial tachycardia with a rate of 190 per minute. The P and T waves are superimposed. (Lipman and Massie: Clinical Scalar Electrocardiography, ed. 5, Chicago, Year Book Pub., 1965)

mate doubling of heart rate. Usually the cardiac beat ranges from about 150 to 250 per minute. Although usually sudden cessation of the episode occurs, sometimes the attack does not appear to stop abruptly. This is because, in spite of the considerable drop in rate at the end of the paroxysm, the sino-atrial rate when the heart resumes normal rhythm is elevated by excitement or otherwise, preventing the obvious sensation of marked change in the cardiac rhythm that occurred at the onset of the attack. Not only is the heart rapid and regular but its rate is very fixed for long intervals of time and cannot be altered by simple procedures like breathing or exercise which affect the rate of the normal heart. If repeated counts of the heart beat taken at the bedside several minutes apart show a significant difference in the rates, it speaks against the diagnosis of paroxysmal atrial tachycardia. The various methods that are used to stop an attack also serve as diagnostic procedures, because there is no other type of rapid heart action that can be made to return to a normal rate by such simple means and so quickly. *If vagus stimulation is produced by pressure* over the carotid sinus or the eyeball in this type of

arrhythmia, the rate either remains unaltered or abruptly falls to the normal sinus range. With normal tachycardia or atrial flutter there is apt to be temporary slowing with gradual return to the previous rate, and when ventricular tachycardia is present vagus stimulation produces no effect. The electrocardiogram is almost invariably diagnostic (see Fig. 16-4), but there are a few puzzling records in which the tracing, unless it is taken at the beginning of the paroxysm, is not adequate to eliminate definitely a rare case of sinus tachycardia or atrial flutter.

Prognosis. The prognosis of paroxysmal atrial tachycardia is usually excellent as to life, but there are rare instances where the tachycardia is so excessive that cardiac failure results even in a normal person. It is always a more important disturbance, however, in the presence of serious heart disease. The cardiac conditions that are prone to be overburdened by this type of tachycardia include mitral stenosis, coronary insufficiency, and cases of enlargement of the left ventricle. The tendency to recurrence of attacks varies greatly from only a few attacks in a lifetime to almost daily paroxysms.

Paroxysmal Atrial Tachycardia with Atrioventricular Block

There is another form of atrial tachycardia which is associated with varying degrees of atrioventricular block. The rising incidence of this arrhythmia and its significance with reference to digitalis intoxication has been gaining attention in recent years. Levine and Lown observed a number of instances of paroxysmal atrial tachycardia with atrioventricular block (PAT with block). In their series originally it was considered that only a comparative few of these patients had attacks in which digitalis intoxication could not be implicated as a causative factor, but as time has gone on, it now appears that, in a certain number of instances, digitalis is not involved. Many of the patients who have developed paroxysmal atrial tachycardia with block have this rhythm precipitated by potassium loss during excessive diuresis.

The electrocardiographic features of PAT with block are as follows:

1. The onset is more gradual than that

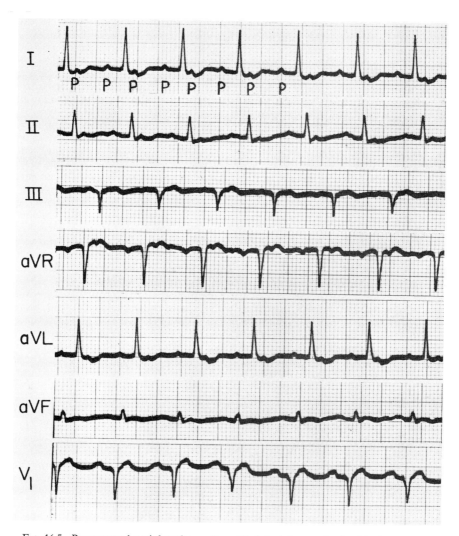

Fig. 16-5. Paroxysmal atrial tachycardia with 2:1 atrioventricular block associated with digitalis intoxication in a man 55 years of age. The rate of the paroxysmal atrial tachycardia is 200 beats per minute, while the ventricular rate is exactly one-half as fast. The symbol P indicates the ectopic atrial beats in lead I. (Massie and Walsh: Clinical Vectorcardiography and Electrocardiography, Chicago, Year Book Pub., 1960)

of supraventricular tachycardia without AV block. The normal P waves become progressively altered in appearance as the ectopic forces stimulate the atrium. Then the rate of this pacemaker speeds up with a 1:1 atrioventricular response initially, followed by the onset of variable atrioventricular block.

2. The differentiation of the atrial flutter pattern from PAT with block may be difficult at times, especially if the atrial rate is approximately 200 beats per minute. The atrial rate in the latter rhythm is usually between 150 and 190 beats per minute, and seldom exceeds 200 beats per minute.

3. The AV block is a constant 2:1 in only 30 per cent of the patients, the remainder showing variable and often inconstant degrees of block. The degree of AV block can be increased by vagal stimulation and decreased by atropine or exercise.

4. Unlike the common form of supraventricular tachycardia, the atrial mechanism in PAT with block, with rare exceptions, cannot be converted to sinus rhythm by carotid sinus stimulation or other simple measures which increase the vagal tone. Generally, its response to various therapeutic agents more closely resembles that of atrial flutter than that of atrial tachycardia. When the P wave is superimposed on the QRS and T deflections, as is often the case, the diagnosis may be overlooked easily. Recognition of the mechanism often depends on a high degree of suspicion, as well as on vagal maneuvers which increase the degree of AV block and uncover the concealed P wave. Suspicion may be aroused by a knowledge of the clinical picture or by the appearance of a newly developed, unexplained, persistent deformity of the QRS complex, the ST segment, or the T wave. Figure 16-5 shows an example of paroxysmal atrial tachycardia with 2:1 atrioventricular block.

ATRIAL FLUTTER

A still higher degree of atrial disturbance is atrial flutter. It is relatively uncommon, its incidence being less than one-twelfth that of atrial fibrillation.

Mechanism. The mechanism producing atrial flutter (and also that causing atrial fibrillation) has been the subject of lively controversy for much of the last decade, and the divergence of opinion is just as marked now as ever. Although investigations in recent years have provided new and important information concerning the genesis of these two rhythms, none of these data incontestably prove or refute any of the theories currently favored. These theories are three in number —the concept of circus movement, the theory of multiple re-entry, and the theory of focal or multi-focal impulse formation.

Atrial flutter is a very rapid regular atrial beat that replaces the normal atrial contraction. A rapid series of impulses is initiated in an ectopic area in either atrium. The atrial rate varies between 200 and 400 beats per minute, but following quinidine administration it may slow to less than 150. Usually the ventricular rate is only a fraction of that of the atria, since junctional tissue cannot conduct impulses so rapidly and a certain degree of atrioventricular block results. In exceptional cases all atrial beats come through to the ventricles; then the heart rate is extremely rapid. Commonly the ratio of atrial to ventricular beats is 2:1 and less often 4:1 or even 5:1 or 6:1. Not infrequently the ventricular response is irregular as a result of a changing atrioventricular block.

Etiology. Unlike paroxysmal atrial tachycardia, which usually occurs in otherwise normal hearts, atrial flutter is apt to be *associated with organic heart disease,* either valvular or myocardial, although it can rarely occur as a purely functional disturbance. Its incidence is probably highest in cases of mitral stenosis, hypertension and coronary heart disease. Occasionally one encounters it in patients with severe thyrotoxicosis. Atrial flutter occurs chiefly in adults, and the exciting factors are the same as those for paroxysmal atrial tachycardia.

Symptoms. Symptoms are produced when the rate of the ventricle is rapid, but are more common in the paroxysmal form of atrial flutter or if heart disease is advanced. The typical symptom is rapid, regular, forceful palpitation subjectively indistinguishable from paroxysmal tachycardia. Symptoms of congestive heart failure may be coincidental or may result from the rapid ventricular action. Pain is rare, although precordial aching may occur. The patient may be made nervous and apprehensive from the alarm occasioned by the attack. If the ventricular rate is very rapid, as in 1:1 rhythm, and the heart rate approaches 300 per minute, dizziness, weakness, and partial or complete syncope may result as a consequence of cerebral anemia and other effects of greatly reduced cardiac output.

Diagnosis. The diagnosis is easily made with the electrocardiogram but with difficulty in any other way. Atrial flutter is characterized at the bedside by long-continued rapid

Fig. 16-6. Atrial flutter with 2:1 atrioventricular block. The atrial rate is 300 and ventricular rate 150 per minute. Note that the atrial waves (F) are represented by small notches in Lead I and by triangular form of P waves in Leads II, III and aVF. (Lipman and Massie: Clinical Scalar Electrocardiography, ed. 5, Chicago, Year Book Pub., 1965)

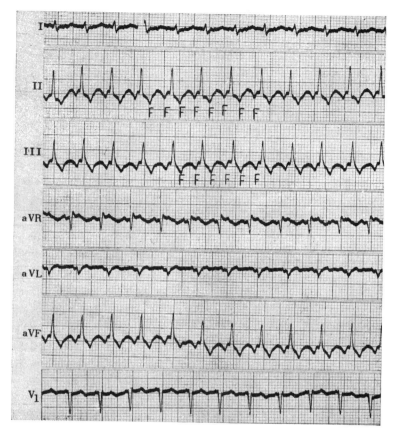

beating at a precise rate. Temporary halving of the heart rate spontaneously, by exercise, or by carotid sinus pressure is suggestive of this arrhythmia. Carotid sinus pressure slows the ventricle in "jumps" because it does not, as a rule, alter the atrial rate but only the ratio of atrial impulses conducted to the ventricle. Upon removal of the carotid sinus pressure the ventricular rate returns to its previous level, but often the return occurs in an irregular although rapid fashion. Severe exercise, on occasion, also causes a sudden change in the ventricular rate which reverts to its original level when the exertion is over. The neck veins always should be inspected for the presence of the rapid regular atrial waves. For this type of examination the patient should be placed in such a position that the neck veins are only partially filled.

The electrocardiograms of atrial flutter are very peculiar and characteristic. In lead I the atrial waves are represented by small notches. In leads II and III the waves have a triangular form. The upstroke is sharp and smooth and the downstroke more prolonged

and notched at its midpoint. The flutter waves are continuous, and as one cycle ends the next begins. They often resemble a tuning-fork record and at other times a picket fence. The rhythm of the atria is strikingly regular. The ventricular rate and rhythm will depend on the degree of heart block. With experience, one learns to detect flutter from the appearance of the electrocardiograms, but if there is any doubt as to the underlying mechanism, slowing of the ventricular rate by vagal stimulation may allow the flutter waves to be more evident. Lead V_1 may be helpful in differentiating questionable cases since it often shows most clearly evidences of atrial activity if carefully examined. Figure 16-6 shows the electrocardiogram of a patient with atrial flutter and 2:1 atrioventricular block.

Prognosis. The prognosis is less favorable than for paroxysmal atrial tachycardia because of the higher incidence of heart disease in association with flutter and because of the longer paroxysms. Sometimes the flutter continues in more chronic form lasting for years.

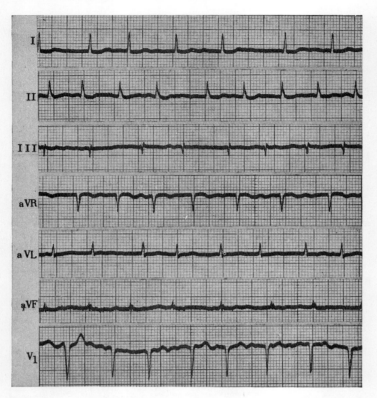

Fig. 16-7. Atrial fibrillation with an irregular ventricular rate of 75 to 110 per minute. (Lipman and Massie: Clinical Scalar Electrocardiography, ed. 5, Chicago, Year Book Pub., 1965)

ATRIAL FIBRILLATION

Atrial fibrillation is closely allied with atrial flutter and has about 12 to 15 times the clinical incidence. It is one of the most common and most important disorders of cardiac rhythm. It probably ranks fourth in frequency as a disturbance of rhythm, sino-atrial tachycardia, premature beats, and paroxysmal atrial tachycardia ranking first, second, and third, respectively. Atrial fibrillation, even of the paroxysmal type, rarely escapes notice and with rare exceptions comes eventually under the scrutiny of a physician.

Mechanism. Atrial fibrillation represents the highest degree of atrial disturbance. In this condition the number of atrial impulses per minute is very great, varying between 350 and 500. The impulses travel in a circus pattern in which the path is impure and irregular. The atria do not actually contract but rather remain distended in diastole and show fibrillary twitching. The speed of the atrial impulses is so great that areas of block or refractory points develop in the circuit, accounting for the irregularity of rate seen in the electrocardiogram. There is no constant pathologic finding in the atria to account for atrial fibrillation; accordingly, it is regarded as a functional derangement accompanying a number of conditions. This arrhythmia can be reproduced in a dog's atrium by a rapid series of faradic stimulations. The number of atrial impulses is so great that only a portion of them can be conducted through the junctional tissue. Consequently, there is always some degree of atrioventricular block associated with this arrhythmia. The ventricular response occurs in a grossly irregular fashion. The peripheral pulse is necessarily irregular both in time and in force. The ventricles respond irregularly, with an average rate of 100 to 140 per minute in untreated cases, but rates above 200 sometimes occur.

Etiology. The condition occurs chiefly in adults of both sexes and is very rare in early childhood. The incidence of atrial fibrillation increases in frequency with increasing years; it is common in old age. The most common conditions with which this arrhythmia is associated are rheumatic valvular disease with mitral stenosis, hypertensive heart disease, coronary artery disease, hyperthyroidism, the various myopathies, atrial septal defects, and

FIG. 16-8. Atrioventricular nodal rhythm with a rate of 108 per minute. The atrial complexes (labeled P in Lead II) are retrograde in nature and may be seen in all the leads. (Lipman and Massie: Clinical Scalar Electrocardiography, ed. 5, Chicago, Year Book Pub., 1965)

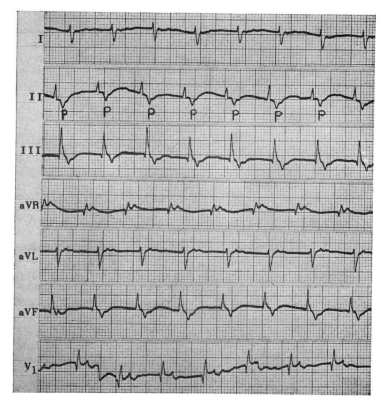

with surgical procedures. It may develop precipitously during acute infections such as pneumonia and in rheumatic fever. It is seen not infrequently during the early stages of an acute coronary thrombosis. Rarely, it develops as a result of excessive digitalis therapy. In addition, there is the important group in which it is present either paroxysmally or permanently in otherwise healthy individuals and without any apparent cause such as organic heart disease or even excesses of tobacco or alcohol. It may follow excitement, trauma, operations or intoxications, particularly in nervously high-strung people.

Symptoms. Symptoms vary with the ventricular rate, the underlying functional state of the heart and the duration of the atrial fibrillation. In the chronic form atrial fibrillation may exist without symptoms. Usually, however, the patient is aware of the irregular heart action and has such sensations as fluttering, skipping, irregular beating or a pounding and heaving action. Palpitation is usually present and may be considered as the characteristic symptom of atrial fibrillation. Dyspnea and pain are much less common, but

they may develop as a part of neurocirculatory asthenia if there is an associated marked psychic element. Although angina pectoris may appear, due to the extra work imposed by rapid heart action on a damaged myocardium, it is comparatively rare in atrial fibrillation, a fact that is best explained by the limitation of activity imposed by the arrhythmia itself and by medical advice. The entire symptomatic picture is particularly striking in the paroxysmal form, and there may also be the more general symptoms of anxiety, nervousness, pallor, cyanosis and collapse. The patient may even harbor feelings of impending death. Successive attacks are apt to cause sufficient psychic trauma that chronic invalidism results even in the absence of signs of heart failure. Congestive failure may be coincidental with, precipitated by, or entirely caused by the rapid irregular ventricular action.

Diagnosis. The bedside recognition of this condition is generally simple. A rapid, apparently grossly irregular heart beat with an appreciable pulse deficit of 10 or more is due to atrial fibrillation in the great majority of cases. In addition, any tachycardia at a rate of over 120 that is grossly irregular is most likely the result of this arrhythmia. When the patient has a history of rheumatic fever and the signs of mitral stenosis, atrial fibrillation occurs frequently and should be suspected if an arrhythmia is found. The electrocardiogram gives immediate evidence of the condition and is of great diagnostic aid when there is a question as to clinical interpretation. The normal P wave in the tracing will be absent, and instead there will be found irregular, rapid undulations (F waves) of varying amplitude, contour, and spacing. These F waves vary in form all the way from being clearly visible in most leads in coarse atrial fibrillation and impure flutter to being imperceptible in fine atrial fibrillation. There is a totally irregular ventricular spacing except in complete atrioventricular block, but, inasmuch as the course of impulses that succeed in reaching the ventricles travel down the normal atrioventricular conduction path, the ventricular complexes are normal in form. Figure 16-7 shows an example of the electrocardiographic finding in atrial fibrillation.

Prognosis. The prognosis in atrial fibrillation depends on the underlying heart condition and the treatment. In the absence of cardiac muscle or valve involvement the prognosis is excellent. The attack, even though subsiding spontaneously, may in some instances recur. In the presence of heart disease the result depends on the severity of the cardiac lesion and upon the ease of controlling the ventricular rate. It is possible to have recurrent episodes of atrial fibrillation over periods of many years in some patients, yet in those cases where the heart is seriously involved an attack may cause death in a matter of hours.

PAROXYSMAL ATRIOVENTRICULAR
NODAL TACHYCARDIA

This arrhythmia is a relatively infrequent variety of paroxysmal tachycardia. It may be diagnosed only by electrocardiographic means, and even then the diagnosis is sometimes difficult. Because of the difficulty of distinguishing between this rhythm and paroxysmal atrial tachycardia, these arrhythmias are frequently grouped together under the term supraventricular tachycardia. Paroxysmal atrioventricular nodal tachycardia is due to rapid impulse formation in the atrioventricular node, both ventricles and atria being controlled from that center. The P waves of the electrocardiogram are inverted and just follow, precede, or occur simultaneously with the QRS complexes. An example is shown in Figure 16-8.

The etiology, symptomatology and prognosis of this arrhythmia are similar to those of paroxysmal atrial tachycardia.

PAROXYSMAL VENTRICULAR
TACHYCARDIA

This arrhythmia is comparatively rare and occurs approximately in the ratio of 1:8 compared with paroxysmal atrial tachycardia.

Mechanism. Paroxysmal ventricular tachycardia may be regarded as a consecutive series of ventricular extrasystoles arising from an ectopic focus in the ventricle. There is much in the nature of this mechanism that resembles a circus motion. Since it starts from an abnormal focus in the ventricle and the impulse travels an abnormal course, the resultant complex will necessarily be unlike the normal configuration. Each individual complex resembles a ventricular extrasystole. The impulses may travel in a retrograde fashion up the junctional tissue and produce atrial contractions. Because the rate is rapid there may be a retrograde block so that only every other ventricular impulse produces an atrial contraction. At other times the atria contract independently and follow their own pacemaker in the sino-atrial node.

Etiology. This arrhythmia occurs in both sexes but, unlike paroxysmal atrial tachycardia, is much more limited to older persons. It appears but rarely in youth. It is a serious condition because of its much higher incidence among patients with important cardiac involvement or toxic states. Precipitating factors include acute myocardial infarction, very toxic doses of digitalis, manipulation during cardiac catheterizations, coronary arteriography, and surgical procedures, particularly those involving manipulation of the heart and great vessels. The author has recently encountered a male patient, age forty-four, who has had recurrent bouts of this arrhythmia associated with subacute lupus erythematosus. Very rarely it may occur transiently in normal people.

Symptoms. The symptomatology resembles that of paroxysmal atrial tachycardia with the exception that these patients are usually seriously ill with some underlying disease; consequently, the tachycardia produces symptoms that are much more accentuated.

Diagnosis. The diagnosis can be made with certainty only by examining the electro-

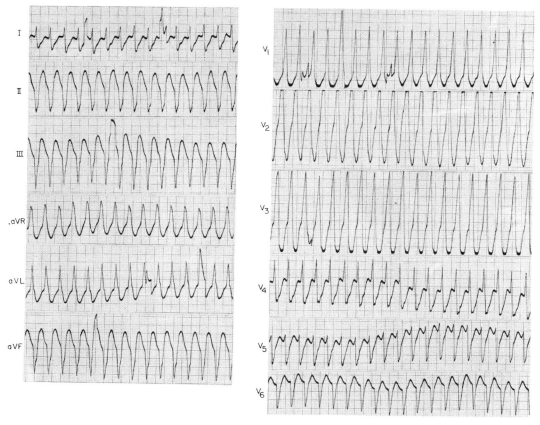

FIG. 16-9. Paroxysmal ventricular tachycardia with a ventricular rate of 188 beats per minute. The ventricular complexes are bizarre in appearance and prolonged in duration. (Massie and Walsh: Clinical Vectorcardiography and Electrocardiography, Chicago, Year Book Pub., 1960)

cardiogram, which reveals abnormally shaped QRS waves resembling repeated ventricular premature beats; the heart rate usually is about 160 to 180 per minute, and very rarely reaches the high levels of 220 or more which occur in atrial tachycardia. The atria beat independently, and the P waves sometimes may be seen clearly superimposed on the QRS and the T waves. Paroxysmal ventricular tachycardia is sometimes difficult to differentiate from paroxysmal atrial tachycardia with bundle branch block when the P waves are hard to identify. A typical electrocardiogram is shown in Figure 16-9.

There are some bedside methods that enable one to suspect the presence of paroxysmal ventricular tachycardia. When paroxysmal, the attacks begin and end suddenly. The rate is rapid, but occasionally slight irregularities can be detected by auscultation, in contrast with atrial tachycardia. The condition may be suspected if the heart rate rises abruptly to a level between 140 to 160 per minute or if the rate is above 160 and the rhythm is slightly irregular. In addition, upon careful examination, slight but suggestive differences in the intensity and the quality of the first sound will be heard in some cases as a result of the different relationship between the ventricular and the atrial systoles in various cycles. Atrial pulsations as seen in the jugular vein are fewer in number than the ventricular rate, but this observation is especially difficult to make. Finally, this type of rapid heart action is not influenced by any of the methods that stimulate the vagus nerve. The duration of the attacks is somewhat like that of paroxysmal atrial tachycardia (that is, minutes or hours, and rarely days).

Prognosis. The prognosis is unfavorable because of the severe underlying heart disease or toxic condition. The occurrence of paroxysmal ventricular tachycardia usually indicates a short life, sometimes only a few hours and infrequently more than a few months or years.

VENTRICULAR FLUTTER AND FIBRILLATION

Ventricular flutter and fibrillation are related in the same way as are their analogous rhythms in the atria. Ventricular flutter is extremely rare. Ventricular fibrillation is, with few exceptions, an irreversible condition found in moribund patients and is one of the causes of sudden death. As in atrial fibrillation, the synergic contractions of the heart are replaced by an incoordinate quivering, each part of the ventricle beating independently. This incoordination directly suspends the pumping action of the heart, and fainting, coma, convulsions and death occur unless the attack quickly subsides. The pulse is absent, and the attack may resemble Adams-Stokes syndrome.

Diagnosis can be made only by electrocardiographic means. Ventricular flutter can be diagnosed in the electrocardiogram when regular continuous waves of large amplitude occur at a rate of over 250 per minute. In these deflections no distinction can be made between the QRS complex and the T wave. Ventricular fibrillation is diagnosed in the tracing by the absence of QRST complexes and the presence of irregular undulations of varying amplitude, contour and spacing. The rate of these may vary from 250 to 500 per minute. The waves are larger than in atrial fibrillation, and no ordinary QRST complexes are seen.

SUMMARY

Palpitation and tachycardia are among the most common complaints that cause patients to seek medical aid. Often, however, the complaint is the most grievous in the presence of the least serious organic disturbance. On the contrary, mild or moderate symptoms may indicate serious underlying disease. Palpitation often results from emotional or psychic disturbance and does not necessarily imply an organic cardiac condition. Increase in the force or the rate of the heart beat and the various cardiac arrhythmias may cause palpitation. Tachycardia, strictly speaking, is a physical sign, but it is often a symptom, the subject complaining not so much of an awareness of the heart beat (palpitation) as of a consciousness that the rate is excessive. Frequent or persistent tachycardia may result from metabolic or hormonal disorders, emotional disturbances, psychic or nervous system disease, infections and other conditions affecting the total organism, as well as from cardiac disease. Every such complaint, therefore, deserves careful study until the mechanism is adequately understood. In this way the proper and logical therapeutic approach should become evident.

BIBLIOGRAPHY

Barker, P. S., Wilson, F. N., and Johnston, F. D.: Mechanism of auricular paroxysmal tachycardia, Amer. Heart J. 26:435–445, 1943.

Beattie, J., Brow, G. R., and Long, C. N. H.: Physiological and anatomical evidence for existence of nerve tracts connecting the hypothalamus with spinal sympathetic centres, Proc. Roy. Soc. [Biol.] 106:253–275, 1930.

Bellet, S.: Current concepts in therapy: Drug therapy in cardiac arrhythmias, II., New Eng. J. Med. 262:979–981, 1960.

———: Clinical Disorders of the Heart Beat, ed. 2, Philadelphia, Lea & Febiger, 1963.

Best, C. H., and Taylor, N. B.: The Physiological Basis of Medical Practice, ed. 8, Baltimore, Williams & Wilkins, 1966.

Bristowe, J. S.: On recurrent palpitation of extreme rapidity in persons otherwise apparently healthy, Brain 10:164–198, 1887.

Burchell, H. B.: Cardiac manifestations of anxiety, Proc. Staff Meet. Mayo Clinic 22:433–440, 1947.

Campbell, M., and Elliott, G. A.: Paroxysmal auricular tachycardia, Brit. Med. J. 1:123–160, 1939.

Cookson, H.: Aetiology and prognosis of auricular fibrillation, Quart. J. Med. 23:309–325, 1930.

Criteria Committee of the New York Heart Association: Nomenclature and Criteria for Diagnosis of Diseases of the Heart and Blood Vessels, ed. 6, Boston, Little, Brown & Co., 1964.

Ernstene, A. C.: Diagnosis and treatment of the cardiac arrhythmias, Cleveland Clin. Quart. 16:185–195, 1949.

Friedberg, C. K.: Diseases of the Heart, ed. 3, Philadelphia, Saunders, 1966.

Goodman, L., and Gilman, A.: The Pharmacological Basis of Therapeutics, ed. 3, New York, Macmillan, 1965.

Katz, L. N., and Pick, A.: Clinical Electrocardiography, Part I., The Arrhythmias, Philadelphia, Lea & Febiger, 1956.

Korth, C.: Production of extrasystoles by means of the central nervous system, Ann. Intern. Med. 11:492–498, 1937.

Levine, S. A.: Clinical Heart Disease, ed. 5, Philadelphia, Saunders, 1958.

Levine, S. A., and Harvey, W. P.: Clinical Auscultation of the Heart, ed. 2, Philadelphia, Saunders, 1959.

Lewis, T.: The Soldier's Heart and the Effort Syndrome, ed. 2, London, Shaw, 1940.

————: The Mechanism and Graphic Registration of the Heart Beat, ed. 3, London, Shaw, 1925.

Lewis, T., Feil, H. S., and Stroud, W. D.: The nature of auricular flutter, Heart 7:191–243, 1920.

Lipman, B. S., and Massie, E.: Clinical Scalar Electrocardiography, ed. 5, Chicago, Year Book Pub., 1965.

Luten, D.: The Clinical Use of Digitalis, Springfield, Ill., Thomas, 1936.

Massie, E., and Walsh, T. J.: Clinical Vectorcardiography and Electrocardiography, Chicago, Year Book Pub., 1960.

Nash, J.: Surgical Physiology, Springfield, Ill., Thomas, 1942.

Oppenheimer, B. S.: Neurocirculatory asthenia and related problems in military medicine, Bull. N. Y. Acad. Med. 18:367–382, 1942.

Prinzmetal, M., Corday, E., Brill, I. C., Oblath, R. W., and Kruger, H. E.: The Auricular Arrhythmias, Springfield, Ill., Thomas, 1952.

Prinzmetal, M., Corday, E., Brill, I. C., Sellers, A. L., Oblath, R. W., Flieg, W. A., and Kruger, H. E.: Mechanism of the auricular arrythmias, Circulation 1:241–245, 1950.

Ravin, A.: Auscultation of the Heart, ed. 2, Chicago, Year Book Pub., 1967.

Rushmer, R. F.: Cardiovascular Dynamics, ed. 2, Philadelphia, Saunders, 1961.

Sodi-Pallares, D., and Calder, R. M.: New Bases of Electrocardiography, St. Louis, Mosby, 1956.

Stroud, W. D.: Diagnosis and Treatment of Cardiovascular Disease, vols. 1 and 2, ed. 3, Philadelphia, Davis, 1945.

Waldman, S., and Moskowitz, S. N.: Treatment of attacks of sinus tachycardia with prostigmin, Ann. Intern. Med. 20:793–805, 1944.

Weiss, E., and English, O. S.: Psychosomatic Medicine, ed. 3, Philadelphia, Saunders, 1957.

White, P. D.: Tachycardia and its Treatment, Modern Concepts of Cardiovascular Disease, New York, Amer. Heart Ass., vol. 9, No. 8, 1940.

————: Neurocirculatory Asthenia (Da Costa's Syndrome, Effort Syndrome, Irritable Heart of Soldiers), Modern Concepts of Cardiovascular Disease, New York, Amer. Heart Ass., vol. 11, No. 8, 1942.

————: Heart Disease, ed. 4, New York, Macmillan, 1951.

Wiggers, C. J.: Mechanism and nature of ventricular fibrillation, Amer. Heart J. 20:399–412, 1944.

Willius, F. A.: Cardiac Clinics, St. Louis, Mosby, 1941.

17

Cough

ROGER S. MITCHELL and JOHN A. PIERCE

Few words imitate the sound of an act with more precision than the word "cough." Like many aspects of pulmonary performance, cough may occur voluntarily, or involuntarily through reflex stimulation. The cough reflex is protective, intended to clear the airway. Since it has no role in the ordinary respiratory cycle, cough always is abnormal. Even though abnormal, cough is acceptable socially because of the ubiquity of respiratory infections and the prevalence of cigarette smoking.

Normal cough may be defined most simply as an explosive expiration. After a short inspiration the glottis is closed; the nasopharynx is also usually partially or completely closed off by the soft palate. A strong expiratory effort is then built up by the abdominal and thoracic muscles. At the end of this pressure build-up, the normal airways are compressed to about 40 per cent of their inspiratory diameter. This narrowing is advantageous because velocity of air flow is increased and material to be removed is less able to escape the blast of air. At this point, the glottis is suddenly opened and air, plus any free material in the airways, will rush out through the mouth. Chest fluoroscopy at this time reveals a rapid contraction of the ribs and especially a rapid ascent of the diaphragm. Even a paralyzed hemidiaphragm shoots up at this time, an observation that indicates that the diaphragm has no *active* expiratory function.

MECHANISM OF COUGH

Cough occurs in three distinct phases. Air drawn into the lungs immediately before cough constitutes an inspiratory phase of the cough. Contraction of the thoracic and abdominal muscles with a closed glottis comprises the compressive phase of cough. Sudden opening of the glottis with abrupt decompression of the intrathoracic gas accomplishes the expulsive phase of the cough. The vigor of the cough is determined by the volume of the precough inspiration, the intensity of the compressive effort, and the rapidity of onset of the expulsive phase of the cough. Although the precough activity of inspiration and compression are essential components, the useful effect of cough occurs only during the expulsive phase.

Understanding the mechanics of cough requires an understanding of the forces involved. Figure 17-1 presents an over-all maximal pressure-volume diagram of the lungs-thorax system. Pressure from the contraction of the thoracic muscles has been measured at the nose, but with the glottis open. It is apparent that muscular contraction produces maximal *positive* intrathoracic pressure (relative to atmospheric pressure) when the lungs are fully inflated. Conversely, maximal *negative* intrathoracic pressure is achieved at levels near full expiration, or residual volume level of lung inflation. At moderate levels of

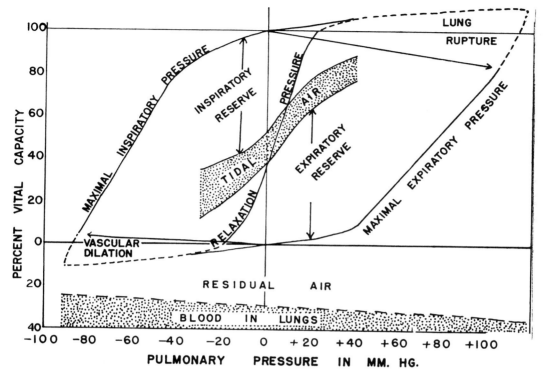

FIG. 17-1. Over-all maximal pressure-volume diagram of the lungs-thorax system. Pressure attained by contraction of thoracic muscles was measured at nose, with glottis open. Note that maximal positive intrathoracic pressure is produced when the lungs are fully inflated; conversely, maximal negative intrathoracic pressure is achieved at levels near full expiration, or residual volume level of lung inflation.

lung inflation, the maximal deviations (from atmospheric pressure) of which the thoracic muscles are capable approximates −60 to +70 cm. of water. It is especially pertinent that the mechanical properties of the lung control the rate of expiratory air flow. The peak rate of flow is no greater during cough than during forced expiration; in fact, it usually is slightly less during cough. The propulsive force of cough accrues from the effects of compression of intrathoracic gas. With compression, the diameter of the airways is decreased, and the linear rate of air travel thus is increased during the expulsive phase of cough. However, the volume of flow is not increased by cough. This illustrates the dominant role of the mechanical properties of the lung in pulmonary performance.

It should be mentioned that all deviations of intrathoracic pressure from atmospheric pressure are imposed on the heart and great vessels. This, naturally, has no relevance to the relationships between thoracic intravascular pressures, as, for example, that between aortic and left atrial pressure. However, these pressures are important in altering the relationships between intra- and extrathoracic pressures within the vessels. A high positive intrathoracic pressure, for example, precludes the entry of blood into the right atrium and, during intense cough compression, may result in an intense facial *cyanosis* due to the regurgitation of blood from the superior vena cava into the facial veins.

It also is pertinent to note that free venous communication exists between intrathoracic and intracranial veins. Cerebrospinal fluid pressure thus parallels intrathoracic pressure. One result of this relationship is *cough syncope.*

At least two types of sensory receptors initiate the cough reflex via afferent fibers in the vagus nerve. Receptors sensitive to mechanical stimulation are especially abundant in the larynx and about the carina. In the trachea, these receptors are mostly in the posterior wall. In the bronchial tree, they are prominent at points of bronchial branching. These receptors are stimulated by direct pressure or deformity of the mucous membrane or by contact with particulate matter. They can be stimulated also through deformity of the trachea from external pressure. They are readily adaptive and they can be blocked selectively by 7.5 to 14.5 per cent ether vapor in the trachea.

The other type of sensory receptors respond to chemical stimuli and initiate the most intractable cough reflex. They are located peripherally, beyond the second bronchial branching. They are exquisitely sensitive to ammonia, sulphur dioxide, ether, and other soluble agents, but not to mechanical or particulate stimulation. Both types of receptors are blocked by cooling the vagus nerve to 7° to 15° C. Although there is some overlap in function of the two types of receptors, the chemical-sensitive receptors are less adaptive than are the pressure receptors.

Cough in both normal and diseased subjects has been studied effectively by cinefluorobronchography. The normal trachea and bronchi, down to the smallest branches visible by this technic, show marked variation in caliber which are dependent upon the transluminal and hence, in part, upon the intrathoracic pressure. However, careful studies do not show any evidence in support of the old concept of true bronchial peristalsis. In chronic bronchitis, especially when it is accompanied by severe diffuse emphysema, the airways tend to collapse excessively upon forced expiration. The collapse is greater in some portions of the bronchial tree than in others, and at the peak of expiratory effort, the collapse may be complete in advanced diffuse emphysema and in severe chronic bronchitis. This phenomenon is probably both due to airway (cartilage) damage and to the high positive extraluminal pressures in these pathologic states. Obviously, the expulsive advantages of a normal degree of airway narrowing are partially lost when any portion of the airway collapses, either excessively or totally.

Cough is only one of the essential physiologic mechanisms for removal of normal bronchial mucus from the tracheobronchial tree. This mucus can be normal or abnormal in both quantity and quality; and it may or may not contain exudate, transudate, bacteria, or foreign material. Other normal removal mechanisms are the ciliated epithelium, the subepithelial lymphatics, and the phagocytes. The normal adult secretes about 100 ml. of bronchial mucus every 24 hours. It is estimated that usually it takes only about 30 to 60 minutes for mucus and/or foreign material to be swept from the levels of the respiratory bronchioles up to the mouth. Cilia do not extend below the respiratory bronchioles; foreign material that penetrates below this point is phagocytized and transmitted up to the cilia-bearing airways via the adjacent lymphatics.

Cough may occur either voluntarily or without conscious effort. Both *voluntary* and *involuntary* cough involve a *reflex arc*. Cough impulses may be stimulated in a number of different ways, including irritation of the tracheobronchial or nasal mucosa; external pressure or pulling upon the trachea; pressure upon the carotid sinus, the liver, the spleen, or the external auditory canal; pleural irritation; or lung congestion. The mucosa of the trachea and main bronchi is the most sensitive area; even a sudden inhalation of cold air may be a sufficient stimulus to induce coughing. Repeated uncontrolled coughing may itself irritate the airway mucosa and thus give rise to more cough stimuli. When cough occurs involuntarily, the stimuli usually must be especially strong, recurrent, or cumulative. The afferent impulses travel via vagal or sympathetic trunks to an area near the olivary bodies in the medulla oblongata. The efferent impulses then descend to the various muscles of expiration and to the glottis.

One supposedly common cause of cough is *postnasal drip* arising from acute or chronic nasal or paranasal sinus inflammation. Pharyngeal and tracheal irritation can be induced in this way, but severe or chronic coughing is probably seldom thus caused. To attribute a severe chronic cough to nasal or sinus pathology is apt to encourage the overlooking of some more serious underlying disease.

The depth or effectiveness of a cough is partially the function of the depth of the initial inspiration. Cough is also obviously under some voluntary control; it can be suppressed, postponed, or made stronger or much weaker by the conscious effort of the individual whose medulla is receiving cough-initiating stimuli. Coughing is more effective in removing material from the large than from the small airways. This is because, the smaller the *total* cross section of the airways at any point in the tracheobronchial tree, the more effective a sudden expiratory effort can be.

A so-called nervous cough is also recognized. Such a cough probably begins with some customary pathology; it becomes chronic perhaps as a result of a subconscious desire for attention, plus the added factor of the chronic mucosal irritation caused by the cough itself. It is doubtful that these psychogenic coughs are due to some pathologic process involving a "cough center" in the brain. The evidence in support of such a center is quite meager.

When coughing is infrequent and not repetitive, when it occurs as part of a natural physiologic progression of events, and especially when it is productive of some material which needs to be removed from the airways, it may be regarded as normal or physiologic. When it is severe, repeated, or uncontrolled, when it is ineffective for any reason such as excessively narrowed or collapsing airways, and especially when it is nonproductive or mostly nonproductive, it should be regarded as abnormal unphysiologic, and potentially harmful.

A therapeutic attack upon coughing can be directed at thinning bronchial secretions or at avoiding or removing abnormal irritation or suppressing the sensitivity of the sites of origin of afferent cough impulses. An intelligent attack upon cough thus requires an accurate knowledge of the cause or causes of the cough in the individual.

NATURE OF THE STIMULI THAT PRODUCE COUGH

The stimuli acting upon the endings of the vagus nerve in the pharynx, the larynx, the trachea, the bronchi (and occasionally in the esophagus) may be inflammatory, mechanical, chemical, or thermal in nature.

INFLAMMATORY STIMULI

These include stimuli initiated by hyperemia or edema of the mucous membrane; by irritation from exudates upon the surface of the mucous membrane, as in diphtheria, Vincent's angina, or that seen in some cases of streptococcal infections of the respiratory mucous membranes. Ulcerations occurring in tuberculosis or syphilis of the larynx, through irritation of nerves or through contraction of scar tissue in the process of healing with resultant traction upon the nerve endings, often provoke coughing.

MECHANICAL STIMULI

The inhalation of dust, smoke, or small foreign bodies is one of the commonest causes of cough. Cigarette smokers often have a chronic cough, produced sometimes by the foreign-body activity (inhaled smoke) present during the period of active smoking, but often present even when the subject is not smoking and resulting from chronic pharyngitis, laryngitis, tracheitis, or bronchitis from prolonged inhalation of smoke. Small particles of any nature present in the inhaled air, or drawn in from the nose or the mouth and suddenly striking the sensitive mucous membranes of the air passages may result in cough.

Miners and other industrial workers exposed to dusty environments commonly are afflicted with chronic cough.

The involuntary inhalation of oral or nasal secretions, or of food particles, or the presence of inflammatory exudates on the mucosal surface of the nasal passages, the pharynx, the larynx, the trachea, or the bronchi may thus act as mechanical stimulants to coughing. The pressure or tension upon structures in the air passages that may result from mediastinal or bronchogenic tumors, aortic aneurysms, the enlarged peribronchial and mediastinal nodes in Hodgkin's disease, tuberculosis, or neoplasms constitute other types of mechanical stimulation. Tension or pressure produced by distortion of the respiratory tract due to pulmonary fibrosis, atelectasis, or pleural effusion may likewise be capable of initiating the stimulus for cough.

CHEMICAL STIMULI

Chemical stimuli that may result in cough are the inhalation of certain irritating gases such as chlorine, bromine, phosgene, chloropicrin, oxychlorcarbon, dichlorethyl sulfide, dichloromethyl ether, and others. The fumes of certain strong chemicals—for example, iodine, sulfuric acid, nitric acid, ammonia—as well as the unpleasant odors of garlic, asafetida, or onion also are capable of producing stimuli that sometimes result in coughing.

Inhaled tobacco smoke contains gases and chemicals that are irritating to the respiratory mucosa; these, as well as the mechanical irritation from inhaled smoke, produce the very common "smoker's cough."

THERMAL STIMULI

Thermal stimuli include the inhalation of very hot or very cold air. However, it is rare for the sudden change in the temperature of the inspired air to be the sole cause of cough production; usually there is pathology somewhere in the respiratory tract that actually initiates the stimulus for coughing, and this is merely accentuated in its action by the temperature change.

PSYCHOGENIC COUGH

Psychogenic cough is not uncommon. It is found (1) in persons who have some organic basis for cough, but either consciously or unconsciously cough excessively. The cough may serve to gain attention and sympathy, to express hostile impulses, etc. It is also found (2) in persons with little or no organic basis for cough in whom it may serve as release of nervous tension during embarrassment, etc. When chronic it may assume the clinical characteristics of a tic, becoming an involuntary reflex.

CHARACTERISTIC TYPES OF COUGH

Few coughs have features of any specific diagnostic importance. As with many other symptoms, cough is more bothersome at night largely because secretions, not being removed as frequently as they are during the day, accumulate and provoke cough, disturbing sleep. Bronchiolitis, or croup, is accompanied by short, rapid, bursts of coughing. Cough occurs upon awakening, and often is productive of a few milliliters of mucoid sputum. Smoker's cough may occur at any time, since the basic respiratory tract inflammation is chronically present; it is characteristically provoked by smoking. Patients with bronchial asthma usually cough during attacks. Occasionally, coughing will precipitate asthmatic bronchospasm. There is often nothing characteristic about the cough of asthma. It may be dry, or productive of thin, watery, or purulent sputum. Wheezing expiratory cough may occur. Rarely, a special syndrome occurs in patients with asthma during the formation of bronchial casts. This is accompanied by a vigorous, intractable, cough and has been called "plastic" bronchitis. It occurs together with exacerbation of the asthmatic symptoms, usually following respiratory tract infection. The sputum always contains bronchial casts, and sometimes *Aspergillus fumigatus* is identified upon culture of the sputum. Acute episodes of pulmonary insufficiency may cause death in some such patients.

Prolonged musical "cat's mew" expiration is characteristic of asthma and is often audible without a stethoscope.

Patients with obstructive pulmonary dis-

ease have a prolonged expulsive phase of cough that is characteristic of their condition. This long, slow cough frequently is accompanied by expiratory wheezing. Such patients commonly laugh in a manner typical for its wheezing character. Local obstruction may be suggested by local wheezing detectible by stethoscope; confirmation is sought by bronchography.

Cough often is troublesome with acute respiratory infections but has no characteristic features. Pneumonia occasionally produces intractable coughing, presumably through stimulation of the peripheral, chemical sensitive receptors. Bronchiectasis is remarkable for the frequent ease with which secretions are produced. Cough in pulmonary infarction secondary to thromboembolism is not often troublesome except for aggravation of pleuritic pain. Pleural friction rubs may persist for several weeks in pulmonary infarction, but usually are more transient when due to other causes.

The most distinctive of all coughs is that encountered in pertussis, because of the characteristic sound of the whoop. The inspiratory whoop of whooping cough is a function of the intensity of the effort of cough and spasm of the laryngeal muscles. The whoop lacks specificity for diagnosis, but it should point out the need for bacteriological methods. In areas in which pertussis continues to be a common infection, the presumptive diagnosis of whooping cough can be made from the whoop.

CONDITIONS IN WHICH COUGH OCCURS

The conditions in which cough may be an important symptom can be classified as follows:

Inflammations
Cardiovascular disorders
Trauma and physical agents
Neoplasms
Allergic disorders
Other causes

INFLAMMATIONS

Acute pharyngitis may be bacterial or viral in origin. A diffuse redness, swelling, and patchy exudate are common in most forms of this disease. In addition, a greyish membrane composed of pus cells, tissue debris, bacteria, and fibrin is generally seen in the bacterial forms (diphtheritic, streptococcal and Vincent's anginal). Although the characteristic appearance of the membrane in these three infections tends to differ slightly, bacteriologic examination of material obtained from the throat is the only reliable method of differentiating them. An acute necrotizing pharyngitis often appears during the course of agranulocytosis. The cough in all forms of acute pharyngitis is apt to be irritative and dry.

Acute laryngitis may occur separately or as a part of a viral or bacterial inflammation of the upper or lower respiratory tract. In addition to hoarseness and cough, these patients often have a sore throat and, especially in *tuberculous laryngitis*, patients are apt also to suffer from very painful swallowing.

Laryngeal tuberculosis is nonspecific in appearance at the outset; as the process progresses, not only the true and false cords but also all adjacent structures become red, swollen, ulcerated, and finally destroyed. Tuberculous laryngitis seldom occurs in the absence of active, infectious pulmonary and/or endobronchial tuberculosis. The diagnosis is best made by biopsy.

Acute tracheobronchitis, due to viral or bacterial agents, may occur as a separate illness or as a part or complication of an acute upper respiratory infection. This syndrome also occurs as a part of a number of specific infections, including influenza, measles, pertussis, and occasionally typhoid fever. Symptoms include fever, dyspnea, substernal pain, and a severe, irritative, often productive cough.

INFLUENZA is a virus infection characterized by an acute inflammation of the upper and lower respiratory tract, and often involving the gastrointestinal tract as well. It is characterized by sudden onset of fever, headache, myalgia, prostration, and weakness. The acute symptoms usually subside in 3 or 4 days. Severe dry cough occurs in most cases. Abdominal pain with diarrhea and/or constipation may occur. The cough may become more prominent as the earlier systemic symptoms diminish. The cough, usually nonproductive, may be productive of small amounts of tenacious mucoid sputum.

Influenza is often complicated by a viral or bacterial pneumonia. It is caused by one of the strains of the influenza virus. If the causative virus belongs to one of the A strains, the disease is apt to be severe, to have a high incidence of complications, and to occur in epidemic or pandemic waves. If the virus belongs to the B, C, or D strains, the influenza is apt to be much less severe and the epidemics are apt to be local rather than widespread.

PERTUSSIS is an acute infectious disease of the entire respiratory tract caused by the *Hemophilus pertussis*. It is called whooping cough because it is characterized by paroxysms of short efforts at coughing with little or no inspiration between them, followed by a sudden forceful "whooping" inspiration. Cough is such a predominant feature of pertussis because the organisms selectively attack the respiratory mucous membranes, in which they cause an intense catarrhal inflammation and interference with ciliary action. The disease is also characterized by inflammatory swelling of the tracheobronchial lymph nodes, a fact that also may play a part in the genesis of the severe cough. Pertussis is frequently complicated by interstitial pneumonia or bronchopneumonia; if these complications are slow in resolving, patchy necrosis of the bronchi and adjacent tissues may lead to the late complication of bronchiectasis.

Chronic bronchitis is defined clinically as a chronic productive cough for at least 3 months of each year for at least 2 consecutive years. It is characterized pathologically by narrowed bronchial lumens due to thickened, inflamed bronchial walls, impairment of ciliary action, overproduction of excessively viscid bronchial mucus, and hypertrophy and increased numbers of bronchial glands and goblet cells. Although its causes are not completely understood, the disease is associated closely with regular frequent inhaling of tobacco smoke, heavy industrial air pollution, cold damp climate and repeated deep viral and bacterial respiratory infections. It is also related at times to chronic episodic allergic bronchial asthma. Patients with chronic bronchitis tend to start their days with an episode of severe dry coughing culminating in the production of some sticky, often mucopurulent mucus. They frequently begin to notice dyspnea on exertion after some 10 to 30 years of coughing; by this time, the disease chronic bronchitis tends to merge into the disease diffuse pulmonary *emphysema* (alveolar wall destruction) and ultimately, in many cases, *cor pulmonale* develops. Repeated attacks of pneumonia are apt to occur during the evolution of these diseases. The attack of pneumonia, often complicated by pulmonary thromboses, frequently abruptly usher in further loss of exercise tolerance.

Bronchiectasis is, by definition, an irreversible destruction of the bronchial walls. It may result from an obstructive or slowly resolving pneumonitis, especially when due to necrotizing microorganisms. Bronchiectasis may also occur following the inhalation of a foreign body and following pertussis. A congenital or developmental form is recognized in which multiple epithelium-lined spaces, reminiscent of bronchogenic cysts, become acutely, and then chronically, infected. The cough in bronchiectasis is usually chronic and is typically worse in the morning. It is characteristically "loose" and relatively productive of large quantities of purulent, often foul, sputum. The sputum tends to settle into 2 or 3 layers upon standing. Patients with bronchiectasis often have severe hemoptysis because the necrotizing process has penetrated into a vessel and because the bronchial vasculature in bronchiectasis often gradually becomes hypertrophied. The diagnosis of bronchiectasis is confirmed by a bronchogram showing localized or widespread dilatation of bronchi and pooling of contrast medium. The dilatations are usually irregular or saccular and often interspersed with areas of narrowing. Smooth cylindrical dilatation, especially when only slight, is a feature of chronic bronchitis, rather than of true bronchiectasis.

Lobar pneumonia is usually caused by *D. pneumoniae*, less commonly by streptococci, staphylococci, and other pus-forming bacteria. This disease occurs after exposure to cold, after an upper respiratory infection, after an alcoholic debauch or without any predisposing cause. Its onset is characteristically sudden, with severe prostration, a teeth-chattering chill, localized severe pleurisy, high fever, and a slight but irritative cough. Within 1 to 2 days the cough tends to become productive of "rusty," frankly bloody or purulent sputum. The cough gradually becomes more severe and finally productive of copious amounts of purulent sputum as the process begins to resolve.

Bronchopneumonia may be caused by the pneumococci, the staphylococci, the streptococci, Klebsiella, and various other bacteria or by various viral agents. Bronchopneumonia is apt to occur in the aged and infirm, following an alcoholic debauch, or in the very young. It is often a complication of influenza or some other severe infection involving the respiratory tract; it may follow the inhalation of food or other foreign material or various irritant gases. When due to one of several different viral agents, it is labelled *viral pneumonia* or *primary atypical pneumonia*. Cough in these pneumonias tends to be relatively dry and irritative at the outset, and only be-

comes severe and frankly productive as the process begins slowly to resolve.

Lung abscess is caused by the inhalation of foreign material (a piece of tonsil following tonsillectomy or a piece of tooth or food), by necrotizing inflammation behind an obstructive neoplasm, by necrosis within a malignant neoplasm or infarct, by blood stream dissemination of a suppurative process elsewhere in the body, by deep, penetrating chest trauma, or by the extension of a subphrenic or liver abscess through the diaphragm into the adjacent lung. During its early, formative phase a lung abscess behaves similarly to an acute severe pneumonia with dry, often relatively mild cough. As soon as necrosis has occurred in the center of the abscess and the fluid contents have gained access to a bronchus, the cough becomes severe and productive of large amounts of foul, purulent, often blood-tinged material. The organisms most commonly involved are Klebsiella, the staphylococci and the pneumococci, but the infections are frequently mixed.

Pulmonary tuberculosis is a chronic inflammatory disease of the lungs often involving the bronchi as well. It is characterized by a recurring sequence of patches of acute pneumonic consolidation followed by necrosis, emptying of necrotic material into a bronchus, leaving an air-containing cavity, and the development of new areas of pneumonitis in which the bacilli-laden necrotic material happens to lodge. Meanwhile, certain more favorable changes may take place, to a greater or lesser extent. The consolidation may resolve entirely or in part. As necrosis begins, the foci may begin to be walled off by a fibrous tissue reaction around them. Necrotic material may inspissate, become too thick to flow down a bronchus, and ultimately calcify. These healing processes may cease without warning, with resumption of the emptying of necrotic foci into nearby bronchi and consequent spread of the disease to new areas. The factors most important in determining how a tuberculous process will behave are host resistance, the virulence of the individual infecting microorganisms, the presence of other diseases and conditions such as diabetes, silicosis, and pregnancy, and the effectiveness of any chemotherapy that may be given. Cough in pulmonary tuberculosis may be due to the presence of exudate in the bronchi, to actual inflammation of the bronchi, usually near an area of parenchymal involvement, to complicating bronchial damage or bronchiectasis, to pleural irritation or to pressure upon bronchi caused by distortion, which is caused in turn by fibrous tissue contraction and/or atelectasis. Cough may be mild or severe, dry or nonproductive. The nature of the cough is dependent upon the status of the disease in the individual. Other symptoms commonly seen in tuberculosis are hemoptysis, pleurisy, weakness, easy fatigability, fever, and weight loss.

Deep fungal infections that are apt to occur in the lungs include especially histoplasmosis and coccidioidomycosis; others are actinomycosis, nocardiosis, blastomycosis, cryptococcosis (torulosis), aspergillosis, and mucormycosis. Pathologically these diseases attack the lung in much the same way as tuberculosis. Cough, caused by the same mechanism as that of tuberculosis, is frequently present. It will be dry or productive depending on whether a necrotic area has begun to slough into an open bronchus.

The x-ray films of the pulmonary fungal diseases are usually not diagnostic and are often quite similar to or even indistinguishable from those of pulmonary tuberculosis. Skin tests and serologic tests are helpful in diagnosing histoplasmosis and coccidioidomycosis.

Histoplasmosis is endemic in the valleys of the Mississippi river and its tributaries. The acute form of the disease is commonly acquired by inhaling dried bat, pigeon, or chicken dung (in caves, old buildings, or especially in abandoned chicken yards). Despite the fact that 50 to 75 per cent of adults in the endemic area have been infected (they have a positive histoplasmin skin test), in most cases the primary infection is inapparent and both the acute and chronic active forms of the disease remain quite uncommon.

Coccidioidomycosis is endemic in various hot arid parts of the world; southern California, New Mexico, and Arizona and western Texas are the endemic areas in the United States. As is true of histoplasmosis, far more persons have the infection than the disease. The disseminated forms are more common in pregnant women and in Filipinos than in the rest of the population. In the acute nondisseminated form the disease is often manifested by a pulmonary nodule or a thin-walled cavity.

Actinomycosis (caused by *Actinomyces bovis*) is apt to spread through natural tissue barriers and thus lead to chronic draining sinuses. Tissue sections and cultures will reveal the characteristic "sulfur granules."

Nocardiosis (due to *Actinomyces aster-oides*) usually attacks debilitated persons and those with other serious pulmonary diseases and is often fatal. The mycelia are faintly acid-fast and may break up into rodlike forms, which can be mistaken for tubercle bacilli.

North American blastomycosis behaves much like actinomycosis. About one-third of cases have pulmonary involvement, usually with patchy pneumonia, cavitation, and fibrosis. The skin and the lymph nodes are commonly involved.

Pulmonary cryptococcosis commonly presents a solitary pulmonary nodule or cavity. A chronic low-grade meningitis, which often ultimately proves fatal, is a common complication.

Aspergillosis occurs most commonly as a saprophytic "fungus ball" or mycetoma in an old inert pulmonary cavity caused by previous tuberculosis, fungus disease, or lung abscess. A severe bronchitis often lasting for two or three months is occasionally seen.

Mucormycosis is a rare, terminal complication seen especially in older persons with severe uncontrolled diabetes.

Parasitic lung diseases may also cause cough due to bronchial irritation; these include paragonimiasis, schistosomiasis, and ecchinococcal disease in particular.

Pleurisy with or without effusion, *pleurodynia*, and *pleural empyema* may all cause cough by irritation of the afferent nerve endings in the pleura, which are involved in the cough reflex arc.

CARDIOVASCULAR DISORDERS

Acute pulmonary edema is usually due to acute left ventricular failure. It may also follow the inhalation of smoke or noxious gases such as NO_2. It is characterized by intense vascular engorgement and by the transudation of fluid from congested capillaries into both the air spaces and interstitial tissues of the lungs. Cough in pulmonary edema is typically frequent, loose, and productive of frothy, often pink, sputum. There is also severe dyspnea and orthopnea. An attack is often ushered in by an attack of paroxysmal nocturnal dyspnea (cardiac asthma). Fine crepitant rales can be heard throughout the lungs. The most common causes of acute left ventricular failure are hypertensive and arteriosclerotic heart disease and aortic regurgitation. A somewhat special form of pulmonary edema is seen in severe mitral stenosis. This form is more chronic and often less severe than others. It may be accompanied by frequent small hemoptyses and, in some cases, by crepitant rales at one or both apices. Other special forms of pulmonary edema are sometimes seen in uremia, in acute rheumatic fever with carditis, after hexamethonium therapy, and rarely in normal persons when exposed to very high altitude and extreme cold. The roentgenographic picture of pulmonary edema is quite diagnostic and is characterized by small to large, symmetrical or asymmetrical patches of ill-defined, cloudy infiltration, especially in the region around the lung roots.

Pulmonary infarction may cause mild to moderate cough, which is usually dry, but sometimes productive of blood or blood-tinged sputum. The patient may or may not also have pleurisy with or without effusion and may or may not have some obvious source of pulmonary emboli.

Aortic aneurysm may cause severe cough by pressure on the trachea, the bronchi, or the lung parenchyma, or by interference with one of the recurrent laryngeal nerves. When an aneurysm presses on the trachea, the cough is apt to have the brassy quality of major airway obstruction.

TRAUMA AND PHYSICAL AGENTS

Foreign bodies of all kinds may be aspirated into the airways. The resulting cough depends on the nature of the foreign material and the location and completeness of the resulting airway obstruction. An obstruction in the trachea or larynx is apt to cause an intense croupy or brassy cough, plus dyspnea, cyanosis, and gagging. After the foreign body has become lodged, the symptoms often tend to subside. A foreign body in one of the main bronchi is apt to cause a continuing irritative cough and wheeze. Obstruction farther down the bronchial tree is very apt to cause severe paroxysmal cough, often followed by pneumonitis, atelectasis, or both. Atelectasis and pneumonia are particularly likely to occur when the inhaled object consists of vegetable matter, such as a peanut, which tends to incite an intense inflammatory reaction in the mucosa with which it remains in contact.

Irritant gases such as phosgene, chlorine, chloropicrin, NO_2, SO_2, ozone, nitro-olefins, tars, oxychlorcarbon, dichlorethyl sulfide, dichlormethylether, and other organic solvents can cause intense inflammation of the respiratory mucosa, a severe irritative cough, and ultimately acute pulmonary edema. Patchy pneumonia is a common complication. If the subject survives the initial insult, later changes such as bronchiolitis obliterans may prove fatal, especially following NO_2 inhalation. Intensely cold air may also act as a mild cough-inducing irritant, especially in persons with some underlying chronic pulmonary pathology. Furthermore, any noxious or irritating gas is considerably more irritating when inhaled through the mouth than when inhaled through the nose, since the nose filters, warms, and moistens inhaled gases to a remarkable degree.

Tobacco smoke contains irritant particulate matter, gases and chemicals which often cause laryngitis and tracheobronchitis, a symptom of which is the very common smoker's cough.

The **pneumoconioses** seldom cause cough unless complicated by extensive fibrosis, chronic bronchitis, or some pulmonary infection. *Beryllium granulomatosis* is a rather special exception in that very intense paroxysmal dry cough, marked weight loss, and alveolar capillary block without much impairment of ventilation are quite typical features. The roentgenographic appearance is very like miliary tuberculosis or miliary sarcoidosis.

NEOPLASMS

Primary bronchogenic carcinoma is a very common cause of cough, especially a severe and/or changing cough. The cough in bronchogenic carcinoma may be caused by partial airway obstruction and by bronchial mucosal irritation either directly or secondary to infection occurring distal to an obstructed bronchus. Cough, chest pain, and hemoptysis form the triad of symptoms so characteristic of this disease. The affected persons usually have been cigarette smokers for many years and often have long been accustomed to a chronic cough, especially in the mornings. When the malignant change takes place, the cough tends to change in some way, to become more or sometimes less productive, to become more persistent or severe, or to change in sound, often to become brassy. The associated chest pain may be pleuritic with or without a clear or bloody effusion, but often is vague and nonpleuritic.

Various other manifestations that should arouse suspicion of bronchogenic cancer in a person with a chronic or changing cough, include personality change or Jacksonian epilepsy suggesting a metastatic focal brain lesion; evidence of involvement of the brachial plexus, or of a recurrent laryngeal, phrenic, or cervical sympathetic nerve; recurrent pneumonitis, especially if in the same cough by pressure upon or invasion of the trachea or the bronchi.

ALLERGIC DISORDERS

Bronchial asthma may be defined as episodic expiratory dyspnea associated with wheezing, not necessarily associated with effort, often induced by contact with a specific substance (antigen), occurring in persons with a family history of allergy and accompanied by blood and sputum eosinophilia. Such patients are apt to show temporary relief after the administration of epinephrine, ephedrine, or some other bronchodilator. Although one may thus describe the so-called extrinsic type of asthma, the intrinsic variety may not exhibit all or even any of these features, but is often related to recurrent deep bronchial infections. The cough in asthma is dry, tight, wheezy, and usually occurs in paroxysms. Chest examination during an attack reveals the suppressed breath sounds of small airway obstruction and musical rales or rhonchi. These signs may be present, but are less evident, between attacks. Status asthmaticus is a protracted attack and is a late and critical phase of asthma in which response is no longer obtained with standard treatment. Death may occur in such an attack. Postmortem examination reveals extensive blocking of the finer airways with inspissated mucus plugs. Bronchial asthma should be differentiated carefully from cardiac asthma and from the various other conditions that cause cough and dyspnea with wheezing due to partial bronchial, tracheal, or laryngeal obstruction.

Hay fever and vasomotor rhinitis may both cause a mild, usually dry cough because of the postnasal drip so frequently accompanying these conditions.

OTHER CAUSES

Other causes of cough include a wide range of conditions involving the lungs and tracheobronchial tree. Calcified parenchymal foci or lymph nodes may ulcerate their way into an adjacent bronchus (*broncholithiasis*) and in so doing cause an intense irritative cough until the material has sloughed out and the patient has expectorated a "lung stone" or chalky material. Hemoptysis frequently accompany this sequence of events. Primary *hemosiderosis* is a rare disease of unknown etiology characterized by cough, frequent small hemoptyses, and progressive dyspnea.

Eosinophilic granuloma (Histiocytosis X) is characterized by diffuse roentgenographic

segment or lobe; or a wheeze which is either made worse or relieved by one or the other lateral recumbent positions. The diagnosis may be confirmed by roentgenologic examination of the chest (including fluoroscopy and tomography), bronchoscopy, bronchography, and sputum cytology. A blind scalene node biopsy is only occasionally helpful, but biopsy of a palpable cervical node, especially when hard and located just behind the medial end of either clavicle, is much more apt to be diagnostic. Sometimes the diagnosis can be established only by open thoracotomy.

Metastatic lung tumors are not prone to cause cough except in two circumstances: when the metastasis occurs in a bronchus or when pulmonary metastasis takes the form of widespread lymphogenous or hematogenous involvement. In these widespread forms, which cause marked alveolar-capillary (diffusion) block, cough is usually quite irritative, severe, and dry.

Bronchial adenoma will compress or invade a bronchial wall and cause severe cough, often with severe hemoptysis.

Bronchiolar or alveolar cell carcinoma, also called pulmonary adenomatosis, usually causes chronic cough. Because this is a tumor of mucus-secreting tissues, affected persons may (but usually do not) expectorate large quantities of clear watery mucoid sputum. The roentgenographic picture frequently simulates an infiltrative process such as tuberculosis.

Primary mesothelioma of the pleura is usually malignant and may cause dry cough, although chest pain and an arthritis-like syndrome (severe pulmonary osteoarthropathy) are much more frequent and suggestive symptoms.

Leukemia may involve the mediastinal and lung root structures and cause a secondary pneumonitis or bronchitis with resultant cough.

Other primary lung tumors that may cause cough are primary *sarcoma*, a very rare tumor; and *bronchogenic cyst*, especially after it has become secondarily infected. Hamartoma, fibroma, lipoma, pulmonary sequestration, and other rare benign tumors seldom if ever cause cough.

Mediastinal Tumors. Tumors of the thyroid or the thymus; teratomas, nerve tissue tumors, lymphomas, aneurysms, inflammatory enlargement of hilar or the paratracheal lymph nodes (due especially to tuberculosis, histoplasmosis, or sarcoidosis) all may cause involvement out of proportion to the mildness of symptoms, which may include cough, episodes of spontaneous pneumothorax, and occasionally diabetes insipidus.

Wegener's granulomatosis is a rare disease characterized by asymmetrical pulmonary infiltrates, often with large nodules that may cavitate; granulomatous involvement of the nasal septum and sinuses causing a severe catarrh; widespread necrotizing angiitis; and a focal glomerulonephritis that causes terminal renal insufficiency.

Sarcoidosis is a relatively common cause of hilar and paratracheal lymph node and/or lung parenchymal involvement that may result in dry cough and dyspnea.

Diffuse interstitial (Hamman-Rich) fibrosis is a rare disease of unknown cause, usually presenting with evidence of diffuse bilateral pulmonary fibrosis, alveolar-capillary block, and relatively little ventilatory impairment.

Alveolar proteinosis is a newly described disease of unknown cause in which the roentgenographic picture is reminiscent of a patchy pulmonary edema. The symptoms at the outset tend to be less severe than would be expected from the appearance of the infiltrate and death usually ensues with evidence of alveolar-capillary block.

Right middle lobe (compression) syndrome also may cause cough because of narrowing of the right middle lobe bronchus with associated atelectasis and pneumonitis. The right middle lobe bronchus is particularly vulnerable to compression by one or more enlarged lymph nodes situated at its origin from the right bronchus. Enlargement of the peribronchial lymph nodes at this site is most often caused by tuberculosis, but histoplasmosis and other infections and bronchogenic carcinoma also may cause this syndrome.

COMPLICATIONS OF COUGH

Cough interferes with normal activity in a number of inconvenient ways. Most of these effects are minor and inconsequential, for example, embarrassment, hoarseness, produced by laryngeal irritation, loss of sleep, or thoracic muscular soreness. However, two rare complications deserve special consideration.

Cough fractures of the ribs occur laterally, at the point of maximal mechanical stress, usually in the middle third of the rib. They occur more commonly in patients with diseases of the bones, such as multiple myeloma, metastatic carcinoma, hyperparathyroidism, or senile osteoporosis. However, they occur also in patients who do not have pre-existing intrinsic disease of the bones. In such instances, the usual history is that an uncommonly vigorous cough effort was accompanied by a sensation of a break, or rupture. Some patients hear the rib break. Pain and soreness follow. Chronic bronchitis is the disease most often associated with "benign" cough fracture of the ribs. The bronchitis should be treated, but the fracture usually requires no therapy.

Cough syncope is another rare but important complication of cough. Chronic bronchitis is, again, the most common associated pulmonary disease. The cause of cough syncope is *cerebral ischemia.* Usually it occurs in obese men past middle life who are heavy smokers of cigarettes. A typical history is of a coughing fit with syncope during cough. The patient is unconscious only a few seconds, but may fall. The potential for accidents is obvious. A convenient aid in establishing the diagnosis of cough syncope is measurement of the intrathoracic pressure. This can be done simply with a blood pressure manometer fitted with a mouthpiece, the nose being occluded.

Cerebral ischemia may result from severe cough through two mechanisms: (1) As intrathoracic pressure exceeds arterial pressure, blood is prevented from entering the cranial vault, since cerebrospinal fluid, and hence intracerebral pressure, parallels intrathoracic pressure. (2) Because cough causes high intrathoracic pressure, blood also is prevented from entering the right atrium, and cardiac output falls. Because cerebral ischemia can be sustained in this manner for several seconds, syncope occurs. Therapy is simple and is directed against the bronchitis. In order to avoid the syncope, the patient need only understand that he must not take a deep breath prior to cough. By avoiding precough inspiration, he limits the amount of pressure developed within the thorax and avoids syncope.

STUDY OF SPUTUM

A discussion of cough is incomplete without consideration of secretions. The study of sputum has primary importance in the evaluation of pulmonary disease. Except for microbiologic examination in pneumonia, fungus disease, and tuberculosis, the study of sputum often is neglected. Patients dislike sputum and dispose of it as promptly as possible since they find it unpleasant esthetically. Its production frequently is denied or minimized by the patient. The physician must not rely entirely on the results of interview for determination of the volume and appearance of sputum.

The exact quantity of tracheobronchial mucus produced daily in healthy people is somewhat uncertain, but may be as much as 100 ml. per day. In the normal subject, mucus is moved rapidly toward the glottis by ciliary action. Only 30 to 60 minutes are required for transit from the level of the respiratory bronchiole to the glottis, at which point its removal from the respiratory tract occurs without notice. This rapid and efficient transit of mucus is a principal factor in maintaining the lower respiratory tract free of microorganisms. Since the ciliated epithelium does not extend beyond the level of the respiratory bronchioles, other mechanisms operate to remove organisms deposited in the peripheral lung parenchyma.

Just as cough always is abnormal, so the production of sputum always is a sign of disease. Smokers accept the production of a few milliliters per day of mucoid sputum as part of their daily lives. The pathology of smoker's bronchitis, a common form of chronic bronchitis, is hyperplasia of the mucus-secreting cells in the respiratory tract. Most parenchymal diseases of the lung lead to sputum production. Persistent daily sputum in a volume exceeding 100 ml. suggests bronchiectasis.

Patients cooperate well in the submission of sputum samples when they learn the physician is interested. Medication vials or clear plastic with a snap-on-cap are convenient for the collection of sputum samples. Ambulatory patients are instructed to collect all sputum from time of awakening until they report. Hospital patients may desire to avoid the sight of sputum samples on the bedside table and find it convenient to place a paper cup upside down over the sample. Some of the more useful studies to be performed on sputum are included in Table 17-1.

SUMMARY

Cough is essentially an explosive expiration. It may be involuntary or voluntary. When involuntary, the reflex are responsible for cough consists of afferent impulses arising from irritation of the laryngeal or tracheobronchial mucosa, pressure or traction on the trachea, pressure upon the carotid sinus, the liver, the spleen, or the external auditory canal, irritation of the pleura, or congestion of the lung parenchyma. These impulses are transmitted by vagal or sympathetic trunks to an area in the medulla oblongata. The efferent impulses then descend to the various muscles of expiration.

The stimuli that can give rise to cough may be inflammatory, mechanical, chemical, or thermal.

The specific diseases that may cause cough were discussed under the following headings: Inflammations, Cardiovascular Disorders, Trauma and Physical Agents, Neoplasms, Allergic Disorders, Other Causes.

Complications of cough, especially cough fractures of ribs and cough syncope, are discussed.

Sputum production and characteristics are described; their study is an important adjunct to the study of cough.

BIBLIOGRAPHY

Bickerman, H. A., and Barach, A. L.: The experimental production of cough in human subjects induced by citric acid aerosols. Amer. J. Med. Sci. 228:156-163, 1954.

Bucher, K.: Pathophysiology and pharmacology of cough. Pharmacol. Rev. 10:43-58, 1958.

Chakravarty, N. K., Matallana, A., Jensen, R., and Borison, H. L.: Central effects of antitussive

TABLE 17-1. Sputum Examination

Collection period:	6-24 hours
Volume:	2-120 milliliters
Appearance:	Clear, buff, yellow, green, red
Layers:	Single gel, single watery, double, triple
pH:	4-8
Purulence:	1+ a few particles of pus in a mucoid gel 4+ pure pus gel
Viscosity:	1+ watery; 4+ solid gel

Peroxidase reaction

Microscopic examination:
a) Unstained: worms, pigmented macrophages, respiratory epithelial cells, and polymorphonuclear leukocytes
b) Wright's stain (or modified Giemsa) for eosinophils, and other cells
c) Papanicolaou: for malignant cells
d) Gram stain: for bacteria
e) NaOH wet preparation for fungi
f) PAS stain: fungi, alveolar proteinosis

Microbiologic examination:
a) Routine culture
b) Anaerobic culture
c) Mycobacterial culture
d) Fungal culture

drugs on cough and respiration, J. Pharmacol. Exp. Ther. 117:127–135, 1956.

Currens, J. H., and White, P. D.: Cough as a symptom of cardiovascular disease, Ann. Intern. Med. 30:528–543, 1949.

Dawes, G. S., and Comroe, J. H.: Chemoreflexes from the heart and lungs, Physiol. Rev. 34:167–201, 1954.

Drinker, C. K.: The function of the nerves in lungs and thoracic wall, Amer. Rev. Tuberc. 58:1–14, 1948.

DiRienzo, S.: Physiopathologie des hustens, Fortschr. Roentgenstr. 72:1–14, 1953.

Fenn, W. O.: Mechanics of respiration, Amer. J. Med. 10:77, 1951.

Leiner, G. C., Abramowitz, S., Small, M. J., and Stenby, V. B.: Cough peak flow rate, Amer. J. Med. Sci. 121:211, 1966.

Ross, B. B., Gramiak, R., and Rahn, H.: Physical dynamics of the cough mechanism, J. Appl. Physiol. 8:264–268, 1955.

Sharpey-Schafer, E. P.: Effects of coughing on intrathoracic pressure, arterial pressure and peripheral blood flow, J. Physiol. 122:351–357, 1953.

———: The mechanism of syncope after coughing, Brit. Med. J. 2:860–863, 1953.

Shane, S. J., Krzyski, T. K., and Copp, E. S.: Clinical evaluation of a new antitussive agent, Canad. Med. Ass. J. 77:600–602, 1957.

Widdicombe, J. G.: Respiratory reflexes, in Fenn, W. O., and Rahn, H. (eds.): Handbook of Physiology, Section 3: Respiration, vol. 1, Washington, D. C., American Physiological Society, 1964.

Whipple, H. E.: Mucous secretions, Ann. N. Y. Acad. Sci. 106: Art. 2, 157–809, 1963.

18

Hemoptysis

JOHN A. PIERCE

Hemoptysis is one of the most alarming and startling of all symptoms. It occurs typically after cough, and frequently recurs over several hours or days. Some patients have hemoptysis daily for many years, whereas others may become exsanguinated in a few seconds. True hemoptysis is defined as the spitting of some quantity of blood, usually more than 2 ml. It is remarkable that hemoptysis is only rarely fatal.

BASIC PATHOPHYSIOLOGY

The basic pathophysiologic mechanisms involved in bleeding into the respiratory tract are (as with bleeding anywhere): (1) disturbances in the integrity of vascular walls (from trauma, inflammation, neoplastic destruction, pressure disruption, vitamin C deficiency, etc.); and (2) disorders in blood clotting mechanisms (platelet deficiency, prothrombin deficiency, lack of antihemophilic factor, etc.). See the chapter on Pathological Bleeding. Two or more of the basic mechanisms often operate together to cause hemorrhage: degenerative vascular changes plus high blood pressure, for example, or pulmonary inflammatory damage plus the trauma of severe coughing.

LOCALIZATION OF BLEEDING SITE

It is always important to localize the origin of pulmonary hemorrhage. Examination of the nose and throat must be done in all patients to determine whether the expectorated blood may have come from the nasal passages or pharynx. Many patients experience a pulling or drawing sensation in the chest with hemorrhage, often localized to the general area of the bleeding. Rales or rhonchi may be localized to one area of the lungs and may aid in establishing the site of hemorrhage. Bronchoscopy during hemorrhage is useful to determine the origin of hemorrhage; however, since blood leaving one lung often is aspirated into the other, the bronchoscopist must see a bleeding point or ascertain an active flow of blood in order to lateralize bleeding. In addition, it should be appreciated that blood may be retained in the lung for some time after it has escaped the vessel. This occurs especially with mild degrees of bleeding and is suggested when expectorated blood is clotted. A fresh hemorrhage from the pulmonary artery may have the dark blue color of unoxygenated blood.

STUDY OF SPUTUM: MICROORGANISMS; CELLS

Years ago, the most frequent cause of hemoptysis in the United States was tuberculosis. Today, hemoptysis is more often caused by pulmonary infarction, bronchogenic carcinoma, lung abscess, or chronic bronchitis than by tuberculosis. The underlying cause of hemoptysis must carefully be sought in each instance. The history, physical examination, and roentgenographic studies frequently permit a presumptive diagnosis to guide the laboratory investigation. Examination of the sputum should be pursued exhaustively whenever the cause of hemoptysis is obscure. In addition to cultural studies for common pathogens, microbiologic examination should include special cultures for **tubercle bacilli** and **fungi.** Anaerobic cultures are likely to be helpful whenever the sputum is foul or putrid.

The importance of **sputum cytology** cannot be overemphasized. This examination, carefully performed, often is positive in patients with bronchogenic carcinoma. We recommend bronchoscopy to localize the site of bleeding, and to obtain washings for cultural, and especially for cytologic examination.

It is important to determine the amount of hemoptysis. Thus, the patient should be instructed to collect all of his sputum so that the volume and appearance can be recorded. Careful examination of the sputum occasionally reveals bits of tumor tissue or calcified particles. The coughing of blood should be observed directly by the physician whenever possible.

CAUSES OF HEMOPTYSIS

The causes of hemoptysis may be classified as follows: (1) trauma, (2) foreign bodies, (3) inflammation, (4) neoplasms, (5) vascular and circulatory conditions, and (6) miscellaneous causes.

TRAUMA

Hemoptysis may result when the lungs are punctured by a fractured rib or lacerated with a stab or gunshot wound. The inhalation of noxious fumes or smoke gives rise to tracheobronchitis, which bleeds when ulcerated. The tracheobronchial tree may be lacerated or fractured by blunt trauma, such as a steering wheel in an automobile collision. Severe protracted coughing may also lead to mucosal lacerations, and thus to hemoptysis.

FOREIGN BODIES

Foreign bodies cause bleeding by direct trauma producing laceration or ulceration of the mucosa of the airways.

INFLAMMATION

Bleeding from infectious lesions may arise in the pharynx, the larynx, the trachea, the bronchi, or the lungs. It is particularly apt to occur with necrotizing infections such as tuberculosis, fungal infections, and pneumonias due to the staphylococci and gram-negative organisms.

Hemorrhage early in **tuberculosis** occurs because necrosis involves the walls of vessels, but it is not uncommon to encounter hemoptysis in patients whose tuberculosis is inactive. Presumably, this occurs because of aneurysmal deformity of vessels, because of bronchiectasis, or because of the erosion of calcific particles through the bronchial mucosa.

Pneumococcal pneumonia often can be diagnosed clinically from the abrupt onset of a shaking chill followed by fever, pleuritic pain, and cough with hemoptysis. Characteristically, the sputum is pink or rust-colored, but hemorrhage at times may be brisk. **Viral pneumonias** may be associated with blood-streaked sputum, but rarely cause significant hemoptysis.

Necrotizing pneumonias often cause hemoptysis. This is apt to occur several days after the onset of the illness and may be abrupt and brisk. Gram-negative organisms are the most frequent causes, but staphylococci also may be responsible. Anaerobic organisms frequently are present in patients with putrid lung abscess. These patients often have advanced periodontoclasia and frequently give a history of dental manipulation shortly prior to the onset of symptoms. Many are alcoholic or epileptic and have inspired regurgited or vomited material.

Fungus infections of the respiratory tract cause bleeding because of tissue necrosis or cavitation. Hemoptysis may occur after the healing of fungal infections, presumably from erosion of calcium deposits, or because of secondary bacterial infection in deformed bronchi.

Parasitic diseases of the lung occasionally cause hemoptysis. An amebic abscess of the liver may erode into the lung through the right hemidiaphragm; the patient may cough up a large volume of thin chocolate-colored fluid, which has been likened to anchovy sauce.

Hemoptysis frequently occurs in patients with **saccular bronchiectasis.** The deformity of the bronchi renders these patients susceptible to persistent bacterial infections, which may from time to time lead to mucosal ulcerations and hemoptysis. The bronchial arteries enlarge considerably with severe bronchiectatic deformity, and hemorrhage from this systemic arterial source may be brisk.

Hemoptysis occurs in patients with **bronchitis.** In such instances, it often is difficult or impossible to identify the site of bleeding. The roentgenogram of the chest often is not helpful, but occasionally will show aspirated blood. The x-ray change almost invariably appears abruptly during a time of active hemoptysis, and may occur with hemoptysis due to any cause. Considerable blood may be aspirated without the production of symptoms. The shadows on the roentgenogram usually disappear within a few days after bleeding stops.

NEOPLASMS

The most common cause of chronic hemoptysis in persons past the age of 45 is **primary bronchogenic carcinoma.** Hemoptysis, together with severe and changing cough, and nondescript chest pain, form the characteristic triad of symptoms of this neoplasm. Unfortunately, all of these symptoms appear very late in the course of this disease. Bleeding in primary bronchogenic cancer may occur because of mucosal ulceration, because of necrosis within the center of a tumor, or secondary to a pneumonic or bronchitic process distal to an obstructing bronchial tumor. Hemoptysis caused by **metastatic cancer** in the lung is rare. Although **primary bronchial adenoma** is not common, when this lesion is present, bleeding is common and apt to be severe. If a bronchoscopist sees what he believes may be a bronchial adenoma, he should not attempt to biopsy it, as the danger of starting an uncontrollable hemorrhage is great.

Hemangioma is a rare tumor of the lung or tracheobronchial tree which may cause severe pulmonary hemorrhage. It may be benign or malignant.

VASCULAR AND CIRCULATORY CONDITIONS

Patients with acute pulmonary edema due to **left ventricular failure** may cough up large quantities of pink frothy sputum. Pulmonary edema due to severe **mitral stenosis** is more often associated with brisk frank hemoptysis. This is an expression of the severe degree of *pulmonary hypertension* that occurs with mitral stenosis.

Pulmonary embolism and thrombosis are extremely common causes of hemoptysis, especially when complicated by true infarction. It should be stressed that many pulmonary emboli occur without hemoptysis or pleurisy and without any obvious source of an embolus. Pulmonary infarction occurs more often in patients with cardiac disease and in hospitalized patients following acute illness and surgery than in healthy people. Whenever frank hemoptysis occurs in a patient with left ventricular failure, a presumptive diagnosis of pulmonary infarction is warranted.

Occasionally, an **aortic aneurysm** erodes into the tracheobronchial tree and causes an exsanguinating hemorrhage.

Patients with hereditary hemorrhagic telangiectasis may have hemoptysis from **pulmonary arteriovenous fistulae.** Typical angiomata often are present on the lips, face, tongue, ears, and fingers. When pulmonary fistulae are present, the patients also have cyanosis, clubbing of the fingers, and a bruit over the fistula. Bleeding may be severe.

MISCELLANEOUS CAUSES

Hemoptysis may occur with any type of **hemorrhagic diathesis.** It occurs with thrombocytopenia, hemophilia, hypoplastic anemia, and leukemia. It may occur with uremia, or in scurvy. The mechanisms involved in these and other clinical disorders are discussed in the chapter on Pathological Bleeding.

Pulmonary hemosiderosis is a rare disease without known cause which usually occurs in young adult males. It is characterized by recurrent episodes of hemoptysis, dyspnea on exertion and with the appearance of a diffuse, almost miliary, infiltrate on the chest roentgenogram.

The right middle lobe syndrome is due to a partial or complete obstruction of the long and narrow right middle lobe bronchus. This causes right middle lobe atelectasis, pneumonitis, or both. The obstruction often is due to scar tissue formation and inflammation, but may result from physical compression of the lumen of the bronchus by an enlarged lymph node. Hemoptysis occasionally accompanies this syndrome.

Lung purpura with nephritis (Goodpasture's Syndrome), **Wegener's granulomatosis,** and **polyarteritis nodosa** are all disorders of obscure etiology that may give rise to hemoptysis.

Pulmonary microlithiasis, pulmonary amyloidosis, chronic lipoid pneumonia, and endometriosis of the lung also are reported causes of hemoptysis.

One should not overlook the fact that certain drugs are capable of inducing hemorrhage, such as **anticoagulants.** These may cause bleeding anywhere, especially if there is an added factor, such as blood vessel fragility or trauma, or infection damaging blood vessels. Therefore, persons receiving anticoagulant drugs who have congestive heart failure, bronchitis, or severe cough or high blood pressure, etc., are particularly prone to hemoptysis.

Severe hypertension, which is so often associated with degenerative changes in small arteries and arterioles, often leads to rupture of these fragile vessels. Bleeding may occur in the brain, the heart, the kidney, the eye, etc. If bleeding occurs in the respiratory tract, hemoptysis may result.

REFERENCES

1. Abbott, O. A.: The clinical significance of pulmonary hemorrhage. Study of 1316 patients with chest disease, Dis. Chest 14:824, 1948.
2. Johnston, R. N., Lockhart, W., Richie, R. T., and Smith, D. H.: Hemoptysis, Brit. Med. J. 1:592, 1960.
3. Sonders, C. R., and Smith, A. T.: The clinical significance of hemoptysis, New Eng. J. Med. 247:791, 1952.

19

Dyspnea

DANIEL S. LUKAS

The term dyspnea implies difficult or uncomfortable breathing. It is the sensation experienced when the act of breathing intrudes upon the conscious sphere as an unpleasant effort. The patient suffering from dyspnea is apt to say: "I'm short of breath"; "I can't catch my breath"; "I'm breathless"; or "I feel like I'm suffocating."

Dyspnea is by no means always a symptom of disease. Normal individuals commonly experience this sensation with vigorous exertion. The level of physical activity provoking the symptom varies widely with age, sex, body size, the state of physical training, the altitude, and the emotional motivation for the task being performed.

Dyspnea indicates disease only when it occurs at levels of activity below those expected to be normally tolerated. In this respect, since the normal range of tolerance for exertion is wide, it is very useful in taking the history to trace the development of the symptom in terms of diminishing ability to perform specific tasks. As an example: A patient may previously have been able to climb three flights of stairs at a moderately fast rate without discomfort, but during the past year has noted progressive difficulty in performing this act and recently has been capable of climbing only one flight of stairs at a very slow rate because of shortness of breath.

Muscular fatigue very often accompanies dyspnea, and, particularly in patients with heart disease, the two symptoms may be inseparable. In some it may be overwhelming fatigue rather than dyspnea which brings activity to a halt. Therefore, an assessment of the tolerance for physical exertion is not complete without inquiry about the specific reactions that limit it. One cannot assume that the patient is dyspneic because he has a disease frequently provoking this symptom or because he manifests tachypnea or hyperpnea. These are *objective* signs of abnormality in breathing and suggest that shortness of breath may be one of his symptoms. Whether it is or not, however, can be answered only by the patient.

Dyspnea is a very important cause of disability in diseases of the lung and the heart. Although several attempts have been made to relate it to a single specific measurable abnormality in cardiac or pulmonary function, none of these applies to all examples of this symptom. The results of many investigations over the years clearly indicate that many factors contribute to dyspnea, but there is no uniform agreement among interested investigators about the relative importance of each disturbance of function in its pathogenesis. A considerable part of the difficulty stems from the fact that the symptom is a subjective one and therefore susceptible to modification by emotional state and drive. It is unlikely on this basis alone that measurements of any single variable or even multiple variables of cardiopulmonary function will correlate satisfactorily with the severity of dyspnea in *all* cases. Another aspect of the problem that is in great need of clarification is the nature of the stimuli, the sensory receptors, and the nerve pathways which participate in the awareness of dyspnea. Little is known about the part played by visceral sensations arising from the pulmonary or cardiovascular structures as opposed to somatic sensations arising from the chest cage and the diaphragm.

The presently available information, which is the product of extensive investigation of cardiopulmonary function, particularly in the recent past, indicates that dyspnea is primarily related to the *ventilatory component* of pulmonary function as opposed to the function of *gas exchange*.

VENTILATORY APPARATUS

The maintenance of an adequate flow of air to the alveoli of the lungs is essential to the normal performance of pulmonary function. The alternate expansion and relaxation of the chest bellows is responsible for this function.

The ability of the chest bellows to pump air into and out of the alveoli may be evaluated by measurement of the maximum breathing capacity (*ventilatory capacity*). This is the maximum volume of air that can be breathed voluntarily in a minute. Maximum breathing capacity normally varies with body size, age, and sex.[1] In young well-trained males it may attain values in the range of 200 liters per minute, whereas in small elderly ladies the normal level may be 60 liters per minute.

Ventilatory capacity measured in this way has been found to be greater than the ventilation attained during maximum exercise or maximum stimulation from carbon dioxide.[2] This clearly indicates that in the capacity of the normal chest bellows to perform there is a margin of reserve that is considerable under normal circumstances and that the ventilatory requirements of most human activities can be met quite adequately.

It is essential to recognize that the chest bellows is a complex apparatus. Its effectiveness in function depends on an intact and mobile rib cage, the health of the diaphragm and other respiratory muscles and their neural control and coordination. Of considerable importance is the patency of the various extrapulmonary and intrapulmonary airways. The elastic resistance of the pulmonary parenchyma and pleura (the resistance of these structures to stretching) is another significant determinant in performance. If the normal state or action of any of these components of the ventilatory apparatus are disturbed sufficiently, decrease in the maximum breathing capacity may ensue. Thus, diaphragmatic paralysis, as in poliomyelitis, is associated with considerable impairment of ventilatory capacity.[3] Obstruction of the airways, particularly the small intrapulmonary segments of this system, as in asthma or emphysema, has a profound slowing effect on the volume rate of air flow in these passages and is a very common clinical cause of a diminished maximum breathing capacity.

Reduction in the ventilatory capacity is perhaps the most common disturbance in pulmonary function encountered among patients with various diseases of the lungs. The severity of dyspnea and the ease with which it is produced by exertion can be correlated fairly well with the degree to which the maximum breathing capacity is impaired. A very close approximation of dyspnea in physiologic terms is obtained when the levels of ventilation are compared with the ability to ventilate. Dyspnea is experienced invariably in normal individuals and in a variety of pulmonary diseases when the ventilation required by a particular activity or metabolic state occupies 30 to 40 per cent of the maximum breathing capacity or, to state the same thing in reverse, when only 60 to 70 per cent of the maximum breathing is not in use and is thus in reserve (breathing reserve).[4] From this relationship it is apparent that a very large ventilation, even though the maximum breathing capacity is normal, may cause dyspnea, and if the breathing capacity is low, relatively slight increases in ventilation from the resting state will produce this symptom. In many conditions not only is the ventilatory *capacity* reduced, but also the ventilatory *requirements* during exercise are abnormally large.

Although it is widely applicable and clinically useful, the definition of the *dyspnea threshold* in terms of ventilation and maximum breathing capacity does not apply without reservation to all conditions provoking dyspnea. Two notable exceptions are pulmonary emphysema and cardiac disease. In emphysema the dyspnea threshold is very variable and the patient may have in use more than 50 per cent of his maximum breathing capacity during exertion without experiencing dyspnea. In heart disease the maximum breathing capacity may be normal and hyperventilation during exercise only mild, yet the patient may experience severe shortness of breath.[5]

MECHANICS AND WORK OF BREATHING

In seeking a physiologic common denominator for dyspnea, considerable attention has been focused on the mechanics of breathing.

The process of breathing is work. By the cyclic changes in intrapleural pressure produced by alternate contraction and relaxation of the respiratory muscles, the following forces must be overcome: the resistance of the lungs to stretch (elastic resistance), which depends on the physical properties of the lung tissues as well as on the surface tension acting at the interface between air and fluid lining the alveoli;[6,7] the resistance to the flow of gas in the airways, related to the geometric dimensions of the air passages; the velocity of gas flow within them; the viscosity and density of the gas;[6,8] and the resistance related to the friction of tissues as they slide over each other or are deformed. In addition, the respiratory muscles must overcome the elastic resistance of the chest wall and the frictional forces developed within the nonpulmonary tissues that are deformed or displaced during breathing. Of the total work expended by the normal subject in breathing at a rate of 15 times per minute, 63 per cent is spent on overcoming the elastic resistance of the lungs and chest wall, 29 per cent on overcoming airway resistance, and only 8 per cent in deforming tissues.[9] With faster rates, overcoming airway resistance requires a progressively larger percentage of the total work. Also, the balance between work in overcoming elastic resistance and that overcoming airway resistance is such that for any given level of alveolar ventilation there is an optimum rate of breathing. Decreasing or increasing the respiratory rate results in increased work expenditure.[9,10]

The work of quiet breathing during the course of a day involves an energy expenditure so small (0.4-0.5 kg. M. per minute) that it can be supplied by 10 Gm. of sugar.[9] With increasing ventilation, the work performed by the respiratory muscles increases, and during maximum ventilation it is approximately 270 kg. M. per minute.[9]

If the lungs are more than normally resistant to stretch (decreased pulmonary compliance) or if airway resistance is increased, the changes in intrapleural pressure and the work which are required to sustain a given level of ventilation are greater than normal. In patients with decreased compliance due to *pulmonary congestion*, the work expended on achieving a given minute volume during exercise may be two to three times normal.[11] In patients with *airway obstruction* due to emphysema, the force and work expended in overcoming resistance to airflow are in-

creased considerably.[12] Disturbances in the chest bellows also may increase the work of breathing. In kyphoscoliosis, work done to move the deformed chest cage in the process of breathing may be five or more times greater than normal.[13] In obesity, the decreased thoracic compliance produced by the encircling girdle of adipose tissue increases the mechanical work of breathing severalfold.[14]

In order to perform their work the respiratory muscles require oxygen. At levels of ventilation within the resting range, 0.5 to 1.0 ml. of oxygen is sufficient to sustain each liter of ventilation.[15]

The oxygen costs of breathing have been shown to increase disproportionately with increase in ventilation,[15] although there is wide scatter among the values reported by different investigators.[15] According to one group of investigators,[16] at a ventilation 25 liters per minute greater than resting ventilation, the cost of each liter of ventilation is 1 ml. of oxygen per minute. At a ventilation in excess of 80 liters per minute, 3.2 ml. of oxygen are needed to support each liter of air breathed. And at 150 liters per minute, 1 liter of oxygen is consumed merely in the act of breathing.

The increased work of breathing in disease requires a greater oxygen supply to the respiratory muscles. A patient with severe pulmonary congestion may need more than three times the normal oxygen supply to support each liter of ventilation in excess of 15 liters per minute above the resting level.[16] A patient with emphysema may require 25 ml. of oxygen per minute to support each liter of ventilation above the resting level.[16] This exceeds the oxygen requirement for maintenance of more than 50 liters per minute in the normal. In kyphoscoliosis and in obesity, the oxygen costs of breathing are increased greatly.[13,17]

Although the data on work, oxygen requirements, and the mechanics of breathing in both the normal state and in disease are far from complete, they do serve to emphasize in a more fundamental manner than otherwise possible the serious defects in the ventilatory apparatus produced by diseases involving the lungs. *Fatigue* of the respiratory muscles resulting from the increased work required of them in sustaining a given level of ventilation may play an important role in the sensation of dyspnea. In disease, not only is the respiratory work for a given level of exertion greater than normal, but the oxygen supply to the muscles of respiration is frequently disturbed by *hypoxemia* and a *restricted blood flow*, thus making them more susceptible to fatigue.

A critical level for the work of breathing at which dyspnea appears has not been found. Actually, in emphysema and mitral stenosis, dyspnea of sufficient severity to cause the patient to stop during exercise has been shown to occur at levels of breathing work considerably less than normal.[18] This may be related to poor oxygen supply to the muscles. Christie[18] has provided evidence that dyspnea severe enough to limit activity occurs when the intrapleural pressure changes required to effect ventilation are large (in the range of 30 cm. of water). He has suggested ". . . that dyspnea is conditioned not by the mechanical work of breathing but by the force which has to be exerted on the lungs in order to increase ventilation in accordance with the demands of exercise." Of interest in this regard is the demonstration that the oxygen cost of breathing is related more closely to the total forve exerted by the respiratory apparatus on the lungs and chest wall than it is to the mechanical work of breathing.[19] If Christie's concept is correct, then dyspnea is related primarily to stimuli arising from stretch receptors in the intrathoracic organs.

Thus, dyspnea is best interpreted as the subjective symptom that arises when the ventilatory apparatus is unduly taxed in meeting a certain requirement for ventilation. In the analysis of this symptom, factors that limit the capacity of the ventilatory apparatus to provide ventilation, or cause it to work excessively in meeting ventilatory requirements, as well as the demands for ventilation imposed on it, must be taken into consideration.

VENTILATION

Relative constancy in the gas composition of the alveolar air is achieved by a cyclic flushing of the alveoli with air from the outside. The rate at which air is moved into and out of the lungs is termed ventilation and is conventionally expressed in liters per minute. At a constant tidal volume it is equal to the tidal volume times the respiratory rate.

Not all of each breath reaches the alveoli to participate in gas exchange. Some of it remains behind in the dead space in which no gas exchange occurs. Anatomically, the dead space consists of the volume of air in the nasopharynx, the trachea, the bronchi, and the nonrespiratory bronchioles. In the normal adult the dead space is from 100 to 150 ml. in size.[20]

Total ventilation is subdivided into two components: alveolar and dead space. The dead space component usually occupies less than 30 per cent of total ventilation.

The relationship between *alveolar ventilation* and carbon dioxide and the rate at which carbon dioxide is manufactured and exhaled from the body is as follows:
Concentration of CO_2 in alveolar air =

$$\frac{CO_2 \text{ output per minute}}{\text{Alveolar ventilation}}$$

Assuming the respiratory exchange ratio (CO_2 output per minute divided by O_2 uptake per minute) to be 1.0, a similar but more complicated relationship exists for oxygen[21]:
Concentration of O_2 in alveolar air =

$$\text{Concentration of } O_2 \text{ in inspired air} - \frac{O_2 \text{ uptake per minute}}{\text{Alveolar ventilation}}$$

From these considerations it is apparent that alveolar ventilation, in relation to metabolic uptake of oxygen and release of carbon dioxide, ultimately determines the gas composition of both the alveolar air and blood flowing from the alveoli. At any given level of metabolism, a decrease below normal in alveolar ventilation will cause the concentration of carbon dioxide in alveolar air to rise and that of oxygen to fall. Increase in the alveolar ventilation will have the opposite effect.

A decision about the appropriateness of ventilation in a given patient may be very difficult without knowledge of the relative sizes of the dead space and the tidal volume, the concentration of oxygen and of carbon dioxide in the arterial blood, and the metabolic rate.

Alveolar ventilation is regulated by complex homeostatic mechanisms,[22,23] and total ventilation may be modified by a host of factors. These mechanisms and factors can be subdivided into chemical, mechanical, physical, cortical, and metabolic.

Chemical Factors. The respiratory control system is exquisitely sensitive to changes in the *concentration of carbon dioxide* in the arterial blood. An increment in carbon dioxide tension as small as 1.5 mm. Hg above the normal of 40 mm. Hg is enough to cause the alveolar ventilation to double.[24,25] Alveolar ventilation increases linearly with increase in arterial carbon dioxide tension, but a limit is reached when carbon dioxide at a level of 9 per cent is inspired. Further increments in carbon dioxide concentration are associated with depression of alveolar ventilation and the mental manifestations related to the narcotic and anesthetic properties of the gas begin to appear.[23]

The respiratory control system is also sensitive to changes in the *concentration of hydrogen ion* in the blood (pH). The increased ventilation that occurs upon breathing carbon dioxide is partly due to the concomitant fall in pH of the blood.[23] For some time it was believed that the respiratory center was much less sensitive to change in hydrogen ion concentration than to change in carbon dioxide tension. This conclusion was based on the fact that the increase in ventilation during carbon dioxide inhalation is much greater than the increase occurring when the pH of the arterial blood is reduced to an equivalent degree by metabolic acidosis, such as may occur following ingestion of ammonium chloride. Thus inhalation of 5 per cent carbon dioxide which may be associated with a change in blood pH from 7.41 to 7.34 results in a 2.68-fold increase in alveolar ventilation. On the other hand, a metabolically induced acidosis with a pH of 7.34 may produce only a 1.09-fold increase in alveolar ventilation. However, Gray[23] has pointed out that in metabolic acidosis the concomitant decrease in carbon dioxide tension of the arterial blood definitely inhibits ventilation. The change in ventilation during metabolic acidosis is therefore the net effect of inhibition due to decrease of carbon dioxide tension and stimulation from increase in hydrogen ion concentration. The change observed upon inhalation of carbon dioxide is due to the additive effect of increase of the two stimuli: carbon dioxide tension and hydrogen ion concentration.

Hyperventilation may become a conspicuous feature of metabolic acidosis. The very deep, usually rapid, respiration of acidosis forms a characteristic clinical picture called *Kussmaul breathing*. Such hyperventilation, often without dyspnea or consciousness of labored respiration, may accompany the ketoacidosis of diabetes, the acidosis of uremia, or the formic acidosis of methyl alcohol poisoning.

Until recently it was not clear whether carbon dioxide tension or hydrogen ion concentration within the cells of the respiratory center is the chief stimulus to respiration. The problem was complicated by the evidence that the sensitivity of the respiratory center may be enhanced by prolonged hypocapnia. The hyperventilation which is a prominent feature of the acclimatization response to altitude has been found to persist upon return to sea level.[23,26] Normal young men passively hyperventilated for 24 hours in a body respirator have been found to have a heightened ventilatory response to carbon dioxide inhalation persisting for as long as 11 days after removal from the respirator.[27]

Decrease in buffering capacity and bicarbonate concentration of the blood follows such prolonged hyperventilation and permits a greater fall in blood pH for a given increase of carbon dioxide tension. However, the phenomenon is not entirely dependent on decreased buffering capacity, since the response of ventilation to increase in hydrogen ion concentration in the blood is also greater.[28] This fact is directly applicable to patients who hyperventilate, since prolonged hyperventilation, regardless of cause, may be self-propagating by virtue of sensitization of the respiratory center. It may partially account for the severe hyperventilation observed in certain patients with pulmonary fibrosis and low blood bicarbonate levels.

On the other hand, prolonged exposure to high concentrations of carbon dioxide diminishes the sensitivity of the respiratory center. This has been observed in normal men after four to six days of exposure to 3 per cent carbon dioxide[29] and is a particularly striking and clinically important feature of patients with severe pulmonary disease and chronic elevations of their alveolar and arterial blood carbon dioxide levels (chronic respiratory acidosis). Again the diminished sensitivity has been shown definitely not to be related entirely to the concomitant increase in blood bicarbonate levels and the greater ability thereby to buffer the acid effect of increases in carbon dioxide tension, since the ventilatory response to change in arterial hydrogen ion concentration is impaired also.[25]

Current evidence indicates that these alterations in the sensitivity of the respiratory center with prolonged hypocapnia or hypercapnia are related to changes in the buffering capacity of the brain.[30] It would appear that the activity of the respiratory center is conditioned by the concentrations within its cells of both carbon dioxide and buffer.[31,32] Indeed, recent experiments by Pappenheimer and his associates indicate that, under normal circumstances, during breathing of carbon dioxide, during chronic acidosis or alkalosis, and during perfusion of the ventriculocisternal space with solutions containing various concentrations of bicarbonate, ventilation is a unique and direct exponential function of the hydrogen concentration of the interstitial fluid surrounding the respiratory neurones.[22] Factors influencing neuronal response to hydrogen ion, such as the concentrations of potassium[33] and other cations in the neurones and the fluid surrounding them, remain to be elucidated.

Reduction in the oxygen tension of the arterial blood stimulates respiration. This effect is mediated by the cells in the carotid and the aortic bodies (peripheral chemoreceptors), which are sensitive to hypoxemia. The effect of hypoxemia on ventilation is not striking. It is not perceptible until the arterial oxygen has fallen to a level of about 65 mm. Hg from a normal of 95.[34] The increase in ventilation in normal men breathing low concentrations of oxygen is quite variable, probably because of variations in the degree of concomitant changes in arterial carbon dioxide tension and the response to them.[34] The fall in blood carbon dioxide tension and rise in pH concurrent with such hyperventilation act to inhibit a further increase in ventilation. When alveolar carbon dioxide tension is held constant, decrease in alveolar oxygen tension from 65 to 35 mm. Hg is capable of evoking a more than sixfold increase in ventilation.[34] Gray[23] has calculated that an oxygen tension of 30 mm. Hg, allowed to act without opposition from a decrease in both carbon dioxide tension and hydrogen ion concentration, would evoke a seven-fold increase in alveolar ventilation.

The importance of hypoxemia in stimulating ventilation in patients with diseases of the lungs or heart is demonstrated by the decrease that occurs with administration of oxygen. This effect may be observed even though the hypoxemia is very slight.

Mechanical and Physical Factors. One of the most fascinating *regulatory mechanisms* of respiration relates to the *work of breathing.* For any given level of alveolar ventilation there is an optimum respiratory rate at which the muscular work of breathing is minimum. Change of breathing frequency in either direction results in the expenditure of larger amounts of work. Such an optimum frequency of breathing originally was predicted by Otis, Fenn, and Rahn[9] from calculations based on the work involved in overcoming the elastic and the airflow resistances of the lungs. Christie and co-workers[35] have measured the work of breathing in normal subjects, have confirmed this optimum frequency (usually 15 per minute, as predicted by Otis, *et al.*), and have demonstrated that it was the frequency naturally chosen by their subjects. Moreover, when the elastic and the airway properties of the lung are modified by disease, as in mitral stenosis or pneumonia, the respiratory frequency at which minimum work is performed in sustaining a particular level of alveolar ventilation is different from normal. It is almost precisely this respiratory rate that the patient selects naturally.[11,36] This remarkable adjustment of respiratory frequency in the interests of body economy in both health and disease apparently is controlled delicately. The mechanisms involved have yet to be elucidated. Meade has presented evidence that respiratory frequency is somewhat more closely adjusted to levels requiring minimum development of transpulmonary pressures and force by the respiratory muscles than it is to levels associated with minimum expenditure of work.[37] He has suggested that vagal afferent impulses arising from stretch receptors in the lungs, and of the type known since the work of Hering and Breuer in 1868, provide the signal for this control of respiratory rhythm.

Stimulation of any afferent nerve may bring about reflex changes.[38] Pain fibers seem to be especially potent, and painful sensations from any source may cause hyperpnea. Occasionally this may be sufficiently prolonged and of sufficient intensity to produce severe hypocapnia and even tetany. Similar although less dramatic effects may be produced through cutaneous nerve fibers by exposure to heat and cold. Stimulation of abdominal viscera at the time of operation may cause moderate hyperpnea. There are numerous examples of the use of reflex stimulation of respiration for the accomplishment of practical clinical results. Mention may be made of spanking the newborn baby to initiate breathing and throwing on cold water or using aromatic spirits of ammonia to arouse a patient from syncope. There is evidence that reflexes originating in the muscles, the tendons, or the joints of moving limbs increase ventilation and may play an important role in the ventilatory adjustments of exericse.[39]

Cerebral Cortical Factors. To a limited extent, normal breathing is under the control of cerebral centers. Gray[23] reminds us

". . . that innumerable daily acts require unconscious interference with the respiratory pattern. Eating, drinking, talking, singing, defecating and threading a needle all involve transitory interference with breathing."

By volition, the alveolar ventilation can be increased to such an extent as to cause a profound fall in alveolar and arterial carbon dioxide tension with consequent fall in pH and tetany. Such voluntary hyperventilation may be continued by determined individuals to the point of unconsciousness. The unconsciousness is due to cerebral ischemia secondary to the decrease in peripheral vascular resistance, the consequent fall in blood pressure, and the constriction of the cerebral vascular bed which results from large, acute decreases in the carbon dioxide tension of arterial blood.[40]

The effect of emotion and of ideational stimuli upon respiration has long been known. Everyone is acquainted with the gasp of horror, the sobbing of grief, the hyperpnea of sexual excitement. On the other hand, the existence of pleasant, peaceful thoughts and of contentment may bring about in excitable, unstable individuals a slight diminution in pulmonary ventilation. Experiments of Finesinger have indicated some of the range of respiratory response to emotion and pain.[41,42] He has shown that unpleasant thoughts tend to augment both the volume and the rate of respiration; the resulting increases in ventilation amounting in some individuals to more than double the preliminary value. Such responses may occur independently of or at least out of proportion to the rate of oxygen consumption. They tend to be maximal in hysteria and in anxiety states. Similarly, painful stimuli produced by the injection of hypertonic saline, repeated pricking, or electrical shock give similar results with maximal effects in hysterical and anxious subjects. Even recollection of painful stimuli in some individuals is sufficient to cause considerable increase in respiration.

Psychogenic dyspnea occurs as a manifestation of various types of psychoneuroses. The complaint is often of "smothering" and/or being "unable to get a deep breath." Meanwhile, the patient is apt to exhibit periodic overbreathing, sometimes punctuated by deep sighing respirations. After the overbreathing there is of course a compensatory normal diminution in rate and depth of respiration. At such times the patient may panic because he "can't get his breath." In its extreme form these manifestations comprise *the hyperventilation syndrome.* The patient hyperventilates chronically. At irregular intervals ventilation is increased even further and the patient experiences sensations of "lightheadedness," dizziness, and numbness or cramping in the hands and feet (tetany). The blood carbon dioxide content, combining power, and tension are low and the pH is alkaline.

It is wise to keep in mind two facts regarding this syndrome: (1) Once initiated and maintained for a period of time, hyperventilation tends to persist because of sensitization of the respiratory center (see above); (2) occasional patients, upon recovery from encephalitis, may manifest involuntary hyperventilation over long periods of time.

Metabolic Factors. Increase in the *metabolic rate* requires an increase in the rate of exchange of oxygen and carbon dioxide by the lungs. In general, alveolar ventilation keeps pace with increased metabolic demands, and the tensions of oxygen and carbon dioxide in the alveolar air and arterial blood are maintained within the normal range.

A considerable number of pathologic states and diseases may cause elevation of the metabolic rate. The presence of fever implies an increased demand for oxygen in accordance with van't Hoff's law, which states that the velocity of chemical reactions is doubled or trebled with each temperature rise of 10° C. Measurements in the presence of fever have indicated an increase in oxygen requirement of approximately 13 per cent for each degree Centigrade rise in body temperature, or 7 per cent for each degree Fahrenheit.[43] In hyperthyroidism the basal metabolic rate may be increased by 10 to 100 per cent. Furthermore, all movements of the thyrotoxic patient are performed clumsily and inefficiently, so that even at bed rest, the daily oxygen requirement of a moderately thyrotoxic patient may be more than twice normal. Among other diseases that are characterized by an increased oxygen utilization are leukemia (plus 20 to plus 80 per cent), pernicious anemia (plus 7 to plus 33 per cent), polycythemia (plus 10 to plus 40 per cent). In each of these states, the increased ventilatory demand that accompanies the metabolic alterations may cause distress in otherwise ill or debilitated individuals.

The increase in ventilation in moderate exercise is directly proportional to the oxygen consumption. In severe grades of exercise, when the oxygen consumption increases beyond 2.0 to 2.5 liters per minute, ventilation rises out of proportion to the oxygen consumption. This has been attributed to the formation of lactic acid and consequent acidosis in severe exercise.[23] Arterial blood gas tensions are maintained at normal levels in moderate exercise, but in severe exercise pH and carbon dioxide tension fall. Even in the most violent exertion, the arterial blood oxygen tension is not decreased.[44,45] In moderate exercise the total ventilation may reach 50 liters per minute; in the severest exercise, 120 liters per minute.

Despite many investigations and numerous reviews of the subject, agreement has not been reached concerning the factors responsible for the control of ventilation during exercise.[39,45,46,47] Much interest has focused on the possible roles of the central blood volume, catecholamines, and chemoreceptors located in the right heart or pulmonary arterial tree which are sensitive to the carbon dioxide tension of mixed venous blood.[45-48] It is of considerable clinical importance that the hyperventilation of exercise is greater in untrained individuals (such as patients whose activity has been restricted) than in individuals who are at the peak of athletic training. The ventilatory response to exercise is increased at altitude and under hot and humid environmental conditions. The type of exercise also influences ventilatory response; thus, at identical oxygen consumptions, ventilation is greater with arm exercise than with leg exercise.[45]

DYSPNEA IN PULMONARY DISEASE

Acute and chronic diseases of the lungs are perhaps the most frequent clinical causes of dyspnea. Only three of the most common diseases are considered here in detail.

PULMONARY EMPHYSEMA

There is a growing accord among pulmonary physiologists that a fundamental defect in this disease is *chronic obstruction* of the small intrapulmonary airways.[49] Initially, obstruction may be due to congestion, edema and hypersecretion of the bronchial mucosa, and spasm of the bronchial muscles. Later, as destruction of alveolar tissue occurs, the important dilating effect that the alveolar septae exert on the bronchioles is lost, thus adding another obstructive factor. When alveolar destruction is extensive, the unsupported bronchioles may collapse completely during expiration.[49] The further diminution

in caliber of the airways during expiration increases the intrapleural and the alveolar pressures to high levels, which in turn tends to collapse more bronchioles. Thus airflow, instead of increasing as it does normally with increase of intrapleural pressure, may actually decrease with increasing pressure.[49] The changes in pulmonary function that are characteristic of emphysema are readily understood if this fundamental obstructive defect is appreciated.

The disturbances in the ventilatory apparatus which result from such obstruction to airflow are frequently severe. Ventilatory capacity is consistently impaired, and the severity of the dyspnea correlates very well with the reduction in this function. With advancing disease, progressive impairment accompanied by increasing disability due to dyspnea is the rule. The maximum breathing capacity may reach such low levels (20 liters per minute) that the ventilatory requirements of even mild exercise cannot be met, and consequently the alveolar gas tensions deviate markedly from normal.

Improvement of the maximum breathing capacity after the administration of a nebulized bronchodilator is usual. The degree of improvement averages about 25 per cent of the prebronchodilator value, but is quite variable.[50]

A sudden increase in the severity of the dyspnea or progressive disability developing over a week or two is usually due to a superimposed bronchial or pulmonary infection with aggravation of airway obstruction. In view of the frequently precarious state of pulmonary function in these patients, such changes in symptoms deserve the utmost attention of the physician.

The work of breathing also is increased. At rest it may be only slightly greater than normal, but upon exercise it is greatly increased. An emphysematous patient breathing 15 liters per minute may be doing as much work in effecting this ventilation as a normal individual breathing 30 to 40 liters per minute.[12] The greatest part of this work is spent on overcoming resistance to airflow in the airways.[12,49] Active participation of the expiratory muscles is required by the augmented resistance during expiration and contributes to the increased work.

Cournand and co-workers[16] have presented some data on the metabolic costs of such disordered breathing. A patient with emphysema and considerable bronchial obstruction manifested an increment in his oxygen consumption of 25 ml. for each liter increase in ventilation above the resting level (normal increase: 1 ml. of oxygen per liter of ventilation per minute). With relief of the reversible component of his bronchial obstruction, the oxygen consumption required to support a liter per minute increase in ventilation fell to 6 ml.

Although in emphysema total ventilation at rest usually is increased slightly, it is only an occasional patient with early emphysema in whom ventilation is greater than normal during exercise. Indeed, in those with severe hypoxemia and chronic respiratory acidosis, ventilation during exercise is usually less than normal, perhaps because of diminished sensitivity of the respiratory center. Therefore, the demands for ventilation made upon the crippled ventilatory apparatus in emphysema usually are not increased. But they require the use of a larger than normal fraction of the breathing capacity, and can be met only at the expense of large swings in intrapleural pressure and considerable muscular effort.

Clinically significant disturbances in gas exchange are common in emphysema and are related to obstruction in the intrapulmonary airways, destruction of alveolar tissue, and consequent uneven distribution of air among the alveoli.[20,51,52] With progression of the disease an increasing number of alveoli are underventilated, which gives rise to progressive lowering of oxyhemoglobin saturation and eventually elevation of the carbon dioxide tension of the arterial blood. The physiologic dead space usually is expanded greatly by parenchymal areas in which the blood supply has been reduced or destroyed. Ventilation to these areas is wasted from the standpoint of gas exchange and may cause effectively functioning alveoli to be deprived of their share of ventilation. As a consequence of alveolar destruction and inhomogeneity of ventilation and perfusion, the area of alveolar capillary membrane available for gas exchange is diminished. The consequent decrease in diffusion capacity is partly responsible for the fall in arterial oxyhemoglobin saturation with exercise.[20,51]

The severe hypoxemia and perhaps the respiratory acidosis are responsible for the muscular fatigue, which is a prominent symptom in such patients and may contribute to fatigue of the respiratory muscles. The intense, oppressive, and alarming sensation of suffocation that they experience during and immediately after exertion is un-doubtedly related to these alterations in the blood gases.

Recent attention has been focused on two types of patients with emphysema.[52-56] One type, designated as Type A[52-55] or "pink puffers,"[56] is characterized by a thin body build, a large emphysematous chest with low diaphragms, little cough and sputum, absence of right heart failure, normal hematocrit, and persistent, disabling dyspnea. In the Type B patient, or "blue bloater," dyspnea fluctuates considerably in severity; he is further characterized by a normal or obese body build, normal position of diaphragm, episodic right heart failure, and high hematocrit. In the Type A patient, arterial oxyhemoglobin saturation and carbon dioxide tension may be normal, whereas the Type B patient manifests marked anoxemia and hypercapnia.[53-54] Briscoe and his co-workers have shown that the differences in blood gases are related to the existence in Type B patients of a smaller total ventilation, a much lower alveolar ventilation-perfusion ratio in poorly ventilated lung spaces (slow space), and a greater diffusing capacity in these spaces.[52] A larger cardiac output in Type B patients may accentuate the ventilation-perfusion abnormalities.[56-57] Although the pathologic differences in the lungs require further investigation, it appears that Type A patients have more extensive anatomic emphysema, whereas Type B patients have more bronchitis and some have little or no emphysema.[52-54]

Cor Pulmonale. The development of cor pulmonale in emphysema usually is accompanied by intensification of dyspnea. The following factors contribute to this change: hypervolemia secondary to polycythemia with consequent alteration in pulmonary blood volume and increased elastic resistance of the lung; inability to increase cardiac output appropriately with exercise and therefore ischemia of the respiratory muscles; aggravation of pre-existing hypoxemia and respiratory acidosis; increase in the degree of pulmonary arterial hypertension with augmented respiratory reflexes arising from the pulmonary artery; and, perhaps most significantly, an underlying pulmomary infection, which is very frequently responsible for precipitating episodes of failure and which increases the disability of the ventilatory apparatus and elevates the rate of metabolic turnover of oxygen and carbon dioxide. The partial reversibility of these untoward developments is revealed by the striking improvement in dyspnea and over-all clinical and physiologic state, which occurs with appropriate therapy.[58,59]

PULMONARY FIBROSIS

Because the nature and the extent of the fibrosis can vary widely, even if produced by the same etiologic agent, the type and the severity of disturbances in pulmonary function are variable.[60] In contrast to the *obstructive* defect present in emphysema, fibrosis produces a *restrictive* defect, which is secondary to the marked decrease in pulmonary compliance. However, bronchial obstruction may complicate the basic disease process.

If fibrosis is extensive, it causes shrinkage of the total lung capacity, particularly of the vital capacity. The maximum breathing capacity, if at all disturbed, is decreased in proportion to, or less than, vital capacity. Hyperventilation is the rule and is particularly in evidence during exercise.

The increased muscular effort and the quite high intrapleural pressures required to hyperventilate the rigid lungs,[20] together with the hyperventilation, are probably the chief abnormalities responsible for the dyspnea.

Tachypnea and hyperventilation are often extreme in the *alveolar capillary block syndrome*.[61] Diseases such as Boeck's sarcoid, miliary tuberculosis of the lungs, pulmonary involvement in rheumatoid arthritis, radiation fibrosis, beryllium granulomatosis, scleroderma, lymphangitic carcinomatosis, and Rich-Hamman's pneumonitis, which produce a diffuse interstitial inflammatory and fibrotic reaction in the alveolar walls, are common causes of this syndrome. The essential physiologic defect is a decrease in diffusion capacity which is both due to increased thickness of the alveolar-capillary membrane and to restriction of its total area.[61,62]

In some areas of the lung, the alveolar walls may be thick enough to block gas exchange completely; blood flowing through these alveoli constitutes a venoarterial shunt.[63] Characteristically, unsaturation of the arterial blood with oxygen is mild or absent at rest but becomes severe during exercise, since diffusion of oxygen at increased rates across the diseased membrane cannot occur without the development of a large oxygen pressure gradient between alveolar air and the blood leaving the alveoli. Because of the hyperventilation and the twenty-fold greater diffusibility of carbon dioxide as compared to oxygen, the pressure of carbon dioxide in the arterial blood and, secondarily, the plasma carbon dioxide content and combining power, may be low (compensated respiratory alkalosis). Respiratory acidosis may appear in very advanced stages of the syndrome when alveolar ventilation becomes inadequate because of disturbances in the distribution of air among the alveoli.

The maximum breathing capacity is remarkably well-preserved and may be greater than normal despite a reduction in vital capacity which is usually very severe. Disability is often out of proportion to the amount of pulmonary involvement visible in roentgenograms of the chest. Therefore, occasional patients with this syndrome have been suspected of being neurotic until studies of function have revealed the severity of the pulmonary insufficiency.

BRONCHIAL ASTHMA

Typical asthma results from interaction of antibodies in the sensitized bronchial mucosa with antigens, either inhaled or carried in the blood. As the result of this immunologic reaction, cholinergic (vagus) fibers in the bronchi are stimulated. In response to this stimulus there occurs (1) *swelling* of the mucosa and the submucosa, (2) *contraction* of bronchial musculature and (3) *excessive secretion* of thick, tenacious mucus. All three of these functional derangements result in narrowing of the total bronchial lumen and even complete occlusion of the smaller bronchioles. The acute asthmatic paroxysm is characterized by obstruction to both inspiratory and expiratory phases of pulmonary ventilation. There is increased respiratory effort with use of the accessary muscles of respiration, which tend to aid inspiration more than expiration. Wheezing and musical rales are heard over the lungs. Breathing is accomplished with the chest in a hyperinflated state in an attempt to overcome the obstruction to the airways. Expiration is prolonged, there is progressive distention of the lungs, and residual volume increases acutely.

An attack terminates when the constricted bronchi widen and the expectoration of mucus plugs is accomplished.

Repeated paroxysms eventually may produce two important changes: (1) hypertrophy of bronchiolar musculature, with increased tonus and permanent narrowing of bronchioles; (2) hypertrophy of bronchial mucous glands. These abnormal glands, instead of secreting small amounts of thin mucus, secrete large amounts of thick, tenacious mucus, which may plug so many bronchioles as to cause death.

Thus both structure and function may be altered in persistent asthma, with, at first, bronchiolar changes and later widespread pulmonary changes and chronic emphysema.

The actions of certain drugs give insight into the mechanisms of asthma. *Iodides* thin the mucous secretions, making cough more effective in clearing the airways. *Epinephrine* and ephedrine relieve bronchospasm and reduce bronchial edema. *Atropine* may reduce cholinergic effects. *Aminophylline* acts directly to relieve spasm of the bronchial musculature.

Since the essential disturbance in this condition is bronchiolar obstruction secondary to spasm of the muscle and edema of the mucosa of the bronchioles, many of the defects of pulmonary function characteristic of pulmonary emphysema occur with varying severity during the acute attack. With subsidence of the acute paroxysm, function improves greatly, although some depression of the maximum breathing capacity, increase in residual volume, hyperventilation, and mild hypoxemia usually persist.[64,65] These residual defects, which are partially or completely reversed by administration of a bronchodilator,[64,65] probably are responsible for the decreased tolerance for exercise manifested between attacks by most asthmatics.

With repeated attacks of bronchiolar obstruction there is a general tendency over the years for all components of pulmonary function to decline, and in many instances the physiologic pattern becomes indistinguishable from emphysema. However, this course is not invariable, particularly with effective therapy.

DYSPNEA IN CARDIAC DISEASE

Although dyspnea may occur in any of the various diseases of the heart, it is most prominent and most disabling in those associated with pulmonary congestion. Left ventricular failure from any cause and mitral stenosis are excellent examples. Hemodynamic studies in these conditions have revealed elevation of pressures in all segments of the pulmonary vascular bed consequent to increase in left atrial pressure.[66,67] The high pressures in the pulmonary veins and the capillaries are particularly noteworthy, since they are responsible for the increased rate

of transudation of fluid into the interstitial tissues and the alveoli and for the consequent expansion of the interstitial fluid volume of the lungs.[68-71] In tight mitral stenosis the pressure at rest in the pulmonary capillaries is usually in the range of the plasma protein osmotic pressure.[72] This indicates that such patients live under the constant threat of pulmonary edema.

Because of gravitational effects, the increase in interstitial fluid volume within the lungs is greater in the lower lobes. The accumulation of edema fluid about the capillaries and small vessels produces an increase in resistance to blood flow in these lobes and a preferential distribution of flow to the upper lobes.[73-75] When pulmonary venous hypertension is more pronounced, perivascular edema and increased vascular resistance are more widespread, and the distribution of pulmonary blood flow tends to revert to the normal pattern.[75]

With long-standing pulmonary venous hypertension, anatomic alterations develop characterized by fibrosis of the alveolar walls and medial hypertrophy and intimal proliferation of the small pulmonary arteries.[76-78] The vascular lesions are responsible for an increase in pulmonary arterial pressure which is greatly disproportionate to the elevation of pulmonary venous pressure.[66,67,72]

The secondary effects on the pulmonary parenchyma of these abnormalities in pulmonary circulation increase the resistance of the lungs to stretch up to three times the normal resistance.[11,79] This alteration in the viscoelastic properties of the lungs is mainly responsible for large swings in intrapleural pressure, increase in the work of breathing, and the large oxygen requirement for each liter of ventilation.[11,16,79]

In a number of patients, the resistance to airflow in the intrapulmonary airways is also greater than normal[79] and is responsible for a further increment in breathing work. Although in the past it has been questioned whether such changes in the mechanical properties of the lungs can occur without the anatomic lesions of pulmonary venous congestion, recent observations leave no doubt that pulmonary engorgement alone results in decreased compliance and increased resistance to airflow of the lungs, and that these abnormalities are accentuated by expansion of pulmonary interstitial fluid volume.[74]

During exercise, the pulmonary vascular pressures of patients with left ventricular disease, and particularly of those with mitral stenosis, rise considerably above the resting level.[66,67,72] Consequently, compliance of the lungs is less than in the resting state. This change in the elastic properties of the lungs is distinctly abnormal since normally pulmonary vascular pressures do not rise, and the dynamic compliance of the lungs increases with exercise.[35]

Hyperventilation of variable degree during both rest and exercise is usually present in patients with pulmonary congestion and serves to increase the burden imposed on the ventilatory apparatus. The degree of hyperventilation is not great and therefore of itself is not responsible for the dyspnea. The hyperpnea is out of proportion to metabolic demands since the arterial carbon dioxide tension is usually low or normal.[5] It is most likely caused by augmented stretch reflexes from the lungs. Hypoxemia also may contribute to the hyperventilation, although it is usually mild in the absence of significant pulmonary edema.

Reduction of cardiac output and inability to increase output appropriately with exercise bear only a general relationship to the severity of dyspnea in patients with pulmonary congestion. In mitral stenosis the symptom may be quite disabling even though the cardiac output is normal. Early fatigue of exercising muscles is perhaps the most common symptom of an inadequate cardiac output. Since the respiratory muscles are performing two to three times as much work as normal in achieving a particular level of ventilation, their early fatigue when blood flow is deficient may be an important contributing factor in the respiratory distress.

Orthopnea is a common symptom of pulmonary congestion. It is the term applied to the phenomenon of dyspnea which occurs at rest in the recumbent, but not the upright or semivertical, position. It usually is relieved by two or three pillows under the head and the back. Marshall and co-workers[11] have observed, in patients with mitral stenosis, considerable decrease in pulmonary compliance in the flat as compared to the upright position. The swings in intrapleural pressure during the respiratory cycle were consequently greater (over 40 cm. of water) and the work of breathing was two to three times greater in recumbency than in the upright position. The respiratory rate also increased to a frequency that corresponded strikingly to the frequency at which the work of venti-

lating the more rigid lungs was at a minimum.

The decrease in compliance upon lying flat probably is related to the fact that more of the lung lies at or below the level of the heart. Thus the increased vascular pressures are distributed throughout a greater portion of the lungs and are augmented in the most dependent regions by the overlying column of blood. In the upright position a greater portion of the lungs lies above the heart. In these regions pulmonary venous and capillary pressures are lowered by hydrostatic effects.

Vigorous movements of the chest bellows are effected more readily in the upright position. This probably explains why some patients with chronic lung disease or bronchial asthma are intolerant of the recumbent position.

Paroxysmal nocturnal dyspnea may occur in mitral stenosis or in any condition that taxes the left ventricle sufficiently to cause it to fail (such as hypertension or aortic insufficiency). The attack may be severe, dramatic, and terrifying.

The patient is aroused from his sleep gasping for air, and must sit up or stand to catch his breath. He may sweat profusely. Sometimes he throws open a window widely in an attempt to relieve the oppressive sensation of suffocation. The chest tends to become fixed in the position of forced inspiration. Both inspiratory and expiratory wheezes, often simulating typical asthma, are heard. In some cases overt *pulmonary edema* occurs, with many moist rales. The acute pulmonary edema rarely terminates fatally. Occasionally the attacks may recur several times a night, necessitating sleeping upright in a chair.

The mechanism of these attacks includes those factors that produce orthopnea, as well as the hypervolemia that occurs during the redistribution of peripheral edema fluid when body position is changed from vertical to horizontal upon retiring.[80] The hypervolemia constitutes an additional burden to the heart and of itself increases pulmonary venous and capillary pressures.[81] The actual attack may be "triggered" by coughing, abdominal distention, the hyperpneic phase of Cheyne-Stokes respiration, a startling noise or anything causing a sudden increase in heart rate and further acute elevation of pulmonary venous and capillary pressures. Usually the attack is terminated by assumption of the erect position and a few deep breaths of air. Cough, an important manifestation of pulmonary congestion, frequently occurs during the attack.

Cardiac Asthma. The asthmatic wheezes often heard in patients with pulmonary congestion have given rise to this term. The wheezes are a manifestation of pulmonary edema, and often are accompanied by other signs of this condition. Reduction in lumen of the small intrapulmonary airways by edema fluid and thickening of bronchiolar walls by edema is responsible for the wheezes. In addition, the high intrathoracic pressure required to overcome the obstruction during expiration tends to narrow the small bronchioles further and even collapse them.[79] Increased resistance to airflow during both inspiration and expiration has been measured in pulmonary congestion,[74,79] and has been found to be especially high (four times normal) in frank pulmonary edema.[82,83] The compliance of the lungs is reduced greatly in pulmonary edema with values as low as one-tenth normal having been recorded. With recovery from edema, very significant reductions in airway resistance and increases in pulmonary compliance occur.[82,83]

Dyspnea Without Pulmonary Congestion. Dyspnea occurs in many forms of heart disease which are not associated with congestion of the lungs. Uncomplicated *pulmonic stenosis* is an excellent example. Probably the symptom is related to an inadequate cardiac output during exercise. In *tetralogy of Fallot*, dyspnea may be severe and often is relieved by assuming a squatting position. In this and other forms of cyanotic heart disease, pre-existing hypoxemia is aggravated by exercise. It is of note that both dyspnea and fatigue appear during exertion when the arterial oxyhemoglobin saturation has fallen significantly below the resting level.

Cheyne-Stokes respiration, or periodic breathing, is a phenomenon that may occur in cardiac failure. It is characterized by alternating periods of hypoventilation and hyperventilation. In its typical form, there is an apneic phase lasting 15 to 60 seconds, followed by a phase during which tidal volume increases with each breath to a peak level, and then decreases in decrescendo fashion to the apneic phase. At the onset of apnea, carbon dioxide tension in brachial or femoral arterial blood is at its lowest. As apnea persists, carbon dioxide tension gradually increases, and respiration is stimulated. Carbon dioxide tension continues to increase

until maximum hyperventilation is attained, after which it and ventilation decrease until apnea again occurs.[84,85] The arterial oxyhemoglobin saturation varies in an inverse manner, being highest at onset of apnea and lowest during midhyperpnea. During the cycle, carbon dioxide tension may vary as much as 14 mm. Hg, and oxyhemoglobin saturation as much as 18 per cent.[84]

One of the factors fundamental to the production of such respiratory oscillations is the circulatory-induced delay in the feedback of information to the brain regarding the effects of ventilation on the pulmonary capillary blood. The circulation time from lung to peripheral artery has been shown to be one-half the length of the Cheyne-Stokes cycle.[85] Thus the oscillating ventilatory pattern produces cyclic variations in the concentrations of respiratory gases in blood passing through the lungs; these cyclic variations eventually reach the respiratory control system but with a temporal phase shift of 180°.

Formerly it was believed that the respiratory center is depressed in Cheyne-Stokes respiration, but more recently it has been shown that respiratory alkalosis frequently is present, that the arterial carbon dioxide tension is lower than normal in both apneic and hyperpneic phases,[84,85] and that the respiratory response to inhalation of carbon dioxide is greater than normal.[84] Plum and his associates[84,86] have called attention to supramedullary dysfunction of the brain in the pathogenesis of Cheyne-Stokes respiration. All of the patients whom they examined had signs of bilateral impairment of the descending motor pathways. The importance of supramedullary neuronal structures in controlling respiration was exemplified by the intense, metronomically regular hyperpnea (central neurogenic hyperventilation) that they have observed in patients with destructive lesions of the central portion of the tegmentum of the pons.[86] In most of these patients, typical Cheyne-Stokes respirations preceded the development of continuous hyperventilation. Cyclic changes in cerebral blood flow also occur during Cheyne-Stokes respiration (flow being greater during hyperpnea), and may account for the fluctuations of mental state, electroencephalographic pattern, and signs of nervous system dysfunction during the cycle.[87]

Cheyne-Stokes respiration is sometimes seen in normal infants, in healthy elderly persons, and in normal individuals at high altitude. It also occurs when certain drugs (such as morphine) are administered; with increased intracranial pressure, in uremia, and in some forms of coma. It has been produced in dogs by prolonging circulation time from the heart to the brain.[88]

DYSPNEA IN ANEMIA

Exertional dyspnea is a common symptom of anemia, and is particularly marked in the more acute and the severe forms. Its pathogenesis is not completely understood.

The supply of oxygen to the tissues is dependent upon transport by hemoglobin. If the hemoglobin concentration and arterial oxyhemoglobin saturation are normal, the mixed venous blood in the resting state is about 75 per cent saturated with oxygen, since the mean extraction of oxygen by the tissues from each 100 ml. of blood is 4 ml. With reduction in hemoglobin concentration, and hence in the amount of oxygen in the arterial blood (normally 19.4 ml. per 100 ml.), the mixed venous blood saturation decreases if extraction of oxygen from each 100 ml. of blood continues as usual. Tissue oxygen tension, which lies between the tension of the arterial and that of the venous blood, therefore falls. This hypoxic effect is greatest in those tissues, such as contracting muscle, in which the extraction rate of oxygen is high.

The hypoxia is prevented partially by an increase in the cardiac output which permits tissue oxygen needs to be met at a lower extraction rate of oxygen from the blood.[89] In severe anemia, the adjustment in output may fall short of the mark. If the hemoglobin concentration is 4 Gm. per 100 ml. of blood, the cardiac output would have to be tripled in order to maintain tissue oxygen exchange at a normal level merely in the basal state.

The heart under these circumstances does not respond normally to stress[90] and may fail. In the production of dyspnea the roles played by the augmented blood flow through the lungs, and by pulmonary congestion resulting from left ventricular failure or strain during exercise,[91] only may be speculated upon.

Although the arterial oxyhemoglobin saturation is within normal limits, the oxygen tension has been demonstrated to be decreased.[92] This may be responsible in part for the hyperventilation that is characteristic of anemia.

SUMMARY

Dyspnea is a subjective symptom related to the effort of breathing and as such must be regarded as originating in the ventilatory apparatus, although the stimuli, the sensory receptors, and the nerve pathways which participate in its appreciation are unknown.

Numerous acute and chronic diseases may affect the various components of the ventilatory apparatus—ribs, spine, respiratory muscles, their peripheral and central nervous control, the extrapulmonary and the intrapulmonary airways, alveolar tissue, pleura, and pulmonary vessels. Such disturbances, if sufficiently severe, decrease the capacity of the apparatus to ventilate and exaggerate the effort necessarily expended to make it function. Alterations in the parenchyma and the airways of the lung produced either by primary lung disease, or secondarily by heart disease, are the most common clinical causes of ventilatory dysfunction and dyspnea.

In many conditions the levels of ventilation required at rest and especially during exercise are greater than normal and serve to overtax a disabled ventilatory apparatus. Severe grades of hyperventilation, such as may occur during vigorous exertion, can provoke dyspnea even in a normal individual.

The rate of alveolar ventilation is adjusted to meet the wide fluctuations in metabolic needs for exchange of oxygen and carbon dioxide which occur in the course of human activity. These adjustments are initiated primarily by alterations in the gas composition and pH of the arterial blood and are designed to minimize such changes. Many additional reflex and emotional factors, which may assume importance in disease, are capable of modifying ventilation.

In order to appraise dyspnea adequately, it is necessary for one to establish the severity of the symptom and the conditions under which it occurs. Through the history and the physical examination, all evidences of disability of the ventilatory apparatus and factors that increase the demands for ventilation must be sought. Detailed studies of pulmonary and cardiac function may be necessary, particularly in those individuals in whom adequate cause for the dyspnea cannot be found or in whom the symptom appears out of proportion to evidences of disease. In most instances, simple studies such as observation of the patient during a simple exercise, radiographic examination of the heart and lungs, determination of blood carbon dioxide content and hematocrit, and an electrocardiogram will suffice.

REFERENCES

1. Baldwin, E. de F., Cournand, A., and Richards, D. W., Jr.: Pulmonary insufficiency. I. Physiological classification, clinical methods of analysis, standard values in normal subjects, Medicine 27:243, 1948.
2. Dripps, R. D., and Comroe, J. H., Jr.: The respiratory and circulatory response of normal man to inhalation of 7.6 and 10.4 per cent O_2 with a comparison of the maximal ventilation produced by severe muscular exercise, inhalation of CO_2 and maximal voluntary hyperventilation, Amer. J. Physiol. 149:43, 1947.
3. Lukas, D. S., and Plum, F.: Pulmonary function in patients convalescing from acute poliomyelitis with respiratory paralysis, Amer. J. Med. 12:388, 1952.
4. Cournand, A., and Richards, D. W., Jr.: Pulmonary insufficiency. I. Discussion of a physiological classification and presentation of clinical tests, Amer. Rev. Tuberc. 44:26, 1941.
5. West, J. R., Bliss, H. A., Wood, J. A., and Richards, D. W., Jr.: Pulmonary function in rheumatic heart disease and its relation to exertional dyspnea in ambulatory patients, Circulation 8:178, 1953.
6. Mead, J.: Mechanical properties of lungs, Physiol. Rev. 41:281, 1961.
7. Pierce, J. A., Hocott, J. B., and Hefley, B. F.: Elastic properties and the geometry of the lungs, J. Clin. Invest. 40:1515, 1961.
8. Fry, D. L., and Hyatt, R. E.: Pulmonary mechanics: a unified analysis of the relationship between pressure, volume and gas-flow in the lungs of normal and diseased human subjects, Amer. J. Med. 29:672, 1960.
9. Otis, A. B., Fenn, W. O., and Rahn, H.: Mechanics of breathing in man, J. Appl. Physiol. 2:592, 1950.
10. Otis, A. B.: The work of breathing, Physiol. Rev. 34:449, 1954.
11. Marshall, R., McIlroy, M. B., and Christie, R. V.: The work of breathing in mitral stenosis, Clin. Sci. 13:137, 1954.
12. McIlroy, M. B., and Christie, R. V.: The work of breathing in emphysema, Clin. Sci. 13:147, 1954.
13. Bergofsky, E. H., Turino, G. M., and Fishman, A. P.: Cardiorespiratory failure in kyphoscoliosis, Medicine 38:263, 1959.
14. Naimark, A., and Cherniack, R. M.: Compliance of the respiratory system and its components in health and obesity, J. Appl. Physiol. 15:377, 1960.
15. Otis, A. B.: The work of breathing, *in* Fenn, W. O., and Rahn, H. (section eds.): Handbook of Physiology, Sec. 3: Respiration, vol. I, Washington, D. C., Amer. Physiol. Soc., 1964.
16. Cournand, A., Richards, D. W., Jr., Bader, R. A., Bader, M. E., and Fishman, A. P.: The oxygen cost of breathing, Trans. Ass. Amer. Physicians 67:162, 1954.
17. Kaufman, B. J., Ferguson, M. H., and Cher-

niak, R. M.: Hypoventilation in obesity, J. Clin. Invest. 38:500, 1959.
18. Marshall, R., Stone, R. W., and Christie, R. V.: The relationship of dyspnoea to respiratory effort in normal subjects, mitral stenosis and emphysema, Clin. Sci. 13:625, 1954.
19. McGregor, M., and Becklake, M. R.: The relationship of oxygen cost of breathing to respiratory mechanical work and respiratory force, J. Clin. Invest. 40:971, 1961.
20. Comroe, J. H., Jr., Forster, R. E., II, Du Bois, A. B., Briscoe, W. A., and Carlsen, E.: The Lung. Clinical Physiology and Pulmonary Function Tests, ed. 2, Chicago, Year Book Pub., 1962.
21. Pappenheimer, J. R., *et al.*: Standardization of definitions and symbols in respiratory physiology, Fed. Proc. 9:602, 1950.
22. Pappenheimer, J. R.: The ionic composition of cerebral extracellular fluid and its relation to control of breathing, Harvey Lect., Ser. 61: 71, 1965–1966.
23. Gray, J. S.: Pulmonary Ventilation and its Physiologic Regulation, Springfield, Ill., Thomas, 1950.
24. Haldane, J. S., and Priestley, J. G.: The regulation of the lung-ventilation, J. Physiol. 32: 225, 1905.
25. Alexander, J. K., West, J. R., Wood, J. A., and Richards, D. W.: Analysis of the respiratory response to carbon dioxide inhalation in varying clinical states of hypercapnia, anoxia and acid-base derangement, J. Clin. Invest. 34:511, 1955.
26. Houston, C. S., and Riley, R. L.: Respiratory and circulatory changes during acclimatization to high altitude, Amer. J. Physiol. 149-565, 1947.
27. Brown, E. B., Jr., Campbell, G. S., Johnson, M. N., Hemingway, A., and Visscher, M. B.: Changes in response to inhalation of CO_2 before and after 24 hours of hyperventilation in man, J. Appl. Physiol. 1:333, 1948.
28. Brown, E. B., Jr., Hemingway, A., and Visscher, M. B.: Arterial blood pH and pCO_2 changes in response to CO_2 inhalation after 24 hours of passive hyperventilation, J. Appl. Physiol. 2:544, 1950.
29. Schäfer, K.-E.: Atmung und Saure-Basengleichwicht bei langdauerdem Aufenthalt in 3% CO_2, Pfluger. Arch. Ges. Physiol. 251:689, 1949.
30. Brown, E. B., Jr.: Changes in brain pH response to CO_2 after prolonged hypoxic hyperventilation, J. Appl. Physiol. 2:549, 1950.
31. Leusen, I. R.: Chemosensitivity of the respiratory center. Influence of changes in the H^+ and total buffer concentrations in the cerebral ventricles on respiration, Amer. J. Physiol. 176:45, 1954.
32. ———: Acid-base equilibrium between blood and cerebralspinal fluid, Amer. J. Physiol. 176:513, 1954.

33. Goldring, R. M., Cannon, P. J., Heinemann, H. O., and Fishman, A. P.: Respiratory adjustment to chronic metabolic alkalosis in man, J. Clin. Invest. 47:188, 1968.

34. Kellogg, R. H.: Central chemical regulation of respiration, in Fenn, W. O., and Rahn, H. (section eds.): Handbook of Physiology, Sec. 3: Respiration, vol. I, Washington, D. C., Amer. Physiol. Soc., 1964.

35. McIlroy, M. B., Marshall, R., and Christie, R. V.: The work of breathing in normal subjects, Clin. Sci. 13:127, 1954.

36. Marshall, R., and Christie, R. V.: The viscoelastic properties of the lungs in acute pneumonia, Clin. Sci. 13:403, 1954.

37. Mead, J.: Control of respiratory frequency, J. Appl. Physiol. 15:325, 1960.

38. Widdicombe, J. G.: Respiratory reflexes in Fenn, W. O., and Rahn, H. (section eds.): Handbook of Physiology, Sec. 3: Respiration, vol. I., Washington, D. C., Amer. Physiol. Soc., 1964.

39. Comroe, J. H.: The hyperpnea of muscular exercise, Physiol. Rev. 24:31, 1944.

40. Burnam, J. F., Hickam, J. B., and McIntosh, H. D.: The effect of hypocapnia on arterial blood pressure, Circulation 9:89, 1954.

41. Finesinger, J. E.: Effect of pleasant and unpleasant ideas on respiration in psychoneurotic patients, Arch. Neurol. Psychiat. 42:425, 1939.

42. Finesinger, J. E., and Mazick, S. G.: Respiratory responses of psychoneurotic patients to ideational and sensory stimuli, Amer. J. Psychiat. 97:27, 1940.

43. Du Bois, E. F.: Basal Metabolism in Health and Disease, Philadelphia, Lea & Febiger, 1936.

44. Himwich, H. E., and Barr, D. P.: Studies in the physiology of muscular exercise and oxygen relationships in the arterial blood, J. Biol. Chem. 57:363, 1923.

45. Dejours, P.: Control of respiration in muscular exercise, in Fenn, W. O., and Rahn, H. (section eds.): Handbook of Physiology, Sec. 3: Respiration, vol. I, Washington, D. C., Amer. Physiol. Soc., 1964.

46. Mitchell, J. H., Sproule, B. J., and Chapman, C. B.: Factors influencing respiration during heavy exercise, J. Clin. Invest. 37:1693, 1958.

47. Yamamoto, W. S., and Edwards, M. W., Jr.: Homeostasis of carbon dioxide during intravenous infusion of carbon dioxide, J. Appl. Physiol. 15:807, 1960.

48. Pi Suner, A.: The regulation of the respiratory movements by peripheral chemoreceptors, Physiol. Rev. 27:1, 1947.

49. Fry, D. L., Ebert, R. V., Stead, W. W., and Brown, C. C.: The mechanics of pulmonary ventilation in normal subjects and in patients with emphysema, Amer. J. Med. 16:80, 1954.

50. Lukas, D. S.: Pulmonary function in health and disease, Med. Clin. N. Amer. 39:661, 1955.

51. West, J. R., Baldwin, E. de F., Cournand, A., and Richards, D. W., Jr.: Physiopathologic aspects of chronic emphysema, Amer. J. Med. 10:481, 1951.

52. King, T. K. C., and Briscoe, W. A.: The distribution of ventilation, perfusion, lung volume and transfer factor (diffusing capacity) in patients with obstructive lung disease, Clin. Sci. 35:153, 1968.

53. Briscoe, W. A., and Nash, E. S.: The slow space in chronic obstructive pulmonary disease, Ann. N. Y. Acad. Sci. 121:706, 1965.

54. Nash, E. S., Briscoe, W. B., and Cournand, A.: The relationship between clinical and physiological findings in chronic obstructive disease of the lungs, Med. Thorac. 2:305, 1965.

55. Burrows, B., Niden, A. H., Fletcher, C. M., and Jones, N. L.: Clinical types of chronic obstructive lung disease in London and in Chicago, Amer. Rev. Resp. Dis. 90:14, 1964.

56. Filey, G. F., Beckwitt, H. J., Reeves, J. T., and Mitchell, R. S.: Chronic obstructive bronchopulmonary disease. II. Oxygen transport in two clinical types, Amer. J. Med. 44:26, 1968.

57. Penman, R. W. B., Howard, P., and Stentiford, N. H.: Factors influencing pulmonary gas exchange in patients with acute edematous cor pulmonale due to chronic lung disease, Amer. J. Med. 44:8, 1968.

58. Harvey, R. M., Ferrer, I., Richards, D. W., Jr., and Cournand, A.: Influence of chronic pulmonary disease on the heart and circulation, Amer. J. Med. 10:719, 1951.

59. Richards, D. W.: The right heart and the lung, Amer. Rev. Resp. Dis. 94:691, 1966.

60. Baldwin, E. de F., Cournand, A., and Richards, D. W., Jr.: Pulmonary insufficiency. II. A study of thirty-nine cases of pulmonary fibrosis, Medicine 28:1, 1949.

61. Austrian, R., et al.: Clinical and physiologic features of some types of pulmonary disease with impairment of alveolar-capillary diffusion. The syndrome of "alveolar-capillary block," Amer. J. Med. 11:667, 1951.

62. Marks, A., Cugell, D. W., Cadigan, J. B., and Gaensler, E. A.: Clinical determination of the diffusion capacity of the lungs: Comparison of methods in normal subjects and patients with "alveolar-capillary block" syndrome, Amer. J. Med. 22:51, 1957.

63. Finley, T. N., Swenson, E. W., and Comroe, J. H., Jr.: The cause of arterial hypoxemia at rest in patients with "alveolar-capillary block syndrome," J. Clin. Invest. 41:618, 1962.

64. Lukas, D. S.: Pulmonary function in a group of young patients with bronchial asthma, J. Allerg. 22:411, 1951.

65. Herchfus, J. A., Bresnick, E., and Segal, M. S.: Pulmonary function studies in bronchial asthma. I. In the control state, Amer. J. Med. 14:23, 1953.

66. Lewis, B. M., Houssay, H. E., Haynes, F. W., and Dexter, L.: The dynamics of both right and left ventricles at rest and during exercise in patients with heart failure, Circ. Res. 1:312, 1953.

67. Lukas, D. S., and Dotter, C. T.: Modifications of the pulmonary circulation in mitral stenosis, Amer. J. Med. 12:639, 1952.

68. Guyton, A. C., and Lindsey, A. W.: Effect of elevated left atrial pressure and decreased plasma protein concentration on the development of pulmonary edema, Circ. Res. 7:649, 1959.

69. Levine, O. R., Mellins, R. B., and Fishman, A. P.: Quantitative assessment of pulmonary edema, Circ. Res. 17:414, 1965.

70. Levine, O. R., Mellins, R. B., Senior, R. M., and Fishman, A. P.: The application of Starling's law of capillary exchange to the lungs, J. Clin. Invest. 46:934, 1967.

71. De Martino, A. G., Kozam, R. L., and Lukas, D. S.: The control of rapidly exchanging water volume of the lung by left atrial pressure, Clin. Res. 12:293, 1964.

72. Araujo, J., and Lukas, D. S.: Interrelationships among pulmonary "capillary" pressure, blood flow and valve size in mitral stenosis. The limited regulatory effects of the pulmonary vascular resistance, J. Clin. Invest. 31:1082, 1952.

73. Dollery, C. T., and West, J. B.: Regional uptake of radioactive oxygen, carbon monoxide and carbon dioxide in the lungs of patients with mitral stenosis, Circ. Res. 8:765, 1960.

74. West, J. B., Dollery, C. T., and Heard, B. E.: Increased vascular resistance in the lower zone of the lung caused by perivascular edema, Lancet 2:181, 1964.

75. Dawson, A., Kaneko, K., and McGregor, M.: Regional lung function in patients with mitral stenosis studied with xenon^{133} during air and oxygen breathing, J. Clin. Invest. 44:999, 1965.

76. Parker, F., Jr., and Weiss, S.: Nature and significance of structural changes in lungs in mitral stenosis, Amer. J. Path. 12:573, 1936.

77. Larrabe, W. F., Parker, R. L., and Edwards, J. E.: Pathology of intra-pulmonary arteries and arterioles in mitral stenosis, Proc. Mayo Clin. 24:316, 1949.

78. Harris, P., and Heath, D.: The Human Pulmonary Circulation. Its Form and Function in Health and Disease, Baltimore, Williams & Wilkins, 1962.

79. Brown, C. C., Jr., Fry, D. L., and Ebert, R. V.: The mechanics of pulmonary ventilation in patients with heart disease, Amer. J. Med. 17:438, 1954.

80. Perera, G. A., and Berliner, R. W.: The relation of postural hemodilution to paroxysmal dyspnea, J. Clin. Invest. 22:25, 1943.

81. Doyle, J. T., Wilson, J. S., Estes, E. H., and Warren, J. V.: The effect of intravenous infusions of physiologic saline solution on the pulmonary arterial and pulmonary capillary pressure in man, J. Clin. Invest. 30:345, 1951.

82. Sharp, J. T., Griffith, G. T., Bunnell, I. L., and Greene, D. G.: Ventilatory mechanics in pulmonary edema in man, J. Clin. Invest. 37:111, 1958.

83. Sharp, J. T., Bunnell, I. L., Griffith, G. T., and Greene, D. G.: The effects of therapy on pulmonary mechanics in human pulmonary edema, J. Clin. Invest. 40:665, 1961.

84. Brown, H. W., and Plum, F.: The neurologic basis of Cheyne-Stokes respiration, Amer. J. Med. 30:849, 1961.

85. Lange, R. L., and Hecht, H. H.: The mechanism of Cheyne-Stokes respiration, J. Clin. Invest. 41:42, 1962.

86. Plum, F., and Swanson, A. G.: Central neurogenic hyperventilation in man, Arch. Neurol. Psychiat. 81:535, 1959.

87. Karp, H. R., Sieker, H. O., and Heyman, A.: Cerebral circulation and function in Cheyne-Stokes respiration, Amer. J. Med. 30:861, 1961.

88. Guyton, A. G., Crowell, J. W., and Moore, J. W.: Basic oscillating mechanism of Cheyne-Stokes breathing, Amer. J. Physiol. 187:395, 1956.

89. Brannon, E. S., Merrill, A. J., Warren, J. V., and Stead, E. A.: The cardiac output in patients with chronic anemia as measured by the technique of right atrial catheterization, J. Clin. Invest. 24:332, 1945.

90. Sharpey-Shafer, E. P.: Transfusion and the anemic heart, Lancet 2:296, 1945.

91. Leight, L., Snider, T. H., Clifford, G. O., and Hellems, H. K.: Hemodynamic studies in sickle cell anemia, Circulation 10:653, 1954.

92. Ryan, J. M., and Hickam, J. B.: The alveolar-arterial oxygen pressure gradient in anemia, J. Clin. Invest. 31:188, 1952.

20

Cyanosis

DANIEL S. LUKAS

Normal Oxygen Relationships

Causes of Cyanosis
   PERIPHERAL CYANOSIS
   PULMONARY CYANOSIS
   RIGHT-LEFT SHUNTS
   ABNORMALITIES OF HEMOGLOBIN

Relationship of Cyanosis to CO_2 Exchange

Effects of Oxygen on Cyanosis

Definition. Cyanosis is the diffuse bluish color that is due to the presence of deoxygenated hemoglobin in increased amounts in the subpapillary venous plexus of the skin. It is not to be confused with the leaden color associated with the presence in the blood of methemoglobin or sulfhemoglobin or with argyria due to deposition of silver after prolonged use of medications containing this metal. Cyanosis is not synonymous with hypoxemia or hypoxia. It does not appear in carbon monoxide poisoning, in which hypoxemia is extreme, in severe anemia, which may be characterized both by hypoxemia and hypoxia, nor in cyanide poisoning, in which there is profound hypoxia without hypoxemia. Thus the presence of cyanosis implies hypoxemia, but the absence of cyanosis does not preclude severe hypoxia.

Pigmentation and thickness of the skin modify the appearance of cyanosis or may hide it completely. The presence in the blood of other pigments, such as methemoglobin or bilirubin, may add to the difficulty of recognition, whereas dilation of surface vessels makes the color more obvious. Cyanosis can best be seen and recognized in places where the skin is thick, unpigmented, and flushed, favorable sites being the lobes of the ears, the cutaneous surfaces of the lips, and the fingernail beds. It is somewhat less apparent in the mucous membranes and in the retina, but these may be important sites for detection of cyanosis in patients with dark skin. The nature of the light under which the subject is examined is of considerable importance in identifying cyanosis; bright daylight is best. Under certain types of fluorescent light, even normal individuals appear cyanotic. The contribution of the vascular contents to the color of the skin is assessed readily by applying sufficient pressure to the skin to empty its vessels.

NORMAL OXYGEN RELATIONSHIPS

Transport of oxygen by the blood is almost entirely dependent on the presence of hemoglobin, because the concentration of oxygen in simple solution under normal conditions is small. When fully saturated with oxygen, each gram of hemoglobin binds 1.34 ml of oxygen; thus, at a normal hemoglobin concentration of 15.0 g/100 ml, the oxygen capacity of blood is 20.1 ml/100 ml. The additional small amount of the gas that is dissolved can be calculated from the oxygen pressure of the equilibrating gas and the solubility coefficient, α for oxygen in blood at the temperature of equilibration. At 37°C, αO_2 is 0.023 ml/ml blood/760 mm Hg of O_2 pressure.

Under normal conditions, blood during passage through the pulmonary capillaries is exposed to an alveolar oxygen tension of approximately 100 mm Hg, and leaves the capillaries in almost complete equilibrium with the alveolar gas. As indicated by the oxyhemoglobin dissociation curves at this tension and at normal pH, hemoglobin is approximately 97 per cent saturated with oxygen. If the hemoglobin concentration is 15 g/100 ml, the concentration of bound oxygen is 19.5 ml/100 ml. Also, at this tension, the concentration of dissolved oxygen is 0.3 ml/100 ml. Thus, normal blood leaves the lungs with an oxygen content of 19.8 ml/100 ml.

As the blood passes through the systemic capillaries, oxygen is removed to meet the metabolic needs of the tissues. The arterio-venous blood oxygen difference for the whole body under resting conditions has been found by the method of cardiac catheterization to be 4.07 ± 0.66 ml/100 ml (mean ± standard deviation).[1] The mixed venous blood in the pulmonary artery therefore contains slightly more than 15 ml of oxygen per 100 ml, which represents an oxyhemoglobin saturation of 75 per cent and an oxygen tension of 40 mm Hg.

Whereas the oxygen tension of blood leaving the pulmonary capillaries is within a fraction of a mm Hg of that in the alveolar air, the oxygen tension of blood leaving the systemic capillaries is not closely equilibrated with that of the tissues. The measurement of average tissue oxygen pressure is of uncertain reliability, but the available values are well below those of simultaneously measured venous oxygen tension, and it is clear that considerable oxygen gradients exist within the tissues.[2] Indeed, in vivo measurements based on the fluorescence of reduced nicotinamide adenine dinucleotide indicate that oxygen tension within the mitochondria, the site at which oxygen acts as the ultimate electron acceptor for the cells, is less than 1 mm Hg.[3] Although this appears to be an extraordinarily low value, it is an astonishing fact that oxidative metabolic processes proceed unimpeded at even lower mitochondrial oxygen tensions, and in the brain, electrical activity ceases only when mitochondrial oxygen tension has decreased to a small fraction of a mm Hg.[4]

Since the classical review by Lundsgaard and Van Slyke,[5] cyanosis has been attributed to the presence in the capillaries of the skin of an average concentration of unoxygenated hemoglobin in excess of 5 g/100 ml. These investigators calculated the average oxyhemoglobin saturation and oxyhemoglobin concentration from simultaneous determinations of arterial and brachial venous-blood oxygen contents and capacity. Newer information regarding anatomic and physiologic aspects of the cutaneous circulation suggests that this concept should be modified.

Because of their anatomic arrangement, the most superficial cutaneous capillaries contribute relatively little to the color of the skin in most areas of the body.[6] These vessels, after originating from the subpapillary arterioles, course perpendicularly to the surface and form tight hair-pin loops in the papillae (see Figure 39-1 in Chapter 39 on Pigmentation of the Skin); when viewed from the skin surface only the small apical segment of these loops is visible.[6,7] In areas in which the skin is thin, only one capillary loop is present in each papilla. The venules into which these capillaries drain form an extensive vascular plexus, which lies immediately beneath the papillae, and which is distributed parallel to the skin surface. It is this subpapillary venous plexus that makes the largest vascular contribution to skin color.[6,8] The vessels of the plexus are thin-walled, and it is believed that they participate in transvascular exchange of gases and other substances.

In the nail folds, the capillary loops are profuse and do lie parallel to the surface; their contents are, therefore, an important source of color in these regions.[6,7] In the nail bed, the capillary loops in each papilla are quite numerous and tortuous, and their density is sufficient to contribute substantially to the color of this region.[8] Arteriovenous anastomoses in the subpapillary plexus are a prominent feature of the skin of the extremities; these communications are under nervous control, and when open are capable of increasing blood flow enormously and shunting blood away from the capillaries.[8,9]

It is clear that brachial venous blood does not drain the capillaries of the skin alone and cannot be used to estimate the oxygen saturation of cutaneous capillary blood. Actually, direct measurements of cutaneous venous oxyhemoglobin saturation are not available. Indirect estimates based on measurements of blood flow and oxygen consumption of the skin indicate that, in general, the skin is relatively overperfused with regard to its metabolic requirements, and that its venous oxygen saturation is high relative to the body as a whole.[9–11] These observations reflect the fact that blood flow to the skin does not subserve the metabolic needs of the skin alone, but is primarily designed to control heat exchange and the temperature of the body. With an increase in ambient temperature, cutaneous blood flow rises sharply, and out of proportion to the accompanying increase in cutaneous metabolic rate.[9,11] In normal subjects in a cool room (17 to 19°C), Roddie and co-workers[12] found that the oxyhemoglobin saturation in the blood from a superficial vein of the forearm was 40 to 72 per cent, and with heating the saturation rose to 85 to 95 per cent. It is well-known that the oxygen saturation and tension of blood obtained from a puncture of the heated ear lobe are almost identical with those of simultaneously sampled arterial blood.[13,14] It is probable that maximum increase in flow upon heating the skin is brought about not only by neurogenically induced vasodilatation, but also by the opening of multiple direct arteriovenous communications.[8,9,10]

Although there is some question regarding the exact concentrations involved, the observations of Lundsgaard and Van Slyke leave no doubt that an increased concentration of deoxyhemoglobin in the cutaneous vessels is responsible for cyanosis. Moreover, their conclusion, drawn from studies of various diseases and of normal subjects under a variety of physiologic conditions (e.g., breathing hypoxic gas mixtures, application of venous tourniquets), that the skin becomes cyanotic when the numerical average of the oxygen deficits in the arterial and venous blood of the arm exceeds 6 to 7 ml/100 ml, stands as an empiric observation.[5,15,16] Such a deficit may arise from two distinct mechanisms: reduction in arterial saturation with normal extraction of oxygen in the cutaneous vessels, or increased extraction in the small vessels with a normal arterial concentration of oxygen. Under certain circumstances, both mechanisms may be operative.

The intensity of cyanosis depends upon the *absolute concentration of deoxyhemoglobin* and not on the ratio of oxy- and deoxyhemoglobin concentrations. Thus, in severe anemia, the concentration of hemoglobin may be too low for cyanosis to appear, despite complete oxygen desaturation of cutaneous blood. Conversely, in polycythemia there is an increased tendency to development of cyanosis, since it appears with lesser degrees of desaturation. At an oxyhemoglobin saturation of 75 per cent, blood with a hemoglobin concentration of 20 g/100 ml contains 5 g of deoxyhemoglobin per 100 ml, whereas at the same saturation, blood with a hemoglobin concentration of 5 g/100 ml contains only 1.25 g of deoxyhemoglobin per 100 ml.

CAUSES OF CYANOSIS

Peripheral cyanosis is due to increased extraction of oxygen in the systemic capillaries. It may arise either from an increased utilization of oxygen, such as occurs in very strenuous muscular exertion, or from a decreased blood flow. The relationships of the oxygen consumed by a particular organ or tissue, the blood flow to it, and the difference in oxygen concentration between the arterial blood supplying it and the venous blood draining it, are stated in the Fick principle:

Blood flow to organ =

$$\frac{\text{rate of O}_2 \text{ consumption by organ}}{\left\{\begin{array}{c}\text{arterial blood O}_2 \text{ content—O}_2 \text{ content of venous blood from organ}\end{array}\right\}}$$

The most common type of cyanosis is dependent upon a decreased blood flow through the peripheral capillary bed. This necessitates the removal of more than the usual amount of oxygen from each unit of blood during its passage through the tissues. This condition may be produced locally in normal persons by chilling or cold applications or by exposure of the body to low environmental temperatures. Under these circumstances, cyanosis is particularly apparent in the nailbeds of the extremities.

At very low temperatures, the metabolism of the skin is inhibited; extraction of oxygen diminishes, and a shift of the oxyhemoglobin dissociation decreases the loss of oxygen in the capillaries. Despite almost complete cessation of cutaneous capillary flow, these events, together with dilation of the vessels, result in the familiar redness of the ears and nose in cold weather.

Slight blueness of the toe nailbeds is common in anxious individuals. Contraction of the superficial vessels is responsible for this phenomenon and for the pale, cold skin that is also frequently present. In polycythemia, the increased viscosity of the blood may result in slower blood flow through peripheral capillaries with resultant cyanosis. The symptom may be a striking feature of Raynaud's disease, in which spasmodic contraction of arteries leads to a diminution of arterial blood flow to the tissues, particularly to the fingers. Cyanosis may occur for analogous reasons in thromboangiitis obliterans or with the endarteritic occlusion of arteriosclerosis. Blood flow in the peripheral capillaries may also be slowed because of obstructed veins, and cyanosis of the affected part may be notable in phlebitis, in thrombosis, and even with varicosities.

Peripheral cyanosis may be a very striking feature of the low output varieties of cardiac failure. The arteriovenous oxygen difference is increased, but at rest is seldom greater than 9 ml/100 ml. In the cyanotic areas the arteriovenous oxygen difference, therefore, must be greater than it is for the body as a whole. This implies a disproportionate reduction of blood flow to these areas. During exercise the arteriovenous difference becomes greater than normal, since cardiac output does not increase appropriately or does not increase at all. Consequently, cyanosis is more apparent during exertion. Pulmonary factors may play an additional role in the cyanosis of cardiac failure when it is accompanied by pulmonary congestion. Unless pulmonary edema is present, however, the hypoxemia is usually mild or absent.[17]

Dilation and prominence of the venules in the skin secondary to a high venous pressure also affect skin color. The relative fullness of the subpapillary venous plexus is particularly important in those diseases in which the venous pressure is markedly and chronically elevated, such as tricuspid insufficiency.[18] In advanced tricuspid valvular disease jaundice may occur together with cyanosis, producing a curious combination of colors, known as icterocyanosis.

The cardiac output is profoundly lowered in shock and cyanosis is observed frequently.

The peripheral cyanosis in cardiac failure with a very low output or in acute reductions of the cardiac output (as when a ball-valve thrombus obstructs the orifice of the mitral valve) is characteristically most marked in distal regions such as the hands, the feet, and the tip of the nose. Peripheral cyanosis from any cause may be differentiated from central cyanosis due to hypoxemia, as Sir Thomas Lewis suggested,[19] by massaging the cyanotic part or applying heat to it. The ensuing increase in blood flow to the part will abolish peripheral, but not central, cyanosis.

Pulmonary Cyanosis. Hypoxemia, and therefore cyanosis, may occur when the normal state of gas exchange between alveolar air and pulmonary capillary blood is disturbed. Such a disturbance may result from an inadequate alveolar ventilation (as in paralysis of the chest cage, depression of the respiratory center, or laryngeal obstruction); from maldistribution of inspired air and blood among the alveoli with consequent underventilation of many alveoli relative to their blood supply (as in emphysema, asthma, or pulmonary edema); from decrease in the diffusion capacity of the alveolar-capillary membrane resulting from destruction of alveoli (as in some forms of emphysema); or thickening of the membrane (as in pulmonary fibrosis, or any condition in which the alveolar septa are infiltrated by inflammatory or neoplastic cells);[20,21] or

from blood flowing through the lungs without coming into contact with alveolar air (pulmonary arteriovenous shunts). The hypoxemia of chronic pulmonary disease frequently is exaggerated by exercise, particularly if the diffusion capacity of the alveolar-capillary membrane is restricted severely. The increase in pulmonary diffusing capacity that occurs normally during exercise is sufficient to satisfy the oxygen requirements of the most vigorous exercise without decrease in arterial oxygenation.

The syndrome of alveolar hypoventilation of sufficient degree to cause hypoxemia, polycythemia and cyanosis with essentially normal function of the lungs may occur when the work of moving the chest bellows is greatly increased, as in advanced kyphoscoliosis or marked obesity.[22] Cyanosis is also seen in patients with impairment of the respiratory muscles due to primary diseases of muscle, a previous attack of poliomyelitis, or other forms of neuritis or neuropathy involving motor nerves. When it is due to primary failure of the respiratory center of obscure origin, the clinical picture may be puzzling, since there is no evidence of lung disease, impairment of the chest bellows, or right-left shunt within the heart or the lungs.[23] In this disorder, arterial oxyhemoglobin saturation, which is decreased, and the carbon dioxide tension, which is increased, both can be brought to normal levels by increasing alveolar ventilation either volitionally or by a mechanical ventilator. A cardinal feature of the condition is a markedly decreased or absent ventilatory response to inhalation of carbon dioxide.

Hypoxemia also occurs when the pressure of oxygen in the inspired air is decreased by a reduction in barometric pressure, such as occurs at high altitude, or by a subnormal concentration of oxygen in air being breathed at sea level. The arterial oxyhemoglobin saturation at an altitude of 17,600 feet is about 68 per cent. The pressure of inspired oxygen at this altitude corresponds to that of 10 per cent oxygen at sea level.

It is essential to bear in mind that when cyanosis is due to arterial hypoxemia alone it is a sign of a very advanced disturbance in gas exchange. Because the upper segment of the oxyhemoglobin dissociation curve is relatively flat, alveolar oxygen pressure may fall as much as 35 mm Hg below the normal value without great change in arterial oxyhemoglobin saturation. Cyanosis may not be apparent until the saturation has dropped to

TABLE 20-1. MIXTURE CALCULATION

SOURCE OF BLOOD	AMOUNT, PARTS	OXYGEN CONTENT, ML/100 ML	OXYHEMOGLOBIN SATURATION, PER CENT
Right-left shunt	1	13.4	66
Pulmonary veins	2	19.8	97
Total (i.e., arterial)	3	17.7	87

85 per cent, and is usually, but not always, discernible at 75 per cent even by well-trained observers.[24] The arterial oxygen tensions at these saturations are 51 and 40 mm. Hg, respectively; about one-half the normal of 95 mm. The consequent loss of pressure-head that drives oxygen into the tissues may be critically important to previously ischemic areas.

Right–Left Shunts. Cyanosis in congenital heart disease is mainly attributable to contamination of the arterial stream by venous blood. Such a right-left shunt may occur through any of the various abnormal communications that may exist between the right and left cardiac chambers or great vessels. Whether or not a shunt exists will depend on the size of the communication and the relationship between the pressures on either side of the communication. Normally both the systolic and the diastolic pressures in the left cardiac chambers and great vessels exceed those in the corresponding right chambers and vessels. In atrial and ventricular septal defects and patent ductus arteriosus, the shunt is from left to right, and cyanosis is absent. If the pressures in the pulmonary artery, right ventricle, and right atrium are increased greatly, as they often are when pulmonary vascular lesions develop or cardiac failure supervenes, the shunt may become bidirectional, or be reversed completely. In pulmonic stenosis, pressures in the right ventricle, and also secondarily in the right atrium, are increased, and may give rise to a right-left shunt through a ventricular septal defect, a patent foramen ovale, or an atrial septal defect. Pressure relationships between the atria may be altered by vigorous crying, the Valsalva maneuver, or heavy exertion, and thereby cause transient reversal of a left–right interatrial shunt.

Several factors determine the presence or absence and degree of cyanosis in congenital heart disease. Most important is the size of the shunt relative to the systemic blood flow. If the systemic blood flow is normal, it is possible for one-third of it to be composed of venous blood without the appearance of cyanosis, since the arterial oxyhemoglobin saturation would be greater than 85 per cent. This is demonstrated in Table 20-1.

Another factor is the oxyhemoglobin saturation of the venous blood. If the systemic blood flow is less than normal in a patient with cyanotic congenital heart disease, the arteriovenous oxygen difference is increased, and the mixed venous blood that is shunted into the arterial circulation is less saturated with oxygen. Under these circumstances, a small shunt may produce a significant degree of hypoxemia. During exercise, the oxyhemoglobin saturation of mixed venous blood normally falls. This change may be exaggerated in cyanotic congenital heart disease because of an inability to increase cardiac output appropriately. This factor, as well as an increase in the size of the shunt, accounts for the exaggerated hypoxemia and cyanosis that develop during exertion. In some patients, cyanosis may not be evident except with exertion. Therefore, observation of the patient during some simple form of exercise constitutes an important part of the examination. In extensive bidirectional shunting through a defect, the saturation of the blood shunted from right to left depends on the ratio of pulmonary and systemic blood flows. If the ratio is high, a large right–left shunt may not produce much arterial desaturation.

Secondary polycythemia occurs frequently and is another factor that is responsible for the very profound degree of cyanosis that is observed in these disorders.

Pulmonary factors ordinarily do not play a role in producing the hypoxemia unless cardiac failure with pulmonary congestion develops. The arterial lesions responsible for the production of marked pulmonary arterial hypertension in some cases of congenital heart disease do not interfere greatly with pulmonary gas exchange, and pulmonary venous saturation in such patients is usually within the normal range. Pulmonary arteriovenous fistula, a congenital vascular lesion, may give rise to cyanosis and polycythemia without disturbing cardiac function. In some cases multiple fistulae occur, and the cyanosis may be pronounced.

The anatomic distribution of cyanosis in the various congenital cardiovascular disorders is like that in arterial hypoxemia of any cause. However, there are instances in which the distribution is not uniform. Cyanosis of the lower extremities, with absence or a lesser degree of cyanosis in the upper extremities, occurs in patent ductus arteriosus when the usual direction of blood flow through the ductus is reversed as a result of severe pulmonary arterial hypertension.[25] Since the ductus is inserted into the aorta distal to the bronchiocephalic arteries, the venous blood is directed mainly into the descending aorta. Occasionally the left hand is more cyanotic than the right because the left subclavian artery, which arises almost opposite the ductus, receives some of the shunt. The differential cyanosis between the upper and lower extremities often is associated with differential clubbing, and is of diagnostic importance. The "machinery" murmur typical of a patent ductus is absent under these circumstances (reversed flow).[25] Reversal of ductus flow also occurs in coarctation of the aorta when a coexisting ductus inserts into the aorta beyond the coarctation.

Normally, a very small quantity of venous blood is shunted into the systemic arterial stream via anastomotic connections between the bronchial and the pulmonary veins, and by drainage of the Thebesian and the anterior cardiac veins into the left heart. This venous admixture does not exceed 1 per cent of the pulmonary blood flow.[26] In some patients with cirrhosis of the liver, venous admixture is increased by the development of anastomoses between the portal, the mediastinal, and the pulmonary veins.[27] This venous admixture, although apparently not large, may contribute to the decreased arterial oxyhemoglobin saturation and the consequent cyanosis that occur in some patients with alcoholic cirrhosis.

Abnormalities of Hemoglobin. Hemoglobin, a metalloprotein of molecular weight 64,500, contains four ferroprotoporphyrin or heme units, each of which is capable of binding a single molecule of oxygen. Truly phenomenal advances in peptide chemistry have resulted in identification of the amino acids and their sequence in the peptide chains that comprise the protein moiety of hemoglobin, and x-ray diffraction studies have revealed the conformation of the entire molecule.[28,29,30] Normal adult human hemoglobin is composed of four polypeptide chains. The sequence of the 141 amino acid residues in each of two of these chains, designated α, is identical, and differs from that of the 146 residues in the other two identical β chains. These chains appear to be crumpled together, and the heme units, which are bonded by their iron atoms to the imidazol nitrogen of histidines at position 87 in the α chains and position 92 in the β chains, are imbedded in them.

It has been known for some time that binding of an oxygen molecule by one of the heme units successively facilitates binding of the gas by the other heme groups in the molecule. This phenomenon, known as the heme-heme interaction, accounts for the distinctive configuration of the oxyhemoglobin dissociation curve, and has been the subject of extensive theoretical analyses in the past.[29] A complete explanation of the phenomenon is still not at hand, but an essential component of the mechanism is a conformational change in the hemoglobin molecule that occurs when it binds oxygen.[30] Hemoglobin is capable of dissociating into two symmetrical dimers, each containing an α and a β chain, and by current theory, the dimer is the primary functional unit. Oxygenation enhances the tendency of hemoglobin to dissociate. Heme-heme interaction is regarded as the result of the effect of oxygen binding on the dissociation of the hemoglobin molecule to dimers and of the rapid exchange of oxygen among dimeric units.[31,32]

Several genetic variants of hemoglobin have been discovered which differ chemically from hemoglobin A only by a substitution of a single amino acid residue in either the α or β peptide chains. The physical properties of these hemoglobins, as in the case of sickle cell hemoglobin (S) or hemoglobin C, differ from those of hemoglobin A. A few of these hemoglobin variants also have an abnormal affinity for oxygen.

One such hemoglobin was obtained from a 14-year-old boy who was completely normal except for cyanosis, which had been present since birth.[33] His hemoglobin showed a striking reduction in its affinity for oxygen; although the arterial blood oxygen tension was normal (100 mm. Hg), the hemoglobin was only 60 per cent saturated with oxygen. Saturation attained a level of 94 per cent during oxygen breathing. Hemoglobin from the patient's mother showed a quantitatively similar decrease in ability to bind oxygen.

This hemoglobin, now designated as *Kansas hemoglobin*, has a threonine residue instead of the normal asparagine residue in position 102 of the β chain, but its primary structure is otherwise identical with that of hemoglobin A.[34] The striking decrease in its affinity for oxygen has been attributed to its increased tendency to dissociate into dimeric units when oxygenated.[34,35] The dissociation constant of the oxygenated tetramer is almost 200 times that of hemoglobin A.[34] Its P50, the oxygen tension at which hemoglobin tension is half saturated with oxygen, is 3.3 times greater than that of normal hemoglobin. The ease with which this hemoglobin unloads its oxygen in the systemic capillaries prevents the development of hypoxia.

Hemoglobin variants with a single amino acid substitution that have been characterized as having increased affinity for oxygen are called Chesapeake, Yakima, Kempsey, Rainier, Hiroshima, and J-Cape Town. All, with the exception of J-Cape Town, are associated with erythrocytosis in members of families who are homozygous for these hemoglobins.[35] The high affinity of hemoglobin Chesapeake for oxygen has been attributed to decreased dissociation of the oxygenated hemoglobin tetramer.[35]

Fetal hemoglobin differs from adult hemoglobin in that it contains two γ peptide chains instead of the two β chains. This hemoglobin constitutes 60 to 90 per cent of circulating hemoglobin at birth, and is gradually replaced by hemoglobin A; by age 4 months, only traces of F persist.[28] Although the oxygen affinity of umbilical cord blood is greater than that of adult blood, this is not an intrinsic property of hemoglobin F, but is related to some factor in the intracellular environment since the difference disappears after dialysis of the protein.[28]

Two hemoglobins associated with a thalassemia-like clinical picture are hemoglobin H and hemoglobin Bart's. All the polypeptide chains in H are β, and in Bart's they are all γ.[28] Both hemoglobins have an abnormally large affinity for oxygen; that for H is ten times normal.[36]

It has been shown recently that certain organic phosphates, especially adenosine triphosphate and 2,3-diphosphoglycerate (2,3-DPG) affect the affinity of hemoglobin for oxygen.[37] This compound is an intermediary product of red cell glycolytic metabolism and is present in relatively high concentration. It binds specifically with deoxyhemoglobin, and consequently reduces affinity of hemoglobin for oxygen. It is believed that the reduction of intracellular concentration of unbound 2,3-DPG which occurs with an increase in deoxyhemoglobin stimulates glyco-lytic production of the compound and raises its total concentration in the cell. Thus, 2,3-DPG might be a cardinal component of a feedback system that relates red cell metabolism to the functional properties of the hemoglobin, and thereby regulates the interaction of hemoglobin and oxygen to a level appropriate for the existing physiologic state.

One of the adaptations to high altitude is a *decreased affinity* of hemoglobin for oxygen (increased P50) which acts to make hemoglobin-bound oxygen more available to the tissues. Recent studies have shown that the increased P50 that occurred in the hemoglobin of intact red cells within 24 hours after ascent to 4,350 meters was accompanied by an increase of more than 50 per cent in the concentration of 2,3-DPG, and that these changes were reversed by descent to sea level.[38] The *marked increase in oxygen affinity* of red cells during storage has been correlated with a drastic fall in red cell 2,3-DPG concentration; this defect can be partially corrected by partial metabolic repletion of erythrocyte 2,3-DPG.[39] Young red cells have a much lower oxygen affinity than old red cells, and this has been attributed to the fact that 2,3-DPG concentration in young cells is 40 per cent greater than that in old cells.[39,40] Increased P50 of erythrocytes has been observed in patients with chronic hypoxemia secondary to either pulmonary disease or congenital heart disease and in patients with chronic low cardiac output[41,42]; it has been suggested that this change may be related to higher intracellular concentrations of 2,3-DPG.

Hemoglobin M is of interest because of its tendency to form methemoglobin. In the several variants of this protein which have been characterized, a single amino acid substitution has been found in the α or β chains, usually at or in proximity to the point of attachment of the heme group.[43] The oxidized or ferric form of the heme units in the abnormal chains resists the action of intracellular enzyme systems that maintain heme iron in the ferrous form, and consequently concentrations of circulating methemoglobin rise to values well above the normal of 2 per cent.[43] Not only is methemoglobin not capable of binding oxygen, but it shifts the dissociation curve of coexisting normal hemoglobin to the left. Patients with methemoglobinemia may experience fatigue, dyspnea, and palpitation, and polycythemia may develop. The skin has a peculiar leaden blue-gray color, and the blood has a chocolate hue.

Hemoglobin M disease should not be confused with another form of congenital methemoglobinemia in which the hemoglobin protein is normal, but which is associated with a deficiency of methemoglobin reductase in the red cell. Reduced nicotinamide adenine dinucleotide diaphorase is the most active enzyme performing this function and is specifically deficient in this disorder.[43]

RELATIONSHIP OF CYANOSIS TO CO_2 EXCHANGE

When hypoxemia is due to an over-all diminution of alveolar ventilation, the tension of carbon dioxide in alveolar air and arterial blood also is increased (see Chapter 19 on Dyspnea). Characteristically, in instances of uneven distribution of air and blood among the alveoli (such as may be caused by obstruction of the intrapulmonary airways in emphysema, asthma, or pulmonary edema), there is an increase in carbon dioxide tension and consequent respiratory acidosis only when many alveolar areas are underventilated and there is already advanced anoxemia. This phenomenon is explained by the fact that other areas of the lung are hyperventilated. Carbon dioxide output from the overventilated alveoli can balance, or even overcompensate for the retention of this gas in the blood of poorly ventilated alveoli because of the steepness of the blood carbon dioxide dissociation curve. On the other hand, the oxyhemoglobin dissociation curve is relatively flat in the usual physiologic range. The additional amount of oxygen that can be bound by the blood in the overventilated alveoli is not sufficient to compensate for the inadequate oxygenation of blood in the underventilated regions.[21]

If the alveolar-capillary membrane is abnormal, hypoxemia may be severe, but because of the much greater diffusibility of carbon dioxide as compared to oxygen, exchange of carbon dioxide is relatively undisturbed unless inadequacy of alveolar ventilation and ventilation/perfusion defects are superimposed.

Until recent years, the clinical importance of carbon dioxide has been poorly appreciated. In high concentrations this gas produces unconsciousness. In lesser concentration, delirium, stupor, and somnolence are common effects. In very high concentrations it can produce death. The exact concentrations at which these phenomena occur is not known. Stupor has been observed in young men breathing 10.4 per cent carbon dioxide for 3 to 4 minutes.[44,45] Patients with pulmonary disease whose arterial carbon dioxide tension rises to the range of 100 mm. Hg frequently become comatose. Normal subjects lose consciousness in 20 to 30 seconds upon breathing a mixture of 30 per cent carbon dioxide and 70 per cent oxygen.[46]

Carbon dioxide is a powerful dilator of the cerebral vessels.[47] The sudden dilatation of these vessels that occurs with increments in arterial carbon dioxide tension causes an abrupt increase in cerebrospinal fluid pressure.[48] This change may be of sufficient degree to produce papilledema.[49] Carbon dioxide directly constricts other systemic vessels and may produce a rise in blood pressure. In high concentrations it may cause cardiac arrhythmias, both auricular and ventricular.[46]

EFFECTS OF OXYGEN ON CYANOSIS

When pure oxygen is breathed, the pressure of oxygen in the alveolar air and arterial blood is increased six-fold. The concentration of oxygen carried in solution consequently rises to 1.8 ml/100 ml; an additional 0.6 ml/100 ml is bound by the hemoglobin, since it becomes fully saturated. The net increase in arterial oxygen content is, therefore, 2.4 ml/100 ml. The additional increase in dissolved oxygen which can be achieved by breathing oxygen under increased pressure in a hyperbaric chamber is directly related to the ambient pressure.

Amelioration of any type of cyanosis will occur on breathing pure oxygen. For example, in peripheral cyanosis, with normal hemoglobin concentration, if the arterial blood oxygen content is raised from 19.8 to 22.2 ml/100 ml and the amount of oxygen extracted by the tissues continues at 12 ml/100 ml the venous blood will be only 9.9 ml/100 ml unsaturated. The average deficit of oxygen in the capillary blood will be 4.4 ml/100 ml (equivalent to 3.3 g/100 ml of deoxyhemoglobin) instead of 6.5 ml/100 ml, and cyanosis will disappear. However, oxygen will not abolish cyanosis when the peripheral blood flow is more restricted, and the arteriovenous oxygen difference in the tissue being examined is consequently greater than that in this example.

In the case of a right–left shunt, breathing of oxygen will also lessen the hypoxemia and relieve cyanosis by increasing the amount of oxygen in both the pulmonary venous blood and in the systemic venous blood that is being shunted. In the mixture calculation described above in the section on congenital heart disease, the pulmonary venous oxygen content will increase to 22.2 ml/100 ml, the right–left shunt content to 15.8 ml/100 ml, and the arterial content to 20.07 ml/100 ml, which corresponds to an oxyhemoglobin saturation of 98 per cent. Although arterial saturation may reach the normal range, oxygen tension will fall far short of 650 mm Hg, the value normally found during oxygen breathing. Measurement of arterial blood oxygen tension while the subject is breathing oxygen is a simple procedure, and the value can be used in a simple shunt formula inter-relating calculated concentrations of dissolved oxygen in pulmonary venous, mixed venous, and arterial blood to estimate the relative magnitude of the shunt. Complete saturation of the arterial blood with oxygen, however, will not occur if the shunt is greater than 40 per cent of the systemic blood flow or if the arteriovenous oxygen difference is greater than normal.

The most dramatic relief of hypoxemia and cyanosis that is achieved by administration of oxygen occurs when gas exchange is impaired by disturbances in pulmonary function. Regardless of whether these disturbances consist of marked generalized alveolar hypoventilation, maldistribution of air and blood among the alveoli, decrease in the pulmonary oxygen diffusing capacity, or a combination of these factors (as is so often the case), administration of oxygen will almost always increase the arterial blood oxyhemoglobin saturation to or near normal. Oxygen therapy is therefore of considerable value, especially in acute conditions like pulmonary edema, pneumonia, chronic pulmonary disease complicated by a respiratory infection and severe asthma. Frequently it is life-saving.

Some reservations about the use of oxygen should be noted. When alveolar ventilation is decreased seriously by respiratory paralysis resulting from poliomyelitis or depression of the respiratory center, oxygen will promptly abolish hypoxemia and cyanosis but it will not correct the coexisting hypercapnia. The patient may be spared the dangers of anoxia while receiving oxygen, but may develop all the serious mental and neurologic consequences of a markedly increased blood carbon dioxide tension and respiratory acidosis. *Mechanical ventilation* is the essential therapy in these conditions, and is the only way to control the concentration of carbon dioxide in the alveolar air and the arterial blood.

In chronic pulmonary disease complicated by chronic hypoxemia and respiratory acidosis, as is often the case in emphysema, oxygen may produce *undesirable* sequelae, especially if it is administered in concentrations approaching 100 per cent. The respiratory centers of such patients are relatively insensitive to carbon dioxide and increase in blood hydrogen ion concentration. A greater than normal portion of central neurogenic drive to respiration arises from hypoxic reflexes originating in the oxygen-sensitive aortic and carotid bodies. Elevation of the arterial oxygen tension to normal or above on breathing oxygen abolishes the hypoxia-induced impulses, and ventilation may drop precipitously. Pre-existing inadequacy of alveolar ventilation is aggravated thereby. Alveolar and arterial carbon dioxide tensions rise sharply, and the various manifestations of the *carbon dioxide narcosis syndrome* may appear.

If oxygen therapy is required, as it often is when the chronic pulmonary insufficiency is acutely aggravated, it is best given in concentrations of *24 to 28 per cent.* Such concentrations will improve arterial oxyhemoglobin saturation substantially without producing intolerable depression of respiratory drive. With judicious use of oxygen-enriched air, guided by careful monitoring of the patient and his arterial blood gas concentrations and supplemented by a vigorous therapeutic attack on underlying bronchial obstruction, pulmonary infection, and cardiac failure, it is usually possible to maintain ventilation without resorting to mechanical respirators.[50,51] The treatment of pulmonary insufficiency, the use of oxygen and mechanical ventilators and their potential dangers are beyond the scope of this chapter; the interested reader is referred to the extensive and growing literature on these subjects.

REFERENCES

1. Schwaber, J. R., and Lukas, D. S.: Hyperkinemia and cardiac failure in the carcinoid syndrome, Amer. J. Med. 32:846, 1962.
2. Foster, R. E.: Diffusion of gases, *in* Fenn, W., and Rahn, H. (eds.): Handbook of Physiology. Respiration, vol. I, Sec. 3, p. 839, Washington, D. C., Amer. Physiol. Soc., 1964.
3. Chance, B., Cohen, P., Jöbiss, F., and Schoener, B.: Intracellular oxidation-reduction states *in vivo*, Science 137:499, 1962.

4. ———: Localized fluorometry of oxidation-reduction states of intracellular pyridine nucleotides in brain and kidney cortex of the anesthetized rat, Science 136:325, 1962.

5. Lundsgaard, C., and Van Slyke, D. D.: Cyanosis, Medicine 2:1, 1923.

6. Rothman, S.: Physiology and Biochemistry of the Skin, Chicago, Univ. of Chicago Press, 1954.

7. Davis, M. J., and Lawler, J. C.: Capillary microscopy in normal and diseased human skin, in Montagna, W., and Ellis, R. A. (eds.): Advances in Biology of Skin. vol. II, Blood Vessels and Circulation, p. 79, New York, Pergamon, 1961.

8. Winkelmann, R. K., Scheen, S. R., Jr., Pyka, R. A., and Coventry, M. B.: Cutaneous vascular patterns in studies with injection preparation and alkaline phosphatase reaction, in Montagna, W., and Ellis, R. A. (eds.): Advances in Biology of Skin. vol. II, Blood Vessels and Circulation, p. 1, New York, Pergamon, 1961.

9. Burton, A. C.: Special features of the circulation of the skin, in Montagna, W., and Ellis, R. A. (eds.): Advances in Biology of Skin. vol. II, Blood Vessels and Circulation, p. 117, New York, Pergamon, 1961.

10. Hertzman, A. B.: Effects of heat on the cutaneous blood flow, in Montagna, W., and Ellis, R. A. (eds.): Advances in Biology of Skin. vol. II, Blood Vessels and Circulation, p. 98, New York, Pergamon, 1961.

11. Greenfield, A. D. M.: The circulation through the skin, in Hamilton, W. F., and Dow, P. (eds.): Handbook of Physiology. Circulation, vol. II, Sec. 2, p. 1325, Washington, D. C., Amer. Physiol. Soc. 1963.

12. Roddie, I. C., Shepherd, J. T., and Whelan, R. F.: Evidence from venous saturation measurements that the increase in forearm blood during body heating is confined to the skin, J. Physiol. 134:444, 1956.

13. Lillienthal, J. L., and Riley, R. L.: On the determination of arterial oxygen saturations from samples of "capillary blood," J. Clin. Invest. 23:904, 1944.

14. Christoforides, C., and Miller, J. M.: Clinical use and limitations of arterialized capillary blood for PO_2 determination, Amer. Rev. Resp. Dis. 98:653, 1968.

15. Lundsgaard, C.: Studies on cyanosis. I. Primary causes of cyanosis, J. Exp. Med. 30:259, 1919.

16. ———: Studies on cyanosis. II. Secondary causes of cyanosis, J. Exp. Med. 30:295, 1919.

17. Carroll, D., Cohen, J. E., and Riley, R. L.: Pulmonary function in mitral valvular disease: Distribution and diffusion characteristics in resting patients, J. Clin. Invest. 32:510, 1953.

18. Sepulveda, G., and Lukas, D. S.: The diagnosis of tricuspid insufficiency. Clinical features in 60 cases with associated mitral valve disease, Circulation 11:552, 1955.

19. Lewis, T.: Diseases of the Heart, London, Macmillan, 1933.

20. Lukas, D. S.: Pulmonary function in health and disease, Med. Clin. N. A. 39:661, 1955.

21. Comroe, J. H., Jr., Forster, R. E., II, DuBois, A. B., Briscoe, W. A., and Carlsen, E.: The Lung. Clinical Physiology and Pulmonary Function Tests, ed. 2, Chicago, Year Book Pub. 1962.

22. Fishman, A. P., Turino, G. M., and Bergofsky, E. H.: The syndrome of alveolar hypoventilation, Amer. J. Med. 23:333, 1957.

23. Rodman, T., Resnick, M. E., Berkowitz, R. D., Fenelly, J. F., and Olivia, J.: Alveolar hypoventilation due to involvement of the respiratory center by obscure disease of the central nervous system, Amer. J. Med. 32:208, 1962.

24. Comroe, J. H., and Botelho, S.: The unreliability of cyanosis in the recognition of arterial anoxemia, Amer. J. Med. Sci. 214:1, 1947.

25. Lukas, D. S., Araujo, J., and Steinberg, I.: The syndrome of patent ductus arteriosus with reversal of flow, Amer. J. Med. 17:298, 1954.

26. Fritts, H. W., Jr., Hardewig, A., Rochester, D. F., Durand, J., and Cournand, A.: Estimation of pulmonary arteriovenous shunt-flow using intravenous injections of T-1824 dye Kr[85], J. Clin. Invest. 39:1841, 1960.

27. Calabresi, P., and Abelmann, W. H.: Portocaval and porto-pulmonary anastomoses in Laennec's cirrhosis and in heart failure, J. Clin. Invest. 36:1257, 1957.

28. Lehmann, H., Huntsman, R. C., and Ager, J. A. M.: The hemoglobinopathies and thalassemia, in Stanbury, J. B., Wyngaarden, J. B., and Frederickson, D. S. (eds.): The Metabolic Basis of Inherited Disease, p. 1100, New York, McGraw-Hill, 1966.

29. Roughton, F. J. W.: Transport of oxygen and carbon dioxide, in Fenn, W., and Rahn, H. (eds.): Handbook of Physiology. Respiration, vol. I, Sec. 3, p. 767, Washington, D. C., Amer. Physiol. Soc., 1964.

30. Muirhead, H., and Perutz, M. F.: A three-dimensional Fourier synthesis of reduced human hemoglobin at 5.5 Å resolution, Nature (London) 199:633, 1963.

31. Benesch, R. E., Benesch, R., and Macduff, G.: Subunit exchange and ligand binding: a new hypothesis for the mechanism of oxygenation of hemoglobin, Proc. Nat. Acad. Sci. U.S.A. 54:535, 1965.

32. Guidotti, G.: Studies on the chemistry of hemoglobin. IV. The mechanism of reaction with ligands, J. Biol. Chem. 242:3704, 1967.

33. Reissmann, K. R., Ruth, W. E., and Nomura, T.: A human hemoglobin with lowered oxygen affinity and impaired heme-heme interactions, J. Clin. Invest. 40:1826, 1961.

34. Bonaventure J., and Riggs, A.: Hemoglobin Kansas, a human hemoglobin with a neutral amino acid substitution and an abnormal oxygen equilibrium, J. Biol. Chem. 243:980, 1968.

35. Bunn, H. F.: Subunit dissociation of certain abnormal hemoglobins, J. Clin. Invest. 48:126, 1969.

36. Benesch, R., Ranney, H. M., and Benesch, R. E.: Some properties of hemoglobin H, Fed. Proc. 20:70, 1961.

37. Benesch, R., Benesch, R. E., and Yu, C. I.: Recriprocal binding of oxygen and diphosphoglycerate by human hemoglobin, Proc. Nat. Acad. Sci. U.S.A. 59:526, 1968.

38. Lenfant, C., Torrance, J., English, E., Finch, C. A., Reyafarje, C., Ramos, J., and Faura, J.: Effect of altitude on oxygen binding by hemoglobin and on organic phosphate levels, J. Clin. Invest. 47:2652, 1968.

39. Bunn, H. F., May, M. H., Kocholaty, W. F., and Shields, S. E.: Hemoglobin function and stored blood, J. Clin. Invest. 48:311, 1969.

40. Edwards, M. J., and Rigas, D. A.: Electrolyte labile increase of oxygen affinity during in vivo aging of hemoglobin, J. Clin. Invest. 46:1579, 1967.

41. Edwards, M. J., Novy, M. J., Walters, C., and Metcalfe, J.: Improved oxygen release: An adaptation of mature red cells to hypoxia, J. Clin. Invest. 47:1851, 1968.

42. Metcalfe, J., Dhindsa, D. S., Edwards, M. J., and Mourdjinis, A.: The oxygen dissociation curve of blood from patients with low rates of peripheral blood flow, Clin. Res. 16:240, 1968.

43. Gerald, P. S., and Scott, E. M.: The hereditary methemoglobinemias, in Stanbury, J. B., Wyngaarden, J. B., and Frederickson, D. S. (eds.): The Metabolic Basis of Inherited Disease, p. 1100, New York, McGraw-Hill, 1966.

44. Haldane, J. S.: Respiration, New Haven, Yale Univ. Press, 1922.

45. Dripps, R. D., and Comroe, J. H., Jr.: The respiratory and circulatory response of normal man to inhalation of 7.6 and 10.4 per cent O_2 with a comparison of the maximal ventilation produced by severe muscular exercise, inhalation of CO_2 and maximal voluntary hyperventilation, Amer. J. Physiol. 149:43, 1947.

46. MacDonald, F. M., and Simonson, E.: Human electrocardiogram during and after inhalation of 30 per cent carbon dioxide, J. Appl. Physiol. 6:304, 1953.

47. Schieve, J. F., and Wilson, W. P.: The changes in cerebral vascular resistance of man in experimental alkalosis and acidosis, J. Clin. Invest. 32:33, 1953.

48. Davies, C. E., and Mackinnon, J.: Neurological effects of oxygen in chronic cor pulmonale, Lancet 2:883, 1949.

49. Simpson, T.: Papilloedema in emphysema, Brit. M. J. 2:639, 1948.

50. Smith, J. P., Stone, R. W., and Muschenheim, C.: Acute respiratory failure in chronic lung disease. Observations on controlled oxygen therapy, Amer. Rev. Resp. Dis. 97:791, 1968.

51. Campbell, E. J. M.: Respiratory failure, Brit. Med. J. 1:1451, 1965.

21

Anorexia, Nausea, and Vomiting

JAMES E. McGUIGAN

Anorexia, nausea, and vomiting are among the most common and distressing symptoms that afflict man. So wide-spread and significant are these symptoms that very commonly patients equate "being sick" with the presence of these symptoms. Anorexia, nausea, and vomiting are associated with a wide variety of clinical disorders, some of which are relatively trivial, others of which may reflect diseases of a most severe and disabling nature. Anorexia, nausea, and vomiting may be evoked by disorders of the gastrointestinal tract but also may reflect psychic, neurologic, or metabolic conditions, or other visceral abnormalities.

INNERVATION OF THE GASTROINTESTINAL TRACT

In order to understand the mechanisms by which nausea and vomiting are provoked it is necessary to discuss that portion of the peripheral and central nervous system which innervates the gastrointestinal tract, regulating and modifying its function.

The gastrointestinal tract receives its extrinsic nerve supply from components of the autonomic nervous system.[1] In purely anatomical terms, autonomic outflow is limited to craniosacral and thoracolumbar spinal segments, craniosacral outflow being designated as parasympathetic and thoracolumbar as sympathetic. Adrenergic nerves act by liberation of norepinephrine or epinephrine; cholinergic nerves liberate acetylcholine. Most sympathetic nerves are adrenergic, whereas most, but perhaps not all, parasympathetic nerves are cholinergic.

Thoracolumbar sympathetic preganglionic fibers synapse with cells in paravertebral ganglia. Postganglionic efferent fibers arising in these ganglia supply most of the gut via the splanchnic nerves. Efferent fibers from the celiac plexus supply the stomach. In addition, the gut is partially supplied through the aortic plexi, the para-aortic nerves, branches from the lumbar portions of the sympathetic trunks, and from fibers carried in the vagus nerves.

Neural plexi extend throughout the alimentary tract. These plexi lie on the surfaces of the pharynx and uppermost esophagus, but in the remainder of the gastrointestinal tract they comprise collections and networks of interconnected ganglion cells located in the submucosa and interspersed between longitudinal and circular smooth muscle layers. In the gut, many adrenergic nerves connect with intramural ganglion cells,[2,3] most of which are cholinergic. Thus, most adrenergic effects on gastrointestinal motility are effected principally by postganglionic cholinergic cells.

With certain exceptions, sympathetic innervation of the gastrointestinal tract is generally inhibitory. Adrenergic receptors have been classified as α and β,[4] α receptors being those that are excited by sympathetic stimulation or sympathomimetic agents, and β receptors being those that are inhibited by these same factors. The ergot alkaloids and haloalkylamines antagonize α receptor responses, whereas β receptor responses are inhibited by propranolol, nethalide, and dichloroisoproterenol. Stimulation of either α or β receptors results in inhibition of intestinal smooth muscle activity.[5] In certain areas of the guinea pig gastrointestinal tract, α receptors are excitatory: these include the esophagus,[6] bile duct,[7] and terminal ileum.[8] In spite of our knowledge of neural circuitry and receptor function, the role of sympathetic activity in the control of gastrointestinal motility is largely unknown.

Parasympathetic activity usually produces increased tone and motility of the gastrointestinal tract, with reinforcement of activity mediated through local nerve plexi.

Efferent parasympathetic innervation of the stomach and most of the intestinal tract (except for its lowermost portions) is supplied by vagal fibers, which follow blood vessels to synapse with cell bodies located in the myenteric and submucosal plexi. The smooth muscle of the gastrointestinal tract is supplied by postganglionic efferent fibers arising in these plexi.

Visceral afferent fibers, with sensory endings in the gut, synapse in gastrointestinal ganglia, muscle layers, or mucosal epithelium. These postganglionic fibers accompany vagal and sympathetic rami to the dorsal roots of the spinal cord. Some afferent fibers pass centrally with the sympathetics through celiac and other ganglia without synapsing. Other afferent fibers synapse in the celiac plexus ganglia, with postganglionic sympathetic fibers constituting the afferent limbs of visceral reflex arcs.

Many gastrointestinal visceral reflexes are conducted without participation of higher central connections. Other reflexes appear to be modified or controlled by medullary and hypothalamic activity. Simultaneous visceral and somatic expression appear to be coordinated by the hypothalamus.[9] Sensory and motor autonomic and somatic functions are connected principally with the cerebral cortex and the cerebellum. It is via these connections that psychic influences modify activity of the gastrointestinal tract.

Currently there is a large amount of investigation being conducted relating to motor activity and neural control of gastrointestinal functions. Our present level of understanding does not permit us to interrelate these investigations, such as observations of electrical activity and changes in intraluminal pressure, with human symptoms in disease states associated with anorexia, nausea, and vomiting. Widespread interest has evolved in the polypeptide hormone gastrin,[10] which has as its principal activity the capacity to evoke gastric secretion of hydrochloric acid powerfully. However, gastrin also exerts effects on motor activity of the stomach and of the small intestine. Similarly, secretin[11] and perhaps other gastrointestinal hormones influence gastrointestinal motility. It remains to be investigated whether these hormones play a significant role in disturbances of motor activity related to anorexia, nausea, and vomiting.

ANOREXIA

Anorexia may be defined as lack or loss of the appetite for food, or as disinterest in the ingestion of food. The concept of appetite is somewhat more elusive, but may be regarded as a favorable disposition toward, or simply as a desire for food. Lack of interest in consumption of a particular variety of food or foods may reflect individual and personal preferences and does not have the same connotation as the somewhat more generalized and at times active disinterest in consumption of all foods, which is termed anorexia. When a man consumes sufficient food, interpreted via complex physiological signals as adequate for his present requirements, a state of satiety is achieved. No further food is then desired, but the subjective sensation is somewhat different from that actively disinterested state, which we define as anorexia. Anorexia is frequently associated with a disinterest in consumption of even those foods toward which the individual may habitually manifest his greatest gustatory interest. Sensations of appetite, hunger, and satiety may be looked upon as normal psychophysiological mechanisms of control of food ingestion. However, in certain states individuals may consume or reject food independent of sensations of appetite, hunger, or satiety.

HUNGER

Hunger has been defined as a craving for food, the driving sensation or urge to eat

PLATE 3

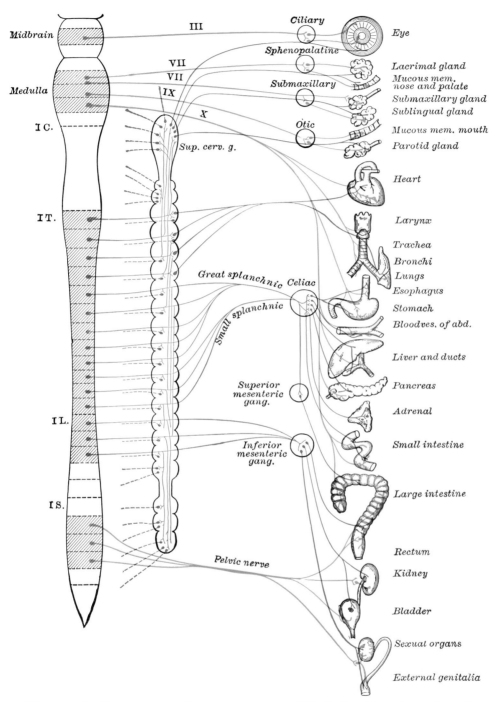

Diagram of efferent autonomic nervous system. (*Blue*) Cranial and sacral outflow, parasympathetic. (*Red*) Thoracolumbar, sympathetic. (*Dotted red line*) Postganglionic fibers to spinal and cranial nerves to supply vasomotors to head, trunk and limbs, motor fibers to smooth muscles of skin and fibers to sweat glands. (Modified after Gottlieb. Gray: Anatomy of the Human Body, ed. 24, Philadelphia, Lea & Febiger)

which follows a period of fasting. Hunger concerns itself with the satisfaction or fulfillment of the requirement for food. Undoubtedly many cultural, physiological, and psychological factors influence the subjective appreciation of hunger. It is well-known that the sensation of hunger often is temporally associated with rhythmic contractions of the stomach,[12] but the speculation that the hunger sensations are the results of these contractions has been largely discarded. Data to the contrary are: humans and experimental animals without stomachs experience hunger; vagally transmitted hunger "pangs" are not correlated in time with gastric contractions; gastric contractions even greater than those observed in the fasting state are observed following ingestion of food; gastrectomized animals are able to regulate their caloric intake. However, the converse is probably a valid physiologic relationship, i.e., hunger causes motor activity of the stomach. Many of the drugs that suppress the intake of food decrease gastric motor activity.

The precise mechanisms by which hunger is produced are not known. Evidence from investigations in experimental animals and correlative clinical states supports the existence of two hypothalamic centers whose function relates to hunger and food ingestion. The first of these, the "feeding center," is located in the ventrolateral portion of the hypothalamus caudolateral to the mamillary bodies. Electrical stimulation of the feeding center results in hyperphagia, whereas ablation of it is associated with reduced food intake, emaciation, and death. The second center, the "satiety center," is located in the ventromedial region of the hypothalamus. Stimulation of this center effects inhibition of food intake, and destruction of it results in excessive food ingestion. There is evidence that the activities of these centers are influenced by blood glucose levels and arteriovenous glucose differences.[13] The satiety center can be inactivated experimentally by administration of goldthioglucose but not by a number of other organic gold compounds. Inactivation of the satiety center, associated with cytotoxicity due to gold, is accompanied by the deposition of gold in cells of the ventromedial hypothalamic area.

It has been proposed that the mechanism determining the expression of hunger or satiety is related to the rate of utilization of glucose, and that this is sensed by glucoreceptors located in the hypothalamus. This hypothesis proposes that large arteriovenous glucose differences stimulate the satiety center and inhibit the feeding center. Low arterial-venous differences in glucose levels, such as those produced by insulin administration, are proposed to produce converse effects. In certain individuals, hypoglycemia may provoke hunger as is seen in states of hyperinsulinism induced in experimental animals, in functional hypoglycemia, and in association with excessive circulating insulin as from β-cell islet tumors. Hunger is also provoked following injection of exogenous insulin in diabetic and nondiabetic patients, in Addison's disease, and in hypoglycemia associated with certain tumors, particularly certain sarcomas. Relief of hunger of this variety promptly follows administration of intravenous glucose. The central nature of stimulation of hunger of this variety was amply demonstrated by its occurrence following insulin injection, even after complete denervation of the gastrointestinal tract.[14] Glucagon administered intravenously reduces hunger, elevates the venous glucose levels, and according to some investigators increases arteriovenous glucose differences.[15] There are several objections to acceptance of the hypothesis that blood glucose levels serve as the sole determinants for hunger. Intravenous glucose does not relieve hunger in normal individuals in the absence of insulin administration. To date, there have not been good correlations between venous glucose levels or arteriovenous glucose differences and hunger in normal individuals. Hunger sensations may follow insulin administration in the absence of substantial differences in arteriovenous glucose levels.

Although blood glucose levels and differences in arteriovenous glucose levels may participate in certain situations in the production of hunger, it is apparent that gastric distention also serves as an important satiety signal. Insertion of nonfood bulk[16,17] (or of food) into the stomach produces short-termed inhibition of eating.

Distention of the stomach produces afferent impulses carried through cervical vagal fibers.[18] Certain of these units respond to as little increase in intragastric pressure as 2 mm. of water. It has been suggested that there are distention-sensitive gastric receptors in the outer layers of the stomach wall, that these units are "in series"[19] with smooth muscle fibers, and that these receptors initiate signals resulting from increases in gastric wall tension as well as from gastric distention or contractions. These mechanoreceptors are present in the walls of the stomach, and of the small and large intestines.[19,20] In experimental animals, increasing gastric distention produces an increase in electrical activity in the hypothalamic satiety center,[21] accompanied by a lack of activity in the region of the hypothalamic feeding center. Intestinal distention produces similar results. In rats, inflation of small intragastric balloons results in decreased food investigative activity.[22] This decrease of food investigation and consumption with gastric distention is eliminated by subtotal vagotomy. Food intake of rats has been demonstrated to be decreased in association with distention of exteriorized small intestinal segments.[23] When these intestinal loops were denervated, decrease in food consumption was inhibited. In addition to the mechanoreceptors, there are also apparently chemoreceptors[24,25] in the wall of the gastrointestinal tract. Glucose perfusion of the stomach and the small intestine of humans and experimental animals produces increased afferent electrical activity in small fiber groups transmitted through fibers contained in mesenteric and splanchnic nerves.

It has been proposed that "long-term" regulation of food intake, as opposed to "short-term" regulation described previously, may be influenced by the magnitude of the adipose tissue reservoir in the organism.[26] This hypothesis is based on observations that rats made hypophagic from hypothalamic lesions reach a plateau of obesity at which food intake falls. If one member of a pair of parabiotic rats is made hyperphagic, the other member progressively loses weight, presumably on the basis of stimulation of its satiety center by the adiposity of its parabiotic mate.

It is apparent from the foregoing discussions that we do not understand completely the mechanisms involved in the production and regulation of hunger. The psychophysiological phenomenon of hunger appears to be influenced by a variety of mechanisms: central regulation mediated through the hypothalamic centers, biochemical alterations in blood and tissue components, and afferent nervous stimuli resulting from mechanical and chemical events occurring in the gastrointestinal tract. The way, or ways, in which these factors are interrelated in their influence upon hunger in the short- and long-term regulation of food intake remain to be defined.

APPETITE

Appetite may be conceived of as an agreeable attitude toward ingesting food, often toward a particular variety or varieties of food. The central nature of appetite is reaffirmed by observations that appetite remains unaffected following autonomic denervation of the stomach, small bowel, and proximal colon. Not only does hunger remain following a gastrectomy, but selective desires for individual foods remain. The parietal and frontal regions of the brain have been known to be associated with appetite. Desire for food is associated with increased rates of gastric hydrochloric acid secretion, with gastric hyperemia, and hypermotility.[27] Anorexia, the absence of hunger or appetite, has been associated with the opposite: decreased gastric hydrochloric acid secretion, with hypomotility of the stomach and pallor of the gastric mucosa. Anorexia may be induced by unpleasant or revolting experiences. Apprehension, fear, or anxiety may result in the sensation of anorexia. However, excitement of pleasurable and desirable types also may be associated with anorexia.

NAUSEA

Nausea is an ill-defined but distinctly unpleasant sensation usually associated with a profound revulsion toward the ingestion of food. Most states proceeding to vomiting are accompanied by anorexia and nausea. Anorexia is commonly followed by nausea, which in turn is followed by vomiting. It must be recognized, however, that any of these three symptoms may be experienced by the patient in the absence of either or both of the other two. Nausea is often but not invariably preceded by anorexia. Nausea without some degree of anorexia is very unusual. Stimuli that evoke anorexia in susceptible persons when amplified will often cause the subjects to become nauseated. Chemical agents, food, drugs, and other stimuli that in small doses produce anorexia will often produce nausea when given in greater doses. The anorectic individual will often become frankly nauseated when confronted with food; his revulsion toward food has been thrust into his consciousness. Both nausea and anorexia are associated with decreased motor activity of the stomach and pallor of the gastric mucosa; the changes are more conspicuous with nausea than with anorexia. In contrast to the hypotonicity of the stomach, there is contraction of the proximal duodenum. It is possible to induce nausea by distention of an airfilled balloon located in the distal esophagus, stomach, or, most especially, in the duodenum. Nausea or vomiting is frequently associated with evidence of diffuse autonomic discharge, including profuse watery salivation, often sudden drenching sweating, and tachycardia. Bradycardia is often experienced concurrently with the act of vomiting.

Patients often have great difficulty in describing the nature of the extremely unpleasant phenomenon that they experience as nausea. The sensation of nausea is commonly described by the patient as a vague unpleasantness located in the epigastrium or diffusely in the abdomen. When nauseated, some patients experience distressing sensations in the region of the throat. The unpleasant abdominal sensations experienced as nausea often have to be distinguished from visceral abdominal pain of mild degree, which is also frequently poorly localized in the abdomen.

The mechanism by which acid secretion is reduced while nausea is experienced has not been defined. The fact that denervation of the stomach does not abolish nausea suggests that the phenomenon is not solely under neural regulation and that other factors,[28] e.g., vascular or hormonal mechanisms, may be involved. The mucosal pallor associated with nausea makes it tempting to speculate that vascular changes within the gastric mucosa are responsible for both reduction in acid secretion and gastric mucosal pallor.

VOMITING

Vomiting may be defined as the sudden forceful peroral expulsion of the contents of the stomach. It often, but not invariably, is preceded by nausea, which may become acutely more severe immediately prior to the act of vomiting.

The vomiting center is believed to be located in the dorsal portion of the lateral reticular formation in the medulla. Destruction of the vomiting center in dogs and cats has been shown to ablate the vomiting response to the usual methods of provocation of vomiting. Apomorphine, an agent capable of inducing vomiting when administered orally or intravenously, when applied to this region of the medulla produces vomiting. A "chemoreceptor zone"[29] has been described adjacent to the vomiting center. From investigations in experimental animals, it has been proposed that this chemoreceptor zone may

be stimulated by humoral agents including certain toxic chemicals, and that stimulation of this chemoreceptor center results in transmission of neural impulses to the vomiting center with resulant vomiting. Afferent stimuli from peripheral sites are believed to be able to stimulate the vomiting center directly through afferent nervous connections with the vomiting center without necessary mediation through the chemoreceptor center.

The Act of Vomiting. Exaggerated and frequently extreme vasomotor phenomena often immediately precede and accompany the act of vomiting. These include abundant watery salivation and sweating, vasoconstriction with pallor, and changes in pulse rate. The patient often may become tremulous, weak, lightheaded, and "dizzy," but seldom experiences true vertigo. A gradually accelerating rate of respiration with some irregularity of breathing may occur immediately prior to the act of vomiting. Retching commonly but not invariably precedes vomiting. The blood pressure may fall just prior to vomiting, and often fluctuates during the act of vomiting. This phenomenon may reflect in part modification of cardiac output resulting from abrupt and marked changes in intrathoracic pressure. The heart rate, which is often rapid prior to vomiting, slows to the point of bradycardia during the act of vomiting. Respirations cease during the act of vomiting.

The sequence of events during the act of vomiting is as follows: the upper half of the stomach and the region of the gastroesophageal sphincter relax. Peristaltic contractions from the midportion of the stomach proceed to the angulus of the stomach, where a violent contraction occurs. The diaphragm undergoes violent descent, with simultaneous contractions of the abdominal muscles expelling gastric contents up into and through the esophagus. Descent of the diaphragm and acute contraction of the abdominal muscles operate in concert to elevate acutely the intra-abdominal pressure. During the forceful expulsion of food up and out through the esophagus the glottis is closed, respirations cease, and the soft palate is thrust upwards against the nasopharynx.

There is no evidence that reverse (cephalad directed) peristalsis occurs in the stomach or plays any part; nor has it been shown that reverse peristalsis in the small intestine plays a significant role in the act of vomiting.[30]

DISTURBANCES ASSOCIATED WITH ANOREXIA, NAUSEA, AND VOMITING

Anorexia, nausea, and vomiting may be observed in a wide variety of psychophysiologic and organic disorders. For purposes of description and discussion causes of vomiting will be classified as associated with psychic and neurological factors, drugs and intoxications, intra-abdominal disorders, and other assorted factors. No classification is satisfactory for these purposes, since one or more of these symptoms may be associated with disturbances of well-being in virtually every disease to which man is prone.

Psychic and Neurological Factors. In many patients, emotional factors play a very important role in the production of anorexia, nausea, and/or vomiting. Life situations that evoke subjective responses of fear, depression, frustration, apprehension, and anxiety may commonly be associated with these symptoms. In not all instances are the predisposing or conditioning emotional responses unpleasant ones. We are all familiar with the loss of appetite associated with apprehension regarding a forthcoming event, even one which may be anticipated with the greatest pleasure. More commonly, however, unpleasant experiences (which may not necessarily be recognized as unpleasant) are associated with these symptoms. However, hyperphagia is a more common symptom of chronic anxiety than loss of appetite. Anorexia is commonly a manifestation of depressed states and may be an early warning signal in the depressed patient. Unpleasant prior life experiences may have conditioned the patient in such a way that he experiences revulsion toward a life situation over which he feels he can exert no control. His response may be to "be sick"—to vomit. Vomiting which is principally on a psychic basis frequently occurs during or shortly after meals. Often it may be unaccompanied by nausea and retching. Vomiting of this variety frequently does not empty the stomach. Following vomiting, the patient may wish to continue to eat and often can do so without immediate recurrence of vomiting.

The ingestion of food for maintenance of adequate nutrition relates to basic needs and requirements for survival. Therefore, it is not surprising that, with subtle or profound psychological disturbances, abnormalities in these primitive attitudes toward food intake and rejection are observed.

Although some patients with severe psychoses may have disturbances of food intake, most such patients do not. The most profound disturbance of impairment of food intake of neuropsychiatric origin has been termed *anorexia nervosa*. This is a state in which there is anorexia and rejection of food of an extraordinary degree.[31] The patient is usually a young woman. The subject may become extremely emaciated. It is not unusual to have patients with anorexia nervosa die of malnutrition. The patient with anorexia nervosa may develop a picture of secondary panhypopituitarism, which has to be distinguished from primary pituitary disease. The secondary hypopituitarism found in these patients may result from nutritional deficiency of amino acid building blocks required for assembly of proteins and polypeptide hormones. Although anorexia is the most conspicuous symptom in patients with anorexia nervosa, their aversion to and revulsion for food may also be manifested by vomiting. Symptoms of anorexia nervosa usually begin before the age of 18 years. The precise basis of the primary psychological disorder associated with the starving state of anorexia nervosa has not been defined.

Vomiting can be induced by the experimental production of hypoxemia of the vomiting center. This fact has been demonstrated in experimental animals in which the carotid arteries have been ligated. Vomiting, which probably reflects oxygen deprivation of the vomiting center, may be seen in association with *severe anemia* of a variety of causes; local or regional *vascular occlusion;* inadequate perfusion of the brain stem, as may be observed acutely following *excessive blood loss;* or in states with *diminished cardiac output.* It has been postulated that the enhanced sensitivity of the vomiting center with the production of vomiting which accompanies *increased intracranial pressure* is a result of impedance of blood flow to the vomiting center, with resultant hypoxia. Inadequate perfusion and oxygenation of the vomiting center with resultant irritability supplies the most likely explanation for the vomiting that often is observed in association with *vascular shock.* Vomiting also may be seen in association with *reductions in environmental oxygen* as in high altitude situations, e.g., mountain climbing or in incompletely pressurized aircraft. It is presumed that vomiting observed with exposure to high altitude, particularly when associated with vigorous oxygen-requiring activity, occurs as a result of relative hypoxemia of the vomiting center.

Increased intracranial pressure often is associated with a "projectile" variety of vomiting. Projectile vomiting associated with increased intracranial pressure commonly is not preceded by nausea, but nausea in some cases may precede the vomiting. Expulsion of the gastric contents is more forceful with projectile vomiting than with other types of vomiting, and may result in hurling gastric contents across the room. Projectile vomiting with increased intracranial pressure may occur with lateral sinus thrombosis, meningitis of any etiology, internal hydrocephalus and various space-occupying intracranial lesions including tumor, hemorrhage, and abscess. One must be cautioned, however, that vomiting in association with increased intracranial pressure is not invariably projectile in nature. At this point it should be emphasized that in addition to the production of vomiting secondary to increased intracranial pressure, certain intracranial tumors may result in a clinical state similar to anorexia nervosa. Tumors involving the hypothalamus, presumably influencing the function of the hypothalamic center(s) participating in the regulation of food intake, have been observed to be associated with anorexia of the severity seen in anorexia nervosa. The clinical syndrome of severe anorexia nervosa has been noted in a child with a tumor in the region of the fourth ventricle.[32] Vomiting is often seen with cerebellar lesions. Some degree of nausea and/or vomiting are very frequent accompaniments of migraine headaches. The mechanism by which vomiting occurs in migraine disorders has not been defined; however, hypoxemia of the vomiting center secondary to vascular changes recognized to occur with migraine has been suggested as the possible mechanism. Nausea and vomiting of this migraine variety may be seen in the absence of headache and with or without abdominal pain. Often the associated visual disturbances afford a clue as to the nature of the vomiting.

Drugs and Toxic Agents. Many chemicals, drugs, and toxic agents possess the capacity to induce nausea and vomiting. Some agents appear to act centrally by stimulation of the medullary chemoreceptor zone, which conveys neural stimulatory impulses to the adjacent vomiting center with the subsequent production of vomiting. Other agents appear to have direct effects on the gastrointestinal organs whereby they induce vomiting. The vomiting center may be stimulated by afferent impulses from the stomach and the small bowel accompanying the vagal nerves.

Mucosal damage of the upper gastrointestinal tract follows ingestion of mercury bichloride, ammonium chloride, copper sulfate, or aminophyllin.[29,33] Ingestion of these compounds commonly is associated with the production of vomiting that probably results from local stimulation of the damaged gastrointestinal organs. It has been concluded that the receptor site for the provocation of emesis observed following oral administration of sodium salicylate is in the upper gut. When copper sulfate is applied to the region of the medullary chemoreceptor zone vomiting can be evoked. Bilateral vagotomy will inhibit the usually observed immediate vomiting seen in dogs in which copper sulfate is placed in the stomach. Vomiting in these vagotomized dogs occurs, but is delayed. The delay in vomiting is interpreted as reflecting the time required for absorption and circulation of copper sulfate until adequate concentration is reached in the medullary chemoreceptor zone to induce nausea of central origin.

Nausea and vomiting are common accompaniments of a variety of febrile infectious diseases. It has been shown experimentally that administration of microgram quantities of staphylococcal enterotoxin and enterobacteriaceal endotoxin induce emesis in cats.[34] The site of action of the staphylococcal enterotoxin in inducing vomiting in the rhesus monkey appears to be located in the abdominal viscera.[35] Sensory responses provoked by stimulation from the staphylococcal toxin in the gastrointestinal tract appear to be transmitted via afferent fibers traveling with the vagus and sympathetic nerves. In rhesus monkeys, following vagotomy and abdominal splanchnicectomy, vomiting is not induced after administration of enterotoxin even in amounts proving lethal to intact animals. The vomiting reflexes in these autonomically denervated monkeys is not suppressed because of a lack of capacity to perform the act of vomiting, since vomiting in response to the emetic agent Veriloid® is maintained in these animals. Vomiting is frequently observed following ingestion of large quantities of alcohol. Gastroscopic examination of such patients frequently shows gastric mucosal hyperemia, and in some instances erosive gastritis. However, in many patients who vomit following the ingestion of alcohol no abnormalities of the gastric mucosa can be visualized. In most instances vomiting following ingestion of alcohol is probably of central origin, since the action of alcohol is similar to other pharmacologically active anesthetic agents, i.e., stimulation of hypothalamic nuclei. A variety of chemical agents including apomorphine, morphine, emetine, histamine, and epinephrine are capable of inducing vomiting when directly applied to the chemoreceptor trigger zone of the hypothalamus. Certain amphetamines and amphetamine derivatives have been widely used to induce anorexia for purposes of weight reduction. These drugs behave as central nervous system stimulants. The mechanisms by which amphetamines reduce appetite is not known. Complete extrinsic denervation of the stomach and intestinal tract does not diminish the effect of amphetamines in reducing appetite.[36]

To date there is no evidence that the vomiting that is seen in association with digitalis glycoside administration is caused by a direct effect on the gastrointestinal tract. In experimental animals digitalis does induce vomiting when applied to the medullary chemoreceptor trigger zone.

INTRA-ABDOMINAL DISORDERS

A wide spectrum of intra-abdominal disorders, a generous portion of which reflect abnormalities of the gastrointestinal tract, may be manifested by anorexia, nausea, and vomiting. The varieties of intra-abdominal abnormalities which may be associated with nausea and vomiting are so numerous that they defy meaningful and worthwhile tabulation and categorization. However, certain intra-abdominal conditions that produce vomiting, as well as certain generalizations regarding abdominal causes of vomiting, merit discussion.

Mechanical Obstruction of the Gastrointestinal Tract. Nausea and vomiting brought to the attention of the physician frequently and appropriately provoke the immediate suspicion that these symptoms may reflect mechanical obstruction of the normal passage of the contents of the gastrointestinal tract. Mechanical obstruction is a relatively uncommon cause of vomiting; however, anorexia, nausea, and vomiting are prominent symptoms of gastrointestinal tract obstruction and may be seen with obstruction at virtually any level. Vomiting found with mechanical obstruction of the gastrointestinal tract is the result of distention of the lumen.[37] This distention activates mechanoreceptors in the gastric and

bowel walls which evoke vomiting through viscerovisceral reflexes and/or activation of the medullary vomiting center via the neural pathways already outlined. Vomiting in association with gastrointestinal visceral distention that is not the result of mechanical obstruction, e.g., paralytic ileus, is believed to be produced by these same mechanisms.

Vomiting with gastrointestinal tract obstruction is seen most commonly when the obstruction is high. Pyloric obstruction, whether associated with congenital hypertrophic pyloric stenosis, pyloric stenosis in the adult, peptic ulcer disease, or tumor, constitutes the major gastric site of obstruction resulting in nausea and vomiting. The nausea and vomiting due to obstruction at the level of the pylorus commonly are observed shortly following eating, and the severity of vomiting often correlates with the acuteness of development and degree of obstruction. With pyloric obstruction, the vomited material often contains undigested food. Bile may be present in the vomitus of patients with pyloric obstruction, even though the ampulla of Vater is distal to the obstructive site. The presence of bile in vomited material from patients with pyloric obstruction reflects incompleteness of the obstruction with regurgitation of intestinal contents. For example, both peptic ulcer disease and tumor may involve the region of the pylorus, producing both relative obstruction and incompetency of the pyloric sphincteric mechanism.

With long-standing pyloric obstruction dilation of the stomach may develop, gradually creating an enormous fluid reservoir; when vomiting occurs it may be of extraordinarily large volumes of material. Associated or preceding symptoms often may supply clues as to the disease responsible for the pyloric obstruction. Examples would be the history of relief of epigastric pain with eating in patients with peptic ulcer disease, or excessive fullness following ingestion of meals of a size previously readily accommodated by the patient who has carcinoma of the stomach.

Intestinal obstruction at virtually all levels, particularly in the upper small intestine, may be associated with vomiting. Fecal vomiting, especially when protracted, is particularly characteristic of obstruction at the intestinal level. Intestinal obstruction may be caused by a large number of abnormalities, including among others tumor, volvulus, intussusception, adhesion, foreign bodies, inflammatory disease, and vascular insufficiency. As in pyloric obstruction, severity of the vomiting due to intestinal obstruction often correlates with the degree of completeness of the obstruction. Acute obstruction more commonly results in vomiting than does chronic incomplete obstruction. Anorexia, nausea, and vomiting are extremely common symptoms with paralytic ileus in which there are dilated nonmotile regions of bowel in the absence of mechanical impedance of the flow of gut contents. Thus, these symptoms do not assist in the differentiation of dilated loops of bowel in either paralytic ileus or mechanical intestinal obstruction. Splanchnic sympathectomy will eliminate vomiting with an intestinal obstruction; however, section of the vagus is required to eliminate the associated anorexia.

Intra-Abdominal Inflammatory Disorders. Inflammatory involvement of virtually any abdominal or pelvic organ may be associated with production of anorexia, nausea, and vomiting. Vomiting in these instances is a result of stimulation of visceral afferent pathways. Stimuli are conducted from the involved organ through the vagi and splanchnic afferent trunks to the vomiting center in the medulla. Their synaptic connections are made with efferent vagal splanchnic and spinal nerves to the pharynx, esophagus, the cardioesophageal junction, the stomach, muscles of the abdominal wall, and the diaphragm. Inflammation with irritation of the visceral peritoneum[38] results in vomiting in the same manner.

Anorexia, nausea, and vomiting are particularly common accompaniments of *acute appendicitis*. Anorexia is usually the initial symptom experienced by patients with acute appendicitis and occurs almost invariably. In acute appendicitis anorexia may be overshadowed later in the course of the symptoms of the attack by acute and sometimes severe abdominal pain.

Vomiting is seen in some patients with viral hepatitis, but this is not the rule. On the other hand, a profound degree of *anorexia*, which usually precedes more overt clinical manifestations, is almost invariably found in patients with *viral hepatitis*. Disappearance of anorexia in patients with viral hepatitis may correlate with morphologic and biochemical evidence of hepatic improvement.

Nausea and vomiting are often found with urinary tract infections, especially when associated with urinary tract obstruction such as is seen with ureteral colic due to impaction of a stone. Obstruction of the ureter may be heralded by severe nausea and vomiting even in the absence of typical colicky pain of the variety usually associated with obstruction of the ureter.

Vomiting is frequent in patients with acute pancreatitis. Vomiting with pancreatitis often may occur in the absence of severe abdominal pain. One must be alert to the possibility that the vomiting in pancreatitis reflects a condition associated with the pancreatitis, and in certain instances may not necessarily be due to the pancreatitis itself. The following are given as examples: the vomiting may reflect biliary tract disease, which so frequently accompanies pancreatitis; hyperparathyroidism with hypercalcemia may be the principal cause of vomiting in certain patients with pancreatitis; peptic ulcer disease, sometimes with penetration of the pancreas and resultant pancreatitis, may result in vomiting.

It must be borne in mind that vascular insufficiency and occlusion of the arterial and venous splanchnic and mesenteric circulation, as well as inferior vena-caval obstruction, may produce anorexia, nausea, and vomiting. In addition, cicatricial stenosis of limited regions of the intestines following episodes of acute vascular insufficiency may produce intestinal obstruction, accompanied by these symptoms.

Nausea and Vomiting of Pregnancy. Nausea is frequently observed in women during the course of pregnancy,[39] and in some pregnant women vomiting may result which may be extremely severe and disabling. The mechanism producing nausea and vomiting in pregnant women in the absence of other demonstrable disease associated with these symptoms is not known. A variety of chemical alterations found in pregnancy have been suspected, but none has been demonstrated to be of importance in the pathophysiology of vomiting. Psychic influences appear to play a part in producing nausea and vomiting in some pregnant women, but whether psychologic factors constitute the entire explanation for this variety of vomiting is not known. Nausea and vomiting are produced in about 10 per cent of women receiving certain oral contraceptives containing norethynodrel.[40] These agents, by their metabolic effects, simulate pregnancy. The intensity, the incidence, and the variability of symptoms among nonpregnant women receiving these agents are similar to those observed in women who are actually pregnant. It is conceivable that steroid hormones elaborated and released during pregnancy may be responsible for the observed nausea and vomiting in a similar manner.

OTHER FACTORS

Nausea and vomiting are common accompaniments of a variety of generalized and systemic disorders. They are particularly common symptoms in children, especially during the course of *febrile illnesses*. There is not a good temporal correlation between the occurrence of fever and vomiting, nor can nausea and vomiting be induced experimentally by production of levels of pyrexia comparable to those observed in certain febrile illnesses. It is conceivable that chemical agents are elaborated and released into the peripheral circulation in association with certain illnesses in which fever is observed, and that these toxic substances, as yet undefined in nature, may induce vomiting by stimulation of the medullary chemoreceptor zone or by action at peripheral sites. Nausea and vomiting commonly occur in patients with *uremia*, as well as in patients with *diabetic ketoacidosis*. The agent or agents responsible for the production of nausea and vomiting in patients with uremia has not been defined, but it appears that it is not urea. However, in uremic patients, anorexia, nausea, and vomiting commonly disappear when effective hemodialysis corrects the grossly disordered biochemical state. Nausea and vomiting associated with diabetic ketoacidosis usually are relieved after the correction of ketoacidosis.

Endocrine Disorders. Anorexia, nausea, and vomiting are common afflictions of patients suffering from Addison's disease. When anorexia, nausea, and vomiting occur in Addison's disease, there are often profound changes in electrolyte levels, with evidence of metabolic alkalosis, hyperkalemia, and elevation of blood urea nitrogen levels. Nausea and vomiting in patients with Addison's disease usually disappear after replacement therapy with required adrenocorticoids.

Hyperparathyroidism may be signaled by profound anorexia, nausea, and vomiting. In many such patients, vomiting is accompanied by abdominal pain, which is often cramping in nature but may be constant. In some patients whose hyperparathyroidism is manifested by anorexia, nausea, and vomiting, abdominal pain is absent. The abdominal distress in certain patients with hyperparathyroidism may be very vague and difficult to distinguish from the nausea that commonly accompanies it. Vomiting is frequently seen in association with hyperthyroidism, particularly in patients in hyperthyroid crisis. It has been postulated that vomiting of patients with hyperthyroidism is a manifestation of the central nervous system irritability, which characterizes hyperthyroidism, and reflects reduction of the threshold of excitation of the medullary vomiting center.

Cardiac Disease. Vomiting with or without abdominal pain is not unusual with actue myocardial infarction. It may occur in association with or distinct from chest and arm pain characteristic of myocardial infarction. Vomiting that is presumed to be secondary to congestion of abdominal viscera may accompany severe congestive heart failure, particularly when it is relatively acute in its development. Other factors may contribute to or be responsible for the vomiting seen in patients with heart disease. These include the administration of drugs that are known to be capable of inducing vomiting, such as digitalis or aminophylline. Severe fluid and electrolyte disturbances, such as may result from too-vigorous use of diuretic agents in patients with heart disease, also may provoke anorexia, nausea, and vomiting.

Malnutrition. Extended periods of fasting or starvation result in anorexia. In certain patients, this effect may be due to the anorexigenic effects of the ketosis that develops secondary to utilization of lipid stores as caloric sources. Protracted periods of malnutrition are associated with multiple deficiencies of nutrients including vitamins, minerals, and sources of calories. It has been shown clearly that anorexia may be produced by administration of a diet deficient in thiamine.[41] It is probable that additional factors, which are in deficient supply to individuals with severe general malnutrition, also contribute to the anorexia so commonly observed.

Motion Sickness. Anorexia, nausea, and vomiting may be the most prominent manifestations of the clinical entity referred to as motion sickness. This distressing constellation of symptoms occurs in susceptible persons during or following transportation by a variety of moving vehicles including trains, planes, ships, cars, etc. As the symptoms develop, the affected individuals become initially anorectic, and then experience profound apathy, salivation, and sweating. These symptoms proceed to their culmination in nausea and vomiting. Similar symptoms can be produced by caloric stimulation of the otic labyrinth. Other factors in addition to labyrinthine stimulation appear to play a part in the production of motion sickness including psychic, tactile, visual, and proprioceptive impulses.

Meniere's Disease. Meniere's disease is a disorder in which there is distention of the membranous labyrinth with degeneration of the organ of Corti. These patients experience genuine vertigo, accompanied by tinnitus and deafness. During or following these acute episodes, nausea and vomiting may be prominent symptoms. Identification of Meniere's disease as the cause of vomiting in such patients usually can be obtained by recognition of the associated symptoms reflecting labyrinthine stimulation, as well as by the acute recurrent nature of the symptoms.

REFERENCES

1. Mitchell, G. A. G.: Anatomy of the Autonomic Nervous System, Edinburgh, E. and S. Livingston, Ltd., 1953.
2. Norberg, K. A.: Adrenergic innervation of the intestinal wall studied by fluorescence microscopy, Int. J. Neuropharmacol. 3:379–382, 1964.
3. Jacobowitz, D.: Histochemical studies of the autonomic innervation of the gut, J. Pharmacol. Exp. Ther. 149:358–364, 1965.
4. Ahlquist, R. P.: A study of the adrenotropic receptors, Amer. J. Physiol. 153:586–600, 1948.
5. Levy, B., and Ahlquist, R. P.: An analysis of adrenergic blocking activity, J. Pharmacol. Exp. Ther. 133:202–210, 1961.
6. Bailey, D. M.: The action of sympathomimetic amines on circular and longitudinal smooth muscle from the isolated esophagus of the guinea-pig, J. Pharm. Pharmacol. 17:782–787, 1965.
7. Crema, A., Benzi, G., Frigi, G. M., and Berte, F.: Occurrence of alpha and beta receptors in the bile duct, Proc. Soc. Exp. Biol. Med. 120:158–160, 1965.
8. Reynolds, D. G., Demaree, G. E., and Heiffer, M. H.: An excitatory adrenergic alpha-receptor mechanism of the terminal guinea pig ileum, Proc. Soc. Exp. Biol. Med. 125:73–78, 1967.
9. Thomas, J. E.: Recent advances in gastrointestinal physiology, Gastroenterology 12:545–560, 1949.
10. Gregory, R. A., and Tracy, H. J.: The constitution and properties of two gastrins extracted from hog antral mucosa. I. The isolation of two gastrins from hog antral mucosa. II. The properties of two gastrins isolated from hog antral mucosa, Gut 5:103–114, 1964.
11. Vagne, M., Stening, G. F., Brooks, F. P., and Grossman, M. I.: Synthetic secretin: Comparison with natural secretin for potency and spectrum of physiological actions, Gastroenterology 55:260–267, 1968.
12. Cannon, W. B., and Washburn, A. L.: An explanation of hunger, Amer. J. Physiol. 29:441–454, 1912.
13. Mayer J.: Genetic, traumatic and environmental factors in the etiology of obesity, Physiol. Rev. 33:472–508, 1953.
14. Grossman, M. I., Cummins, G. M., and Ivy, A. C.: The effect of insulin on food intake after vagotomy and sympathectomy, Amer. J. Physiol. 149:100–106, 1947.
15. Magee, D. F.: Gastro-intestinal Physiology, p. 194, Springfield, Ill., Charles C Thomas, 1962.
16. Janowitz, H. D., and Grossman, M. I.: Some factors affecting the food intake of normal dogs and dogs with esophagostomy and gastric fistula, Amer. J. Physiol. 159:143–148, 1949.
17. ———: Effect of prefeeding, alcohol and bitters on food intake of dogs, Amer. J. Physiol. 164:182–186, 1951.
18. Iggo, A.: Gastrointestinal tension receptors with unmyelinated afferent fibers in the vagus of the cat, Quart. J. Exp. Physiol. 42:130–143, 1957.
19. ———: Tension receptors in the stomach and the urinary bladder, J. Physiol. 128:593–607, 1955.
20. Paintal, A. S.: Responses from mucosal mechanoreceptors in the small intestine of the cat, J. Physiol. 139:353–368, 1957.
21. ———: A study of gastric stretch receptors: their role in the peripheral mechanism of satiation of hunger and thirst, J. Physiol. 126:255–270, 1954.
22. Chernigovsky, V. N.: The significance of interoceptive signals in the food behavior of animals, in Conference on Brain and Behavior, 2d, Los Angeles, 1962. Brain and Behavior. II. The Internal Environment and Alimentary Behavior, pp. 319–348, Washington, American Institute of Biological Sciences, 1962.
23. Sharma, K. N.: Alimentary receptors and food intake regulation, in Kare, M. R., and Maller, O. (eds.): The Chemical Senses and Nutrition, p. 286, Baltimore, Johns Hopkins Press, 1967.
24. Iggo, A.: Gastric mucosal chemoreceptors with vagal afferent fibers in the cat, Quart. J. Exp. Physiol. 42:398–409, 1957.
25. Sharma, K. N., and Nasset, E. S.: Electrical activity in mesenteric nerves after perfusion of gut lumen, Amer. J. Physiol. 202:725–730, 1962.
26. Magee, D. F.: Gastro-intestinal Physiology, p. 195, Springfield, Ill., Charles C Thomas, 1962.
27. Wolf, S., and Wolff, H. G.: Human Gastric Function, p. 111, London, Oxford, 1947.
28. Grossman, M. I., Woolley, J. R., Dutton, D. F., and Ivy, A. C.: The effect of nausea on gastric

secretion and a study of the mechanism concerned, Gastroenterology 4: 347–351, 1945.

29. Borison, H. L., and Wang, S. C.: Physiology and pharmacology of vomiting, Pharmacol. Rev. 5: 193–230, 1953.

30. Gregory, R. A.: Changes in intestinal tone and motility associated with nausea and vomiting, J. Physiol. 105: 58–65, 1946.

31. Bruch, H.: Anorexia nervosa and its differential diagnosis, J. Nerv. Ment. Dis. 141: 555–566, 1965.

32. Udvarhelyi, G. B., Adamkiewicz, Jr., J. J., and Cooke, R. E., "Anorexia nervosa" caused by a fourth ventricle tumor, Neurology 16: 565–568, 1966.

33. Wolf, S.: Studies on nausea. Effects of ipecac and other emetics on the human stomach and duodenum, Gastroenterology 12: 212–218, 1949.

34. Martin, W. J., and Marcus, S.: Relation of pyrogenic and emetic properties of enterobacteriaceal endotoxin and of staphylococcal enterotoxin, J. Bact. 87: 1019–1026, 1964.

35. Sugiyama, H., and Hayama, T.: Abdominal viscera as site of emetic action for staphylococcal enterotoxin in the monkey, J. Infect. Dis. 115: 330–336, 1965.

36. Harris, S. C., Ivy, A. C., and Searle, L. M.: The mechanism of amphetamine-induced loss of weight, J.A.M.A. 134: 1468–1475, 1947.

37. Herrin, R. C., and Meek, W. J.: Afferent nerves excited by intestinal distension, Amer. J. Physiol. 144: 720–723, 1945.

38. Walton, F. E., Moore, R. M., and Graham, E. A.: The nerve pathways in the vomiting of peritonitis, Arch. Surg. 22: 829–837, 1931.

39. Hall, M. B.: Nausea and vomiting of pregnancy, Amer. J. Med. Sci. 205: 869–875, 1943.

40. Bakker, C. B., and Dightman, C. R.: Side effects of oral contraceptives, Obstet. Gynec. 28: 373–379, 1966.

41. Williams, R. D., Mason, H. L., Wilder, R. M., and Smith, B. F.: Observations on induced thiamin deficiency in man, Arch. Intern. Med. 66: 785–789, 1940.

22

Constipation and Diarrhea

MALCOLM L. PETERSON

When a patient describes a change in bowel habit the physician must try to determine the specific pathophysiology involved in the disturbance of intestinal absorption and motility. Diagnosis is facilitated by the development of such information. Rational therapy is possible only if the doctor has a sound understanding of the factors that regulate intestinal transit.

To avoid a pitfall of history-taking, the physician should ask for a specific description of bowel habit and stool characteristic rather than phrase the question in terms of "normal." (*Constipation* to one may simply be *less diarrhea* to another.) In most American and European populations, the usual bowel habit is passage once daily of a plastic, intact fecal mass measuring 150 to 300 gm. (about the shape of a thin, medium-sized potato or often in the form of one to several segments shaped like small bananas). Normally the stool, although appearing to be a soft solid, contains about 70 per cent water. Form, color, odor, and consistency are subject to some variation resulting from dietary and bacterial influences, but the familiar olive drab stool is usually only slightly odoriferous and remains intact in the toilet bowl. Significant and sustained variation from this pattern is worthy of medical attention.

It is important at the outset of this discussion to define in what sense the terms constipation and diarrhea will be used, since the patient's statements of these complaints often cannot be taken at face value. This is particularly true with regard to constipation, because individuals vary widely in their concept of what constitutes normal bowel action. Does the patient mean that he does not have a bowel action every day; that the stool is too hard, or too small; or that he never has a feeling of complete evacuation? The details may reveal that he needs reassurance rather than a laxative. Before attempting a precise definition, therefore, it is necessary to discuss the normal physiology concerned with the formation of feces.

NORMAL PHYSIOLOGY OF FOOD AND RESIDUE PROPULSION

RATE OF TRANSIT

Within a few minutes after food enters the stomach, some of it passes into the duodenum. The rate of gastric emptying depends upon a number of factors, among them the quantity and the quality of the food, the emotional state of the individual, his nutritional status, and the time interval since the previous food intake. On the average, after an ordinary mixed meal, the stomach is empty in 3 to 4 hours. With a meal containing much fat there may be a delay of 6 hours or more.

In the small intestine, the rate of passage of chyme is relatively rapid in the duodenum and jejunum, slowing considerably in the ileum, particularly in the distal 12 to 14 inches. The residue of a mixed meal will begin to pass through the ileocolic sphincter in from 2 to 3 hours after it is consumed and will have completed its passage into the cecum in from 6 to 9 hours. A great deal of the water content is absorbed, including the fluid derived from mucus, but the consistency of the contents of the distal small gut is still semiliquid.

Transit of the colon involves a more variable period between different persons, and in the same person under diverse conditions. From cecum to sigmoid, the transit time is normally several hours to 24 to 48 hours. In diarrhea the time may be minutes, in constipation it may be days.

Even when there is little or no fluid ingested, there is a large volume of fluid secreted into the gastrointestinal tract. The various types of secretion and their production in quite large quantities are essential to normal distal propulsion of gastrointestinal contents and to physiologic digestion and absorption. The sources and volumes in an average adult are approximately:

Saliva	1,500 ml.
Gastric secretions	2,500
Bile	500
Pancreatic juice	700
Total digestive secretions	5,200 ml.

Absorption of all but about 500 ml. of this fluid, plus ingested water, is complete in the small bowel. Another 200 to 350 ml. of water is absorbed in the colon.

NERVE CONTROL

Under normal conditions the vagus, the splanchnic and the pelvic nerves may play a significant role in transmitting impulses between the central nervous system and the viscera. These connections are shown in Plate 3. The parasympathetic efferent supply of the small bowel and the proximal third of the colon are supplied via the vagus and that of the remainder of the colon via the lower sacral segments of the spinal cord, through the pelvic nerves. The splanchnic nerves supply the sympathetic innervation. The afferent autonomic nerve distribution is also through the vagus, the splanchnic, and the pelvic nerves (see Plate 3).

Of the several types of muscular activity encountered in the small intestine, the segmenting and pendular movements (movements of mixing and churning) are inherent in the muscle itself. The peristaltic contractions are accomplished through local myenteric reflexes,[1] but it is usually considered that they may be augmented by vagus and pelvic efferent impulses and inhibited by splanchnic efferent impulses. Augmentation and inhibition effects are likewise exerted by these nerves on the tone of the intestine. The sympathetic fibers are believed to exert a continuous inhibitory effect, whereas the vagal impulses are intermittent.

Similarly, in the colon, the chief effect of sympathetic activity is inhibition, although this may not be apparent in postsympathectomy patients except under conditions of stress. Hence the tone and the peristaltic activity of the small bowel and colon may be profoundly affected by impulses received through their extrinsic nerves—impulses that may originate in the higher nerve centers or in the cord as part of a reflex arc.

NEUROHORMONAL CONTROL

The influence of the nervous system cannot be understood without consideration of the substances that are released when these nerves are stimulated. *Acetylcholine*, produced at the terminals of the parasympathetic postganglionic fibers, increases tone and activity of the intestine. It is also the mediator in transmission of all preganglionic and some sympathetic postganglionic impulses.[2] Most sympathetic postganglionic nerves release *norepinephrine* (and perhaps epinephrine) and therefore are termed "adrenergic." Much recent work suggests that *serotonin* (5-hydroxytryptamine), found in large quantities in the intestinal tract, alters intestinal motility in the direction of increased activity. The release of serotonin probably is not controlled by extrinsic nerves,[3] since its site of action is distal to the ganglionic synapse. Its release may possibly be controlled by neural elements within the intestinal wall.[4] At present the available evidence indicates that serotonin helps to regulate peristaltic activity by mediating pressure reception in the mucosa. Other chemicals may be important in normal intestinal motor function—certainly *potassium* plays a role in the functioning of nerve and muscle cells within the gut wall.

DEFINITIONS

Constipation may be considered as simply undue delay in the evacuation of feces. This usually results in the passage of hard dry stools, or no stool at all for an inordinate number of days. The evacuation of hard stools is accomplished only with some difficulty involving excessive use of the voluntary muscles. The definition here given does not imply that there need normally be a bowel movement every 24 hours. There are healthy persons who pass a well-formed stool of normal consistency once every two or even three or more days. They are not constipated. The definition does not imply that the constipated stool is small, although it may be if it contains less water and fiber. Neither does it imply that there need be a feeling of gratification, of complete evacuation, after defecation, although this normally occurs. A feeling of incomplete evacuation may be due to local conditions in the rectum or, more frequently, to psychic factors.

Diarrhea, as the opposite of constipation, means undue rapidity in the passage of the feces, with resultant discharge of loose stools. It may, or may not, be accompanied by abdominal cramping or tenesmus. The number of stools does not enter into the definition of diarrhea, although commonly the frequency of the bowel movements is increased.

In regard to both of these definitions it has been suggested that the disorder must be habitual before it can be considered either constipation or diarrhea. This technicality can be disposed of if the modifying adjectives, acute and chronic, are used.

Dysentery is a term misused by many persons to describe any severe diarrhea. The term should be restricted to inflammations of the intestine characterized by severe diarrhea with frequent passage of mucus and blood and accompanied by systemic disturbances, such as fever, etc. The most common forms are bacillary dysentery and amebic dysentery.

CAUSES OF CONSTIPATION

The volume of laxatives and "natural regulators" sold in the United States would suggest that constipation tends to be a national preoccupation. The reported symptom, undue delay in fecal evacuation, demands careful individual study by the physician before he can accept the complaint as significant.

TABLE 22-1. CAUSES OF CONSTIPATION

Neurogenic

  Cortical, voluntary or involuntary delay of evacuation
  Central nervous system lesions
    Multiple sclerosis
    Cord tumors
    Tabes dorsalis
    Traumatic spinal cord lesions
  Postganglionic disorders
    Hirschsprung's disease (congenital megacolon)
    Opiate effect
    Anticholinergic drugs

Muscular

  Atony
    (1) Laxative abuse
    (2) Severe malnutrition
  Metabolic defects
    (1) Hypothyroidism
    (2) Hypercalcemia
    (3) Potassium depletion
    (4) Porphyria
    (5) Hyperparathyroidism

Mechanical

  Bowel obstruction
    Neoplasm
    Volvulus
    Diverticulitis
  Extra-alimentary tumors, including pregnancy
  Rectal lesions
    Lymphogranuloma venereum
    Thrombosed hemorrhoids
    Fissure-in-ano
    Perirectal abscess

Many persons without disease have only one stool every two to three days, but in others *a change* in bowel habit from one stool daily to such a schedule can be a very important clue to disease. The normal stimuli to evacuate the sigmoid colon initiate such basic reflexes that relatively few factors can appreciably postpone fecal elimination.

Causes of constipation can be neurogenic, muscular, or mechanical. As with any physiologic classification based on imperfect knowledge, some overlapping will occur, and an etiologic factor, if completely elucidated, might account for disturbances under several of these functional headings. In Table 22-1, etiologies are classified under the pathophysiologic processes believed to be primarily operative.

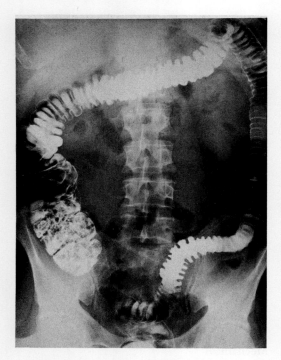

FIG. 22-1. Often this type of hypertonic or "spastic" colon is associated with constipation, due to failure of normal transit in the descending colon.

NEUROGENIC BASIS

Central Constipation

Voluntary Retention. Certainly the most common cause of delayed evacuation is voluntary restriction of defecation. When stool enters the rectum in sufficient quantity to stimulate the pressure receptors, the patient is aware of the need to defecate but is able to overcome the need by voluntary contraction of the external sphincter and associated muscles. The rectum then adjusts itself to the increased tension and ceases to send out afferent impulses, or the rectum may actually return stool into the sigmoid. If this is done habitually, the reflex ceases to function.

The signal in most normal persons occurs shortly after the first meal of the day and is initiated by the *gastrocolic reflex*. Students, office employees, factory workers, and others who must leave home soon after breakfast often learn to disregard signals to move the bowels. The signal may be repeated, perhaps after a midmorning coffee break, and again perhaps after lunch. If repeatedly *consciously* disregarded, the impulse to evacuate

may become *unconsciously* blocked. The affected person, not understanding the origin of his problem, often considers himself to be constipated and becomes involved in the laxative habit, which leads to further constipation.

Remarkable conscious or unconscious disregard of the impulse to defecate is possible. Everyone uses this control occasionally; infrequent inhibition of the impulse is not harmful. Combat troops and travelers find control of the urge essential. Facility for conditioning of the reflex has been built into the training of some of the Soviet cosmonauts. Children often develop constipation in deliberate efforts to manipulate their parents.

Excessive Tone. Another large group of constipated persons suffers from excessive tone of the circular muscle of the intestines, particularly of the distal colon, induced by an imbalance of the autonomic nervous system. Experimentally, markedly increased contraction of the colon has been observed with a wide variety of stressful situations, such as exposure to cold, pain, compression of the head, and discussion of troublesome life situations.[5] Further, patients with *spastic colons* overreact to prostigmine. Since it is well-known that excessive tone (spasm) interferes with the propulsive motility, it is easy to understand why these patients have difficulty with constipation, and why the stool produced is usually small in character and segmented. This is a central type of constipation, since it must be presumed that cortical and subcortical impulses travel to parasympathetic centers, with resultant activation of sacral, and possibly vagal, fibers supplying the colon (Fig. 22-1).

Psychogenic. Constipation may result from certain types of acute emotional disturbances (grief, anger, abject fear), which cause increased epinephrine production with inhibition of peristalsis.[6] Paranoid psychoses often are accompanied by constipation.

Spinal Cord Lesions

Traumatic lesions and organic diseases of the nervous system, such as tabes dorsalis, multiple sclerosis, brain and cord tumors, meningitis, and the like, may produce constipation. Stimuli from the higher nerve centers may influence bowel activity directly. Such influences are evident from both clinical and experimental studies. Cord involvement is, however, more likely to upset gastrointestinal motility than are diseases of the brain, possibly because the effect may be on only one set of autonomic nerves, leaving the "opposing" set in control. For example, tabes dorsalis may activate parasympathetic nerve fibers and produce severe hypertonus, which interferes with peristaltic activity. Traumatic lesions may destroy efferent nerves concerned with the defecation reflex. When the spinal cord is unable to recognize the presence of stool in the rectum there is no stimulus to start the reflex. At the higher level, again, many patients with strokes are unable to recognize the pressure produced by rectal stool accumulation. These patients are usually constipated at first, and are then likely to have involuntary liquid stools as the spinal cord takes over the reflex.

Postganglionic Disorders

Megacolon. In Hirschsprung's disease, regions of the bowel, usually in the colon, are congenitally without myenteric or submucosal plexuses.[7] Blockage occurs because peristalsis cannot pass through this section. Further, this segment is narrowed because the smooth muscle contracts when separated from the nearest ganglion cell.

The functional blockade is overcome only by forceful propulsion from above the affected segment, and there may be long intervals between defecations. Evacuation often requires enemas. Diagnosis demands careful assessment of history, proctoscopic findings, barium enema, and bowel wall biopsy.

The aganglionic segment may be located just inside the anal margin only or may extend upward into the rectum, or even into the sigmoid. Portions of small intestine have in some instances been shown to lack myenteric ganglion cells.

Typically the condition involves the rectum and is observed in infants with severe constipation and huge abdomens. The narrow, usually empty rectum connects by a short conical portion with a greatly dilated descending colon. Rarely, the transverse colon also is dilated. The distended bowel segments have normal myenteric ganglia, normal propulsive activity, and hypertrophic muscular coats; they usually are filled with puttylike feces.

Removal of the congenitally aganglionic segment can accomplish cure.

Acquired megacolon sometimes occurs as a late complication of Chagas' disease (South American trypanosomiasis). Tissue reaction to the parasite destroys the ganglia.

Drugs. A few drugs, given orally or parenterally, delay the passage of intestinal contents. Opiates and meperidine compounds are notorious constipating agents. Addicts usually are constipated while using these drugs.

Morphine and, to a lesser extent, *codeine*, increase the tone of the small intestine and the colon, decreasing propulsive motility. In the small intestine this is followed by atony in about 1 hour. The colon becomes atonic in 3 or 4 hours. Efforts to block the effect of morphine by various means have shown that its spasmogenic action is mediated through postganglionic fibers of the extrinsic intestinal nerves, but whether by stimulation of the cholinergic fibers or by blocking the adrenergic inhibitory supply is not known. The latter is suggested by in vitro experiments.[8]

Anticholinergic drugs, usually only in doses that already have produced other atropine-like effects, can produce constipation. In peptic ulcer patients, constipation often results from side effects of the common therapy with anticholinergic drugs and aluminum-containing antacids. The latter also tend to have a constipating action, via an unknown mechanism.

Atropine decreases motility by functionally paralyzing parasympathetic nerves. So do the synthetic parasympathetic drugs, such as tricyclamol,[9] propantheline, etc. Tetraethylammonium chloride, which paralyzes both parasympathetic and sympathetic nerves, produces almost complete inertness of the bowel, as does dibutoline, which, like atropine, is parasympatholytic, but also has a direct inhibitory action on smooth muscle.

MUSCULAR BASIS

The bowel may be unable to move the stool distally in the usual length of time because of weakness of the bowel muscles or weakness of the voluntary muscles of defecation. In these situations, there may be no abnormal reflex activity nor any disturbing impulses directly from the central nervous system.

Muscular Atony from Laxative Abuse. Perhaps the most vexing type of constipation to manage is the end-stage of laxative abuse. This problem results from muscular atony. Patients, many of whom are started on this road by well-intentioned physicians, take increasing amounts and varied types of laxatives, until even various potent plant extracts are less and less effective. The subject may be sent to a specialist and often is referred with the diagnosis of Hirschsprung's disease. Patient and physician are frustrated by the

TABLE 22-2. CAUSES OF DIARRHEA

Malabsorption	**Neuromuscular**
Malabsorption of fats	*Autonomic system imbalance*
Maldigestion secondary to lipase insufficiency	Postvagotomy
Pancreatitis	Diabetic enteropathy
Carcinoma of the pancreas	Irritable colon syndrome*
Mucoviscidosis	Narcotic withdrawal*
Kwashiorkor	*Hormonal and pharmacologic influence*
Zollinger-Ellison syndrome	Serotonin (chromaffin tumors)
Maldigestion secondary to bile salt deficiency	Thyroxin (thyrotoxicosis)
Resection or disease of distal ileum	Gastrin (Zollinger-Ellison tumor)
(depletion)	Histamine (mastocytosis)
Regional enteritis	Pholine iodide
Ileectomy for tumors or inflammatory	
disease	**Mechanical**
Bacterial growth (deconjugation)	*Incomplete obstruction*
Postgastrectomy afferent loop syndrome	Neoplasm
Jejunal diverticulosis	Adhesions
Malassimilation secondary to defective paths	Stenosis
of absorption	*Fecal impaction*
Acanthocytosis	*Muscular incompetency*
Celiac disease	Scleroderma
Intestinal lymphangiectasia	
Whipple's disease	**Inflammatory Basis and Direct Irritants**
	Infections
Malabsorption of carbohydrates	Parasites
Primary lactase deficiency	Giardia lamblia
Primary sucrase deficiency	Endameba histolytica
Secondary disaccharidase deficiencies	Helminths
Defective glucose transport system	Bacterial
	Salmonella
Malabsorption of water	Shigella
Interference with absorption	Staphylococcus
Mucosal cell damage	Tuberculosis
X-ray	Viral
Metallic poisons	*Nonspecific*
Gluten	Jejunitis (tropical sprue)
Colchicine*	Regional enteritis
Mesenteric vascular occlusion*	Ulcerative colitis
Osmotic effects of nonabsorbable solutes	Postantibiotic proctitis
and ions (mannitol, Mg++, etc.)	"Turista"*
	Amyloidosis
Excessive secretion	Diverticulitis
Cholera	*Cathartics: cascara, senna, etc.*
Villous adenoma	*Poisons: mercury, arsenic, etc.*
Bile acid toxicity in colon	

* Assignment of this diagnosis to the indicated category is based upon incomplete evidence or crass speculation.

necessarily protracted therapeutic program to solve a problem that was years in development. Success is usually possible by making clear to the patient the cause of the trouble and by use of stepwise reduction of daily doses of senna alkaloids over many weeks or months.

Weakness of the voluntary muscles occurs with cachexia, obesity, emphysema, pregnancy, and ascites. Because of the important role of the abdominal, the pelvic, and the diaphragmatic muscles in initiating and completing defecation in man, diseases affecting the strength of these muscles obviously will make evacuation difficult. This is seen most conspicuously in the stretching and thinning of muscle tissue associated with severe rectocele. An additional mechanical factor here involved is the angulation of the ampulla, causing the propulsive force to be directed against the perineum rather than toward the anus.

MECHANICAL BASIS

An abnormal physical state of the bowel content or actual physical obstruction of various degrees may retard propulsion.

Obstruction of Lumen. Actual physical,

anatomic, or mechanical narrowing of the lumen of the colon which develops slowly may cause *obstipation* (severe refractory constipation). This may result from constricting neoplasms, inflammatory lesions, etc., especially lymphogranuloma venereum. Two types of pathophysiologic process are involved: (1) actual physical blockade, and (2) reflex inhibition of the gut above the lesion.

Occasionally painful rectal conditions (hemorrhoids, fissures, abscesses, etc.) can cause excessive sphincter tone, resultant failure to evacuate, and consequent constipation. An additional factor, understandably enough, is apt also to be operative: voluntary failure to defecate so as to avoid extreme pain.

Mechanical obstruction, of such a degree that even strong intestinal and abdominal muscles cannot force the intestinal content through it, usually is acute. A gradually developing stenosis is more likely to produce constipation through inhibition of reflexes. Common causes of acute obstruction are strangulated hernia, intussusception, and volvulus.

Large extra-alimentary tumors, e.g. fibroids, ovarian cysts, pregnancy, etc., are associated with constipation, but this effect may be more a consequence of loss of mechanical advantage of voluntary muscles than any direct influence on the gut itself.

CAUSES OF DIARRHEA

By definition, any factor that hastens evacuation of the feces may be a cause of diarrhea. However, hypermotility in the small bowel and the proximal colon can be compensated for by slightly longer retention and dehydration in the distal colon. Furthermore, hypermotility in the distal colon may result in little abnormality if the stool is already of normal consistency. It is helpful to recall in this regard that a liquid stool contains only about 10 per cent more water than the hardest scyballum, so that addition or removal of relatively small amounts of fluid can alter physical characteristics of excreta tremendously.

It is not surprising that excessive stool production can be ascribed to any of many possible causes when we realize that in the normal person about 10 liters of fluid pass the ligament of Treitz (at the duodenal-jejunal junction) every day. Anything that can influence the complex processes involved

in water, solute, or fat absorption can initiate a series of malabsorptive events which will result in diarrhea. Austin Flint's definition in 1880 of the term diarrhea, "to denote morbid frequency of intestinal dejections which are also liquid or morbidly soft, and often otherwise altered in character," is still useful, because diarrhea (Gr. διαρροια, a flowing through) means many different things in lay *and* medical argot. Some patients emphasize stool frequency and others note stool consistency; physicians may translate the term through their own personal as well as medical experience.

From the patient's description of alterations in his stools, useful clues can be selected in directing the physician's attention to one or the other of the possible causes of diarrhea. Age, sex, race, exposure (travel, epidemic, etc.), dietary relationships, associated symptoms, presence of other diseases, and use of specific drugs are aspects of the history which may be the key in establishing the cause of diarrhea. In Table 22-2 are listed the categories and some of the specific conditions that can result in diarrhea.

As with constipation, so with diarrhea, many classifications have been suggested. None is completely satisfactory because it is impossible to include all of the many factors involved, such as the etiology, pathology, chemistry, clinical picture, and characteristics of the excreta.

MALABSORPTION

Malabsorption may involve water primarily or fat, protein, or carbohydrate, or various combinations of these. With these absorptive deficiencies there also may be significant failure in uptake and excretory losses of certain other nutritive elements (vitamins, minerals, etc.).

Basic Pathophysiology

There are a number of possible basic causes of malabsorption, especially these:

1. A defect in the mucosa of the small intestine which may be (a) of genetic origin (congenital celiac disease), or (b) acquired (nontropical sprue, gluten-induced enteropathy), or (c) acquired by cell injury from inadequate blood supply or toxins, chemicals, or radiation.

2. Temporary inflammatory changes in the intestinal mucosa (from toxins, chemicals, viruses, bacteria, parasites, etc.) which limit absorption.

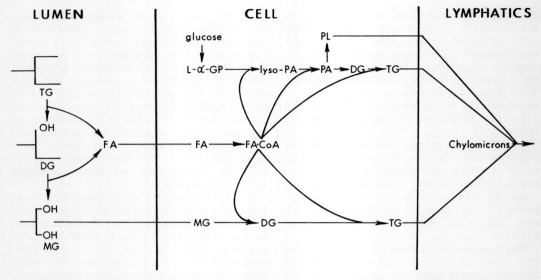

FIG. 22-2. Scheme of fat digestion and absorption. The dietary triglyceride (TG) is hydrolyzed in the lumen into α,β diglyceride (DG) and then β-monoglyceride (MG) and fatty acids (FA) by pancreatic lipase. These lipolytic products enter the cell where the coenzyme A-activated fatty acids (FA-CoA) are reassembled into TG via intermediate steps involving synthesis of phospholipid (PL), glycerophosphate (Lα-GP), lypophosphatidic acid (lyso-PA), and phosphatidic acid (PA) or addition to partial glycerides. Then the dietary fat is circulated as chylomicrons via the lacteal and thoracic duct.

3. Factors that cause excess secretion by the mucosa (cholera, villous adenoma, bile acid toxicity).

4. Derangement of bile salt activity.

5. Lack of certain digestive enzymes from pancreas or intestinal mucosa.

6. Osmotic effects (mannitol, magnesium ion, etc.).

Malabsorption of Fat

Obviously, whenever the ingested or secreted contents of the gut cannot be absorbed, changes in bowel habit ensue. Failure to absorb fat results in a pasty stool, which has a relatively high water content. It is often malodorous, light-colored, and floats, making it difficult to flush the stool down the toilet.

Pancreatic lipase hydrolyzes digested triglycerides (see Fig. 22-2) into free fatty acids and β monoglycerides.[10] These relatively more polar lipids can form macromolecular aggregates with bile salts, and they are dispersed as mixed micelles in a fashion that permits the products of enzymatic lipolysis to approach and, presumably, dissolve in the lipid membrane of the microvilli (see Fig. 22-3). Triglyceride cannot be so readily dispersed and is, therefore, not available for absorption in the absence of lipase. Lipase acts by cleaving off first the α and then the α' acyl groups, leaving a β monoglyceride, which can be absorbed. This lipolytic action is optimum at slightly basic pH, and diminished lipase activity will result if the duodenal pH is lowered. Thus, gastrin-producing tumors provoke such profound gastric acid secretion that the bicarbonate-rich pancreatic secretions fail to neutralize the duodenal contents, and the reduction in lipase activity in this acidified milieu causes steatorrhea.

Pancreatic destruction must be relatively extensive to result in enzyme deficiency sufficient to cause steatorrhea. This does not usually occur in acute pancreatitis, but may be a permanent dysfunction after prolonged and recurrent attacks of pancreatitis. Blockade of the ducts or replacement of the pancreas by tumor also must be fairly complete to prevent release of sufficient amounts of lipase from the gland. On the other hand, an insufficiency of lipase is common in mucoviscidosis, leading to a need for exogenous pancreatic enzymes. Since pancreatic enzyme synthesis is one of the major drains on amino acid pools, it is not surprising that pancreatic insufficiency is an expression of protein malnutrition, as seen in kwashiorkor.

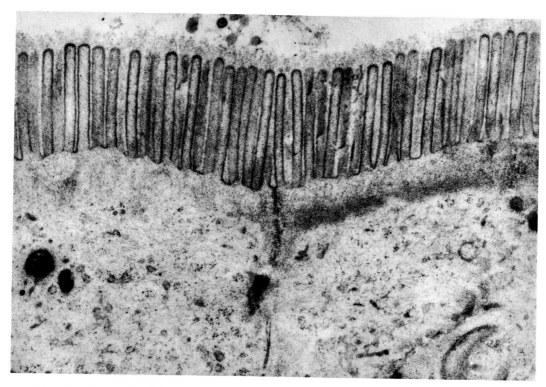

Fig. 22-3. Microvilli of human jejunal epithelial cells. This electron micrograph of normal gut mucosa shows the palisade of microvillous projections of the luminal surface of these epithelial cells. The micrograph is taken at the junction of two cells. The terminal web is visible in the apex of the cell on the right.

Bile Salt Disorders

Even in the presence of normal pancreatic function malabsorption of fat can occur in states of deficiency of the essential cofactors for micellar dispersion of the lipolysis products.[11] In the human liver, two primary bile acids, cholic and chenodeoxycholic acid, are synthesized from cholesterol. These, together with secondary bile acids, chiefly deoxycholic acid formed by dehydroxylation of primary bile acids by intestinal bacteria, are conjugated by the liver with glycine or taurine. At proper concentrations of these conjugated salts (and at the appropriate pH and temperature) polar lipids can be brought from immiscible two-phase systems into crystal-clear micellar dispersions of the water-insoluble phase. Such conditions exist in the gut, favoring fat absorption in the upper small bowel. The *bile salts* are reabsorbed in the distal ileum by an active transport system, but if they are deconjugated by various intestinal bacteria, the *bile acids* are less completely absorbed by passive diffusion throughout the length of the small bowel. This enterohepatic recirculation from liver to gut to portal circulation and back to liver normally cycles the entire bile salts pool six times daily.

Various abnormalities of the bowel have been shown to result in altered bile salt metabolism, leading to steatorrhea and attendant alterations in bowel habit. Depletion of the bile salt pool in situations that prevent conservation of the bile salts by reabsorption has been shown to occur in resection of the distal ileum or in disease states that affect the distal small bowel, especially *regional enteritis*. Not only does steatorrhea occur on the basis of inadequate amounts of bile salts, but the nonabsorbed bile salts can be deconjugated by colonic bacteria to free bile acids, which are toxic to the mucosa of the large intestine and thus cause a choleretic diarrhea. Under experimental conditions in normal subjects, deconjugated bile acids infused into the colon can cause significant watery diarrhea.

In circumstances in which *bacterial overgrowth* high in the small intestine occurs (jejunal diverticulosis, afferent loop after Bilroth II gastrectomy, and perhaps intestinal atony on neuropathic bases) there may be deconjugation of bile salts into free bile acids, which are far less effective in micelle formation. Thus, steatorrhea has been found to be associated with presence of free bile acids and high counts of jejunal organisms in patients with gastrectomy. In conjunction with a reduction in jejunal bacterial population and disappearance of unconjugated bile acids from the jejunum, the diarrhea

has been reversed by administration of oral antibiotics.

Steatorrhea may be a consequence of *blockade* of any of the pathways of intestinal assimilation of fat. Even though the mechanisms of hydrolysis of triglyceride or of micellar dispersion of the fatty acids and monoglycerides are intact, lipids taken up by the cells may not be moved through the intracellular resynthesis process, the lymphatics may be obstructed, or there may be insufficient cell surface for completion of the absorptive process before the fat has traversed the gut. In patients with a-beta-lipoproteinemia (acanthocytosis), the intestinal mucosa cells are engorged with fat

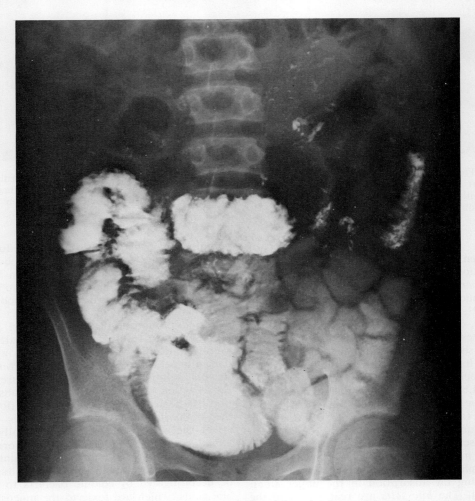

FIG. 22-4. The characteristic roentgenologic picture in the malabsorption states. Dilated loops of small bowel are divided into sausage-shaped segments. Fluid and fat are not absorbed adequately by the flattened, shortened villi, and a bulky, foamy stool results.

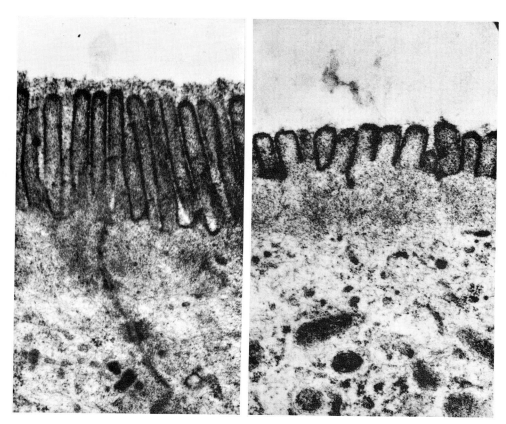

Fig. 22-5. Microvilli of human jejunal epithelium from a normal person (left) and a patient with celiac disease (right). These electron micrographs at the same magnification show the changes in brush borders which effect a loss of absorptive surface in celiac disease. The beautiful architecture of the tall microvilli gives way to a stunted pattern. Since the microvilli provide the route of passive absorption of lipids and contain the disaccharidases, it is clear why such changes are associated with diarrheal states characterized by steatorrhea and carbohydrate intolerance. (courtesy of Dr. William Black)

and no postprandial chylomicronemia is observed. Since dietary fat is incapable of being released from the mucosal cell, essentially all absorption from the lumen is blocked and steatorrhea results. Apparently a similar blockade of fat movement away from the gut accounts for the steatorrhea seen in intestinal lymphangiectasia.[12] In this instance the fat passes through the mucosal cells, but then it cannot move away from the villi because the lymphatics are only blind sacs. Indeed, reverse flow of chlyomicrons from distended lymph channels is suggested by the observation that chyle could be aspirated from the gut of a child with this congenital anomaly of the lymph system. Steatorrhea results whenever the available intestinal mucosal surface is

insufficient for fat absorption to be complete before the stream of luminal contents passes the absorptive regions. This is the rule in patients who have surgically shortened intestines, or extensively diseased mucosa with limited remaining absorptive area, e.g., in sprue or celiac disease (see Figs. 22-5 and 22-6), or in widespread infiltrative or inflammatory disease.

Malabsorption of Carbohydrates

Since most ingested carbohydrate is presented to the mucosal cell as disaccharide (maltose from amylolytic action on starch, lactose in milk products, or sucrose in sweetened foods), absence of the respective disaccharidases can result in sugar malabsorption. Whenever such osmotically active molecules

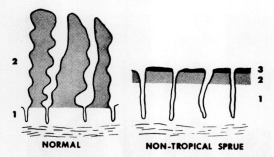

NORMAL   **NON-TROPICAL SPRUE**

FIG. 22-6. Epithelial zonation in the human jejunum. The zonation of the normal and abnormal intestinal epitheliums is derived from histochemical characteristics. Zone 1 comprises the crypts, and this germinal region is more extensive in nontropical sprue. Zone 2 represents the villous epithelium; in sprue this area is considerably smaller. Zones 1 and 2 in sprue are identical histochemically to Zones 1 and 2, respectively, of the normal intestine. Zone 3 is the location of the peculiar surface epithelium of sprue, and it shows striking deviations from the normal absorptive epithelium. (Padykula, Gastroenterology 40:738)

remain in the gut lumen, the entrapped water will appear in the stool. The characteristic clinical picture of malaise, nausea, borborygmi, distention, flatulence, and watery stools follows shortly after eating sufficient quantities of the offending carbohydrate. The rare patient with sucrase deficiency,[13] a recessive genetic error, may give a lifelong history of postprandial diarrhea correlated with dietary sucrose loads. On the other hand, patients with lactase deficiency do not develop this enzyme deficiency until adult years. The precise basis on which lactase deficiency and resulting milk intolerance is acquired is not clear, but genetic influences are suggested by the observation that almost all Orientals, American Indians, and members of only certain African tribes are affected. In the U. S. the frequency of lactase deficiency is relatively low, of the order of 5 per cent for Caucasians. Negroes have a higher frequency, about 25 per cent. The implications of this knowledge for surplus food export programs and anthropological studies is still being assessed, but from the clinical standpoint there is no doubt about the relevance of this diagnosis to the management of the deficiency state.

Primary deficiency of a single enzyme usually will result in a rather clear picture of the influence of dietary carbohydrates on the patient's bowel habit, but secondary deficiencies, which are not limited to intolerance of a single sugar, occur in generalized mucosal diseases such as celiac disease, tropical sprue, and Whipple's disease. Improvement in the underlying disease will be associated with return of disaccharidase activity, so that only temporary attention to dietary restriction of carbohydrate is necessary. In patients with isolated lactase deficiency, ingestion of milk and ice cream can be restricted to relieve symptoms. Primary sucrase deficiency is more difficult to treat because isomaltose, released by starch hydrolysis, is digested by sucrase. Thus, withholding dietary sucrose, a difficult regimen to follow because of patterns of commercial food preparation, is not sufficient to overcome the problem. Exogenous sucrase replacement does alleviate the annoying symptoms.

Malabsorption of Water

Deficit in water uptake is usually secondary to mucosal cell damage. Impaired sodium transport or carbohydrate maldigestion in the small bowel has been demonstrated following exposure to ionizing radiation, certain toxins (including gluten in patients with celiac disease), and in circumstances of vascular insufficiency. Injury that results in failure to transport these solutes is followed by watery diarrhea. Sometimes blood may be prominent in the stool because of the severity of the mucosal destruction.

Watery diarrhea in the absence of mucosal disease can be osmotically induced by mannitol, magnesium salts (including those intended primarily as antacids rather than laxatives), and other poorly absorbed molecules. Secretion of water to produce watery stools is the basis of choleretic diarrhea resulting from the toxicity of deconjugated bile acids on colonic mucosa. The incredible water losses in cholera are felt to be on the basis of a toxin elaborated by the *Vibrio comma*, which poisons the barrier to egress of extracellular fluid into the gut. Exactly what that barrier is and how the material from the bacteria affects it is not yet known. Active secretion of mucus by a villous adenoma in the rectosigmoid can cause watery diarrhea, which may be accompanied by hypokalemia and hypoproteinemia.

Malabsorption syndromes are better understood in recent years largely because of the relative ease with which biopsies of the small bowel can now be obtained. Familiar now are the short, blunt villi and lengthened dilated crypts in the mucosa of these patients, and the fact that the rates of mucosal cell loss and cell renewal are significantly increased (see Figs. 22-5 and 22-6). Nevertheless, the cause of these anatomic changes is still obscure. Celiac disease may be a complex metabolic disorder, genetically transmitted, with disturbed enzymatic pathways.[14] As a result there is defective absorption of electrolytes, water, protein, lipids, and vitamins, not only because of decreased mucosal surface, but also because of deficiency in the chemical organization of absorptive cells, especially in relation to active transport.

Secondary malabsorption syndromes occur with diseases that lead to impaired or incomplete digestion and absorption from the small bowel, e.g. regional enteritis, amyloidosis, scleroderma, radiation enteritis, intestinal lipodystrophy, lymphoma, jejunal diverticulosis, internal fistulas, the blind loop syndrome, and others. It is apparent that a number of factors may be involved in the diarrhea that is associated with these disorders, but basically the stimuli are the same—an increase in fecal bulk due to unabsorbed water, fat, or solute—perhaps compounded by metabolic consequences of the changes in small intestinal bacterial content. Of particular interest are the patients with small-intestinal diverticulosis, who have been intensely studied. Heavy growth of bacteria in the diverticula may convert conjugated bile salts to toxic unconjugated salts which may interfere further with fat and water absorption. And lastly, the microorganisms may utilize nutrients such as vitamin B_{12} at the expense of the patients' nutritional status. It is this last factor apparently that accounts for the anemia so commonly found in a number of the secondary malabsorption states.

Neuromuscular Origins of Diarrhea

The normal synergism of the components of the autonomic nervous system facilitates the transit and absorption of intestinal contents. Dysfunction of the sympathetic system, the parasympathetic system, or the muscular tissue can result in altered absorption and transit time. Generally there is a direct relationship between intestinal motility and absorption, i.e., agents or circumstances that produce atony usually impair water absorption, whereas increased motility may be associated with prolonged transit time. Since motility is under both neural and endocrine control, it is not surprising that a variety of disease states and medications can influence bowel habits.

After complete vagotomy, gastric motility is severely diminished, but intestinal motility is not markedly affected. Nevertheless, a certain number of patients have transient diarrhea after vagotomy. Whether this is only a reflection of interrupted parasympathetic innervations or some other indirect consequence of the operation is not clear. Parallel observations in other states of neuropathy, e.g., diabetic enteropathy, have led to the speculation that surgical or metabolic parasympathetic denervation results in diminished motility with corresponding reduction in absorption. The fact that these states of diarrhea sometimes can be reversed by use of Urecholine (a parasympathomimetic drug) further suggests that they are mediated by the autonomic system.

Irritable colon syndrome has manifestations of autonomic dysfunction when pharmacologic studies of intestinal motility have been carried out. The common history is one of episodes of watery diarrhea occurring during or just after periods of stress. Often the pressure of unusual situations in occupation, home, or school will be associated with the symptoms. With the diarrhea the patient experiences abdominal discomfort, often located in the left upper quadrant, giving rise to the term "splenic flexure syndrome." The stool volume usually is not very great, but the patient experiences urgency and frequency of defecation. Often the stools are more watery or numerous after midday, but patients with this disorder rarely are awakened by an urge to move their bowels. In the absence of blood in the stools, constitutional symptoms, and dietary relationship of the diarrhea, the diagnosis of irritable colon syndrome is very likely. Confirmation is afforded by finding normal mucosa upon sigmoidoscopy and obtaining relief of symptoms with administration of diphenoxylate (Lomotil), but sometimes the distinction between lactase deficiency and irritable colon syndrome can be very difficult.

Narcotic addiction usually is associated with constipation attributed to neuromuscular effects of the drug. Conversely, diarrhea is associated with the withdrawal syndrome, but whether this represents compensatory rebound phenomena in the nervous or muscular tissues has not been assessed.

Many hormones affect the gut, but their mechanisms of action are not well-understood. In overproduction of serotonin by chromaffin tumors, diarrhea can be a prominent symptom. Characteristically, hyperfunction of the thyroid gland is accompanied by increased frequency of defecation without marked change in the quality of stool. Although there are multiple reasons for the diarrhea associated with Zollinger-Ellison syndrome, this altered bowel habit may result from the excitatory function of gastrin on smooth muscle. Histamine has a profound effect on smooth muscle, and in patients with mastocytosis this substance may affect colonic contractions in such a fashion that diarrhea results.

Diarrhea can be an undesirable side-effect of numerous drugs. Excessive dosage of

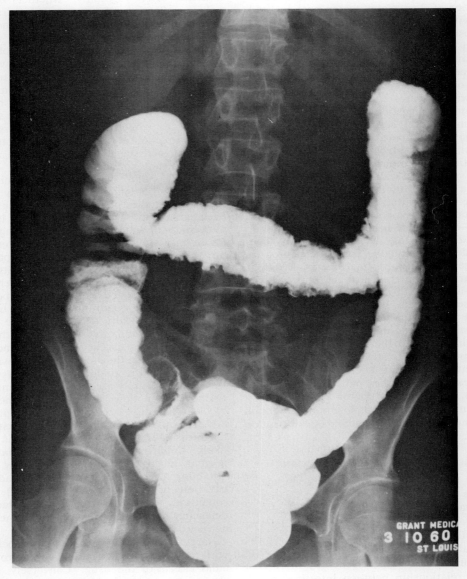

Fig. 22-7. The colon in acute ulcerative colitis, with barium clearly outlining many of the ulcers. Admixture of mucus, pus and blood to the mushy fecal content results in a characteristic type of diarrhea.

colchicine, quinidine, and various alkylating agents often is signaled by appearance of diarrhea. Therapeutic doses of certain medications can produce diarrhea. For example, the organophosphorus compound echothiophate (phospholine iodide) currently is being used as eye drops for patients with glaucoma. This potent cholinesterase inhibitor can produce diarrhea resulting from the accumulation of acetylcholine in the neuromotor end-plates of the intestinal muscles, especially the colon.

MECHANICAL DIARRHEA

For reasons that may be more complicated than we now realize, incomplete obstruction of the bowel may be associated with diarrhea. Stenosis of the large bowel associated with inflammatory changes, extraluminal constriction by adhesions, or invasion by tumor can produce diarrhea. Whether these conditions create circumstances that enhance bacterial overgrowth, resulting in bile salt deconjugation and choleretic diarrhea has not been clarified. Clearly, the evaluation

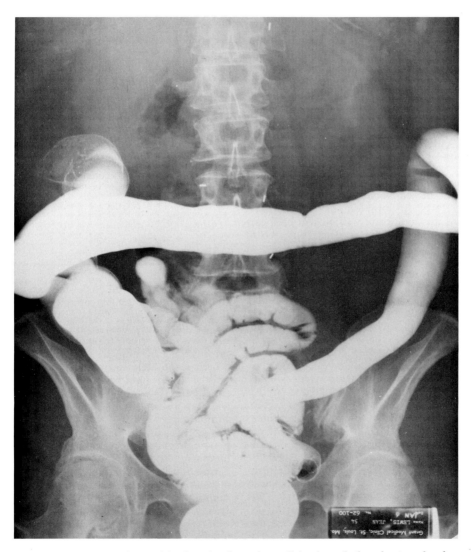

FIG. 22-8. In the patient with chronic ulcerative colitis the tubular shortened colon discharges the fecal content in the same mushy state in which it is received from the ileum. Because of extensive damage to the mucosal cells very little water can be absorbed.

of any patient with diarrhea demands a rectal examination, which may disclose fecal impaction, a common cause of diarrhea in elderly, bedridden, postoperative, or malnourished patients.

Scleroderma can be associated with diarrhea. In such instances histological study of the intestinal muscle shows that there is considerable atrophy and replacement by collagen. Resulting atony probably causes impairment of water absorption and diarrhea.

INFLAMMATORY DIARRHEA

Mucosal damage from organisms or their toxins can produce diarrhea which may be brief and self-limited but can be so profuse that dehydration and death ensue. In the usual instance, pathogenic bacteria are not cultured from the stool, although *Shigella* and *Salmonella* are frequently found.

Salmonellosis is increasingly a public health problem, since food processing methods result in dissemination of contaminated sources such as dried egg powder. The clustering of patients with watery stools in families, schools, or institutions can lead one to suspect this ubiquitous problem.

Turista, an explosive diarrhea, which affects a large proportion of international travelers, has long been the subject of speculation. The cause is unknown, but recent studies have suggested that qualitative or quantitative alterations in the colonic bacterial population may be involved.[15] "Traveler's diarrhea" (turista, Montezuma's revenge, etc.) is not restricted to tropical climes. Controlled studies show that prevention by use of various antibiotics is not feasible.

"Intestinal flu" is a very common epidemic dysentery. Many types of enteroviruses, including ECHO and Coxsackie viruses, have been established as capable of causing this sudden, usually brief illness.

Regional enteritis commonly produces diarrhea, particularly if it involves the distal ileum, blocking the enterohepatic recirculation of bile salts. Other factors may be responsible for the diarrhea if the inflammation has resulted in a secondary disaccharidase deficiency or in rectal irritability. The stools are usually watery and contain blood; sometimes steatorrhea is a prominent feature if bile salt deficiency is severe.

Ulcerative Colitis. The diarrhea that characterizes ulcerative colitis is bloody, watery, and associated with urgency and tenesmus. Since not every patient with ulcerative colitis

TABLE 22-3. DIAGNOSTIC TECHNIQUES IN EVALUATION OF DIARRHEA

History

Physical examination (including rectal examination and sigmoidoscopy)

Roentgenologic examination of alimentary tract

Examination of stool
  Inspection
  Microscopic examination for ova and parasites
  Culture
  Fecal fat measurements (3-day on known fat intake)

Examination of duodenal or jejunal contents
  Microscopic examination
  Culture
  Secretin test

Examination of tissue
  Jejunal biopsy
  Rectal biopsy
    Light microscopy
    Electron microscopy
    Disaccharidase assay

Blood tests
  Disaccharide tolerance test
  Serological test for amebiasis
  Serum gastrin assay
  Serum carotene

Urine tests
  Xylose absorption test
  5-hydroxyindolacetic acid
  Histamine

has blood in the stool (or even diarrhea), this diagnosis is worthy of consideration in dealing with a variety of gastrointestinal, hepatic, or dermatological complaints. Occasionally patients given certain *broad-spectrum antibiotics* develop a pattern of diarrhea which resembles that seen in mild ulcerative colitis. Even upon proctoscopic examination, the distinction may be impossible to make, so that reliance on history plus the self-limited course of the antibiotic effect may be the only basis of differentiation. For roentgenologic characteristics of acute and chronic ulcerative colitis see Figs. 22-7 and 22-8.

Amebiasis. Although colonic amebiasis is a relatively uncommon problem, it is endemic in the U. S. In addition, world travelers and returning military personnel add to this constant background level of amebic infestation.

Giardiasis is recognized as a cause of a malabsorptive pattern of diarrhea much more frequently. Reports of outbreaks, such as the recent episodes in the resort town of

Aspen, Colorado, should lead to search for *Giardia lamblia* (a flagellate protozoon) in the jejunal aspirates of the diarrhea victim who has been exposed.[16,17]

Tropical sprue remains an enigma today, but there is little question that it is the cause of diarrhea in many native and foreign residents of certain tropical areas. The frequency of jejunitis in Americans assigned to Pakistan or Southeast Asia approaches 40 per cent, but ascribing diarrhea to this cause is untenable in the absence of jejunal biopsy and proper diagnostic evaluation for other causes.

Cathartics are variously classified as saline, emollient, bulky, or irritant. In fact, most mechanisms of action are poorly understood.

The saline cathartics, such as magnesium sulfate and magnesium citrate, exert osmotic effects because the cations are not absorbed well. They retain water ingested with them in the bowel and even increase the water bulk. Mineral oil, certain surfactants and cellulose laxatives exert action by entrapping bile salts and other amphipathic materials, thereby increasing stool volume.

DIAGNOSTIC ASSESSMENT OF DIARRHEA

If one uses his knowledge of the pathophysiology of diarrheal states, he finds that the history can provide the information necessary to establish the correct diagnosis in most instances. The physical examination can uncover important diagnostic leads, such as the characteristic indolent perianal fistula associated with regional enteritis, the erythema nodosum, pyoderma, or uveitis associated with ulcerative colitis, or the dermographia of mastocytosis (urticaria pigmentosa). Careful inspection and palpation of the rectum and proctoscopic examination should be carried out in every patient with diarrhea. The proctoscopic appearance in patients with amebiasis, ulcerative colitis, regional enteritis, or bacterial enteritis should be distinctive enough to permit confirmation or elimination of these diagnostic considerations. Patients with irritable colon syndrome may show persistent spasms of the rectosigmoid, causing considerable difficulty in passing the sigmoidoscope.

Roentgenologic examination of the gut with special attention to the small bowel can show flocculation and moulage pattern that is nonspecific in states of malabsorption from various causes. Study of roentgenograms after barium enema can usually facilitate the distinction between regional enteritis of the colon (granulomatous colitis) and ulcerative colitis.

Inspection of the stool by the physician is mandatory if he is to assess the basis of the diarrhea with confidence. These observations and tests usually should be done before the radiologist has given the patient barium sulfate. Odor, color, consistency, presence or absence of mucus, pus, or blood, and the recognition of parasites or undigested food can be reliably determined only by first-hand observation. Microscopic examination for ova and parasites should be done on very fresh warm specimens or those preserved in polyvinyl alcohol. Culture of fresh stools on selective media and appropriate subcultures or fermentative classification tests should be done as early as possible in the evaluation. Analysis of fecal fat levels is valid only when the patient is continuously fed a 100-Gm. fat diet and a 72-hour stool collection is carefully done. Less than 21 Gm. of fat (van de Kamer method) is normally excreted in a 3-day period under these conditions. Substitutes for this rather tedious determination are not reliable, so that use of radioiodinated absorption studies or spot checks for visible or chemical fat is of no great diagnostic benefit.

In rare instances, duodenal or jejunal contents may be examined usefully, especially for *Giardia lamblia* or for overgrowth of bacteria in postgastrectomy diarrheal states. A secretin test may provide chemical or cytologic evidence for pancreatic dysfunction or neoplasm.

One of the most useful studies for differentiation of causes of the malabsorptive state is the jejunal biopsy; however, without proper care of the tissue in mounting, sectioning, and staining, little reliable assistance can be expected. The characteristic appearance of celiac disease, intestinal lymphangiectasia, Whipple's disease (especially on PAS stain and under electron microscopy), and acanthocytosis will be apparent readily. Assay of a small portion of the tissue for lactase, sucrase, and maltase provides the most useful evidence for primary or secondary disaccharidase deficiencies.

Rectal biopsy can show granulomata (regional enteritis), schistosomiasis, amyloidosis, or the mucosal ulcers seen in ulcerative colitis (unfortunately these are not specifically characteristic).

The observation that blood levels of glucose do not change significantly following ingestion of disaccharides is less useful than the direct enzyme assay in establishing the diagnosis of disaccharidase deficiency. Nevertheless, disaccharide tolerance tests, done with great care, can be informative, especially if the diarrhea and other symptoms are provoked by the carbohydrate test meal. Other blood tests of use in evaluating causes of diarrhea include the red-cell agglutination test of serum antibodies to *Endamoeba histolytica* (available through the U.S.P.H.S. Communicable Disease Center), which has been found to be especially useful in diagnosis of amebic abscess of the liver. Radioimmunoassay for serum gastrin can establish the diagnosis of Zollinger-Ellison syndrome. Serum levels of carotene are low in malabsorptive states, but this test is of much less use than fecal fat measurement and is no more specific as to the cause of lipid malabsorption.

Urine levels of xylose following ingestion of 25 Gm. of this pentose may be low (less than 5 Gm. in 5 hours) if there is impaired mucosal water absorption reflecting intestinal epithelial disease. Unfortunately, this test can be falsely positive if gastric emptying is delayed and falsely negative if there is renal disease or only limited bowel involvement.

Urinary levels of 5-hydroxyindolacetic acid can be of use in establishing the diagnosis of a serotonin-producing neoplasm. Histamine levels in urine have been grossly elevated in patients with diarrhea associated with mastocytosis.

REFERENCES

1. Bülbring, E., Lin, R. C. Y., and Schofield, G.: An investigation of the peristaltic reflex in relation to anatomic observations, Quart. J. Exp. Physiol. 43:26–35, 1958.
2. Thomas, J. E.: The autonomic nervous system in gastrointestinal disease, J.A.M.A. 157:209–212, 1955.
3. Lee, C. Y.: The effect of stimulation of extrinsic nerves on peristalsis and on the release of 5-hydroxytryptamine in the large intestine of the guinea-pig and of the rabbit, J. Physiol. 152:405, 1960.
4. Haverback, B. J., and Davidson, J. D.: Serotonin and the gastrointestinal tract, Gastroenterology 35:570–578, 1958.
5. Almy, T. P., Hinkle, L. E., Jr., Berle, B., and Kern, F., Jr.: Alteration in colonic function in man under stress, Gastroenterology 12:437–444, 1949.
6. Grace, W. J., Wolf, S., and Wolff, H. G.: Life situations, emotions and colonic function, Gastroenterology 14:93–108, 1950.
7. Fisher, J. H., and Swenson, O.: Aganglionic lesions of the colon, Amer. J. Surg. 99:134–136, 1960.
8. Daniel, E. E., Sutherland, W. H., and Bogoch, A.: Effects of morphine and other drugs on motility of the terminal ileum, Gastroenterology 36:510–523, 1959.
9. Fink, S., and Friedman, G.: The differential effect of drugs on the proximal and distal colon, Amer. J. Med. 28:535–540, 1960.
10. Peterson, M. L.: On the re-esterification of fatty acids during absorption of fat, Gastroenterology 44:774, 1963.
11. Hofmann, A. F.: A physicochemical approach to the intraluminal phase of fat absorption, Gastroenterology 50:56, 1966.
12. McGuigan, J. E., Purkerson, M. L., Trudeau, W. L., and Peterson, M. L.: Studies of the immunologic defects associated with intestinal lymphangiectasia with some observations on dietary control of chylosis ascites, Ann. Intern. Med. 68:398, 1968.
13. Peterson, M. L., and Herber, R.: Intestinal sucrase deficiency in adults, Trans. Ass. Amer. Physicians 80:275, 1967.
14. Padykula, H. A., Strauss, E. W., Ladman, A. V., and Gardner, F. H.: A morphologic and histochemical analysis of the human jejunal epithelium in non-tropical sprue, Gastroenterology 40:735–765, 1961; Frazer, A. C.: Pathogenetic concepts of the malabsorption syndrome, Gastroenterology 38:389–398, 1960; di Sant' Agnese, P. A., and Jones, W. O.: The celiac syndrome (malabsorption) in pediatrics, J.A.M.A. 180:308–316, 1962.
15. Kean, B. H., Schaffner, W., Brennan, A. B., and Waters, S. R.: The diarrhea of travelers, J.A.M.A. 180:367–371, 1962.
16. Moore, G. T., Cross, W. M., McGuire, D., et al.: Epidemic giardiasis at a ski resort, New Eng. J. Med. 281:402, 1969.
17. Veazie, L.: Epidemic giardiasis, New Eng. J. Med. 281:853, 1969.

23

Hematemesis and Melena

LEON SCHIFF

GENERAL CONSIDERATIONS

Definitions. *Hematemesis* is the vomiting of blood, whether fresh and red or digested and black.

Melena, by derivation, means black, and is usually used to describe the passage of black "tarry" stools, with the coal-black, clotted gummy appearance of tar. However, melena is used clinically in a wider sense to describe the passage of blood in the stools, whether the color is visibly altered or not and whether the color is light, reddish, or (as is more common) dark brown or blackish.

Pathogenesis. Bleeding in the gastrointestinal tract may result from:

1. Disease of, or trauma to, tissue, with secondary erosion or rupture of blood vessels.

2. Primary disorders affecting the walls of the blood vessels (increased capillary fragility, varices, aneurysm, arteriosclerosis, etc.).

3. Disturbance of the blood-clotting mechanism.

In general, any of the disorders discussed in the chapter on Pathologic Bleeding may result in the presence of some blood in the gastrointestinal tract, but only when fairly large amounts are present does hematemesis occur or does melena become obvious. These will not be discussed here.

SOURCE OF HEMORRHAGE

The vomiting of large amounts of blood or the passage of tarry stools are symptoms that usually appear with dramatic suddenness. They may supervene in patients with pre-existing digestive disturbances or may, of themselves, prove the harbingers of disease. Their occurrence may clarify the significance of existing symptoms, or may constitute the sole evidence of disease. It is well-known that they occur most commonly in a number of disorders, which will be considered separately. The occurrence of hematemesis indicates a bleeding point proximal to the ligament of Treitz. The appearance of the vomitus, whether resembling coffee-grounds or bright red and obviously bloody, has proved of little diagnostic value.

Melena without Hematemesis. Although it is generally true that the occurrence of melena (tarry stools) without hematemesis indicates a lesion distal to the pylorus (usually a duodenal ulcer), this is not invariably so. We have seen melena without hematemesis in cases of ruptured esophageal varix associated with hepatic cirrhosis and in cases of gastric cancer. Ratnoff and Patek[1] noted 9 instances of melena without hematemesis in 386 cases of hepatic cirrhosis. Benedict[2] reported melena alone in 5 of 20 cases of hemorrhage from gastritis. Jones[3] observed melena only in 6 fatal cases of bleeding gastric ulcer. A common feature of these 6 cases was their extremely poor general condition, and it was suggested that the patients may have been too weak to vomit.

Color of Stools. While the presence of bright blood in the stools usually indicates a bleeding point low in the intestine, this is not an infallible sign. In the presence of hypermotility, the blood may be swept through the intestinal tract so rapidly as to appear unaltered in the feces. The presence of bright blood in the stools has been noted in 3 individuals 4 to 17 hours after they were given 1,000 ml. of citrated human blood intragastrically; none of them passed a tarry stool.[4] Tarry stools are said to occur when blood is introduced in the cecum, particularly in the presence of delayed colonic motility.[5] The author has seen truly tarry stools in hemorrhage arising just distal to the ileocecal valve; but not when bleeding took place beyond this area. According to Hilsman,[5] the color of the stools (whether bright red, dark red, brown, or tarry) depends more on the time the blood remains in the intestine than on the level at which the bleeding occurs.

CHARACTERISTICS OF MELENA

Amount of Blood Necessary. Daniel and Egan[6] reported the occurrence of tarry stools after the oral administration of 50 to 80 ml. of fresh human blood. The writer and his associates have reported the occurrence of tarry stools after the oral administration of 100 ml. of citrated human "bank" blood. These observations indicate that the passage of a tarry stool does not necessarily indicate severe blood loss.

Duration of Tarry Stools. Tarry stools may be passed for 3 to 5 days following the intragastric administration of 1,000 to 2,000 ml. of citrated human blood to human subjects.[4] This indicates that the passage of a tarry stool is no proof that hemorrhage is continuing. The number of tarry or bloody stools that follow the intragastric administration of blood is not necessarily related to the quantity of blood introduced.

Duration of Occult Blood. Hesser[7] has pointed out that occult blood is usually present in the stools for about 2 to 3 weeks following hematemesis or melena in patients with bleeding peptic ulcer. We have been able to confirm this experimentally, upon oral or intragastric administration of citrated human blood. The persistence of a positive test for occult blood is, therefore, not necessarily an indication that hemorrhage is continuing.

SEVERITY OF HEMORRHAGE

It is difficult to estimate the quantity of blood lost by judging from the amount apparently present in the vomitus: first, because of the admixture of gastric contents; second, because only part of the effused blood is vomited. One not infrequently hears a patient proclaim that he has vomited a gallon or two of blood! As Cullinan and Price[8] have well put it, the amount of blood vomited varies with the patient's imagination.

It may be difficult to estimate the severity of the bleeding when the patient is first seen clinically, for, as Black[9] has stated, the rate of blood loss may influence the patient's appearance. Thus, "the rapid loss of a small amount of blood may produce as much appearance of circulatory failure" as the gradual loss of a larger quantity. The pulse rate may be misleading, as Wallace and Sharpey-Schafer[10] have shown, because the heart rate may be slowed, increased or unchanged after the rapid removal of up to 1,150 ml. of blood in control subjects. We have been impressed with the frequency of a normal pulse rate in the presence of a rather marked fall in blood pressure soon after massive hematemesis or melena. The hemoglobin percentage may prove unreliable shortly after hemorrhage, since the lowest values are usually obtained from 6 to 48 hours later[9] as a result of dilution of the blood by tissue fluids. Wallace and Sharpey-Schafer[10] obtained maximum blood dilution (and lowest hemoglobin percentage) from 3 to 90 hours after the rapid removal of as much as 1,150 ml. of blood in control subjects. They found the time of maximal dilution to vary in the same individual on different occasions.

Ebert, Stead and Gibson[11] removed amounts ranging from 760 to 1,220 ml. of blood from six normal subjects in 6 to 13 minutes. They found a sharp drop in plasma volume immediately after hemorrhage; thereafter the plasma volume gradually increased, until, at the end of three to four days, it was greater than the original plasma volume by an amount approximately equal to the volume of red cells removed. After the first two hours, the change in plasma volume was much more accurately reflected by the hemaocrit value than by the protein concentration. "If the difference between the original hematocrit reading and that made 72 hours after venesection is taken as 100 per cent, it is found that 14 to 36 per cent of this drop occurred in two hours, 36 to 50 per cent in eight hours, and 63 to 77 per cent in 24 hours."

Howarth and Sharpey-Schafer[12] describe three low-blood-pressure phases after hemorrhage. The first phase is that of sudden vasovagal reaction, with bradycardia and muscle vasodilatation, which develops suddenly during or after bleeding. The second phase is associated with increased heart rate, low right-auricular pressure, and low cardiac output. Large transfusions raise right-auricular pressure, cardiac output, and blood pressure. The third phase "takes time to develop and persists over long periods. Severe anemia may be a causal factor in this phase. Right auricular pressure and cardiac output are increased. Large transfusions may be dangerous from overloading." I have seen instances of pulmonary edema following blood transfusions in patients with severe gastroduodenal hemorrhage, who were probably in phase 3 of Howarth and Sharpey-Schafer, and in whom the cardiac output probably fell as the result of the transfusion (instead of increasing as it would normally, according to Sharpey-Schafer[13]).

AZOTEMIA

The frequent occurrence of azotemia following hematemesis and melena has been confirmed by numerous observers, since it was first pointed out by Sanguinetti,[14] in 1933, in cases of bleeding gastric and duodenal ulcer. The writer and his associates[15] reported an elevation of the blood urea nitrogen to 30 mg. per cent or more in about two-thirds, and elevation of 50 mg. per cent or more in one-fifth of 135 cases of hematemesis or melena due to various causes. Following a single nonfatal hemorrhage, the blood urea nitrogen may increase within a few hours, and usually reaches a maximum within 24 hours, dropping sharply to normal by the third day[16] (Fig. 23-1).

The rate of subsidence of the azotemia can be increased by slow-drip blood transfusion, but not by infusion of plasma in a comparable amount.[17] In cases in which there is a second (nonfatal) hemorrhage, there is a secondary increase within 24 hours, with a drop to normal by the third day. In cases in which repeated hemorrhages occur and ultimately prove fatal, there is an increasingly or persistently high level of the urea nitrogen in the blood. The kidneys have generally been found normal at autopsy.

The mechanism of the azotemia is not the same as that associated with high intestinal obstruction, because it occurs in the absence of any vomiting (that is, in the presence of melena alone) and is associated with a nor-

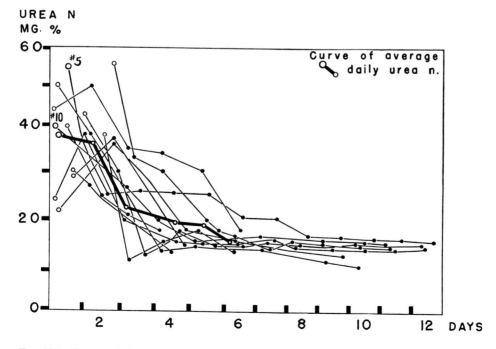

FIG. 23-1. Repeated determinations of the value for blood urea nitrogen in 12 cases of single hemorrhage followed by recovery. (Arch. Int. Med. 64:1239–1251)

mal or increased blood chloride concentration and a normal carbon dioxide combining power of the blood.

Other things being equal, the degree of azotemia is determined by the amount of blood entering the intestinal tract in a given period of time. The time factor is important, since it has been shown that, if a given quantity of blood is introduced into the gastrointestinal tract over a period of days, the maximum elevation of the blood urea nitrogen obtained on any single day may be much less than if a fraction of the blood is given quickly. (Thus, the administration of 250 ml. of citrated human blood daily to a control subject for 8 days yielded a maximum blood urea nitrogen value of 26 mg. per cent; whereas giving 1,000 ml. of blood intragastrically during a half hour yielded a maximum elevation of 47 mg. per cent[18] (Fig. 23-2). The time element may explain the disparity between the degree of anemia and the level of the blood urea nitrogen in some patients with hematemesis. Thus, if a patient loses 2,000 ml. of blood over a period of 8 days, one might not expect the same degree of elevation of the blood urea nitrogen which would follow the

sudden loss of this quantity of blood, although comparable degrees of anemia might develop.

The azotemia occurs irrespective of the cause of hemorrhage into the upper digestive tract. It does not appear in hemorrhage from the colon, a fact that may prove of value in differential diagnosis. It does not follow the sudden withdrawal of as much as 1,150 ml. of blood in control subjects, except in the presence of renal impairment.[10]

The factors that may influence the azotemia include *dehydration, shock, impairment of renal function, increased catabolism of tissue protein*, and *absorption of products of decomposition of the blood liberated into the intestinal tract.* Observations on both man and animals indicate the importance of the digestion and the absorption of the blood liberated into the intestinal tract in the production of the azotemia.[18,19,20,21,22] Black,[9] although admitting the role of the blood in the intestinal tract, nevertheless believes that functional renal failure, resulting from a fall in the pressure and the amount of the blood supplied to the kidneys, plays an important role at the time the blood urea nitrogen is ris-

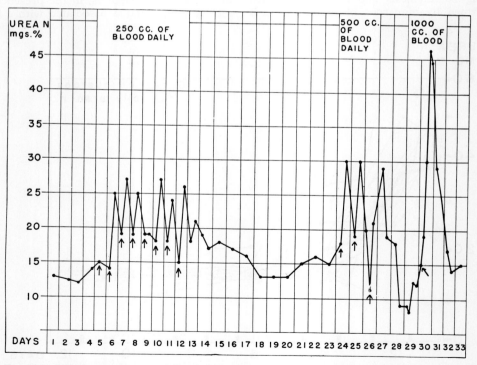

Fig. 23-2. Blood urea nitrogen following intragastric administration of varying quantities of citrated blood in one patient. (Am. J. Digest. Dis. 6:597–602)

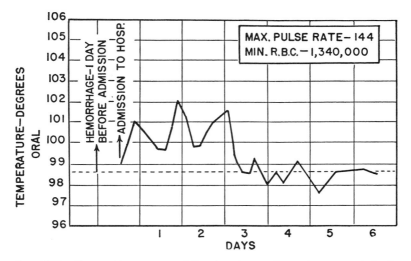

FIG. 23-3. Temperature curve following hemorrhage in case of J. P. (bleeding gastric ulcer).

ing. He believes that the rise of the blood urea which follows the giving of large amounts of blood by mouth is smaller and slower in onset than the azotemia of severe hematemesis. The observations of Gregory *et al.*[22] in experimental animals indicate that the azotemia may be due to decreased renal function caused by low blood pressure and dehydration or to absorption of digested blood protein. They found the rise in the blood urea nitrogen that followed mainte- nance of a low blood pressure through bleed-

ing to be slower and more sustained than that which followed the giving of blood by stomach tube.

Although functional renal failure may oc- cur in the presence of shock, it is not essential to the genesis of the azotemia. This is sub- stantiated by the production of azotemia through the intragastric administration of blood to individuals without obvious renal disease (producing in some instances a curve almost exactly the same as that which fol- lowed hematemesis in the same subject), by

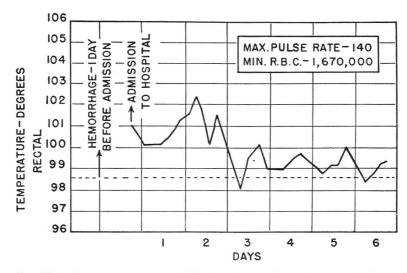

FIG. 23-4. Temperature curve following hemorrhage in case of J. W. (bleeding duodenal ulcer).

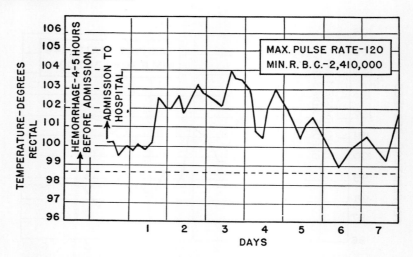

FIG. 23-5. Temperature curve following hemorrhage in case of L. G. (gastric carcinoma).

the demonstration that the introduction of such blood does not cause impairment of renal function, and by the demonstration of normal renal function in the presence of azotemia.[23]

We thoroughly endorse Black's statement that "the level to which the blood urea nitrogen rises is of value in judging the severity of gastroduodenal hemorrhage and repeated estimation a good measure of progress." In a series of 135 cases, the writer and his associates[15] reported a maximum blood urea nitrogen of less than 30 mg. per cent to be a favorable prognostic sign in patients with hematemesis due to peptic ulcer, hepatic

cirrhosis, or undetermined cause. Exceptions noted were two cases of ruptured aortic aneurysm and one of perforated peptic ulcer. (Subsequent observations include a fatal case of bleeding peptic ulcer without significant elevation of the blood urea nitrogen, in which death was due to pneumonia.) The presence of a maximum blood urea nitrogen content of 50 mg. per cent or more was followed by a fatal outcome in *one third* of the cases, whereas an elevation of 70 mg. per cent or more was accompanied by a fatal outcome in about *two thirds* of the cases. In interpreting azotemia in a given case, one should keep in mind that the blood urea nitrogen

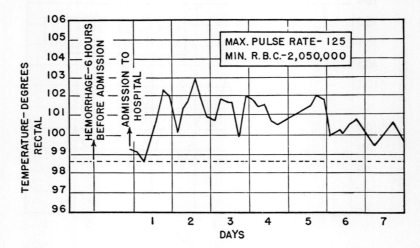

FIG. 23-6. Temperature curve following hemorrhage in case of F. W. (hepatic cirrhosis with ruptured esophageal varix).

level may be affected by such complicating factors as starvation, dehydration, alkalosis, or pre-existing renal disease. In our experience, a blood urea nitrogen content of over 100 mg. per cent has been found to indicate pre-existing kidney disease. Evidently the functional renal failure and the amount of blood entering the intestinal tract are, clinically, not sufficient to produce a degree of azotemia above this level.

FEVER

Fever occurs in the majority of patients with hematemesis and melena, irrespective of the cause of hemorrhage (Figs. 23-3 to 23-6). It usually appears within 24 hours, lasts from a few days to a week or slightly longer, and may reach a maximum of 103°. It more frequently follows massive or moderately severe than mild hemorrhage.

The cause of the fever is not known. Ac-

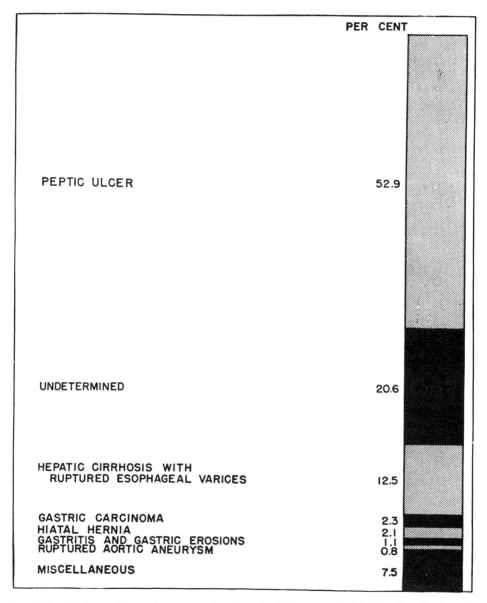

FIG. 23-7. Etiology of hematemesis and melena in 640 cases admitted to the Cincinnati General Hospital over a 10-year period.

TABLE 23-1.

ETIOLOGY OF UPPER GASTROINTESTINAL BLEEDING IN 5,192 CASES—12 AUTHORS—YEARS 1950-57*

	PEPTIC ULCER	ESOPHAGEAL VARICES	GASTRITIS	GASTRIC CANCER	HIATUS HERNIA	OTHER	UNDETER- MINED
Average	65%	9%	11%†	1%	2%	2%	10%

* Data from Gray, S. J., *et al.*: Med. Clin. N. Am. 41:1327.
† Acute ulceration gastroscopically observed; not seen by x-ray.

TABLE 23-2. CAUSES OF BLEEDING (1,400 PATIENTS WITH UPPER-GASTROINTESTINAL HEMORRHAGE) 1946-1969*

	NO. OF PATIENTS	% OF PATIENTS
Duodenal ulcer	388	27.71
Varices	262	18.71
Gastric ulcer	176	12.57
Gastritis	174	12.43
Esophagitis	93	6.64
Esophagogastritis	16	1.14
Mallory-Weiss syndrome	72	5.14
Anastomotic ulcer	42	3.00
24 other diagnoses	79	5.64
Undetermined or incorrect	98	7.00
Total	1,400	99.98

* Palmer, E. D.: The vigorous diagnostic approach to upper-gastrointestinal tract hemorrhage, J.A.M.A. 207: 1477, 1969.

cording to Dill and Isenhour,[24] numerous factors have been invoked, including absorption of blood decomposition products, reduction in blood volume, anemia, associated gastritis, or increased lability of the heat-regulating center as a result of asthenia or shock. The absorption of blood decomposition products has been considered the most likely cause by a number of European observers. Black[9] suggests that the fever may possibly be related to the endogenous breakdown of the body protein which may occur after hemorrhage. However, the experimental observations of Dill and Isenhour, both in man and animals, and our own observations in man[25] indicate that the intragastric administration of large quantities of citrated blood is not followed by any significant elevation of temperature. Incidentally, no change in the white-blood-cell count followed the administration of such blood.

ETIOLOGY

Vomiting of blood or the passage of tarry stools may be due to a variety of disorders. The most common of these is bleeding peptic ulcer. Alsted[26] has pointed out that reports on the etiology of gastrointestinal hemorrhage coming from various clinics seem to fall into two groups. In the first, the cause of the hemorrhage was almost always determined, with peptic ulcer comprising about three-fourths of the cases; in the second, the cause of the hemorrhage was undetermined in from one-fourth to one-half of the cases. He indicates that the patients in the first group were admitted to institutions treating selected chronically ill patients, whereas those of the second group entered municipal hospitals dealing largely with acutely ill patients.

In our own experience with 640 cases of hematemesis and melena admitted to the Cincinnati General Hospital over a ten-year period (1937-1947), peptic ulcer comprised 339, or 52.9 per cent of the causes; the cause was undetermined in 132, or 20.6 per cent; hepatic cirrhosis was present in 80, or 12.5 per cent; gastric carcinoma in 15, or 2.3 per cent; hiatal hernia in 14, or 2.1 per cent; gastritis with mucosal erosions in 7, or 1.1 per cent; aortic aneurysm rupturing into the esophagus in 5, or 0.8 per cent; and miscellaneous causes were found in 48, or 7.5 per cent (Fig. 23-7).

The etiologic factors in other series of cases[27,28] are listed in Tables 23-1 and 23-2. In Palmer's series, the diagnoses were based on the author's "vigorous diagnostic approach," which consists of ice water lavage of the stomach as soon as the history and physical examination have been completed, followed by immediate esophagogastroscopic and contrast roentgenologic examinations. Using this type of approach, Palmer reports a diagnostic accuracy of 87.1 per cent in 650 patients, as compared with an accuracy of 34.9 per cent obtained in 212 patients using the classical approach. The advantage of Palmer's method lies in the greater frequency with which bleeding can be traced, as contrasted with the mere demonstration of a lesion capable of explaining bleeding.

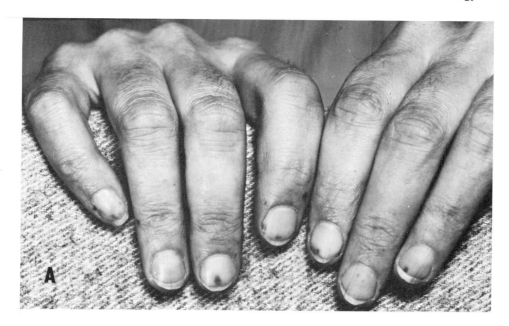

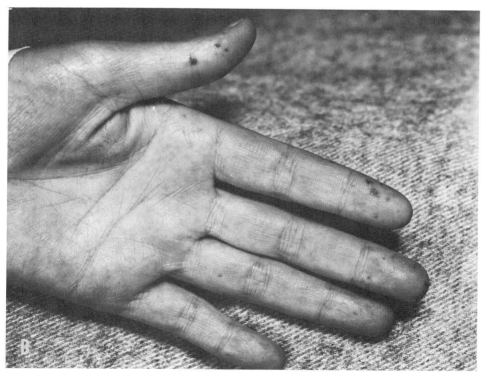

Fig. 23-8. Osler's disease. Telangiectatic lesions with characteristic punctate areas on the palmar surface of the fingers and the typical diffuse, sometimes linear spots under the nails. These ordinarily do not have very sharply defined margins. (Bean, W. B.: Vascular Spiders and Related Lesions of the Skin, Springfield, Ill., Thomas)

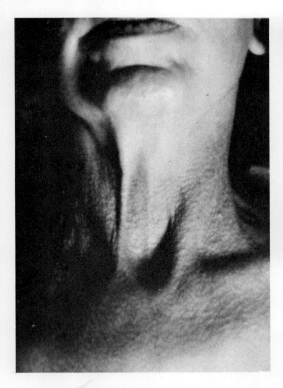

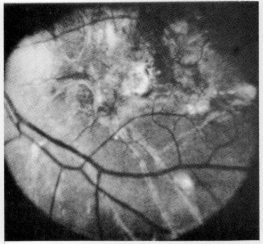

Fig. 23-10. Angioid streaks and proliferative changes in fundus oculi. (McKusick, V. A.: Heritable Disorders of Connective Tissue, ed. 2, St. Louis, Mosby)

Fig. 23-9. Pseudoxanthoma elasticum, revealing the leathery, ridged, yellowish skin of the anterior portion of the neck. (Bean, W. B.: Vascular Spiders and Related Lesions of the Skin, Springfield, Ill., Thomas)

HISTORY AND PHYSICAL EXAMINATION

Inquiry should be made regarding bleeding tendencies during childhood and early adulthood which, if present, should suggest a blood dyscrasia. A family history of gastrointestinal bleeding is suggestive of hemophilia or Osler-Rendu-Weber disease. Questioning should be directed toward eliciting a history of ingestion of drugs capable of inducing gastrointestinal bleeding, such as steroids, aspirin, butazolidin, and rauwolfia alkaloids. A history of alcoholism should favor erosive gastritis or bleeding esophageal varices. The passage of possible tarry stools should be checked by inquiry regarding concomitant faintness or weakness, ingestion of iron and bismuth compounds, and the eating of licorice candy or foods which may discolor the stools. The typical peptic ulcer syndrome may frequently be absent prior to ulcer bleeding. *Prominent heartburn* and belching and epigastric or low substernal discomfort or pain,

particularly in the recumbent position and brought on by large meals or by stooping over as in lacing one's shoes, should suggest the presence of a hiatal hernia.

The examination of a patient with massive hematemesis or melena must, of necessity be cursory. Attention should be concentrated on pulse rate, blood pressure, and general appearance. Icterus, if present, should direct attention to disease of the liver, as should the presence of vascular spiders on the face, neck, upper trunk, or upper limbs. Search should be made on the skin of the face, the lips, the mucocutaneous junction, and the mucous surfaces of the mouth for the brownish, freckle-like melanin spots of the Peutz-Jeghers syndrome. The telangiectasia of the Osler-Rendu-Weber syndrome are usually reddish (occasionally purplish) and are commonest on the lips, the tongue, the ears, the fingers, and the toes, and frequently can be demonstrated to pulsate (Fig. 23-8). Also to be looked for are the skin changes characteristic of pseudoxanthoma elasticum: the yellowish discoloration and the lax, redundant and relatively inelastic quality with thickening and a grooved appearance of "coarse Moroccan leather."[29,30] According to McKusick, the regions prone to be involved are the face, the neck, the axillary folds, the cubital areas, the inguinal folds, and the periumbilical area[31] (Fig. 23-9). Examination of the ocular fundi may reveal the angioid streaks of pseudoxanthoma elasti-

Fɪɢ. 23-11. Photograph of x-ray film showing esophageal varices in a case of hepatic cirrhosis (patient R. R.).

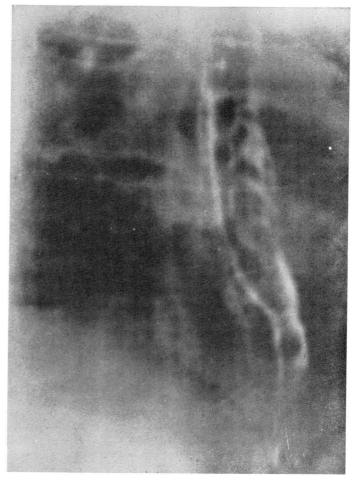

cum.[31] These streaks are brownish or gray, are four or five times wider than veins, and resemble vessels (Fig. 23-10). The left supra-clavicular space should be felt for the presence of "sentinel glands." The time-honored practice of palpating the abdomen gently and briefly in cases of upper digestive tract hemorrhage for fear of reinducing bleeding by the usual form of palpation is no longer tenable. It is indeed difficult to picture dislodgement of a clot from an esophageal varix by pressing on the abdomen. Hemostasis in the capillary bleeding of erosive gastritis and esophagitis is said to be accomplished by the prevention of filling of the injured capillaries through the opening of arteriovenous shunts of the mucosal vascular system, rather than by clot formation.[28] Furthermore, the importance of surface clotting in the hemostasis of bleeding peptic ulcer has been seriously questioned.[28]

A palpable liver of increased consistency should strongly suggest the presence of hepatic cirrhosis, as should the presence of splenomegaly, ascites, vascular spiders, or distended veins over the chest and the abdomen. It should be remembered that the spleen contracts after hemorrhage, and thus, for a time may not be palpable. It is needless to add that the presence of an abdominal tumor should suggest carcinoma. Search for the characteristic continuous murmur of splenic arteriovenous fistula should be made over the lower left posterolateral ribs in young patients with suspected portal hypertension and hypersplenism in the absence of hepato-megaly and abnormal liver function tests.[32]

X-RAY EXAMINATION

The great value of x-ray examination in furnishing direct evidence of peptic ulcer or gastric cancer need only be mentioned in

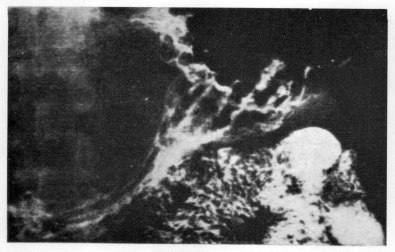

Fig. 23-12. Film showing a lobulated mass at the esophagogastric junction.
(Karr, S., and Wohl, G. T.: New England J. Med. 263:667)

passing. Unfortunately, the roentgenogram has proved to be of little value in the diagnosis of gastritis.[33] Gastric erosions are rarely demonstrated roentgenologically. Roentgen examination may prove of particular value in the diagnosis of esophageal varices (Fig. 23-11), and may furnish the sole anatomic evidence of hepatic cirrhosis.[34]

In an excellent discussion of the subject, Schatzki[34] points out that the principle of roentgen visualization of esophageal varices rests on the fact that the dilated veins bulge into the lumen of the esophagus and produce an "uneven wormlike surface." Large varices may be detected fluoroscopically, whereas small ones may be visible only on a roentgenogram. Occasionally varices may be seen in the cardiac end of the stomach and be mistaken for the enlarged folds of a localized hypertrophic gastritis, or even for a tumor[35]

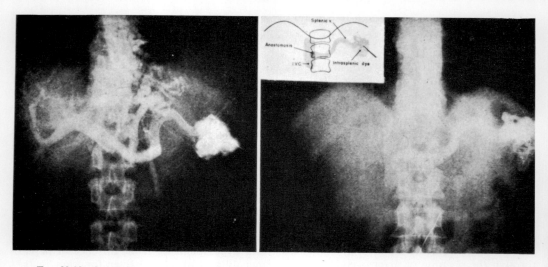

Fig. 23-13. Splenoportogram in Laennec's cirrhosis with bleeding varices. (*Left*) Preoperative study. The coronary and short gastric veins are dilated and there are gastric and esophageal varices. There is backflow into the inferior mesenteric vein. The portal radicles in the liver are attenuated. Intrasplenic pressure 28.5 cm. (*Right*) Repeat study two months after portacaval shunt. The anastomosis is patent and there is no collateral filling. Splenic pressure, 16 cm. (Ann. Int. Med. 52:782)

(Fig. 23-12). He advises that the examination be made with the patient in the horizontal position, as varices become smaller in the erect position. He uses a suspension of equal parts of barium and water, and advises coating the inner surface of the esophagus with only a thin layer of barium, because filling the organ with a large amount of the opaque medium will obliterate the protruding vessels. Films should be taken in several projections after slight inspiration, since during this phase the lower end of the esophagus is stretched slightly, thus avoiding misinterpreting of tortuous folds in a slack esophagus. Nelson[36] recommends the admixture of carboxymethylcellulose (0.25 to 0.75 per cent) to increase the adherence of the barium to the esophageal and gastric mucosa, or the administration of atropine, 0.5 to 1.0 mg., subcutaneously 30 minutes before the examination. He stresses the value of the Valsalva maneuver in demonstrating varices and states that the Müller maneuver may occasionally show varices when all other methods have failed. Barium studies of the esophagus are much less reliable than either esophagoscopy or splenoportography for the demonstration of esophageal varices.[47] It has been estimated that the radiologist is only able to visualize varices in about 30 to 50 per cent of the cases.[36] Even when special techniques are employed, only 70 per cent are said to be demonstrated.[37]

It was formerly customary to defer roentgenologic examination of the upper digestive tract in patients with hematemesis or melena until two or three weeks after the hemorrhage. The reason for this delay was the fear of reinducing hemorrhage through the manipulation of the abdomen. The disadvantage of deferring the examination has been twofold: (1) an ulcer may heal within one to three

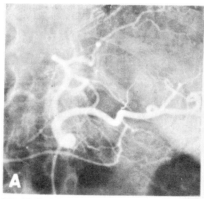
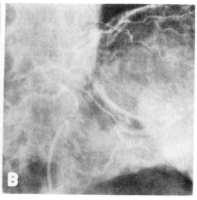
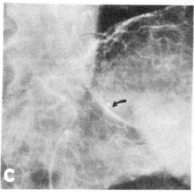

Fig. 23-14. Arteriographic demonstration of gastric bleeding secondary to a peptic ulcer. (A) Early arterial phase of the celiac arteriogram demonstrating excellent filling of the splenic, right and left gastric arteries. The hepatic artery had an anomalous origin from the superior mesenteric artery. (B) In the midarterial phase a crescent-like accumulation of contrast material extends from a branch of the left gastric artery in the upper portion of the body of the stomach. (C) At the end of the arterial phase residual contrast material can be seen within the stomach (arrow) indicating the site of bleeding.

At surgery a large 2 cm. benign gastric ulcer was found with an edematous 2 cm. border on each side. At the base of the ulcer crater was a large arterial bleeder. (Baum, Stanley et al.: Clinical application of selective celiac and superior mesenteric arteriography, Radiology 84:279, 1965)

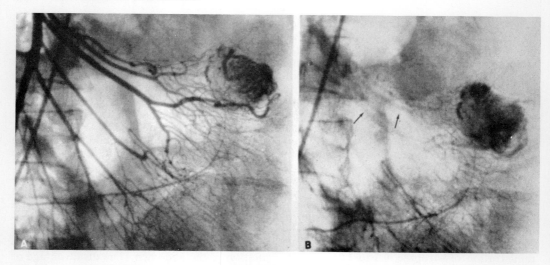

Fig. 23-15. Superior mesenteric angiography in a 54-year-old woman with a jejunal leiomyoma. (A) Early arterial phase. Anteroposterior projection. Branches of the first and second jejunal arteries supply the markedly vascular lesion. Distorted vessels and newly formed vascular spaces are seen. (B) Late arterial phase. Anteroposterior projection. A well circumscribed area of contrast accumulation is present. Early venous drainage is indicated by arrows. (Boijsen, Erick et al.: Angiography in diagnosis of chronic unexplained melena, Radiology 89:413, 1967)

weeks after hemorrhage (Benedict,[2] Hampton,[38] Jones[3] and Schiff[39]) and thus escape detection, and (2) it withholds the means of establishing promptly the diagnosis of peptic ulcer in patients past 50 years of age with

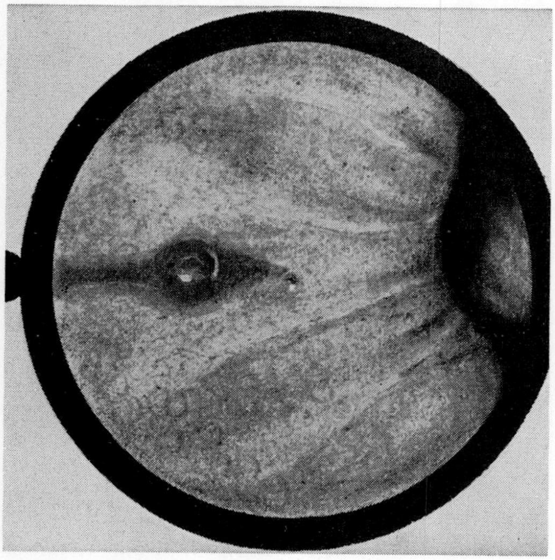

Fig. 23-16. Photograph of drawing of a bleeding mucosal erosion seen at gastroscopy. There was associated hypertrophic gastritis as evidenced by the polygonal pattern of the nearby mucosa.

massive hemorrhage, in whom emergency surgery may be contemplated.

Hampton[38] devised a technique for the roentgenologic demonstration of bleeding duodenal ulcers in which neither abdominal palpation nor compression is used, in order to obviate the danger of reinducing hemorrhage if such existed.

At the Cincinnati General Hospital, the Hampton technique has been carried out since 1938 in many patients with severe hematemesis and melena, often within a few hours after admission to the hospital. The procedure has proved to be quite safe and of great value in establishing an early diagnosis in cases of severe gastroduodenal hemorrhage. In a series of unselected cases[40] examined by this method during a one-year period, a diagnostic accuracy of 86 per cent was obtained. Early radiologic examination of the upper digestive tract has been carried out with a portable x-ray apparatus.[41] Four ounces of barium suspension are drunk as rapidly as possible by the patient, who is then turned into the right lateral position with the film cassette and grid beneath him. An exposure is made in this position, followed in quick succession by right anterior oblique, right posterior oblique, and anteroposterior projections.

Esophageal varices may also be demonstrated by means of percutaneous spleno-portal venography (Fig. 23-13).

Angiography is being used increasingly in the localization of bleeding sites in the gastro-intestinal tract as well as in the detection of lesions producing hemorrhage[42-46] (Figs. 23-14 and 23-15).

A radiopaque tube progressively passed through the intestinal tract with suction induced at various levels, followed by introduction of an x-ray opaque medium when aspirated material gives a positive test for occult blood, may reveal sites of bleeding which escape detection when conventional methods are used.[47,48]

ESOPHAGOSCOPY AND GASTROSCOPY

The mere demonstration of esophageal varices by x-ray examination or endoscopy prior to an episode of bleeding is no proof that they are the actual source of hemorrhage. The purpose of performing esophagoscopy in the presence of upper gastrointestinal hemorrhage is not only to determine the presence (or absence) of esophageal varices, but to see if they are bleeding. The hazard incurred by the procedure has been exaggerated. In the hands of the particularly interested and experienced esophagoscopist it is minimal.[28,49] As Smith[49] has indicated, "esophagoscopy in the presence of actively bleeding esophageal varices is not for the occasional endoscopist."

In addition to being prerequisite in the clinical diagnosis of gastritis, gastroscopy is particularly valuable in revealing erosions or small superficial or acute ulcers that usually are not demonstrable on roentgen examina-

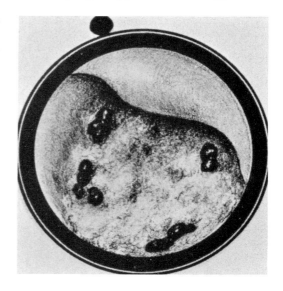

Fig. 23-18. Photograph of drawing made at gastroscopy of a large benign gastric ulcer containing several large clots (patient C. F.). There was no antecedent history of hematemesis or melena. The lesion disappeared following medical therapy.

tion (Figs. 23-16 and 23-17). In some cases of gastritis, there may be oozing from the mucosa without definite erosion (Benedict,[50] Schindler[51]), and in others, fresh or old blood may be seen without demonstrable erosion (Benedict[50]). Schindler[52] believed that hemorrhagic erosions may occur in the absence of demonstrable gastritis, and our experience would confirm this view. The erosions are

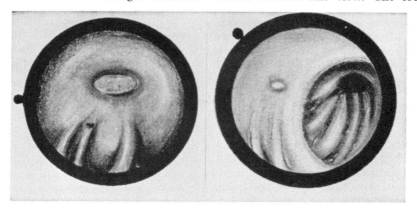

Fig. 23-17. (*Left*) Photograph of drawing of superficial gastric ulcer made at gastroscopy 3 days after massive hematemesis. (*Right*) Gastroscopic findings after 15 days on Meulengracht diet. Note marked reduction in size of ulcer.

small, usually less than 5 mm. in diameter, and deep. They may be reddish, grayish-red or brownish-red in color. Occasionally a gastric ulcer containing clots may be seen without an antecedent or subsequent history of hemorrhage (Fig. 23-18).

Mucosal hemorrhages may not necessarily be significant, since they may be present in the normal stomach. Ruffin and Brown[53] believe that they may result when suction is employed prior to introduction of the gastroscope. In this connection, the important observations that Wolf and Wolff[54] made in their experimental subject must be kept in mind, namely, that acceleration of acid production and motor activity were always accompanied by hyperemia and engorgement of the mucosa. When vascular engorgement was prolonged, the rugae became intensely red, thick, and turgid, presenting the picture of what has been called hypertrophic gastritis. In this state, the mucosa was unusually fragile, hemorrhages and small erosions resulting from the most minor traumata.

Since it is known that erosions may heal within a few days and that peptic ulcers may heal within two weeks, it is most desirable to perform gastroscopy within two or three days after hemorrhage. Jones[3] performed successful gastroscopy mainly between the third and tenth day following hemorrhage in 116 out of 217 cases without radiologic proof of peptic ulcer (the so-called acute lesion group). A gastric ulcer was found in 65 of these cases, and valuable diagnostic information was obtained in 31 additional instances.

BLEEDING PEPTIC ULCER

According to Crohn[55] and Hurst,[56] the frequency of hemorrhage in peptic ulcer is probably about 10 per cent, if patients who are not admitted to the hospital as well as hospital patients are included. Hemorrhage in patients with peptic ulcer is generally due to erosion of an artery lying at the base of the ulcer. Ulcers on the posterior wall of the superior portion of the duodenum are unusually prone to bleed. In some cases, the stomach itself may be eroded as the result of an associated gastritis (Benedict,[2] Alsted[26]). Chronic gastric ulcers are apt to bleed more severely than duodenal ulcers, probably because of erosion of larger-sized arteries, i.e., the main trunks of the right or the left gastric arteries, as compared with branches of the gastroduodenal or pancreaticoduodenal arteries.[57]

In discussing cases of bleeding peptic ulcer, Jones[3] states:

At necropsy it was usual to find one large open vessel in the floor of the ulcer, and it was remarkable that death had occurred usually not quickly but after several recurrent bleedings in the course of as many days. Bleeding with acute collapse must have occurred from the large exposed vessel, not once but perhaps six times. It would seem probable that in most cases bleeding from such a large vessel could have occurred for only a short period, perhaps 10 to 15 minutes, and then ceased. At operation the vessel usually did not begin to spurt until it was manipulated.

If the loss of blood is severe, there is a prompt fall in blood pressure, which in itself, if not too great, is advantageous, since it helps curtail further bleeding. Clotting of the blood serves to close the opening in the blood vessel. Effectual sealing of the vascular wall is furthered by the retraction of the open end of the artery. Only after a few days does the clot begin to harden. It is apparent that if the eroded artery is sclerotic it may not be able to retract sufficiently to prevent further bleeding, which may prove fatal.

It is generally agreed that during hunger the stomach exhibits active contractions, and it is conceivable that such contractions may dislodge the clot. The administration of food has a quieting effect on these hunger contractions (Christensen[58]). This fact, among others, led Meulengracht[59] to begin the immediate feeding of patients suffering from bleeding peptic ulcers. Most reports, including our own,[60] indicate that immediate feeding has resulted in a substantial reduction in mortality and a shortening of hospital stay.

The relative frequency of hematemesis versus melena varies in different statistics. In hospital cases, hematemesis accompanied by melena occurs more frequently than melena alone. This may be explained by the fact that melena may be unnoticed or disregarded by the ambulatory patient, whereas hematemesis is more apt to cause him to seek hospital care.

Hemorrhage is an indication of activity of the ulcerative process. It is said to occur rarely in patients under strict treatment. In most cases, ulcerlike symptoms precede hemorrhage for varying periods of time, usually for many years. In some cases, however, there are no antecedent symptoms, or symptoms have been present for only a few days or weeks.

Disappearance of pain for weeks or longer

following hemorrhage has been pointed out by Hurst[56] and has been quite striking in our experience. The cause of this phenomenon is not clear. In some instances it has been found to be associated with actual healing of the ulcer. It is possible that the lack of gastric tone occurring as a result of the anemia may play a role (Carlson[61]). Bonney and Pickering[62] suggest that the blood in the crater may increase the thickness of the protective layer of slough, which may cover the pain nerve endings and hinder their excitation by the hydrochloric acid. Another explanation of the initial loss of pain may be the neutralizing effect of the blood in the stomach on the gastric acidity.[63]

The symptoms of bleeding peptic ulcer depend upon the severity of the hemorrhage. In mild cases there may be little more than hematemesis or melena. In more severe hemorrhage there may be weakness, dizziness, faintness, excessive perspiration, thirst, or actual syncope and shock. Headache may be quite severe; in several of our patients, this was relieved by inhalation of oxygen or by a blood transfusion. Hematemesis may precede or follow the passage of loose tarry stools. Syncope, not infrequently, takes place in the bathroom, and may be due to a fall in blood pressure upon assumption of the erect position. In this connection, Wallace and Sharpey-Schafer[10] reported syncope fol-lowing assumption of the erect position as long as 5 or 6 hours after venesection in some of their control subjects. They found that the rapid removal of from 900 to 1,150 ml. of blood resulted in an exaggerated "postural response" in every instance immediately following the removal.

In one patient with duodenal ulcer and a rather severe hemorrhage manifesting itself by melena, the first complaint was marked shortness of breath, which she experienced after climbing two flights of stairs on her way to dinner. Earlier in the day she fainted at the hairdresser's, and she had felt faint on two other occasions. She had passed a tarry stool the day before the attack of dyspnea, but recalled this only after passing several more tarry stools the following day. Another patient felt a little weak and sweated a little after a round of golf on a cool October day. He was driven home by a friend. Before entering his home, he sat on the porch, but grew weaker and became frightened. He called his family physician, who advised a suppository. He noticed that his stool was black, but he went to bed without notifying anyone. He passed three black stools during the night, and the following morning fainted in the bathroom. Another patient, not included in this study, became a little faint and sweated as he was dictating a letter to his stenographer. That night he passed

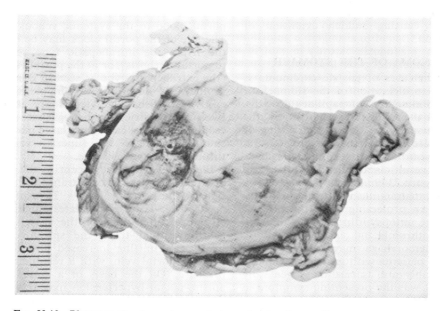

Fig. 23-19. Photograph of specimen of stomach showing malignant gastric ulcer with a gaping sclerotic artery in its base (patient J. S.).

be bleeding from esophageal varices, and were less apt to be bleeding from sites other than varices, than those who bled without hepatic decompensation. Bleeding in patients who have had a recent portacaval shunt may not necessarily indicate recurrence of esophageal varices, but rather prove to be due to a peptic ulcer developing following the shunt.[102,103] In dogs, the secretion of hydrochloric acid from a Heidenhain pouch has been shown to increase greatly after portacaval transposition. This may be due to the increased effect of a humoral secretagogue that originates in the abdominal viscera and is normally inactivated by the liver.

Panke and his associates[104] have stressed the value of determining the intrasplenic pulp pressure (a measure of the portal venous pressure) in patients with upper digestive tract hemorrhage. In a series of 130 patients, they found that bleeding esophagogastric varices were never associated with a splenic pulp pressure below 250 mm. of water. Contrariwise, bleeding from other lesions was never associated with pressures above 290 mm. of water. Variceal bleeding was associated with high splenic pulp pressures regardless of the presence of shock. They reported a 90 per cent accuracy in determining the presence or absence of varices.

GASTRITIS AND ESOPHAGITIS

Gastritis has long been recognized as a cause of varying degrees of hemorrhage, particularly by European observers. This relationship has been stressed, among others, by Faber,[105] Moutier,[106] Henning,[107] and Benedict.[2] In a series of 42 cases of hemorrhage from gastritis, Benedict reported a mild degree of hemorrhage in 7, a moderate degree in 14, and a severe degree in 21. The bleeding occurring in chronic gastritis usually takes place from erosions in the mucous membrane (Figs. 23-20, 23-21), which most commonly occur on the crests of the folds. In some cases there may be oozing from the mucosa without definite erosion (Benedict,[2] Schindler[51]). Schindler believed that most of the profuse hemorrhages in gastritis occur, in the chronic hypertrophic form, from an ulceration eroding a small blood vessel. Among the 42 cases reported by Benedict, the gastritis was superficial in 13, hypertrophic in 12, atrophic in 2, "postoperative" in 5, and mixed in 10. This author stresses excessive use of alcohol as the most important etiologic factor in massive bleeding from gastritis. According to Palmer, ingestion of large amounts of alcohol during a brief period produces an acute gastritis with frequently demonstrable erosions and with return of the gastroscopic appearance to

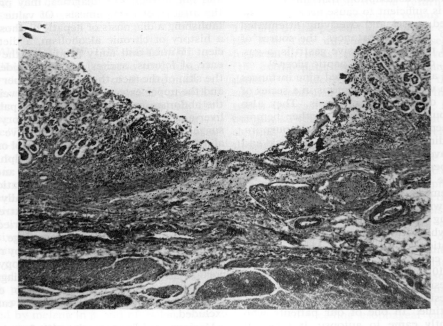

Fig. 23-20. Photomicrograph of a gastric mucosal erosion which produced fatal hemorrhage. × 30. A blood clot covers the erosion. (Dr. Ralph Fuller)

FIG. 23-21. Biopsy at edge of erosion in case of erosive esophagitis. The hemorrhage stopped about half an hour before the specimen was taken. No clot has formed on the erosion's surface, in the mucosa's capillaries, or in the other vessels. (Palmer, E. D.: Diagnosis of Upper Gastrointestinal Hemorrhage, Springfield, Ill., Thomas)

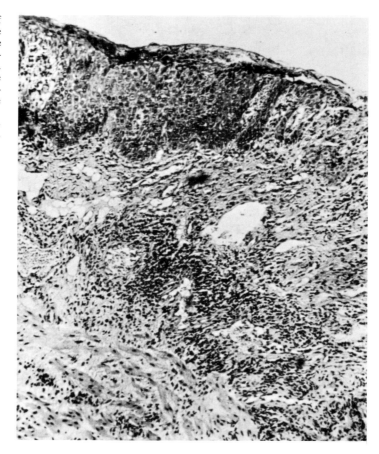

normal soon after avoidance of alcohol.[108]

Benedict[50] believes that gastritis may reasonably be assumed to be the cause of hematemesis if no other pathologic changes have been found and there is gastroscopic evidence of severe gastritis. Although we realize that this view may be correct, we have been hesitant to follow it in the absence of demonstrable erosions. In this connection, it must be realized that one is particularly apt to be in error if the gastroscopic examination is made, as is customary, two or three weeks after the hemorrhage, since erosions may heal within a few days.

The relatively high incidence of subacute erosive esophagitis and acute erosive gastritis as a cause of upper digestive tract hemorrhage in Palmer's series of cases is testimony to the diagnostic value of early endoscopy, particularly in cases where roentgenographic examination is apt to prove negative. Palmer recommends a swallow of 10 per cent fluorescin several minutes before the procedure to improve the visualization of both esophageal and gastric erosions, particularly following ice-water lavage.

HIATAL HERNIA

Bleeding in cases of hiatal hernia may be due to congestion of the blood vessels in the herniated portion of the stomach, gastritis, or ulceration.[109] There may be ulceration of the esophagogastric junction, or there may be a gastric ulcer adjacent to the neck of the sac where it passes through the diaphragm. The symptoms of hiatal hernia have been well-described.[110,111,112] At the time of admission it may be difficult to prove the hiatal hernia as the cause of the bleeding. Esophagoscopy and gastroscopy may prove helpful. In some instances presumptive proof may be based on the lack of recurrence of bleeding following repair of the hernia.

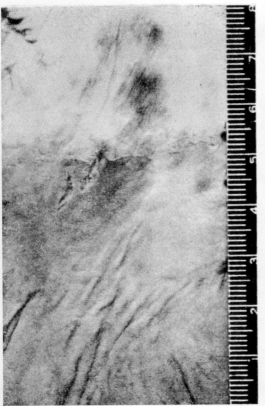

Fig. 23-22. Specimen showing two small 1 cm. lacerations just inferior to the gastro-esophageal junction. (Decker, J. P. *et. al.*: New England J. Med. 249:957)

HEMATEMESIS AND MELENA DUE TO MISCELLANEOUS CAUSES

Miscellaneous causes of hematemesis and melena found in 43 patients (48 cases) of a series of 640 cases seen at the Cincinnati General Hospital are listed in Table 23-3. Other causes include hemorrhage from localized arteriosclerosis of gastric vessels,[113] hereditary telangiectasia,[114,115,116] tumors of the small intestine,[117] rupture of aneurysm of the hepatic artery[118] or splenic artery,[119] aortic stenosis,[120] pseudoxanthoma elasticum,[29,30,31] ruptured aortic aneurysm, periarteritis nodosa,[121] jejunal diverticulosis,[122] multiple hemangiomas of the jejunum,[123] and gastric carcinoid.[124] Bleeding may also arise from Meckel's diverticulum or diverticulitis of the colon.

Hematemesis and melena have been ascribed to aspirin ingestion.[125-137] Muir and

TABLE 23-3. CAUSES OF HEMATEMESIS AND MELENA IN MISCELLANEOUS GROUP OF 43 PATIENTS OVER A 10-YEAR PERIOD

CAUSE OF HEMORRHAGE	NUMBER OF PATIENTS
Acute esophagitis with pancreatic necrosis	1
Banti's syndrome (extrahepatic block)....	2
Benign tumor of the stomach	1
Blood dyscrasia	8
Carcinoma of the esophagus	3
Chronic relapsing pancreatitis	1
Cirrhosis with esophageal diverticulum...	1
Cholecystoduodenal fistula	1
Curling's ulcer	1
Erosive esophagitis and/or erosive gastritis associated with liver disease	8
Erosion of the aorta due to periaortitis ...	1
Gastric varices	1
Lymphosarcoma of the stomach	1
Malignancy eroding the gastrointestinal tract	3
Mesenteric thrombosis	5
Prolapsed gastric mucoa	1
Ulcerative esophagitis	3
Ulcerated heterotopic gastric tissue	1

Cossar[138] found that 72 out of 157 patients admitted with upper gastrointestinal hemorrhage had taken aspirin within 24 hours of the onset of bleeding. Overt bleeding, on the other hand, may follow the ingestion of a single tablet of aspirin. Slight to intense hyperemia, and even a submucous hemorrhage, have been reported at gastroscopic examinations made upon patients following the ingestion of three crushed aspirin tablets.[126] Acute gastric erosions attributed to salicylates have been described at gastroscopy[127,128,139,140] and laparotomy.[135]

Muir and Cossar gave aspirin shortly before partial gastrectomy, and found less reaction in the resected specimens when soluble aspirin was given as contrasted with ordinary aspirin. In one case, a half aspirin tablet was found imbedded in the mucosa of the greater curvature, lying beneath overlapping edematous and congested rugae.[138] According to Winkelman and Summerskill,[131] factors involved in mucosal damage and resistance seem more important than hydrochloric acid secretion in relation to gastrointestinal bleeding following the consumption of aspirin. Aspirin is reported either to have no effects on gastric secretion of humans or animals, or, if anything, to lower gastric secretory activity.[141,142]

In experiments conducted on both dogs and rats, Menguy[143] found that aspirin administered so that the compound did not enter into contact with the gastric mucosa profoundly decreased the rate of mucous secretion. It also altered the composition of mucus in such a way as to render it theoretically less efficient as a protective barrier. "It is entirely possible then that the altered mucus production represents simply the result of aspirin-induced cellular injury which in turn might render the cells more friable, with ensuing appearance of superficial erosions." The mechanism of aspirin-produced gastric injury still requires further elucidation.

Hemorrhage from gastroesophageal lacerations at the cardiac orifice of the stomach—the so-called Mallory-Weiss syndrome[144,145]—is an uncommon cause of massive bleeding (Fig. 23-22). It occurs in alcoholics and is usually preceded by violent or protracted retching and vomiting. It may occur in the absence of alcoholism, as in the vomiting of pregnancy or even obstructing ulcer.[28] There may be one laceration,[28] or two to four as originally described. Mallory and Weiss[144] reported the lesions to be arranged characteristically around the circumference of the cardiac opening, along the longitudinal axis of the esophagus. In their report, the size of the lesions varied from 3 to 20 mm. in length and from 2 to 3 mm. in width. According to Palmer, the laceration is found at gastroscopy to be a straight cleft running roughly parallel to the esophageal axis. The cleft is usually an estimated centimeter in length and rarely may extend for as many as 4 centimeters. A characteristic feature of the laceration is rather steep elevation of its edges, with fairly wide gaping. The cleft is always filled with clot and it is presumed that the ridge-like elevation is due to bleeding beneath the laceration's edges. Mallory and Weiss considered the pressure changes in the stomach during the disturbed mechanism of vomiting, together with regurgitation of the gastric juice and the corrosive effect of alcohol, to be responsible for the lesions described in their cases.

Heuer[146] reported a case in which the pathologist failed to find any erosion of the mucosa of the stomach or duodenum, but, upon injecting the gastric artery with saline from a pressure bottle, he was able to observe a jet of fluid from the mucosal lining. Serial sections of the area showed a small ruptured aneurysm concealed by overlying, mucosal folds. It appears quite plausible that this type

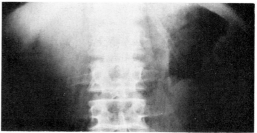

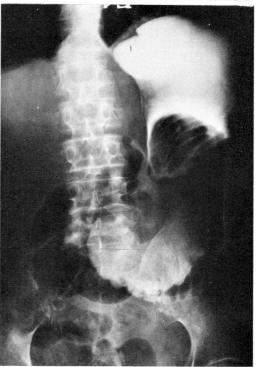

Fig. 23-23. (*Top*) A lobulated mass is shown projecting into the lumen of the distal stomach. (*Bottom*) Following a barium swallow, the mass in the stomach shows valvulae conniventes on its surface. There is obstruction of the duodenum and proximal jejunum secondary to the intussusception.

of lesion may be the underlying cause of hemorrhage in some otherwise unexplained cases.

Retrograde jejunogastric intussusception occurs more often in women than in men, is much more frequent after gastroenterostomy than after gastric resection, and may occur as long as 18 years after the operation, with an average interval of 6 years[147] (Fig. 23-23). In the majority of cases, vomiting of food and bile precedes hematemesis. A mass may be palpable above and to the left of the umbilicus in more than half of the cases. The x-ray finding within the lumen of the stomach of a partially moving filling defect simulating the normal pattern of small intestinal folds (Kerckring folds or valvulae conniventes) is characteristic.

Fistulization between the intestinal tract and an abdominal aortic prosthesis is a common cause of late graft failure and usually occurs at suture lines that are contiguous with bowel loops.[148] "Any massive gastrointestinal hemorrhage after an abdominal aortic operation should be considered of aortic origin until proved otherwise."[148]

Massive gastrointestinal bleeding may result from hemorrhage into the bile ducts.[149-153] Hemobilia, as this condition has been called, is most commonly due to aneurysm of the hepatic artery or liver trauma. Sparkman[150,151] stressed the triad of abdominal injury, gastrointestinal hemorrhage and biliary colic as highly suggestive of traumatic hemobilia. The pain is characteristic of biliary colic and the patient, having previously experienced such pain before bleeding, may rightly warn the physician that he is about to bleed again. Transient jaundice is a common accompaniment. An intrahepatic cavity that periodically empties its contents into the biliary tract is the basis of the syndrome. According to Schatzki,[153] scintillating scanning of the liver may reveal that the hepatic cavity is acting as the source of the bleeding. In a recent case report, the bleeding originated in an hepatic abscess.[154]

Pseudoxanthoma elasticum should be recognized by the characteristic skin changes and the angioid streaks in the retina. Superficial ulceration has been observed at gastroscopy and in the resected stomach. In some cases, gastroscopy soon after hematemesis has been negative.[155] The bleeding point may be in the duodenum, or there may be multiple bleeding points in other part of the intestine.

SUMMARY

Bleeding into the gastrointestinal tract may be brought to the attention of the patient and the physician through vomiting of blood (hematemesis) or through the detection of blood in the stools (melena).

Pathogenic mechanisms include (1) conditions involving the tissues of the walls of the gastrointestinal tract, (2) disorders of blood vessel walls, and (3) disturbances of blood clotting.

The most common clinical causes are peptic ulcer, esophageal varices associated with hepatic cirrhosis, gastric cancer, hiatus hernia, gastritis, and esophagitis. Examination by roentgenography and by gastroscopy and esophagoscopy is of great assistance in the differential diagnosis of the more usual causes of gastrointestinal bleeding.

Among the less frequent causes are blood dyscrasias, the Mallory-Weiss syndrome, mesenteric thrombosis, gastrointestinal neoplasms other than gastric carcinoma, diverticula of the alimentary tract, pseudoxanthoma elasticum, and a few rare miscellaneous conditions.

Bleeding into the gastrointestinal tract is of serious import, whether acute and dramatic or chronic and obscure. Discovery of the cause should be as prompt as possible so that proper therapy can be used to prevent death, various complications, or chronic disability.

REFERENCES

1. Ratnoff, O. D., and Patek, A. J., Jr.: The natural history of Laennec's cirrhosis of the liver; an analysis of 386 cases, Medicine 21:207, 1942.
2. Benedict, E. B.: Hemorrhage from gastritis; a report based on pathological, clinical, roentgenological and gastroscopic findings, Amer. J. Roentgen. 47:254, 1942.
3. Jones, F. A.: Haematemesis and melaena with special reference to bleeding peptic ulcer, Brit. Med. J. 2:441; 477, 1947.
4. Schiff, L., Stevens, R. J., Shapiro, N., and Goodman, S.: Observations on the oral administration of citrated blood in man; II, The effect on the stools, Amer. J. Med. Sci. 203:409, 1942.
5. Hilsman, J. H.: The color of blood-containing feces following instillation of citrated blood at various levels of the small intestine, Gastroenterology 15:131, 1950.
6. Daniel, W. A., Jr., and Egan, S.: Quantity of blood required to produce a tarry stool, J.A.M.A. 113:2232, 1939.
7. Hesser, S.: Über die Dauer von Magengeschwürblutungen, Acta Med. Scand. (supp. 59) p. 367, 1934.
8. Cullinan, E. R., and Price, R. K.: Haematemesis following peptic ulceration; prognosis and treatment, St. Barth. Hosp. Rep. 65:185, 1932.
9. Black, D. A. K.: Critical review; azotaemia in gastro-duodenal haemorrhage, Quart. J. Med. 11:77, 1942.
10. Wallace, J., and Sharpey-Schaefer, E. P.: Blood changes following controlled haemorrhage in man, Lancet 2:393, 1941.
11. Ebert, R. V., Stead, E. A., Jr., and Gibson, J. G., II: Response of normal subjects to

acute blood loss, with special reference to the mechanism of restoration of blood volume, Arch. Intern. Med. 68:578, 1941.

12. Howarth, S., and Sharpey-Schafer, E. P.: Low blood-pressure phases following haemorrhage, Lancet 1:18, 1947.

13. Sharpey-Schafer, E. P.: Transfusion and the anaemic heart, Lancet 2:296, 1945.

14. Sanguinetti, L. V.: Curvas azohemicas en las hemorragias retenidas del tubs digestiva, Arch. Argent. Enferm. Apar. Dig. y Nutr. 9:68, 1933.

15. Schiff, L., Stevens, R. J., and Moss, H. K.: The prognostic significance of the blood urea nitrogen following hematemesis or melena, Amer. J. Dig. Dis. 9:110, 1942.

16. Schiff, L., and Stevens, R. J.: Elevation of urea nitrogen content of the blood following hematemesis or melena, Arch. Intern. Med. 64:1239, 1939.

17. Black, D. A. K., and Smith, A. F.: Blood and plasma transfusion in alimentary haemorrhage, Brit. Med. J. 1:187, 1941.

18. Schiff, L., Stevens, R. J., Goodman, S., Garber, E., and Lublin, A.: Observations on the oral administration of citrated blood in man; I, The effects on the blood urea nitrogen, Amer. J. Dig. Dis. 6:597, 1939.

19. Kaump, D. H., and Parsons, J. C.: Extrarenal azotemia in gastro-intestinal hemorrhage; II, Experimental observations, Amer. J. Dig. Dis. 7:191, 1940.

20. Chunn, C. F., and Harkins, H. N.: Experimental studies on alimentary azotemia; I, Role of blood absorption from the gastrointestinal tract, Surgery 9:695, 1941.

21. ———: Alimentary azotemia due to whole blood absorption from the gastrointestinal tract, Proc. Soc. Exp. Biol. Med. 45:569, 1940.

22. Gregory, R., Ewing, P. L., and Levine, H.: Azotemia associated with gastrointestinal hemorrhage; an experimental etiologic study, Arch. Intern. Med. 75:381, 1945.

23. Stevens, R. J., Schiff, L., Lublin, A., and Garber, E. S.: Renal function and the azotemia following hematemesis, J. Clin. Invest. 19:233, 1940.

24. Dill, L. V., and Isenhour, C. E.: Observations on the incidence and cause of fever in patients with bleeding peptic ulcers, Amer. J. Dig. Dis. 5:779, 1939.

25. Schiff, L., Shapiro, N., and Stevens, R. J.: Observations on oral administration of citrated blood in man; III. The effect on temperature and the white blood cell count, Amer. J. Med. Sci. 207:465, 1944.

26. Alsted, G.: Changing Incidence of Peptic Ulcer, Copenhagen, E. Munksgaard, 1939.

27. Gray, S. J., Olson, T. E., and Manrique, J.: Hematemesis and melena, Med. Clin. N. Amer. 41:1327, 1957.

28. Palmer, E. D.: Diagnosis of Upper Gastrointestinal Hemorrhage, Pub. 443, Amer. Lect. Series, Springfield, Ill., Thomas, 1961.

29. Strandberg, J.: Pseudoxanthoma elasticum, Zbl. Haut. Geschlechtskr. 31:689, 1929.

30. McKusick, V. A.: Heritable Disorders of Connective Tissue, ed. 2, St. Louis, Mosby, 1960.

31. Grönblad, E.: Angioid streaks—pseudoxanthoma elasticum: verläüfige mitheilung, Acta Ophthal. 7:329, 1929.

32. Murray, M. J., Thal, A. P., and Greenspan, R.: Splenic arteriovenous fistulas as a cause of portal hypertension, Amer. J. Med. 29:849, 1960.

33. Ansprenger, A., and Kirklin, B. R.: The roentgenologic aspects of chronic gastritis; a critical analysis, Amer. J. Roentgen. 38:533, 1937.

34. Schatzki, R.: Roentgen demonstration of esophageal varices; its clinical importance, Arch. Surg. 41:1084, 1940.

35. Karrs, S., and Wohl, G. T.: Clinical importance of gastric varices, New Eng. J. Med. 263:665, 1960.

36. Nelson, S. W.: The roentgenologic diagnosis of esophageal varices, Amer. J. Roentgen. 77:599, 1957.

37. Leevy, C. M., Cherrick, G. R., and Davidson, C. S.: Medical progress. Portal hypertension, New Eng. J. Med. 262:397-403, 451-456, 1960.

38. Hampton, A. O.: A safe method for the roentgen demonstration of bleeding duodenal ulcers, Amer. J. Roentgen. 38:565, 1937.

39. Schiff, L.: Unpublished observation.

40. Knowles, H. C., Felson, B., Shapiro, N., and Schiff, L.: Emergency diagnosis of upper digestive tract bleeding by roentgen examination without palpation ("Hampton Technic"), Radiology 58:536, 1952.

41. Chandler, G. N., Cameron, A. D., Nunn, A. H., and Street, D. F.: Early investigations of haemetemesis, Gut 1:6, 1960.

42. Nusbaum, M., Baum, S., Blakemore, W. S., and Finkelstein, A. K.: Demonstration of intra-abdominal bleeding by selective arteriography, J.A.M.A. 191:389, 1965.

43. Nusbaum, M., and Baum, S.: Radiographic demonstration of unknown sites of gastrointestinal bleeding, Surg. Forum 14:374, 1964.

44. Annes, G., Caplan, L. H., and Heimlich, H.: Upper gastrointestinal hemorrhage—undetected site localized by selective arteriography, Arch. Surg. 94:44, 1967.

45. Boijsen, E., and Reuter, S. R.: Angiography in diagnosis of chronic unexplained melena, Radiology 89:413, 1967.

46. Baum, S., Roy, R., Finkelstein, A. K., and Blakemore, W. S.: Clinical application of selective celiac and superior mesenteric arteriography, Radiology 84:279, 1965.

47. Raskin, H.: Personal communication.

48. Morrison, J.: Personal communication.

49. Smith, H. W.: Esophagoscopy during active upper gastrointestinal hemorrhage, Conn. Med. 23:519, 1959.

50. Benedict, E. G.: Personal communication.

51. Schindler, R., in discussion on Benedict, E.

B.: Hemorrhage from gastritis; a gastro-scopic study, Amer. J. Dig. Dis. 4:657, 1937.

52. Schindler, R.: Gastroscopy, The Endoscopic Study of Gastric Pathology, ed. 2, p. 223, Chicago, Univ. of Chicago Press, 1950.

53. Ruffin, J. M., and Brown, I. W., Jr.: The significance of hemorrhagic or pigment spots as observed by gastroscopy, Amer. J. Dig. Dis. 10:60, 1943.

54. Wolf, S., and Wolff, H. G.: Human Gastric Function, ed. 2, p. 149, New York, Oxford, 1947.

55. Crohn, B. B.: Affections of the Stomach, Philadelphia, Saunders, 1927.

56. Hurst, A. F., and Stewart, M. J.: Gastric and Duodenal Ulcer, London, Oxford, 1929.

57. Shapiro, N., and Schiff, L.: Ten years' experience with bleeding peptic ulcer with emphasis on 45 fatal cases, Surgery 31:327, 1952.

58. Christensen, O., cited by Meulengracht, E.: Behandlung von Hämatemesis und Meläna mit uneingeschränkter Kost, Wien. klin. Wschr. 49:1481, 1936.

59. Meulengracht, E.: Treatment of haematemesis and melaena with food; the mortality, Lancet 2:1220, 1935.

60. Schiff, L.: The Meulengracht diet in treatment of bleeding peptic ulcer, J. Amer. Diet. Ass. 18:298, 1942.

61. Carlson, A. J.: Personal communication.

62. Bonney, G. L. W., and Pickering, G. W.: Observations on mechanism of pain in ulcer of stomach and duodenum; nature of the stimulus, Clin. Sci. 6:63, 1946.

63. Van Liere, E. J., Sleeth, C. K., and Northrup, D.: Effect of acute hemorrhage on emptying time of the stomach, Amer. J. Physiol. 117:226, 1936.

64. McLaughlin, C. W., Baker, C. P., and Sharpe, J. C.: Bleeding duodenal ulcer complicated by myocardial infarction, Nebraska Med. J. 25:266, 1940.

65. Blumgart, H. L., Schlesinger, M. J., and Zoll, P. M.: Multiple fresh coronary occlusions in patients with antecedent shock, Arch. Intern. Med. 68:181, 1941.

66. McKinlay, C. A.: Coronary insufficiency precipitated by hemorrhage from duodenal ulcer, J. Lancet 63:31, 1943.

67. Kinney, T. D., and Mallory, G. K.: Cardiac failure associated with acute anemia, New Eng. J. Med. 232:215, 1945.

68. Rasmussen, H., and Foss, M.: The electrocardiogram of acute hemorrhage from stomach and intestines, Acta Med. Scand. 111:420, 1942.

69. Scherf, D., Reinstein, H., and Klotz, S. D.: Electrocardiographic changes following hematemesis in peptic ulcer, Rev. Gastroent. 8:343, 1941.

70. Master, A. M., Dack, S., Grishman, A., Field, L. E., and Horn, H.: Acute coronary insufficiency: an entity; shock, hemorrhage and pulmonary embolism as factors in its pro-duction, J. Mount Sinai Hosp. N. Y. 14:8, 1947.

71. Davies, D. T., and Wilson, A. T. M.: Personal and clinical history in haematemesis and perforation, Lancet 2:723, 1939.

72. Gainsborough, H., and Slater, E.: A study of peptic ulcer, Brit. Med. J. 2:253, 1946.

73. Rivers, A. B.: Hemorrhage from the stomach and duodenum, in Eusterman, G. B., and Balfour, D. C. (eds.): The Stomach and Duodenum, p. 759, Philadelphia, Saunders, 1935.

74. Palmer, W. L.: Peptic ulcer, in Portis, S. A. (ed.): Diseases of the Digestive System, ed. 2, p. 208, Philadelphia, Lea & Febiger, 1944.

75. Schiff, L.: Unpublished observation.

76. Smyrniotis, F., Schenker, S., O'Donnell, J., and Schiff, L.: Lactic dehydrogenase activity in gastric juice for the diagnosis of gastric cancer, Amer. J. Dig. Dis. 7:712, 1962.

77. Snell, A. M., and Butt, H. R.: Chronic atrophy of the liver, in Barr, D. P. (ed.): Modern Medical Therapy in General Practice, p. 2,386, Baltimore, Williams & Wilkins, 1940.

78. Linton, R. R.: The surgical treatment of bleeding esophageal varices by portal systemic venous shunts, with a report of 34 cases, Ann. Intern. Med. 31:794, 1949.

79. Whipple, A. O.: Portal Bed Block and Portal Hypertension, in Advances in Surgery, vol. 2, p. 155, New York, Interscience, 1949.

80. Garrett, N., Jr., and Gall, E. A.: Esophageal varices without hepatic cirrhosis, Arch. Path. 55:196, 1953.

81. Tisdale, W. A., Klatskin, G., and Glenn, W. W. L.: Portal hypertension and bleeding esophageal varices. Their occurrence in the absence of both intrahepatic and extrahepatic obstruction of the portal vein, New Eng. J. Med. 261:209, 1959.

82. Liebowitz, H. R.: Bleeding Esophageal Varices, Portal Hypertension, Springfield, Ill., Thomas, 1959.

83. Snodgrass, R. W., and Mellinkoff, S. M.: Bleeding varices in the upper esophagus due to obstruction of the superior vena cava, Gastroenterology 41:505, 1961.

84. Felson, B., Zeid, S., and Schiff, L.: Unpublished observations.

85. Campbell, G. S., Bick, H. D., Paulsen, E. P., Lober, P. H., Watson, C. J., and Varco, R. L.: Bleeding esophageal varices with polycystic liver, New Eng. J. Med. 259:904, 1958.

86. Sedacca, C. M., Perrin, E., Martin, L., and Schiff, L.: Polycystic liver: An unusual cause of bleeding esophageal varices, Gastroenterology 40:128, 1961.

87. Liebowitz, H. R.: Pathogenesis of esophageal varix rupture, J.A.M.A. 175:874, 1961.

88. Wangensteen, O. H.: The ulcer problem (Listerian oration), Canad. Med. Ass. J. 53:309, 1945.

89. Chiles, N. H., Baggenstoss, A. H., Butt, H. R., and Olsen, A. M.: Esophageal varices: Comparative incidence of ulceration and spon-

taneous rupture as a cause of fatal hemorrhage, Gastroenterology 25: 565, 1953.

90. Child, C. G., III, and Donovan, A. J.: Surgical treatment of portal hypertension, Amer. J. Dig. Dis. 3: 114, 1958.

91. Rolleston, H. D., and McNee, J. W.: Diseases of the Liver, Gall-Bladder and Bile Ducts, ed. 3, New York, Macmillan, 1929.

92. Morlock, C. G., and Hall, B. E.: Association of cirrhosis, thrombopenia and hemorrhagic tendency, Arch. Intern. Med. 72: 69, 1943.

93. Preble, R. B.: Conclusions based on sixty cases of fatal gastro-intestinal hemorrhage due to cirrhosis of the liver, Amer. J. Med. Sci. 119: 263, 1900.

94. Young, P. C., Burnside, C. R., Knowles, H. C., Jr., and Schiff, L.: The effect of the intragastric administration of whole blood on the blood ammonia, blood urea nitrogen and non-protein nitrogen in patients with liver disease, J. Clin. Invest. 35: 747, 1956.

95. White, F. W., and Chalmers, T. C.: The problem of gross hematemesis in a general hospital, Trans. Ass. Amer. Physicians 61: 253, 1948.

96. Zamcheck, N., Chalmers, T. C., White, F. W., and Davidson, C. S.: The bromsulphalein test in the early diagnosis of liver disease in gross upper gastrointestinal hemorrhage, Gastroenterology 14: 343, 1950.

97. Stahl, J., and Bockel, R.: L'ammoniémie dans le diagnostic de hémorrhagies digestives, Strasbourg Med. 7: 389, 1956.

98. McDermott, W. V., Jr.: A simple discriminatory test for upper gastrointestinal hemorrhage, New Eng. J. Med. 257: 1161, 1957.

99. Belkin, G. A., and Conn, H. O.: Blood ammonia concentration and bromsulfalein retention in upper gastrointestinal hemorrhage, New Eng. J. Med. 260: 530, 1959.

100. Atkinson, M., Barnett, E., Sherlock, S., and Steiner, R. E.: The clinical investigation of the portal circulation, with special reference to portal venography, Quart. J. Med. 24: 77, 1955.

101. Merigan, T. C., Jr., Hollister, R. M., Gryska, P. F., Starkey, G. W. B., and Davidson, C. S.: Gastrointestinal bleeding with cirrhosis, New Eng. J. Med. 263: 579, 1960.

102. Clarke, J. S., Ozeran, R. S., Hart, J. C., Cruze, K., and Crevling, V.: Peptic ulcer following portacaval shunt, Ann. Surg. 148: 551, 1958.

103. Dubuque, T. J., Jr., Mulligan, L. V., and Neville, E. C.: Gastric secretion and peptic ulceration in the dog with portal obstruction and portacaval anastomosis, Surg. Forum 8: 208, 1958.

104. Panke, W. F., Moreno, A. H., and Rousselot, L. M.: The diagnostic study of the portal venous system, Med. Clin. N. Amer. 44: 727, 1960.

105. Faber, K.: Gastritis and Its Consequences, London, Oxford, 1935.

106. Moutier, F.: Traité de gastroscopie et de pathologie endoscopique de l'estomac, Paris, Masson, 1935.

107. Henning, N.: Die Entzündung des Magens, Leipzig, Barth, 1934.

108. Palmer, E. D.: Gastritis: a revaluation, Medicine 33: 199, 1954.

109. Sahler, O. D., and Hampton, A. O.: Bleeding in hiatus hernia, Amer. J. Roentgen. 49: 433, 1943.

110. Jones, C. M.: Hiatus esophageal hernia; with special reference to a comparison of its symptoms with those of angina pectoris, New Eng. J. Med. 225: 963, 1941.

111. Harrington, S. W.: Diagnosis and treatment of various types of diaphragmatic hernia, Amer. J. Surg. 50: 377, 1940.

112. Olsen, A. M., and Harrington, S. W.: Esophageal hiatal hernias of the short esophagus type; etiologic and therapeutic considerations, J. Thorac. Surg. 17: 189, 1948.

113. Frank, W.: Hematemesis associated with gastric arteriosclerosis; review of literature with case report, Gastroenterology 7: 231, 1946.

114. Griggs, D. E., and Baker, M. Q.: Hereditary hemorrhagic telangiectasia with gastrointestinal bleeding, Amer. J. Dig. Dis. 8: 344, 1941.

115. Kushlan, S. D.: Gastro-intestinal bleeding in hereditary hemorrhagic telangiectasia; historical review and case report with gastroscopic findings and rutin therapy, Gastroenterology 7: 199, 1946.

116. Bean, W. B.: Enteric bleeding in rare conditions with diagnostic lesions of the skin and mucous membrane, Trans. Amer. Clin. Climat. Ass. 69: 72, 1957.

117. Segal, H. L., Scott, W. J. M., and Watson, J. S.: Lesions of small intestine producing massive hemorrhage, with symptoms simulating peptic ulcer, J.A.M.A. 129: 116, 1945.

118. Gordon-Taylor, G.: Rare causes of severe gastro-intestinal haemorrhage, with note on aneurysm of hepatic artery, Brit. Med. J. 1: 504, 1943.

119. Murphy, B.: Aneurysm of splenic artery; death from haematemesis, Lancet 1: 704, 1942.

120. Williams, R. C., Jr.: Aortic stenosis and unexplained gastrointestinal bleeding, Arch. Intern. Med. 108: 859, 1961.

121. Lee, H. C., and Kay, S.: Primary polyarteritis nodosa of the stomach and small intestine as a cause of gastro-intestinal hemorrhage, Ann. Surg. 147: 714, 1958.

122. Denkewalter, F. R., Molnar, W., and Horava, A. P.: Massive gastro-intestinal hemorrhage in jejunal diverticulosis, Ann. Surg. 148: 862, 1958.

123. Evans, A. L., Cofer, O. S., and Gregory, H. H.: Multiple hemangiomas of the jejunum as a cause of massive gastrointestinal bleeding, J. Med. Ass. Georgia 47: 600, 1958.

124. Schoenfeld, R., Cahan, J., and Dyer, R.: Gastric carcinoid tumor—An unusual cause of hematemesis, Arch. Intern. Med. 104: 649, 1959.

125. Aspirin poisoning, symposium section, Internat. Med. Dig. 56:54, 1950.

126. Douthwaite, A. H.: Some recent advances in medical diagnosis and treatment, Brit. Med. J. 1:1143, 1938.

127. Douthwaite, A. H., and Lintott, G. A. M.: Gastroscopic observation of the effect of aspirin and certain other substances on the stomach, Lancet 2:1222, 1938.

128. Hurst, A. F.: Aspirin and gastric hemorrhage, Brit. Med. J. 1:768, 1943.

129. Hurst, A. F., and Lintott, G. A. M.: Aspirin as a cause of haematemesis; a clinical and gastroscopic study, Guy Hosp. Rep. 89:173, 1939.

130. Crismer, R.: Gastric hemorrhage provoked by acetylsalicylic acid, Acta Clin. Belg. 2:193, 1947.

131. Winkelman, E. I., and Summerskill, W. H. J.: Gastric secretion in relation to gastrointestinal bleeding from salicylate compounds, Gastroenterology 40:56, 1961.

132. Allibone, A., and Flint, F. J.: Gastrointestinal haemorrhage and salicylates, Lancet 2:1121, 1958.

133. Kelly, J. J., Jr.: Salicylate ingestion: A frequent cause of gastric hemorrhage, Amer. J. Med. Sci. 232:119, 1956.

134. Lange, H. F.: Salicylates and gastric hemorrhage. II. Manifest bleeding, Gastroenterology 33:773, 1957.

135. Muir, A., and Cossar, I. A.: Aspirin and gastric haemorrhage, Lancet 1:539, 1959.

136. Waterson, A. P.: Aspirin and gastric haemorrhage, Brit. Med. J. 2:1531, 1955.

137. Pierson, R. N., Jr., Holt, P. R., Watson, R. M., and Keating, R. P.: Aspirin and gastrointestinal bleeding. Chromate[51] blood loss studies, Amer. J. Med. 31:259, 1961.

138. Muir, A., and Cossar, I. A.: Aspirin and ulcer, Brit. Med. J. 2:7, 1955.

139. Douthwaite, A. H.: Effect of aspirin on the stomach, Lancet 2:917, 1954.

140. Weiss, A., Pitman, E. R., and Graham, E. C.: Aspirin and gastric bleeding, Amer. J. Med. 31:266, 1961.

141. Lynch, A., Shaw, H., and Milton, G. W.: Effect of aspirin on gastric secretion, Gut 5:230, 1964.

142. Winkelman, E. I., and Summerskill, W. H. J.: Gastric secretion in relation to gastrointestinal bleeding from salicylate compounds, Gastroenterology 40:56, 1961.

143. Menguy, R.: Gastric mucosal injury by aspirin, Gastroenterology 51:430, 1966.

144. Mallory, G. K., and Weiss, S.: Hemorrhages from lacerations of the cardiac orifice of the stomach due to vomiting, Amer. J. Med. Sci. 178:506, 1929.

145. Decker, J. P., Zamcheck, N., and Mallory, G. K.: Mallory-Weiss syndrome. Hemorrhage from gastroesophageal lacerations at the cardiac orifice of the stomach, New Eng. J. Med. 249:957, 1953.

146. Heuer, G. J.: The surgical aspects of hemorrhage from peptic ulcer, New Eng. J. Med. 235:777, 1946.

147. Foster, D. G.: Retrograde jejunogastric intussusception—a rare cause of hematemesis. Review of the literature and report of two cases, Arch. Surg. 73:1009, 1956.

148. Cordell, A. R., Wright, R. H., and Johnston, F. R.: Gastrointestinal hemorrhage after abdominal aortic operations, Surgery 48:997, 1960.

149. Sandblom, P.: Hemorrhage into the biliary tract following trauma: "Traumatic hemobilia," Surgery 24:571, 1948.

150. Sparkman, R. S.: Massive hemobilia following traumatic rupture of liver: Report of a case and review of the literature, Ann. Surg. 138:899, 1953.

151. Sparkman, R. S., and Fogelman, M. J.: Wounds of the liver. Review of 100 cases, Ann. Surg. 139:690, 1954.

152. Ferguson, L. K., and Nusbaum, M.: Idiopathic massive hemobilia, Amer. J. Surg. 102:109, 1961.

153. Schatzki, S. C.: Hemobilia, Radiology 77:717, 1961.

154. Karam, J. H., and Jacobs, T.: Hemobilia: Report of a case of massive gastrointestinal bleeding originating from a hepatic abscess, Ann. Intern. Med. 54-319, 1961.

155. Stokes, J. F., and Jones, F. A., *in discussion of* Edwards, H.: Haematemesis due to pseudoxanthoma elasticum, Gastroenterologia 89:345, 1958.

24

Jaundice

LEON SCHIFF

Jaundice, or icterus, is the condition recognized clinically by a yellowish discoloration of the plasma, the skin, and the mucous membranes caused by staining by bile pigment. It may be the first, and sometimes the sole, manifestation of disease. It is detected best in the peripheral portions of the ocular conjunctivae and can be observed also in the mucous membrane of the hard palate or in the lips when compressed with a glass slide. It may be overlooked in poor or artificial light. Attention may be first directed to it by a laboratory report of "serum icteric."

BILIRUBIN METABOLISM

It is now generally accepted that the formation of bilirubin from hemoglobin occurs mainly in the cells of the reticuloendothelial system. Studies with erythrocytes labeled with Cr[51] and Fe[59] have shown that the principal sites of hemoglobin catabolism are the bone marrow, the spleen, and the liver, whereas the kidneys, the lungs and the intestines play a minor role.[1,2]

In the normal individual, 1/120 of the total circulating erythrocytes are destroyed daily.

In the adult this represents 7.5 Gm. of hemoglobin. The released hemoglobin is broken down into heme and globin; the latter being further catabolized into its constituent amino acids, which are reutilized. The heme is broken down into inorganic iron and protoporphyrin; the protoporphyrin being further catabolized into bilirubin. The daily breakdown of hemoglobin (7.5 Gm.) should result in the formation of 300 mg. of bilirubin.

The over-all metabolism of bilirubin by the liver cell involves three processes: (1) transport of bilirubin from the plasma to the liver (uptake); (2) conjugation of bilirubin, primarily with glucuronic acid; and (3) excretion of the water-soluble conjugate into the biliary system. Jaundice can result from interference with any of these three processes, or from obstruction of bile flow thru the ductal system.

Since unconjugated bilirubin is almost insoluble at a physiologic pH, it is transported in the blood tightly bound to albumin. The maximum binding capacity is 2 moles bilirubin/1 mole albumin,[3] which is equivalent

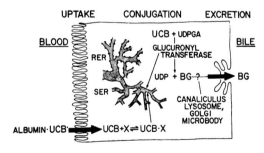

FIG. 24-1. Schematic representation of current concept of the hepatic metabolism of bilirubin. BG, bilirubin glucuronide; RER, rough endoplasmic reticulum; SER, smooth endoplasmic reticulum; UCB, unconjugated bilirubin; UDP, uridine diphosphate; UDPGA, uridine diphosphate glucuronic acid; X, cytoplasmic acceptor of UCB. (Arias, I. M.: Postgrad. Med. 40:15)

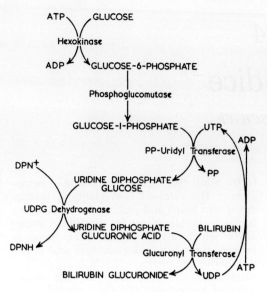

FIG. 24-2. A possible mechanism for the conjugation of bilirubin with glucuronic acid. (Billing, B. H., and Lathe, G. H.: Am. J. Med. 24:111)

in the normal adult to a plasma unconjugated bilirubin concentration of 60 to 80 mg./100 ml. There is little likelihood that the binding capacity of the plasma would become saturated in the jaundiced patient. Under normal conditions, bilirubin is removed from the circulation by the liver, so that the serum bilirubin level usually remains below 1 mg./100 ml. Isotope studies indicate that this is an extremely rapid process involving first the detachment of the albumin at the cell surface.[4] The pigment is then accepted by one or more intracellular proteins —not albumin—present in the cell sap.[5]

Approximately 15 per cent of the bilirubin formed each day is derived from sources other than the destruction of mature circulating erythrocytes and is responsible for the early-labeling peak of bile pigments.[6] This peak consists of erythropoietic and hepatic components.[7] Animal experiments have shown that the hepatic component of the early labeled peak is increased after surgery, and so may contribute to the rise in serum bilirubin frequently observed in the immediate postoperative period.[8]

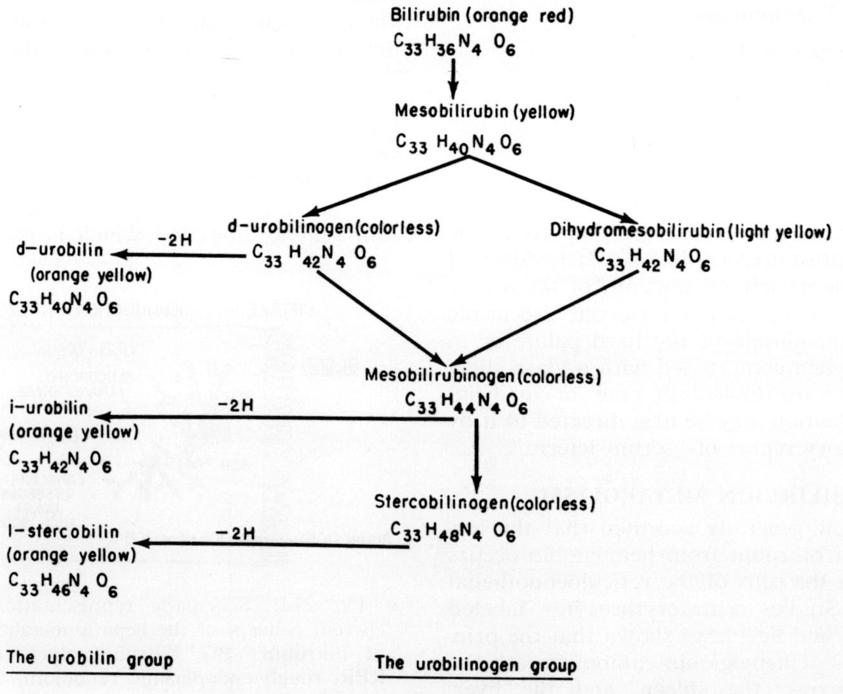

Bilirubin (orange red)
$C_{33}H_{36}N_4O_6$

Mesobilirubin (yellow)
$C_{33}H_{40}N_4O_6$

d−urobilinogen(colorless)
$C_{33}H_{42}N_4O_6$

Dihydromesobilirubin(light yellow)
$C_{33}H_{42}N_4O_6$

−2H

d−urobilin
(orange yellow)
$C_{33}H_{40}N_4O_6$

Mesobilirubinogen(colorless)
$C_{33}H_{44}N_4O_6$

i−urobilin
(orange yellow)
$C_{33}H_{42}N_4O_6$

−2H

Stercobilinogen(colorless)
$C_{33}H_{48}N_4O_6$

l−stercobilin
(orange yellow)
$C_{33}H_{46}N_4O_6$

−2H

The urobilin group   **The urobilinogen group**

FIG. 24-3. The bacterial reduction of bilirubin by the human intestinal flora. (Watson, C. J., Lowry, P., Collins, S., Graham, A. and Ziegler, N. R.: Tr. A. Am. Physicians 67:242)

In its passage through the liver cell, unconjugated ("indirect-reacting") bilirubin is converted into a water-soluble ("direct-reacting") conjugated form, which is then excreted into the bile.[9,10,11,12] Uridine diphosphate glucuronic acid (UDPGA) acts as the glucuronyl donor for the conjugation of bilirubin; the conjugating enzyme, glucuronyl transferase, being located in the microsomes of the liver cells, located predominantly in the smooth and also in the rough portions of the endoplasmic reticulum.[13] The series of enzymic reactions involved in the synthesis of bilirubin glucuronide is given in Figure 24-2. Other conjugates of bilirubin, such as the sulfate,[14,15] have been detected, but there have been no reports of increases in alternate types of conjugation to compensate for a reduction in glucuronide formation.

Recent studies have suggested that the excretion of the conjugated bilirubin (bilirubin glucuronide) may be under hormonal control, since hypophysectomized animals have a decreased ability to excrete conjugated bilirubin, which can be corrected by treatment with pituitary hormone and thyroxine.[16] Organic anions as well as such drugs as the anabolic steroids[17] will compete with bilirubin glucuronide for excretion, and thus may cause jaundice.

In normal subjects, bilirubin is rarely excreted in the urine. In fresh specimens of icteric urine, only the conjugated pigments can be detected. There is a poor correlation between the concentration of conjugated bilirubin in the plasma and that in the urine, particularly in viral hepatitis, in which, at the onset of the disease, bilirubin may appear in the urine with serum levels of 2 to 3 mg./100 ml.; however, during convalescence, it often fails to appear with levels of 6 to 8 mg./100 ml.[18] Conjugated bilirubin is excreted in the urine mainly by glomerular filtration.[19,20,21,22] Although bilirubin glucuronide can be shown histochemically to accumulate in renal tubules, most investigators now believe that bile pigments are probably not secreted by the tubules[20,23] as was formerly thought.

After it enters the small intestine, the bilirubin is reduced to urobilinogens (Fig. 24-3), which are partially reabsorbed and re-excreted into the intestine (Fig. 24-4). It is now generally accepted that the urobilinoid pigments are formed from conjugated bilirubin in the intestine by the bacterial flora. The presence of conjugated, rather than free, bilirubin appears to be necessary,[24] and although the individual enzyme systems have not been isolated, in-vitro studies have shown that fecal bacteria, such as the Clostridium-like

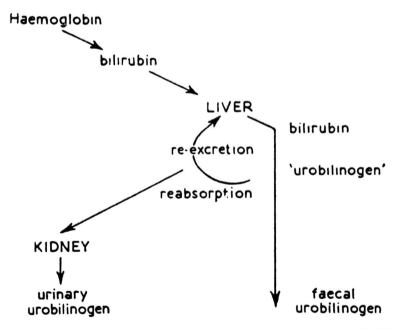

FIG. 24-4. Fate of bilirubin after excretion into the gut. (Gray, C. H.: The Bile Pigments, London, Methuen)

organism G62 and *E. coli*, are capable of carrying out the conversion of bilirubin to urobilinogen.[25,26] Attempts to determine the relative proportions of urobilin IX$_a$, stercobilin, and d-urobilin and their precursors in fecal urobilin have, for the most part, been unsuccessful because of difficult and unsatisfactory analytic procedures, and conflicting results have been obtained. More recently, Watson[27] concluded that the composition of the urobilin group in urine, bile, and feces at any time is controlled by the mobility of the intestinal contents and the rate of filling of the colon, and appears to depend on the efficiency of bacterial reduction and the site of absorption in the colon. He was unable to correlate the composition of the fecal urobilin with the state of health or disease; and although urobilin IX$_a$ predominated in some subjects, stercobilin was the dominant pigment in others. The administration of broad-spectrum antibiotics resulted in d-urobilin becoming the dominant pigment in feces, bile, and urine. However, this pigment was found in appreciable quantities in some subjects who had never received antibiotic therapy, and may be normally present in all subjects in small amounts, which are not detected by our present technics.

McMaster and Elman[28] postulated, as the result of experiments with dogs, that urobilinogen was normally reabsorbed from the intestine and re-excreted by the liver, and that in the presence of liver damage re-excretion was impossible, so that the pigment passes instead to the kidney and is excreted in the urine. The form in which reabsorbed stercobilinogen is normally excreted in the bile is unknown, because it is only in the presence of infection that appreciable amounts of urobilinoids and bile pigments, other than bilirubin, can be detected. Urobilinogen excretion correlates well with urinary pH, both in normal subjects and in patients with hepatic dysfunction or hemolytic disease, higher values being recorded in alkaline than in acid urines.[29] The significance of urinary urobilinogen determinations in these conditions thus can be assessed only if allowance is made for urinary pH.

CLASSIFICATION AND MECHANISMS

The fact that various classifications of jaundice have been proposed would indicate the lack of an ideal one. With advances in knowledge of cellular structure, increasing interest in cellular physiology, and the dis-

TABLE 24-1. CLASSIFICATION OF JAUNDICE

1. Hemolytic
2. Hepatocellular
   A. Without features of biliary obstruction
   B. With features of biliary obstruction (cholestatic jaundice)
   C. Congenital
3. Obstructive

covery of the conjugation of bilirubin, more attention is being focused on the liver cell itself in the pathogenesis of icterus.

McNee's classification[30] into (1) obstructive hepatic, (2) toxic and infective hepatic and (3) hemolytic types has maintained its clinical usefulness. Watson's[31] division of regurgitation jaundice into the cancerous, calculous, and parenchymal types, based largely on the extent of biliary obstruction, has been of further help in clinical practice. Watson considers biliary obstruction to be complete when the daily fecal excretion of urobilinogen is less than 5 mg. (normal range is 40 to 280 mg.). Factors that diminish urobilinogen production in the intestine, such as diarrhea and ingestion of antibiotics, must of course be excluded. Watson found complete biliary obstruction in 92 per cent of his cancerous cases, in contrast with only 3.5 per cent of the parenchymal and 11.5 per cent of the calculous groups.

The author prefers the clinical classification of jaundice shown in Table 24-1. The hepatocellular type comprises the various forms of hepatitis and hepatic cirrhosis and includes the intrahepatic cholestatic forms of hepatitis (which are chiefly of viral or drug origin) and the hereditary hyperbilirubinemias. The obstructive form includes biliary obstruction due to neoplasm, gallstones, stricture, cholangitis, or contiguous inflammatory processes or cysts.

HEMOLYTIC JAUNDICE

In hemolytic disease there is an increased production of bilirubin, most of which is excreted by the liver. Therefore, an elevated fecal urobilinogen excretion occurs, and excessive amounts of urobilinogen may appear in the urine. Unconjugated bilirubin is the main pigment found in the serum of these patients. Therefore, bilirubinuria is not usually observed. Occasionally, if hepatic dysfunction is present, conjugated bilirubin appears in the plasma.[32] On the other hand, marked hemolysis can be accompanied by considerable quantities of conjugated bilirubin in the blood (and by bilirubinuria) due to overloading of the excretory capacity of an otherwise normal liver.[33]

OBSTRUCTIVE AND HEPATOCELLULAR JAUNDICE

Controversy still exists regarding the mechanisms of the development of jaundice. It has generally been accepted that obstructive jaundice is caused by hydrostatic dilatation and rupture of the bile capillaries with leakage of bilirubin back from the biliary system into the lymphatics of the liver, and thence to the blood stream. Gonzalez-Oddone[34] observed the prompt appearance of bilirubin (mainly of the prompt-reacting type) in the thoracic duct lymph after ligature of the common duct in dogs. On the other hand, Grafflin and Chaney[35] studied the excretion of fluorescent substances by the liver after ligature of the common duct in white mice, and were unable to visualize any suggestion of rupture or leakage of the dye ("and so presumably of bile") into the blood or the lymph. By fluorescence microscopy, Hanzon[36] observed the movement of uranin injected into living rats with ligated bile ducts. The canaliculi became much dilated with uranin, which was then observed to flow abruptly into the blood.

Various other mechanisms have been invoked to explain regurgitation of bile into the blood. These include (1) increased permeability of the bile capillaries, especially at the ampullae (the point at which the canaliculi emerge from the liver cords),[37] (2) necrosis of liver cells,[38] (3) swelling of the parenchymal cells of the liver with obstruction of the bile canaliculi,[39] (4) swelling of the liver cords, edema of the spaces of Disse and fibrosis of the portal areas,[40] (5) obstruction of the intralobular canaliculi by bile thrombi,[41,42] and (6) compression or rupture of the canals of Hering in the region of the periportal fields as a result of exudative processes.[43] With the use of the electron microscope Popper and Schaffner[44] have more recently pointed out dilatation of the bile canaliculi with diminution and distortion of the microvilli, and rupture of the canaliculus into the surrounding tissue space both in intrahepatic cholestasis and extrahepatic obstructive jaundice. Decrease in the microvilli and dilatation of the canaliculi may interfere with the normal hydration of bile, thus favoring cholestasis.

Where the injured liver cells appear to be histologically normal, particularly in instances of hepatocellular jaundice, the studies of Hanzon[36] suggest an impairment of the unidirectional transport mechanism of the hepatic cell affecting its permeability, and thereby permitting regurgitation of the bile through the cell from the canaliculi.

Cholestatic jaundice has proved to be the main stumbling block to an entirely satisfactory classification of jaundice. This type of icterus is characterized by biochemical and clinical features usually found in obstructive jaundice, but without demonstrable obstruction. It occurs most commonly following the use of such drugs as arsenicals, chlorpromazine, methyl testosterone, oral contraceptives, and norethandralone, but may also occur in viral hepatitis[45] (so-called cholangiolitic hepatitis). It may appear in pregnancy and recur in subsequent pregnancies. The primary pathophysiologic basis may well prove to be an impairment in bilirubin transport accompanied by changes in permeability of the liver cell, permitting reflux of conjugated bilirubin from the cells and canaliculi into the lymph spaces and sinusoids.

HEREDITARY HYPERBILIRUBINEMIAS
(IN THE ADULT)

Gilbert's Syndrome (Constitutional Hepatic Dysfunction), Idiopathic Unconjugated Hyperbilirubinemia. The term Gilbert's syndrome usually comprises a heterogenous group of benign disorders, which are characterized by mild unconjugated hyperbilirubinemia not attributable to overt hemolysis and which are seen most commonly in young males. Jaundice may be present from birth, or may be noted first in adult life and persist into old age, tending to lessen with age. The icterus fluctuates in degree and may be increased by fatigue, emotional tension, excessive intake of alcohol, or intercurrent infection. Neither hepatomegaly nor splenomegaly is present. Hepatic function is usually normal, except for an impaired bilirubin tolerance, and the liver is usually normal on histologic examination, although fatty infiltration of the liver has been reported.

The majority of patients have an unconjugated bilirubinemia of 1 to 4 mg./100 ml. It has been postulated that a defect in the uptake of bilirubin by the liver cell is responsible for the jaundice in these patients. Analysis of plasma bilirubin disappearance curves, following an injection of bilirubin, tends to substantiate this hypothesis.[46]

Patients with hyperbilirubinemia greater than 5 mg./100 ml. are rare, and it seems likely that, in these subjects, there may be a defect in glucuronide formation such as is seen in infants with the Crigler-Najjar syndrome, but to a varying extent.[47] Fecal urobilinogen excretion is usually decreased. The administration of ACTH or prednisolone does not appear to affect the degree of jaundice in these patients.[48] Phenobarbital administration will lower the serum bilirubin concentration in these cases.[49]

It is important to bear in mind that chronic unconjugated hyperbilirubinemia, in the absence of overt hemolysis, may exist in a number of disease states, including cardiac disorders, fatty liver, malignant tumors, infections, and cirrhosis.[50] Unconjugated hyperbilirubinemia may follow a bout of viral hepatitis[51,52] and may occasionally represent a hemolytic state.[53] It may also occur at high altitudes,[54] in thyrotoxicosis,[55] or following a portacaval shunt.[56]

Chronic Idiopathic Jaundice (Dubin-Johnson Syndrome). This disorder, which was first described independently by two groups of workers, Dubin and Johnson[57] and Sprinz and Nelson,[58] is a chronic or intermittent form of jaundice with both free and conjugated bilirubin in the plasma. It is characterized by the presence of large amounts of a yellow-brown, lipofuscin-like pigment in the liver cells. The pigment has the physical and chemical characteristics of melanin.[59-61]

As in Gilbert's syndrome, this disorder manifests itself as a form of chronic or intermittent jaundice most commonly seen in young people, and frequently familial in occurrence. According to Dubin[57] most patients complain of abdominal pain in the region of the liver, and the liver is palpable and tender in about one-half of the cases.

Corriedale sheep have been found to have both morphologic and functional defects similar to those of patients with the Dubin-Johnson syndrome.[62] They exhibit impairment in biliary excretion of bilirubin and dyes, which are organic anions, but excrete bile acids and cations normally, which indicates that different mechanisms are involved in the excretion of these two groups of compounds.[63]

A striking feature is the failure of the gallbladder, although normal, to visualize on oral cholecystography. The liver is normal except for the pigment in its cells, which may be so abundant as to discolor

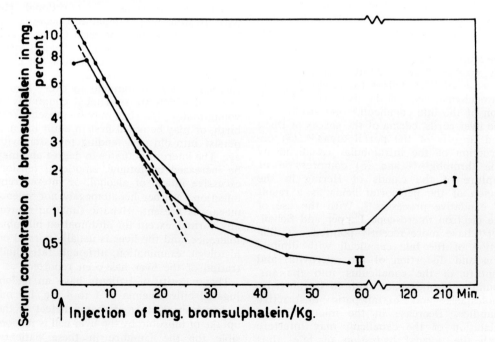

Fig. 24-5. Bromsulphalein disappearance curve. (I) Case III, (II) Normal subject. (Mandema, E., de Fraiture, W. H., Nieweg, H. O., and Arends, A.: Am. J. Med., 27:47)

it green, slate blue, or black. This gross discoloration may be detected in a needle biopsy specimen.

Jaundice may be precipitated or aggravated by many factors, including pregnancy, surgical operations, severe physical strain, alcoholism, and infectious diseases.[57] The icterus may be mistaken for the obstructive variety because of abdominal pain, dark urine, pale stools, increase in direct-reacting bilirubin, and a nonvisualizing gallbladder. Prognosis is excellent, as indicated by the long duration of the disease and the absence of progressive hepatic damage in cases of long standing.[57]

Except for the presence of pigment, the hepatic cells appear to be histologically normal. The serum proteins, transaminases, bile acids, alkaline phosphatase, and flocculation tests are usually within normal limits, but may be raised slightly. On the other hand, all patients show a marked retention of such dyes as bromsulphalein,[57,64] rose bengal,[65] indocyanine green,[66] and methylene blue,[67] which appears to be due to a defect in excretion by the hepatic cells. During the first 30 minutes after the injection, the dye is cleared from the plasma at a rate similar to or slightly reduced from that seen in the normal subject. The level of the dye in the plasma then rises again and remains elevated for many hours, so that it can still be detected after 48 to 72 hours (Fig. 24-5). With bromsulphalein, the proportion of dye conjugated with glutathione in the plasma gradually rises, and an appreciable amount of the injected dye can be recovered from the urine.

Measurements of serum bilirubin show elevation of both the conjugated (direct) and the total levels. These levels tend to fluctuate under the influence of the factors mentioned above, and range from normal to 19 mg./100 ml. of plasma. Approximately 60 per cent of the cases have total bile pigment concentrations under 6 mg./100 ml. of plasma.

The occurrence of unconjugated hyperbilirubinemia in some instances of Dubin-Johnson syndrome,[68,69] and even alternating increases in the conjugated and unconjugated serum bilirubin have been reported.[70]

Rotor's Syndrome.[71,72] Although this disorder was described by Rotor and associates in 1948, it is only within recent years that interest in familial non-hemolytic jaundice with conjugated bilirubin in the serum has been renewed.

The disease appears to be familial in occurrence, with both sexes probably equally represented, and is characterized by a chronic, relatively mild jaundice, fluctuating in degree. As in Gilbert's syndrome, the icterus may increase with fatigue, emotional upsets, or respiratory infections.[73] In one patient the icterus was said to diminish during each of 3 pregnancies,[73] in direct contrast with behavior of cases of the Dubin-Johnson syndrome.[57] In one of Rotor's cases, ingestion of fatty foods was said to deepen the jaundice. Abdominal pain is usually absent, and the liver and the spleen are not enlarged.

The disorder is chronic, not incapacitating, requires no treatment and appears to be compatible with a normal life. In contrast with the Dubin-Johnson syndrome, the oral cholecystogram is normal, and no pigment is present in the liver cells. However, the bile ducts may fail to visualize roentgenologically following the intravenous injection of iodipamide,[72,75] although shown to be patent and otherwise normal at peritoneoscopy and laparotomy.[76,77] Davis and Young have observed coincidental gallbladder calculi.[76] The liver biopsy specimen is essentially normal on light microscopy and fluorescence microscopy and probably so on electron microscopy.[72] In the case studied by Arias[74] the pericanalicular lysosomes appeared to be increased in numbers and in dispersion throughout the cell as examined with the electron microscope.

Information based on the few cases studied would indicate that the cephalin flocculation test is sometimes abnormal, but the thymol turbidity, zinc sulfate turbidity, total lipids, serum proteins, and serum transaminases are within normal limits. The serum alkaline phosphatase activities may tend toward the low side of normal; the level of the serum trihydroxy and dihydroxy bile acids may be within normal range.

There is abnormal retention of bromsulphalein in the plasma, and the appearance of the dye in the bile following intravenous injection may be somewhat delayed. The retained bromsulphalein has been found to be almost entirely in the unconjugated form[72,75] at 45 minutes after injection of the dye, but at 100 minutes, Arias has found that most of the dye in the serum is conjugated. He found the hepatic storage of bromsulphalein to be normal and the hepatic

Tm (transport maximum) for bromsulphalein to be markedly reduced.

The serum bilirubin levels fluctuate and are usually less than 10 mg. per cent, with the free and conjugated pigments present in about equal proportion. Bile pigments can be detected in the urine, provided that the level of conjugated pigments is sufficiently high. Abnormal amounts of urinary urobilinogen are usually not present, although they have been reported. The fecal urobilinogen is not increased.

CLINICAL APPROACH

The clinician usually has little difficulty in distinguishing hemolytic from hepatocellular and obstructive jaundice. His usual task is to differentiate jaundice due to primary liver disease from that due to obstruction of the extrahepatic bile ducts. In the differentiation of the various forms of jaundice, he has available four methods of approach, short of surgical intervention or peritoneoscopy: (1) the history and the physical examination, (2) laboratory tests, (3) x-ray examination, (4) response of the serum bilirubin to steroid administration, (5) duodenal drainage, and (6) needle biopsy of the liver in selected cases.

HISTORY

Family History. The familial occurrence of icterus should suggest the possibilities of congenital hemolytic jaundice, Gilbert's syndrome, the Dubin-Johnson syndrome and Rotor's syndrome. A history of consanguinity of parents should arouse suspicion of Wilson's disease.

Occupation. The increased likelihood of hepatic cirrhosis in bartenders and brewery workers and the predisposition to Weil's disease among workers in rat-infested premises are well-known.

Recent contact with a jaundiced individual should suggest the possibility of infectious hepatitis, as should a history of recent travel or ingestion of raw oysters or raw or steamed clams.[78,79]

The ingestion or the administration of or exposure to hepatotoxic drugs, particularly carbon tetrachloride, thorazine, methyl estosterone, norethandralone, oral contraceptives, and mono-amine-oxidase inhibitors ould suggest the possibility of a toxic or ig induced hepatitis.

eedle puncture or transfusion from 6 s to 6 months prior to the onset of jaundice should lead to suspicion of serum hepatitis.

A history of a recent gallbladder operation should lead to suspicion of a residual common duct stone or stricture as the cause of icterus, but careful inquiry should be made as to the transfusion of blood or plasma at the time of surgery in order to exclude serum hepatitis.[80]

History of Resection of a Malignant Tumor. If the interval between resection of the tumor and the appearance of icterus is more than 3 or 4 years, an unrelated cause of the icterus should be considered. Metastatic tumor of the liver is more apt to appear within 2 or 3 years.[81]

While **chills and fever** in a jaundiced patient are usually indicative of cholangitis, it is well to remember that they may be prominent during the preicteric phase of infectious hepatitis and may occur in thorazine or other drug-induced hepatitis.

Pruritus. As George Budd pointed out over 100 years ago, pruritus is most pronounced in cases of occlusion of the common bile duct, particularly by tumor. According to Schoenfield, pruritus occurs with extrahepatic obstruction in 75 per cent of patients with malignant lesions and in 50 per cent of those with benign disorders. He finds that itching occurs in 20 per cent of patients with hepatitis and in 10 per cent of those with portal cirrhosis, associated presumably with intrahepatic cholestasis. About 75 per cent of patients with bile duct stricture or primary biliary cirrhosis have pruritus. Although an increase in serum bile acids has long been suspected as the cause of the pruritus, a parallel relationship need not exist.[82,83] The concentration of bile acids in the skin is greater in hepatobiliary disorders associated with pruritus than in subjects with similar disorders without itching, and may exceed the concentration in the blood.[82] Itching occasionally occurs in viral hepatitis, and in nutritional cirrhosis.

Abdominal pain is usually inconspicuous in patients with viral hepatitis or hepatic cirrhosis. In cases of *common duct stone*, the pain is generally colicky and is accompanied by nausea and vomiting and usually requires an opiate for relief.

It is well recognized that pain occurs in most cases of *pancreatic carcinoma*. Although the nature of the pain is not pathognomonic, it is usually located in the epigastrium, is often described as boring in nature and frequently radiates to the back. As pointed out by Chauffard,[84] it is worse when the patient lies on his back and is lessened by turning on one side and drawing up the knees, by changing to the prone position, or by sitting up and bending forward. It is frequently so severe as to require an opiate. An atypical pain pattern may be produced by *peritoneal tumor implants.*

Abdominal pain is usually prominent in cases of *malignant tumor of the liver,* primary more than metastatic. It is usually localized to the right hypochondrium and may be dull or sharp and intermittent in character. It may radiate to the right infrascapular area or right flank and may be increased by deep breathing, coughing, exertion, or changes in posture. It is presumably due to invasion or stretching of the liver capsule by the neoplasm.

PHYSICAL EXAMINATION

Age and Sex. The age and the sex of the patient are of diagnostic help. Infectious hepatitis and active chronic hepatitis are seen most commonly in young adults, whereas common duct stone and neoplastic jaundice usually occur in middle-aged or older individuals. Weil's disease, at least in this country, is said to be rare in females and in children.[85] Portal cirrhosis, hepatoma, pancreatic cancer, and primary hemochromatosis predominate in the male, while common duct stone, primary biliary cirrhosis, and carcinoma of the gallbladder are more prevalent in the female.

Vascular Spiders.[86] These structures should be looked for carefully with the aid of a good light. Inspection with a hand lens may be necessary to distinguish them from small papular lesions. They may pulsate and can be obliterated by pressing on their central point with the end of a pencil. They usually indicate the presence of hepatic cirrhosis.

Breath. A peculiar sickly sweetish breath (hepatic foetor) is characteristic of severe hepatic disease with necrosis.[87] According to Hoffbauer,[88] hepatic foetor is sometimes detected on the breath of patients with well-compensated hepatic cirrhosis, or it may follow the therapeutic use of large quantities of pure methionine. Methyl mercaptan has been isolated from the urine of patients with hepatic foetor,[89] and this, coupled with a high plasma level of methionine, suggests that the mercaptan arises by hydrolytic or reductive fission of the sulfur-carbon bond in methionine.

Cervical lymphadenopathy should suggest the presence of viral hepatitis or infectious mononucleosis.

Prominent superficial abdominal veins are observed most often in patients with hepatic cirrhosis but may occur in the presence of peritoneal tumor implants, obstruction of the portal vein by tumor, or in cases of inferior caval obstruction. In portal hypertension the blood flow in the abdominal veins is radially away from the umbilicus, whereas in inferior caval obstruction it is always upward over the abdominal wall.[90] Normal veins may be made more prominent by stretching and thinning of the overlying skin as a result of abdominal distention in the absence of portal hypertension.

Liver. The normal liver is soft, smooth, and frequently tender. It has a sharp edge which may not be palpable or may be felt 1 to 2 fingerbreadths below the right costal margin. Although a reliable method for estimating liver size is not available, it is safe to assume that a liver that extends 3 fingerbreadths or more below the right costal margin is probably enlarged (and hence the seat of disease), provided that one may exclude downward displacement by right pleural cavity fluid or marked pulmonary emphysema, and that the body habitus is not hyposthenic. Variations in the shape and the position of the liver appear to accompany body types. In a stocky person, the liver may often extend to the left lateral abdominal wall with its lower edge lying relatively high; it may not be palpable beneath the costal margin. In a lanky individual, the normal liver, including the left lobe, may lie entirely in the right abdomen and may extend 5 fingerbreadths below the costal margin.[91]

A liver that is unduly firm is apt to be diseased, as is one with a blunted edge or an irregular contour. An irregular, firm, nodular liver is most commonly indicative of intrahepatic malignant neoplasm. However, the large regenerating nodules of postnecrotic cirrhosis may produce an irregularity of contour which may closely simulate that produced by tumor. The same may hold true in the fatty or cystic liver.

The liver may not extend below the right costal margin in cases of hepatitis or cirrhosis. It is usually found from 1 to 2 (or

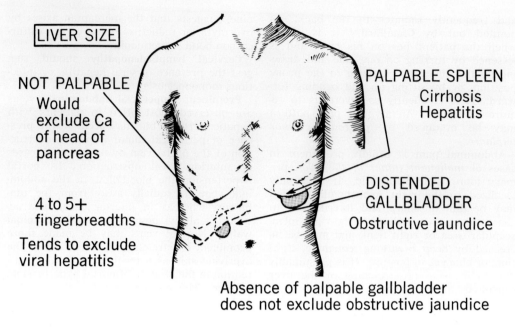

LIVER SIZE

NOT PALPABLE
Would exclude Ca of head of pancreas

4 to 5+ fingerbreadths
Tends to exclude viral hepatitis

PALPABLE SPLEEN
Cirrhosis
Hepatitis

DISTENDED GALLBLADDER
Obstructive jaundice

Absence of palpable gallbladder does not exclude obstructive jaundice

FIG. 24-6. Abdominal findings in various forms of jaundice. (Schiff, L.: Postgrad. Med. 41:39)

2 to 3) fingerbreadths below the right costal margin in viral hepatitis and is frequently tender in this disease. A very large liver (one extending 4 to 5 fingerbreadths or more below the right costal margin) is usually indicative of fatty vacuolization, cirrhosis, tumor, amyloidosis, or congestive failure, and is most unusual in viral hepatitis (Fig. 24-6). Enlargement of the left lobe of the liver should suggest hepatic syphilis, but may be caused by primary or metastatic tumor or by abscess.

The presence of a friction rub over the liver is most commonly indicative of a malignant tumor (invading or breaking through the liver capsule); it may follow percutaneous liver biopsy. A harsh (arterial) murmur over the liver has been reported in hepatoma and alcoholic hepatitis.[92] It is apparently due to locally increased arterial blood flow and should be contrasted with the venous hum arising in collateral venous channels.

The absence of a palpable liver in a patient who has had jaundice for 2 to 3 weeks or more would tend to exclude neoplastic obstruction of the bile ducts, since sufficient bile stasis should result, by this time, to produce detectable hepatic enlargement.[93]

Gallbladder. The presence of a smooth, nontender, distended gallbladder in a jaundiced patient is almost always indicative of neoplastic obstruction of the common bile duct, in accordance with Courvoisier's law. It is found much more frequently at operation or necropsy than it is on physical examination; a discrepancy accounted for by the overlying right lobe of the liver or, less frequently, by a thick abdominal wall. Painless distention of the gallbladder may be encountered in patients who have been vomiting and not ingesting fats.[94]

Spleen. In the absence of hemolytic jaundice, a palpable spleen is usually indicative of hepatocellular jaundice. The spleen is palpable in about one-half of patients with hepatic cirrhosis, in about 10 to 15 per cent of patients with viral hepatitis, and about 20 per cent of cases of hepatic neoplasm.[95] It is well to bear in mind that in obstructive jaundice of long standing, splenomegaly may be a manifestation of obstructive cirrhosis. In cancer of the body and the tail of the pancreas, splenic enlargement may result from encroachment of the tumor on the splenic vein.[96] Splenomegaly is also encountered occasionally in the periampullary tumor.

Ascites. The presence of ascites in a jaundiced patient is usually indicative of hepatic cirrhosis, but may also be observed in massive or subacute hepatic necrosis, in the presence of peritoneal tumor implants, or following invasion of the portal vein by tumor.

Palmar Erythema. Patek[97] and Perera[98] have pointed out the frequency of a symmetric erythema—so-called palmar erythema—involving the eminences of the palms and the digits of the hands in patients with hepatic cirrhosis.

"Routine" Tests

Blood Count. According to Havens,[99] the white cell count is usually reduced during the preicteric and normal during the icteric phase of infectious hepatitis, although Jones and Minot[100] reported leukocytosis within the first few days of the disease. The chief value of a white cell count in a patient with jaundice is in helping to distinguish uncomplicated viral hepatitis, in which there is usually no leukocytosis, from conditions in which leukocytosis is found frequently, such as toxic hepatitis, amebic hepatitis, metastatic hepatic neoplasm, common duct stone (with cholangitis), and Weil's disease. The presence of eosinophilia should suggest toxic hepatitis.

Blood Urea Nitrogen. Elevation of the blood urea nitrogen in a patient with jaundice should suggest the possibility of Weil's disease or exposure to a hepatotoxic agent which is also injurious to the kidney, such as, for example, carbon tetrachloride. Renal failure complicating liver disease must also be considered.

Urine Analysis. The presence of albuminuria should suggest the possibility of Weil's disease, although it may occur in the preicteric and the early icteric phases of viral hepatitis. Since jaundice may occur in amyloidosis, the simultaneous occurrence of marked albuminuria should also arouse suspicion of this disorder.

Stool Examination. Strongly positive tests for occult blood in the stools should arouse suspicion of an ulcerating periampullary lesion or a pancreatic cancer eroding the stomach or the duodenum.

Serum Lipids. Increase in serum lipids should suggest biliary cirrhosis, fatty liver, or Zieve's syndrome.[101]

Liver Profile

The writer and his associates have employed the following profile in the differential diagnosis of jaundice: (1) serum bilirubin (method of Malloy and Evelyn as modified by Ducci and Watson); upper limit for 1-minute bilirubin, 0.25 mg. per cent, and for total bilirubin, 1.50 mg. per cent,[102,103] (2) cephalin-cholesterol flocculation (method of Hanger[104] 1 to 2+ in 24 hours considered normal); (3) thymol turbidity (Shank and Hoagland's modification[105] of Maclagan's method,[106]) with normal range of 0 to 5 units; (4) zinc sulfate turbidity (method of Kunkel[107]) with normal values of 12 units or less; (5) thymol flocculation (Neefe), 1+ flocculation considered normal;[108] (6) serum alkaline phosphatase (Bodansky method[109]), with normal for adults 0 to 4 units per 100 ml.; (7) serum glutamic oxaloacetic[110] (SGOT) and serum glutamic pyruvic transaminase[111] (SGPT), normal range 4 to 40 units; (8) 5-nucleotidase,[112] normal value 0.3 to 3.2 units per 100 ml.

In *hepatocellular jaundice* there usually are a positive cephalin-cholesterol flocculation, increased thymol and zinc turbidity, positive thymol flocculation, and little or no increase in the serum alkaline phosphatase (less than 10 Bodansky units per 100 ml. or 30 to 35 King-Armstrong units). By contrast, we note that the usual findings in cases of *obstructive jaundice* are a negative cephalin-cholesterol flocculation, normal thymol and normal or decreased zinc turbidity, negative (or 1+) thymol flocculation, and increase in the serum alkaline phosphatase of more than 10 Bodansky units per 100 ml. (or more than 30 to 35 King-Armstrong units).

Although obstructive jaundice is virtually always accompanied by an increase in the serum alkaline phosphatase, this increase may be of moderate degree, less than 10 Bodansky units per 100 ml., even in cases of biliary obstruction due to neoplasm.[113] A steadily rising concentration of both serum alkaline phosphatase and serum bilirubin, coupled with a negative cephalin flocculation test, constitute a most reliable index of obstructive jaundice.[114] One may exclude increases in the enzyme concentration attributable to bone disease by determining the concentration of serum 5-nucleotidase, which is not influenced by osseous factors.[112] On the other hand, the serum 5-nucleotidase may rarely be increased in the face of a normal serum-alkaline phosphatase concentration.

Determination of the serum glutamic oxaloacetic (SGOT) and serum glutamic pyruvic (SGPT) transaminase levels may be of value in the distinction between hepatocellular and obstructive jaundice. In ob-

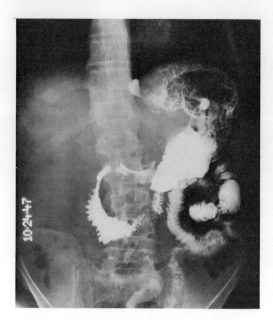

FIG. 24-7. (P.M.) Carcinoma of the head of the pancreas, producing extrinsic pressure on bulb and smoothing of inner border of duodenum. (Schiff, L.: Clinical Approach to Jaundice, Springfield, Ill., Thomas)

structive jaundice the concentration of these enzymes is usually not greater than 300 to 400 units, whereas in the very early stages of hepatitis, an increase of 1,000 or more units is frequent. However, we have seen a patient with obstructive jaundice due to carcinoma of the head of the pancreas in whom the serum transaminase (SGPT) was reported to be 750 units, and a case of carcinoma of the ampulla of Vater with a value of approximately 600 units. The diagnostic value of these enzyme determinations decreases with increase in the duration of jaundice. The most marked increases occur in the very early stages of hepatitis. Thus, in patients first seen 2 or 3 weeks after the onset of symptoms, the enzyme concentration may have fallen to the levels ordinarily observed in obstructive jaundice.[113] A persisting increased thymol turbidity at such a time would favor hepatocellular jaundice.

The application of immunologic techniques in the differentiation of obstructive from other forms of jaundice appears promising. A recent study would indicate the value of elevation of the serum IgM in distinguishing some patients with intrahepatic cholestasis from those with obstructive jaundice.[115,116]

Sera of patients with primary biliary cirrhosis produce granular cytoplasmic staining in unfixed tissue sections using fluorescein conjugates of antihuman gamma-globulin and anticomplement in the double layer immunofluorescent technique. This test appears to be consistently positive in primary biliary cirrhosis, and consistently negative in extrahepatic obstructive jaundice.[117,118]

It is well recognized that most of the individual laboratory tests constituting the so-called liver profile are not specific liver function tests, and hence may be positive in the absence of liver disease. The importance of the clinical examination in the interpretation of the results of these liver function tests becomes evident. As Himsworth[39] has stated so well, "There is yet no test which approaches in value a careful clinical assessment of the patient and none which can be interpreted without it." This is well exemplified by increases in the serum alkaline phosphatase which occur in the presence of osseous lesions, such as Paget's disease and hyperparathyroidism, and by positive cephalin flocculation tests observed in infectious mononucleosis, hemolytic jaundice, disseminated lupus erythematosus, pernicious anemia, acute leukemia, chronic malaria, and diffuse diseases of the reticuloendothelial system.[114]

PROTHROMBIN RESPONSE TO VITAMIN K[119,120,121]

Four of the clotting factors in plasma appear to be synthesized exclusively in the liver, namely, prothrombin, Factor VII (pro-SPCA or proconvertin), Factor X (Stuart-Power factor), and Christmas factor (plasma thromboplastin component). Their formation depends on the normal absorption of vitamin K from the intestine and the functional integrity of the liver cells. Three of these factors (prothrombin, Factor VII, and Factor X) influence the one-stage prothrombin time. Thus, a long prothrombin time may be due to the exclusion of bile from the intestine and/or severe liver injury. If the prothrombin time of the blood of an icteric patient is markedly prolonged (that is, if the "prothrombic activity" is under 40 per cent of normal) and becomes normal within 24 hours after parenteral administration of vitamin K, it is probable that liver cell function is reasonably good and that the jaundice is due to extrahepatic obstruction. The failure of the prothrombin time to shorten under these circumstances

FIG. 24-8. (R.R. 32331). Carcinoma of the ampulla of Vater. Spot film showing defect in descending duodenum. (Schiff, L.: Clinical Approach to Jaundice, Springfield, Ill., Thomas)

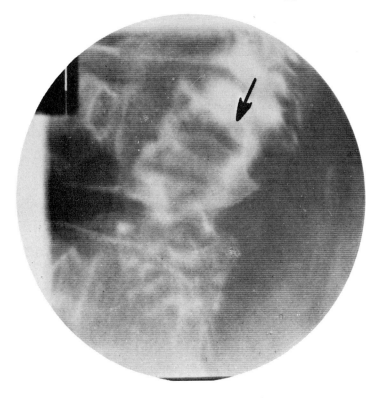

would indicate the presence of parenchymal liver disease. An adequate amount of vitamin K is provided by 10 mg. of menadione sodium bisulphite (Hykinone) given subcutaneously. In order to exclude intrinsic errors in the test itself, it is best to determine the blood prothrombin time on two separate days, both before and after the administration of the vitamin K. A recent case of common duct stones presented itself with purpura and a marked hypoprothrombinemia, which responded to vitamin K administration. No other clinical features of common duct stone were present.

RESPONSE TO STEROIDS

The response of the serum-bilirubin to steroid therapy may prove to be helpful in the differential diagnosis of jaundice in spite of earlier conflicting reports.[122,126a] A period of 4 or 5 days is usually chosen during which ACTH or corticosteroids are given and the effects on the serum bilirubin concentration observed. The ACTH is usually administered intramuscularly in doses of 60 to 120 units per day, whereas the corticosteroids are given in the form of 30 to 60 mg. of prednisone daily. A drop in serum

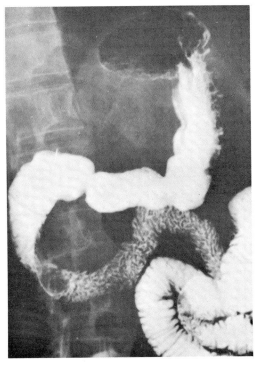

FIG. 24-9. (E. T. 158725). Defect in descending duodenum.

bilirubin concentration of 40 to 50 per cent or more is strongly indicative of hepatitis; the drop is rapid in the first 24 to 48 hours, and is followed by a slower fall. In obstructive jaundice (and cirrhosis) the drop is less marked, and when treatment is discontinued, the value promptly returns to pretreatment levels or no further change occurs. Unfortunately, variations in response and overlapping of effects make the test unreliable in individual cases.[122] Nevertheless, a definite response to the initial test followed by continued improvement with (or without) further therapy would argue strongly for hepatitis.

The mechanism of the resulting decrease in serum bilirubin is not known. It is not that of increased biliary excretion, increased renal clearance of bile pigments, or decrease in the rate of red cell breakdown. An additional metabolic pathway for bilirubin has been suggested,[126] as has inhibition of hepatic bilirubinogenesis.[127]

DUODENAL DRAINAGE

Duodenal drainage may be helpful in the differential diagnosis of jaundice by furnishing material for clinical, microscopic and cytologic examinations.[128]

ROENTGEN EXAMINATION

X-ray examination has been of limited value in the differential diagnosis of jaundice, largely because of four factors: (1) inability to furnish direct evidence of hepatitis, (2) inadequacies of present-day technics in the demonstration of tumors producing jaundice, (3) limitations of cholecystography and intravenous cholangiography, and (4) lack of proof that gallstones are the cause of jaundice by their mere demonstration.

X-ray changes caused by tumors producing icterus depend largely on pressure or displacement effects upon contiguous structures resulting from expansion of the neoplasm, and may not be present during the early stages of tumor growth. A carcinoma

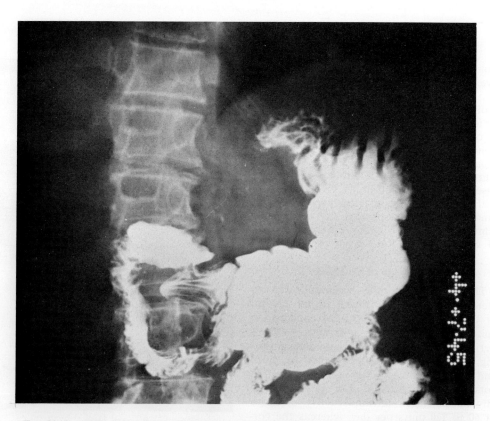

FIG. 24-10. (W.B. 539). Reversed-3 sign in the descending portion of the duodenum with clinical evidence suggestive of carcinoma of the ampulla of Vater. (Schiff, L.: Differential Diagnosis of Jaundice, Chicago, Year Book Pub.)

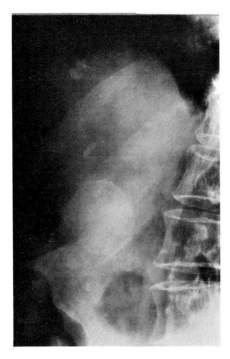

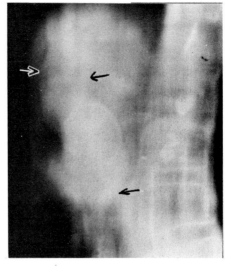

FIG. 24-11. (*Left*) Large calculus demonstrated by 4-day dye (Telepaque) test not previously revealed on plain film or after attempt at intravenous cholangiography. (*Right*) Calculus shown in common bile duct following intravenous cholangiograph performed immediately after demonstration by 4-day technique. Upper arrows indicate degree of dilatation of common bile duct. Lower arrow indicates narrowing of duct distal to the calculus.

of the head of the pancreas producing jaundice may not be large enough to bulge appreciably on the surface of the gland, and therefore may escape detection on roentgen examination.

Cholecystography has been of little diagnostic value in cases of hepatocellular or obstructive jaundice, since the gallbladder may fail to visualize because of the liver's impaired ability to excrete the dye.

Despite its limitations, the roentgen examination may be helpful in the diagnosis of the cause of jaundice. A plain film may reveal enlargement of the liver and the spleen, a stone in the common bile duct, a ground-glass appearance suggestive of ascites, or an elevated right diaphragm indicative of hepatic tumor or abscess. Esophageal varices may be visualized in cases of hepatic cirrhosis or hepatoma. By revealing the presence of a primary neoplasm in the alimentary canal or other body system, the roentgen examination may help to confirm the diagnosis of a metastatic hepatic tumor; or, by failing to reveal a primary site elsewhere, it may strengthen the clinical impression of hepatoma. It may furnish evidence of an enlarged liver by demonstrating displacement of the stomach posteriorly and/or

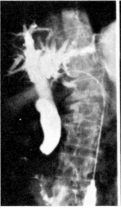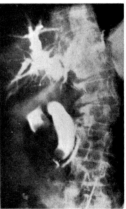

FIG. 24-12. (*Left*) Cholangiogram taken immediately after transhepatic injection of contrast material. Failure of common bile duct to fill completely and nipplelike appearance at lower end of contrast column are consistent with obstruction caused by stricture or neoplasm. (*Right*) Patient erect, 15 minutes later. Common bile duct is now filled and large solitary stone clearly demonstrated. Note upward convexity of contrast column above obstructing gallstone and reflux filling of distal pancreatic duct. (Zinberg, S. S., et al.: Percutaneous transhepatic cholangiography, Amer. J. Dig. Dis. 10:54, 1965)

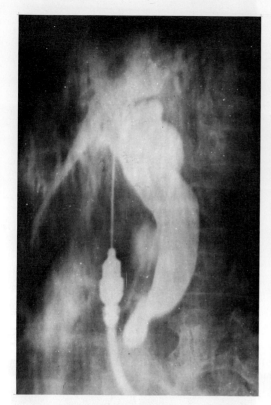

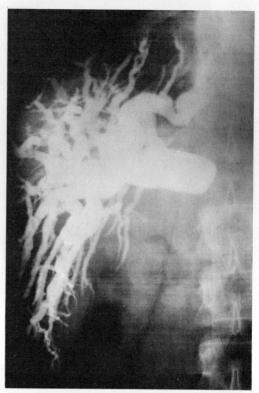

FIG. 24-13. Transhepatic cholangiogram showing periampullar carcinoma. Dilated common bile duct with concave termination. (Schiff, L.: Postgrad. Med., 41:39)

FIG. 24-14. (B.K.) Transhepatic cholangiogram showing biliary tract dilatation associated with carcinoma of head of pancreas. (Schiff, L.: Diseases of the Liver, ed. 2, Philadelphia, Lippincott)

to the left, or displacement of the hepatic flexure of the colon downward.

A pancreatic tumor may produce anterior displacement of the duodenal loop, downward displacement of the duodenal-jejunal juncture, compression or invasion of the duodenum or the stomach, or widening of the duodenal loop (Fig. 24-7). Periampullary tumor may produce a filling defect in the descending duodenum (Figs. 24-8 and 24-9) or Frostberg's reversed-3 sign (Fig. 24-10).

By demonstrating calcification in the pancreas, the roentgen examination may lead to the diagnosis of relapsing pancreatitis as a cause of icterus.

Intravenous cholangiography may be employed successfully when the serum bilirubin has dropped to 3 mg. per cent or less (Fig. 24-11), or when bromsulphalein retention is less than 15 to 30 per cent.[129,130] The common duct is demonstrated best within the first hour. It is well to remember that the normal common bile duct measures up to 10 mm. in diameter on the roentgenogram, and that following cholecystectomy the common duct may dilate up to 16 mm. in diameter. More marked dilatation or persistent opacification on 2- or 3-hour films is indicative of obstructive disease.

Oral cholangiography may be accomplished by repeating the dose of iopanoic acid (Telepaque), giving it on the evening before and again on the morning of the x-ray examination,[131] or by administering iopanoic acid in doses of 1.0 Gm. (2 tablets) after each meal for a 4-day period, with the patient on a relatively fat-free diet.[132,133] On the morning of the fifth day, roentgenograms are taken with the patient fasting. By this technic, opacification of radiolucent biliary calculi may result from deposition of the Telepaque on the surface of the stones (Fig. 24-11, *left*).

FIG. 24-15. (W.J.) Operative cholangiogram showing common duct stone. (Schiff, L.: Clinical Approach to Jaundice, Springfield, Ill., Thomas)

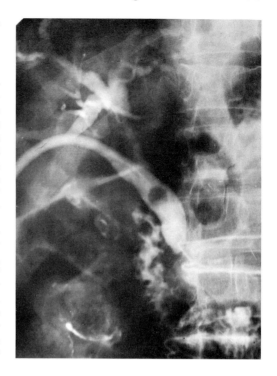

Percutaneous transhepatic cholangiography[134-140] is being used increasingly for demonstrating the presence of obstructive jaundice and indicating the site and nature of the obstructing lesion. One particular advantage is that it may be used when intravenous cholangiography is contraindicated, i.e., when the serum bilirubin is over 3 mg. per cent. It is the best means presently available for distinguishing intrahepatic cholestasis from extrahepatic obstructive jaundice.

If bile is aspirated following the introduction of a 19- or 20-gauge needle (usually about 6 inches long) through the abdominal wall into the liver substance, the presence of dilation of the bile ducts secondary to biliary tract obstruction is usually indicated. When bile is thus obtained, an x-ray contrast medium is injected through the needle in order to visualize the dilated ducts, as well as the site of obstruction. A convex appearance of

FIG. 24-16. (W.J.) Note shift of stone on comparing with Fig. 24-15. Upper arrow points to pancreatic duct. (Schiff, L.: Clinical Approach to Jaundice, Springfield, Ill., Thomas)

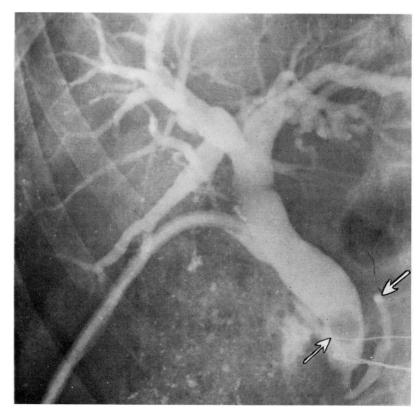

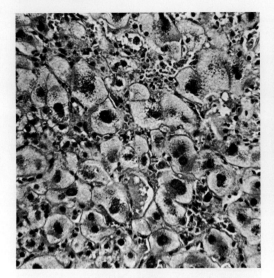

FIG. 24-17. Acute viral hepatitis. A high-power view, demonstrating swollen parenchymal elements ("balloon cells") with ground-glass cytoplasm and amitotic nuclear division. Focal inflammatory aggregates are evident, but the liver cells exhibit no fatty vacuolization. (Schiff, L.: Diseases of the Liver, ed. 2, Philadelphia, Lippincott)

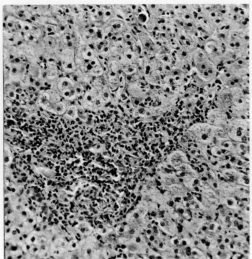

FIG. 24-18. Infectious (viral) hepatitis. A portal area is the seat of marked infiltration with lymphocytes and monocytes, but shows no other significant alteration. Hepatic cells are swollen, pale staining, granular, and often multinucleated. Near the upper center of the photograph is a single cell which has become shrunken, rounded, hyperchromatic, and separated from its neighbors. (Weisbrod, F. G., Schiff, L., Gall, E. A., Cleveland, F. P., and Berman, J. R.: Gastroenterology 14:56)

the termination of the visualized common bile duct is very suggestive of obstruction by stone (Fig. 24-12), whereas a concave termination is usually indicative of neoplastic obstruction (Figs. 24-13 and 24-14). The surgeon is alerted in advance of the procedure, so that if bile is aspirated, a laparotomy is performed on the same day to avert bile peritonitis. If no bile is aspirated after introducing the needle in several different directions, the presence of hepatocellular jaundice is assumed; however, the procedure may fail to detect dilated ducts in about 20 per cent of the cases. It requires further evaluation of reliability and hazards.

The importance of operative and postoperative cholangiography in the detection of stones in the common and the intrahepatic ducts is well-known (Figs. 24-15 and 24-16). It has been estimated that common duct calculi may be overlooked by ordinary methods in some 10 to 30 per cent of patients operated upon. The necessity for meticulous technic and intimate teamwork on the part of the anesthetist, the roentgenologist, and the surgeon has been stressed. For details, the reader is referred to the monographs of Mirizzi,[141,142] Norman[143] Partington and

Sachs,[144] and to the studies of Isaacs and Daves.[145]

NEEDLE BIOPSY OF THE LIVER

The use of needle biopsy of the liver should be confined to selected, unsolved cases of jaundice for many reasons: (1) the diagnosis of the cause of jaundice can be made in 85 to 90 per cent of cases on the basis of the clinical examination and the results of laboratory tests;[40,113,146] (2) the diagnostic use of steroids has decreased the need for needle biopsy in the jaundiced patient, particularly when definite decrease of the icterus results, and the steroids are then continued therapeutically; (3) marked increases of the serum glutamic transaminases (of an order of 1,000 units or more) justify deferment of the biopsy because of the likelihood of hepatitis; (4) there is the added danger of hemorrhage and, in cases of obstructive jaundice, bile peritonitis.[147] Nevertheless, in carefully selected patients who are observed closely after the procedure and treated promptly when indications arise, the danger is slight. The overall risk of

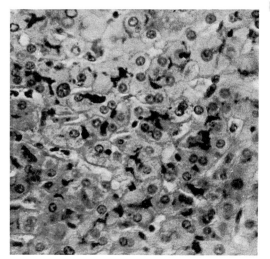

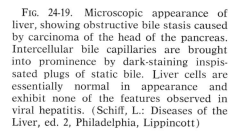

FIG. 24-19. Microscopic appearance of liver, showing obstructive bile stasis caused by carcinoma of the head of the pancreas. Intercellular bile capillaries are brought into prominence by dark-staining inspissated plugs of static bile. Liver cells are essentially normal in appearance and exhibit none of the features observed in viral hepatitis. (Schiff, L.: Diseases of the Liver, ed. 2, Philadelphia, Lippincott)

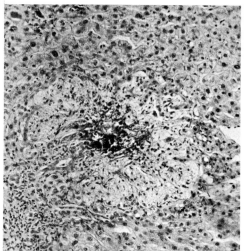

FIG. 24-20. Microscopic appearance of liver showing obstructive bile stasis, with a bile lake pathognomonic of extrahepatic biliary obstruction. Characteristic is a central pool of extravasated bile surrounded by a radial zone of degenerated parenchyma exhibiting a peculiar feathery reticulated appearance. (Weisbrod, F. G., Schiff, L., Gall, E. A., Cleveland, F. P., Berman, J. R.: Gastroenterology 14:56)

needle biopsy of the liver includes a mortality of 0.1 per cent and a complication rate of 0.32 per cent, according to the reviews of Terry[148] and Zamcheck and Klausenstock.[149] Lindner reports a death rate of 0.013 per cent, based on 97 replies to a questionnaire covering a total of 77,721 percutaneous liver biopsies made with the Menghini needle.[150]

Actually, the procedure probably will *be indicated* in less than 10 per cent of cases of jaundice, and includes the following situations:

When Difficulty Exists in Distinguishing Medical from Surgical Cases. Needless surgery may be averted by demonstrating the presence of hepatitis (Figs. 24-17 and 24-18); conversely, surgical therapy may be expedited in cases of obstructive jaundice (Figs. 24-19 and 24-20).

It should be emphasized that the biopsy specimen is almost of no help in determining the cause of extrahepatic obstruction; hence, needle biopsy of the liver should not be performed when the jaundice is obviously due to extrahepatic obstruction! Instead, surgery should be carried out.

The Presence of an Obscure Systemic Dis- order. Unsuspected granulomatous disease may be revealed in the biopsy specimen.

Suspicion of Metastatic Neoplasm of the Liver. In over 100 cases of proved neoplasm of the liver, the specimens obtained by needle biopsy were positive for tumor in 74 per cent; and, interestingly enough, the positive incidence was as high with the transthoracic as with the transabdominal approach.[151] In an experience which now covers the procurement of needle specimens in about 200 cases of malignant neoplasms of the liver, the high percentage of positive yields remains unaltered, and the risk of procedure has not been increased by the presence of neoplasm. This has also been the experience of Fenster and Klatskin.[95] Whether or not preliminary photoscans of the liver to help determine the proper or most promising site of needle biopsy will increase the positive yields in the needle specimens awaits further study.

Hepatomegaly of Undetermined Cause. A fatty liver may be discovered in a patient thought to have cirrhosis, neoplasm, or hepatitis. Histologic changes of obstructive jaundice may be found in patients with suspected hepatitis, and vice versa.

CONCLUSION

As was so well-stated more than a century ago,

Jaundice is rather a symptom of disease than a disease itself, and may arise from various causes which it is very important that we should be acquainted with; because knowledge of the cause, or of the circumstances under which the jaundice arose in any particular case, often gives us an insight into its real nature, which we could scarcely obtain from considering the symptoms merely.*

Excluding the hemolytic and hereditary varieties, most cases of jaundice comprise the various forms of hepatitis and cirrhosis or obstructive types due to gall stones or neoplasms. In the interpretation of the significance of jaundice, even in the present-day laboratory age, the physician will derive greatest help from the clinical approach. Nevertheless, he should be wary lest certain diagnostic clues prove misleading. These pertain particularly to the age of the patient and a history of alcoholism, which, although favoring certain causes of jaundice, do not of themselves exclude others. Similarly, the physician should bear in mind that *exposure* to an hepatotoxic agent does not necessarily establish a causal relationship, since there is at present no specific means of proving such a relationship in the form of a reliable skin test or by the demonstration of specific circulating antibodies. He should also realize that obstructive jaundice due to neoplasm, particularly that arising in the bile ducts, may sometimes endure for several years, and may even escape detection at laparotomy. Since jaundice is rarely, if ever, a surgical emergency, biding one's time may prove of help in diagnosis as the result of variations in the intensity of the icterus or its actual disappearance.

In the past few decades, aids in the diagnosis of the cause of jaundice have been provided through the introduction of new biochemical tests, advances in roentgenologic technics, and the procurement of needle specimens of the liver. As time passes, additional advances will be forthcoming; however, as those of the past, all will undoubtedly have their limitations, some their risks, and none will replace the clinical examination of the patient. It is hoped that these advances will soon include isolation of the hepatitis virus or viruses. We also need serologic tests for viral hepatitis and for specific immunologic changes of direct aid in the documentation of drug-induced hepatitis. Such aids, now lacking, would better enable the clinician to meet the challenge posed by the appearance of jaundice.

* George Budd, On Diseases of the Liver, 1846.

REFERENCES

1. von Ehrenstein, G., and Lockner, D.: Physiologischer erythrozytenabbau, Acta Haemat. 22:129, 1959.
2. Hughes-Jones, N. C., and Cheney, B.: The use of Cr^{51} and Fe^{59} as red cell labels to determine the fate of normal erythrocytes in the rat, Clin. Sci. 20:323, 1961.
3. Ostrow, J. D., Schmid, R., and Samuelson, D.: The protein binding of C^{14}-bilirubin in human and murine serum, J. Clin. Invest. 42:1286, 1963.
4. Brown, W. R., Grodsky, G. M., and Carbone, J. V.: Intracellular distribution of tritiated bilirubin during hepatic uptake and excretion, Amer. J. Physiol. 207:1237, 1964.
5. Grodsky, G.: Studies in the uptake and intrahepatic transport of H^3 bilirubin, *in* Bouchier and Billing (eds.): Bilirubin Metabolism, p. 99, Oxford, Blackwell Scientific Pub., 1967.
6. London, I. M., West, R., Shemin, D., and Rittenberg, D.: On the origin of bile pigment in normal man, J. Biol. Chem. 184:351, 1950.
7. Yamamoto, T., Skanderberg, J., Zipursky, A., and Israels, L. G.: The early appearing bilirubin: Evidence for two components, J. Clin. Invest. 44:31, 1965.
8. Israels, L. G., Levitt, M., Novak, W., and Zipursky, A.: The early bilirubin, Medicine 45:517, 1966.
9. Billing, B. H.: The Role of Conjugation in the Excretion of Bilirubin, Amsterdam, Elsevier Monograph, 1961.
10. Billing, B. H., Cole, P. G., and Lathe, G. H.: The excretion of bilirubin as a diglucuronide giving the direct van den Bergh reaction, Biochem. J. 65:774, 1957.
11. Schmid, R.: The identification of "direct-reacting" bilirubin as bilirubin glucuronide, J. Biol. Chem. 229:881, 1957.
12. Talafant, E.: Properties and composition of the bile pigment giving a direct diazo reaction, Nature 178:312, 1956.
13. White, A. E.: The distribution of glucuronyl transferase in cell membranes, *in* Bouchier and Billing (eds.): Bilirubin Metabolism, p. 183, Oxford, Blackwell Scientific Pub., 1967.
14. Noir, B. A., Groszman, R. J., and de Walz, A. T.: Studies on bilirubin sulphate, Biochim. Biophys. Acta 117:297, 1966.
15. Noir, B. A., de Walz, A. T., and Rodriguez Garay, E.: Studies on bilirubin sulphate in human bile, *in* Bouchier and Billing (eds.): Bilirubin Metabolism, p. 99, Oxford, Blackwell Scientific Pub., 1967.

16. Gartner, L. M., and Arias, I. M.: Pituitary regulation of bilirubin excretion by the liver, J. Clin. Invest. 45:1011, 1966.

17. Arias, I. M.: Personal communication.

18. Nosslin, B.: The direct diazo-reaction of bile pigments in serum, Scand. J. Clin. Lab. Invest. vol. 12, suppl. 49, 1960.

19. Ali, M. A. M., and Billing, B. H.: Effect of acid-base changes in renal clearance of bile pigments, Clin. Sci. 30:543, 1966.

20. Fulop, M., and Brazeau, P.: The renal excretion of bilirubin in dogs with obstructive jaundice, J. Clin. Invest. 43:1192, 1964.

21. Hoenig, V., and Schück, O.: Dialysability of conjugated bilirubin from plasma of jaundiced dogs and patients, Lancet 2:1297, 1964.

22. Wallace, D. K., and Owen, E. E.: An evaluation of the mechanism of bilirubin excretion by the human kidney, J. Lab. Clin. Med. 64:741, 1964.

23. Ali, M. A. M., and Billing, B. H.: Renal excretion of bilirubin by the rat, Amer. J. Physiol. 214:1340, 1968.

24. Watson, C. J., Campbell, M., and Lowry, P. T.: Preferential reduction of conjugated bilirubin to urobilinogen by normal fecal flora, Proc. Soc. Exp. Biol. Med. 98:707, 1958.

25. Gustafsson, B. E., and Lanke, L. S.: Bilirubin and urobilins in germfree, ex-germfree and conventional rats, J. Exp. Med. 112:975, 1960.

26. Matusi, K.: Studies on the reduction products of bilirubin in the small intestine, Igaku Kenkyu 29:1086, 1959.

27. Watson, C. J.: Composition of the urobilin group in urine, bile, and feces and the significance of variations in health and disease, J. Lab. Clin. Med. 54:1, 1959.

28. McMaster, P. D., and Elman, R.: Urobilin physiology and pathology, Ann. Intern. Med. 1:68, 1927.

29. Bourke, E., Milne, M. D., and Stokes, G. S.: Mechanisms of renal excretion of urobilinogen, Brit. Med. J. 2:1510, 1965.

30. McNee, J. W.: Jaundice: a review of recent work, Quart. J. Med. 16:390, 1922-23.

31. Watson, C. J.: Regurgitation jaundice: clinical differentiation of the common forms, with particular reference to the degree of biliary obstruction, J.A.M.A. 114:2427, 1940.

32. Tisdale, W. A., Klatskin, G., and Kinsella, E. D.: The significance of the direct-reacting fraction of serum bilirubin in hemolytic jaundice, Amer. J. Med. 26:214, 1959.

33. Schalm, L., and Weber, A. P.: Jaundice with conjugated bilirubin in hyperhaemolysis, Acta Med. Scand. 176:549, 1964.

34. Gonzalez-Oddone, M. V.: Bilirubin, bromsulfalein, bile acids, alkaline phosphatase and cholesterol of thoracic duct lymph in experimental regurgitation jaundice, Proc. Soc. Exp. Biol. Med. 63:144, 1946.

35. Grafflin, A. L., and Chaney, V. E., Jr.: Studies of extrahepatic biliary obstruction in the white mouse by fluorescence microscopy, Bull. Hopkins Hosp. 93:107, 1953.

36. Hanzon, V.: Liver cell secretion under normal and pathologic conditions studied by fluorescence microscopy on living rats, Acta Physiol. Scand. supp. 101, 28:1, 1952.

37. Watson, C. J.: The bile pigments, New Eng. J. Med. 227:705, 1942.

38. Rich, A. R.: The pathogenesis of the forms of jaundice, Bull. Hopkins Hosp. 47:338, 1930.

39. Himsworth, H. P.: Lectures on the Liver and Its Diseases, ed. 2, Cambridge, Mass., Harvard, 1950.

40. Watson, C. J.: An approach to the distinction of medical and surgical jaundice, Minnesota Med. 32:973, 1949.

41. Eppinger, H.: Die Leberkrankheiten: Allgemeine und Spezielle Pathologie und Therapie der Leber, Vienna, Springer, 1937.

42. Lucke, B.: The pathology of fatal epidemic hepatitis, Amer. J. Path. 20:471, 1944.

43. Steigmann, F., and Popper, H.: Intrahepatic obstructive jaundice, Gastroenterology 1:645, 1943.

44. Popper, H., and Schaffner, F.: Response of the liver to injury, in Popper and Schaffner (eds.): Progress in Liver Disease, p. 86, New York, Grune and Stratton, 1961.

45. Watson, C. J., and Hoffbauer, F. W.: The problem of prolonged hepatitis with particular reference to the cholangiolitic type and to the development of cholangiolitic cirrhosis of the liver, Ann. Intern. Med. 25:195, 1946.

46. Billing, B. H., and Williams, R. S.: Unpublished data.

47. Arias, I. M.: Panel: Bilirubin metabolism, Gastroenterology 36:166, 1959.

48. McMahon, F. G.: Effect of prednisolone, physical activity, fat intake and choleretic agents on the serum bilirubin level in a case of constitutional hepatic dysfunction (Gilbert's disease), Gastroenterology 32:325, 1957.

49. Whelton, M. J., Krustev, L. P., and Billing, B. H.: Reduction in serum bilirubin by phenobarbital in adult unconjugated hyperbilirubinaemia: is enzyme induction responsible? Amer. J. Med. 45:160, 1968.

50. Levine, R. A., and Klatskin, G.: Unconjugated hyperbilirubinemia in absence of overt hemolysis, Amer. J. Med. 36: 541, 1964.

51. Hult, H.: Cholemic simple familial (Gilbert) and posthepatitic states without fibrosis of the liver, Acta Med. Scand. (supp. 244) 138:1-96, 1950.

52. Kalk, H., and Wildhirt, E.: Die posthepatitische hyperbilirubinamie, Z. Klin. Med. 155:547, 1959.

53. Foulk, W. T., Butt, H. R., Owen, C. A., Jr., and Whitcomb, F. F., Jr.: Constitutional hepatic dysfunction (Gilbert's disease): its natural history and related syndromes, Medicine 38:25, 1959.

54. Berendsohn, S.: Hepatic function at high altitudes, Arch. Intern. Med. 109:256, 1962.

55. Greenberger, N. J., Milligan, F. D., De Groote, L. V., and Isselbacher, K. J.: Jaundice and thyrotoxicosis in the absence of congestive heart failure, Amer. J. Med. 36:840, 1964.

56. de Silva, L. C., Jamra, M. A., Maspes, V., Pontes, J. F., Pieroni, R. R., and de Ulhóa Cintra, A. B.: Pathogenesis of indirect reacting hyperbilirubinemia after portacaval anastomosis, Gastroenterology 44:117, 1963.

57. Dubin, I. N.: Chronic idiopathic jaundice: a review of 50 cases, Amer. J. Med. 24:268, 1958.

58. Sprinz, H., and Nelson, R. S.: Persistent non-hemolytic hyperbilirubinemia associated with lipochrome-like pigment in liver cells: Report of four cases, Ann. Intern. Med. 41:952, 1954.

59. Bynum, W. T.: Mavero-hepatic icterus (black liver jaundice), Gastroenterology 33:97, 1957.

60. Caroli, J.: International Association for the Study of Liver Disease, 1st Mtg., London, Apr. 1960, Lancet 1:1066, 1960.

61. Wegmann, R., Weinmann, S., and Rangier, M.: Infra-red spectrography of the black pigment extracted from the spleen. Rev. Med. Mal. Foie 35:95, 1960.

62. Cornelius, C. E., Arias, I. M., and Osburn, B. I.: Hepatic pigmentation with photosensitivity: a syndrome in Corriedale sheep resembling Dubin-Johnson syndrome in man, J. Amer. Vet. Med. Ass. 146:709, 1965.

63. Arias, I. M., Bernstein, L., Toffler, R., Cornelius, C., Novikoff, A. B., and Essner, E.: Black liver disease in Corriedale sheep: a new mutation affecting hepatic excretory function, J. Clin. Invest. 43:1249, 1964.

64. Mandema, E., de Fraiture, W. H., Nieweg, H. O., and Arends, A.: Familial chronic idiopathic jaundice (Dubin-Sprinz disease) with a note on bromsulphalein metabolism in this disease, Amer. J. Med. 28:42, 1960.

65. Wolf, R. L., Pizette, M., Richman, A., Dreiling, D. A., Jacobs, W., Fernandez, O., and Popper, H.: Chronic idiopathic jaundice; a study of 2 afflicted families, Amer. J. Med. 28:32, 1960.

66. Shaldon, S., and Caeser, J. J.: Personal communication.

67. Calderon, A., and Goldgraber, M. B.: Chronic idiopathic jaundice: a case report, Gastroenterology 40:244, 1961.

68. Sageld, W., Dolgaard, O. Z., and Tygstrup, N.: Constitutional hyperbilirubinemia with unconjugated bilirubin in the serum and lipochrome-like pigment granules in the liver, Ann. Intern. Med. 56:308, 1962.

69. Schoenfield, L. J., McGill, D. B., Hunton, D. B., Foulk, W. T., and Butt, H. R.: Studies of chronic idiopathic jaundice (Dubin-Johnson syndrome). I. Demonstration of hepatic excretory defect, Gastroenterology 44:101, 1963.

70. Satler, J.: Another variant of constitutional familial hepatic dysfunction with permanent jaundice and with alternating serum bilirubin relations, Acta Hepatosplen. 13:38, 1966.

71. Rotor, A. B., Manahan, L., and Florentin, A.: Familial non-hemolytic jaundice with direct van den Bergh reaction, Acta Med. Philipp. 5:37, 1948.

72. Schiff, L., Billing, B. H., and Oikawa, Y.: Familial nonhemolytic jaundice with conjugated bilirubin in the serum; a case study, New Eng. J. Med. 260:1315, 1959.

73. Haverback, B. J., and Wirtschafter, S. K.: Familial non-hemolytic jaundice with normal liver histology and conjugated bilirubin, New Eng. J. Med. 262:113, 1960.

74. Arias, I. M.: Studies of chronic familial non-hemolytic jaundice with conjugated bilirubin in the serum with and without an unidentified pigment in the liver cells, Amer. J. Med. 31:510, 1961.

75. Peck, O. C., Rey, D. F., and Snell, A.: Familial jaundice with free and conjugated bilirubin in the serum and without liver pigmentation, Gastroenterology 39:625, 1960.

76. Davis, W. D., and Young, P. C.: An unusual type of hyperbilirubinemia with bromsulfalein retention and microscopically normal liver, Gastroenterology 37:206, 1959.

77. Charbonnier, A.: Personal communication.

78. Koff, R. S., Grady, G. F., Chalmers, T. C., Mosley, J. W., Swartz, B. L., and the Boston Inter-Hospital Group: Viral hepatitis in a group of Boston hospitals. III. Importance of exposure to shellfish in a non-epidemic area, New Eng. J. Med. 276:703, 1967.

79. Koff, R. S., and Sear, H. S.: Internal temperature of steamed clams, New Eng. J. Med. 276:737, 1967.

80. Schiff, L.: Homologous serum hepatitis: clinical implications, New Orleans Med. Surg. J. 99:611, 1947.

81. ———: Diagnostic significance of the time interval between resection of a malignant tumor and the appearance of jaundice, Amer. J. Dig. Dis. 5:573, 1960.

82. Schoenfield, L. J.: The relationship of bile acids to pruritus in hepatobiliary disease, presented at a conference on bile salt metabolism sponsored by the U. of Cincinnati Med. Center, Cincinnati, Sept. 28 and 29, 1967 (to be published).

83. Spiegel, E. L., Schubert, W., Perrin, E., and Schiff, L.: Benign recurrent intrahepatic cholestasis, with response to cholestyramine, Amer. J. Med. 39:682, 1965.

84. Chauffard, M. A.: Le cancer du corps de pancréas, Bull. Acad. Nat. Med. 60:242, 1908.

85. Ashe, W. F., Pratt-Thomas, H. R., and Kumpe, C. W.: Weil's disease: a complete review of American literature and abstract of the world literature; 7 case reports, Medicine 20:145, 1941.

86. Bean, W. B.: The cutaneous arterial spider: a survey, Medicine 24:243, 1945.
87. Watson, C. J.: The prognosis and treatment of hepatic insufficiency, Ann. Intern. Med. 31:405, 1949.
88. Hoffbauer, F. W.: Bedside diagnosis of jaundice, Northwest Med. 48:757, 1949.
89. Challenger, F., and Walshe, J. M.: Foetor hepaticus, Lancet 1:1239, 1955.
90. Sherlock, S.: Cirrhosis of the liver, Postgrad. Med. J. 26:472, 1950.
91. Fleischner, F. G., and Sayegh, V.: Assessment of the size of the liver; roentgenologic considerations, New Eng. J. Med. 259:271, 1958.
92. Clain, H., Wartuoby, K., and Sherlock, S.: Abdominal arterial murmurs in liver disease, Lancet 2:516, 1966.
93. Schiff, L.: Absence of a palpable liver: a sign of value in excluding obstructive jaundice due to pancreatic cancer, Gastroenterology 32:1143, 1957.
94. Jones, C. M.: Personal communication.
95. Fenster, L. F., and Klatskin, G.: Manifestations of metastatic tumors of the liver: a study of 81 patients subjected to needle biopsy, Ann. Med. 31:238, 1961.
96. Duff, G. L.: The clinical and pathological features of carcinoma of the body and tail of the pancreas, Bull. Hopkins Hosp. 65:69, 1939.
97. Patek, A. J., Jr.: *Quoted by* Perera: J.A.M.A. 119:1417, 1942.
98. Perera, G. A.: A note on palmar erythema (so-called liver palms), J.A.M.A. 119:1417, 1942.
99. Havens, W. P., Jr.: Infectious hepatitis, Medicine 27:279, 1948.
100. Jones, C. M., and Minot, G. R.: Infectious (catarrhal) jaundice, an attempt to establish a clinical entity; observations on excretion and retention of bile pigments and on blood, Boston Med. Surg. J. 189:531, 1923.
101. Zieve, L.: Jaundice, hyperlipemia and hemolytic anemia: a heretofore unrecognized syndrome associated with alcoholic fatty liver and cirrhosis, Ann. Intern. Med. 48:471, 1958.
102. Zieve, L., Hill, E., Hanson, M. C. L., Falcone, A. B., and Watson, C. J.: The serum bilirubin, Bull. Univ. Minn. Hosp. 22:14, 1951.
103. ———: Normal and abnormal variations and clinical significance of the one-minute and total serum bilirubin determinations, J. Lab. Clin. Med. 38:446, 1951.
104. Hanger, F. M.: Serological differentiation of obstructive from hepatogenous jaundice by flocculation of cephalin-cholesterol emulsions, J. Clin. Invest. 18:261, 1939.
105. Shank, R. E., and Hoagland, C. L.: A modified method for the quantitative determination of the thymol turbidity reaction of serum, J. Biol. Chem. 162:133, 1946.
106. Maclagan, N. F.: Thymol turbidity test; a new indicator of liver dysfunction, Nature 154:670, 1944; The thymol turbidity test as an indicator of liver dysfunction, Brit. J. Exp. Path. 25:234, 1944.
107. Kunkel, H. G.: Estimation of alterations of serum gamma globulin by a turbidimetric technique, Proc. Soc. Exp. Biol. Med. 66:217, 1947.
108. Neefe, J. R., Gambescia, J. M., Gardner, H. T., and Knowlton, M.: Symposium on viral hepatitis; comparison of the thymol, cephalincholesterol flocculation and colloidal red tests in acute viral hepatitis, Amer. J. Med. 8:600, 1950.
109. Bodansky, A.: Phosphatase studies: II. Determination of serum phosphatase; factors influencing the accuracy of the determination, J. Biol. Chem. 101:93, 1933.
110. Cabaud, P., Leeper, R., and Wroblewski, F.: Colorimetric measurement of serum glutamic oxaloacetic transaminase, Amer. J. Clin. Path. 26:1101, 1956.
111. Wroblewski, F., and Cabaud, P.: Colorimetric measurement of serum glutamic pyruvic transaminase, Amer. J. Clin. Path. 27:235, 1957.
112. Young, I. I.: Serum 5-nucleotidase: characterization and evaluation in disease states, Ann. N.Y. Acad. Sci. 75:357, 1958.
113. Schenker, S., Balint, J., and Schiff, L.: Differential diagnosis of jaundice: a perspective study of 61 proved cases, Amer. J. Dig. Dis. 7:449, 1962.
114. Hanger, F. M.: The meaning of liver function tests, Amer. J. Med. 16:565, 1954.
115. Bevan, G.: Personal communication.
116. Fahey, J. L., and McKelvey, E. M.: Quantitative determination of serum immunoglobin in antibody-agar plates, J. Immun. 94:84, 1965.
117. Kantor, F. S., and Klatskin, G.: Serological diagnosis of primary biliary cirrhosis: a potential clue to pathogenesis, Trans. Ass. Amer. Physicians 80:267, 1967.
118. Walker, J. G., Doniach, D., Roitt, I. M., and Sherlock, S.: Serological tests in the diagnosis of primary biliary cirrhosis, Lancet 1:827, 1965.
119. Giansiracusa, J. E., and Althausen, T. L.: Diagnostic management of patients with jaundice, J.A.M.A. 134:589, 1947.
120. Lord, J. W., Jr., and Andrus, W. DeW.: Differentiation of intrahepatic and extrahepatic jaundice: response of the plasma prothrombin to intramuscular injection of menadione (2 methyl-1, 4-naphthoquinone) as a diagnostic aid, Arch. Intern. Med. 68:199, 1941.
121. Turner, R. H.: *Quoted by* Schiff, L.: Differential Diagnosis of Jaundice, p. 250, Chicago, Year Book Pub., 1946.
122. Chalmers, T. C., Gill, R. J., Jernigan, T. P., Svec, F. A., Jordan, R. S., Waldstein, S. S., and Knowlton, M.: Evaluation of a 4-day ACTH test in the differential diagnosis of jaundice, Gastroenterology 30:894, 1956.

123. Ingelfinger, F.: Differential Diagnosis of Jaundice, DM, Nov. 1958, Chicago, Year Book Pub.

124. Solem, J. H.: The value of ACTH administration in the differential diagnosis of jaundice, Gastroenterologia 87:23, 1957.

125. Summerskill, W. H. J., Clowdus, B. F., Bollman, J. L., and Fleisher, G. A.: Clinical and experimental studies on the effect of corticotropin and steroid drugs on bilirubinemia, Amer. J. Med. Sci. 241:555, 1961.

126. Williams, R., and Billing, B. H.: Action of steroid therapy in jaundice, Lancet 2:392, 1961.

126a. Schiff, L.: The use of steroids in liver disease, Medicine 45:565, 1966.

127. Katz, R., Ducci, H., and Alessandri, H.: Influence of cortisone and prednisolone on hyperbilirubinemia, J. Clin. Invest. 36:1370, 1957.

128. Schiff, L. (ed.): Diseases of the Liver, ed. 3, Philadelphia, J. B. Lippincott, 1969.

129. Berk, J. E., and Feigelson, H. H.: Current status of intravenous cholecystography and cholangiography, Southern Med. J. 50:421, 1957.

130. Johnson, G., Jr., Pearce, C., and Glenn, F.: Intravenous cholangiography in biliary tract disease, Ann. Surg. 152:91, 1960.

131. Twiss, J. R., and Gillette, L.: Oral cholangiography; a method of visualizing the "nonvisualized" gallbladder, J.A.M.A. 169:1275, 1959.

132. Salzman, E., and Warden, M. R.: Telepaque opacification of radiolucent biliary calculi; the "rim sign," Radiology 71:85, 1958.

133. Watkins, D. H., and Salzman, E.: Opacifying gallstones, Arch. Surg. 80:986, 1960.

134. Atkinson, M., Happey, M. G., and Smiddy, F. G.: Percutaneous transhepatic cholangiography, Gut 1:357, 1960.

135. Kaplan, A. A., Traitz, J. J., Mitchell, S. D., and Block, A. L.: Percutaneous transhepatic cholangiography, Ann. Intern. Med. 54:856, 1961.

136. Santos, M., Figueroa, L., and Lopez, O.: Percutaneous transhepatic cholangiography in the diagnosis of posthepatic jaundice, Surgery 48:295, 1960.

137. Shaldon, S., Barber, K. M., and Young, W. B.: Percutaneous transhepatic cholangiography, a modified technique, Gastroenterology 42:371, 1962.

138. Flemma, R. J., and Shingleton, W. W.: Clinical experience with percutaneous transhepatic cholangiography, Amer. J. Surg. 111:13, 1965.

139. Glenn, F., Evans, J. A., Mujahed, A., and Thorbjarnarson, B.: Percutaneous transhepatic cholangiography, Ann. Surg. 156:451, 1962.

140. Zinberg, S. S., Berk, J. E., and Plasencia, H.: Percutaneous transhepatic cholangiography: Its use and limitations, Amer. J. Dig. Dis. 10:154, 1965.

141. Mirizzi, P. L.: Fisiopathologia del Hepato-Coledaco: Colangio-grafia operatoria, vol. 26, Buenos Aires, Ateneo, 1939.

142. ——: La cholangiographie operatoire. Quinze annes d'experience, Lyon Chir. 43:385, 1948.

143. Norman, O.: Studies on the hepatic ducts in cholangiography, Acta Radiol. (supp. 84) pp. 1-81, 1951.

144. Partington, P. F., and Sachs, M. D.: Cholangiography, in Carter, B. N. (ed.): Monographs on Surgery, p. 75, New York, Nelson, 1951.

145. Isaacs, J. P., and Daves, M. L.: Technique and evaluation of operative cholangiography, Surg., Gynec. Obstet. 111:103, 1960.

146. Hanger, F. M.: Diagnostic problems of jaundice, Arch. Intern. Med. 86:169, 1950.

147. Gallison, D. T., Jr., and Skinner, D.: Bile peritonitis complicating needle biopsy of the liver, New Eng. J. Med. 243:47, 1950.

148. Terry, R.: Risks of needle biopsy of the liver, Brit. Med. J. 1:1102, 1952.

149. Zamcheck, N., and Klausenstock, O.: The risk of needle biopsy, New Eng. J. Med. 249:1062, 1953.

150. Lindner, H.: Limitations and dangers in percutaneous liver biopsies with the Menghini needle, Recent Advances in Gastroenterology, Proc. 3rd World Congr. of Gastroenterology 3:373, 1966.

151. Ward, J., Schiff, L., Young, P., and Gall, E. A.: Needle biopsy of the liver: IX. Further experiences with malignant neoplasm, Gastroenterology 27:300, 1954.

25

Fever

*ELISHA ATKINS**

Regulation of Body Temperature

Body Temperature in Health

Limits of Body Temperature Compatible
with Life

Fever: Types and Terminology

Pathogenesis of Fever

Metabolism in Fever

Complications of Fever

Spurious Fever

Effects of Fever

Clinical Causes of Fever

Definition. Fever is an elevation of body temperature due to disease.

Evaluation of the significance of fever requires some knowledge of the mechanisms of temperature control and of the various ways in which that control may be disturbed. In this chapter, after outlining the principal factors concerned with maintenance of a steady body temperature, we shall consider the kinds of conditions in which fever occurs. In most instances the actual pathogenesis of this important manifestation of disease is not fully known.

REGULATION OF BODY TEMPERATURE

In order to maintain a relatively constant body temperature, a fine balance between heat loss and heat production must be maintained, so that a slight increase or decrease of one is promptly compensated by a similar increase or decrease of the other. Maintenance of body temperature within the normal range is accomplished by a number of physiologic processes, involving both chem-

ical and physical transfer of heat. The operation of these mechanisms is integrated by the central nervous system.

SOURCES OF BODY HEAT

Small, and usually inconsequential quantities of heat may be derived from external sources: by radiation from the sun or a heating fixture, by conduction from an electric heating pad or hot water bottle, or from ingestion of hot foods or fluids.

The principal source of heat is combustion of food within the body. The contribution of various organ systems to the total heat production varies greatly according to circumstances. During rest, the proportions are approximately as follows: respiration and circulation one-tenth; brain and muscle metabolism, each two-tenths; abdominal viscera (mainly the liver) one-half. During physical work, one generates much additional heat in the muscles.[1]

Heat production in the muscular system is of special importance in temperature regulation because it is adapted to maintaining uniform body temperature, being readily increased or decreased according to need.

HEAT ELIMINATION

Three forms of heat elimination are of importance: radiation, vaporization, and convection. In addition to these, a small amount of heat is lost by conduction to cooler objects and by the warming of ingested food.

Radiation is the process by which energy is transferred from warmer objects to cooler ones by means of electromagnetic waves. Under ordinary conditions about 60 per cent of the body heat is eliminated in this way.

Vaporization of water from the surface of the body takes place constantly, even in the absence of sweating, just as water gradually leaves any moist object that is exposed to the air. Evaporation also occurs in the respiratory passages. Since heat is required

* The author is grateful to Dr. P. B. Beeson, who generously has allowed the incorporation of major sections of his text from the third edition of this chapter.

may be useful in explaining an otherwise puzzling fever.

Digestion of Food. Some workers have recorded rise of body temperature of 0.2 to 0.5° F. in experimental subjects after ingestion of a meal.[41] The elevation began in 20 to 30 minutes and reached its peak within 90 minutes. These findings could not be substantiated in the later studies of Mellette et al.[37]

Warm Environment. The average temperature becomes measurably higher in persons who move from temperate to tropical climates. Temporary change to a warm environment may also raise the temperature level slightly. In one experiment it was found that the rectal temperatures of a group of normal subjects rose from an average of 98.06° F. to 99.32° F. when the room temperature was raised from 68.0° to 86.0° F.[42] It is a common experience in hospitals to find that on very hot days many patients who have no other cause for fever register oral temperatures of 99.0° F. or more.

Cold Environment. Exposure to cold causes only a slight reduction in the body temperature of a normal adult, but induces a somewhat greater change in an infant or in an old person.

Menstrual Cycle. There is a rhythmic variation in body temperature associated with the menstrual cycle. Immediately before the onset of menstruation the temperature falls 0.5° to 0.75° F. below its previous level. This relatively low temperature is maintained until the time of ovulation, which is usually about the thirteenth or the fourteenth day of the cycle. Then there is a rise of 0.5° to 0.75° F., which is maintained until just before the next menstrual period. Such variations may be exaggerated in women who have fever from another cause, such as pulmonary tuberculosis. Amenorrheic women have no cyclic temperature change, and in them it has been reported that estrogen therapy depresses body temperature whereas progesterone provokes a rise. Therefore it has been assumed that endogenous estrogens and progesterone are responsible for the biphasic basal temperature of the menstrual cycle. However, certain clinical observations indicate that body temperature change does not always coincide with any narrow phase of the ovarian follicle cycle.[43]

Pregnancy. Early in pregnancy there is a slight rise in average temperature. About the fourth month of gestation a gradual fall begins, and this continues until parturition, when there is a quick return to the normal level.[44]

LIMITS OF BODY TEMPERATURE COMPATIBLE WITH LIFE

Low Temperatures

Formerly it was believed that life would cease if the body temperature fell below about 90.0° F. Smith and Fay[45] have shown, however, that by administering sedatives and then applying cold, the body temperature can be reduced to 75.0° to 80.0° F. and maintained there for days without evident harm. An extreme example of hypothermia is reported by Laufman.[46] The subject, under influence of alcohol, lay unconscious for many hours out of doors in cold weather. When brought to a hospital the rectal temperature, obtained 90 minutes after warming had begun, was 64.4° F. It was calculated that on admission the rectal temperature must have been in the vicinity of 61° F. This is the lowest recorded internal body temperature in a patient who survived.

Profound hypothermia with a fall in rectal temperature to 87.8° F. has been reported in a patient with disseminated lupus erythematosus treated with cortisone.[47] There were signs of active heat loss with sweating and vasodilatation despite the low temperature, which was felt to be caused by the action of steroid on the thermoregulatory center. ACTH and cortisone also have a marked antipyretic effect in many febrile states, presumably due, like that of other antipyretics, to a direct action on the hypothalamus. Certain of these drugs affect normal body temperature as well and several (such as chlorpromazine) have been used, in conjunction with physical methods, to induce hypothermia in surgery.[48]

High Temperatures

In the medical literature there are reports of fantastic fevers, 130° F. or even 150.0° F. These are undoubtedly the results of fraud or error on the part of either the patients or the physicians. Experiments in animals and acceptable observations in human beings indicate that living tissues are irreversibly damaged at temperatures above the region of 115.0° F. Richet placed the upper possible limit at 114.8° F. (46.0° C.), and this has been endorsed by MacNeal[49] after a careful study of the evidence. There are a number of acceptable reports of temperatures as high as 112.0° or 113.0° F. with recovery. In a case

FIG. 25-1. Rat-bite fever, due to infection with *Spirillum minus.* An example of a relapsing fever. Short febrile periods are separated by two or three days of normal temperature.

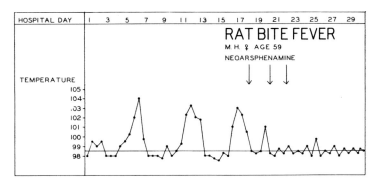

of staphylococcal septicemia the fever ranged between 104.0° F. and 112.0° F. continuously for three months.[50]

As has been pointed out by DuBois,[51] there is a sort of temperature "ceiling" in most febrile disease, at about 105° or 106° F. It would appear that the body's thermostat can rarely be disturbed sufficiently to permit an elevation beyond this level. Of special interest is DuBois' analysis of actual temperature readings in 357 patients with febrile diseases. Although the level seldom exceeded 106° F., readings in the range of 104° to 105° F. were obtained more frequently than 103° to 104° F., and twice as frequently as the 102° to 103° F. range. This seems to point to a "secondary thermostat setting" of thermoregulation, operating best in the range of 104° to 105° F.

FEVER: TYPES AND TERMINOLOGY

Fever is an elevation of the body temperature due to disease. It is, of course, only a symptom and, as is discussed subsequently, occurs in a wide variety of pathologic conditions.

Pyrexia is a term usually considered synonymous with fever, although some writers have used it to indicate elevations not due to infection.

Hyperpyrexia and hyperthermia usually refer to high fever, 105.0° F. or more.

Habitual hyperthermia has been used to designate a condition in which the average temperature is slightly above the accepted "normal" limit.

An intermittent or quotidian fever is one in which the temperature falls to normal and rises again each day.

In a remittent fever there is a marked variation in the temperature level each day, but the low point is still above the normal line.

A relapsing fever is one in which short febrile periods are interspersed by periods of one or more days of normal temperature. Figure 25-1 illustrates this in a case of rat-bite fever.

A hectic or septic fever is an intermittent fever in which the daily oscillations are very large; it often is associated with chills and sweating.

PATHOGENESIS OF FEVER

A satisfactory explanation of the genesis of fever must encompass two facts: (1) Fever is a manifestation of many kinds of disease processes, not only infectious diseases, but also injuries, neoplastic diseases, vascular accidents, metabolic disorders, etc. The most obvious common factor in them is tissue injury. (2) Fever occurs in disease of practically any tissue of the body.

Several theories of the mechanism of the production of fever have been proposed. One is that an abnormal distribution of body water, with hemoconcentration, causes a rise of body temperature by interfering with the transfer and the dissipation of heat.[52] Clinical observations do not support this hypothesis. Although some hemoconcentration usually occurs when the temperature is rising, it is probably only a concomitant process. Certainly there is no constant pattern of temperature variation associated with rapid change in fluid and electrolyte balance. Some workers have sought to explain fever as the result of overfunction of the adrenals and the thyroid, because of histologic evidence of intense activity in these glands following induction of fever in animals.[53] However, fever occurs in animals whose adrenals or thyroid have been destroyed, as well as in patients with Addison's disease or myxedema. An endocrine mechanism clearly cannot explain all of the known phenomena.

Clinical observation of febrile disorders

suggests strongly that cerebral thermoregulation is faulty.[54] As will be seen below, there is now good evidence that the activity of these centers is modified by some product or products of tissue injury.

Most experimental work on the pathogenesis of fever has been carried out with bacterial pyrogens. These substances, also known as endotoxins, are complex lipopolysaccharides of high molecular weight (approximately 1×10^6) which form part of the cell wall of Gram-negative bacteria and, in conjunction with protein, comprise the somatic 'O' antigen. Because of their ubiquity and ability to withstand autoclaving as well as to pass through filters, endotoxins readily contaminate biologic materials and are very difficult to remove from them. Endotoxins are extremely potent pharmacologic agents. In minute amounts they produce a wide variety of reactions in both animals and man, including fever, leukopenia, alterations in blood coagulation and, with large doses, shock and death.[56] Given intravenously, as little as 0.002 gamma of purified material per kg. body weight regularly produces a pyrogenic response in man.[57]

Two features of the febrile response caused by endotoxins seem relevant to their probable mechanism of action. First, after intravenous inoculation there is a variable latent period (from 15 to 30 minutes in rabbits and up to an hour or more in man) before the onset of fever. Second, during this period, circulating granulocytes virtually disappear from the blood stream due to their adherence to the walls of blood vessels throughout the body. These features of endotoxin-induced fever have given rise to the belief that endotoxins do not act directly on the thermoregulatory center of the brain, but release an intermediary pyrogen from a tissue source within the body, presumably from the granulocyte. A considerable body of evidence in support of this view has been accumulated in recent years.[58]

A material with pyrogenic properties has been recovered from saline extracts of rabbit granulocytes.[59] This material has been purified and appears to be a protein with a molecular weight of 10,000 to 20,000.[60] It therefore is clearly different from endotoxin. Originally, polymorphonuclear leukocytes were thought to be the only source of this substance; however, a more recent study indicates that extracts of many other normal tissues are similarly pyrogenic.[61]

A substance known as endogenous pyrogen (EP), with biological properties similar to leukocyte pyrogen, appears in the blood of a number of animals,[62] including humans,[63] given endotoxin intravenously. The febrile response corresponds closely with the amount of this material in the circulation. Conversely, when circulating leukocytes are abolished by nitrogen mustard, animals do not develop fever to ordinary doses of endotoxin, presumably because such animals cannot release EP.[64] However, these leukopenic animals respond normally when injected with EP. In vitro studies have confirmed that blood and exudate leukocytes derived from either animals or man release an EP upon addition of endotoxin.[58] This effect presumably is largely due to the granulocytes in such preparations. More recent work, however, indicates that components of the reticuloendothelial system, including rabbit alveolar[65] and exudate macrophages,[66] and Kupffer cells of the liver,[67] as well as human blood monocytes[68] also may be activated in vitro to produce EP.

There is evidence that EP plays a role in fevers produced by a number of agents other than the endotoxins of Gram-negative bacteria. Pyrogenic substances, which resemble endotoxin-induced EP in their biologic effects, are present in a number of human pathologic fluids[69,70] and also in the circulation of animals inoculated intravenously with myxoviruses, or with a variety of Gram-positive bacteria.[71] Similarly, fevers resulting from the reaction of microbial antigens with antibodies in specifically sensitized hosts appear to be caused by a circulating endogenous pyrogen, though its cellular source remains uncertain.[65,72] In man, buffy coat incompatibilities[73] and certain immune hemolytic reactions[74] are associated with marked leukopenias and fevers resembling those produced by endotoxins. Finally, in studies of fever accompanying peritoneal infections with pneumococci, it has been shown that pyrogen is rapidly liberated by cells in the inflammatory exudate and subsequently reaches the blood by way of the thoracic duct lymph.[75,76]

In all of these experimental situations it seems clear that an intermediary pyrogen, liberated from tissues of the host, plays a major role in producing the febrile response. Furthermore, when the brain is perfused directly with this substance, accelerated and augmented fevers are obtained, suggesting that EP has a direct and immediate action on the thermoregulatory centers of the brain.[77,78]

Studies by Wood and his colleagues[79,80] and Fessler *et al.*[81] have provided information of great interest concerning the factors that modify release of pyrogen from granulocytes. The production of this material by granulocytes appears to be an active metabolic process, dependent upon temperature and intact cellular structure, and may be blocked by certain enzyme inhibitors. The composition of the medium is important in determining the amount of pyrogen released from exudate granulocytes. Ions such as K+ and Ca++ prevent its release, presumably by maintaining certain functions of the cell membrane. On the other hand, the inhibiting effects of these ions may be circumvented by a variety of conditions, including phagocytosis, and the addition of endotoxins or agents in inflammatory exudates, all of which have been found to activate granulocytes to produce pyrogen in vitro.

These studies indicate the subtle balance that probably exists between various activators and inhibitors in the body. When the balance is disturbed by certain influences, there is production and release of EP, which in turn causes fever.

Unsolved Questions. It is apparent from this discussion that many questions concerning the pathogenesis of fever remain unanswered. Is there more than one type of endogenous pyrogen? Are phagocytic leukocytes (granulocytes and monocytes) and tissue macrophages the only source of EP? Although EP seems to be the chief factor in producing fever of microbial origin, nothing is known about the cause of fever in malignant tumors, lymphomas, collagen diseases, or certain metabolic diseases such as gout and porphyria. In some of these conditions, factors known to contribute to fever in various infectious diseases, such as inflammation and hypersensitivity, may play a role.

Also, little is known of the location or precursors of EP in the cell or of the specific mechanism by which EP is activated or disposed of in the body. No attempt has been made as yet to determine if this substance has other physiologic properties, although there is one study that strongly suggest that EP can evoke inflammation.[82] Whether EP plays any part in conferring nonspecific resistance to various microbes or their products is unknown, although it seems unlikely that the temperature-elevating effect of EP serves any directly useful role in combating infection.

Finally, the mechanism by which EP stimulates the hypothalamus to produce an increase in body temperature is unknown.

METABOLISM IN FEVER

The basal metabolism is elevated in fever, in proportion to the height of the temperature—roughly 7 per cent for each degree Fahrenheit. In other words, the effect of fever on the metabolic rate follows the principle of van't Hoff: that the velocity of chemical reactions is proportional to the temperature at which they occur. At a temperature of 105.0° F. the basal metabolism is approximately 50 per cent above normal.

The biochemical disturbances that have been noted in fever are not very distinctive. During the first week or two of a febrile disease, there is always some destruction of body protein, evidenced by negative nitrogen balance. Fever often is accompanied by mild to severe dehydration. The biochemical disturbances characteristic of dehydration may become evident: passage of Na and Cl into cells: loss of K, P, and N from cells; and loss of cell water as well as of extracellular (plasma and interstitial) water (Chap. 35). Achlorhydria is usually present in persons with high fever, but gastric secretion of acid is resumed when the temperature falls. Mild acidosis is common during infectious fevers.

As stated, the endocrine, metabolic, and biochemical evidences of fever are not distinctive but appear to be shared by many conditions associated with stress. In general, fever and the disorders that cause fever also stimulate the hypothalamic-pituitary-adrenocortical system. Thus, adrenocortical hyperactivity is not part of the mechanism that produces fever; it is an important part of the *response* to fever.

COMPLICATIONS OF FEVER

Herpes Simplex. Herpetic lesions about the mouth occur so frequently in certain febrile diseases that they are described in textbooks as manifestations of those diseases. Meningococcal meningitis and pneumococcal pneumonia are particularly likely to be so complicated, whereas, peculiarly, typhoid fever, typhus fever, and primary atypical pneumonia are accompanied only rarely by herpes. Actually, "fever blisters" are due to a separate infection by the virus of herpes simplex, which apparently is activated by the rise in body temperature. The purest example of the association with fever is found in persons who are given artificial fever therapy; in them the incidence of labial herpes may be as high as 46 per cent.[83] The lesions appear 30 to 48 hours after a treatment.

Albuminuria. Albumin is frequently present in the urine of patients with fever. In many cases this is certainly due to a direct effect of the disease on the kidneys; consequently, there has been some controversy as to whether or not fever alone may cause albuminuria. Welty, however, by studying a group of patients being treated with fever in the Kettering Hypertherm, found that alubuminuria occurred solely from the artificially induced rise in body temperature. He reported "true febrile albuminuria" in more than three-fourths of his patients.[84]

Chills. In a chill, or rigor, the subject suddenly begins to feel cold. His skin becomes pale, cyanotic, and covered with "gooseflesh." Even though covered by several blankets and warmed by hot water bottles, he cannot get warm. His whole body shivers and his teeth chatter—so that the bed shakes and he speaks with difficulty. This state continues for a period of about 10 to 40 minutes, and then gradually he feels less cold, his skin becomes pink and warm, and there may be sweating. During the "cold" phase there is a rapid rise in body temperature, of some 2° to 7° F.

Depending upon the underlying process there may or may not be a rapid return of temperature toward normal. The temperature rise is due to a great increase in heat production; the heat elimination remains about normal.[85] The most common cause of a chill is the introduction of some foreign substance into the blood stream—either living infectious agents or their products, bacterial pyrogens. However, chills can occur in the absence of extraneous substances; for example, they may be experienced by patients with lymphoma or hypernephroma.

When the time at which the chill-producing substance enters the circulation is known, as when typhoid vaccine is injected intravenously, there is always a lapse of approximately one hour before the onset of the chill. Similarly, a period of time elapses between instrumentation of infected tissues and subsequent chills. Very probably the lag period is the time necessary for tissue injury to occur, with release of endogenous pyrogen, which in turn alters the function of the thermoregulatory centers. This time relationship often is not appreciated, and the taking of blood cultures is sometimes postponed until "the height of the chill." Actually, the "ideal" time would be about one hour before the chill. Since this is not predictable, the best practice is to take a series of blood cultures, at 30- or 60-minute intervals.

Perera noted that sympathectomized limbs participate in the tremor of a chill but that they do not exhibit the vasoconstriction present in other parts of the body.[86] He found also that in persons with hemiplegia the paralyzed limbs exhibit tremor during chills, and he concludes from this that the efferent tract from the "chill center" is by way of an extrapyramidal pathway in the spinal cord and the motor nerves.

During a chill the rectal temperature rises steadily, while the skin usually remains cool. Microscopic study of the circulation in the capillaries in the nail folds at this time reveals that the flow of blood almost ceases.[87] This results in more nearly complete removal of oxygen from the blood and is the reason for the characteristic cyanosis. Other observations of the circulatory changes during chill and fever have been reviewed by Altschule and Freedberg.[88]

A sharp drop in the blood leukocyte count occurs during and shortly after a chill; therefore, a leukopenia immediately after a chill may have no diagnostic significance in relation to the primary disease.

In some infectious diseases, it is common to have a series of chills. These include brucellosis, typhus fever, malaria, many acute viral diseases such as influenza, and such pyogenic infections as pyelonephritis, acute osteomyelitis and postpartum infection. In pneumococcal pneumonia, on the other hand, it is unusual to have more than one chill which occurs at the onset, because the fever is sustained thereafter. However, if an antipyretic drug is given to a patient with pneumonia, his temperature will fall and then may rise again, with a chill.

Sweating. Sweating is the counterpart of the chill. It facilitates heat loss and tends to produce a rapid fall in temperature. It is usually combined with a rich circulation to the skin, which permits rapid dissipation of heat by vaporization. Sweating is particularly common in diseases associated with intermittent fever, such as tuberculosis, acute brucellosis, or rheumatic fever. In contrast, it does not occur during the febrile period of pneumonia, unless the patient is given an antipyretic drug. When a patient complains of "night sweats" we may suspect that he has an intermittent fever, although it is true that some persons, particularly when convalescing from prolonged illnesses, may have night sweats without fever.

Convulsions. Convulsions may occur at the onset of infectious diseases. This phenomenon is limited to children and in them it appears to be dependent largely on the rapidity with which the temperature rises. Wegman experimented with kittens and noted that they frequently had convulsions if subjected to rapid rise in body temperature; adult cats under the same conditions seldom had convulsions.[89]

The question which is not yet settled is whether febrile convulsions are essentially benign or whether they indicate some abnormality in the central nervous system. Some follow-up studies have provided evidence that children who have suffered febrile convulsions are liable to nonfebrile seizures later, or to exhibit signs of cerebral damage suggestive of conditions such as birth trauma or encephalitis.[90,91]

Delirium. Fever and delirium are often associated. In general, it may be said that delirium seldom is present when the fever is less than 104.0° F., although in exceptional instances and in elderly patients it may accompany only a moderate elevation of the temperature. The reason is that delirium depends on several factors: not only the degree of the fever, but also on the temperament of the patient, his previous health, drugs he has received, and the nature of his underlying disease.

SPURIOUS FEVER

MacNeal has described some of the ways in which high temperature has been faked by patients.[49] The most common method is to heat the thermometer with a hot water bottle or other source of heat. This is especially easy if the patient has previously obtained a spare thermometer to substitute for the one given him. Another trick is to hold the bulb of the thermometer tightly between the fingers and rub it against the bedclothes. Skilled malingerers can raise the reading by tapping the bulb end of the thermometer, jarring the mercury upward. In addition to these methods it is said that some individuals are able to warm the thermometer simply by friction with the tongue or anal sphincter. We have already noted that vigorous chewing motion can raise the mouth temperature by as much as 1.0° F. To detect trickery, it is recommended that simultaneous temperatures be taken in the axilla, the rectum and the mouth, with a different observer holding each thermometer in place.

Useful clues from the patient's chart for detecting this state have been summarized by Petersdorf and Bennett and include failure of the temperature curve to follow normal diurnal variation and the absence of correlation of the fever pattern with pulse rate or sweats.[92]

EFFECTS OF FEVER

It is often said that fever assists the host in combating infection. There is no question of the value of fever in neurosyphilis and in certain other types of infection, such as those due to the gonococcus. Moreover, some bacteria and spirilla suffer attenuation of virulence at febrile temperatures. It has also been observed that failure to develop fever in the presence of a severe infection usually signifies a grave prognosis. On the other hand, it is probable that in infections the actual presence of fever has little bearing on the outcome, since most organisms do not induce changes in body temperature which would destroy them.[93] The fever that accompanies noninfectious conditions does not appear to serve any useful purpose and may at times be harmful. In malignant disease, for example, high temperature only accelerates weight loss and causes malaise. Likewise, fever that follows myocardial infarction increases the metabolic rate, thereby placing an extra load on the weakened myocardium. The hyperpyrexia of heat stroke may cause irreversible damage or death.

CLINICAL CAUSES OF FEVER

INFECTIONS

Infections are certainly the most frequent causes of fever. In general it may be said that any known infection may cause fever; to list a large number of infectious diseases would serve no purpose here. Instead, a few instances will be cited wherein certain infections cause fevers that are particularly characteristic. These are less commonly observed now than formerly, because effective chemotherapy alters their natural courses.

In typhoid and parathyroid fevers there is a classical temperature course; it consists of a "staircase" rise for several days, a plateau of remittent fever for one to three weeks, then a steplike return to normal temperature.

Typhus fever produces a fairly uniform temperature curve. After a sudden elevation

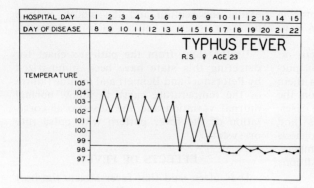

HOSPITAL DAY	1	2	3	4	5	6	7	8	9	10	11	12	13	14	15
DAY OF DISEASE	8	9	10	11	12	13	14	15	16	17	18	19	20	21	22

TYPHUS FEVER
R.S. ♀ AGE 23

Fig. 25-2. The typical temperature course in a case of murine typhus fever. There is a remittent fever for about 10 days, then a fall by lysis, usually reaching normal between the 14th and 18th days of illness.

there is a sustained high fever for nine or ten days, then a fall by lysis, returning to normal about the fourteenth to the eighteenth day of disease. An example of this is shown in Figure 25-2.

Gonococcal endocarditis may have a unique fever: two steeplelike rises and falls in each 24-hour period—double quotidian.[94] This also is described as a feature of kala-azar. It may be present occasionally in other severe infections. We have seen a double quotidian fever in miliary tuberculosis.

In dengue a "saddle-back" temperature curve is typical. By this is meant a fever that rises rapidly, declines somewhat during the succeeding two or three days, then rises again to a peak on about the sixth day, after which it subsides quickly.

Localized collections of pus, as in subdiaphragmatic abscess or osteomyelitis, frequently lead to a hectic type of fever, associated with chills and sweating. This may also be seen in patients with pyelonephritis, ascending cholangitis (Charcot's biliary fever), and thrombophlebitis.

Diseases that cause relapsing fevers are not very frequent in the United States. The following diagnostic possibilities should receive special consideration: (1) malaria; (2) rat-bite fever, caused by either *Spirillum minus* or *Streptobacillus moniliformis* (Fig. 25-1); (3) relapsing fever, caused by *Spirillum recurrentis;* and (4) chronic meningococcemia.

DISEASES OF THE CENTRAL NERVOUS SYSTEM

Head Injury. Fever is nearly always present after head injury, and the height of the temperature may be of some value in estimating prognosis. In slight concussions there is a rise to 101° F. or less, whereas in more serious cases the fever is often higher, and in the most severe injuries there may be

a rapid ascent to a hyperthermic level before death. Erickson states that following middle meningeal hemorrhage, a person may be more or less poikilothermic, his body temperature fluctuating markedly with changes in the environmental temperature.[95]

Cerebral Vascular Accident. Hemorrhage or thrombosis in the vessels of the brain is usually attended by a moderate fever—100° to 102° F. In large hemorrhages very high fever may develop just before death.

Neurogenic Hyperthermia. Following surgical operations in the region of the pituitary fossa and the third ventricle, a serious hyperthermia sometimes occurs. The rectal temperature rises steadily during the first few hours after operation. The skin of the extremities is cold, while that of the trunk is relatively warm. There is complete absence of sweating. Energetic treatment of the fever is indicated: application of ice bags, alcohol rubs, cold air fan, etc.[95]

Degenerative Disease. Disturbances in temperature regulation are occasionally noted after recovery from encephalitis. Children who have sustained cerebral trauma in a birth injury often have faulty temperature regulation. Approximately 50 per cent of cases of multiple sclerosis have a low fever at some time.[96]

Spinal Cord Injury. Holmes made a study of the effects of spinal cord injuries and observed that injury to the cervical cord was frequently followed by severe disturbance of temperature regulation. Injury to the lower cervical cord usually resulted in very low body temperature, whereas patients with upper cervical cord injury often had high, irregular fevers.[97] The cause of this temperature disturbance probably is the interruption of the tracts leading to and from the hypothalamus.

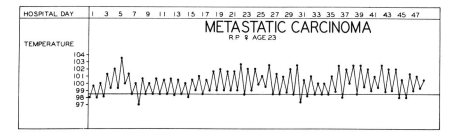

FIG. 25-3. Temperature chart of a young woman with fever due to carcinoma of the pancreas with metastasis to the liver.

NEOPLASMS

Malignant growths frequently cause fever.[98] Sometimes, for example, in carcinoma of a bronchus, this fever may be the result of an associated infection; but often the tumor alone appears to be responsible. Hypernephroma is notorious in this respect; it may even cause a hectic fever with chills and sweats. Primary or metastatic carcinoma in the liver is also frequently attended by fever. Figure 25-3 shows the temperature chart of a patient with primary carcinoma of the pancreas, with metastasis to the liver. Harsha has reviewed the literature on fever in malignant disease, and reports a case in which there was dramatic cessation of a hectic fever after removal of a retroperitoneal malignant tumor.[99] Similar defervescence has followed extirpation of mesotheliomata of the pleura.[100] The cause of the fever in malignancy is thought to be the liberation of products from the tissue destroyed by the invading neoplasm but there is, in fact, a poor correlation between the degree of fever and the extent of tissue necrosis. Infection and obstruction are a more frequent cause of fever in malignancy than the disease itself.[101] The fever of malignancy presents no characteristic features, although low-grade or regularly recurrent fevers seem more common in tumors not associated with infection.[102]

Lymphoma. Fever is an almost constant accompaniment of this group of neoplastic diseases and is often the first symptom. Consequently, such conditions as Hodgkin's disease, lymphosarcoma, and leukemia always must be considered in investigating cases of obscure fever. A few persons with Hodgkin's disease exhibit a peculiar relapsing fever, in which periods of about seven to ten days of normal temperature alternate with equal periods of fever. This is called the Pel-Ebstein fever. An example is shown in Figure 25-4.

BLOOD DISEASES

Acute leukemia is usually a febrile disease, even in the absence of discernible infection.[103,104] Certain acute hemolytic anemias also are associated with fever, especially those due to an immunological process or sickle-cell anemia in crisis.[105] Hemorrhagic disorders, such as thrombocytopenic purpura,

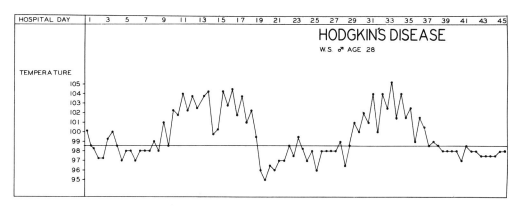

FIG. 25-4. An example of the Pel-Ebstein type of fever in a case of Hodgkin's disease.

hemophilia, and scurvy, may cause fever if there is hemorrhage into the tissues. Severe anemia from chronic blood loss is not a cause of fever. Chronic aplastic anemia, chronic lymphocytic leukemia (in the absence of infection), and myelofibrosis are rarely febrile diseases, but high fevers often are present in acute agranulocytosis.

EMBOLISM AND THROMBOSIS

Embolism or aseptic thrombosis in a large artery or vein often is associated with fever. This probably depends on the occurrence of tissue necrosis (and attendant inflammation) due to interference with the nutrition of the part supplied by the vessel. In myocardial infarction, for example, low fever is expected during the first few days, and elevations as high as 103° to 104° F. sometimes are seen.

Septic thrombophlebitis in postpartum patients occasionally may give rise to persistent spiking fevers with either positive or negative blood cultures, but without local signs of infection. The fever often responds dramatically to anticoagulants after trials with various antibiotics have been unsuccessful.[105a]

HEAT STROKE

Heat stroke is a serious condition characterized by high fever, coma, and absence of sweating. It should not be confused with heat cramp or heat exhaustion, neither of which causes a change in body temperature. Heat stroke is induced by prolonged high environmental temperature; it occurs most commonly in old people, or in those who have been consuming alcohol. Apparently the fault here is failure of the cerebral centers of heat regulation. The onset of symptoms is usually sudden, with loss of consciousness. The affected person ceases to sweat just prior to his collapse. Ferris and his associates carried out an excellent study on 44 patients with heat stroke during a single period of hot weather.[106] The body temperatures of their patients ranged from 104° to 112° F. Absence of sweating was noted in all of them. Biochemical studies revealed normal blood chlorides, but there was some acidosis and hemoconcentration. The reason for the sudden cessation of sweating could not be ascertained. Seventeen of the 44 patients died. It was concluded that energetic measures must be employed in an effort to reduce the body temperature quickly; the procedures recommended were ice-water tubbing combined with massage.

Patients with heat stroke may present with numerous other complications including jaundice, acute renal failure, myocardial infarction, and hematologic complications.[107,107a,107b]

DISTURBANCES IN FLUID BALANCE

Dehydration is commonly held to be responsible for fever. However, there is little evidence that this is true in adults and the best clinical practice is to search for some other cause.

There can be little doubt that infants during the first few days of life can have temperature elevation due to lack of water—the so-called dehydration or inanition fever. Administration of adequate fluid is followed by prompt cessation of the fever. The mechanism of this is obscure.

Fever may be observed in severe diabetic acidosis, and some persons have ascribed this to dehydration. Himwich produced acidosis and high fever in depancreatized dogs by withholding water and insulin; then by giving fluids he found that the temperature returned to normal. Insulin alone did not have this effect.[108] However, the temperature is frequently normal or subnormal in diabetic acidosis; consequently the presence of fever should stimulate a search for some other disease process.

HEART FAILURE

Some degree of fever is often present in patients with congestive heart failure, but there is usually some associated complication which could cause it, such as bronchopneumonia, pulmonary infarction, rheumatic fever, myocardial infarction, or thrombophlebitis. Nevertheless, there are many instances in which no such complication is obvious and where fever appears with failure and disappears when compensation is regained. Steele studied this problem experimentally and concluded that a slowing blood flow to the surface of the body could interfere with heat dissipation sufficiently to bring about an elevation of body temperature.[109] This hypothesis was supported by the results of experiments of Stewart et al., employing rapid digitalization.[110] Kinsey and White, on the other hand, studied 200 cases of congestive heart failure and concluded that fever could usually be attributed to complications. They stated that decompensation alone would not be likely to cause a temperature elevation of more than 1.0° F.[111]

THYROID DISEASE

It is common to find a slight temperature elevation—99.5° to 100.5° F.—in persons who have thyrotoxicosis. This is probably due to the excessive heat production which accompanies the increased metabolism. In a thyroid crisis, which may appear spontaneously or may occur immediately after surgery on the thyroid (occasionally also after other surgical procedures), there is a rapid rise in body temperature to 104° F. or higher, accompanied by tachycardia, thready pulse, restlessness, sometimes mania, and eventually stupor.

STEROID FEVER

There is a poorly defined group of diseases in which fever occurs either at regular or irregular intervals (so-called "cyclic" or "periodic" fever, respectively.[112] The febrile episodes often are associated with bouts of aseptic arthritis or peritonitis. Although symptoms may recur for years, patients generally remain healthy and the prognosis is benign in most instances. Recently, evidence has accumulated that "periodic disease" may include several distinct diseases of varying etiology.

In Familial Mediterranean fever, a form of periodic febrile disease that is associated with amyloidosis and appears to be almost entirely restricted to Jews and Armenians, no cause for the fever has been determined as yet.[113]

A number of steroid metabolites of the pregnene and etiocholane type, when given by either intravenous or intramuscular routes, produce marked pyrogenic responses in man, associated with leucocytosis, headache, myalgia, and arthralgia.[114] One of these hormones, the urinary ketosteroid, etiocholanolone, has been detected in the blood during febrile episodes in some patients with recurrent fevers.[115] At present, the mechanism by which these agents cause fever is unknown, but since there is a prolonged delay before onset of fever, it seems doubtful that they act directly on the thermoregulatory center. Human leucocytes can be stimulated by etiocholanolone *in vitro* to release EP.[116] This action appears to be highly specific, since minor structural modifications of the molecule abolish its pyrogenic properties both *in vivo* and *in vitro*. These similarities between *in vitro* and *in vivo* activity suggest that pyrogenic steroids may act like other fever-inducing agents by releasing an intermediate pyrogen from leucocytes. These steroids appear to produce fever only in man, and hence may be distinguished clearly from various pyrogens of microbial origin which, as noted previously, are effective in a number of animals.

At present, none of these compounds, with the possible exception of etiocholanolone, has been shown to play a role in fevers occurring clinically. Recent unpublished studies indicate that plasma levels of etiocholanolone may be elevated in patients with a wide variety of diseases, during both febrile and afebrile periods. However, since many transformation products of endogenous adrenocortical and gonadal hormones, as well as some bile acids, are pyrogenic, these agents well may be implicated in certain hitherto unexplained fevers associated with various hepatic and endocrine disorders.

LIVER DISEASES

Various diseases of the liver are prone to produce fever. Liver abscess, amebic or bacterial, may cause a hectic type of fever. The frequency of temperature elevation in neoplastic disease of the liver already has been mentioned. McCrae and Caven noted fever in 80 per cent of their cases of syphilis of the liver.[117] About one-half of all patients with cirrhosis of the liver have temperature elevations, which are typically moderate and prolonged in uncomplicated cases.[118]

MISCELLANEOUS DISEASES AFFECTING THE HEART

Fever almost invariably accompanies either acute or subacute endocarditis.[119] Certain clinical features of this disease, including fever, anemia, petechiae, peripheral embolic phenomena, and changing cardiac murmurs may be mimicked closely by myxomas of the left auricle.[120] A febrile illness associated with a pleuropericardial inflammatory reaction may follow shortly after extensive closed heart surgery, involving either mitral valvulotomy or pericardiotomy. Originally this syndrome was attributed to reactivation of rheumatic fever, but as it may occur in patients undergoing cardiac surgery without other evidence of this disease, as well as in other patients after nonpenetrating chest injuries[121] or myocardial infarction,[122] it has been suggested that the symptoms are due to an auto-immune reaction.[123-125]

Another febrile syndrome has been described in a small number of patients undergoing open-heart surgery with cardiopulmonary bypass through a pump oxygenator.

These patients develop a viral-like illness that resembles infectious mononucleosis, with fever, splenomegaly, and atypical lymphocytes.[126,127] The fever, which usually begins several weeks after operation, follows an intermittent daily course and gradually subsides after a month or so. Recently, this illness has been found to be caused by infection with cytomegalic virus.[128]

Patients undergoing rejection of transplanted organs may respond with fever one or two weeks after operation, presumably because of a hypersensitivity reaction of the delayed type to homologous tissue. Since the immune mechanisms of such patients have been suppressed by various agents, infection remains an important possible cause of fever in these instances.[129]

SARCOID

Nearly half of the patients with sarcoid, a granulomatous disease of unknown etiology involving the lymph nodes, liver, spleen, eyes, and skin, present with a significant degree of fever. The cause of fever in such patients is obscure and, since it follows no characteristic pattern, fever is unfortunately of little help in diagnosis.[130]

TISSUE TRAUMA

Crushing injuries and fractures of large bones usually are followed by some rise in body temperature. Also, a moderate elevation is to be expected during the first day or two after an extensive surgical procedure.[131] The inflammation resulting from release of products of damaged tissue is probably the cause of these fevers.

PEPTIC ULCER

European physicians have reported fever in 8 to 25 per cent of patients with uncomplicated peptic ulcer.[132] The elevation seldom exceeds 100.5° F. Dill and Isenhour, in this country, investigated the subject.[133] They found fever in 46 per cent of a group of patients with uncomplicated peptic ulcer, but the significance of the finding was somewhat clouded by the fact that the same criteria for fever were satisfied in 37 per cent of their control group—persons with digestive symptoms but without demonstrable organic lesions. Upon the basis of the available evidence, the statement that uncomplicated peptic ulcer is a cause of fever is still open to question.

Massive hemorrhage from a peptic ulcer results in fever in at least 80 per cent of cases. Attempts to produce this type of fever in normal subjects by the introduction of large quantities of blood into the intestinal tract were unsuccessful.[134] One could speculate that the fever in bleeding ulcer is due to increased heat produced by the specific dynamic action of a large quantity of protein absorbed from the intestinal tract in a subject whose means of heat dissipation is handicapped by the circulatory embarrassment of blood loss. One factor, which perhaps is not appreciated sufficiently in evaluating fever after gastrointestinal hemorrhage, is the effect of blood transfusions that these patients receive. The findings of Selesnick and White indicate that the fever of gastrointestinal hemorrhage rarely exceeds 100° F. except after transfusion.[135]

ABNORMALITIES OF THE SKIN

Persons who have congenital absence of the sweat glands or other generalized skin disease may be handicapped seriously in hot weather, when vaporization is the principal means of heat loss. Under such conditions they may develop fever.[136] Woodyatt reported this in the case of a woman with extensive ichthyosis. In the winter she was able to work normally, but in summer she would develop fever and symptoms resembling those of effort syndrome.[137]

SERUM SICKNESS AND ALLERGY

Serum sickness, with fever, arthralgia, and urticaria, may occur from five to ten days after administration of an animal serum to a human being and apparently results from a violent immune reaction to the foreign protein. The temperature elevation may be considerable—103° to 105° F. Presumably the syndrome is due to factors released by the patient's tissues following an antigen-antibody reaction. Circulating endogenous pyrogen has been detected in sensitized rabbits that develop fever after intravenous injection of HSA.[138] Fevers perhaps caused by a similar mechanism include those characteristically present in many collagen diseases of so-called auto-immunity (acute rheumatic fever, lupus erythematosus, rheumatic arthritis, polyarteritis, etc.).[139,140]

It has been suggested that allergy may cause certain obscure fevers, but there is not a great deal of evidence to support the idea. Rowe, however, has reported a case in which the evidence was strong that a prolonged obscure fever was due to food allergy.[141]

PAROXYSMAL TACHYCARDIA

Patients occasionally have fever during paroxysms of tachycardia, in the absence of any other disease.[142] This may be due to the combined effect of impaired circulation and extra heat production resulting from the muscular activity of the heart.

ANESTHESIA

Because it is usually thought that the body temperature tends to fall during anesthesia, the temperature of operating rooms is usually kept rather warm, and patients are often wrapped in blankets during the immediate postoperative hours. In many cases this practice is illogical. Burford followed the temperature of 50 patients during operations and found that instead of a fall there was a moderate elevation in 33 of them.[143]

Dangerous hyperthermia is an occasional complication of anesthesia. This is a special hazard in the case of young children, and the danger is increased in operations about the face, e.g., for cleft palate.[144,145] Burford believes that the production of hyperthermia is as follows: on a warm day the environmental temperature is so high that heat loss can be accomplished only by vaporization; high humidity decreases the efficiency of this mechanism which is further impaired by the patient's mask and drapes. The anesthetic depresses the function of the temperature-regulating centers in the brain. With this combination of circumstances, heat loss cannot keep pace with heat production, and body temperature rises. This aggravates matters, since heat production is increased with a rise in temperature, according to van't Hoff's law. The temperature continues to rise following the operation and within a few hours there is high fever and collapse. This syndrome closely resembles neurogenic hyperthermia, including the absence of sweating and the coldness of the skin of the extremities. Death may ensue. Mangiardi reported on three such cases in adults, and advocated therapy with oxygen inhalation, alcohol sponging and continuous intravenous administration of 50 per cent dextrose solution.[146]

More recent articles on fulminating hyperthermia with anesthesia suggest uncoupling of oxidative phosphorylation as a possible cause of the fever.[147,148]

DRUG FEVERS

A number of drugs may cause fever after prolonged administration. Some of the important ones are antihistamines, atropine, barbiturates, bromides, butazolidin, dilantin, iodides, mercurials, morphine, p-amino-salicylic acid (PAS), penicillin, quinidine, salicylates, streptomycin, sulfonamides, and thiouracil. Drug fevers caused by antibacterial agents may be difficult to identify because they occur in persons who already have fever due to something else. In most cases, drug fevers are due to hypersensitivity, and since they often are associated with skin eruptions, the simultaneous appearance of rash and fever may make the diagnosis easy. The various causes and manifestations of drug fevers have been reviewed comprehensively by Cluff and Johnson.[149]

Temperature elevations of as much as 2° F. may occur when morphine is withheld from an addict.[150]

Another type of febrile reaction which occurs in the therapy of syphilis is known as the Jarisch-Herxheimer reaction. It may result from treatment either with an arsenical or with penicillin and is undoubtedly related to the effect on the syphilitic infection. Within a few hours after the first injection, the patient develops fever and malaise; these may be associated with an intensification of a skin eruption or severe pain in a syphilitic lesion of bone. The symptoms seldom last more than 24 to 48 hours.

Other drugs that may induce fever under certain conditions are epinephrine, dinitrophenol (DNP) and lysergic acid diethylamide (LSD), an inhibitor of serotonin.[149,151] Both serotonin and norepinephrine are normally present in high concentration in the region of the hypothalamus and are capable of modifying thermoregulation when injected directly into the cerebral ventricles of various animals.[152,153] Although their role in producing fever has not been established, it seems likely that alterations in the stores of these amines in the CNS may influence the febrile response to other pyrogens.[154]

Patients with pheochromocytoma characteristically have a moderate elevation in temperature during an attack and may occasionally have signs that simulate overwhelming infection.[155]

Little is known about the mechanisms by which these agents produce fever and it seems probable that some are direct stimulants to the central nervous system, whereas others, such as DNP and epinephrine, act peripherally rather than on the thermoregulatory center itself. The relationship between central and peripheral roles of endogenous sympathetic amines in modifying body temperature deserves further investigation, as does the possibility that these substances contribute (through alterations in their concentration in the brain) to other naturally occurring or experimental fevers.

Fever Due to Heavy Sedation

It is not unusual for fever to occur in persons who have received heavy sedation (amytal narcosis for psychiatric therapy, barbiturate intoxication in suicide attempt, patients being treated for delirium tremens or tetanus). This temperature elevation suggests a pulmonary complication, such as atelectasis or pneumonia.[156] Clinical experience shows that the sedation alone may cause fever, since there is frequently no sign of any other complication.

Pyrogens

Chill and high fever occasionally follow the intravenous administration of saline solutions, serums, and other biologic preparations, because of the presence of bacterial pyrogens (discussed previously), which gain access through contamination of the material at some stage of preparation. Special precautions must be taken to avoid pyrogen contamination of any material that is to be given intravenously. Pyrogens are exceedingly difficult to remove from biologic preparations, because they can pass through bacterial filters and can withstand autoclaving.[56]

Cotton-Dust Fever

Persons who handle raw cotton, in mills or in making mattresses, are subject to a febrile disorder. Toward the end of the day there is malaise, chilliness, and fever of 100° to 102° F. The symptoms subside during the night, and the person usually feels well enough to return to work the next day. A tolerance develops within a few days, so that there are no symptoms as long as employment is continued. However, tolerance is lost when the worker takes a short vacation. Studies have indicated that the febrile reaction is related to the presence of a species of *Aerobacter cloacae* in the cotton fibers. This organism has been shown to be a potent pyrogen producer, and the presumption is that the symptoms are caused by absorption of the pyrogen from the respiratory mucosa.[157]

Metal-Fume Fever

Workers in certain metal industries are subject to illness of the type just described for cotton workers, including the development of tolerance. The workers particularly susceptible are those exposed to fumes containing zinc oxide.[158] It has been impossible to produce fever in animals exposed to the same fumes. The suggestion has been offered that in man the metal fumes cause increased absorption of bacterial products from the respiratory mucosa. However, the fever (which also occurs after inhalation of certain polymer fumes)[159] may be due to an immunologic response[160] or to absorption of finely divided particles per se, as in some experimental fevers.[71]

"Catheter Fever"

Occasionally the passage of a catheter or other instrument through an infected urethral tract is followed in an hour or two by the development of fever, sometimes with a chill. It has been shown that this fever is caused by a bacteremia, which is usually transient. A similar fever may follow digital dilation of a rectal stricture.

Teething

Lay people regard teething as a frequent cause of fever in children, whereas physicians are somewhat reluctant to take this view. However, most pediatricians believe that now and then, especially when there is swelling and inflammation of the gum over the erupting tooth, teething may cause a rise in temperature.

"Milk Fever"

In the last century, when puerperal infection was more frequent than it is today, physicians were so accustomed to the appearance of fever about the third day after delivery that they came to regard engorgement of the mother's breasts as a process that could cause fever. However, modern obstetricians now believe that fever which occurs coincidentally with the onset of lactation is probably due to some undetected infection.

NEUROCIRCULATORY ASTHENIA

Friedman studied a group of soldiers with the syndrome of neurocirculatory asthenia and found that 11 of 30 of these individuals were subject to occasional temperature elevations. The average maximal temperature in the 11 men was 99.8° F., whereas it was 98.6° F. in 11 normal control subjects during the same period of time.[161]

HABITUAL HYPERTHERMIA

Reimann was interested in the problem of persons whose temperatures are set at a level slightly above the average normal (habitual hyperthermia) and reported on a group of 16 such cases.[162] Each one was subjected to thorough examination and was observed over a period of years, without finding evidence of organic disease. Reimann believed that such people are not rare and often are improperly managed because of the assumption that even a slight fever means disease. He thought that certain persons, particularly those with neurotic dispositions, maintain a body temperature that is always slightly above normal, and that long-continued low-grade fever in them should not be interpreted as an indication of infection or other febrile disease. All physicians are familiar with this clinical problem,[163] and after a thorough work-up to eliminate the possibility of organic disease, it seems advisable to make a positive diagnosis of habitual hyperthermia at times, in order to spare these patients the anxiety and expense of repeated examinations and treatment.

PSYCHOGENIC FEVER

Most physicians are convinced that under certain conditions an emotional stimulus may induce an elevation of temperature. Dunbar has reviewed the evidence on the subject.[164] The slight rise so often observed at the time of admission to a hospital appears to be an example of psychogenic fever. We have all noticed that occasionally a patient who has no apparent cause for fever will show a slight elevation on the day of admission, but a normal temperature thereafter. Similarly, in pediatric wards it is not unusual to find a number of slight elevations immediately after visiting hours.

Wynn took the temperatures of 40 nurses immediately before and immediately after the writing of a state board examination and found that the average was 98.9° F. before, and 98.3° after the examination. Similarly, he found that among 324 draftees who were awaiting physical examination for the Army, the average temperature was 99.3° F. Indeed, 17 per cent of the men had temperatures above 100.0° F. He attributed these elevations to anxiety and excitement.[165]

Wolf and Wolff[166] reported another interesting example of psychogenic fever; their patient, a man, had had periodic bouts of fever for 13 years. He had suffered from migraine previously, and with the appearance of the fever his migraine ceased. After extensive negative studies for other causes of fever, therapy directed toward certain personality disorders seemed to relieve him of both the fever and the headaches.

FEVER OF UNKNOWN ORIGIN

One of the most intriguing and difficult problems of diagnosis in medicine is the fever of unknown origin (F.U.O.). The causes of most such fevers of short duration are probably infectious diseases, especially viral. Other pyrexic states, which follow a more prolonged course (2 or 3 weeks or longer), are due to a variety of causes, as is evident by the number of diseases which may present at some time or other with fever. A point stressed in one large series is that most patients with F.U.O. are not suffering from rare diseases, but have unusual manifestations of common illnesses.[167] In over one third of the patients in this series the fevers were found after careful study to be of infectious origin and nearly two thirds of these patients recovered or benefited from specific treatment. One clearly must make every effort to arrive at a correct diagnosis before blindly subjecting such patients to various therapeutic trials.

There appears to be little difference in the relative contribution of various disease categories (infectious, neoplastic and collagen) in the several series of F.U.O. reported over the past 30 years. However, within the fevers of obscure origin due to infectious diseases there has been a diminution of those caused by Gram-positive cocci and a corresponding increase in Gram-negative enteric infections. Tuberculosis continues to cause many a chronic obscure fever. Discussions of the problems of diagnosis and treatment of patients with F.U.O. are presented in a number of recent reviews of this subject.[167-174] It seems likely that with our many new diagnostic technics we shall remove a higher percentage of cases from the unknown category.

SUMMARY

Body temperature is maintained relatively constant by centers in the hypothalamus which regulate heat production and loss through the central nervous system. Body heat is derived principally from combustion of food in the liver and voluntary muscles. Heat is lost by radiation, convection, and vaporization. Under normal conditions, the nervous system is able to keep body temperature stable simply by varying the caliber of peripheral blood vessels and hence regulating the loss of heat from the surface of the body.

There is no set "normal" body temperature. The temperature varies considerably in different parts of the body; furthermore, there are small differences in rectal temperatures among healthy individuals. In all persons there is a diurnal variation, amounting to as much as 3° F., the peak usually being attained in the evening, the low point during sleep in the early morning hours.

Certain physiologic conditions influence the body temperature; among these are exercise, digestion of food, ovulation, and pregnancy. Knowledge of the possible effect of exercise may be of particular importance to clinicians in evaluating "fever" in children.

Elevation of body temperature is caused by increased heat production or impairment of heat elimination. In rare instances this may be brought about by a direct peripheral effect on voluntary muscles or vasculature, but in the great majority of cases fever is caused indirectly by an effect on the temperature-regulating centers in the brain. In infections, neoplastic diseases, and other conditions associated with cell injury and inflammation, it seems probable that an endogenous pyrogen liberated from the host's tissues affects these hypothalamic centers. A fever-producing substance has been isolated from polymorphonuclear leucocytes, monocytes, and macrophages (including fixed cells of the reticuloendothelial system). Such a substance is presumed to be the circulating pyrogen detected in the sera of animals during a variety of experimentally induced fevers.

Many different types of disease cause fever. Among the most important are infections, diseases of the central nervous system, neoplasms, and vascular accidents. An understanding of the characteristics and mechanisms of fever is of great value in the study of disease.

REFERENCES

1. Bazett, H. C.: The regulation of body temperatures *in* L. H. Newburgh (ed.): Physiology of Heat Regulation and the Science of Clothing, pp. 109-192, Philadelphia, Saunders, 1949.
2. Burton, A. C., and Bronk, D.: The motor mechanism of shivering and of thermal muscular tone, Amer. J. Physiol. (Proc.) 118:284, 1937.
3. Burton, A. C.: Range and variability of blood flow in human fingers and vasomotor regulation of body temperature, Amer. J. Physiol. 127:437, 1939.
4. Barbour, H. G.: Die Wirkung unmittelbarer Erwärmung und Abkühlung der Wärmezentra auf die Körpertemperatur, Arch. Exp. Path. Pharmakol. 70:1, 1912.
5. Isenschmid, R., and Schnitzler, W.: Beitrag zur Lokalisation des der Wärmerregulation vorstehenden Zentralapparates im Zwischenhirn, Arch. Exp. Path. Pharmakol. 76:202, 1914.
6. Ranson, S. W.: *in* Hypothalamus and central levels of autonomic function, Nerv. Ment. Dis. Monog. 20:342, 1940.
7. Keller, A. D.: Separation in the brain stem of the mechanisms of heat loss from those of heat production, J. Neurophysiol. 1:543, 1938.
8. Nakayama, T., Hammel, H. T., Hardy, J. D., and Eisenman, J. S.: Thermal stimulation of electrical activity of single units of preoptic region, Amer. J. Physiol. 204:1122, 1963.
9. Hellon, R. F.: Thermal stimulation of hypothalamic neurones in unanaesthetized rabbits, J. Physiol. 193:381, 1967.
10. Ström, G.: Central nervous regulation of body temperature, *in* Field, J., Magoun, H. W., and Hall, V. E. (eds.): Handbook of Physiology, Sec. 1, Neurophysiology, vol. 2, p. 1173, Washington, D.C., Amer. Physiol. Soc. 1960.
11. Cooper, K. E.: Temperature regulation and the hypothalamus, Brit. Med. Bull. 22:238, 1966.
12. Benzinger, T. H., Pratt, A. W., and Kitzinger, C.: The thermostatic control of human metabolic heat production, Proc. Nat. Acad. Sci. U.S.A. 47:730, 1961.
13. Sherrington, C. S.: Notes on temperature after spinal transection, with some observations on shivering, J. Physiol. 58:405, 1924.
14. Pickering, G.: Regulation of body temperature in health and disease, Lancet 1:1, 59, 1958.
15. Hammel, H. T., Hardy, J. D., and Fusco, M. M.: Thermoregulatory responses to hypothalamic cooling in unanesthetized dogs, Amer. J. Physiol. 198:481, 1960.
16. Hardy, J. D.: Physiology of temperature regulation, Physiol. Rev. 41:521, 1961.
17. von Liebermeister, C.: Handbuch der Pathologie und Therapie des Fiebers, Leipzig, Vogél, 1875.

18. Macpherson, R. K.: The effect of fever on temperature regulation in man, Clin. Sci. 18: 281, 1959.

19. Cooper, K. E., Cranston, W. I., and Snell, E. S.: Temperature regulation during fever in man, Clin. Sci. 27: 345, 1964.

20. Andersen, H. T., Hammel, H. T., and Hardy, J. D.: Modifications of the febrile response to pyrogen by hypothalamic heating and cooling in the unanesthetized dog, Acta Physiol. Scand. 53: 247, 1961.

21. Bard, P., and Woods, J. W.: Central nervous region essential for endotoxin fever, Trans. Amer. Neurol. Ass. 87: 37, 1962.

22. Thompson, R. H.: Influence of environmental temperature upon pyrogenic fever, Dissertation, Philadelphia, Univ. of Penn., 1959. (Quoted in Ref. 16)

23. Jackson, D. L.: A hypothalamic region responsive to localized injection of pyrogens, J. Neurophysiol. 30: 586, 1967.

24. Wells, J. A., and Rall, D. P.: Mechanism of pyrogen induced fever, Proc. Soc. Exp. Biol. Med. 68: 421, 1948.

25. Grant, R.: Nature of pyrogen fever; effect of environmental temperature on response to typhoid-paratyphoid vaccine, Amer. J. Physiol. 159: 511, 1949.

26. DuBois, E. F.: Fever and the Regulation of Body Temperature, Springfield, Ill., Thomas, 1948.

27. Horvath, S. M., Menduke, H., and Piersol, G. M.: Oral and rectal temperatures of man, J.A.M.A. 144: 1562, 1950.

28. Reimann, H. A.: Habitual hyperthermia; a clinical study of four cases with long-continued low grade fever, Arch. Intern. Med. 55: 792, 1935.

29. Gerbrandy, J., Snell, E. S., and Cranston, W. I.: Oral, rectal, and oesophageal temperatures in relation to central temperature control in man, Clin. Sci. 13: 615, 1954.

30. Eichna, L. W., Berger, A. R., Rader, B., and Becker, W. H.: Comparison of intracardiac and intravascular with rectal temperatures in man, J. Clin. Invest. 30: 353, 1951.

31. Eichna, L. W.: Thermal gradients in man. Comparison of temperatures in the femoral artery and femoral vein with rectal temperatures, Arch. Phys. Med. 30: 584, 1949.

32. Rubin, A., Horvath, S. M., and Mellette, H. C.: Effect of fecal bacterial activity on rectal temperature of man, Proc. Soc. Exp. Biol. Med. 76: 410, 1951.

33. Reader, S. R., and Whyte, H. M.: Tissue temperature gradients, J. Appl. Physiol. 4: 396, 1951.

34. Horvath, S. M., and Hollander, J. L.: Intra-articular temperature as a measure of joint reaction, J. Clin. Invest. 28: 469, 1949.

35. Petrakis, N. L.: Temperature of human bone marrow, J. Appl. Physiol. 4: 549, 1952.

36. Bazett, H. C., Love, L., Newton, M., Eisenberg, L., Day, R., and Forster, R.: Temperature changes in blood flowing in arteries and veins in man, J. Appl. Physiol. 1: 3, 1948-1949.

37. Mellette, H. C., Hutt, B. K., Askovitz, S. I., and Horvath, S. M.: Diurnal variations in body temperatures, J. Appl. Physiol. 3: 665, 1951.

38. Kleitman, N.: Biological rhythms and cycles, Physiol. Rev. 29: 1, 1949.

39. Van der Bogert, F., and Moravec, C. L.: Body temperature variations in apparently healthy children, J. Pediat. 10: 466, 1937.

40. Searcy, H. B.: Chewing gum fever, J. Med. Ass. Alabama 13: 266, 1944.

41. Benedict, F. G., and Slack, E. P.: A Comparative Study of Temperature Fluctuations in Different Parts of the Human Body, Carnegie Institution of Washington, Publication No. 155, 1911.

42. Lee, F. S., and Edwards, D. J.: The action of certain atmospheric conditions on body temperature and the vascular system, Proc. Soc. Exp. Biol. Med. 12: 72, 1915.

43. Whitelaw, M. J.: Hormonal control of the basal body temperature pattern, Fertil. & Steril. 3: 230, 1952.

44. Seward, G. H., and Seward, J. P., Jr.: Changes in systolic blood pressure, heart rate, and temperature before, during, and after pregnancy in healthy woman, Human Biol. 8: 232, 1936.

45. Smith, L. W., and Fay, T.: Observations on human beings with cancer, maintained at reduced temperatures of 75°-90° Fahrenheit, Amer. J. Clin. Path. 10: 1, 1940.

46. Laufman, H.: Profound accidental hypothermia, J.A.M.A. 147: 1201, 1951.

47. Kass, G. H.: Hypothermia following cortisone administration, Amer. J. Med. 18: 146, 1955.

48. Dripps, R. D. (ed.): The Physiology of induced hypothermia: Proceedings of a Symposium, Washington, D. C., Nat. Acad. Sci.-Nat. Res. Council 1956 (pub 451).

49. MacNeal, W. J.: Hyperthermia, genuine and spurious, Arch. Intern. Med. 64: 800, 1939.

50. MacNeal, W. J., Ritter, H. H., and Rabson, S. M.: Prolonged hyperthermia; report of a case with necropsy, Arch. Intern. Med. 64: 809, 1939.

51. DuBois, E. F.: Why are fever temperatures over 106° F. rare?, Amer. J. Med. Sci. 217: 361, 1949.

52. Barbour, H. G.: Heat-regulating mechanism of the body, Physiol. Rev. 1: 295, 1921.

53. Cramer, W.: Fever, infections and the thyroid-adrenal apparatus, Brit. J. Exper. Path. 7: 95, 1926.

54. Welch, W. H.: The Cartwright Lectures. On the general pathology of fever, Med. News 52: 365, 393, 539, 565, 1888.

55. Nowotny, A. (ed.): Molecular biology of gram-negative bacterial lipopolysaccharides, Ann. N.Y. Acad. Sci., 133: 277–786, 1966.

56. Bennett, I. L., Jr., and Cluff, L. E.: Bacterial pyrogens, Pharm. Rev. 9:427, 1957.

57. Westphal, O.: Pyrogens, in Springer, G. F. (ed.): Polysaccharides in Biology, p. 115, New York, Macy, 1957.

58. Snell, E. S., and Atkins, E.: The Mechanisms of fever, in Bittar, E. E. (ed.): The Biological Basis of Medicine, vol. II, pp. 397–419, Academic Press, London, 1968.

59. Bennett, I. L., Jr., and Beeson, P. B.: Studies on the pathogenesis of fever. 1. The effect of injection of extracts and suspensions of uninfected rabbit tissues upon the body temperature of normal rabbits, J. Exp. Med. 98:477, 1953.

60. Kozak, M. S., Hahn, H. H., Lennarz, W. J., and Wood, W. B., Jr.: Studies on the pathogenesis of fever. XVI. Purification and further chemical characterization of granulocytic pyrogen, J. Exp. Med. 127:341, 1968.

61. Snell, E. S., and Atkins, E.: The presence of endogenous pyrogen in normal rabbit tissues, J. Exp. Med. 121:1019, 1965.

62. Atkins, E., and Wood, W. B., Jr.: Studies on the pathogenesis of fever. II. Identification of an endogenous pyrogen in the blood stream following the injection of typhoid vaccine, J. Exp. Med. 102:499, 1955.

63. Snell, E. S., Goodale, F., Jr., Wendt, F., and Cranston, W. I.: Properties of human endogenous pyrogen, Clin. Sci. 16:615, 1957.

64. Herion, J. C., Walker, R. I., and Palmer, J. G.: Endotoxin fever in granulocytopenic animals, J. Exp. Med. 113:1115, 1961.

65. Atkins, E., Bodel, P., and Francis, L.: Release of endogenous pyrogen in vitro from rabbit mononuclear cells, J. Exp. Med. 126:357, 1967.

66. Hahn, H. H., Char, D. C., Postel, W. B., and Wood, W. B., Jr.: Studies on the pathogenesis of fever. XV. The production of endogenous pyrogen by peritoneal macrophages, J. Exp. Med. 126:385, 1967.

67. Dinarello, C. A., Bodel, P., and Atkins, E.: The role of the liver in the production of fever and in pyrogenic tolerance, Trans. Ass. Amer. Physicians 81:334, 1968.

68. Bodel, P., and Atkins, E.: Release of endogenous pyrogen by human monocytes, New Eng. J. Med. 276:1002, 1967.

69. Snell, E. S.: Pyrogenic properties of human pathologic fluids, Clin. Sci. 23:141, 1962.

70. Bodel, P. T., and Hollingsworth, J. W.: Pyrogen release from human synovial exudate cells, Brit. J. Exp. Path. 49:11, 1968.

71. Atkins, E., and Freedman, L. R.: Studies in staphylococcal fever. I. Responses to bacterial cells, Yale J. Biol. Med. 35:451, 1963.

72. Bodel, P. T., and Atkins, E.: Studies in staphylococcal fever. IV. Hypersensitivity to culture filtrates, Yale J. Biol. Med. 37:130, 1964.

73. Brittingham, T. E., and Chaplin, H., Jr.: Febrile transfusion reactions caused by sensitivity to donor leukocytes and platelets, J.A.M.A. 165:819, 1957.

74. Jandl, J. H., and Tomlinson, A. S.: Destruction of red cells by antibodies in man. II. Pyrogenic, leukocytic and dermal responses to immune hemolysis, J. Clin. Invest. 37:1202, 1958.

75. Bennett, I. L., Jr.: Studies on the pathogenesis of fever. V. The fever accompanying pneumococcal infection in the rabbit, Bull. Hopkins Hosp. 98:216, 1956.

76. King, M. K., and Wood, W. B., Jr.: Studies on the pathogenesis of fever. V. The relation of circulating endogenous pyrogen to the fever of acute bacterial infections, J. Exp. Med. 107:305, 1958.

77. King, M. K., and Wood, W. B., Jr.: Studies on the pathogenesis of fever. IV. The site of action of leucocytic and circulating endogenous pyrogen, J. Exp. Med. 107:291, 1958.

78. Cooper, K. E., Cranston, W. I., and Honour, A. J.: Observations on the site and mode of action of pyrogens in the rabbit brain, J. Physiol. 191:325, 1967.

79. Kaiser, H. K., and Wood, W. B., Jr.: Studies on the pathogenesis of fever. X. The effect of certain enzyme inhibitors on the production and activity of leucocytic pyrogen, J. Exp. Med. 115:37, 1962.

80. Berlin, R. D., and Wood, W. B., Jr.: Molecular mechanisms involved in the release of pyrogen from polymorphonuclear leucocytes, Trans. Ass. Amer. Physicians 75:190, 1962.

81. Fessler, J. H., Cooper, K. E., Cranston, W. I., and Vollum, R. L.: Observations on the production of pyrogenic substances by rabbit and human leucocytes, J. Exp. Med. 113:1127, 1961.

82. Moses, J. M., Ebert, R. H., Graham, R. C., and Brine, K. L.: Pathogenesis of inflammation. I. The production of an inflammatory substance from rabbit granulocytes in vitro and its relationships to leucocyte pyrogen, J. Exp. Med. 120:57, 1964.

83. Warren, S. L., Carpenter, C. N., and Boak, R. A.: Symptomatic herpes; a sequela of artificially induced fever; incidence and clinical aspects; recovery of a virus from herpetic vesicles, and comparison with a known strain of herpes virus, J. Exp. Med. 71:155, 1940.

84. Welty, J. W.: Febrile albuminuria, Amer. J. Med. Sci. 194:70, 1937.

85. Barr, D. P., and DuBois, E. F.: Clinical calorimetry; the metabolism in malarial fever, Arch. Intern. Med. 21:627, 1918.

86. Perera, G. A.: Clinical and physiologic characteristics of chill, Arch. Intern. Med. 68:241, 1941.

87. Fremont-Smith, F., Morrison, L. R., and Makepeace, A. W.: Capillary blood flow in man during fever, J. Clin. Invest. 7:489, 1929.

88. Altschule, M. D., and Freedberg, A. S.: Cir-

culation and respiration in fever, Medicine 24:403, 1945.

89. Wegman, M. E.: Factors influencing the relation of convulsions and hyperthermia, J. Pediat. 14:190, 1939.
90. Peterman, M. G.: Febrile convulsions, J. Pediat. 41:536, 1952.
91. Lennox, W. G.: Significance of febrile convulsions, Pediatrics 11:341, 1953.
92. Petersdorf, R. G., and Bennett, I. L., Jr.: Factitious fever, Ann. Intern. Med. 46:1039, 1957.
93. Bennett, I. L., Jr., and Nicastri, A.: Fever as a mechanism of resistance, Bact. Rev. 24:16, 1960.
94. Futcher, P. H.: The double quotidian temperature curve of gonococcal endocarditis; a diagnostic aid, Amer. J. Med. Sci. 199:23, 1940.
95. Erickson, T. C.: Neurogenic hyperthermia (a clinical syndrome and its treatment), Brain 62:172, 1939.
96. McKenna, J. B.: The incidence of fever and leukocytosis in multiple sclerosis, Arch. Neurol. Psychiat. 24:542, 1930.
97. Holmes, G.: Goulstonian lectures on spinal injuries of warfare; II. The clinical symptoms of gunshot injuries of the spine, Brit. Med. J. 2:815, 1915.
98. Hoeprich, P. D.: The fever of neoplasia, Gen. Pract. 38:115, 1968.
99. Harsha, W. N.: Fever in malignant disease, Amer. Surgeon 18:229, 1952.
100. Clagett, O. T., McDonald, J. R., and Schmidt, H. W.: Localized fibrous mesothelioma of the pleura, J. Thorac. Surg. 24:213, 1952.
101. Browder, A. A., Huff, J. W., and Petersdorf, R. G.: The significance of fever in neoplastic disease, Ann. Intern. Med. 55:932, 1961.
102. Boggs, D. R., and Frei, E., III: Clinical studies of fever and infections in cancer, Cancer 13:1240, 1960.
103. Silver, R. T., Utz, J. P., Frei, E., III, and McCullough, N. B.: Fever, infection and host resistance in acute leukemia, Amer. J. Med. 24:25, 1958.
104. Raab, S. O., Hoeprich, P. D., Wintrobe, M. M., and Cartwright, G. E.: The clinical significance of fever in acute leukemia, Blood 16:1609, 1960.
105. Margolies, M. P.: Sickle-cell anemia. A composite study and survey, Medicine 30:357, 1951.
105a. Dunn, L. J., and Van Voorhis, L. W.: Enigmatic fever and pelvic thrombophlebitis. Response to anticoagulants, New Eng. J. Med. 276:262, 1967.
106. Ferris, E. B., Jr., Blankenhorn, M. A., Robinson, H. W., and Cullen, G. E.: Heat stroke; clinical and chemical observations on 44 cases, J. Clin. Invest. 17:249, 1938.
107. Knochel, J. P., Beisel, W. R., Herndon, E. G., Jr., Gerard, E. S., and Barry, K. G.: The renal, cardiovascular, hematologic and serum electrolyte abnormalities of heat stroke, Am. J. Med. 30:299, 1961.
107a. Gilat, T., Shibolet, S., and Sohar, E.: The mechanism of heatstroke, J. Trop. Med. Hyg. 66:204, 1963.
107b. Gottschalk, P. G., and Thomas, J. E.: Heat stroke, Proc. Mayo Clin. 41:470, 1966.
108. Himwich, H. E.: The metabolism of fever, with special reference to diabetic hyperpyrexia, Bull. N.Y. Acad. Med. 10:16, 1934.
109. Steele, J. M.: Elevation of rectal temperature following mechanical obstruction to the peripheral circulation, Amer. Heart J. 13:542, 1937.
110. Stewart, H. J., Evans, W. F., Brown, H., and Gerjuoy, J. R.: Peripheral blood flow, rectal and skin temperature in congestive heart failure: The effects of rapid digitalization in this state, Arch. Intern. Med. 77:643, 1946.
111. Kinsey, D., and White, P. D.: Fever in congestive heart failure, Arch. Intern. Med. 65:163, 1940.
112. Reimann, H. A.: Periodic diseases. Oxford, Blackwell, 1963, pp. 41-69.
113. Sohar, E., Gafni, J., Pras, M., and Heller, H.: Familial Mediterranean fever. A survey of 470 cases and review of the literature, Amer. J. Med. 43:227, 1967.
114. Kappas, A., and Palmer, R. H.: Selected aspects of steroid pharmacology, Pharmacol. Rev. 15:123, 1963.
115. Bondy, P. K., Cohn, G. L., and Gregory, P. B.: Etiocholanolone fever, Medicine 44:249, 1965.
116. Bodel, P., and Dillard, M.: Studies on steroid fever. I. Production of leukocyte pyrogen *in vitro* by etiocholanolone, J. Clin. Invest. 47:107, 1968.
117. McCrae, T., and Caven, W. E.: Tertiary syphilis of the liver, Amer. J. Med. Sci. 172:781, 1926.
118. Tisdale, W. A., and Klatskin, G.: The fever of Laennec's cirrhosis, Yale J. Biol. Med. 33:94, 1960.
119. Kerr, A., Jr.: Subacute Bacterial Endocarditis, Springfield, Ill., Thomas, 1955.
120. Goodwin, J. F., Stanfield, C. A., Steiner, R. E., Bentall, H. H., Sayed, H. M., Bloom, V. R., and Bishop, M. B.: Clinical features of left atrial myxoma, Thorax 17:91, 1962.
121. Goodkind, M. J., Bloomer, W. E., and Goodyer, A. V. N.: Recurrent pericardial effusion after nonpenetrating chest trauma. Report of two cases treated with adrenocortical steroids, New Eng. J. Med. 263:874, 1960.
122. Dressler, W.: Post-myocardial-infarction syndrome: report on forty-four cases, Arch. Intern. Med. 103:28, 1959.
123. Engle, M. A., and Ito, T.: Postpericardiotomy syndrome, Amer. J. Cardiol. 7:73, 1961.
124. Drusin, L. M., Engle, M. A., Hagstrom, J. W. C., and Schwartz, M. S.: The postpericardiotomy syndrome. A six-year epidemiologic study, New Eng. J. Med. 272:597, 1965.

125. Goodyer, A. V. N., and Glenn, W. W. L.: Management of the circulatory, inflammatory and metabolic complications of mitral valvulotomy, New Eng. J. Med. 257:735, 1957.

126. Seaman, A. J., and Starr, A.: Febrile post-cardiotomy lymphocytic splenomegaly: A new entity, Ann. Surg. 156:956, 1962.

127. Wheeler, E. O., Turner, J. D., and Scannell, J. G.: Fever, splenomegaly and atypical lymphocytes. A syndrome observed after cardiac surgery utilizing a pump oxygenator, New Eng. J. Med. 266:454, 1962.

128. Lang, D. J., Scolnick, E. M., and Willerson, J. T.: Association of cytomegalovirus infection with the post-perfusion syndrome, New Eng. J. Med. 278:1147, 1968.

129. Rifkind, D., Marchioro, T. L., Waddell, W. R., and Starzl, T. E.: Infectious diseases associated with renal homotransplantation. I. Incidence, types and predisposing factors, J.A.M.A. 189:397, 1964.

130. Nolan, J. P., and Klatskin, G.: The fever of sarcoidosis, Ann. Intern. Med. 61:455, 1964.

131. Wise, R. I.: Fever in the postoperative period, Amer. J. Cardiol. 12:475, 1963.

132. Bang, S.: Fever in gastric and in duodenal ulcer, Arch. Intern. Med. 41:808, 1928.

133. Dill, L. V., and Isenhour, C. E.: Observations on the incidence and cause of fever in patients with bleeding peptic ulcers, Amer. J. Dig. Dis. 5:779, 1939.

134. Schiff, L., Shapiro, N., and Stevens, R. F.: Observations on the oral administration of citrated blood in man; III. The effect on temperature and the white blood cell count, Amer. J. Med. Sci. 207:465, 1944.

135. Selesnick, S., and White, B. V.: Body temperature in persons with bleeding peptic ulcer, Gastroenterology 20:282, 1952.

136. Stiles, F. C., and Weir, J. R.: Ectodermal dysplasia presenting as fever of unknown origin, J.A.M.A. 158:1432, 1955.

137. Woodyatt, R. T.: Ichthyosis, fever and effort syndrome, Trans. Ass. Amer. Physicians 50:105, 1935.

138. Root, R. K., and Wolff, S. M.: Pathogenic mechanisms in experimental immune fever, J. Exp. Med. 128:309, 1968.

139. Harvey, A. McG., Shulman, L. E., Tumulty, P. A., Conley, C. L., and Schoenrich, E. H.: Systemic lupus erythematosus: Review of the literature and clinical analysis of 138 cases, Medicine 33:291, 1954.

140. Calabro, J. J., and Marchesano, J. M.: Fever associated with juvenile rheumatoid arthritis, New Eng. J. Med. 276:11, 1967.

141. Rowe, A. H.: Fever due to food allergy, Ann. Allerg. 6:252, 1948.

142. Lian, C., Facquet, J., and Brawerman: Fièvre et tacycardies paroxystiques, Arch. Mal. Coeur 32:566, 1939.

143. Burford, G. E.: Hyperthermia following anesthesia; a consideration of control of body temperature during anesthesia, Anesthesiology 1:208, 1940.

144. Bigler, J. A., and McQuiston, W. O.: Body temperatures during anesthesia in infants and children, J.A.M.A. 146:551, 1951.

145. Pickrell, H. P.: Hyperpyrexia pallida and its prevention, Aust. & New Zeal. J. Surg. 21:261, 1952.

146. Mangiardi, J. L.: Experiences with post-operative temperatures above 108° F, Amer. J. Surg. 81:189, 1951.

147. Stephen, C. R.: Fulminant hyperthermia during anesthesia and surgery, J.A.M.A. 202:178, 1967.

148. Wilson, R. D., Dent, T. E., Traber, D. L., McCoy, N. R., and Allen, C. R.: Malignant hyperpyrexia with anesthesia, J.A.M.A. 202:183, 1967.

149. Cluff, L. E., and Johnson, J. E., III: Drug fever, Progr. Allerg. 8:149, 1964.

150. Vogel, V. H., Isbell, H., and Chapman, K. W.: Present status of narcotic addiction; with particular reference to medical indications and comparative addiction liability of the newer and older analgesic drugs, J.A.M.A. 138:1019, 1948.

151. von Euler, C.: Physiology and pharmacology of temperature regulation, Pharmacol. Rev. 13:361, 1961.

152. Feldberg, W., and Myers, R. D.: Effects on temperature of amines injected into the cerebral ventricles. A new concept of temperature regulation, J. Physiol. 173:226, 1964.

153. Feldberg, W., Hellon, R. F., and Lotti, V. J.: Temperature effects produced in dogs and monkeys by injections of monoamines and related substances into the third ventricle, J. Physiol. 191:501, 1967.

154. Giarman, N. J., Tanaka, C., Mooney, J., and Atkins, E.: Serotonin, norepinephrine, and fever, Advances Pharm. 6A:307, 1968.

155. Fred, H. L., Allred, D. F., Garber, H. E., Retiene, K., and Lipscomb, H.: Pheochromocytoma masquerading as overwhelming infection, Amer. Heart J. 73:149, 1967.

156. Swank, R. L., and Smedal, M. I.: Pulmonary atelectasis in stuporous states; a study of its incidence and mechanism in sodium amytal narcosis, Amer. J. Med. 5:210, 1948.

157. Ritter, W. L., and Nussbaum, M. A.: Occupational illnesses in cotton industries; "cotton fever," Mississippi Doctor, p. 96, Sept. 1944.

158. Sayers, R. R.: Metal fume fever and its prevention, Public Health Rep. 58:1080, 1938.

159. Harris, D. K.: Polymer-fume fever, Lancet 2:1008, 1951.

160. McCord, C. P.: Metal fume fever as an immunological disease, Industr. Med. Surg. 29:101, 1960.

161. Friedman, M.: Etiology and pathogenesis of neurocirculatory asthenia. I. Hyperthermia as one of the manifestations of neurocirculatory asthenia, War Med. 6:221, 1945.

162. Reimann, H. A.: The problem of long-continued, low-grade fever, J.A.M.A. 107: 1089, 1936.

163. Richardson, J. S.: Pyrexia of uncertain origin and psychogenic fever, Practitioner 170: 61, 1953.

164. Dunbar, H. F.: Emotions and Bodily Changes, ed. 2, New York, Columbia, 1938.

165. Wynn, F. B.: The psychic factor as an element in temperature disturbance; shown by some observations in the selective draft, J.A.M.A. 73: 31, 1919.

166. Wolf, S., and Wolff, H. G.: Intermittent fever of unknown origin; recurrent high fever with benign outcome in a patient with migraine and notes on "neurogenic" fever, Arch. Intern. Med. 70: 293, 1942.

167. Petersdorf, R. G., and Beeson, P. B.: Fever of unexplained origin: report on 100 cases, Medicine 40: 1, 1961.

168. Oppel, T. W., and Berntsen, C. A., Jr.: The differential diagnosis of fevers: the present status of the problem of fever of unknown origin, Med. Clin. N. Amer. 38: 891, 1954.

169. Keefer, C. S., and Leard, S. E.: Prolonged and Perplexing Fevers, Boston, Little, Brown, 1955.

170. Reid, J. V. O.: Pyrexia of unknown origin: study of a series of cases, Brit. Med. J. 2: 23, 1956.

171. Bennett, I. L., Jr., and Hook, E. W.: Fever of unknown origin, Disease-a-Month, Nov. 1957.

172. Geraci, J. E., Weed, L. A., and Nichols, D. R.: Fever of obscure origin—the value of abdominal exploration in diagnosis. Report of seventy cases, J.A.M.A. 169: 1306, 1959.

173. Pettersson, T.: Fever of obscure origin. A follow-up investigation of 88 cases, Acta Med. Scand. 171: 575, 1962.

174. Sheon, R. P., and Van Ommen, R. A.: Fever of obscure origin. Diagnosis and treatment based on a series of sixty cases, Amer. J. Med. 34: 486, 1963.

175. Fransén, H., and Böttiger, L. E.: Fever of more than two weeks' duration, Acta Med. Scand. 179: 147, 1966.

26

Lymphadenopathy and Disorders of the Lymphatic System

OTHMAR CHARLES SOLNITZKY and HAROLD JEGHERS

INTRODUCTION

The lymphatic system is involved in many diseases, both local and systemic, and there are various types of involvement. In addition, lymph nodes are affected by primary disease of both the lymphatic and the reticuloendothelial systems, as well as by cancer. The lymphatic system, particularly the lymph nodes, may become diseased in the following ways: (1) carcinomatous invasion, (2) infectious adenopathy, (3) infiltration by foreign substances, (4) disturbances of metabolism, especially of lipids (storage type of adenopathy), and (5) primary hematopoietic disorder.

Many of the lymph nodes of the body thus affected are amenable to palpation, biopsy, and roentgen ray studies. The character of the lymph node enlargement, the degree and extent of the involvement of the nodes, and the character of the histologic changes within them are of great importance, not only in diagnosis, but also in treatment.

Diagnostically, involved lymph nodes can give a clue to the site of origin and, in many cases, to the nature of the causative agent.

A knowledge of the drainage areas of the various regional lymph nodes of the body is essential in planning adequate treatment, whether by radiation or by radical surgical dissection.

RELATION OF LYMPHATIC SYSTEM TO OTHER CIRCULATORY SYSTEMS

There are three major circulatory systems: (1) the blood vascular, (2) the cerebrospinal, and (3) the lymphatic (Fig. 26-1). The *blood vascular system* is a closed vascular ring provided with a pump, the heart. The function of this system is to ensure that blood reaches all parts of the body in order that each cell may receive nourishment in accordance with its functional needs. Blood flows away from the heart in the arteries and arterioles to reach the capillaries, which not only permit the escape into the tissue spaces of nutrient fluid, but also reabsorb some of the tissue fluid. From the capillaries, the blood is returned back to the heart by the veins. Thus, in the blood vascular system, blood flows in two directions: from and to the heart.

The *cerebrospinal fluid circulatory system* is also a closed system of channels, containing the cerebrospinal fluid. It consists of the ventricles and the cerebral aqueduct of the brain, the central canal of the spinal cord, and the subarachnoid space. Normally, the cerebrospinal fluid, elaborated chiefly by the choroid plexuses of the brain ventricles, flows in one direction: from the ventricles through the foramina of Luschka and Magendie into the subarachnoid space, from which it is transferred across the arachnoid villi into the dural venous sinuses and finally into the internal jugular vein to be returned to the right side of the heart. Thus, cerebrospinal fluid does not enter the venous system directly, but across the meningeal barrier represented by the arachnoid villi and the dura mater.

The *lymphatic system*,[1] unlike the first two, is not closed, but communicates directly with the venous system at the root of the neck. It consists of a system of blindly beginning capillaries, which pick up tissue fluid not absorbed through the blood capillaries, and of a series of collecting vessels of increasing size which eventually drain the contained fluid, called lymph, into the subclavian veins. In the lymphatic system the flow of lymph is always in one direction only, that is, to the heart. A characteristic of the lymphatic system is the interpolation along its main vessels of filters—the lymph nodes—through which lymph must first pass before being transferred to the veins.

FUNCTIONS OF LYMPHATIC SYSTEM

The lymphatic system performs several important functions[2]:

1. Lymphatic vessels furnish preformed tubes for the passage of lymph. These vessels can also serve for the transport of viruses and bacteria. Microorganisms may be introduced directly into lymphatic capillaries or vessels by puncture or incised wounds, or they may enter the lymphatics from a suppurative focus. In either case, there may occur a consequent infection of the lymphatic channels (*tubular lymphangitis*), or of the lymph nodes (*lymphadenitis*). If the lymph nodes break down, the infective organism can then enter the blood stream (*septicemia*). At times, infection may be limited to the superficial reticular lymphatics of the skin (e.g., *erysipelas*).

2. Production of lymphocytes. Lymphocytes are produced in the germinal centers of lymph nodes and leave the nodes through their efferent vessels. The ultimate fate of these lymphocytes is not known.

3. Production of antibodies. Immune substances can be extracted from lymphocytes. Lymphocytes contain at least one globulin, which is identical with blood globulin. Immune bodies are linked in the blood with globulins.

4. Phagocytosis. This function is performed by the reticuloendothelial cells lining the lymph sinuses of lymph nodes.

5. Hemopoiesis. Under normal conditions, the lymphatic system is concerned only with production of lymphocytes, but under pathologic conditions, the reticuloendothelial component of the lymphatic system has the capacity to revert to the function of blood formation.

6. By a process of absorption through its capillaries, the lymphatic system returns to the blood stream both fluid and chemical substances that escaped from the blood stream across the walls of the blood capillaries. A considerable amount of protein escapes in this manner into the extravascular tissue spaces, from which it is partly ab-

sorbed into the lymphatic system and thence returned to the blood stream.

7. Absorption of fats and fat-soluble materials from the intestine. This function can be demonstrated easily by giving the patient, by mouth, olive oil stained with Sudan IV or some other dye. The dye will appear in the thoracic duct lymph approximately 1.5 hours after the ingestion of the dye-labeled olive oil. This procedure is utilized as a clinical diagnostic method to locate tears of the thoracic duct in cases of chylothorax.

8. Drainage of lymph via a thoracic duct cannula has been reported to reduce blood urea nitrogen in uremic patients as well as increase allograft acceptance for renal transplantation.[238]

A number of monographs and review articles can be consulted for detail.[239,240,241,242,253]

THE FORMATION OF LYMPH

Tissue fluid is derived both from blood plasma and tissue cells. It represents a balance between the rate of its filtration at the arterial ends of the blood capillaries and its resorption at the venous ends.[3,4,5] Ordinarily, there is little tissue fluid.

Substances in true solution in the blood plasma, such as glucose, inorganic salts, amino acids, etc., exert little or no effective osmotic pressure within the blood capillaries. Their molecules are so small that they pass easily through the blood capillary walls into the tissue spaces. As a result, nutritive material from the blood plasma can easily reach the tissue cells, and waste products also can easily reach the blood for excretion. On the other hand, the blood plasma proteins, because of the larger size of their molecules, cannot readily pass through the blood capillary walls. Of the three plasma proteins (albumin, globulin fraction, and fibrinogen), albumin has the smallest molecule, and hence passes into the tissue spaces in greater amounts than the globulins and fibrinogen. The formation of tissue fluid is regulated by two pressures: the hydrostatic and the osmotic.

The forces that regulate the exchange between blood capillaries and tissue spaces are the same as those that regulate the formation of lymph. Any condition that enhances the filtration of fluid from the blood capillaries tends to increase the flow of lymph. The lymphatic capillaries are far more permeable than the blood capillaries and offer little resistance to the passage of proteins or crystalloids. The lymphatic capillaries have the very special function of removing extravascular protein, which cannot be absorbed by the blood capillaries and which, in the absence of normally functioning lymphatic capillaries, would accumulate in the tissue spaces and lead to edema. From this point of view, the lymphatic capillaries play a major role in protein metabolism and nutrition. The lymphatic capillaries can also take up from the tissue fluid particulate matter, such as microorganisms.

The formation of lymph depends upon: (1) the amount of free fluid in the tissue spaces and (2) influences that empty draining lymphatics and permit further absorption of raw material by lymphatic capillaries.

The formation and flow of lymph can be increased as follows:[3,4,5]

1. Increase in capillary pressure consequent to increased venous pressure from venous obstruction. Where the tissues are firm and resistant, little edema develops. In areas with much loose areolar tissue, a considerable degree of edema will develop early.

2. Increase in permeability of the capillary wall by heat or a rise in temperature, reduced oxygen supply, and certain drugs, such as histamine.

3. Increased metabolic activity resulting from both muscular and glandular activity. Little lymph is formed under conditions of absolute rest or anesthesia. Active muscular contractions also exert a pumping effect upon the lymph, driving it along toward the thoracic duct and the blood stream.

4. Passive movement and massage.[6] The bedridden patient with cardiac edema delivers very little edema fluid to the blood vascular system via the lymphatics. Massage and passive movement not only augment the blood flow and the capillary pressure, but also aid in propelling the lymph along the lymphatic vessels.

5. Hypertonic solutions. Hypertonic solutions of glucose, sodium chloride, or sodium sulfate, introduced intravenously, enhance the volume of lymph in the thoracic duct. Isotonic solutions also increase the formation and flow of lymph, since they bring about a dilution of the blood plasma colloids, with the resulting rise in filtration through the capillary walls.

ANATOMY AND CHEMICAL COMPOSITION OF LYMPH

Lymph has certain basic similarities with blood. Like the latter, it consists of a fluid medium and certain corpuscular elements.

The fluid portion of lymph, derived from

blood plasma by a process of filtration, carries to the tissue spaces both oxygen and various nutritive substances (salt, proteins, hormones, enzymes, etc.). The tissue cells, in turn, discharge into the tissue spaces various metabolites. Hence, the chemical composition of lymph will necessarily vary at different times and in different parts of the body. Ordinarily, lymph from the greater part of the body is colorless. After a fatty meal, lymph in the thoracic duct contains a high content of absorbed emulsified fat, and hence appears milky. Such milky lymph is called chyle.[7]

The proteins of tissue fluid and lymph are derived chiefly from blood plasma. In addition, the liver constantly forms new plasma protein, which eventually reaches the blood stream by way of the lymphatics. The proportion of albumin to globulin is greater in lymph than in blood plasma because of the freer passage of the smaller albumin molecule through the walls of the blood capillaries. The chlorides tend to be higher in lymph, whereas the calcium concentration is lower. Lymph contains fibrinogen in very low concentrations, as well as prothrombin. It clots more slowly than blood plasma because of the lack of blood platelets. Like blood plasma, lymph contains 26 to 28 m.Eq./liter carbon dioxide and follows the reaction of the blood.

Cellular Elements. The lymph of the thoracic duct contains mostly lymphocytes. The cell count varies from 2,000 to 20,000 lymphocytes/cu. mm. In the case of lymph nodes, the lymphocytes are more numerous in the *efferent* than in the afferent vessels. The cell count can be increased by massage over the lymph nodes. In general, the lymphocyte count of the lymph is greater in the young than in the old.

It has been estimated that under normal conditions an average of 200,000,000 lymphocytes enter the blood stream from the lymphatic system per hour. Nevertheless, the lymphocyte count of the blood remains constant, with the exception of slight fluctuations. The problem of what happens to this large number of lymphocytes has not been solved. There are two main views as to the nature of the lymphocyte: (1) the lymphocyte is an embryonic cell capable of metaplastic transformation into the cellular elements of the blood, such as granulocytes; and (2) the lymphocyte is a special end product of cellular differentiation with specific functions. Most of the evidence so far favors the second view. *Early dissolution under pituitary-adrenal controls seems to be the most likely fate of the lymphocytes.* Such dissolution contributes to the protein content of the blood.

In addition to lymphocytes, lymph may occasionally contain polymorphonuclear leukocytes and macrophages.

Rarely, lymph may contain a few erythrocytes. This occurs in cases in which the lymphatic drainage includes areas of inflammation and congestion. In such cases, there is probably direct leakage from blood capillaries that are in direct contact with lymphatic capillaries.

VOLUME OF LYMPH

It has been estimated that in a resting human adult the average flow of lymph from the thoracic duct amounts to 0.93 ml./minute or 1.38 ml./kg. of body weight per hour. The maximum rate of flow induced by a heavy meal was 3.9 ml./minute, whereas the minimum was 0.38 ml./minute.[7] The rate of flow can be increased by the ingestion of food or water, or by abdominal massage. In a report of a thoracic duct fistula in a carefully studied patient, the lymph flow varied from 1.06 to 1.86 ml/kg./hour.[8]

FLOW OF LYMPH

Under normal conditions, the direction of the flow of lymph is toward the heart. It resembles the flow of venous blood in that it depends on the presence of neighboring structures, chiefly contracting muscles, which force the flow of lymph in a direction determined by the valves of the lymphatic capillaries, vessels and collecting ducts.[9] The propulsive action of the heart does not directly affect the flow of lymph.

Factors Affecting Movement of Lymph. Specifically, the factors that affect the movement of lymph are the following[10]: (1) The remitting compression of lymph vessels by surrounding structures, especially contracting muscles. (2) Respiratory movements. Through such movements, lymph is propulsed from the cisterna chyli into the thoracic duct. (3) Propulsive action of the smooth muscles contained in the wall of the lymphatic vessels, the lymph nodes, and the collecting ducts. (4) Arterial pulsations. Most of the lymphatic vessels course with the regional blood vessels. The deep lymphatic vessels accompany not only the veins but also arteries, the pulsations of which can be transmitted to the lymph vessels. (5) The negative pressure in the great vessels at the root of the neck determines the flow of lymph from the terminal parts of the jugular, the subclavian, the bronchomediastinal, and the thoracic ducts into them. (6) Peristaltic contractions of the intestines. (7) Capillary blood pressure. (8) The force of gravity.

UNCOMMON MODES OF LYMPH FLOW

Shortcircuiting. Although, as a rule, lymph transmitted by the lymphatic vessels must traverse at *least one group of lymph nodes before reaching the thoracic* duct and the blood stream, there are cases in which it may bypass one or more groups of lymph nodes as the result of anastomotic connections between afferent and efferent vessels. Such *anomalous connections* provide the anatomic basis for the tragic cases in which a small septic scratch results in *rapid septicemia* and death within a short time. This shortcircuiting of lymphatic vessels past lymph nodes also explains the cases of *rapid metastasis* of certain cancers. Thus, although breast cancer usually metastasizes to the axillary nodes, and the enlargement may act as a warning signal to the patient, there are cases in which the lymphatic vessels from the mammary gland bypass the axillary nodes and drain directly across the costocoracoid membrane to the deeply situated infraclavicular nodes (nodes that are not palpable, even when enlarged); hence the cancer emboli can reach the blood stream quickly (see Fig. 26-14).

Retrograde Lymphatic Spread. The direction of spread of cancer emboli by lymphatics depends upon the direction of the lymph flow. When all, or a majority of the lymph channels draining a certain area *become blocked, a retrograde flow of lymph will take place.*[11,12]

The question of retrograde spread of cancer is an important one, since it directly affects the choice of surgical procedures. There is ample evidence to show that radical procedures result in fewer recurrences. The higher incidence of recurrences in less radical operations may be due to a preoperative retrograde spread.

Retrograde spread may not be grossly detectable. In such cases, histologic examination will show distention of intramural lymphatics with cancer cells. Retrograde spread may be indicated grossly by the presence of many hyperplastic nodes, not necessarily invaded by metastases, below the level of the main cancer site, or by the presence of actual gross metastases below this level.

Common examples of retrograde spread are the following:

In blockage of the para-aortic abdominal nodes, cancer cell emboli from *ovarian or testicular primary cancer may reach the iliac nodes in a retrograde manner without* involvement of the inguinal nodes, which receive no lymph from the ovary or testis unless cancer in these organs breaks through their capsules.

In case of blockage of the axillary nodes, cancer cell emboli from mammary cancer may reach the pulmonary lymphatics and thus invade the mediastinal nodes. Conversely, in lung cancer, in the presence of adhesions between the visceral and the parietal pleura, lymph from the lung may pass to the axillary or the para-aortic nodes, with spread of cancer to these locations (see Fig. 26-12).

In case of cancer of the stomach with blockage of the mediastinal nodes, retrograde flow may lead to annular carcinomatous constriction of segments of the bowel.[11]

Crossed Spread. The spread of cancer cell emboli from one side of the body to the other may occur in one of the following ways:

1. Lymphatic efferents from an organ may terminate in the regional lymph nodes of both sides. This is particularly true of cancer of the tongue and the lip.

2. Communications across the mid-line of cutaneous lymphatics. This is of particular significance in the case of the cutaneous lymphatics of the mammary gland and of the perineum (see Figs. 26-11 and 26-14).

3. Direct cross anastomoses of the regional lymph nodes of the two sides. Thus, although cancer of the ovary, the testis, the kidney, the bladder and the suprarenal will at first metastasize to the homolateral para-aortic nodes and remain unilateral for a time, eventually it will spread to the other side, since the right and the left para-aortic nodes communicate with each other by cross anastomoses.

4. Anomalous division and termination of the thoracic duct. Thus, the thoracic duct may divide terminally into two or more branches, emptying partly into the left and partly into the right jugulosubclavian junction. Or the thoracic duct may terminally veer to the right and empty wholly into the right jugulosubclavian junction.[13]

LYMPHATICOVENOUS COMMUNICATIONS

For a long time it has been postulated that there are direct communications between the lymphatic system and the venous system other than the termination of the thoracic duct into the internal jugular or the subclavian vein. Pressman and Simon[184] have demonstrated such communications by the injections of saline into a lymph node, immediately followed by the injection of air at the same site. This method demonstrated direct communications between the lymph node and the immediately adjacent and easily observable veins of the area.

Threefoot, Kent and Hatchett,[185] by means of plastic corrosion models, demonstrated in rats the existence of both lymphaticovenous and lymphaticolymphatic communications. Lymphaticovenous communications have been described also in cats, dogs, and monkeys. They have been demonstrated by Threefoot and Kossover[257] in certain anatomic areas in man by postmortem lymphography with radioactive radiopaque media. Their paper reviews the background of this interesting and important subject.

Under normal conditions, lymphaticovenous communications cannot be demonstrated unequivocally. It is only under conditions of stress, i.e., conditions that impose some obstruction or stress on the lymphatic system, that such connections become evident.

AREAS LACKING LYMPHATIC DRAINAGE

There are large areas of the body which lack lymphatics. The most important of these are[14]:

1. *The central nervous system (brain and spinal cord) and the meninges.* The central nervous system contains a circulatory system peculiar to itself, as described previously.

2. *Nonvascular tissues,* such as the epidermis of the skin, the epithelial lining of mucous membranes, hair, nails and cartilage.

3. *Liver.* Although lymphatic vessels accompany the hepatic artery, portal vein and bile ducts, the hepatic lobules are not provided with lymphatic capillaries. The latter are confined to the perilobular connective tissue septa. The hepatic lymphatic capillaries absorb not only material carried by the hepatic artery and portal vein, but also protein released directly into the extravascular tissue by the hepatic parenchymal cells.

4. *Spleen.* Lymphatic capillaries and vessels are here confined to the capsule and the larger trabeculae. There is no direct connection between these capsular and trabecular lymphatic channels and the blood sinusoids of the spleen.

5. *Bone marrow.*

6. *Muscles.* Lymphatic vessels here lie only in the intermuscular fascial planes. There is no evidence of their presence within the muscle fiber bundles.

7. *Eyeball.* Although there are no true lymphatic vessels in the eyeball, this organ contains in its anterior and posterior chambers a fluid similar to lymph, which is elaborated by the ciliary bodies of the choroid and drained into the canal of Schlemm, which in turn empties its contents into the venous system of the eyeball.

LYMPHATIC CAPILLARIES

In its peripheral portion, the lymphatic system is represented by lymphatic capillaries, which begin blindly in the tissue spaces. They have no direct communication with the blood capillaries. They are larger and more variable in caliber than the blood capillaries.

Structurally, lymphatic capillaries consist of endothelial tubes to which are attached externally both reticular and elastic fibers, continuous with the surrounding connective tissue. These fibers serve to prevent collapse of the lymphatic capillaries whenever the fluid in the intercellular spaces increases, as in inflammatory states. The pressure of the fluid places tension on the reticular and elastic fibers, and thus tends to keep the capillaries open. On the other hand, whenever lymphatic capillaries are damaged, these fibers, by traction, prevent rapid healing, which occurs in the case of tears in blood capillaries. Nevertheless, lymphatic capillaries are highly elastic and can undergo considerable distention without rupture.

Lymphatic capillaries anastomose freely with one another to form lymphatic capillary plexuses. Such plexuses are found in glands and under the body surfaces; they also occur in the skin, the mucous membranes of the respiratory, the digestive, and the genitourinary tracts, as well as in serous membranes (pleura, peritoneum), and synovial membranes (bursae, joints). In the skin and the mucous membranes, these plexuses are usually arranged in a superficial and a deep set.

The lymphatic capillaries of the small intestine particularly are well-developed in the villi, in which they are called lacteals. These capillaries play an important part in the transportation of fat. Almost two-thirds of the fat absorbed from the intestine enters the lacteals, and is carried by them as emulsified fat to the lymphatic vessels, and eventually to the thoracic duct.

There is no evidence that the caliber of lymphatic capillaries is affected directly by vasoconstrictors such as epinephrine or pituitary hormones.

The lymphatic capillaries are concerned with the primary functional capacity of the tubular portion of the lymphatic system, namely, absorption.

LYMPHATIC VESSELS

Lymphatic vessels are interposed between the lymphatic capillaries and the larger collecting lymphatic ducts. They are characterized also by the interpolation of lymph nodes in their path.

They frequently anastomose and tend to travel in company with veins. Occasionally, veins are surrounded by a web of lymphatic channels. Their walls are made up of collagenous, reticular, and elastic fibers, as well as smooth muscle. The proportions and the disposition of these vary considerably, depending upon the size and location of the vessel. Structurally, they resemble veins, but they do not possess clearly defined layers in their walls. They also show less tendency than do veins to unite into large vessels. By co-ordinated contraction of circular and longitudinal muscle, effective propulsive movements may result.

A conspicuous feature of lymphatic vessels is the abundance of valves. These are bicuspid, occasionally tricuspid. They project into the lumen in the direction of the flow of lymph. Under physiologic conditions, the intralymphatic pressure is low, so that the valves seem to be the most important factor in controlling direction of lymph flow. They are responsible for the uneven or beaded appearance of lymphatic vessels. The vessel wall is dilated just proximal to the site of the valve. Valves are absent in the superficial capillaries. They usually make their appearance in the deep capillary plexuses. They increase in number in the lymphatic vessels in which they are most nu-

merous just before reaching a lymph node.

Usually lymphatic vessels are disposed in two sets, superficial and deep. This is particularly true of the lymphatic vessels of the extremities. The superficial set lies in the dermis and the superficial fascia. The lymphatic vessels of this set accompany the superficial veins (cephalic and basilic in the upper extremity; lesser and greater saphenous in the lower). The deep set lies beneath the deep fascia and runs with the deep arteries and their accompanying veins in the intermuscular planes. Usually there is little communication between the superficial and the deep lymphatic vessels, except where the superficial vessels pierce the deep fascia to empty into the deep lymph nodes. Since the lymphatic vessels accompany both the superficial and the deep veins and the deep arteries, the lymphatic and venous drainages coincide closely. This is of practical value from the surgical point of view, since veins and arteries can be seen easily, whereas lymphatic vessels cannot.

LYMPHANGITIS

Lymph vessels may be affected by acute, subacute or chronic inflammatory processes. Lymphangitis usually arises from superficial wounds, such as punctures, small abrasions, cuts and scratches. Consequently, it affects primarily the superficial lymphatic vessels.

Lymphangitis involving the lymphatic capillary plexuses of the skin is called capillary or reticular lymphangitis. Streptococci and pyogenic staphylococci are the most common causative organisms in lymphangitis. **Capillary (reticular) lymphangitis** may occur in any part of the body. It is seen most characteristically in erysipelas. Capillary lymphangitis is marked by an intense hyperemia, with exudation about the rich cutaneous lymphatic capillary plexuses. The lymphatic capillaries themselves may become plugged by clotting of the lymph within them. There is accompanying intense heat, moderate swelling and redness of the skin. Pain may be present or absent. The face is the area most commonly involved. If the infection occurs in the extremities, the capillary lymphangitis may be the starting point of a tubular lymphangitis. As a rule, the condition is self-limited, ending after a few days without suppuration or necrosis. Occasionally it may be very virulent and rapidly fatal.

Tubular lymphangitis occurs almost exclusively in the extremities.[15,16] It is due to infection of lymphatic vessels that drain a wounded, infected area. The wound may be very slight and often is not noticed or is forgotten. It is characterized by the appearance, some time after the infliction of the wound, of subcutaneous red streaks coursing up an extremity from the area of the wound to the nearest regional lymph nodes. If the involved lymph vessels are large, they may be felt as tender cords upon palpation. The lymph nodes into which the inflamed vessels drain also react and become enlarged, tender and painful. Toxemia is often severe in such cases. The lymph node reaction may not occur until the acute tubular lymphangitis has subsided, so that errors in diagnosis may arise, particularly if the initial wound has healed.

The involved lymph vessels are surrounded by a zone of hyperemia and exudate. The vessels may become obstructed by an accumulation of desquamated endothelial cells, leukocytes, and coagulated lymph. Local abscesses may develop. A diffuse cellulitis may complicate the lymphangitis. Usually, prompt resolution follows the early and adequate treatment of the initial wound. On the other hand, with injudicious treatment or inability of the regional lymph nodes to cope with a particularly virulent organism (usually the streptococcus), the infection may rapidly develop within 48 hours into a serious, often fatal, systemic involvement, from the entrance into the blood stream of the infecting organism and its toxins, which constitutes the condition known as septicemia.

Chronic tubular lymphangitis may follow acute lymphangitis, but it more often is the result of repeated subacute attacks of infection.

DILATATION OF LYMPHATIC CAPILLARIES AND VESSELS

Dilatation of lymphatic vessels is found as lymphangiectasis, capillary lymphangioma, cavernous lymphangioma and solitary lymph cyst.

Acquired dilatation of lymphatic vessels is due to obstruction of the main collecting lymphatics.

Lymphangiectasis may involve various parts of the body and lead to enlargement of the affected part. It is most commonly seen in the tongue (macroglossia)[17] and lip (macrocheilia).[18] It may occasionally involve the subcutaneous lymphatics of an extremity (Milroy's disease).[19]

Capillary lymphangioma occurring in the skin is known as lymphatic nevus. This consists of brownish papules covered with small vesicles containing lymph.

Cavernous lymphangioma consists of an aggregation of lymphatic cysts. This condition is found most often in the neck and in the axilla. In the neck it is usually known as cystic hygroma, and should be differentiated from lymphadenopathy.[20] Here it appears during early infancy, or may be present at birth. Typically, the cystic hygroma occupies the lower part of the neck and may extend upward to the ear or downward behind the clavicle, where it comes into relation with the cervical pleura. Cavernous lymphangioma is due to lack of communication, during development, between the primitive lymphatic system and the collecting lymphatic vessels, or with the venous system.

OBSTRUCTION OF LYMPHATIC VESSELS

Lymphatic vessels may undergo obstruction from various causes. The end result is lymphatic edema, which involves the region drained by the obstructed vessels. Lymphatic edema is characterized by little tendency to pit upon pressure (so characteristic of venous obstruction), and by brawny induration of the subcutaneous tissues. Eventually, the skin becomes coarse and rough and the part involved often undergoes tremendous swelling (elephantiasis). Sometimes, lymphatic vesicles develop in the affected area, which may rupture and lead to ulceration and recurrent infection. Leakage of lymph is known as *lymphorrhea*.[21]

Primary lymphedema may result from lymphangiectasis, as already described, or may be due to other congenital changes.[246] Acquired obstruction[22] may result from the following:

1. Surgical procedures, such as radical mastectomy, extensive removal of the axillary lymph nodes, and the division of lymphatic vessels, may result in massive lymphatic edema of the upper extremity. Similar effects may follow radiation therapy. Factitial proctitis is an example of a localized disorder by which radium therapy of malignancy of the cervix uteri may occasionally, as a complication, destroy the lymphatics of the rectum, producing lymphatic block, lymphedema, and an annular type of rectal constriction.[186]

2. Inflammation, followed by fibrosis of

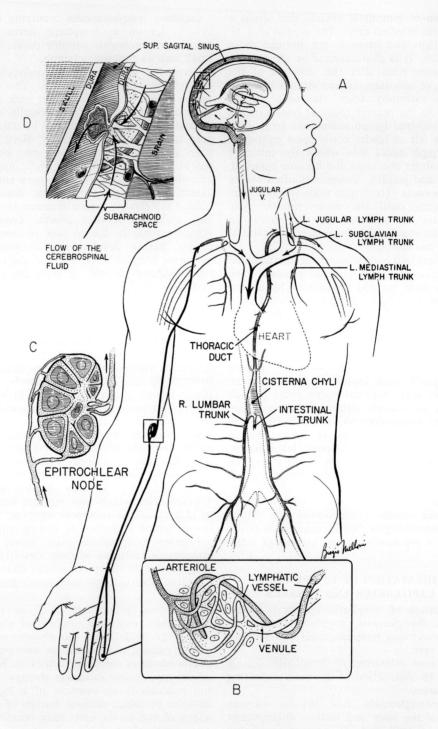

FIG. 26-1. (A) Relation of lymphatic and cerebrospinal fluid systems to venous system. (B) Diagram of the magnified view of the peripheral origin of the lymphatic vessels. (C) Diagram of enlargement of lymph node intercalated in the lymphatic channels. (D) Diagram of magnified view of a subarachnoid villus.

the lymphatic vessels. This may occur following an attack of acute lymphangitis, recurring erysipelas, or certain persistent chronic infections, for example, tropical ulcers.

3. Neoplastic invasion of lymphatic vessels. Thus, in the case of breast cancer, obstruction of the subcutaneous lymphatics through their permeation by cancer cells leads to the formation of discrete nodules in the skin (orange peel or *peau d'orange*). Likewise, the brawny arm, which develops some months or years after radical mastectomy for cancer, may occur from lymphatic permeation by malignant cells. Invasion of the lymphatics of the ligaments of Cooper of the breast eventually results in gross retraction of the skin.

It is well to remember that rarely unilateral lymphedema may be the presenting manifestation of neoplasm, especially in older adults. The most frequent example of this is swelling of one lower extremity as a result of a lymphoma, or carcinoma of the prostate,[187] or other malignant tumor.[243,244]

4. Parasitic infections. The most dramatic form of elephantiasis occurs in connection with infections by *Filaria sanguinis hominis*. The resulting lymphatic edema affects particularly the scrotum or the vulva and the lower extremity, and there is enormous thickening of the subcutaneous tissues.

THE MAIN LYMPHATIC DUCTS

ANATOMY

The main lymphatic ducts include the following: (1) the right and the left jugular trunks, (2) the right and the left subclavian trunks, (3) the right and the left bronchomediastinal trunks, (4) the right lymphatic duct, (5) the intestinal trunk, (6) the right and the left lumbar trunks, and (7) the thoracic duct[14,54] (see Figs. 26-1 and 26-12).

The jugular trunk is formed on each side of the *union of the efferents from the inferior deep cervical lymph nodes*. It terminates at the junction of the subclavian and the internal jugular veins. Instead of emptying independently into the systemic venous circulation, it may join with the subclavian trunk to form the right lymphatic duct; on the left side, it may join the thoracic duct. The jugular trunk receives lymph from the inferior and the superior deep cervical nodes, the axillary nodes, the back of the scalp, the skin of the arm, and the pectoral region. The jugular trunk thus

is concerned with the lymphatic drainage of the head, the neck, the arm, and part of the thorax.

The subclavian trunk is formed on each side by the union of the efferents from the apical axillary (infraclavicular) lymph nodes. It terminates on the right side, in the subclavian vein or joins the right jugular trunk to form the right lymphatic duct; on the left side, it either joins the thoracic duct or empties independently into the left subclavian vein. The subclavian trunk receives lymph by way of the axillary nodes from the upper extremity, the posterior surface of the thorax, the mammary gland, the front of the chest, and the lateral wall of the chest.

The bronchomediastinal trunk is formed on each side by the union of the efferents from the tracheobronchial and the superior mediastinal nodes. Although it usually terminates in the subclavian vein, it may join the right lymphatic or the thoracic duct. The bronchomediastinal trunk receives lymph from the lungs, the bronchi, the trachea, the esophagus, and the heart.

The right lymphatic duct is formed on the right side, at the root of the neck, by the junction of the right jugular, the right subclavian and the right bronchomediastinal ducts. It may be absent if one or more of these open independently into the right internal jugular, the right subclavian or the left innominate veins, respectively.

The right lymphatic duct is concerned with the lymphatic drainage of the right half of the head and neck, the right upper extremity and mammary gland, and the right half of the thorax. When present, it is about half an inch long. Its tributaries normally communicate with the thoracic duct. Its importance thus lies in the fact that it provides an alternate route for passage of lymph into the systemic venous circulation in cases of obstruction of the thoracic duct.

The intestinal trunk is a single short trunk extending from the celiac preaortic nodes to the cisterna chyli. It may enter the latter independently, but often joins the right or the left lumbar trunk. It receives lymph from the preaortic nodes (celiac, superior and inferior mesenteric), and hence is concerned with the lymphatic drainage of the lower part of the esophagus, the stomach, the liver and the gallbladder, the pancreas, and the small and large intestines, exclusive of the anal canal.

The lumbar trunks, right and left, are

two short lymphatic vessels extending from the upper para-aortic nodes on each side of the abdominal aorta to the cisterna chyli. The left lumbar trunk passes behind the abdominal aorta. They are concerned with the lymphatic drainage of the lower extremities, the perineum, the pelvis and the pelvic organs, the kidneys, the suprarenals and the deep structures of the abdominal walls.

The thoracic duct is the main collecting duct of the lymphatic system.[2] It transports lymph to the systemic venous system from both lower extremities, the perineum, the pelvic and the abdominal organs, the abdominal walls, and the right half of the body above the xiphisternal junction.

The thoracic duct extends from the cisterna chyli to the root of the neck. The cisterna chyli is a lymph sac about 2 inches long, lying in front of the first and the second lumbar vertebrae, beneath the diaphragm. It is formed mainly by the confluence of the intestinal and the two lumbar lymphatic ducts.

The thoracic duct measures 16 to 18 in. (40 to 45 cm.) in length and approximately ⅛ in. (0.3 cm.) in width. However, its caliber is not uniform.

Structurally, the thoracic duct resembles a vein, differing from the latter by a greater content of smooth muscle and a greater number of bicuspid valves.

In its ascending course from the cisterna chyli, the thoracic duct is in close proximity to large arteries, whose pulsations aid considerably in propelling the flow of lymph toward the root of the neck. Thus, the thoracic duct enters the posterior mediastinum by passing through the aortic hiatus of the diaphragm. Here it lies between the azygos vein and the aorta, the right border of which overlaps it. In the posterior mediastinum, it ascends in or near the mid-line, lying here on the thoracic vertebrae behind the esophagus and close to the right border of the descending thoracic aorta.

At about the level of the fourth or the fifth thoracic vertebra, it turns to the left and enters the superior mediastinum to ascend along the left border of the esophagus and behind the left subclavian artery. Upon reaching the root of the neck, it curves to the left behind the left common carotid artery, the vagus and the internal jugular vein. After a short downward course, it joins the beginning of the left innominate vein. Near its termination, the thoracic duct is joined by the left bronchomedias-

tinal, the left subclavian and the left jugular lymphatic trunks. The mouth of the thoracic duct is guarded by a sentinel valve, which prevents the entrance of blood into it during life. After death, this valve no longer functions, so that at autopsy the terminal part of the thoracic duct may contain a variable amount of blood.

The tributaries of the thoracic duct are as follows:

1. In the abdomen it receives the intestinal and the right and the left lumbar trunks, and efferents from the intercostal lymph nodes of the lower six intercostal spaces.

2. In the thorax, it receives: (A) afferents from the right and the left para-aortic and the retroperitoneal lymph nodes, which enter it after passing through the crura of the diaphragm, (B) efferents from the posterior mediastinal nodes, and (C) efferents from the intercostal lymph nodes of the upper five or six intercostal spaces.

On the other hand, the thoracic duct sends afferents to the superior mediastinal nodes and has communications with the azygos system of veins. Both of these types of anastomoses are found chiefly above the level of the eighth thoracic vertebra. Below this level, the thoracic duct is a single tube. Therefore, traumatic injuries of the thoracic duct below the level of the eighth thoracic vertebra are prognostically far more serious and may prove fatal, unless the torn duct is ligated.

The thoracic duct may show important anomalies.[55] Thus, it may veer to the right and open into the right innominate vein. Or it may bifurcate, one branch opening into the left and the other into the right innominate vein.

CHYLOUS EFFUSIONS

Since the thoracic duct drains lymph from the greater part of the body, its severance entails a considerable loss of fluid, fat and protein, and lymphocytes.[56] Hence such injuries are followed by: (1) dehydration producing excessive thirst, decreasing urinary output, and dry skin; (2) loss of weight because of rapid depletion of body fat depots; (3) marked weakness; (4) loss of fat-soluble vitamins A and D absorbed from the gastrointestinal tract; (5) striking drop in number, or complete disappearance of lymphocytes in the circulating blood. This marked drop in the lymphocyte count can be of great diagnostic value, especially in accident cases with chest injury but no evidence of injury to the thoracic duct; (6) loss of protein.

To these would be added the effects of compression by the accumulation of the extravasated lymph or chyle.

Extravasated lymph or chyle usually does not clot like blood; hence the wound may not heal. Consequently, life may be endangered unless operative repair or ligation of the duct is carried out. Because of the bacteriostatic action of lymph, severance of the thoracic duct is not accompanied by infection unless this is introduced by the traumatic agent.

Rupture of the thoracic duct may result from trauma, operative procedures, or obstruction. It may occur in the cervical, the thoracic or the abdominal segments of the thoracic duct.

Chylous effusions into the root of the neck may result from trauma and embolism, as well as operations on the neck by the anterior approach. The extravasated lymph or chyle accumulates in the lower part of the neck, and since it does not clot, it forms a doughy swelling. Cervical chylous effusions rarely are associated with thrombosis of the neck veins.

Rupture of the duct in its thoracic course may be due to trauma or certain operations, such as thoracic sympathectomy, pneumonectomy, rib resection, and thoracolysis. In such cases, the chylous effusion first involves the mediastinum, and finally one or both pleural cavities, with resulting chylothorax.[56] The chylous effusion usually assumes such proportions that compression of one or both lungs leads to serious embarrassment of respiration. Compression of the thoracic vessels may lead to vascular collapse, resembling shock from hemorrhage. Chyle extravasated into the pleural cavity causes an inflammatory reaction, resulting in thickening of the pleura, with loss of its elasticity and deposition on its surface of heavy exudate.

In the abdominal cavity, chylous effusions usually are due to obstruction, with consequent increase in the intraductal pressure, dilatation, and rupture of the distal afferents of the thoracic duct. The chylous effusion may enter the peritoneal cavity, with resulting chylous ascites (chyloperitoneum), or may enter the urinary passages, with the occurrence of chyluria.[57]

Chylous fluid obtained by aspiration in cases of chylous effusions has the following

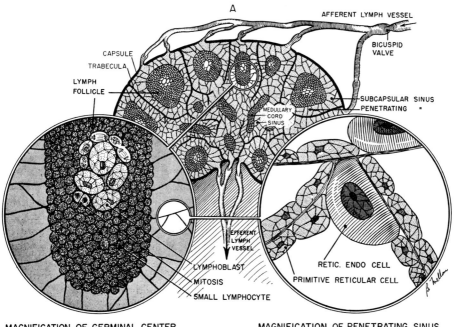

FIG. 26-2. Diagram of the structure of a lymph node.

characteristics; it is a milklike fluid, which forms three layers upon standing; an upper "cream" layer, a middle "milk" layer, and a lower sediment layer, consisting chiefly of cellular elements. Upon standing for a long time, a small coagulum forms. The specific gravity varies from 1.016 to 1.025. The protein content varies from 3 to 6 Gm./100 ml.[56]

STRUCTURE OF LYMPH NODES

A lymph node is made up of (1) a connective tissue framework, (2) lymphoid tissue, (3) reticuloendothelial tissue, and (4) a system of sinuses (see Fig. 26-2).

The connective tissue framework consists of a capsule, trabeculae, and a groundwork of reticular fibers. The capsule forms a dense envelope for the node peripherally. It is particularly well-developed at the hilus, at which point it may extend for some distance into the medullary portion of the node. The capsule is made up chiefly of collagenous fibers with some fibroblasts, and a smaller amount of elastic fibers. It also contains smooth muscle, particularly at the sites of entry and exit of the afferent and the efferent vessels. The trabeculae extend into the cortical portion of the node from the deep surface of the capsule. In the medullary portion of the node, the trabeculae anastomose into a meshwork, which fuses with the hilar portion of the capsule. The groundwork consists of a fine mesh of reticular fibers, which penetrate all parts of the node, forming especially dense networks about the lymph follicles, blood vessels, and on the deep surface of the capsule.

The lymphoid tissue of the node is disposed in two forms: the lymph follicles and the medullary cords. The follicles are aggregated under the capsule and constitute the cortex of the node. Each follicle contains a central pale area—the germinal center, and a darker peripheral zone. The germinal center contains lymphoblasts, and a few macrophages. It is concerned with the production of lymphocytes by mitotic division. Follicle size and degree of mitotic activity depend upon the age, the state of nutrition, etc., of the organism. They may be absent, and later form *de novo*. The peripheral part of the follicle consists of densely packed lymphocytes, which continually leave the follicle to enter the lymph sinuses of the node, and thus leave the node through the efferent vessels. The medullary cords consist of lymphoid tissue. They branch and anastomose to form a wide-meshed network. The cords are continuous with the follicles peripherally; at the hilus they end freely.

The reticuloendothelial cells line all the lymph sinuses of the nodes, covering not only their walls, but also the fine trabeculae of reticular fibers crossing their lumen. These cells function particularly in the phagocytosis of invading microorganisms, cancer emboli, and substances of various types which may come in contact with them as they course with the lymph through the sinuses. These cells may multiply and enlarge, become free, and act as wandering macrophages. Through their phagocytic action, they play an important part in the defense of the body against disease.

The lymphatic sinuses of the node consist of (1) subcapsular or marginal sinus, (2) the penetrating or the trabecular sinuses, and (3) the medullary sinuses. All of these sinuses communicate with one another. The subcapsular sinus lies just beneath the capsule. It receives lymph from the afferent vessels of the node and transmits it to the penetrating or trabecular sinuses. The latter accompany the trabeculae. The medullary sinuses are particularly wide and surround the medullary cords. From them the lymph passes into the efferent vessels. All of the lymph sinuses are traversed by myriads of interconnecting reticular fibers, which transform the sinuses into labyrinthine passages in which the flow of lymph is slowed markedly.

Lymph Vessels. Lymph is conducted to the node by afferent and from it by efferent lymph vessels. *The afferent vessels,* several in number, enter the capsule at various points of its periphery and discharge their contained lymph into the subcapsular sinus, the entrance area for a system of intranodal sinuses. The points of entry are guarded by bicuspid sentinel valves, which prevent backward flow. *The efferent vessels,* one or more, are larger than the afferent. They receive lymph from the medullary sinuses. The speed of flow is accelerated here because of the reduction in the combined cross-sectional area of the stream. The mouths of the efferent vessels also are guarded by bicuspid sentinel valves, which prevent a retrograde flow of lymph into the node when the vessels contract by activation of their own musculature or when they are compressed by neighboring muscles.

The blood supply of lymph nodes is derived chiefly from arteries which enter the node through its hilus. Some small arteries enter the node through the capsule. The smaller arteries and the veins course through the medullary cords to the follicles, at which point they break up into a dense capillary network. The larger vessels pass along the trabeculae. The venous drainage roughly parallels the arterial system.

Nerves to the lymph node are both sensory and motor. Sensory nerves ramify within the capsule; rapid enlargement of a node may produce pain. The motor nerves are postganglionic sympathetic fibers. They enter at the hilus with the blood vessels and follow these throughout. The reader is referred to standard histology texts for more detailed information.

AGE CHANGES IN LYMPHOID TISSUE

The amount of lymphoid tissue and general distribution of lymph nodes bear a definite relation to age.[35] The rate of growth of lymphoid tissue is highest in infancy, and continues at a high level throughout childhood. It reaches its peak at about puberty, and declines thereafter. At two years of age, the child has 50 per cent of the lymphoid tissue of a 20-year-old person; at four years, 80 per cent; at eight years, 120 per cent; at 12 years, 190 per cent; at 16 years, 120 per cent. The maximal development of lymphoid tissue occurs during the time when acute infections of the respiratory and the alimentary tracts are most common, and during the period of greatest increase in weight and height. This suggests that it is part of a natural defense mechanism. During infancy and childhood, moreover, lymphoid tissue responds characteristically to infection by prompt and excessive swelling and hyperplasia. With advancing age, such dramatic changes become less frequent.

Lymph nodes are more numerous and larger in children than in adults. There is marked hypertrophy during childhood, and involution during adult life. However, there is no real atrophy, as a rule, since at any age local or generalized infections may induce hypertrophy. Involutional changes in the lymph nodes consist of reduction in the size of the nodes and of the germinal centers, accompanied by infiltration with fat.

The fact that certain groups of lymph nodes disappear in adult life and that certain areas of lymphoid tissue, although they do not disappear, undergo involution, is of practical significance, since it serves to explain the relative incidence of certain pathologic conditions with reference to age. Perhaps the most significant diseases from this point of view are: adenoiditis, tonsillitis, retropharyngeal abscess, appendicitis, and mesenteric adenitis.

Adenoid tissue is present in the nasopharynx at birth. It increases in size, and reaches its maximum at three to five years of age. Hypertrophy during infancy is a normal physiologic process and must not be interpreted as pathologic, unless there is evidence of infection (*adenoiditis*). A regressive process eliminates the adenoid tissue of the nasopharynx (pharyngeal tonsil) as a source of obstruction in older children.

The palatine tonsils are present in the newborn. They gradually increase in size during the second and the third years, and become relatively smaller after the age of five years. This corresponds with the marked reduction in the incidence of *tonsillitis* after this age.

Retropharyngeal abscess occurs most commonly in infants up to the age of two and one-half or three years, and more rarely in older children. Such abscesses are due to pyogenic infections of the small retropharyngeal lymph nodes, which lie on either side of the mid-line between the posterior wall of the pharynx and the prevertebral fascia. These nodes undergo involution early in life.

Appendicitis occurs most commonly in childhood, adolescence, and early adulthood. In childhood, it is an important pathologic condition, being the most common lesion requiring intra-abdominal surgery. It is rare during infancy, but becomes more common after the age of two years. This relation between the incidence of appendicitis and age definitely is correlated with the fact that in early life the appendix contains much lymphoid tissue, disposed in the form of a circumferential aggregation of lymph follicles, which is especially prone to infection. The subsequent atrophy of this tissue accounts to a high degree for the markedly reduced frequency of appendicitis in later years.

The mesenteric nodes are more hyperplastic in childhood and adolescence than in adult life. Correspondingly, *mesenteric adenitis*, both acute and chronic, usually occurs between the ages of three and 13 years.

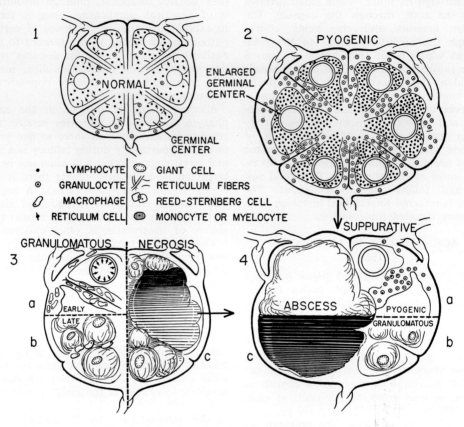

FIG. 26-3. Diagrammatic schema of lymph node pathology.

1. The normal lymph node shows the subcapsular and the medullary lymphatic spaces that also traverse the cortical zone (in white). The capsule and the fibrous supporting septa are in heavy black. The lymphoid pulp is indicated by dots, which represent various stages of lymphocytes from lymphoblasts to small lymphocytes. The germinal centers are shown in the cortex as circles. (See legend for explanation of symbols depicting various types of cells to be referred to later.)

2. Acute pyogenic lymphadenitis. In this diagram the lymphatic sinuses of the node are dilated and engorged with granulocytes (polymorphonuclear leukocytes) represented by small circles with a central dot. The germinal centers are moderately hyperplastic, indicated by double circles. The lymphocytes in the pulp are packed more tightly. The architecture of the lymph node is intact.

3. Granulomatous lymphadenitis. The various stages of development of granulomatous reaction. In segment **a,** the dilated lymphatics are filled with histiocytes or macrophages. The germinal centers are preserved and enlarged slightly. The pulp contains reticulum cells, the forerunner of the histiocytes, and these also are increased in the germinal centers. Often this is referred to as a reactive lymph node. In segment **b,** the architecture of the node is replaced entirely by granulomas having a tubercle or tuberclelike structure. These are represented by ball-like masses with a central giant cell (small circles with peripheral dots for nuclei). In segment **c,** the granulomatous masses are being replaced by caseation necrosis (lighter parallel lines) which, in the upper portion is undergoing liquefaction necrosis (heavier parallel lines).

4. Suppurative lymphadenitis. This usually occurs as an end stage in certain types of acute pyogenic lymphadenitis and perhaps occasionally in granulomatous adenitis, as indicated by the arrows. To the left is shown abscess formation. To the right, 4 **a,** is shown the transition of abscess from pyogenic lymphadenitis; below, 4 **b,** from granulomatous lymphadenitis.

5. **a.** Chronic hyperplastic lymphadenitis. This represents the hyperplastic response to chronic nonsuppurative infection. The germinal centers are increased in number and enlarged. This is indicated by the double circle. The pulp is increased in amount and

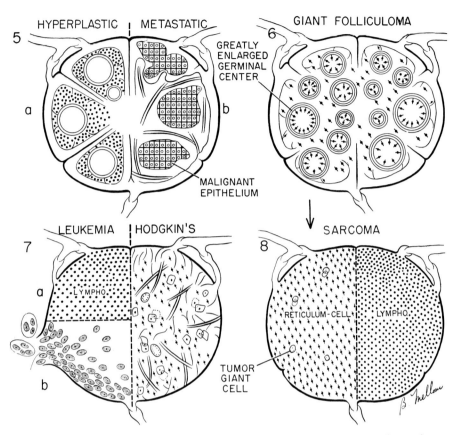

crowded with lymphocytes. Polys might occur in the sinuses. **b.** Metastatic carcinoma. *Above:* An early stage of metastasis is shown with epithelial cells infiltrating the subcapsular lymphatics. *Below:* Islands of malignant epithelial cells are replacing the normal lymphoid architecture and are stimulating fibrosis.

6. Giant folliculoma or Brill-Symmers disease. This is a low-grade malignancy. The germinal centers are increased tremendously in size and number, enlarging the node, at times, to giant size. Reticulum cells are increased in both the germinal centers and the pulp. Ultimately the entire node is replaced by reticulum cells, giving rise to full-blown reticulum-cell sarcoma, as indicated by the arrow. Occasionally the node may assume the character of lymphosarcomatous Hodgkin's disease.

7. This diagram shows leukemic infiltration of the lymph node to the left, and Hodgkin's disease to the right, both of which are malignant. Leukemia (*Left*, **a** and **b**). The entire lymph node is replaced by various types of white cells. These may be myelocytes, lymphocytes, monocytes, or more malignant blast forms, referred to as stem cells. Plasma-cell myeloma or plasma-cell leukemia may also show similar infiltration. The capsule is invaded and the surrounding fat is infiltrated. Hodgkin's disease (*Right*). This is the most variable histologic picture seen in the lymph node, with destruction of the pre-existing normal architecture. The stromal or ground substance of the lymph node is increased, as shown by the irregular black bands. Germinal centers and lymphoid pulp are replaced by malignant reticulum cells, which differentiate to macrophages or histiocytes, many of them binucleated to form a characteristic tumor giant cell, known as the Reed-Sternberg cell. The latter are indicated in the diagram by double or overlapping cytoplasmic squares with enlarged nuclei. The cytoplasm is often indistinct. The identity of the malignant reticulum cells is disputed, and sometimes they are referred to as retrothelial cells. Typical foreign body giant cells also may be present. An increased number of eosinophils infiltrate the node in a minority of the cases.

8. Reticulum cell sarcoma (*Left*). The lymph node is replaced completely by a diffuse

(*Continued on following page*).

MODES OF INVOLVEMENT OF LYMPHATIC SYSTEM AND PATHOLOGIC CHANGES

The lymphatic system, particularly the lymph nodes, may become involved in the following ways: (1) carcinomatous invasion; (2) infectious adenopathy; (3) infiltration by foreign substance; (4) disturbance of metabolism, especially of lipids (storage type of adenopathy); and (5) primary hematopoietic disease.

CARCINOMATOUS INVASION

Primary carcinoma of the lymphatic system is unknown. Consequently, the presence of carcinoma in a lymph node must be considered as secondary to cancer of some organ drained by the involved nodes. Carcinoma has a special tendency to spread by the lymphatic system, as evidenced by the preponderance of metastases to the regional lymph nodes; therefore, meticulous node extirpation is part of surgical treatment. Lymphosarcoma, unlike sarcoma, also spreads by the lymphatic system.

Spread of cancer by the lymphatic route may occur by permeation or cancer cell emboli.[24] In permeation, the cancer cells, after reaching the lymphatic capillaries, invade their lumina and then spread along the lymph streams. Embolic spread is the predominant form of lymphatic spread of cancer. The emboli are filtered from the lymph stream by the lymph nodes. At first, they become arrested in the subcapsular sinus, but eventually the metastatic cancer may completely replace the node[25] (Fig. 26-3). The metastatic cancer has the same morphologic characteristics as the primary cancer. Metastatically involved nodes are subject to secondary changes, such as necrosis and fibrosis. Cancer cells in lymphatic channels also may reach the venous system by means of lymphaticovenous shunts.[25B]

It must be emphasized that the clinical examination of lymph nodes is not sufficient to determine the presence or the absence of lymph node metastases.[26] An enlarged lymph node is not necessarily involved metastatically; lymph nodes often show reactive hyperplasia before they are invaded by cancer emboli. Such reactive hyperplasia is due to phagocytosis of cellular debris, resulting from necrosis of the primary growth. This is the so-called *foreign body reaction*. The affected lymph node presents the picture of *granulomatous lymphadenitis*. The primary cancer may also serve as an entrance site for infection leading to infectious lymphadenopathy. It occurs particularly in lymph nodes at some distance from the primary cancerous focus. Lymph nodes in the immediate vicinity of the cancerous focus may show no reactive hyperplasia, and therefore may not be enlarged, and yet may contain cancer emboli. Enlargement of lymph nodes due to reactive hyperplasia without cancer emboli represents a basis for considerable improvement in prognosis.

Atypical lymph nodes may be reached by metastases through lymphatic vessels that drain an organ that has become involved secondarily by cancer through the hematogenous route.[27]

INFECTIOUS ADENOPATHY

The lymphatic system may be invaded by acute or chronic infectious processes, which may affect both the lymphatic vessels and the nodes.

The involvement may be due to the entrance into the lymph stream of viruses, bacteria, or parasites, or to transportation of toxic substances from foci of infection.

The morphology of the inflammatory reaction chiefly depends upon the nature of the infecting organism and the resistance of the patient.

In acute inflammation, the lymph nodes become enlarged, tender, soft, and elevated.[28] The overlying skin is reddened and surrounding tissues are edematous and infiltrated. The lymph nodes present the histologic picture of acute pyogenic lymphadenitis (Fig. 26-3). Upon section, the nodes are hyperemic and bulge above the cut surfaces. There may be small hemor-

---

(*Continued from preceding page*).
proliferation of reticulum cells, with the occasional formation of tumor giant cells. Lymphosarcoma (*Right*). The lymph node is replaced entirely by a proliferation of lymphocytes or, at times, lymphoblasts. The identical picture is seen in the lymph nodes in cases of lymphocytic or lymphoblastic leukemia. (Diagrams and legends prepared by Dr. Charles F. Geschickter, Department of Pathology, Georgetown University School of Medicine.)

rhages or areas of necrosis. The lymph sinuses of the involved node contain polymorphonuclear leucocytes from the blood stream and macrophages derived from the reticuloendothelial cells. Both may contain bacteria, dead cells, or tissue fragments. If the infection is overcome, regressive changes will take place. On the other hand, the infective process may lead to suppuration and abscess formation.[29] If suppuration occurs, sinuses may open on the surface and the infection may spread to the next group of nodes, and eventually reach the systemic venous circulation. Suppurative lymphadenitis may represent the terminal stage of an acute pyogenic lymphadenitis or a granulomatous lymphadenitis (Fig. 26-3).

In chronic infections, the enlarged lymph nodes are often not accompanied by edema and tenderness. The nodes are more or less firm, depending upon the degree of fibrosis. The lymph sinuses contain a large number of phagocytes and fewer polymorphonuclears. Among the lymphocytes are found mononuclears and plasma cells. Mitoses are frequent. Reticulum cells also proliferate. There are various degrees of fibrosis. The germinal centers are enlarged.[30]

Granulomatous Lymphadenitis. In various infections caused by bacteria (e.g., tuberculosis, leprosy, typhoid fever), fungi (e.g., histoplasmosis, actinomycosis, blastomycosis, sporotrichosis, cryptococcosis, torulosis and coccidioidomycosis), and viruses (e.g., lymphopathia venereum, ? cat-scratch disease), the histologic picture presented by the involved lymph nodes is that of granulomatous lymphadenitis, characterized by the replacement of the architecture of the node by granulomas having a tubercle or tuberclelike structure. The granulomas consist of firm nodules of newly-formed connective tissue. Macrophages enlarge to form epithelioid cells, some of which may fuse to form Langhans giant cells. If several granulomas coalesce, the center may undergo necrosis, the surrounding structures being stimulated to form new blood vessels and connective tissue. Eventually, there is scarring.[31]

Infiltrative Invasion

This type of involvement of the lymphatic system occurs predominantly in the respiratory system and is associated with the inhaling of dust particles (coal, silica, etc.).[32] Such dust particles are removed from the pulmonary alveoli by macro-

phages. The dust-laden macrophages then migrate into the interalveolar septa and enter the interlobular and the perivascular lymphatics. In time, the lymphatics of the lung become filled with the dust-laden macrophages with the development of an obstructive lymphangitis. Many of these macrophages eventually migrate to the bronchial lymph nodes. Upon degeneration of the macrophages, the freed dust particles are now taken up by the reticuloendothelial cells of the nodes. Because of reactive changes, a slow proliferation of fibroblasts and formation of a considerable quantity of collagenous fibers follow. Eventually, there is not only extensive replacement of the lung parenchyma, but also obstruction of the pulmonary circulation.

Infiltrative adenopathy is seen particularly in anthracosis, silicosis, and chalicosis. The histologic picture of the affected nodes is that of *granulomatous lymphadenitis* (Fig. 26-3).

Metabolic Disturbances

In certain pathologic states associated with disturbances in metabolism of lipids, the reticuloendothelial cells of lymph nodes (and other organs) become engorged with various types of lipids.[33] Such lipoid-storing reticuloendothelial cells are very characteristic. They are large and their cytoplasm is filled with globules of lipid, giving the cell a vacuolated appearance. Hence, these cells are called "foam" cells. The lipids chiefly involved are cerebroside, phosphatide, and cholesterol. Since these pathologic states are characterized by hyperplasia of the reticulum cells filled with lipid granules, the condition may be called a lipidosis, lipid histiocytosis, or lipid reticulosis. Since the accumulations of lipid-laden macrophages impart to the organs in which they occur a yellow discoloration, the lipidoses also are referred to as xanthomatoses.

The clinical anatomic features of the various types of lipidoses are dominated by the specific lipid involved, by the disturbed fat metabolism, and by the effects of the xanthomatous accumulations in the tissues of the body. The altered lipid metabolism may be secondary or primary.

In the primary lipidoses, the anatomic and functional changes related to the lipoid storage are so constant and specific that they are recognized as disease entities. There are two well-defined primary lipidoses: (1) Gaucher's disease, and (2) Niemann-Pick's disease. Both are congenital and familial, and occur almost exclusively in Jewish infants and children. Both pursue a course that is ultimately fatal.

In Gaucher's disease, the essential lipid disturbance affects the metabolism of the galactolipin kerasin.[34] This lipid is a cerebroside and is stored in the reticuloendothelial cells of the body. Although the accumulations of the foam cells are focal, they are generalized in distribution. The foam cells are very large, contain one or more nuclei, and the cytoplasm has a peculiar fibrillary or weblike structure, seen in no other lipidosis. Accumulation of foam cells leads to generalized enlargement of lymph nodes, both superficial and deep. The spleen becomes enlarged enormously. Foam cells fill the lymph sinuses of the nodes. Here they are not distributed diffusely, but tend to form nodular accumulations. The germinal centers are hyperplastic. Since the pathologic picture is essentially a storage phenomenon, there are no mitoses visible. The architecture of the nodes is not disturbed. The lipid kerasin cannot be demonstrated histologically by ordinary neutral fat dyes. It also does not rotate the plane of polarized light. Eventually, the foam cells disintegrate, and the liberated kerasin stimulates the proliferation of fibroblasts, with consequent development of granulomatous lymphadenitis.

In Niemann-Pick's disease there is a pronounced cholesterolemia (over 500 mg. per 100 ml.). The lipid chiefly and specifically involved in this type of lipidosis is the phosphatide lecithin.[23,33] The foam cells are large and pale yellow. Their cytoplasm is filled with small round drops of lecithin arranged in a typical mulberry-like crustation. The stored lipid stains a dark dirty red with Sudan III and is anisotropic. The foam cells fill the lymph sinuses of lymph nodes.[33] There is no alteration of the architecture of the nodes except that the foam cells are distributed in nodular collections. There is enlargement of the superficial nodes. In addition, the intra-abdominal lymph nodes particularly (especially the hepatic, the pancreatic, the splenic, and the mesenteric) are filled with foam cells, and hence are considerably enlarged. There are no mitoses.

Two other diseases have been classified as lipid storage disease: the Hand-Schüller-Christian and Letterer-Siwe's diseases. In Hand-Schüller-Christian disease the lymph nodes are enlarged moderately, although marked lymphadenopathy may occur.[36] The lesions in the nodes and elsewhere are filled with large mononuclear cells containing much cholesterol and fatty acids. However, there are several factors that indicate that this disease is not a lipid storage disease. The level of cholesterol in the blood plasma is normal; there is absence of evidence of lipid storage early in the disease; the early lesions are granulomatous in character; and finally the lesions eventually heal by connective tissue replacement. These findings favor the view that Hand-Schüller-Christian disease is an inflammatory granuloma.[37] However, so far, no causative organism has been found by bacteriologic and animal inoculation studies.

Letterer-Siwe's disease also is not a true lipid storage disease.[38] Although there is generalized lymphadenopathy, the essential pathologic change is a diffuse granulomatous process, which is identical in all important respects with the early lesion in Hand-Schüller-Christian disease. Letterer-Siwe's disease is thus apparently a more acute and severe form of Hand-Schüller-Christian disease.

Eosinophilic granuloma[39] is a condition similar in gross pathology and microscopic appearance to Hand-Schüller-Christian disease. The etiology of these three conditions and their relation to each other is not clear.[40]

Secondary lipidosis may occur in connection with diabetes mellitus, jaundice, or nephritis. Whenever cholesterolemia occurs in diabetes mellitus, typical foam cells containing cholesterol or cholesterol esters may appear in the lymph nodes and other organs. In obstruction of the biliary passage for a considerable time, as in chronic pancreatitis, the blood cholesterol becomes raised, with lipid (cholesterol) storage in the reticuloendothelial cells.

Hypercholesterolemia also can be produced experimentally by the administration of large quantities of cholesterol in the food, with the appearance of large depots of cholesterol in the reticuloendothelial cells.

Primary Hematopoietic Disease

Primary disease may involve the lymphatic, the leukocytic, or the erythrocytic divisions of the hematopoietic system. Lymph nodes may become involved by primary tumors of lymphoid tissue (primary

peripheral lymph vessels are fine in caliber (usually less than 1 mm. in diameter), run parallel to the superficial veins (demonstrable by phlebography), and present a characteristic beaded appearance because of the presence of valves (Fig. 26-4). The lymphatic vessels bifurcate and anastomose with each other. They are of uniform diameter until they reach the pelvis, at which point they increase slightly in diameter. Ordinarily, when the injection is made unilaterally, lymphatics crossing over to the opposite side are demonstrable in the upper sacral and lumbar regions, in the case of the lower extremity. This feature is highly significant in the planning and follow-up of radical surgery and therapy in the retroperitoneal region.

Normal lymph nodes, although usually present singly or in groups at certain locations, do not show a constant pattern. They vary both in number and size from patient to patient. There is also a dissimilarity between the two sides in the same patient. In size, nodes may measure up to 1.5 to 2 cm. in maximum diameter. The peripheral contour is regular and there is usually a slight indentation in the region of the hilus. In shape, normal nodes appear as globular or reniform. Usually, eight to 12 afferent vessels enter the node, the efferent vessels being fewer in number. The opacification of the normal node by the contrast medium is homogeneous, giving the node a fine reticular pattern in the roentgenogram.

Irregularities of nodal architecture, simulating neoplastic disease, may be observed in nodes in the absence of disease. Such irregularities consist primarily of filling defects produced by fatty infiltration or fibrous replacement consequent to previous infections. Such defects are seen most frequently in the femoral and the inguinal lymph nodes, which represent the primary drainage from the lower extremity. However, they may also occur in the iliac and para-aortic nodes. Small defects may be caused by hilar vessels, by superimposition of separate nodes, or by wrapping of the node around a blood vessel. Oblique and stereoscopic roentgenograms can often clarify the situation under such circumstances.

The Abnormal Lymphogram. Abnormalities of the lymphatic channels are observed in primary and secondary lymphedema and in lymphatic obstruction. Kinmonth *et al.*[197]

described four types of lymph vessel abnormality in idiopathic lymphedema; hypoplasia, aplasia, dilatation, and varicosity of lymphatic vessels.

Various roentgenographic abnormalities are produced by disease of the lymph nodes. Briefly, these consist of enlargement, filling defects, and irregularities of the marginal outline. These abnormalities are significant not only in the determination of the type of disease, but also of its extent.

Inflammatory Nodes. In nodes involved only by inflammatory processes, the significant roentgenographic findings are: (1) enlargement, the nodes usually measuring 2 to 4 cm. in diameter; (2) regularity of peripheral contours; (3) normality of architecture. Although opacification is not homogeneous, as is the case with normal nodes, intrinsically the inflammatory nodes present a finely reticular architecture.

Metastatic Nodes. Early metastatic lesions may not cause any abnormality. As a rule, a metastatic lesion, to be visible on the roentgenogram, must attain a diameter of at least 4 mm. If the node is completely filled with metastases, it is not visualized on the roentgenogram. However, its presence will nevertheless be revealed by deviating afferent vessels. Nodes that are partially occupied by metastases of sufficient size are characterized by: (1) filling defects along the margin of the node, so that the border presents a distinct irregularity in outline; and (2) dilatation of the afferent lymph vessels. Metastatic nodes may be normal in size or only slightly enlarged (Fig. 26-5). As a rule, not all of the nodes of a particular group are visualized. This in itself is indicative of metastatic replacement.

Lymphomatous Nodes. In general, lymphomatous nodes are characterized by enlargement and preservation of the normal marginal outlines. Various lymphomas affect the internal architecture differently. Thus, lymphosarcoma is associated with a foamy or lacy pattern, in addition to enlargement and normal peripheral contours. In Hodgkin's disease, enlargement is often great and the internal architecture presents scattered, punched-out areas of replacement within the center of the node. In chronic lymphatic leukemia, the roentgenogram shows areas of increased collection of opaque medium.

There is now an extensive literature on lymphography which can be consulted for more detail.[263-266]

Complications.[198,199] As a rule, the use of lymphography is not attended by significant complications. It has been shown repeatedly that lymphography is not associated with any functional or anatomical changes in the lymphatic vessels and lymph nodes. The minor complications, which may occur occasionally, consist of (1) transient lymphangitis, (2) local wound infection, and (3) fine pulmonary embolization. Perhaps the most serious complications are pulmonary embolization and hemoptysis.[259] The latter may be of a delayed type.

A possible complication that has been mentioned is the spread of tumor emboli caused by the lymphographic procedure itself. Its occurrence would be very difficult to substantiate. Iodine sensitivity from the radiopaque media used is another possible complication. The literature should be consulted for detail on these and other rarer complications.

Advantages of Lymphography. Lymphography has these distinct advantages:

1. It makes possible a more exact location of involved lymph nodes and indicates the status of such nodes.

2. It helps to demonstrate involved nodes in case of unsuspected disease.

3. It demonstrates unsuspected extension of malignancy.

4. It determines the feasibility of radical surgery.

5. It helps assess the degree of thoroughness of radical surgery.

6. Since opacification of abnormal nodes persists for a long time, lymphography helps to follow the progress of the malignant nodal disease following radiotherapy or chemotherapy.

7. It aids in the detection of metastatic lesions in the absence of palpable nodes.

8. In urologic cases, it demonstrates the cause of displacement of the kidney and the ureters.[200]

9. It aids in the study of abnormalities of the thoracic duct.

10. It aids in differentiating between primary and secondary lymphedema.

SCINTIGRAPHY

Lymph nodes can be visualized not only roentgenographically, after the intralymphatic injection of contrast medium, but also by the introduction of various radioisotopes. Intralymphatic injection of radioiodinated lipoids or colloidal radiogold[201] or interstitial injection of the [198]Au colloid[202] allows imaging (scintigraphy) of the lymph nodes that drain the area by conventional radioisotope scanners, or the more recent scintillation cameras. The patterns of lymph node uptake demonstrate anatomic, functional, and pathological pathways of lymphatic drainage. Scintigraphy permits serial observation of lymph node pickup over a period of at least seven days. Secondary and variable routes of lymph node drainage also can be demonstrated.

For the diagnosis of malignant involvement of regional lymph nodes, scintigraphy, which primarily demonstrates the pattern of lymph flow, is, according to Lang,[202] a less reliable tool than lymphography, which additionally visualizes the architecture of the nodes. Recent experience[253,253a] indicates that lymph node scanning, after subcutaneous injection of [198]Au or [99m]Tc (technetium) sulfur colloid, remains a valuable diagnostic tool in a variety of circumstances.

The hope that cancericidal doses of radiation could be delivered to the regional nodes draining a tumor[204] or involved with malignant lymphoma[204a] seems unrealistic in view of the demonstration[203] that cancerous nodes, even with lymph node elements present, often do not sequester radioactive colloids, and metastases may so alter flow patterns that the site of deposition is unpredictable.

Following intravenous injection of ^{75}Se-methionine, a radioselenium analog of methionine, concentration in malignant lymphomas has been recorded.[254] This observation has been extended and comparison with lymphography[254a] shows general agreement in detecting intra-abdominal lymphomas, with some false negative studies in each group. Apparently the high rate of protein synthesis in these nodes accounts for the incorporation of the amino acid analog in high concentration. Interpretation must be cautious because of the normal high hepatic and intra-intestinal concentrations. Sequential imaging has discriminated artifactual uptake from lymphomatous disease. The high diagnostic yield from the simple radioisotope study recommends it when intra-abdominal lymphoma is suspected.

REGIONAL LYMPHADENOPATHY

In the following sections, lymphadenopathy involving various regions will be described, its pathologic physiology analyzed, and its clinical significance discussed.

LYMPH NODES OF HEAD AND NECK

Group I—Clinically Important and Readily Palpable

Of the numerous lymph nodes of the head and the neck, only the following are easily palpable when enlarged: (1) occipital, (2) posterior auricular, (3) anterior auricular, (4) "tonsillar" and other superior deep cervicals, (5) superficial cervicals, (6) sub-maxillary, (7) submental, (8) posterior cervical, (9) inferior deep cervicals, including the supraclavicular nodes, jugulo-omohyoid (tongue node), etc. The scalene nodes, although not palpable, belong in this group.

Any regional group of nodes may, of course, be involved in a disease producing a generalized lymphadenopathy, which fact will not be mentioned under each region, unless of special importance. Generalized

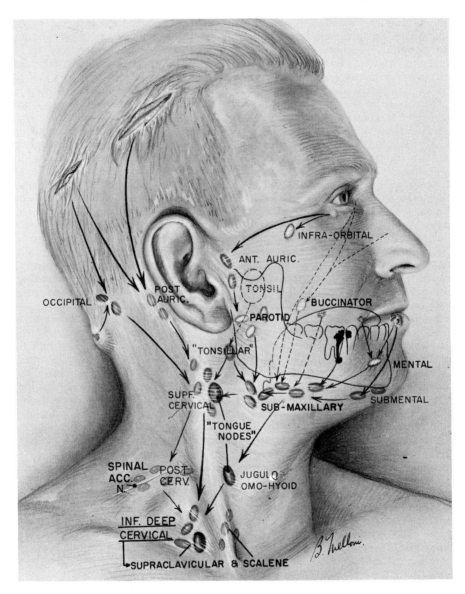

FIG. 26-6. Diagrammatic view of the lymph nodes of the head and the neck with directions and channels of lymph flow. Nodes indicated in dark color are those generally palpable clinically. Nodes in lighter color (infraorbital, parotid, buccinator, and mental) are either less constant or deeper and generally not detectable clinically.

lymphadenopathy will be discussed separately later. The sections under head and neck nodes will stress, instead, the clinical significance of enlargement of nodes in each area or certain combination of areas. Reference to Figure 26-6 while reading this section will help visualize the anatomic locations of nodes and their drainage areas.

1. The Occipital Nodes. ANATOMY. The occipital nodes, one to three in number, lie midway between the external occipital protuberance and the mastoid process, in close relation to the great occipital nerve, near the occipital insertion of the semispinalis capitis muscle. Enlarged occipital nodes may cause pressure on this nerve and neuralgia in its distribution. These nodes receive afferents from the back of the scalp and the back of the head and drain into the deep cervical nodes.

CLINICAL SIGNIFICANCE. Any infectious lesion in the scalp of this drainage area, whether localized or diffuse, may produce isolated occipital lymphadenopathy which, depending upon the nature and the extent of the primary infection, may be unilateral or bilateral. A small primary lesion may be easily overlooked when the hair is heavy. Pediculosis capitis, which may be suspected from the presence of nits in the hair, and ringworm of the scalp are particularly common initiating conditions in children.

Being so readily detectable, occipital lymphadenopathy may be a conspicuous part of a generalized lymphadenopathy, and for this reason is often the first node enlargement to be detected. At one time, painless occipital nodes, and also epitrochlear nodes without local reason, were considered suggestive of systemic syphilis. This is now a rare cause. Cancer with primary site in this drainage area is quite rare.

2. The Posterior Auricular Nodes. ANATOMY. The posterior auricular nodes, usually two in number, lie on the mastoid process behind the pinna of the external ear, on the insertion of the sternocleidomastoid muscle. They receive afferents from the external auditory meatus and the skin of the back of the pinna and of the temporal region of the scalp. They drain into the upper part of the superficial cervical nodes.

CLINICAL SIGNIFICANCE. Comments made about the occipital nodes with relation to scalp infections apply also to posterior auricular lymphadenopathy. If the primary scalp lesion of the drainage area is overlooked, pain, fever and local tenderness behind the ear may stimulate mastoiditis, especially if the middle ear is injected or chronically infected. The auditory meatus as a site for an infectious process (or rarely, a neoplasm) should not be overlooked. The Ramsay-Hunt syndrome of herpes zoster may involve the auditory meatus with lymphadenopathy.

Enlargement of posterior auricular lymph nodes generally has been considered a characteristic and often diagnostically suggestive finding in rubella, accompanied at times by suboccipital and posterior cervical lymphadenopathy, and less commonly by axillary and inguinal adenopathy. This may not always be true, as shown by the study of Kalmansohn,[58] who found posterior cervical lymphadenopathy to be more common and often more marked in 100 adults with this disorder. At any rate, the frequent presence of marked posterior auricular lymphadenopathy in rubella (German measles) and the rarity of this sign in regular measles, is a finding of considerable diagnostic value.

3. Anterior Auricular Nodes. ANATOMY. The anterior auricular nodes lie immediately in front of the tragus, superficial to the parotidomasseteric fascia. They receive afferents from the lateral portion of the eyelids and its palpebral conjunctivae, from the skin of the temporal region, the external auditory meatus, and the anterior surface of the pinna of the external ear.

CLINICAL SIGNIFICANCE. The skin drainage area of this node is limited and conspicuously apparent, so that any infectious or neoplastic process is readily detected early. Particularly significant as primary lesions in this area are rodent ulcer, epithelioma, primary syphilitic chancre, or any infectious skin disorder of the face. Erysipelas may at times produce significant lymphadenopathy because of its common initiation about the upper cheek and the eyelids.

Herpes zoster ophthalmicus commonly produces unilateral enlargement of the anterior auricular nodes[59] which, in fact, is considered part of the clinical picture. It has been noted at times before the appearance of the skin eruption and results from the primary viral infection, although subject to exacerbation when the skin vesicles become infected secondarily.

Diagnostically peculiar to this area is the association of lesions of eyelids and conjunctivae with anterior auricular lymphadenopathy, a clinical complex known as the *oculoglandular syndrome*.

Kalmansohn[58] noted anterior auricular lymphadenopathy in 52 per cent of adults in a large outbreak of German measles, coupled at times with ocular complaints and palpebral conjunctivitis.

Rice[60] reported a 27 per cent incidence of anterior auricular lymphadenopathy in a large series of 112 cases of trachoma with lid activity.

Oculoglandular Syndrome. It is well-known that a wide variety of infecting organisms (especially the gonococcus) may produce acute purulent conjunctivitis endangering sight. The process as a rule is acute and regional lymphadenopathy is not prominent. Of particular interest is the ability of the intact conjunctiva to be the site of entrance of a number of infectious agents, which may produce a more chronic disorder characterized by involvement of the conjunctiva and significant lymphadenopathy of the anterior auricular nodes. Sometimes these disorders are characterized under the name "oculoglandular syndrome" or "Parinaud's syndrome" (not to be confused with the neurologic syndrome of Parinaud). The early description of a disorder in this group was that of a glandular type of conjunctivitis associated with painful and enlarged anterior auricular nodes with minimal systemic symptoms. A leptothrix organism was demonstrated in some cases by Verhoeff[61] in 1933. There may be mild irregular fever, minimal systemic symptoms associated at times with mild blood eosinophilia. Lymphadenopathy commonly is limited to the anterior auricular group, which becomes painfully enlarged, and rarely, as is true for all disorders in this group, involves nodes in the neck area, particularly in the submaxillary nodes, which drain the inner aspect of the eyelids. Rarely the facial nodes and the infraorbital nodes may become involved also.

The virus of lymphopathia venereum may rarely be a cause of this syndrome.[62] Specific diagnosis by use of the Frei test is possible. Tularemia may occur as a pure oculoglandular syndrome[63] when the *Bacillus tularensis* enters the body through an intact conjunctiva. Nodular conjunctivitis, often ulcerative, followed by marked anterior auricular lymphadenopathy, extending at times to include the cervical nodes, follows. The systemic response and the ocular disability may last for weeks to months. Diagnosis by bacterial culture and agglutination tests usually firmly establishes the etiology. As a rule, the systemic response of this form of tularemia is less marked than the usual type, with a consequent lower mortality.

A significant advance in explaining obscure instances of the oculoglandular syndrome has been the demonstration that *cat-scratch fever*[64,205] may be manifested by conjunctivitis, with granulation, followed by anterior auricular lymphadenopathy and the usual systemic features of this disorder. A history of contact with cats is common. Diagnosis is possible by a specific skin test with antigen prepared from pus. The propensity of this type of lymphadenopathy to suppuration is well-known.

Not to be overlooked is the possibility of tuberculosis, syphilis, or sporotrichosis, which occasionally produce this syndrome and, more rarely still, other unusual infections such as glanders, chancroid, etc.[65-68] Neoplasm of the eyelid with regional anterior auricular metastasis can closely simulate the oculoglandular syndrome, particularly if the primary lesion on the eyelid is infected.

The viral disorder *epidemic keratoconjunctivitis*[69] produces an oculoglandular syndrome, commonly unilateral. The more acute form is of about two weeks duration accompanied by conjunctivitis with a watery discharge containing demonstrable lymphocytes. The absence of purulent discharge, in the presence of acute bulbar and palpebral conjunctival inflammation, occasionally with a pseudomembrane, with multiple cases occurring in an epidemic and the absence of a detectable organism in the eye by the usual bacteriologic technics are suggestive diagnostic criteria. A definitive diagnosis depends on special laboratory studies. The edematous erythema of the skin about the eye suggests infection of the reticular lymphatics and resembles erysipelas. In some cases, corneal involvement damages sight. Anterior auricular nodes are large and tender in over 90 per cent of cases; such changes are occasionally followed by submaxillary and cervical lymphadenopathy. If present, systemic features are mild, but rarely may be marked.[70]

The recently described pharyngoconjunctival fever of adenoidal-pharyngeal-conjunctival (APC) viral etiology is characterized by fever, various systemic complaints, nasopharyngitis and lymphadenopathy of cervical or submaxillary and occasionally anterior auricular groups of nodes.[71] It can be added to the already large group of disorders manifesting the oculoglandular syndrome.

Eyelid edema, occasional enlargement of lacrimal gland, slight conjunctival reaction, anterior auricular and occasionally submaxillary lymphadenopathy, all unilateral, may be an early phase of Chagas' disease of South America, and is known as the oculonodal complex (sign of Chagas-Romaña).[72] In this syndrome, the eye is apparently the inoculation site for the etiologic agent contained in the excreta of the reduviid bug vector.[73]

In summary, the intact conjunctiva may serve as the portal of entrance for a variety of etiologic infectious agents carried to the area by finger contact, fomites, kissing, spray droplets, contact with cats, etc., producing conjunctivitis and regional anterior auricular lymphadenopathy, with spread at times to cervical nodes and with varying systemic features. The submaxillary nodes, draining, as they do, the inner aspect of the eyelids, often are involved coincidently when the anterior auricular nodes are involved and should be searched for, since they are less conspicuous clinically. The nature of the primary inoculation makes unilateral involvement much more common than bilateral.

4. The Superior Deep Cervical Nodes, Including the "Tonsillar" and the "Tongue" (Jugulodigastric) Nodes. ANATOMY. The tonsillar node, the main node of the tonsil, belongs to the superior deep cervical nodes. This node lies below the angle of the mandible, between the internal jugular and the common facial veins, at the posterior side of the posterior belly of the digastricus.

The jugulodigastric node is an important node in the lymphatic drainage of the tongue, receiving afferents from the greater part of the tongue, with the exception of the apex. It lies just below the great cornu of the hyoid bone, close to the bifurcation of the common carotid artery.

CLINICAL SIGNIFICANCE. The tonsillar node undergoes enlargement with infections of the palatine tonsil and, to some degree, of the pharynx. The jugulodigastric node undergoes enlargement because of neoplastic invasion by cancer involving the margins, the central and the posterior portions of the tongue.

5. Superficial Cervical Nodes. ANATOMY. The superficial cervical nodes lie on the external surface of the sternomastoid muscle, in close relationship to the external jugular vein as it emerges from the parotid gland. They receive afferents from the pinna of the external ear and the parotid region and send efferents around the anterior border of the sternomastoid muscle to the superior deep cervical nodes.

CLINICAL SIGNIFICANCE. The superficial cervical nodes have the same clinical significance as the posterior and the anterior auricular and the parotid nodes.

6. Submaxillary Nodes. ANATOMY. The submaxillary nodes lie within the submaxillary fascial compartment, surrounded by the deep cervical fascia. Some of the nodes are imbedded within and others lie on the submaxillary gland. In cancer, removal of submaxillary nodes necessitates removal of the submaxillary salivary gland. One of the nodes, the node of Stöhr, lying in relation to the external maxillary artery, is concerned particularly in lymphatic drainage of the tongue. These nodes receive efferents from the submental nodes. The submaxillary nodes receive afferents from the sides of the tongue, the gums, the lateral part of the lower lip, the entire upper lip, the angle of the mouth and the cheek, and the medial angle of the eye. Since the submaxillary nodes drain not only cutaneous areas but also parts of the mucous membrane of the lips and the mouth, their efferents drain not only into the superficial but also into the deep cervical lymph nodes.

CLINICAL SIGNIFICANCE. Enlargement follows infection or neoplasm primarily in the drainage area. The initial lesion in the mouth may not always be readily detectable upon clinical inspection and may require palpation of the mouth with the gloved hand. Infections of dental origin are very common as a cause of submaxillary lymphadenopathy and may require dental and roentgen examination for evaluation. The lip, the tongue, or the inside of the mouth are common locations for primary syphilitic chancre or for neoplasm. Rarely, the inside of the mouth is the site of primary oral tuberculosis.[206]

Submaxillary lymphadenopathy may be confused readily with mumps of the maxillary salivary glands, especially when the parotids are not involved.

One should not overlook that the area of the medial aspects of the conjunctiva and the eyelids drains to the submaxillary lymph nodes, which may be enlarged along with the anterior auricular nodes as part of the oculoglandular syndrome.

7. The Submental Notes. ANATOMY. The submental nodes lie in the submental triangle, bounded by the inferior border of the mandible, the anterior bellies of the two digastric muscles, and the hyoid bone. They usually lie near the mid-line. They drain the central part of the lower lip, the floor of the mouth, the tip of the tongue, the skin of the chin, and their efferents pass either to the submaxillary nodes or to the deep cervical nodes.

CLINICAL SIGNIFICANCE. Enlargement follows infection or neoplasm which is primary in the drainage area. The initial lesion in this area is easily seen, or at least detectable, by palpation of the mouth with the gloved hand. Infections of dental origin are very common as a cause of submental lymphadenopathy.

Submental lymphadenopathy should not be confused with sublingual mumps. In all instances in which the submental and the submaxillary nodes are enlarged, the physician should palpate the drainage areas within the mouth with his gloved hand to detect a primary infection or a neoplastic lesion not clinically observable.

8. Posterior Cervicals. ANATOMY. The posterior cervical nodes belong to the deep cervical nodes, but often are palpable as a separate group. They are located in the occipital triangle, above the level of the inferior belly of the omohyoid. They are related intimately to the spinal accessory nerve, which crosses this triangle.

CLINICAL SIGNIFICANCE. The posterior cervical nodes are commonly involved in scalp infections, pediculosis and tuberculosis. Other infections and neoplasms are more rarely the cause. Because of their close relationship to the spinal accessory nerve, removal of these nodes in the surgical treatment of tuberculous cervical adenitis or biopsy of these nodes in suspected primary or secondary neoplasms often entails damage to this nerve, with consequent spinal accessory nerve paralysis.[74]

Although generalized lymphadenopathy is common in African trypanosomiasis, bilateral enlargement of the posterior cervical nodes is especially prominent and constitutes a diagnostic feature of this disease, known as Winterbottom's sign.[75]

9. The Inferior Deep Cervicals. ANATOMY. The inferior deep cervical nodes lie in the lower part of the neck, below the level of the inferior belly of the omohyoid muscle. Some of these nodes lie behind the sternomastoid muscle, in the fat covering the anterior scalene muscle; these are known as the scalene nodes. Others lie beyond the posterior border of the sternomastoid muscle in the supraclavicular triangle (the supraclavicular nodes) (Virchow's node).

The inferior deep cervical nodes receive afferents from the back of the scalp and of the neck, from many of the superior deep cervical nodes, from some of the axillary nodes, and even from vessels directly from the skin of the arm and from the pectoral region. Altogether, therefore, the inferior cervical nodes receive a great deal of the lymphatic drainage of the entire head and neck, plus some drainage from the arm and the superficial aspects of the thorax.

CLINICAL SIGNIFICANCE. Because of their wide connections, the inferior deep cervical nodes may be involved in carcinoma originating anywhere in the head or the neck; in addition, the supraclavicular nodes may be involved by carcinoma originating within the abdomen or the thorax. The nodes on the left are involved more frequently, probably because of their relationship to the thoracic duct, whereas the nodes on the right usually are involved only when there are tumors in the thorax. The supraclavicular and the scalene nodes will be discussed separately.

A number of papers present excellent general information on the problem of cervical lymphadenopathy.[209,210,211,212,245] Persistent jugular lymph sac must be differentiated from cervical lymphadenopathy.[255] A massive lymphadenopathy, especially of the cervical area, is a prominent feature of the recently described disorder of sinus histiocytosis with massive lymphadenopathy.[273]

The Jugulo-omohyoid (Tongue Node). The jugulo-omohyoid node belongs to the inferior deep cervical group. It is situated in relation to the internal jugular vein and the common carotid artery, just above the point at which these vessels are crossed by the superior belly of the omohyoid muscle. It receives lymph from the apex of the tongue by lymphatics that bypass the submental nodes.

Cancer originating in the apex of the tongue may spread by lymphatics to the submental nodes, but also by a direct route to the jugulo-omohyoid node (tongue node).[76] This node should not be confused with the large node of the superior deep cervical group, often called the "main tongue node" (jugulodigastric), located at the level of the bifurcation of the common artery, just below the great cornu of the hyoid bone, which becomes involved from cancer of the margin and the posterior part of the tongue. (See reference to these two tongue nodes on Fig. 26-6.)

Supraclavicular Nodes. The supraclavicular nodes on each side are essentially part of the homolateral deep cervical node group and when enlarged are usually palpable behind the clavicular insertion of the sternomastoid muscle. The Valsalva maneuver may aid in detecting a supraclavicular lymphadenopathy not readily palpable.[256] Being intercalated in the drainage system from the head, the arm, the chest wall, and the breast, frequently they are involved in infectious and neoplastic processes developing in these drainage areas.

The particular interest of the supraclavicular nodes, especially those on the left, centers in their occasional and peculiar metastatic involvement from neoplasms originating within the abdominal cavity,

and, for that matter, rarely from lesions located anywhere in the drainage area of the thoracic lymphatic duct. Because its lymphatic drainage is from the lungs and the mediastinum, the right supraclavicular node is enlarged primarily from metastases from the lung and the esophagus. It has been reported to be involved from cancer of the pancreas,[77] and rarely from other intra-abdominal tumors, probably as a result of lymphatic crossover in the mediastinum.

Excluding a nonvisceral site for a malignancy, metastatic involvement of the supraclavicular nodes has been accepted as diagnostic of distant intrathoracic or intra-abdominal neoplasm and is known by various special names, such as sentinel node, signal node, and the eponyms, Virchow's node and Troisier's node.[77] Although this sign was introduced in 1848 by Virchow as associated with cancer of the stomach,[78] its present meaning is much broader. In an extensive study of supraclavicular metastases, Viacava and Pack[77] noted them in 28

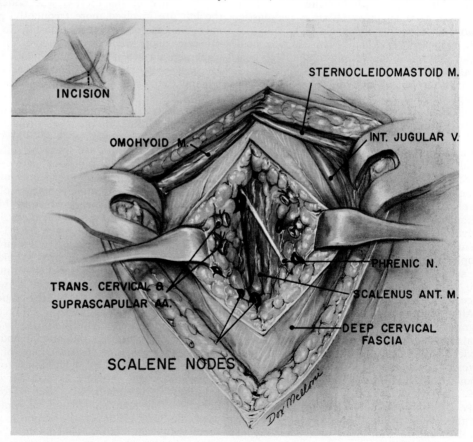

FIG. 26-7. Diagram to illustrate anatomic location and relations of scalene nodes.

per cent of 4,365 cases of cancer. The order of the primary site was 13.27 per cent from the lung; 8.1 per cent pancreas; 7.1 per cent esophagus; 6.9 per cent kidney; 6.1 per cent ovary; 4.8 per cent testicle, and 2.6 per cent stomach. These figures indicate that this diagnostic sign is not particularly common, and when present is of ominous prognostic interest rather than of helpful early diagnostic value. It is actually infrequent in cancer of the stomach, the neoplasm with which it is usually thought to be commonly associated. McKusick,[78] in an interesting report, stresses that the Virchow-Troisier node may be a noticeable metastatic lesion with cancer of the gallbladder.

In general, a *right-sided* or *bilateral* supraclavicular node is suggestive of a *lung* or an *esophageal* lesion, whereas an isolated *left* supraclavicular metastasis suggests a primary site in the *kidney,* the *ovary,* the *testes,* the *gallbladder,* or the *stomach.*[77,78] Controversy has centered in whether tumor spreads to the supraclavicular nodes by lymphatic permeation or by embolization. To support the former view are reports of lymphatic ducts completely filled with tumor cells.[79] Some interesting experimental studies by Zeidman[80] support the tumor emboli theory and indicate strongly that tumor emboli can reach the supraclavicular node from the thoracic duct through afferent branches and need not be explained by retrograde passage through efferent channels. In one study, there was a positive correlation between supraclavicular metastasis and the presence of neoplastic cells in the thoracic duct lymph.[207]

One should not overlook the fact that any intra-abdominal infection, especially if of chronic nature, such as tuberculous peritonitis, may produce a left supraclavicular infectious lymphadenopathy.[78] Patients vaccinated against smallpox in the left deltoid region may develop a noticeable postvaccinal lymphadenitis of the left supraclavicular lymph node.[270] If its cause is overlooked, the enlarged supraclavicular node may be confused with a lymphoma, an aspect effectively discussed by Hartsock[274] and Bellanti.[270]

Scalene Nodes and Scalene Node Biopsy. Extensive studies[81-83] have firmly established the value of the scalene node biopsy, a procedure introduced by Daniels[84] in 1949 for the diagnosis of intrathoracic disease. This operation can be performed under local anesthesia and is neither complicated, dangerous, nor prolonged. Figure 26-7 indicates in diagrammatic fashion the anatomic relations of the scalene nodes. This operation permits entrance to a fat-filled space bound medially by the internal jugular vein; laterally by the omohyoid muscle, below by the subclavian vein and overlying the scalenus anticus muscle. The fat pad in this space constantly contains several lymph nodes, even if not enlarged enough to detect upon physical examination. The scope of operation can be extended to include exploration of the upper part of the mediastinum.[81]

The report by Harken *et al.*[81] adds much data supporting the diagnostic importance of this procedure and emphasizes especially the value of *exploration of the upper mediastinum,* since approximately half of their positive results came from tissue removed from the mediastinum when the scalene node biopsy was negative. The authors reported a positive histologic diagnosis of 45 of 142 cases (31.7 per cent) with the use of this complete technic. Anatomic peculiarities of the lymph drainage of the right and the left lung into the hilar area and to the scalene nodes must be understood to secure the best results (see Fig. 26-12). Homolateral biopsy can be utilized in all cases with the exception of lesions in the left lower lobe, a point emphasized by Harken *et al.*[81] Figure 26-12 shows clearly that the left lower lobe has lymphatic drainage via the intertracheal-bronchial nodes to both lateral chains. Bilateral scalene node and upper mediastinal node biopsies are indicated when a primary site is suspected to be in the left lower lobe. Positive results of about 40 per cent in carcinoma of the lung can be expected when these anatomic factors are considered.

Shefts, Terrill, and Swindell,[82] in a report of 314 biopsies in 293 patients, secured a positive histologic diagnosis in 102 patients (35 per cent). Included in their series of cases were 60 with Boeck's sarcoid, bronchogenic carcinoma 20, tuberculosis 9, primary lymphoma 7, metastases to lung 4. Cuykendall[83] has reported such biopsies valuable in 41 cases.

Lillington and Jamplis[208] and others[268,269] have reviewed this subject and the reader is referred to these sources for critical discussions of its present status. An extensive literature exists on this procedure. Aside from malignancy, the procedure has proved particularly valuable by frequently proving Boeck's sarcoid to be the cause of obscure lung and hilar node pathology. It has also shown that silicosis can involve the scalene node. The curative potential of surgery for lung cancer often can be evaluated more correctly when scalene node biopsy results are available.

Group II—Less Clinically Important and Not Readily Palpable

In the anterior part of the face are several groups of nodes not ordinarily searched for or detectable routinely, but which may occasionally become clinically significant and produce signs and/or symptoms. These include the infraorbital, the facial, the parotid, and the mental.

Here we shall not discuss other nodes of the head and the neck, such as the anterior cervicals, the retropharyngeal, and the many deep neck nodes likely to be encountered only in surgical procedures, especially radical dissections, since such nodes are detectable only indirectly through clinical manifestations or biopsies.

1. Infraorbital Nodes. ANATOMY. The infraorbital nodes lie just below the orbit; they help drain the outer aspect of the eyelids and the conjunctiva. Their efferents join the anterior auricular, as well as the submaxillary nodes.

CLINICAL SIGNIFICANCE. This node sometimes becomes enlarged and tender from infections of the conjunctiva and the eyelid, and therefore may constitute part of the oculoglandular syndrome.

2. The Facial Lymph Nodes. ANATOMY. The superficial facial lymph nodes (buccinator nodes) lie on the buccinator muscle and are inconstant. They drain the medial aspect of the eyelids, the conjunctiva, the nose and the cheek, and send efferents to the submaxillary nodes.

CLINICAL SIGNIFICANCE. These nodes are rarely detectable, since they are inconstant and lie in the deep and not readily palpable areas.[85] If enlarged, they may be detected by bimanual palpation of the cheek with one hand gloved for examination within the mouth, and are more rarely present as a detectable lump in the cheek which, according to Bailey,[86] must be differentiated from a lipoma of the sucking pad and tumor or cyst of a molar gland.[87] A suppurating gland can leave a scar on the cheek.

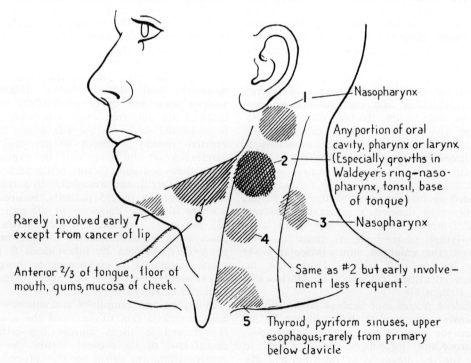

Rarely involved early 7 except from cancer of lip

Anterior 2/3 of tongue, floor of mouth, gums, mucosa of cheek.

1 — Nasopharynx

Any portion of oral cavity, pharynx or larynx (Especially growths in Waldeyer's ring—nasopharynx, tonsil, base of tongue)

3 — Nasopharynx

Same as #2 but early involvement less frequent.

5 Thyroid, pyriform sinuses, upper esophagus; rarely from primary below clavicle

FIG. 26-8. Various lymph node groups with the most likely sites of the primary lesion that may cause the metastases. (Martin, H., and Morfit, H. M.: Surg. Gynec. Obstet. 78:133-159)

3. The Parotid Group. ANATOMY. The parotid group is fairly large, containing usually from ten to sixteen nodes. They lie within the parotid fascial compartment, enclosed by the superficial layer of the deep cervical fascia. Some of the nodes are imbedded within the substance of the parotid, and others are outside of the parotid, but within the parotid fascial compartment. The intraparotid nodes receive afferents from the eyelids, the external auditory meatus, the skin of the temporal and the frontal regions, and the tympanic cavity. The deep parotid nodes drain the back of the nose and the nasopharynx, as well as the parotid gland.

CLINICAL SIGNIFICANCE. These nodes are not commonly palpable. Occasionally pain or enlargement in the parotid area may be explained by some infection or tumor in the drainage area, which includes locations not readily accessible to clinical inspection, such as the back of the nose and the nasopharynx, best studied by endoscopic or mirror examination.

4. Mental Node. ANATOMY. This node lies in relation to the mental foramen of the mandible. It helps to drain the lower lip, the tip of the tongue, and the floor of the mouth. Although its efferents drain chiefly into the submaxillary nodes, some of these efferent lymphatic channels enter the mandibular foramen.

CLINICAL SIGNIFICANCE. This node permits cancer emboli to involve the mandible in metastatic cancer from the lip or the tip of the tongue. This is the reason for *combining hemimandibulectomy with radical neck dissection in treatment* of cancer of the lip and the tongue.[88]

Cancerous Metastasis to Head and Neck Nodes. Any of the head and the neck nodes may be involved with metastatic cancer, the primary site of which lies externally on the scalp or the face, or from the oral, the nasal and the pharyngeal areas. Martin and Morfit[89] have emphasized the importance of always considering this etiology when any of these nodes manifest a chronic enlargement characterized by unilateral location and firmness to touch with absence of pain. Figure 26-8 from Martin and Morfit[89] shows the more common sites for such metastatic lesions. If an infectious focus can be excluded, the drainage area of the in-

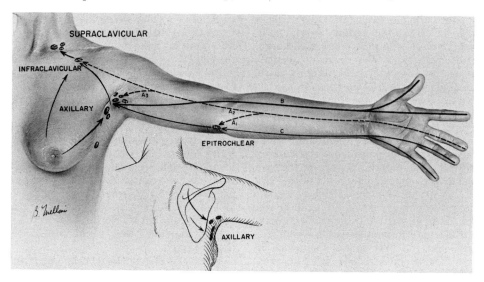

FIG. 26-9. Lymphatic drainage of the upper extremity. The lymphatic vessels draining the fingers and the hand converge on the dorsum of the hand. From here the lymphatic drainage pursues three courses. The lymph vessels draining the ulnar aspect (little finger and ring finger) accompany (C) the basilic vein and drain into the epitrochlear nodes and thence into the axillary nodes. The lymph vessels draining the thumb and the index fingers (D) bypass the epitrochlear nodes and go directly to the axillary nodes. The lymph vessels (A) draining the middle fingers may drain into the epitrochlear (A₁), the axillary (A₂, A₃), or may bypass both of these groups of nodes to drain directly into the infraclavicular, and thence into the supraclavicular, and finally into the bloodstream. The axillary nodes also receive lymph from the posterior scapular region (insert).

volved node should be searched for a primary site of a neoplasm.

Cancerous lymphadenopathy in the neck may present a difficult diagnostic problem, since it must be differentiated from such benign masses as chronic infectious lymphadenopathy, sebaceous cyst, lipoma, thyroglossal cyst, branchiogenic cyst, etc.[90]

THE AXILLARY NODES

Anatomy. The axillary nodes are subdivided into five groups: lateral, posterior, central, anterior and apical.

The lateral axillary nodes lie near the junction of the axillary and the brachial veins on the medial aspect of the humerus, and constitute the main termination of afferent channels of the superficial and the deep lymphatics of the upper extremity. Although their efferents drain mostly into the central and the apical nodes, some channels pass directly to the supraclavicular group. *The posterior axillary nodes* lie along the axillary border of the scapula, in relation to the subscapular vein, receiving afferent lymph channels from the upper extremity and the posterior thoracic wall, and draining efferently into both the lateral and the central axillary nodes. *The central axillary nodes* lie in the deep fat of the axilla or between layers of the axillary fascia at its base, receiving afferents from the lateral, the posterior, and the anterior axillary nodes and terminating their efferents in the apical axillary nodes. *The anterior axillary nodes*, situated along the lower border of the pectoralis major, in relation to the lateral thoracic vein, drain the greater part of the lymph from the mammary gland and also receive efferents from the anterior chest wall. The efferents end in the central and the apical axillary nodes. *The apical axillary or the infraclavicular nodes* lie along the upper part of the axillary vein in the interval between the costocoracoid membrane anteriorly, the axillary vein posteriorly, and the first intercostal space inferiorly. These nodes receive afferents from the other axillary nodes, as well as direct afferents from the superior part of the *subclavian trunk* (see Fig. 26-9).

Clinical Significance. Axillary lymphadenopathy is a common clinical problem and suggests mainly an infectious process or neoplasm in the drainage area, which includes part of the hand and the arm, chest wall, upper and lateral abdominal wall, and part of the breast (Fig. 26-9). It may follow

lesions in the drainage area of the epitrochlear nodes if the pathologic condition spreads beyond this lymph node barrier. Evaluation is made more difficult in that nodes may be palpated, at times, in supposedly "normal" persons.[213] There are many reports on the value of careful study of axillary lymphadenopathy.[214,215]

In most instances, infectious lymphadenopathy is responsible for axillary node involvement, since the fingers and the arm are subject to so many potentially infected traumatic episodes. Likewise many infectious systemic diseases commence by inoculation in this drainage area, producing axillary lymphadenopathy with one or more satellite nodes prior to systemic invasion. Representative examples include extragenital chancre of syphilis, brucellosis in veterinarians, inoculation tuberculosis, tularemia, cat-scratch disease, sporotrichosis, etc. The axillary nodes are especially likely to be involved in streptococcal infections of the hand with tubular lymphangitis. Axillary nodes commonly suppurate in certain types of infections. They may enlarge in rheumatoid arthritis of the arm.[248]

Although any skin neoplasm primary in the drainage area, particularly malignant melanoma and epidermoid carcinoma, may metastasize to the axillary nodes, special attention in these nodes centers about the frequency with which they are involved with *carcinoma primary in the female breast.* Presence of axillary nodes gravely influences the prognosis and the type of surgical resection. It is well to note that metastasis to the supraclavicular lymph nodes from carcinoma of the breast is unusual unless the axillary nodes are also invaded.[91] Occasionally, axillary metastasis from breast cancer is striking when the primary lesion is small and readily overlooked.[92,93] Rarely, lymph-node enlargement of infectious nature, if located very anteriorly in the axilla, may simulate a cancer of the breast.

Accessory breast tissue may occur in the axillary area and may be confused readily with axillary lymphadenopathy, especially when such breast tissue is the site of painful enlargement during or after pregnancy.

Prophylactic vaccines, BCG vaccine and serum, are often injected in the shoulder area and may occasionally initiate axillary lymphadenopathy of marked degree on the same side,[94,95] followed rarely by suppuration. BCG vaccine used in infancy

FIG. 26-10. Lymphatic drainage of lower extremity, genitalia, and lower abdomen. I. Lymphatic drainage of medial and middle aspects of foot (B), heel and outer aspect of foot (A). Channel B shows superficial drainage of inner and middle aspects of foot, leg, genitalia, perineum, and lower abdomen to superficial inguinal nodes.

II. Channel A shows superficial drainage of small toe and outer aspect of foot, heel, and knee to the popliteal nodes with major lymphatic channel deep along femoral vein to deep inguinal nodes.

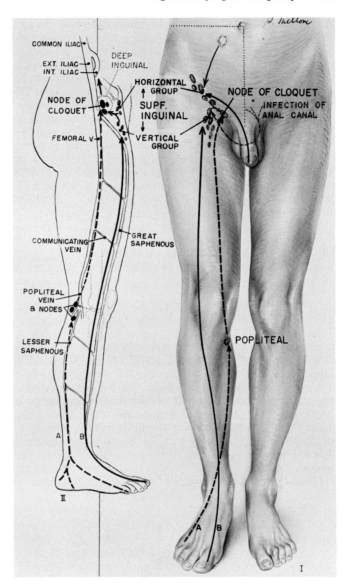

may lead to calcification of the axillary nodes, a finding readily detected on the roentgenogram of the chest area.[96]

Also worth noting is the rare presence of Irish nodes[216]; nodes beneath the lateral edge or deeper in the left axilla in the absence of similar nodes on the right side. They have a diagnostic significance for cancer of the stomach, similar to the Virchow node.

Rarely an anomalous axillary pectoral muscle (Langer's arch) may present as an axillary mass[217] and cause a diagnostic problem.

Subpectoral Abscess (Suppurative Infra- **clavicular Lymphadenitis).** Acute subpectoral abscess is an unusual and relatively uncommon clinical entity produced by suppuration of the infraclavicular apical axillary nodes on one side of the body, a result usually of infection with a *hemolytic streptococcus*. When infected, these nodes become enlarged and may suppurate to involve the surrounding fat in a suppurative, necrotic process. Because it is enclosed in tight fascia-lined pockets, the infectious process produces a severe disability characterized by high fever, a toxic state, tenderness to palpation over the affected area, and much pain in the region of the shoulder, especially upon abduction of the arm.[97,98] If not treated, the pus dissects extensively along the fascial planes and may reach the axilla with spontaneous drainage, or may cause septicemia.

The infraclavicular nodes are most likely to become involved in those persons with an infection of the middle finger in whom the lymphatic drainage is directly to the infraclavicular nodes without passage through the epitrochlear or axillary nodes (see A-A4 in Fig. 26-9). It may also follow failure of inadequate defense reaction of the latter nodes in cases in which they are intercalated in the lymphatic pathway to the infraclavicular nodes. The initial infection may originate elsewhere on the hands, the arms, or the shoulder. There is a close analogy between *acute infraclavicular adenitis* and *deep inguinal adenitis*.

THE EPITROCHLEAR (SUPERFICIAL CUBITAL OR SUPRATROCHLEAR) NODES

Anatomy. The epitrochlear nodes lie on the back of the elbow, in the superficial fascia above the medial epicondyle of the humerus and in relation to the basilic vein. Their afferents drain lymph from the little, the ring, and the ulnar half of the middle finger (but not from the thumb and the index fingers), and also from the ulnar part of the palm of the hand and the forearm. Their efferents terminate in the axillary nodes.

Clinical Significance. Acute enlargement of the epitrochlear nodes in one arm, as a result of local infection or of neoplasm primary in the drainage area, is common and well-understood. More difficulty may be encountered when the drainage area in one arm is the inoculation site for an infectious agent capable of producing a systemic disease, in which the epitrochlear lymph node is only a satellite response in a more complex picture. Representative examples would include lesions such as extragenital chancre of syphilis, tularemia, cat-scratch disease, inoculation tuberculosis, etc.

Being intercalated in the drainage to the axillary nodes, enlargement of the latter nodes may follow epitrochlear adenopathy if the defense mechanism at this level fails.

Of course, epitrochlear nodes may be involved in any disease capable of producing a generalized lymphadenopathy. Being easily palpated, enlargement of these nodes is readily detected clinically. Much interest has centered in the older literature concerning the frequency and the diagnostic significance of bilateral painless epitrochlear lymphadenopathy with regard to the systemic phase of syphilis.[99,100] However, any diagnostic value assigned to this finding must be conditioned by the fact that lymph node enlargement in this region is often a chronic nonspecific lymphadenitis resulting from repeated minor trauma and infections in the drainage area, being more common in men than women, and more frequent and striking in those doing manual labor.[100,101]

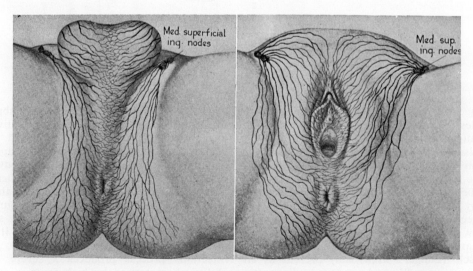

FIG. 26-11. Diagram of the cutaneous lymphatics of the perineum (*Left*—male. *Right*—female) showing their communication across the mid-line and drainage into the superficial inguinal nodes. (Pack, G. T., and Rekers, P.: Amer. J. Surg. 56:545-565)

It has been noted with rheumatoid arthritis.[248] Epitrochlear involvement is said to
be minimal or absent with generalized tuberculous lymphadenopathy,[102] and less frequent in Hodgkin's disease than in lymphosarcoma.[47]

THE INGUINAL LYMPH NODES

Anatomy. The inguinal lymph nodes are
arranged in two groups: superficial and deep
(Fig. 26-10). *The superficial inguinal nodes*
lie in the superficial fascia and are disposed
in an upper horizontal and a lower vertical
group. *The horizontal group* lies parallel to
the inguinal ligament, below the attachment
of the fascia of Scarpa to the fascia lata.
These nodes drain lymph from the skin of
the anterior abdominal wall below the umbilicus, the skin of the penis and the scrotum
in the male, the skin of the vulva and the
mucosa of the vagina in the female, the skin
of the perineum and the gluteal region
(Fig. 26-11), and the lower part of the anal
canal. They receive no lymph from the testis
or the ovary. *The vertical group* lie on either
side of the upper part of the greater saphenous vein. They receive all of the superficial
lymphatic vessels of the lower extremity
which accompany the greater saphenous vein.
They do not receive the lymphatic vessels
accompanying the shorter saphenous vein;
these end in the popliteal nodes. In addition, the vertical group also receives lymph
from the penis, the scrotum, and the gluteal
region. The superficial inguinal nodes drain
into the deep inguinal nodes (Figs. 26-10 and
26-13).

The deep inguinal nodes, one to three
in number, lie beneath the fascia lata, on
the medial side of the femoral vein and
below the femoral canal. One node *(node
of Cloquet)* lies within the fat of the
femoral canal. The deep inguinal nodes
receive the deep lymphatic vessels accompanying the femoral vein, including those
draining the popliteal nodes. They also receive lymph from the glans penis or the
glans clitoris and from the superficial inguinal nodes. They drain into the external
iliac nodes by efferents which partly traverse the femoral canal and partly course
in front of and lateral to the femoral sheath.

Clinical Significance. Persistent enlargement of the superficial inguinal nodes of
minimal degree is a common clinical finding, and represents the effect of chronic
hyperplasia of these nodes from constant
and often unnoticed or forgotten minor

infections and irritations in the drainage
areas, to which most people are subjected
at various times. For this reason, a minimal degree of superficial inguinal lymphadenopathy is difficult to evaluate. Physicians learn to accept a so-called "usual
life" baseline degree of groin lymphadenopathy. Diagnostic interest should be aroused
when the nodes are (1) increasing in size
under observation, (2) larger than expected,
(3) painful, or (4) suppurating.

Significant lymphadenopathy of the superficial inguinal nodes is related most
commonly to: (1) local infectious process
of the drainage area; (2) systemic infection
in which the infectious agent enters the
body in the drainage region; or (3) primary neoplasm in this area, chiefly a malignant melanoma or an epidermoid carcinoma. The number of disorders possible in
the large and anatomically complicated
drainage area is infinitely greater than in
the axillary node drainage area.

The ease with which a local infection or
small primary neoplasm can be overlooked
if located on the scrotum, between the buttocks, on the labia, under the prepuce, in
the umbilicus, the cutaneous zone of the
anus, or between the toes is well-known,
since these areas are not examined as frequently and thoroughly as the upper extremities or head and neck.

Lesions of the penis which are especially
important include: syphilitic chancre, gonorrhea, lymphopathia venereum, chancroid,
and malignancy. Granuloma inguinale is
not a lymph node disease but may predispose to secondary infectious lymphadenitis.

Minor but often overlooked causes include pediculosis pubis, tinea crurum of
the inguinal area, ringworm between the
toes, and the irritation incident to wearing
a truss to restrain a hernia.

An infectious or neoplastic lesion is not
easily overlooked on the legs, the lower
abdomen, the buttocks, or the lower back,
but may readily be missed if present on
the scrotum, the perineum, the anus, or
the labia. Tumors of the testis metastasize
directly to the upper para-aortic nodes
(Fig. 26-13) and involve the superficial inguinal nodes only when the tumor breaks
through the capsule of the testicle to invade the scrotum (Figs. 26-10 and 26-11).

All infections or neoplastic lesions primary in these skin areas do not necessarily
involve the superficial inguinal nodes. The
skin of the heel and the posterior half of

the outer aspects of the foot drain into the popliteal nodes, and from these, directly to deep inguinal nodes (see Fig. 26-10 and discussion in the following section on popliteal nodes). In an occasional anomaly, lymphatics from upper posterior thigh and lower buttocks penetrate the fascia and reach the common iliac nodes along the sciatic nerve sheath,[103] thus permitting lesions in this drainage area to bypass the superficial inguinal nodes. Lesions of the glans penis or the glans clitoris may drain, not only to the superficial inguinals, but also directly into the deep inguinal and the other deep nodes.[103] There is also possibility of drainage of the penis to the prepubic lymph nodes, and thence to the external iliac lymph nodes, without passage to the superficial inguinals.[103] Therefore, absence of palpable superficial inguinal nodes does not rule out infections or tumor metastases from these areas. See the excellent paper by Pack and Rekers[103] for a detailed discussion of this subject.

Several infectious systemic diseases in which the etiologic agent enters the drainage area of the superficial inguinal nodes may produce a satellite enlargement in these nodes, or, if lymphadenopathy is general, exaggeration of the nodes in this location. This is particularly likely to occur with bubonic plague, scrub typhus, rat-bite fever, and filariasis. Superficial inguinal adenitis has been noted in swamp fever (due to leptospirae).[104] This suggests the possibility that the infection was acquired through the skin of the leg. Atypical mycobacterial infection of the genital region in a female child was reported as a cause of bilateral inguinal adenitis.[249]

Superficial inguinal adenitis may be noted in infants and small children when the thigh is used as a site for subcutaneous prophylactic inoculation with vaccines against the various diseases of childhood, smallpox vaccination, or BCG vaccine.[94,95,105] In infants, suppuration of the superficial inguinal nodes with thigh injections was much more frequent than suppuration of the axillary nodes when comparable injections of BCG vaccine were given in the shoulder area.[105] A possible explanation is that in infants the superficial inguinal nodes are already under continuous phagocytic stress because of constant irritation and soilage from urine and feces in the diaper area and are unable to accept the added phagocytic load resulting from the vaccination. Inguinal lymphadenopathy has

been reported following the administration of live attenuated measles virus vaccine injected in the buttock.[252]

In contrast with the paucity of subcutaneous masses in the axillary area capable of simulating lymphadenopathy are the variety of conditions present in the groin. Tumefactions in the groin which must be distinguished from lymphadenopathy are: hernia, varix, lipoma, aneurysm, tuberculosis of bursa of short head of rectus femoris muscle, psoas abscess, ectopic testis, ectopic spleen, inguinal endometriosis, etc.[103,106,107,218] For this reason, the differential diagnosis of masses in the groin is not always easy and must be considered carefully before a palpable "lump" is called an enlarged node.

In females, a primary lesion of lymphopathia venereum deep in the vagina or the fornix does not produce superficial lymphadenopathy. Instead, the lymph drainage is to the lymphatics about the rectum, with production of a periproctitis, which may eventuate in a rectal stricture.[62]

Acute Iliac Lymphadenitis. Although the nodes are classified as in the retroperitoneal group, suppuration of the external iliacs bears a closer relationship to infections of the extremities, and will be better understood if viewed in this light.

Suppuration of the external iliac nodes,[108-110] most commonly unilateral, may manifest a striking analogy to subpectoral abscess (suppurative infraclavicular lymphadenitis). These nodes, located retroperitoneally deep in the iliac fossa, adjacent to the external and the common iliac vessels and anterior to the psoas muscle, receive drainage from the superficial and the deep inguinals, the penis, the urethra, the prostate, the bladder, the uterus, the deep lymphatics of the abdominal wall and the upper thigh. The nodes enlarge to a clinically significant degree two or three weeks after onset of an infection primary in one of the drainage sites, usually due to *hemolytic staphylococcus* or *hemolytic streptococcus*. Such lymphadenitis is most common in children and young adults and may occur without obvious involvement of the superficial inguinal nodes. The clinical picture is one of high fever, leukocytosis, occasionally bacteremia, lower abdominal pain but without sign of peritoneal irritation, psoas muscle spasm limiting extension of the leg on the involved side, abdominal tenderness with rectus muscle spasm. At times, the greatly enlarged nodes are detectable as a palpable tender mass just above Poupart's ligament. Often the nodes suppurate to form an extraperitoneal abscess requiring surgical drainage.

THE POPLITEAL NODES

Anatomy. The popliteal nodes, five or six in number, lie under the deep fascia in the fat around the popliteal vessels in the popliteal fossa. They receive lymph vessels from the knee joint and skin of the lateral side of the lower part of the leg, foot, and heel. They receive lymph from the deep structures of the leg and foot by lymphatic vessels coursing along the anterior and posterior tibial arteries and veins. Their efferents drain into the deep inguinal nodes by lymphatic vessels which accompany the popliteal and femoral veins. An inconstant anterior tibial node may be intercalated be-

tween the heel area and the popliteal node, but is only rarely clinically important.

Clinical Significance. Except for the previously described drainage area, infections and neoplasms of the foot and the lower leg spread lymphatically directly to the superficial inguinal lymph nodes without filtering through the popliteal nodes. Infections of the knee joint and lesions on the heel and the outer side of the posterior half of the foot drain into the popliteal nodes (see channel A, Fig. 26-10). Popliteal nodes are not easy to palpate unless greatly enlarged, because of their subfascial location. It is well to remember that the afferent lymphatic channels from the popliteal nodes course along with the femoral artery to drain directly into the deep femoral and the external iliac nodes, bypassing completely the superficial inguinal nodes.[103] It is a practical clinical point that the absence of enlarged su-

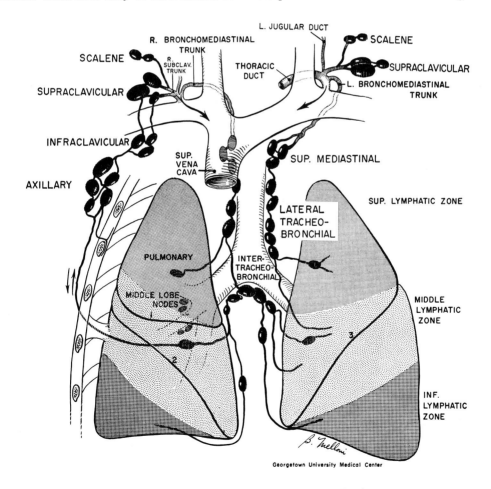

Georgetown University Medical Center

FIG. 26-12. Lymphatic drainage of lungs and mediastinum.

perficial inguinal nodes does not rule out spread beyond the popliteal nodes of a tumor of heel and outer foot. Radical resection of malignant melanoma is influenced by this anatomic fact.

THE MEDIASTINAL LYMPH NODES

Anatomy. The mediastinum contains a large number of nodes, the most important of which may be divided into two groups: (1) the superior mediastinal and (2) the tracheobronchial (Fig. 26-12).

THE SUPERIOR MEDIASTINAL nodes lie in front of the aortic arch, in relation to the large arterial trunks arising from the aortic arch, and also to the innominate veins. They receive afferents from the thymus, the pericardium, the heart, the esophagus, and the trachea, as well as from the parasternal nodes. Their efferents join with those from the tracheobronchial, on each side, to form the corresponding bronchomediastinal trunk.

THE TRACHEOBRONCHIAL NODES include some of the largest nodes in the body. They may be subdivided into (1) the lateral tracheobronchial, (2) the intertracheobronchial, and (3) the pulmonary.

The lateral tracheobronchial nodes lie in relation to the trachea and lateral to the primary bronchi.

The intertracheobronchial nodes lie at the bifurcation of the trachea, between the primary bronchi.

The pulmonary nodes are both extrapulmonary and intrapulmonary in location. The extrapulmonary nodes lie in the hilum of each lung; these are the so-called *hilar nodes*. The intrapulmonary nodes lie along the secondary branches of the primary bronchi and are related to the lobes of the lungs. Of these, the nodes related to the right middle lobe are of special importance, since they drain not only the middle but also the lower lobe of the right lung and almost completely surround the secondary middle lobe bronchus. Consequently, when enlarged, these nodes are very likely to compress this bronchus and thus interfere with the drainage of both the middle and the lower lobes.

It is to be noted that the lymphatic drainage of the lung *does not conform* to the anatomic division of the lobes. Hence, in the surgical treatment of cancer of the lung, pneumonectomy and not lobectomy is indicated. The pulmonary nodes drain into the intertracheobronchial and the lateral tracheobronchial nodes, which in turn drain into the superior mediastinal nodes. From the mediastinal nodes of each side, the lymph passes through the corresponding bronchomediastinal trunk into the venous system. Blockage of the mediastinal nodes leads to retrograde flow, and, in the presence of pleural adhesions, cancer may spread to the axillary nodes. Similarly, with blockage of the axillary nodes, retrograde flow will carry cancer emboli across the chest wall to the mediastinal nodes.

The tracheobronchial nodes drain lymph from lungs, bronchi, thoracic portion of the trachea, heart, esophagus and liver; their efferents join the bronchomediastinal lymphatic trunk.

Clinical Significance—Mediastinal Lymphadenopathy. Only rarely does a clinically significant degree of hilar lymphadenopathy follow ordinary bacterial infections of the lung, such as pneumonia or reinfectious type of pulmonary tuberculosis. Diffuse staphylococcal or streptococcal bronchopneumonias, multiple lobe bronchiectasis, or abscess formation may rarely produce a bilateral form, whereas unilateral hilar lymphadenopathy may occasionally follow bronchiectasis, lung abscess, or viral infection. Tuberculosis, in sharp contrast, whether as a primary complex or in hematogeneous form, often involves the hilar lymph nodes on one or both sides, with persistence for long periods, and termination by healing and constriction, calcification, or rarely caseation. A lung infection that has cleared may leave a hilar adenitis which persists for a time. Coccidioidomycosis, histoplasmosis, and especially sarcoidosis may produce bilateral symmetrical mediastinal lymph-node enlargement, the latter being a particularly common benign type.[111-113]

Silicosis and other pneumoconioses, asbestosis and beryllium intoxication may all manifest by chest roentgenogram evidence of both bilateral lymphadenopathy and pulmonary (lung field) involvement.[112] The pathology of the nodes in these conditions is one of an infiltrative nature.

Bilateral mediastinal lymphadenopathy, often without pulmonary involvement, occasionally with arthralgia, commonly is associated with erythema nodosum.[111,114,219] Although various etiologies for this syndrome have been proposed, much attention centers on sarcoidosis as one of the interesting causes.[115,116]

In sarcoidosis the enlarged hilar lymph nodes are bilateral, never calcify, occur early in the course, are harmless as such, and generally regress.[220] Rare causes of bilateral mediastinal lymphadenopathy without lung changes are infectious mononucleosis and the collagen diseases.

Metastasis to hilar nodes, irregularly unilateral, especially from the lungs and more rarely from distant organs such as the kidney and the testis, may occur. Lymphatic leukemia and the lymphomata group of disorders are more likely to produce a bilateral but often asymmetrical mediastinal lymphadenopathy.

Mediastinal lymph node hyperplasia may rarely simulate a thymoma.[221,222]

Mediastinal lymph node enlargement may or may not cause symptoms:

1. ASYMPTOMATIC. The use of routine chest roentgenograms, in miniature or standard size, in mass population surveys for chest disease, pre-employment examination, induction station surveys, upon admission to many hospitals, etc., has resulted in detection of many instances of hilar adenopathy which are apparently asymptomatic. Perhaps the majority fall in the asymptomatic group. However, an extensive literature based on the study of certain cases admitted to hospitals indicates that a variety of signs and symptoms may be produced by various forms of hilar lymphadenopathy. A study of these clinical observations is important in understanding the mechanism of their production and often indicates the basic pathology responsible.

2. SYMPTOMATIC. *A. Cough.* Regional nodes about the trachea and the bronchi, when sufficiently enlarged, are said to produce a cough by an irritative process or by pressure; often it is of a type commonly called "brassy." The exact mechanism in any instance is difficult to evaluate since many of these people also have intrinsic lung and bronchial diseases. Pulmonary or bronchial infection, granulation tissue, neoplasm, and bronchial lithiasis are other possible mechanisms for the production of the cough.

B. Obstructive phenomena. Early partial bronchial obstruction by lymph nodes may cause obstructive emphysema because the bronchial lumen is greater upon inspiration than expiration, and the inspiratory phase is more forceful. Ingress is thus easier than egress. This condition is more common in children because their bronchial structure is compressed more easily and the lymph node enlargement is proportionately greater in that age group. The resulting physical signs are usually lobar in distribution rather than generalized, because of the nature of the process initiating the lymph node enlargement.

Partial obstruction, particularly if persistent for long periods, may lead to bronchiectasis, perhaps by preventing proper ciliary movement of secretions, and thus causing a situation readily predisposing to low-grade persistent infection. Chronicity leads to slow progression of the infectious process, which as in emphysema usually is localized and segmental. More rarely lung abscess may follow partial bronchial obstruction.

Complete bronchial obstruction or partial obstruction with lumen-contained secretions may lead to complete *atelectasis* productive of the usual physical and roentgen findings. At times, atelectasis may result from intraluminal rupture of suppurated mediastinal nodes or extrusion of a broncholith into the lumen. Some feel that atelectasis on this basis may be the explanation for most cases of epituberculosis among infants and children. At this age tuberculosis is especially likely to involve bronchial and hilar nodes primarily, with the lung involvement being atelectatic from mechanical compression of the lumen, and not parenchymal.

However, it should be pointed out that edema and inflammation of the bronchial wall alone may lead to bronchial obstruction, and that extrinsic pressure is not necessary.[116]

Although such obstruction from lymph node pressure may occur in any lobe of the lung, the bronchus of the right middle lobe is peculiarly susceptible to compression because it is surrounded by a group of lymph nodes draining both the adjacent lower lobe and the middle lobe, an anatomic situation first stressed by Brock *et al.*[118,119] Therefore, infection in either of these two lobes can predispose to lymph node changes in this particular anatomic group. The small lumen size of the middle lobe bronchus and its almost right angle drainage into intermediate bronchi constitute further peculiar hazards to drainage of this lobe.[117] The clinical features produced by obstruction of the right middle lobe bronchus have become popularly known as the *"middle lobe syndrome"* as the result of the description by Graham, Burford and Mayer.[120] Clinical features are often chronic and most characteristically include obstructive phenomena of the right middle lobe with wheezing, pneumonitis or bronchiectasis, chest pain, periodic hemoptysis and demonstrable roentgen findings.[117,120] This syndrome of extrinsic bronchial obstruction of the right middle lobe should not be confused with obstruction of intraluminal origin such as that produced by a bronchial tumor, granulomatous lesion of the bronchus, etc.

C. Hemoptysis. Next to cough, this is probably the most common indirect manifestation of hilar and bronchial lymphadenopathy. Mechanisms include friability of granulation tissue, mechanical erosive process, chronic obstruction with bleeding produced by associated infections (i.e., bronchiectasis, lung abscess, etc.), and the irritating and cutting effects of broncholithiasis with rupture of bronchial pulmonary vessels. Periodic hemoptysis is especially characteristic of the "middle lobe syndrome."[117,120]

D. Calcification of Lymph Nodes. A variety of mechanisms may predispose to calcification of intrathoracic lymph nodes. Calcification of lymph nodes is commonly due to tuberculosis or histoplasmosis, but may be caused by fungus infection, coccidioidomycosis, etc. Large calcified lymph nodes in the hilar area can produce any of the features discussed in this section. However, there are certain clinical features peculiar to calcified nodes.[121-124] They show a propensity to penetrate the bronchial wall, possibly by erosive action of the calcified node against a bronchial wall in constant motion.[122] Extrusion of the calcified node into the lumen of a bronchus may produce bronchial obstructive symptoms of various types, occasionally an intractable localized wheeze, paroxysms of coughing productive of gritty particles and even of the broncholith itself, hemoptysis, and other features. Calcified nodes may compress a bronchus and cause atelectasis, produce a traction diverticulum of the esophagus, cause dysphagia, or even rarely compress the superior vena cava.[223] Bronchoscopic examination and roentgen studies are helpful. Reports of 41 cases by Schmidt, Clagett, and McDonald[125] indicate that broncholithiasis is by no means rare. Storer and Smith[223] have reviewed this intriguing subject.

Calcification of an entire lymph node should not be confused with peripheral calcification, the so-called "eggshell calcification," considered as diagnostic of silicosis of mediastinal lymph nodes, but perhaps very rarely seen in other conditions, such as sarcoidosis.[111]

E. Caseation of hilar nodes may lead to traction diverticulum of the esophagus, with its attendant disturbance of swallowing and of the morphology of this organ.[126]

F. Mediastinitis. Infectious lymphadenopathy of the hilar area may lead to mediastinitis. However, considering the great frequency of infections of hilar nodes from various pulmonary infections, mediastinitis due to this cause is a rare complication.

G. Superior Vena Caval Obstruction. Hilar lymphadenopathy may rarely produce superior vena caval obstruction. This may be a late feature resulting from cicatrization of tissue about the superior vena cava from mediastinal infection of lymph node origin, or obstruction may result from compression. Compression occurs particularly from lymph node enlargement as a result of metastasis from a bronchial carcinoma, commonly on the right, because of the peculiar anatomic relationships in that area.

H. Hoarseness is an uncommon manifestation. It may occur with lymph node metastasis from cancer, particularly of the breast, compressing the recurrent laryngeal nerve, or it may possibly result from venous obstruction of the superior vena cava, producing edema of the larynx.

I. Bronchoesophageal fistula is an unusual complication, which may result from an infectious erosive process originating in tuberculous lymph nodes and resulting in the formation of a fistulous tract between a bronchus and the esophagus. A coughing spell which comes on a short interval after swallowing is diagnostically suggestive. A coughing paroxysm from aspirating food or fluid into the larynx due to an upper esophageal difficulty in swallowing comes on at once without the latent interval necessary for esophageal peristalsis to carry food or fluid to the fistulous opening into the bronchus.

J. Dysphagia is likewise an unusual feature, sometimes caused by bronchoesophageal fistula,[127] traction diverticula of the esophagus or enlarged mediastinal nodes.

K. Chest pain has been neither severe nor common with mediastinal lymphadenopathy. It may result from broncholithiasis, traction diverticula of the esophagus, or bronchoesophageal fistula.

L. Roentgen studies give much helpful information in evaluating mediastinal lymphadenopathy.[128,129]

M. A palpable swelling of the chest wall in the region of the second and the third intercostal spaces near the sternum may rarely occur when a lymphoma involves the sternal nodes.[47,130]

Occasionally in neoplasm of the breast, and very rarely from primary tumors elsewhere, there may be metastases to the parasternal nodes.[224] It is well to carefully pal-

pate each of the upper five intercostal areas, on both sides, close to the sternum, as part of a search for nodal metastases. This is an area easily overlooked in the physical examination; hence, the reason for the added emphasis.

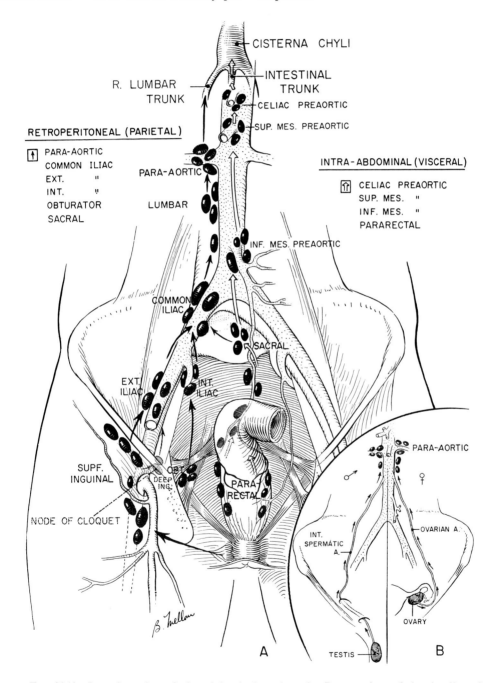

FIG. 26-13. Lymph nodes of the abdominal cavity. A. Retroperitoneal (parietal) and intra-abdominal (visceral) nodes. B. Lymphatic drainage of ovary or testis directly to upper para-aortic nodes without passage through the lower retroperitoneal nodes.

ABDOMINAL LYMPH NODES

Anatomy. The lymph nodes of the abdominal cavity are divided into two large groups: (1) the intra-abdominal or visceral and (2) the retroperitoneal or parietal.[54] Reference to Figure 26-13 will be helpful in understanding this section. A more detailed description can be obtained from standard sources.[14]

THE INTRA-ABDOMINAL NODES OR VISCERAL NODES consist of a large number of nodes which are located in the various peritoneal ligaments (lesser and greater omentum, gastrosplenic ligament, mesentery, and mesocolon) and at the root of the large visceral branches of the aorta. The latter are called the preaortic nodes and are subdivided into the celiac, the superior mesenteric, and the inferior mesenteric.

The celiac preaortic nodes are disposed about the origin of the celiac artery. They receive lymph from the organs supplied by the branches of the celiac artery, namely, the lower part of the esophagus, the liver, the gallbladder, the stomach, the spleen, the pancreas, and the duodenum. Lymph from these organs first passes through nodes which are located close to these organs within the peritoneal ligaments traversed by the nutritive branches of the celiac artery. Such nodes include the gastric nodes (in the lesser and the greater omenta), the hepatic and the cystic nodes (in the lesser omentum), and the pancreaticolienal nodes (in the gastrosplenic ligament).

The superior mesenteric preaortic nodes lie about the origin of the superior mesenteric artery. The inferior mesenteric preaortic nodes surround the origin of the inferior mesenteric artery. These two groups of nodes receive lymph from the small and the large intestines, not directly, but indirectly, after its passage through a series of nodes located within the mesentery and the mesocolon. The latter nodes are collectively known as the mesenteric nodes. They are arranged in two groups: (1) the proximal, lying about the arterial arcades formed by the branches of the superior and the inferior mesenteric arteries, and (2) the distal, located along the wall of the gut beside the vasa recta, branches of the arterial arcades.

The efferents of the preaortic nodes unite to form a single trunk, the intestinal trunk, which joins the cisterna chyli.

THE RETROPERITONEAL OR PARIETAL NODES comprise (1) the sacral, (2) the internal iliac, (3) the external iliac, (4) the common iliac, and (5) the para-aortic.

The sacral nodes lie in the hollow of the sacrum, in relation to the middle and the lateral sacral arteries. They receive lymph from the rectum, the posterior wall of the pelvis, the prostate, and the cervix of the uterus. Their efferents join the internal iliac and the para-aortic nodes.

The internal iliac nodes are disposed about the internal iliac vessels and their branches. A special group is located about the obturator canal and constitutes the obturator nodes. They receive a large part of the lymph from the rectum, the bladder, the urethra, the prostate, the uterus, and the buttocks. Their efferents drain into the common iliac nodes.

The external iliac nodes are located about the external iliac vessels, just behind the inguinal ligament, and in relation to the genitofemoral nerve. They receive lymph from superficial and deep inguinal nodes, internal iliac nodes, deep structures of the anterior abdominal wall below the level of the umbilicus, glans penis or glans clitoris, bladder, cervix and body of the uterus, upper part of the vagina, prostate, and membranous urethra. Their efferents join the common iliac nodes.

The common iliac nodes are disposed about the common iliac vessels. They receive afferents from the external iliac, the internal iliac, and the sacral nodes. In addition they also receive lymph directly from the rectum, the vagina, the uterus, and the prostate. Their efferents empty into the right and the left para-aortic nodes.

The para-aortic nodes form an almost continuous chain on each side of the abdominal aorta. They rest on the psoas major muscle. Those on the right side also are related to the inferior vena cava. They receive the efferents of the common iliac nodes (hence the lymph from the lower extremities, the external genitalia and most of the lymph from the pelvis). In addition, they receive lymph from the lateral abdominal wall by lymphatics accompanying the lumbar arteries, the kidneys, the suprarenals, the testes, the ovaries, the fallopian tubes, and the body of the uterus. Their efferents unite on each side to form the right and the left lumbar lymphatic trunks, which unite to form the cisterna chyli. Some of the efferents join the preaortic nodes, as well as some relatively unimportant nodes, behind the abdominal aorta (retroaortic nodes). Still other efferents, instead of joining the lumbar trunks, pass through the crura of the diaphragm to join the thoracic duct directly. Lymphography and echographic technics[271] have been used to study retroperitoneal lymph node enlargement.

Clinical Significance. The lymph nodes of the abdomen and the pelvis constitute the largest group of nodes of the body. These nodes drain lymph not only from the lower extremities, but also from all of the pelvic and the abdominal organs which are frequently subject to infectious and neoplastic processes. Because of their anatomic proximity to blood vessels and nerve plexuses of the abdominal cavity and to the various segments of the gastrointestinal tract, their enlargement from neoplastic or infectious involvement produces a rich symptomatology,[131-134] the analysis of which is of great value in diagnosis.

Clinically, the most important symptoms are: abdominal discomfort, digestive disturbances, abdominal pain, backache, and fever. Less frequent in occurrence, but nevertheless significant, are the following: constipation, ascites, edema, chyloperitoneum, urinary disturbances, jaundice, and intestinal obstruction. Although the clinical picture is characterized by a variety of symptoms, the physical signs of neoplastic involvement of the abdominal nodes are few and consist of demonstration of palpable nodes, localized tenderness, and occasionally of abnormal bruits.[131,132]

1. ABDOMINAL DISCOMFORT occurs as soreness, sense of heaviness or fullness in the epigastric region after meals and inability to eat a full meal. It is caused by the crowding of the stomach and the intestine by enlarging para-aortic and intra-abdominal nodes. The stomach and intestines are unable to expand as their contents increase with the ingestion of meals. There is also delay in emptying of the stomach and passage of food down the intestine because of impaired peristaltic activity.[132]

2. DIGESTIVE DISTURBANCES. *Bloating* and *belching* may be the only symptoms and may be misinterpreted as due to cholecystitis, peptic ulcer, neurasthenia, or even malingering. *Nausea* and *vomiting* are less frequent and may occur irregularly or become constant and progressive with rapid loss of weight. *Diarrhea* is not common. When it occurs, it may be irregular or may continue indefinitely. It has a tendency to

increase progressively in severity. It is associated with loss of weight and strength in spite of a normal or ravenous appetite. Usual therapeutic measures are unavailing, and whatever improvement may be obtained proves to be only temporary. Diarrhea may be associated with melena; it usually sets in when the intramural lymphoid tissue of the bowel (solitary lymph follicles, patches of Peyer, and annular follicles of the appendix) become involved by the neoplastic process.[131,132]

3. ABDOMINAL PAIN. The para-aortic and the pelvic retroperitoneal, as well as the preaortic intra-abdominal lymph nodes, are associated intimately with the abdominal autonomic nervous system, which contains parasympathetic, sympathetic, and pain fibers. The parasympathetic fibers regulate the motility and the secretory activity of the gastrointestinal tract. The sympathetic fibers are concerned especially with regulation of vasomotor tone of the blood vessels of the gut. The pain fibers relay pain impulses from all of the abdominal and the pelvic organs. After passing through the abdominal autonomic nervous system, which is intimately related to the whole length of the abdominal aorta and its branches, the pain impulses are finally transmitted to the spinal cord by the lumbar and the thoracic splanchnic nerves.

The intra-abdominal lymph nodes, located within the lesser and the greater omenta, the mesentery, and the mesocolon also are related intimately to the branches of the celiac, the superior and the inferior mesenteric arteries, which are accompanied throughout their course by the peripheral fibers of the parasympathetic and sympathetic nerves and by pain fibers.

Enlarged retroperitoneal, as well as intra-abdominal lymph nodes, may irritate both autonomic and pain fibers and thus lead not only to impairment of the secretory and motor activity of the gastrointestinal tract, but also to pain. Pain may be caused in another way by the effects of direct neoplastic infiltration of the wall of the digestive tube, gaseous distention, and excessive motor activity ("spastic" pain).

Pain due to compression by enlarged lymph nodes is at first characteristically dull in character and felt as soreness. Its distribution depends entirely upon the nerves involved by the pressure. Thus, enlarged para-aortic or preaortic nodes compressing the pain fibers coursing through the abdominal autonomic nerves related to the aorta may produce pain suggestive of disease of various organs such as the gallbladder, the pancreas, or the appendix. If the pain is severe, the clinical picture may suggest an acute abdominal emergency. Surgery in such cases may bring temporary relief. However, the underlying neoplastic process is relentless in its progress, so that the pain may recur with even greater intensity. With progressive enlargement of the nodes, the pain may be so severe as to simulate the intractable pain of interstitial pancreatitis. The distribution of the pain will become more extensive as more and more of the para-aortic and the preaortic nodes become enlarged.

"Spastic pain" is cramplike or colicky, and occurs in waves. Pressure on the ureter may lead to ureteral spastic pain, simulating pain from ureteral stone.[135] In mesenteric adenitis, the spastic pain occasionally may be due to ileocecal intussusception.[134]

4. BACKACHE. This type of pain is especially characteristic of pressure by enlarged para-aortic and mesenteric nodes on branches of the lumbar and the sacral plexuses and may be felt at various levels of the trunk or in the lower extremities. Depending on the particular nerve irritated, it may be localized in the hip, the thigh, the knee, the ankle or the feet. It may first be felt in the hip and then extend to the foot, simulating sciatic neuritis. It may be unilateral or bilateral. At first, the pain is dull in character. Later, when the nerves become infiltrated with cancer metastases, or when metastases to the pubic bones or to the bones of the lower extremities have occurred, the pain becomes boring and severe.[132]

5. FEVER. Often enlargement of the para-aortic and intra-abdominal nodes in Hodgkin's disease and lymphosarcoma is characterized by fever, which is conspicuously absent if the lymphadenopathy in these diseases is confined to the cervical nodes. Fever also develops with involvement of mediastinal nodes. Usually the fever is continuous, but occasionally may be of the relapsing or intermittent Pel-Ebstein type. Irradiation of the abdomen may cause the fever to diminish or disappear within one to three weeks. This therapeutic test is helpful in the diagnosis of abdominal lymphadenopathy due to Hodgkin's disease or lymphosarcoma.

6. CONSTIPATION. Enlargement of both para-aortic and intra-abdominal (mesenteric) nodes may lead to mechanical interference with the motor activity of the gut, and thus cause constipation which is proportional to other preceding or concomitant symptoms, such as abdominal pain, backache, bloating, and belching. It is characteristic of this type of constipation that it often diminishes or disappears with retrogression of the enlarged nodes following irradiation, to reappear when the nodes enlarge again with advance of the neoplastic process.

7. ASCITES. Ascites may be caused by portal vessel compression from lymph nodes or by metastases to peritoneal surfaces, the latter being more common.

8. EDEMA. Enlargement of the iliac and the pelvic retroperitoneal nodes may compress the iliac veins, especially the external iliac, with resulting edema of the lower extremities. However, this is rarely of a degree to involve an entire lower extremity. Usually, the edema first appears in the feet and the ankles. Compression of the common iliac vein by enlarged common iliac nodes results in edema not only of the lower extremity, but also of the scrotum, penis, pubic region, and lower abdomen. Deep palpation of the iliac region may reveal a nodular mass of enlarged nodes or a matted mass, tender to pressure.

9. CHYLOPERITONEUM. Marked enlargement of the celiac preaortic or of the para-aortic nodes in the immediate vicinity of the celiac artery may block the cisterna chyli with the production of chyloperitoneum. At the same time, such blockage, because of retrograde flow, may result in cancerous infiltration of the stomach and the duodenum associated with gastrointestinal bleeding.

10. URINARY DISTURBANCES. Such disturbances, when present, usually take the form of increased frequency of urination and hematuria. Urinary disturbances are not a common complication. They may be due to compression of the ureter by enlarged iliac nodes, resulting in hydronephrosis or pyonephrosis. However, urinary disturbances may also result from cancerous infiltration of the ureter by the lymphatic spread from the primary cancer or by direct extension from involved adjacent para-aortic nodes.

11. JAUNDICE. Jaundice, occurring with intra-abdominal lymphoid tumors or lymph node metastases, usually indicates liver metastases, and only rarely results from lymph node obstruction of extrahepatic

biliary passages, as indicated by paucity of even isolated case reports in the literature.[136,137]

12. INTESTINAL OBSTRUCTION. Such obstruction may involve the duodenum, the cecum, or the other parts of the intestine, and is either due to compression by enlarged nodes adjacent to these structures or to actual infiltration of the bowel by the neoplastic process affecting the nodes. The intestinal obstruction is accompanied by pain of increasing severity, nausea, and vomiting.

13. PHYSICAL SIGNS. The physical signs associated with enlarged retroperitoneal and intra-abdominal nodes are scanty and usually consist of the demonstration of the enlarged nodes by palpation and the elicitation of tenderness upon pressure over the nodes. Occasionally, abnormal bruits may be heard.

Physical signs are conspicuously absent in the early stages, and may also be absent in cases in which the clinical symptoms are marked. Evidence of nodes may be obscured by cancerous involvement of the gastrointestinal tract, the liver, and the spleen, as well as by peritoneal carcinomatosis.

As a rule, the physical signs do not become apparent until the involved nodes have reached a certain size. Under such conditions, by careful palpation through relaxed abdominal walls, over the iliac region or over the course of the abdominal aorta, the enlarged nodes can be felt as nodular masses of irregular size. Should the nodes be matted together, only a deep resistance may be felt upon deep palpation. This must not be mistaken for muscular rigidity. The palpable nodes or resistance may be confined to one side. This is particularly true with lymphadenopathy associated with cancer of the testis or the ovary. In such cases, the palpable nodes are always confined to one side or the other, depending upon the site of the primary cancer, since, with cancer of these organs, the spread is always to the homolateral nodes at first. The enlarged nodes are situated high in the abdomen at the level of the renal vessels, because the lymphatics from the testis or the ovary follow the internal spermatic or the ovarian vessels, respectively, and drain into the upper para-aortic nodes (see Fig. 26-13). Later, with retrograde involvement of the iliac para-aortic nodes, the palpable nodular mass extends vertically toward the iliac region.

Palpable, enlarged para-aortic nodes are fixed characteristically, and show practically no mobility, not even with respiration. By contrast, enlarged intra-abdominal nodes, particularly the mesenteric or the mesocolic, display a noticeable degree of mobility and shifting and may give the impression of a pedicled mass. At the same time, the mass gives a sensation of solidity and lack of resilience. If these physical aspects of enlarged para-aortic and intra-abdominal nodes are kept in mind, their confusion with enlarged liver, spleen, or kidney can be avoided. The liver and the spleen may be displaced forward and downward by greatly enlarged para-aortic nodes.

The palpable enlarged nodes may vary in size at intervals. This is particularly true in cases of abdominal lymphadenopathy due to Hodgkin's disease or lymphosarcoma. In these diseases, there is an abnormal predisposition to respiratory infections. With each infection there occurs a rapid enlargement of the nodes. With subsidence of the infection, the nodes may regress in size, but the enlargement seldom disappears. Eventually, there is progressive enlargement, although there are cases in which the nodes remain small throughout the disease.

In lymphoblastoma, there may be enlargement of all retroperitoneal and intra-abdominal nodes, but in addition all aggregations of lymphoid tissue of the small and large bowel may become infiltrated with neoplastic cells. Also, there is a marked tendency for retroperitoneal nodes of the two sides to become matted together along the whole length of the abdominal aorta. In the majority of cases of lymphoblastoma, however, definite masses cannot be felt.

Enlarged nodes may be demonstrated not only by abdominal palpation, but also by rectal or vaginal examination. In women, enlarged pelvic nodes must be differentiated from uterine fibroids, ovarian cysts, or pyosalpinx. At the same time, it must be remembered that these conditions may be coincidental.

In palpating for enlarged retroperitoneal and intra-abdominal nodes, careful attention must be paid to certain procedural details. The patient must be placed in the recumbent position; the head should be flexed on the chest; and the arms should be relaxed and placed by the side of the body. In order to relax the anterior wall as completely as possible, the patient should be encouraged to breathe through the mouth. Further relaxation may be achieved by placing a pillow under the small of the back.

The second significant physical sign of enlarged nodes is tenderness elicited by pressure. Such tenderness is usually slight or moderate.

Abnormal Bruits. Enlarged para-aortic nodes may interfere with normal expansion of the aorta and thus produce abnormal bruits. Constriction of the abdominal aorta may also result from either bilateral or unilateral enlargement of the para-aortic nodes.

Clinical Syndromes of the Intra-Abdominal Nodes. 1. The Sprue Syndrome. Lymphomatous involvement of the lymphatic system of the abdomen may lead to the syndrome of secondary sprue in several ways.[138,139]

Infiltration of the wall of the gastrointestinal tract may block the intestinal lacteals and result in malabsorption, with the development of a nutritional deficiency state.

Enlarged lymphomatous nodes, through pressure on the gut or the pain fibers, may produce pain related to meals. Under such circumstances, often the patient will resort to a simple monotonous diet, usually low in proteins, and again suffer from nutritional deficiency.

The lymphomatous process may interfere with the motor functions of the gut and lead to diarrhea. If this is marked, there will be loss of fluid, electrolytes, and nutritive elements.

2. Syndrome of Calcified Intra-Abdominal Lymph Nodes. Calcified intra-abdominal nodes may produce no symptoms and be discovered upon routine x-ray examination or as an incidental finding in x-ray studies of the urinary or the genital tracts. Such asymptomatic calcified nodes may cause confusion in the presence of renal, ureteral, and vesical calculi.

However, calcified intra-abdominal nodes in the mesentery may cause symptoms that suggest the advisability of x-ray studies of the gastrointestinal tract. Such nodes are particularly the mesenteric nodes near the ileocecal junction. Almost invariably, such symptomatic calcified nodes are due to tuberculosis. In addition to the calcified nodes, the patient may show evidences of a tuberculous process involving the wall of the gut itself. The calcified nodes are tender upon pressure, usually slightly movable. Since they are associated intimately with blood vessels and nerves coursing through the mesentery, there is usually distortion of the affected segments of the blood vessels. The mesentery itself often shows scarring and puckering, interfering with normal motor function of the intestine.[140]

Clinically, the syndrome of calcified mesenteric nodes is characterized by repeated attacks of abdominal pain in the right lower quadrant, accompanied by nausea, vomiting, and weakness. There is no elevation of temperature and no leukocytosis during the attack. There is usually a history of underweight and lack of endurance, in spite of good appetite, of repeated visits to a physician, and of slow convalescence following various attacks of infections.

Roentgenographic studies show not only the calcified nodes, but barium studies demonstrate spasm of the loop of the intestine at the site of the calcified nodes, delay in emptying of the ileum, and reversed peristalsis.[141]

3. Syndrome of Tuberculous Mesenteric Lymphadenitis. This condition is usually secondary to tuberculosis elsewhere. The process begins in the patches of Peyer and the solitary lymph follicles of the ileum. These lymphoid structures enlarge, fuse, caseate, and ulcerate. The ulcers enlarge laterally since the tuberculous process follows the intestinal lymphatics, which course at right angles to the longitudinal axis of the bowel. Accompanying this process there is massive involvement of the mesenteric lymph nodes.[142,143] As a rule, tuberculous mesenteric lymphadenitis is confined to the ileum. However, in some cases, it may also involve the jejunum and the duodenum as well as the cecum and the colon. The nodes may remain discrete or become matted together to form large masses. Eventually, gradual calcification of the involved nodes takes place.

Some cases are asymptomatic. Calcified nodes may be seen on routine roentgenograms of the gastrointestinal or urinary tracts. When the infection is active, there is fever, malaise, loss of weight, and abdominal pain. Since the mesenteric nodes near the ileocecal junction are involved most often, the pain and associated tenderness in the right iliac fossa may simulate that of appendicitis. The nodes are usually not palpable unless they are enlarged considerably.

The tuberculous nodes may break down

and discharge their contents into the peritoneal cavity, with resulting localized peritonitis (cold abscess), or generalized tuberculous peritonitis. Fistulas may develop between different segments of the small intestine. The enlarged, fused nodes may also produce multiple obstructions of the bowel[144,145]

4. SYNDROME OF ACUTE NONSPECIFIC MESENTERIC LYMPHADENITIS. This syndrome is characterized by recurring abdominal pain and tenderness in the right iliac fossa, associated with enlarged mesenteric (intra-abdominal) nodes.[146,147] It is seen most commonly in children and subsides by the time of puberty. Since it simulates acute appendicitis, diagnosis is usually made at laparotomy.

In the early stages, there is discrete enlargement only of the nodes within the mesentery. It is characteristic of this condition that the mesenteric nodes near the ileocecal junction are involved constantly. This is not true of acute appendicitis. The nodes are red and swollen. Upon culture, they prove to be sterile.[147] Histologically, the nodes show a nonspecific inflammatory reaction and cellular hyperplasia. Although many cases of nonspecific mesenteric adenitis are associated with upper respiratory tract infection, the reactive lymphadenopathy probably is due to absorption of toxins from the intestinal tract. Gambill[225] has discussed its status as a clinical entity. Suppuration of the affected nodes occurs rarely.[247]

There is generalized abdominal pain, intermittent and colicky in nature, and centered about the umbilical region. Usually, it is more severe than the initial pain in acute appendicitis. There is tenderness in the right iliac fossa. The point of tenderness shifts to the left when the patient is turned on the left side (Brennan's sign). This shift in tenderness does not occur in acute appendicitis and is due to the positional shift of the mesentery and its contained enlarged nodes. There is also moderate elevation of temperature and occasionally nausea, vomiting, and anorexia. There is an initial polymorph leukocytosis which, however, subsides rapidly in two to three days.

5. SYNDROME OF PERITONITIS FROM LYMPH NODE SUPPURATION. Very rarely, peritonitis may follow suppuration of an intra-abdominal lymph node.[148]

LYMPH NODE SYNDROMES

A considerable literature attests to the wide interest in lymph node disease. In the section to follow, a number of characteristic lymph node syndromes are briefly described. The reader is also referred elsewhere to representative articles, which discuss various classifications and clinical features of, and give fuller details about, various types of lymphadenopathy.[149-156]

In addition to the regional types of lymphadenopathy, related mostly to local area disease as already described, are other clinical states not so easily classified. The following groupings of syndromes have been found by us to be a helpful method of presenting certain of the lymphadenopathies.

SYNDROME OF PRIMARY SORE OR
ENTRANCE LESION ON AN EXTREMITY,
REGIONAL LYMPHADENOPATHY,
FEVER, AND SYSTEMIC SYMPTOMS

A number of diseases, mostly infections, fit into a clinical pattern or syndrome characterized by a primary sore or entrance lesion on an extremity, regional (satellite) lymphadenopathy, fever, and systemic symptoms with or without a rash. The initial inoculation of the infectious agent, although much more common on the more exposed limb, may occur occasionally on the chest or the abdomen, with axillary or superficial inguinal lymphadenopathy, respectively, with a similar clinical picture.

The best-known syndrome consists of a wound or abrasion at site of entry, with tubular lymphangitis and septicemia due to *Streptococcus hemolyticus*,[157] referred to in the past by the old-fashioned term "blood poisoning." It is now rare since the advent of sulfa and antibiotic therapy. The unusual occurrence of a primary syphilitic chancre and regional lymphadenopathy, not yet subsided, simultaneously with the presence of the systemic features of the secondary stage of syphilis, fits into this category. The nonvenereal site of extragenital chancre (e.g., the finger of a dentist or a physician) often makes the diagnosis confusing.[158] Rarely, primary inoculation of tuberculosis in the skin of an extremity in a person who is tuberculin-negative may produce an indolent ulcer at the inoculation site, lymphangitis, and satellite lymphadenopathy. There is usually only minimal systemic reaction and fever, but there is transition of the tuberculin test to positive as healing occurs.[159,160]

In a sense this constitutes, by analogy with the primary lung infection, a dermatologic, primary Ghon tubercle, with a primary skin lesion and its satellite adenopathy forming a complex like the Ghon pulmonary complex.[160]

Sporotrichosis of the lymphangitic type may commence as indolent ulcers at the inoculation site, with chronic nodular and often painless lymph channel involvement, but without marked regional lymphadenopathy or systemic symptoms.[161]

Anthrax usually commences as a firm red papule, progressing through vesicular formation to a painless ulcer surrounded by a zone of erythema and edema, followed by tender regional lymphadenopathy with severe systemic symptoms, often with bacteremia.[162,163]

Inoculation of the skin by the *Erysipelothrix rhusiopathia*, commonly from handling fish or dead animal matter, may produce a local lesion, lymphangitis, and regional adenitis, with variable systemic symptoms and constitute the clinical picture of the occupational disease known as *erysipeloid* of Rosenbach.[164]

A sensitive ulcer on a finger, regional lymphadenopathy, fever, systemic symptoms, with or without a rash, often with bacteremia, in a person who has handled rabbits, constitute a picture classic for the ulceroglandular type of *tularemia*.[165,166]

Bubonic plague is another classic example of this syndrome. A vesicle forms at the site of bite of an infected flea, followed by very large painful regional adenitis, often suppurative or hemorrhagic, with severe systemic symptoms.[167]

Several rickettsial diseases fit into this pattern. Best known, as a result of World War II experiences, is *scrub typhus* due to *R. orientalis*.[168] A black eschar forms at the site of a mite bite, followed by regional adenopathy (usually without lymphangitis), systemic spread, fever, and rash. At times lymphadenopathy becomes generalized. *Boutonneuse fever* (due to *R. conorii*) carried by a dog tick, *South African tick bite fever*, and possibly *Kenya typhus* have an initial sore, lymph node enlargement, and a systemic picture similar to scrub typhus. *Rickettsialpox* (due to *R. akari*), a relatively new American rickettsial disease, is somewhat similar, manifesting an initial painless lesion at the site of the infecting mite bite, painful regional adenitis, systemic spread, fever, and a characteristic rash.[169]

Filariasis does not entirely fit this syndrome. Usually the legs are involved, but fail to show a primary entrance lesion. However, lymphangitis, regional lymphadenopathy, and various systemic symptoms may occur.

Rat-bite fever is characterized by a late local lesion at the rat-bite site, followed by lymphangitis, regional lymphadenopathy, systemic symptoms, rash, and fever, all of which may show remissions and relapses.[170,171] The *Spirillum minus* organism does this more strikingly than the *Streptobacillus moniliformis*.

Cat-scratch disease (nonbacterial regional lymphadenitis) is now known to be a frequent cause of this syndrome. Commonly, but not always, a cat scratch causes a local inoculation lesion (? due to virus), regional lymphadenitis (often large and suppurating), and systemic symptoms with occasional transitory rash.[172] Absence of bacteria in the pus and a positive skin test with "cat-scratch antigen" help establish the diagnosis.

Although all of these syndromes are infectious, one never should overlook the fact that a *primary neoplasm* may occur on an extremity, cause regional metastasis, and manifest systemic symptoms and fever as a result of visceral metastases.

Syndrome of Diseases Originating in the Oropharynx with Cervical Satellite Lymphadenopathy, Fever, and Systemic Symptoms

In a sense, the usual bacterial infections of the throat (especially of the tonsils) such as streptococcal sore throat, scarlet fever, diphtheria, etc., belong to this category. Lymphadenopathy in throat infections of viral etiology is usually less striking than it is for bacterial infections. Most characteristic of diseases illustrating this syndrome is infectious mononucleosis, when associated with a severe sore throat. Weil's disease occasionally produces cervical adenopathy as part of the total clinical picture.

Cat-scratch disease[172] occasionally may have an oropharyngeal site of origin, with striking lymph node enlargement of the neck, progressing at times to suppuration. An oral cavity syphilitic chancre with regional neck lymphadenopathy, followed by the secondary systemic phase, is especially classic of this syndrome. Likewise is cervical node tuberculosis, which may rarely manifest a systemic spread.

Syndrome of a Genital Lesion, Groin Lymphadenopathy, Fever, and Systemic Symptoms

Of course, many of the diseases described under the first section for an extremity site of origin could occur if the inoculation site of the infectious agent is on the genitalia instead of an extremity. In general, however, infectious disorders with a primary genital site are of venereal origin and include primarily syphilis, gonorrhea, chancroid, and lymphopathia venereum. Rarely, a tuberculous infection may be responsible. Cancer of the penis with regional groin metastases and systemic metastatic spread fits into this pattern quite readily.

Generalized Lymphadenopathy

Generalized lymph node enlargement obviously can occur as a result of various diffuse skin disorders which permit infectious and toxic multiple regional lymph node involvement of a chronic reactive type. A specific syndrome (lipomelanotic reticular hyperplasia of lymph nodes) usually related to erythematous and exfoliative types of pruritic dermatosis, in which the lymphadenopathy is characterized by lipid and melanin infiltration and reticulum cell reaction (at times suggesting a lymphoma),[173,174] can be identified specifically in this general category.

Superficial lymphadenopathy is one of the features of the Sézary syndrome, a rare disorder, presenting with an exfoliative erythroderma in association with some striking systemic clinical manifestations, as well as a characteristic cell in the peripheral blood.[226]

By common understanding, the term "generalized lymphadenopathy" has come to mean involvement of two and preferably three regionally separated lymph node groups in which enlargement results from a systemic disorder acting on lymphoid tissue, generally by one of the mechanisms described previously under modes of involvement. Although the basic stress is generalized, enlargement of nodes often occurs in irregular fashion and need not appear simultaneously and to an equal degree in all body areas.

Generalized lymphadenopathy of infectious origin may occur in addition to a more prominent regional adenopathy in the drainage area of the inoculation site in a number of the disorders described in the preceding sections 1, 2, and 3, such as cat-scratch disease,[172] infectious mononucleosis, tularemia,[166] plague,[167] secondary syphilis, postvaccinal lymphadenitis,[270] etc. Children often manifest a greater degree of generalized lymph node response to a particular infection than do adults for reasons commented upon previously (e.g., in measles, rubella, rheumatic fever, scarlet fever, etc.). Although some of the infectious diseases that produce a generalized type of lymphadenopathy are well-known, others are less understood: for example, brucellosis,[175,176] generalized peripheral lymphadenopathy of tuberculous origin,[177] certain tropical diseases,[178] and others.[250]

Generalized lymph node enlargement may be primary in lymphoid or reticular endothelial tissue of lymph nodes, as in Hodgkin's disease, lymphosarcoma, and lymphatic leukemia; or secondary to primary involvement of the hemopoietic system as in myelogenous or monocytic leukemia, sickle cell and hemolytic anemia. General lymph node enlargement may be of metabolic origin, as in Niemann-Pick's disease, Gaucher's disease, etc. These are all well-known and adequately described in many excellent articles and standard texts.

Less well-understood is the generalized lymphadenopathy so common in sarcoidosis,[179] serum sickness,[180] and status lymphaticus. Generalized lymphadenopathy may occur in some of the disorders of the collagen tissues. Particularly well-documented are rheumatoid arthritis,[181] Still's disease,[181] dermatomyositis, and disseminated lupus erythematosus.[182,183]

Particular attention should be paid to patients with suspected systemic disease if the original biopsy diagnosis of a superficial lymph node is reported as hyperplasia. One should carefully follow the clinical course of this type of patient, whether the nodes are regional or generalized, for possible development of a recognizable serious illness, particularly a disease of collagen tissue or malignancy.[227] This sequence appears to be rather common when looked for.

Generalized lymphadenopathy may occur occasionally in the adult acquired form of toxoplasmosis, and the entire syndrome may resemble, to a remarkable degree, acute infectious mononucleosis. One should suspect toxoplasmosis especially if this picture occurs in a person exposed to certain birds and mammals, including the domestic dog. The diagnosis can be confirmed by the toxoplasma dye test and toxoplasma complement fixation test.[228] At times, the lymphadenitis may be relapsing.[229] Rarely,

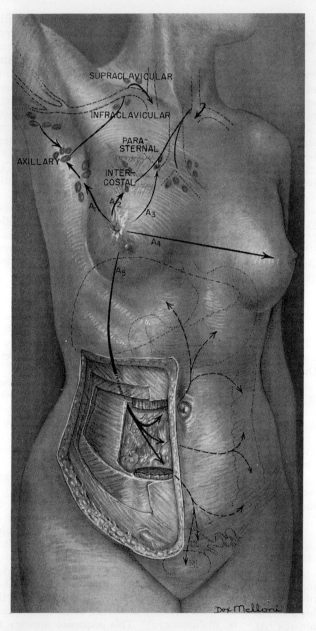

Fig. 26-14. Lymphatic drainage of the mammary gland. Metastases from cancer of the mammary gland may follow several lymphatic pathways: A_1. Upper outer quadrant to axillary, infravicular, supraclavicular nodes, etc. A_2. Upper inner quadrant to intercostal and parasternal nodes. A_3. Upper inner quadrant directly to parasternal nodes. A_4. Directly across mid-line to opposite breast. A_5. Lower quadrants, particularly inner aspect, through pectoralis major, external oblique and linea alba, to subperitoneal lymphatic plexus, followed by abdominal and pelvic spread.

leishmaniasis may be localized to lymph nodes and cause enlargement at multiple sites.[239] Generalized adenopathy occurs in "Ardmore disease,"[231] characterized also by upper respiratory infection, enlarged and painful liver, splenomegaly, and a prolonged course of several months. Posterior cervical nodes were reported as enlarged in 95 per cent of cases with this disease.

Rarely, some of the hydantoin type of anticonvulsant drugs may cause lymphadenopathy, mimicking a lymphoma clinically and even pathologically, but reversible upon cessation of their use.[232,233,267] Histiocytic medullary reticulosis, a rapidly fatal reticuloendothelial proliferative disorder, should be included among the unusual causes of generalized lymphadenopathy. A characteristic clinical picture, coupled with bone marrow findings, may serve to establish antemortem diagnosis.[234,235] "Rademacher's disease," is another rare condition capable of causing generalized lymphadenopathy.[236] Other rare causes may occur.[272]

SYNDROMES OF LYMPHATIC METASTASES FROM CANCER OF BREAST

Cancer of the mammary gland may metastasize by several lymphatic pathways (see Fig. 26-14). Cancer arising in the upper outer quadrant of the gland metastasizes to the axillary nodes (A_1), the infraclavicular and the supraclavicular nodes. From here, cancer emboli can reach the venous system via the jugular trunk. Cancer metastazing in this manner has the most favorable prognosis. Supraclavicular lymph node metastases may develop after radical mastectomy as the first clinical evidence of recurrence. This circumstance is often a sign of widespread dissemination.[251]

In the upper inner quadrant it may metastasize first to the intercostal, then to the parasternal nodes (A_2), or it may reach the parasternal nodes directly (A_3). The parasternal nodes drain into the mediastinal nodes, from which cancer emboli can

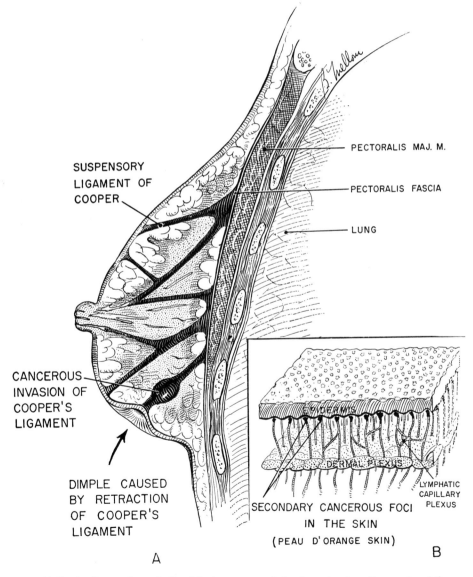

SUSPENSORY LIGAMENT OF COOPER

PECTORALIS MAJ. M.

PECTORALIS FASCIA

LUNG

CANCEROUS INVASION OF COOPER'S LIGAMENT

DIMPLE CAUSED BY RETRACTION OF COOPER'S LIGAMENT

EPIDERMIS

DERMAL PLEXUS

LYMPHATIC CAPILLARY PLEXUS

SECONDARY CANCEROUS FOCI IN THE SKIN
(PEAU D'ORANGE SKIN)

A

B

FIG. 26-15. A. Retraction of the skin in cancer of the breast when ligaments of Cooper contract following cancer invasion. B. Secondary cancerous foci in skin producing *peau d'orange* skin.

reach the venous system by way of the bronchomediastinal trunk. Because of the involvement of the mediastinal nodes, cancer spreading by this route has a dangerous prognosis. Parasternal nodes (A_3) should be searched for by careful palpation in the upper five intercostal spaces, on both sides, close to the sternum.[224]

The lymphatics of the skin of one mammary gland communicate directly across the mid-line (A_4) with those of the opposite side. Hence, unilateral cancer may become bilateral by this lymphatic route. Contralateral axillary metastases indicate a poor prognosis.[260]

Cancer developing in the lower quadrants, particularly the lower inner, may spread by lymphatics that traverse the pectoralis major, the external oblique, and the upper thin part of the linea alba and communicate with the subperitoneal lymphatic plexus (A_5). Thus, cancer emboli may reach the peritoneal cavity and set up secondary foci on any of the abdominal organs. Cancer cells may also drop by gravity from the peritoneal cavity into the pelvic cavity, and thus give rise to secondary pelvic metastases. Because of the possibility of invasion of the peritoneal cavity, this type of spread has the most dangerous prognosis. Furthermore, because of this possible mode of metastasis, every patient with breast nodules should have careful rectal and vaginal examination.

The mammary gland and its overlying skin is anchored to pectoral fascia covering the pectoralis major by bands of fibrous tissue called the ligaments of Cooper. When these ligaments become invaded by cancer emboli, contraction occurs along them. As a result, the skin of the breast may become attached to the subjacent neoplastic growth, so that the skin cannot be pinched up from the tumor. With further extension of the cancer, the entire breast may be bound to the pectoral fascia, so that it can no longer move in the long axis of the pectoralis major. Finally, with continued contraction of the involved ligaments of Cooper, there is dimpling of the skin or the nipple of the mammary gland (Fig. 26-15A).

The lymphatic vessels draining the skin over the mammary gland may become blocked with consequent stagnation of lymph and edema of the skin. Since the hair follicles are attached more firmly to the underlying superficial fascia, the edematous skin projects in between the hair follicles. This skin thus presents pitting. This

TABLE 26-1. IMPORTANT CAUSES OF SUPPURATION OF LYMPH NODES

Streptococcal pharyngitis
Streptococcal wound infection
Tuberculous lymphadenitis
Staphylococcal lymphadenitis
Lymphopathia venereum
Coccidioidomycosis
Anthrax
Cat-scratch disease
Chancroid
Sporotrichosis
Plague
Tularemia

condition is called *peau d'orange* (Fig. 26-15B). *Peau d'orange* may occur in other parts of the body in which blockage of the skin lymphatics occurs, e.g., ischiorectal abscess.

SUPPURATION OF LYMPH NODES

A distinctive phenomenon, which occasionally follows infectious lymphadenopathy, occurs when the infecting organism overwhelms the local defensive mechanism within the node to produce excess cellular reaction and collection of pus. Suppuration may subside spontaneously, or it may require incision and drainage or lead to destruction of the node with spontaneous rupture and drainage. This may occur in a single node or lead to coalescence of multiple nodes with suppuration, at times from several sites.

The nodes most likely to suppurate are the cervical and superficial inguinal, occasionally the axillary, and much less often the epitrochlear or popliteal. The rarity of suppuration of the intrathoracic and the intra-abdominal nodes deserves comment, considering the frequency of involvement of these nodes.

Of the many regional and systemic infections leading to adenopathy, relatively few produce lymph node suppuration with any regularity. Those most commonly responsible are listed in Table 26-1.

Hemolytic streptococcus infections of the pharynx and tonsils, producing cervical and more rarely retropharyngeal suppuration (most commonly in children under age five), were the most common forms prior to the sulfonamide era. There is some question whether the occasional peritonsillar abscess or cellulitis of the neck complicating tonsillitis is due to another superimposed bacterial infection. Streptococcus infections in extremity wounds often produce tubular lymphangitis (characterized by painful red streaks) and suppurative regional lymphadenitis, the pus often being thin, possibly because of the presence of the enzymes, streptokinase and streptodornase. Staphylococcus infection is manifested by a thick yellow-white type of pus. Lymphopathia venereum (of viral origin), especially in the male, and chancroid (due to *Bacillus ducreyi*) are common genital infections predisposing to suppurative superficial inguinal adenitis. Cervical tuberculous lymphadenitis with suppurative scrofula, now rare in Europe and America, was in past years a classic and common form of cervical node suppuration with localization at a lower level in the neck than streptococcus adenitis. Pediculosis of the scalp, probably by permitting secondary infection, occasionally may produce suppuration of occipital and posterior neck nodes.

Anthrax and plague represent serious systemic disorders with regional nodes draining the entrance area manifesting marked suppuration, which occasionally may be hemorrhagic or manifest necrotic liquefaction. Fungus infections, especially sporotrichosis (usually on an extremity), and coccidioidomycosis (cervical area), occasionally may produce suppuration. Cat-scratch disease (nonbacterial regional lymphadenitis), of probable virus etiology, has been found to be a common cause of lymph node suppuration, most common in the groin or the axilla, occasionally epitrochlear, and rarely cervical.[172] Early, the enlarged nodes may simulate a lymphoma. Following suppuration they simulate tularemia. Bacteriologically negative pus, history of contact with cats, and use of the cat-scratch antigen skin test assist in diagnosis.

An unusual cause is the disorder of serious prognosis which occurs in infants and young children, with a possible genetic predilection for males. It is an inborn abnormality of phagocytic function. It is characterized by chronic suppurative lymphadenitis (cervical in location), along with pulmonary infiltrations, hepatosplenomegaly, and a characteristically distributed eczematoid dermatitis. Pathologically, there is a generalized granulomatous process and hypergammaglobulinemia.[237] This disorder is well-documented in the literature.[261] Of special interest is evidence that the neutrophil white blood cells do not have normal bactericidal function.[262]

BCG vaccination in infants may lead to suppuration of the axillary nodes when the shoulder is the site of injection, and suppuration of the superficial inguinal nodes when the thigh is the injection site. Suppuration may not take place until months following the injection and appears related to the dosage. Groin suppuration is much more common than axillary suppuration for reasons explained in the section on inguinal adenitis.

REFERENCES

1. Drinker, C. K., and Yoffey, J. M.: Lymphatics, Lymph and Lymphoid Tissue: Their Physiological and Clinical Significance, Cambridge, Mass., Harvard, 1941.
2. Drinker, C. K.: The functional significance of the lymphatic system, Bull. N. Y. Acad. Med. 14:231–251, 1938.
3. Landis, E. M., Jonas, L., Angevine, M., and Erb, W.: The passage of fluid and protein through the human capillary wall during venous congestion, J. Clin. Invest. 11:717–734, 1932.
4. Markowitz, C., and Mann, F. C.: The role of the liver in the formation of lymph, Amer. J. Physiol. 96:709–712, 1931.
5. McMaster, P. D.: Condition in skin influencing interstitial fluid movement, lymph formation and lymph flow, Ann. N. Y. Acad. Sci. 46:743–787, 1946.
6. Ladd, M. P., Kottke, F. J., and Blanchard, R. S.: Studies of effect of massage on flow of lymph from foreleg of dog, Arch. Phys. Med. 33:604–612, 1952.
7. Bierman, H. R.: Characteristics of the thoracic duct lymph in man, J. Clin. Invest. 32:632–649, 1953.
8. Crandall, L. A., Jr., Barker, S. B., and Graham, D. G.: A study of the lymph flow from a patient with thoracic duct fistula, Gastroenterology 1:1040–1048, 1943.
9. Henry, C. S.: Studies on the lymphatic vessels and on the movement of lymph in the ear of the rabbit, Anat. Rec. 57:263–278, 1933.
10. Smith, R. O.: Lymphatic contractility; possible intrinsic mechanism of lymphatic vessels for transport of lymph, J. Exp. Med. 90:497–509, 1949.
11. Heller, E. L.: Carcinoma of the stomach with multiple annular metastatic intestinal infiltrations, Arch. Path. 40:392–394, 1945.
12. Glover, R. P., and Waugh, J. M.: The retrograde lymphatic spread of carcinoma of the "rectosigmoid region"; its influence in surgical procedures, Surg. Gynec. Obstet. 82:434–448, 1946.
13. Pernis, van, P. A.: Variations of the thoracic duct, Surgery 26:806–809, 1949.

14. Rouvière, H.: Anatomy of the Lymphatic System, Tobias, M. J. (trans.), Ann Arbor, Mich., Edwards Brothers, Inc., 1938.
15. Weeks, A., and Delprat, G. D.: Superficial abrasion with secondary infection and lymphangitis, Surg. Clin. N. Amer. 14:1537–1545, 1934.
16. Steel, W. A.: Acute lymphangitis, Amer. J. Surg. 36:37–43, 1937.
17. Hendrick, J. W.: Macroglossia or giant tongue, Surgery 39:674–677, 1956.
18. Archer, W. H.: Lymphangioma of lips; report of 2 cases, Oral Surg. 5:170–171, 1952.
19. Allen, E. V.: Lymphedema of the extremities: classification, etiology and differential diagnosis: a study of three hundred cases, Arch. Intern. Med. 54:606–624, 1934.
20. Gross, R. E., and Goeringer, C. F.: Cystic hygroma of the neck, Surg. Gynec. Obstet. 69:48–60, 1939.
21. Fishback, F. C.: Lymph leakage (lymphorrhea): a complication of saphenous vein ligation, with suggestions for treatment, Surgery 22:834–836, 1947.
22. Martorell, F.: Chronic edema of the lower limbs, Angiology 2:434–460, 1951.
23. Menten, M. L., and Welton, J. P.: Lipid analysis in a case of Niemann-Pick disease, Amer. J. Dis. Child. 72:720–727, 1946.
24. Gilchrist, R. K., and David, V. C.: Lymphatic spread of carcinoma of the rectum, Ann. Surg. 108:621–642, 1938.
25. Black, M. M., Kerpe, S., and Speer, F. D.: Lymph node structure in patients with cancer of the breast, Amer. J. Path. 29:505–521, 1953.
26. Lachman, E.: Common and uncommon pathways in the spread of tumors and infections, Surg. Gynec. Obstet. 85:767–775, 1947.
27. Batson, O. V.: Function of the vertebral veins and their role in the spread of metastases, Ann. Surg. 112:138–149, 1940.
28. Edwards, H. C.: Acute lymphangitis and acute lymphadenitis, Practitioner 136:281–288, 1936.
29. Price, L. W.: The pathology of lymph node enlargement, Postgrad. Med. J. 23:401–425, 1947.
30. Hadfield, G.: General pathology of lymphadenopathies, Ann. Roy. Coll. Surg. Eng. 5:89–105, 1949.
31. Quinland, W. S.: Some types of lymphadenopathy with emphasis on lymphosarcoma, J. Nat. Med. Ass. 43:113–121, 1951.
32. Lanza, A. J.: Silicosis and Asbestosis, New York, Oxford, 1938.
33. Thannhauser, J.: Lipidosis; Disease of the Cellular Lipid Metabolism, ed. 2, New York, Oxford, 1950.
34. Medoff, A. S., and Bayrd, E. D.: Gaucher's disease in 29 cases: Hematologic complication and effect of splenectomy, Ann. Intern. Med. 40:481–492, 1954.
35. Scammon, R. E.: A summary of the anatomy of the infant and child, in Abt, I. A. (ed.): Pediatrics, vol. I, ch. 3, pp. 277–278, Philadelphia, Saunders, 1923.
36. Freund, M., and Ripps, M. L.: Hand-Schüller-Christian disease: a case in which lymphadenopathy was a predominant feature, Amer. J. Dis. Child. 61:759–769, 1941.
37. Hansen, P. B.: Relationship of Hand-Schüller-Christian syndrome, Letterer-Siwe's disease and eosinophilic granuloma of bone with report of five cases, Acta Radiol. 32:89–112, 1949.
38. Abt, A. F., and Denenholz, E. J.: Letterer-Siwe's disease. Splenohepatomegaly associated with widespread hyperplasia of non-lipoid-storing macrophages; discussion of so-called reticulo-endothelium, Amer. J. Dis. Child. 51:499–522, 1936.
39. Jaffe, H. L., and Lichtenstein, L.: Eosinophilic granuloma of bone, Arch. Path. 37:99–118, 1944.
40. Lichtenstein, L.: Histiocytosis: X. Integration of eosinophilic granuloma of bone, "Letterer-Siwe disease," and "Schüller-Christian disease" as related to manifestations of a single nosologic entity, Arch. Path. 56:84–102, 1953.
41. Pund, E. R., and Stelling, F. H.: Lymphosarcoma, Amer. J. Surg. 52:50–54, 1941.
42. Sugarbaker, E. D., and Craver, L. F.: Lymphosarcoma: a study of 196 cases with biopsy, J.A.M.A. 115:17–23, 112–117, 1940.
43. Clarke, R. G., and Simonds, J. P.: Primary lymphosarcoma of the appendix, Cancer 4:994–998, 1951.
44. Currie, D. J., and Luke, J. C.: Giant follicular hyperplasia of the rectum showing malignant degeneration, Can. Med. Ass. J. 63:150–152, 1950.
45. Baehr, G., and Klemperer, P.: Giant follicle lymphoblastoma; benign variety of lymphosarcoma, New York J. Med. 40:7–11, 1940.
46. Jackson, H., Jr., and Parker, F., Jr.: Hodgkin's disease: clinical diagnosis, New Eng. J. Med. 234:103–110, 1946.
47. Goldman, L. B.: Hodgkin's disease: An analysis of 212 cases, J.A.M.A. 114:1611–1616, 1940.
48. Warren, S., and Picena, J. P.: Reticulum-cell sarcoma of lymph nodes, Amer. J. Path. 17:385–394, 1941.
49. Wilkie, D.: Reticulum-cell sarcoma of small intestine with perforation, Brit. J. Surg. 41:50–53, 1953.
50. Wintrobe, M. M.: Clinical Hematology, ed. 5, Philadelphia, Lea & Febiger, 1961.
51. Isaacs, R.: Correlation of clinical and laboratory data in diseases of lymph nodes, J. Mich. Med. Soc. 37:1072–1073, 1938.
52. Herbert, P. A., and Miller, F. R.: Histopathology of monocytic leukemia, Amer. J Path. 23:93–123, 1947.

53. Whitby, L. E. H., and Britton, C. J. C.: Disorders of the Blood, ed. 9, London, Churchill, 1963.

54. Solnitzky, O.: Anatomical factors influencing the spread of cancer, Bull. Georgetown Univ. Med. Center 3:176-193, 1950.

55. Davis, H. K.: A statistical study of the thoracic duct in man, Amer. J. Anat. 17:211-244, 1915.

56. Hoffman, E., Ivins, J. L., and Kern, H. M.: Traumatic chylothorax, A.M.A. Arch. Surg. 64:253-268, 1952.

57. Little, J. M., Harrison, C., and Blalock, A.: Chylothorax and chyloperitoneum, Surgery 11:392-401, 1942.

58. Kalmansohn, R. B.: Rubella (German measles); observations on an epidemic, with particular reference to lymphadenopathy, New Eng. J. Med. 247:428-429, 1952.

59. Edgerton, A. E.: Herpes zoster ophthalmicus: report of cases and review of literature, Arch. Ophthal. 34:45-64, 114-153, 1945.

60. Rice, C. E.: A note on the frequency of involvement of the anterior auricular lymph nodes in trachoma, Amer. J. Ophthal. 18:651, 1935.

61. Verhoeff, F. H., and King, M. J.: Leptothricosis conjunctivae (Parinaud's conjunctivitis), Arch. Ophthal. 9:701-714, 1933.

62. Koteen, H.: Lymphogranuloma venereum, Medicine 24:1-69, 1945.

63. Francis, E.: Oculoglandular tularemia, Arch. Ophthal. 28:711-741, 1942.

64. Cassady, J. V., and Culbertson, C. S.: Cat scratch disease and Parinaud's oculoglandular syndrome, A.M.A. Arch. Ophthal. 50:68-74, 1953.

65. Tassman, I. S.: The Eye Manifestations of Internal Diseases (Medical Ophthalmology), St. Louis, Mosby, 1951.

66. Sorsby, A.: Systemic Ophthalmology, St. Louis, Mosby, 1951.

67. Allen, J. H.: Lids, lacrimal apparatus and conjunctiva: review of recent literature, A.M.A. Arch. Ophthal. 45:100-119, 1951.

68. Hartmann, K.: Ectogenous conjunctival tuberculosis due to bovine tubercle bacilli; treatment by electrocoagulation; contribution to Parinaud's symptom complex, Klin. Mbl. Augenheilk. 113:20-28, 1948.

69. Sanders, M., Gulliver, F. D., Forcheimer, L. I., and Alexander, R. C.: Epidemic keratoconjunctivitis; clinical and experimental study of an outbreak in New York City; further observations on the specific relationship between a virus and the disease, J.A.M.A. 121:250-255, 1943.

70. Curry, J. J., and Lowell, F. C.: Epidemic keratoconjunctivitis: report of a case with marked systemic manifestations, New Eng. J. Med. 231:11-13, 1944.

71. Ryan, R., O'Rourke, J. F., and Iser, G.: Conjunctivitis in adenoidal-pharyngeal-conjunctival virus infection, A.M.A. Arch. Ophthal. 54:211-216, 1955.

72. Weinman, D.: Chagas' disease, Oxford Syst. Med. 5:860(55)-860(107), 1950.

73. Moseley, V., and Miller, H.: South American trypanosomiasis (Chagas' disease), Arch. Intern. Med. 76:219-229, 1945.

74. Munslow, R. A., and Capps, J. M.: Droop shoulder following cervical node biopsy, Texas J. Med. 48:706-707, 1952.

75. Strong, R. P.: Stitt's Diagnosis, Prevention and Treatment of Tropical Diseases, p. 187, Philadelphia, Blakiston, 1942.

76. Looney, W. W.: Lymphatic drainage of the head and neck—emphasizing special structures, Ann. Otol. 44:33-41, 1935.

77. Viacava, E. P., and Pack, G. T.: Significance of supraclavicular signal node in patients with abdominal and thoracic cancer: a study of one hundred and twenty-two cases, Arch. Surg. 48:109-119, 1944.

78. McKusick, V. A.: Virchow-Troisier node: an occasional conspicuous manifestation of gallbladder cancer, Southern Med. J. 46:965-967, 1953.

79. Willis, R. A.: The spread of tumours in the human body, p. 32, London, Butterworth, and St. Louis, Mosby, 1952.

80. Zeidman, I.: Experimental studies on the spread of cancer in the lymphatic system. III. Tumor emboli in thoracic duct, the pathogenesis of Virchow's node, Cancer Res. 15:719-721, 1955.

81. Harken, D. E., Black, H., Clauss, R., and Farrand, R. E.: A simple cervicomediastinal exploration for tissue diagnosis of intrathoracic disease with comments on the recognition of inoperable carcinoma of the lung, New Eng. J. Med. 251:1041-1044, 1954.

82. Shefts, L. M., Terrill, A. A., and Swindell, H.: Scalene node biopsy, Amer. Rev. Tuberc. 68:505-522, 1953.

83. Cuykendall, J. H.: Use of prescalene lymph node biopsy in absence of palpable supraclavicular nodes: report of forty-one cases, J.A.M.A. 155:741-742, 1954.

84. Daniels, A. C.: A method of biopsy useful in diagnosing certain intrathoracic diseases, Dis. Chest. 16:360-366, 1949.

85. Bailey, H.: Demonstrations of Physical Signs in Clinical Surgery, ed. 12, p. 88, Baltimore, Williams & Wilkins, 1954.

86. Bailey, H.: Adenitis of facial lymph gland, Practitioner 125:618-620, 1930.

87. Fifield, L. R.: Mixed tumours of the molar glands, Lancet 2:652, 1927.

88. Polya, A. E., and Navrath, D. V.: Untersuchungen über die Lymphbahnen der Wangenschleimhaut, Deutsch. Z. Chir. 66:122-175, 1902.

89. Martin, H., and Morfit, H. M.: Cervical lymph node metastasis as the first symptom of cancer, Surg. Gynec. Obstet. 78:133-159, 1944.

90. Martin, H., and Romieu, C.: The diagnostic significance of a lump in the neck, Postgrad. Med. 11:491–500, 1942.

91. Carey, J. M., and Kirklin, J. W.: Extended radical mastectomy: a review of its concepts, Proc. Mayo Clin. 27:436–440, 1952.

92. Weinberger, H. A., and Stetten, D. W.: Extensive secondary axillary lymph node carcinoma without clinical evidence of primary breast lesions, Surgery 29:217–222, 1951.

93. Cogswell, H. D.: Hidden carcinoma of the breast, Arch. Surg. 58:780–789, 1949.

94. Lapin, J. H., and Tuason, J.: Immunization adenitis, J.A.M.A. 158:472–474, 1955.

95. Guld, J., Magnus, K., Tolderlund, K., Biering-Sorensen, K., and Edwards, P. O.: Suppurative lymphadenitis following intradermal B.C.G. vaccination of the newborn: a preliminary report, Brit. Med. J. 2:1048–1054, 1955.

96. Stein, S. C., and Sokoloff, M. J.: Calcification of regional lymph nodes following B.C.G. vaccination, Amer. Rev. Tuberc. Pul. Dis. 73:239–245, 1956.

97. Lawrence, K. R., and Anglem, T. J.: Acute subpectoral abscess: A surgical emergency, New Eng. J. Med. 237:390–395, 1947.

98. Straus, D. C.: Subpectoral abscess (suppurative infraclavicular lymphadenitis, with report of 3 cases), Int. Surg. Dig. 20:259–273, 1935.

99. Evans, G.: Palpable epitrochlear glands: their value as a physical sign, Lancet 2:256–257, 1937.

100. Beeson, P. B.: Epitrochlear adenopathy in secondary syphilis, Arch. Derm. Syph. 32:746–749, 1935.

101. Martin, L.: Palpable epitrochlear gland: incidence and relation to syphilis, Lancet 1:363–364, 1947.

102. Chanarin, I.: Epitrochlear adenopathy in the Bantu, S. Afr. Med. J. 23:960–962, 1949.

103. Pack, G. T., and Rekers, P.: The management of malignant tumors in the groin: a report of 122 groin dissections, Amer. J. Surg. 56:545–565, 1942.

104. Spain, R. S., and Howard, G. T.: Leptospirosis due to Leptospira grippotyphosa, J.A.M.A. 150:1010–1012, 1952.

105. Gaisford, W., and Griffiths, M.: B.C.G. vaccination in the newborn, preliminary report, Brit. Med. J. 2:702–705, 1951.

106. Cole, P. P.: Inguinal swellings, Med. Press 207:91–96, 1942.

107. Cohn, I.: Masses in groin, Int. Clin. 2:229–256, 1935.

108. Carson, M. J., and Hartman, A. F.: Diagnosis and management of severe infections in infants and children: A review of experiences since the introduction of sulfonamide therapy; VI. Acute iliac lymphadenitis, J. Pediat. 29:183–188, 1946.

109. Irwin, F. G.: Acute iliac adenitis, Arch. Surg. 36:561–570, 1938.

110. Hyman, A.: Suppurative retroperitoneal pelvic lymphadenitis, Ann. Surg. 91:718–723, 1930.

111. Hodgson, C. H., Olsen, A. M., and Good, C. A.: Bilateral hilar adenopathy: Its significance and management, Ann. Intern. Med. 43:83–99, 1955.

112. Dawber, T. R., and Hawer, L. E.: Diseases of the Chest, pp. 123–145, 363–375, Baltimore, Williams & Wilkins, 1952.

113. Katz, S.: The etiology of mediastinal lymphadenopathy, Gen. Pract. 8:64–65, 1953.

114. Favour, C. B., and Sosman, M. C.: Erythema nodosum, Arch. Intern. Med. 80:435–453, 1947.

115. Wynn-Williams, N., and Edward, G. F.: Bilateral hilar lymphadenopathy; its association with erythema nodosum, Lancet 1:278–280, 1954.

116. Löfgron, S., and Lundback, H.: The bilateral hilar lymphoma syndrome: a study of the relation of tuberculosis and sarcoidosis of 212 cases, Acta Med. Scand. 142:265–273, 1952.

117. Lindskog, G. E., and Spear, H. C.: Middle-lobe syndrome, New Eng. J. Med. 253:489–495, 1955.

118. Brock, R. C., Cann, R. J., and Dickinson, J. R.: Tuberculous mediastinal lymphadenitis in childhood. Secondary effects on lungs, Guy. Hosp. Rep. 87:295–317, 1937.

119. Brock, R. C.: The Anatomy of the Bronchial Tree with Special Reference to the Surgery of Lung Abscess, New York & London, Oxford, 1946.

120. Graham, E. A., Burford, T. H., and Mayer, J. A.: Middle lobe syndrome, Postgrad. Med. 4:29–34, 1948.

121. Ziskind, M. M.: Effects of calcified lymph nodes perforating the bronchial tree, New Orleans Med. Surg. J. 104:640–644, 1952.

122. Halle, S., and Blitz, O.: Eroding calcified mediastinal lymph nodes, Amer. Rev. Tuberc. 62:213–218, 1950.

123. Maurer, E. R.: The surgical significance of calcified parabronchial and paratracheal lymph glands, J. Thorac. Cardiovasc. Surg. 23:97–110, 1952.

124. Head, J. R., and Moen, C. W.: Late nontuberculous complications of calcified hilus lymph nodes, Amer. Rev. Tuberc. 60:1–14, 1949.

125. Schmidt, H. W., Clagett, O. T., and McDonald, J. R.: Broncholithiasis, J. Thorac. Surg. 19:226–245, 1950.

126. Katz, H. L.: Traction diverticula of the esophagus in middle lobe syndrome, Amer. Rev. Tuberc. 65:455–464, 1952.

127. Coleman, F. P., and Bunch, G. H., Jr.: Acquired non-malignant esophagotracheobronchial fistula, J. Thorac. Surg. 19:542–558, 1950.

128. McCort, J. J.: Radiographic identification of lymph node metastases from carcinoma of the esophagus, Radiology 59:694–711, 1952.

129. McCort, J. J., and Robbins, L. L.: Roentgen diagnosis of intrathoracic lymph node metastases in carcinoma of lung, Radiology 57:338–359, 1951.

130. Sicher, K.: Sternal swelling as presenting sign of Hodgkin's disease, Brit. Med. J. 2:824, 1948.

131. Wilensky, A. O.: General abdominal lymphadenopathy; with special reference to non-specific mesenteric adenitis, Arch. Surg. 42:71–125, 1941.

132. Desjardins, A. U.: Retroperitoneal lymph nodes; their importance in cases of malignant tumors, Arch. Surg. 38:714–754, 1939.

133. Webster, D. R., and Madore, P.: Mesenteric lymphadenitis; a clinical and experimental study, Gastroenterology 15:160–165, 1949.

134. Ferguson, G.: Acute non-specific mesenteric lymphadenitis: possible mechanism pain illustrated by 2 cases, A.M.A. Arch. Surg. 65:906–911, 1952.

135. Marshall, V. F., and Schnittman, M.: Iliac lymphadenopathy as a cause of ureteral obstruction, Surgery 23:542–549, 1948.

136. Bower, J. S., and Coca-Mir, R.: Jaundice in acute subleukemic-lymphatic leukemia due to obstruction of the common duct by portal nodes, J.A.M.A. 146:987–988, 1951.

137. Berkowitz, D., Gambescia, J. M., and Thompson, C. M.: Jaundice with signs of extra-hepatic obstruction as presenting symptom of bronchogenic carcinoma, Gastroenterology 20:653–657, 1952.

138. Sleisenger, M. H., Almy, T. P., and Barr, D. P.: Sprue secondary to lymphoma of the small bowel, Amer. J. Med. 15:666–674, 1953.

139. Adlersberg, D., and Schein, J.: Clinical and pathological studies in sprue, J.A.M.A. 134:1459–1467, 1947.

140. Auchincloss, H.: Clinical study of calcified nodes in mesentery, Ann. Surg. 91:401–415, 1930.

141. Golden, R.: Observations on small intestinal physiology in the presence of calcified mesenteric lymph nodes, Amer. J. Roentgen. 35:316–323, 1936.

142. Blacklock, J. W. S.: Tuberculosis in infancy and childhood, Brit. Med. J. 2:324–328, 1936.

143. ———: Surgical tuberculosis of bovine origin, Ann. Roy. Coll. Surg. Eng. 2:93–103, 1948.

144. Marshak, R. H., and Dierling, D.: Duodenal obstruction due to tuberculous lymphadenitis, Radiology 44:495–497, 1945.

145. Culligan, J. M.: Intestinal obstruction due to calcified mesenteric glands, Minnesota Med. 21:482–483, 1938.

146. Klein, W.: Nonspecific mesenteric adenitis, Arch. Surg. 36:571–585, 1938.

147. Postlethwait, R. W., and Campbell, F. H.: Acute mesenteric lymphadenitis, Arch. Surg. 59:92–100, 1949.

148. Studley, H. O.: Intra-abdominal rupture of retroperitoneal tuberculous lymph node, Ann. Surg. 115:477–480, 1942.

149. Held, I. W., and Goldbloom, A. A.: Lymphadenopathy, a clinical interpretation, Med. Clin. N. Amer. 18:633–702, 1934.

150. McGuinness, A. E.: The significance of lymphadenopathy, Med. J. Aust. 1:285–288, 1953.

151. McGovern, V. J.: The significance of generalized lymph node enlargement, Med. J. Aust. 1:288–330, 1953.

152. Poncher, H. G., and Pierce, M.: Chapter 57, pp. 583–596 in Grulee, G. G., and Eley, R. C. (eds.): Child in Health and Disease, Baltimore, Williams & Wilkins, 1952.

153. Craver, L. F.: The significance of enlarged lymph nodes, Amer. J. Dig. Dis. 11:65–70, 1944.

154. Wiseman, B. K.: The lymphadenopathy question, Publ. No. 13, pp. 20–26, Washington, D. C., Amer. Assoc. Advancement Sci., 1940.

155. Murray, N. A., and Broders, A. C.: Pathology of lymph nodes: diagnosis and prognosis, Amer. J. Clin. Path. 13:450–463, 1943.

156. Kastlin, G. J.: A clinical résumé of cervical lymph gland disease, Penn. Med. J. 43:801–808, 1940.

157. Ghormley, R. K., and Hoffmann, H. O.: Lymphangitis and lymphadenitis, Amer. J. Surg. 50:728–731, 1940.

158. Tobias, N.: Extragenital chancres: A clinical study, Amer. J. Syph. Neurol. 20:266–274, 1936.

159. Carter, B. N., and Smith, J.: Tuberculous lymphadenitis secondary to inconspicuous healed traumatic cutaneous tuberculous lesions, J.A.M.A. 105:1839–1842, 1935.

160. O'Leary, P. A., and Harrison, M. W.: Inoculation tuberculosis (Review), Arch. Derm. Syph. 44:371–390, 1941.

161. Gastineau, F. M., Spolzar, L. W., and Haynes, E.: Sporotrichosis: Report of six cases among florists, J.A.M.A. 117:1074–1077, 1941.

162. Gold, H.: Studies of anthrax (Clinical report of ten human cases), J. Lab. Clin. Med. 21:134–152, 1935-36.

163. Lebowich, R. J., McKillip, B. G., and Conboy, J. R.: Cutaneous anthrax; pathologic study with clinical correlation, Amer. J. Clin. Path. 13:505–515, 1943.

164. Klauder, J. V.: Erysipeloid as an occupational disease, J.A.M.A. 111:1345–1348, 1938.

165. Pullen, R. L., and Stuart, B. M.: Tularemia, analysis of 225 cases, J.A.M.A. 129:495–500, 1945.

166. Kavenaugh, C. N.: Tularemia (123 cases), Arch. Intern. Med. 55:61–85, 1935.

167. Meyer, K. F.: Plague, Med. Clin. N. Amer. 27:745–765, 1943.

168. Sayan, J. J., Pond, H. S., Forrester, J. S., and Wood, F. S.: Scrub typhus in Assam and Burma, 616 cases, Medicine 24:155–214, 1946.

169. Greenberg, M., Pellisseri, O., Kleim, J. F., and Huebner, R. J.: Rickettsialpox (clinical description), J.A.M.A. 133:901–906, 1947.

170. Brown, T. M., and Nunemaker, J. C.: Ratbite fever; review of American cases with reevaluation of etiology; report of cases, Bull. Hopkins Hosp. 70:201–327, 1942.

171. Watkins, C. G.: Ratbite fever, J. Pediat. 28:429–448, 1946.

172. Daniels, W. B., and MacMurray, F. G.: Catscratch disease, J.A.M.A. 154:1247–1251, 1954.

173. Laippy, T. C., and White, C. J.: Dermatitis with lipomelanotic reticular hyperplasia of lymph nodes, A.M.A. Arch. Derm. Syph. 63:611–618, 1951.

174. Nairn, R. C., and Anderson, T. E.: Erythrodermia with lipomelanic reticulum-cell hyperplasia of lymph nodes (dermatopathic lymphadenitis), Brit. Med. J. 1:820–824, 1955.

175. Spink, W. W., and Anderson, D.: Studies relating to the differential diagnosis of brucellosis and infectious mononucleosis; clinical, hematologic, and serologic observations, Trans. Ass. Amer. Physicians 64:428–434, 1951.

176. Bloomfield, A. L.: Enlargement of the superficial lymph nodes in brucella infection, Amer. Rev. Tuberc. 45:741–750, 1942.

177. Rosencrantz, E.: Generalized tuberculous lymphadenitis, Amer. Rev. Tuberc. 41:806–808, 1940.

178. Ash, J. E.: The lymph node in tropical diseases, Amer. J. Trop. Med. 27:483–491, 1947.

179. Longcope, W. T., and Freiman, D. G.: A study of sarcoidosis (based on a combined investigation of 160 cases including 30 autopsies from the Johns Hopkins Hospital and Massachusetts General Hospital), Medicine 31:1–132, 1952.

180. Kojis, F. G.: Serum sickness and anaphylaxis, Amer. J. Dis. Child. 64:93–143, 313–350, 1942.

181. Motulsky, A. G., Weinberg, S., Saphir, O., and Rosenberg, E.: Lymph nodes in rheumatoid arthritis, A.M.A. Arch. Intern. Med. 90:660–676, 1952.

182. Fox, R. A., and Rosahn, P. P.: The lymph nodes in disseminated lupus erythematosus, Amer. J. Path. 19:73–99, 1943.

183. Harvey, A. M., Shulman, L. E., Tumulty, P. A., Conley, C. C., and Schoenrick, E. H.: Systemic lupus erythematosus; review of the literature and clinical analysis of 138 cases, Medicine 33:291, 1954.

184. Pressman, J. J., and Simon, M. B.: Experimental evidence of direct communications between lymph nodes and veins, Surg. Gynec. Obstet. 113:537–541, 1961.

185. Threefoot, S. A., Kent, W. T., and Hatchett, B. F.: Lymphaticovenous and lymphaticolymphatic communications demonstrated by plastic corrosion models of rats and by post-mortem lymphangiography in man, J. Lab. Clin. Med. 61:9–22, 1963.

186. Wenzel, J. F.: Factitial proctitis: the role of lymphatic destruction, Amer. J. Surg. 92:678–682, 1956.

187. Spittell, J. A., Jr., Smith, R. D., Harrison, E. G., Jr., and Schirger, A.: Unilateral secondary lymphedema. A clue to malignant disease, Proc. Mayo Clin. 38:139–144, 1963.

188. Kinmonth, J. B., Taylor, G. W., and Harper, K.: Lymphangiography; technique for its use in lower limbs, Brit. Med. J. 1:940–942, 1955.

189. Wallace, S., Jackson, L., Schaffer, B., Gould, J., Greening, R. R., Weiss, A., and Kramer, S.: Lymphangiograms: their diagnostic and therapeutic potential, Radiology 76:179–199, 1961.

190. Fischer, H. W., Lawrence, M. S., and Thornbury, J. R.: Lymphography of the normal adult male. Observations and their relation to the diagnosis of metastatic neoplasm, Radiology 78:399–406, 1962.

191. Ditchek, T., Blahut, R. J., and Kittleson, A. C.: Lymphadenography in normal subjects, Radiology 80:175–181, 1963.

192. Malamos, B., Moulopoulos, S. A., and Sarkas, A.: Lymphadenography: its uses in haematology, Brit. Med. J. 2:1360–1361, 1959.

193. Wallace, S., Jackson, L., and Greening, R. R.: Clinical applications of lymphangiography, Amer. J. Roentgen. 88:97–109, 1962.

194. Viamonte, M., Jr., Altman, D., Parks, R., Blum, E., Bevilacqua, M., and Recher, L.: Radiographic-pathologic correlation in the interpretation of lymphangioadenograms, Radiology 80:903–916, 1963.

195. Pomerantz, M., and Ketcham, A. S.: Lymphangiography and its surgical applications, Surgery 53:589–597, 1963.

196. Greening, R. R., and Wallace, S.: Further observations in lymphangiography, Radiol. Clin. N. Amer. 1:157–173, 1963.

197. Kinmonth, J. B., Taylor, G. W., Tracy, G. D., and Marsh, J. D.: Primary lymphoedema: clinical and lymphangiographic studies of a series of 107 patients in which the lower limbs were affected, Brit. J. Surg. 45:1–9, 1957.

198. Fuchs, W. A.: Complications in lymphography with oily contrast media, Acta Radiol. 57:427–432, 1962.

199. Bron, K. M., Baum, S., and Abrams, H. L.: Oil embolism in lymphangiography. Incidence, manifestations, and mechanism, Radiology 80:194–202, 1963.

200. Schaffer, B., Gould, R. J., Wallace, S., Jackson, L., Iuker, M., Leberman, P. R., and Fetter, T. R.: The urologic applications of lymphangiography, J. Urol. 87:91–96, 1962.

201. Sage, H. H., Kizilay, D., Miyazaki, M., Shapiro, G., and Sinha, B.: Lymph node scintigrams, Amer. J. Roentgen. 84:666–672, 1960.

202. Lang, E. K.: Demonstration of blockage and involvement of the pelvic lymphatic system by tumor with lymphangiography

and scintiscanograms, Radiology 74:71–73, 1960.

203. Thomas, C. G., Jr.: Lymphatic dissemination of radiogold in the presence of lymph node metastases, Surg. Gynec. Obstet. 103: 51–56, 1956.

204. Seitzman, D. M., Wright, R., Halaby, F. A., and Freeman, J. H.: Radioactive lymphangiography as a therapeutic adjunct, Amer. J. Roentgen. 89:140–149, 1963.

204a. Seitzman, D. M.: Lymphangiography, Gen. Pract. 23:117, 1965.

205. Margileth, L. M.: Cat scratch disease as a cause of oculoglandular syndrome of Parinaud, Pediatrics 20:1000–1005, 1957.

206. Editorial: Primary tuberculosis of the mouth, Brit. Med. J. 2:147, 1956.

207. Watne, A. L., Hatiboglu, I., and Moore, G. E.: A clinical and autopsy study of tumor cells in the thoracic duct lymph, Surg. Gynec. Obstet. 110:339–345, 1960.

208. Lillington, G. A., and Jamplis, R. W.: Review: Scalene node biopsy, Ann. Intern. Med. 59:101–110, 1963.

209. Sage, H. H.: Palpable cervical lymph nodes, J.A.M.A. 168:496–498, 1958.

210. Snapper, I.: The bedside diagnosis of cervical lymphadenopathies. Med. Clin. N. Amer. 46:627–639, 1962.

211. Brandow, E. C., Jr., Volk, B. M., and Olson, K. B.: The significance of a lump in the neck, Postgrad. Med. 2:401–410, 1957.

212. Jones, P. G.: Swellings in the neck in childhood, Med. J. Aust. 1:212–214, 1963.

213. McNair, T. J., and Dudley, H. A. F.: Axillary lymph nodes in patients without breast carcinoma, Lancet 1:713–715, 1960.

214. Pierce, E. H., Gray, H. K., and Dockerty, M. B.: Surgical significance of isolated axillary adenopathy, Ann. Surg. 145:104–107, 1957.

215. Atkins, H., and Wolff, B.: The malignant gland in the axilla, Guy. Hosp. Rep. 109:1–6, 1960.

216. Aaron, A. H.: in the discussion of Bacon, H. E.: Extra-rectal metastatic growths from upper abdominal and mammary cancer: report of seventeen cases, J.A.M.A. 112:808–814, 1939.

217. Saitta, G. F., and Baum, V.: Langer's axillary arch: an unusual cause of axillary mass, J.A.M.A. 180:690, 1962.

218. Dormandy, T. L.: Inguinal endometriosis, Lancet 1:832–834, 1956.

219. Winn-Williams, N.: On erythema nodosum, bilateral hilar lymphadenopathy and sarcoidosis. Tubercle 42:57–63, 1961.

220. Smellie, H., and Hoyle, C.: The hilar lymphnodes in sarcoidosis: with special reference to prognosis, Lancet 2:66–70, 1957.

221. Castleman, B.: Localized mediastinal lymph node hyperplasia resembling thymoma, Cancer 9:822, 1956.

222. Inada, K., and Hamajaki, M.: Localized mediastinal lymph-node hyperplasia resembling thymoma: a case report, Ann. Surg. 147:409–413, 1958.

223. Storer, J., and Smith, R. C.: The calcified hilar node: its significance and management, Amer. Rev. Resp. Dis. 81:853–867, 1960.

224. Smithies, D. W., and Rigby-Jones, P.: Clinical evidence of parasternal lymph node involvement in neoplastic disease, Acta Radiol. (supp.) 188:235–247, 1959.

225. Gambill, E. E.: So-called mesenteric adenitis—a clinical entity or wastebasket diagnosis? Minnesota Med. 43:614–616, 1960.

226. Taswell, H. F., and Winkelmann, R. K.: Sézary syndrome—a malignant reticulemic erythroderma, J.A.M.A. 177:465–472, 1961.

227. Moore, R. D., Weisberger, A. S., and Bowerfind, E. S., Jr.: An evaluation of lymphadenopathy in systemic disease, Arch. Intern. Med. 99:751–759, 1957.

228. McCreanor, J. D.: Lymphadenopathy in toxoplasmosis, New Zeal. Med. 61:18–20, 1962.

229. Harrison, R. J., Broomfield, B. E., and Kippax, P. W.: Toxoplasmosis with relapsing lymphadenitis, Lancet 1:247–248, 1963.

230. Bell, D. W., Carmichael, J. A. G., Williams, R. S., Holman, R. L., and Stewart, P. D.: Localized leishmaniasis of lymph nodes: report of four cases, Brit. Med. J. 1:740–744, 1958.

231. Wilson, W. L., Williams, C. D., Sanders, S. L., and Warner, R. P.: Ardmore disease, Arch. Intern. Med. 100:943–950, 1957.

232. Saltzstein, S. L., and Ackerman, L. V.: Lymphadenopathy induced by anticonvulsant drugs and mimicking clinically and pathologically malignant lymphomas, Cancer 12:164–182, 1959.

233. Bajoghli, M.: Generalized lymphadenopathy and hepatosplenomegaly induced by diphenylhydantoin, Pediatrics 28:943–945, 1961.

234. Greenberg, E., Cohen, D. M., Pease, G. L., and Kyle, R. A.: Histiocytic medullary reticulosis, Proc. Mayo Clin. 37:271–283, 1962.

235. Zak, F. G., and Rubin, E.: Histiocytic medullary reticulosis, Amer. J. Med. 31:813–819, 1961.

236. Clinicopathologic Conference: Recant, L., and Hartroft, W. S. (eds.): Rademacher's disease: diminished immunity of an unusual form complicated by lymphadenopathy, Amer. J. Med. 32:80–95, 1962.

237. Bridges, R. A., Berendes, H., and Good, R. A.: A fatal granulomatous disease of childhood: the clinical, pathological and laboratory features of a new syndrome, Amer. J. Dis. Child. 97:387–408, 1959.

238. Fitts, T. C., Williams, A. V., Graber, C. D., Artz, C. P., and Hargest, T. S.: Thoracic duct lymph: Its significance in dialysis and immunology, Surg. Clin. N. Amer. 49:533, 1969.

239. Courtice, F. C.: Lymphatic function: Concepts old and new, Med. J. Aust. 1:379, 1968.

240. Rusznyzák, I., Földi, M., and Szabó, G.: Lymphatics and Lymph Circulation, New York, Pergamon Press Ltd., 1960.

241. Yoffey, J. M., and Courtice, F. C.: Lym-

phatics, Lymph and Lymphoid Tissue, Cambridge, Harvard University Press, 1956.

242. Mayerson, H. S.: Observations and reflections on the lymphatic system, *in* Transactions & Studies of the College of Physicians of Philadelphia, Fourth Series, vol. 28, no. 3, pp. 109–127, January, 1961.

243. Shieber, W.: Lymphographic detection of undiagnosed neoplasms causing edema of lower extremity, Arch. Surg. 94:380, 1967.

244. Smith, R. D., Spittell, J. A., Jr., and Schirger, A.: Secondary lymphedema of the leg: Its characteristics and diagnostic implications, J.A.M.A. 185:80, 1963.

245. Fisch, U.: Lymphography of the Cervical Lymphatic System, p. 179, Philadelphia, Saunders, 1968.

246. Craig, O.: Primary lymphedema and lymphatica porosa, Radiology 92:1216–1222, 1969.

247. Asch, M. J., *et al.*: Suppurative mesenteric lymphadenitis: A report of two cases and review of the literature, Amer. J. Surg. 115: 570–573, 1968.

248. Robertson, M. D., *et al.*: Rheumatoid lymphadenopathy, Ann. Rheum. Dis. 27:253–260, 1968.

249. Andringa, C. L., and Cherry, J. D.: Bilateral inguinal adenitis due to a nonphotochromogenic atypical Mycobacterium, J.A.M.A. 198: 209–211, 1966.

250. Barta, I.: Differential diagnosis of acute generalized lymphadenopathy and chronic abdominal lymph-node disease, Acta Med. Acad. Sci. Hung., 24:1–12, 1967.

251. Jackson, S. M.: Carcinoma of the breast—the significance of supraclavicular lymph node metastases, Clin. Radiol. 17:107–114, 1966.

252. Dorfman, R. F., and Herweg, J. C.: Live, attenuated measles virus vaccine: Inguinal lymphadenopathy complicating administration, J.A.M.A. 198:230–231, 1966.

253. Kazem, I., Antonaides, J., Brady, L. W., Croll, M. N., and Lightfoot, D.: Clinical evaluation of lymph node scanning utilizing Colloidal Gold 198, Radiology 90:905–911, 1968.

253a. Hauser, W., Atkins, H. L., and Richards, P.: Lymph node scanning with ^{99m}Tc-Sulfur Colloid, Radiology 92:1369–1371, 1969.

254. Herrera, N. E., Gonzales, R., Schwarz, R. D., Diggs, A. M., and Belsky, J.: ^{75}Se-methionine as a diagnostic agent in malignant lymphoma, J. Nucl. Med. 6:792–804, 1965.

254a. Spencer, R. P., Montana, G., Scanlon, G. T., and Evans, O. R.: Uptake of selenomethionine by mouse and in human lymphomas, with observations on selenite and selenate, J. Nucl. Med. 8:197–208, 1967.

255. Steinberg, I., and Watson, R. C.: Lymphangiographic and angiographic diagnosis of persistent jugular lymph sac, New Eng. J. Med. 275:1471–1474, 1966.

256. Kuiper, D. H., and Papp, J. P.: Supra-

clavicular adenopathy demonstrated by the Valsalva maneuver, New Eng. J. Med. 280: 1007–1008, 1969.

257. Threefoot, S. A., and Kossover, M. F.: Lymphaticovenous communications in man, Arch. Intern. Med. 117:213–223, 1966.

258. O'Brien, P. H., Sherman, J. O., and Beal, J. M.: Lymphatics and malignant disease, Med. Clin. N. Amer. 51:249–261, 1967.

259. Jackson, R. J. A.: Complications of lymphography, Brit. Med. J. 1:1203–1205, 1966.

260. Devitt, J. E., and Michalchuk, A. W.: Significance of contralateral axillary metastases in carcinoma of the breast, Canad. J. Surg. 12:178–180, 1969.

261. Azimi, P. H., Bodenbender, J. G., Hintz, R. L., and Kontras, S. B.: Chronic granulomatous disease in three female siblings, J.A.M.A. 206:2865–2870, 1968.

262. Holmes, B., *et al.*: Fatal granulomatous disease of childhood: An inborn abnormality of phagocytic function, Lancet 1:1225–1228, 1966.

263. Solnitzky, O. C.: Lymphography, Georgetown Med. Bull. 17:214–228, 1964.

264. Chavez, C. M.: Lymphangiography, Amer. J. Med. Sci. 248:225–245, 1964.

265. Love, L., and Kim, S. E.: Clinical aspects of lymphangiography, Med. Clin. N. Amer. 51: 227–248, 1967.

266. Takahashi, M., and Abrams, H. L.: The accuracy of lymphangiographic diagnosis in malignant lymphoma, Radiology 89:448–460, 1967.

267. Bjornberg, A., and Holst, R.: Generalized lymphadenopathy as a drug reaction to hydantoin, Acta Neurol. Scand. 43:399–402, 1967.

268. Palumbo, L. T., and Sharpe, W. S.: Scalene node biopsy: Correlation with other diagnostic procedures in 550 cases, Arch. Surg. 98:90–93, 1969.

269. Conn, J. H., *et al.*: A critical evaluation of scalene lymphadenectomy in 500 patients, Amer. Surg. 35:125–129, 1969.

270. Hartsock, R. J., and Bellanti, J. A.: Postvaccinal lymphadenitis, Gen. Pract. 39:99–105, 1969.

271. Asher, W. M., and Freimanis, A. K.: Echographic diagnosis of retroperitoneal lymph node enlargement, Amer. J. Roentgen. 105: 435–445, 1969.

272. Theodoropoulas, G., Makkous, A., and Constantonlakis, M.: Lymph node enlargement after a single massive infusion of iron dextran, J. Clin. Path. 21:492–494, 1968.

273. Rosai, J., and Dorfman, R. F.: Sinus histiocytosis with massive lymphadenopathy: A newly recognized benign clinical pathological entity, Arch. Path. 87:63–70, 1969.

274. Hartsock, R. J.: Postvaccinal lymphadenitis: Hyperplasia of lymphoid tissue that simulates malignant lymphomas, Cancer 21:632–649, 1968.

27

Pathologic Bleeding

ROBERT GOLDSTEIN

Definition. For the purpose of this chapter pathologic bleeding is defined as hemorrhage resulting from impaired hemostatic mechanisms with consequent loss of the normal ability to terminate blood loss.

Obviously, the mechanisms of hemostasis may be normal yet inadequate to meet the demands imposed by trauma or disease. Examples of such situations are: bleeding peptic ulcer, ruptured aneurysm, laceration of major vessels, erosions of vessels by malignant tumor or other pathological processes. Although in most such instances, the causes of bleeding are usually evident, the physician is not infrequently called upon to distinguish such conditions from those in which the hemostatic mechanisms are primarily at fault or to determine whether or not any derangement of the hemostatic mechanisms is contributing to the hemorrhages. Hemostasis is a complex phenomenon, and although our understanding of the mechanisms involved is far from complete and concepts are still the subject of considerable controversy, notable advances in our knowledge have been made so that the patient with disordered hemostasis can benefit enormously by a rational approach to his disease.

NORMAL HEMOSTASIS

The various mechanisms concerned in hemostasis may be considered as involving extravascular, vascular, and intravascular factors all of which are interrelated. For more detailed and extensive discussion of hemostasis and hemorrhagic diseases the reader is referred to monographs and reviews.[1-10]

Extravascular and Anatomic Factors. The extent of hemorrhage which follows a vascular injury is dependent not only upon the severity of the injury and the size of the vessel involved, but also upon the blood pressure within the vessel (Fig. 27-1) and the counter-pressure which is built up in the adjacent extra-vascular tissue by the accumulation of extravasated blood (Fig. 27-2). Bleeding into firm tissue or a "solid" organ rapidly results in progressively increasing extravascular pressure, which in turn decreases the flow of blood from the injured vessel, enabling other mechanisms of hemostasis to function more effectively. The degree of tamponade developed depends upon the distensibility, denseness and elasticity of the surrounding tissues. Thus, in bone, hemorrhage into the matrix is practically impossible, whereas injury to a vessel of similar size in muscular tissue would result in more hemorrhage but still considerably less than that which would occur in regions where structures are loose, as in the subcutaneous tissues of the infraorbital regions, of the neck or the axillae. An injury to a vessel of comparable size in the mucous membrane of hollow organs, such as the gastrointestinal, the respiratory, or the genitourinary tracts, might be life-endangering, since there is so little supporting tissue that blood can escape freely. Conditions affecting supporting tissue, such as debility, advanced age, Ehlers-Donlos syndrome, or prolonged corticosteroid therapy will also increase blood loss.

Most, if not all, tissues contain clot-promoting substances called tissue thromboplastin. It is probable that injury to the vessel wall and extravasation of blood into surrounding tissues results in the release of this thromboplastic substance which may play a role in hemostasis by accelerating platelet massing at the site of injury (described below) and coagulation of the extravasated blood, both of which aid in sealing the injured vessel. Since there is wide variation in thromboplastic activity among tissues, the relative amounts of thromboplastin released may account in part for the differences noted in bleeding tendency in different areas of the body.

Vascular Factors. The vascular factors which are concerned in hemostasis are vessel size, elasticity, strength, tone and contractility. By virtue of their thick walls containing muscular and elastic tissue, arteries can withstand more stress and trauma than arterioles, capillaries, venules or veins. Once perforated or ruptured, however, the egress of blood is great, due to the high intravascular pressure in relation to the low extravascular tissue tension. Under such circumstances, hemostatic mechanisms must act rapidly to prevent catastrophe. The vessel retracts longitudinally and circularly, undergoes segmental spasm, which decreases blood flow, and the

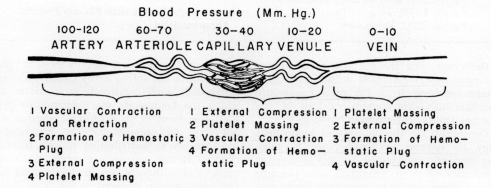

FIG. 27-1. Probable order of importance of the components of hemostasis in different vessels. (Tocantins: Ann. Surg. 125:292)

aperture is decreased by puckering of the intima. In addition, drop in blood pressure and vascular collapse may supervene. Though temporary, these reactions may retard blood flow sufficiently to permit initiation and completion of coagulation which will plug the hole. It is thus evident that, at this level of the circulation, losses in elasticity of the artery from any cause—arteriosclerosis, aneurysms, etc.—may seriously jeopardize hemostasis. Also, it is clear that hypertension may impose an additional increment of strain on the hemostatic mechanism when arterial bleeding occurs.

The situation regarding veins is quite different. They, too, react to trauma with spasm and retraction. But since venous pressure is low, tamponade from extravascular tissue pressure is more effective in stemming the flow of blood, provided sufficient tissue surrounds the open vessel. However, under some pathologic conditions, such as portal obstruction, congestive heart failure, phlebarteriectasia or varicose veins, venous pressure may be abnormally high, which may lead to excessive hemorrhage. Also, veins are more easily traumatized than arteries because of the relative thinness of the venous wall.

At the microscopic level of the vascular tree there is proportionally much less muscle and elastic tissue in the vessel walls than in the large vessels, and it decreases progressively from arterioles, to venules, to capillaries. Therefore, in these smaller vessels and particularly in the capillaries, vascular strength is dependent in large part upon the endothelial structure and basement membrane plus support from surrounding tissue. It is these vessels whose strength is so impaired by vitamin C deficiency, allergic, immunologic, inflammatory and drug reactions, infectious diseases, and thrombocytopenia. The role of platelets in the maintenance of the strength of the capillary wall remains unknown, and equally unexplained is the mechanism by which corticosteroids can decrease the capillary fragility seen in thrombocytopenia without increasing the

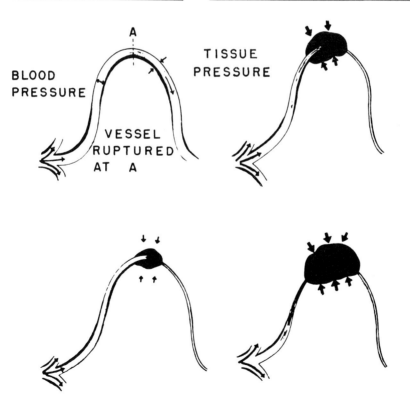

Fig. 27-2. Diagram showing hydrostatic dynamics of hemorrhage from small blood vessels. (Tocantins: Ann. Surg. 125:292)

platelet level. Clinically, capillary fragility is determined by subjecting the capillaries to increased physical stress either by means of a tourniquet (thus increasing intracapillary pressure to a predetermined level for a measured period of time) and noting the number of petechiae, or by application of negative pressure for a one minute period and determining the relative pressure which first produces petechiae.[13]

Extravascular tissue pressure is most effective in controlling bleeding from these small vessels because of the relatively low intravascular pressures. (Figs. 27-1 and 27-2.) At the arteriocapillary junction pressure is approximately 30 mm. of mercury and at the capillary venule junction about 10 mm. It should be pointed out that in the instances of an arteriole supplying a plexus of capillaries, obstruction of the flow in one or several of the capillaries by the increase in tissue pressure will result in back-pressure equal only to that of the arteriole—approximately 30 mm. of mercury. However, if all the capillaries from arterioles are obstructed, the pressure within the capillaries rises until it either overcomes the obstruction or becomes equal to that of the arterial supply. Thus, capillary bleeding may become very extensive despite high tissue pressures unless the break in the vessel is repaired.

The response of arterioles, venules and capillaries to trauma is very important in the mechanism of hemostasis, since by far the greatest number of traumatic incidents —cuts, bruises, abrasions, puncture wounds, etc.—involve this region of the vascular tree. It has been emphasized by Macfarlane,[12] Tocantins[11] and others that under normal conditions puncture of a capillary is followed by prompt disappearance of the vessel and cessation of bleeding. Since this occurs even in the presence of increased intracapillary pressure, it is unlikely that it is due to passive collapse of the punctured vessel. It is felt by some observers[12] that disappearance of the capillaries represents an active constriction of the capillaries in response to the stimulus mediated through the Rouget cells in the capillary wall. However, microscopic evaluation would indicate that true capillaries are simple endothelial tubes with no contractile ability, which branch from the meta-arterioles and have a sphincter at their origin. Trauma could cause constriction of the meta-arterioles or of the "precapillary

sphincter" which would reduce the flow of blood into the capillaries and cause "plasma skimming" in which fluid without red cells traverses the capillary, with the result that the vessel becomes invisible. Whether or not there is true constriction of the capillaries, or only constriction of the meta-arterioles and venules in response to injury, certain findings are difficult to explain. Disappearance of capillary loops following trauma fails to occur in the absence of platelets (thrombocytopenia). The role platelets play in vasoconstriction remains obscure, for although they do contain serotonin, a vasoconstrictor, which is released when they are damaged or take part in coagulation, and which may be released when platelets adhere to the vessel wall at the point of injury, it has been reported that both the bleeding time and capillary fragility remained normal despite prolonged depletion of platelet serotonin induced by reserpine.[14] Recently it has also been reported that a plasma protein which has no coagulation activity also plays some role in the vascular response to injury. The prolonged bleeding time found in patients with von Willebrand's disease has been thought to be due to a primary vascular defect characterized by capillaries which may appear distorted and which fail to disappear in response to trauma. Nilsson et al.[15] have reported that the bleeding time can be reduced to normal by injection of fraction I-0 from either normal or hemophilic plasma but not with a similar fraction obtained from the plasma from a patient with von Willebrand's disease. The mode of action of this fraction is not known. The active material is distinct from fibrinogen and AHF (factor VIII) and has no corrective effect upon the prolonged bleeding time of thrombocytopenia.

It has been generally accepted that the bleeding time, whether done by the Duke[16] or Ivy[17] method, reflects the hemostatic response of the capillaries to trauma. However, it is more than likely that arterioles and venules are also involved and that the bleeding time primarily reflects their hemostatic response to trauma.

Intravascular Factors—Platelets and Coagulation. That platelets and coagulation are important in the hemostatic mechanism is amply demonstrated by the hemorrhagic manifestations encountered in patients with thrombocytopenia or derangements of blood coagulation due to deficiency of one or more of the plasma coagulation factors. Until about 15 years ago there was little distinction made between the role of platelets and blood clotting in hemostasis. Since then a better understanding has been achieved of the platelet and coagulation reactions which are coordinated into the hemostatic process.

PLATELETS. Platelets are produced in the bone marrow by the megakaryocytes and normally are maintained at a level of 150,000 to 350,000 per cubic mm. in the peripheral blood. Relatively little is known about the regulation of platelet production. Evidence indicates that a factor or factors (thrombopoietin) present in plasma increases the number of megakaryocytes formed from precursor cells, accelerates their maturation, and increases the release and production of platelets. Under normal conditions platelets maintain a discoid shape in the peripheral blood. About two-thirds of the platelets circulate systemically and the remainder are pooled in the spleen. Splenomegaly is associated with an increase in splenic pooling which may amount to as much as 80 to 90% of the platelet mass. By a variety of radioisotope tagging techniques the normal platelet life span in the human has been estimated to be 9 to 11 days. There is disagreement amongst investigators as to whether platelet survival studies indicate a linear or an exponential loss of platelets from the peripheral blood. A linear loss would be consistent with the concept of a finite platelet life span and removal of senescent platelets similar to what happens to red cells. However, this would not be compatible with the concepts that platelets are being continually utilized to maintain the integrity of the microcirculation and the endothelium and also by slow continuous intravascular clotting. Under these conditions an exponential survival curve would be anticipated, indicative of random platelet loss. Evidence has accumulated that the young platelets in the peripheral blood are larger, are metabolically more active and are "stickier" and adhere to collagen more readily than "older" platelets. It is suggested that it is the younger platelets which are most active in the maintenance of vascular integrity and hemostasis. The random removal of these platelets from the circulation for these purposes may be missed by the usual techniques employed in determining platelet survival.

Electron microscopy reveals that the platelet membrane possesses a surface coat which is acquired during platelet formation in the

TABLE 27-1. PLATELET FACTORS OR ACTIVITIES WHICH MAY PLAY A ROLE IN HEMOSTASIS

Platelet factor 1: Plasma factor V-like activity

Platelet factor 2: Accelerator of the conversion of fibrinogen to fibrin by thrombin-fibrinoplastic activity

Platelet factor 3: Platelet thromboplastin activity

Platelet factor 4: Anti-heparin activity

Platelet factor 5: Clottable factor, fibrinogen or fibrinogen-like protein clotted by thrombin

Platelet factor 6: Anti-fibrinolytic activity

Platelet factor 7: ? factor VII-like activity

Clot retraction activity—probably due to a contractile protein in platelets similar to actomyosin of muscle, contracts in the presence of Ca^{++} or Mg^{++} and ATP

Vascular factor—action on capillary fragility and vasoconstriction

Serotonin

megakaryocytes. This surface coat which consists of sulfated acid-mucopolysaccharide appears to be continuous with the outer layer of the platelet membrane and probably is of great importance in the adhesion and cohesion reactions of the platelets and of the selective absorption of coagulation factors onto the platelet surface. The surface area is significantly increased by microcanalicular invaginations of the membrane. These microcanaliculae in addition to increasing surface area, give the platelet a sponge-like character, so that in effect the platelet carries with it some plasma with its content of coagulation factors to sites of platelet adhesion and cohesion. A lipoprotein component of the membrane frequently referred to as *platelet factor 3* promotes coagulation as described below. Microtubular structures have been described within the platelet. They appear to form a marginal bundle around the circumference of the plasma membrane. It has been postulated that these microtubules are actually rigid and under tension in the intact platelet and can be thought of as a cytoskeletal system responsible for maintaining the discoid shape of the platelet in the circulation. It has also been postulated that these microtubules are composed of microfibrils made up of the contractile protein, *thrombosthenin*, present in the platelet. Whether or not thrombosthenin makes up part of the microtubular structure, it is thought to be responsible for clot retraction and platelet pseudopodia formation. The platelets also

TABLE 27-2. PLASMA COAGULATION FACTORS

INTERNATIONAL NOMENCLATURE	TERMINOLOGY FREQUENTLY USED IN LITERATURE
PRO-COAGULANTS	
Factor I	Fibrinogen
Factor II	Prothrombin
Factor III	Thromboplastin, Thrombokinase, Prothrombinase
Factor IV	Calcium
Factor V	Labile Factor, Proaccelerin, Plasma Accelerator Globulin (AC-G), Plasma Prothrombin Conversion Accelerator, Plasmatic Co-factor of Thromboplastin
Factor VI	not used
Factor VII	Serum Prothrombin Conversion Accelerator (SPCA), Proconvertin, Stable Factor, Cothromboplastin, Autoprothrombin I
Factor VIII	Antihemophilic Factor (AHF) Antihemophilic Factor A (AHFA) Antihemophilic Globulin (AHG) Platelet Co-factor I, Thromboplastinogen
Factor IX	Plasma Thromboplastin Component (PTC), Christmas Factor, Antihemophilic Factor B (AHFB), Platelet Co-factor II, Autoprothrombin II
Factor X	Stuart Factor*, Prower Factor*
Factor XI	Plasma Thromboplastin Antecedent (PTA), Antihemophilic Factor C (AHFC)
Factor XII	Hageman Factor, Antihemophilic Factor D (AHFD), Glass Factor, Contact Factor
Factor XIII	Fibrin-Stabilizing Factor, Fibrinase
INHIBITORS	
	Anti-thromboplastin, Antithrombin, ? Heparin, Heparin Co-factor

*Factors VII and X were first clearly differentiated in 1957. Prior to that time the terms listed for Factor VII actually could refer to either Factor VII or X or both.

contain mitochondria, glycogen particles and many granules. At least a portion of the platelet granules are lysosomes since the hydrolytic enzymes, acid phosphatase, beta-glucuronidase, and cathepsin have been identified in platelets and in isolated platelet granules. In common with other cells, platelets require a constant supply of ATP for their metabolic activities. The primary source of energy is glucose, which the platelet can metabolize both aerobically and anaerobically. Enzymes of the Embden-Meyerhof pathway, citric acid cycle, and the hexose-monophosphate shunt are present in the platelet. Since platelets contain no DNA and relatively little RNA, it is unlikely that

the enzyme systems can be renewed. The short life-span of the platelet may be related to mitochondrial senescence, leading to decrease in ATP supplied by enzymes of the Krebs cycle and respiratory chain associated with mitochondria.

A number of activities which appear to be concerned with hemostasis and coagulation have been attributed to platelets. These activities may be classified into two major groups: (1) those which are intrinsic constituents of the platelets and are not found in plasma, and (2) those which are also present in plasma. In the former group are: (A) platelet factor 2, a protein which accelerates the clotting of fibrinogen by thrombin;

(B) platelet factor 3, a lipoprotein present in the platelet membrane and the membranes of granules which accelerates blood clotting; (C) platelet factor 4, a protein with anti-heparin activity; (D) platelet factor 6, a protein with anti-fibrinolytic activity; and (E) a contractile protein, thrombosthenin, which probably is involved in clot retraction. In the second group all the procoagulants of plasma may be included. Some of these coagulation factors such as fibrinogen, Factors V, XI, and XIII appeared to be adsorbed onto the surface of the platelet or are within the platelet and cannot be removed from intact platelets by repeated washing. In the case of fibrinogen there is evidence that fibrinogen of plasma origin is adsorbed onto the surface of the platelet but does not enter into the cell, suggesting that the intercellular portion of platelet fibrinogen is probably synthesized in the megakaryocyte. Whether this is also the case for Factors V, XI and XIII remains obscure. Factor V activity of platelets has been designated as platelet factor 1, and platelet fibrinogen as platelet factor 5. The other plasma coagulation factors (factors II, VII, VIII, IX, X, XII) and plasminogen can be washed off intact platelets with varying degrees of ease. They presumably coat the platelet and fill the microcanaliculae along with the other plasma proteins and provide the "periplatelet atmosphere." Normally all the serotonin in the blood is in the platelets. Platelets and megakaryocytes do not *synthesize* serotonin, but platelets *concentrate* it by an active transport mechanism. Epinephrine and norepinephrine are also taken up by platelets by an active transport mechanism which is not the same as that for serotonin, and they are not concentrated to the same extent as is serotonin. Histamine is normally not concentrated by human platelets.

How the platelets affect the strength of the capillary wall and reduce capillary fragility is not known, nor is it understood how corticosteroids decrease capillary fragility in the absence of platelets. However, there is considerable experimental data on the role of platelets in the formation of the hemostatic plug in vascular injury.[26-28] When a small vessel such as an arteriole or venule is severed or lacerated, constriction occurs within a few seconds, but this is not sufficient to stop the flow of blood, and in the absence of platelets the vasoconstriction does not persist. Almost immediately platelets begin to adhere to the injured vascular wall and to each other. Thus, a loose platelet aggregate is formed both inside and outside the vessel wall, the so-called white thrombus. Such an aggregate of platelets may suffice to stop bleeding from a smaller vessel with low intravascular pressure. However, on the arterial side of the circulation parts of the platelet plug may be carried away by the blood stream but these are rapidly replaced. In these vessels blood continues to ooze through the loose platelet plug until it is made more solid by changes which take place within it (viscous metamorphosis of the platelets, the laying down of fibrin by the process of coagulation, and clot retraction).

Evidence now available indicates that the platelets do not adhere to damaged endothelial cells but rather to connective tissue exposed by injury. It is the *collagen* component of connective tissue that is primarily involved in the reaction. The mechanism of this reaction between collagen and platelets is not known, but it results in important biochemical and morphological alterations in the platelet. Adenosine diphosphate, serotonin and other platelet components are released from the platelet, platelet factor 3 is made available for the coagulation process (see below) and the intracellular granules disappear. The aggregation of platelets which follows the initial reaction between platelets and connective tissue or collagen is thought to be mediated through the release of ADP from the platelets, perhaps reinforced by release of ADP from other damaged cells in the area. The mechanism by which ADP causes platelet aggregation is poorly understood. ADP also causes further release of ADP from newly-aggregated platelets, thus in part explaining the continued aggregation of platelets at the site of vascular injury. The released serotonin and epinephrine may also play a role in platelet aggregation and release of ADP. Such aggregates are relatively unstable and disaggregation may occur unless further reactions take place which are dependent upon the formation of thrombin. The formation of thrombin is favored in these platelet aggregates because platelet factor 3 is more available for the coagulation process. Thrombin in trace amounts also causes platelet aggregation through release of ADP from the platelet. In addition it causes platelet degranulation, with release of intracellular contents and increased availability of platelet factor 3, thus further accelerating thrombin formation. Thrombin may also be formed via the extrinsic pathway (see below) by the release of tissue thromboplastin at the site of vascular injury. The other effect of thrombin, of course, is the conversion of fibrinogen to fibrin and it is the laying down of fibrin which converts the relatively fragile platelet aggregates into the more stable hemostatic plugs. Other factors in or on the surface of the platelets favor fibrin formation within the platelet aggregates. Platelet factor 2 accelerates the conversion of fibrinogen to fibrin by thrombin. The clottable protein in the platelets and the fibrinogen on their surface ensure the presence of fibrinogen for conversion to fibrin within the hemostatic plug. The presence of plasma coagulation factors in or on the surface of the platelets, whether they are intrinsic constituents of the platelets or not, favors coagulation by supplying the necessary factors for both the intrinsic and extrinsic coagulation pathways. Thrombosthenin, the actomysin-like protein in platelets that contracts in the presence of divalent cations (Ca^{++}, Mg^{++}) and ATP, is undoubtedly responsible for retraction of the fibrin-clot, thus strengthening the hemostatic plug. The antiheparin activity neutralizes any heparinlike substances which may be released from the injured vessel wall (thus favoring coagulation) and the antifibrinolytic activity of the platelets may well prevent premature dissolution of the hemostatic plug by the normal mechanism of clot lysis. The vasoconstriction caused by vascular injury is of short duration, but with the aggregation of platelets there is reinforcement and prolongation of the vasoconstriction. Whether this is due to the release of serotonin or some other factor from the platelets or to the formation of some vasoconstrictor during coagulation is not known.

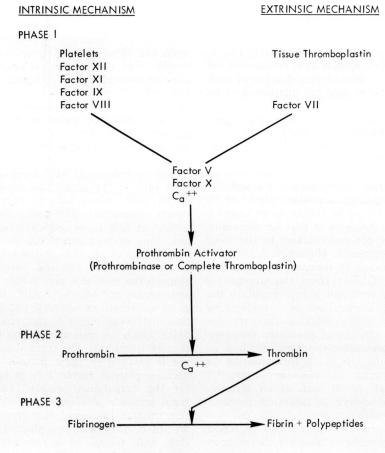

FIG. 27-3. Blood coagulation.

BLOOD COAGULATION

Although the bleeding time may be normal and minor injuries (such as that inflicted for the determination of the bleeding time) may not cause immediate excessive loss of blood in patients with severe coagulation defects other than thrombocytopenia, delayed or secondary bleeding often occurs, indicating a defect in the hemostatic plug which is probably due to faulty fibrin formation. When somewhat larger vessels are injured in which platelet aggregates (white thrombi) alone are ineffective, bleeding may continue indefinitely or until the coagulation defect is corrected. Identification of such defects is, therefore, important both in the diagnosis and the treatment of pathologic bleeding. For a rational approach to diagnosis and treatment, an understanding of present concepts of the coagulation mechanism is fundamental.

The coagulation of blood is a complex phenomenon, and although many aspects of it are poorly understood, recent advances have brought about considerable agreement in and clarification of our concepts. At the present time 10 plasma factors, which are believed by most investigators to be distinct and separate plasma proteins, have been identified as procoagulants that interact with each other, and with calcium and platelets in the process of coagulation. Considerable confusion has arisen in the past from the multiplicity of terms used to identify these factors. An International Committee on Nomenclature has attempted to bring some order to this chaos and has suggested the use of Roman numerals to identify the plasma clotting factors. Some *platelet* factors have been designated by Arabic numbers (see Table 27-1) and this may cause confusion. The plasma factors are listed in Table 27-2 by the Roman numerical system together with the most common synonyms.

For a practical clinical approach, coagulation can best be considered as proceeding by two different mechanisms. One, designated as *intrinsic*, refers to the coagulation of whole blood or plasma as it proceeds without the addition of tissue extracts (tissue thromboplastin) which accelerate coagulation whereas the other designated as *extrinsic* refers to the coagulation process as it proceeds in the presence of such tissue extracts. Both the intrinsic and extrinsic mechanisms may be thought of as occurring in three phases. Phase 1: The evolution of

prothrombin activator (prothrombinase or "complete" thromboplastin). Phase 2: The conversion of prothrombin to thrombin by the activator developed in phase 1. Phase 3: Conversion of fibrinogen to fibrin by thrombin. Intrinsic and extrinsic coagulation differ primarily in the first phase, which is the most complex. The coagulation scheme in Figure 27-3 illustrates the differences between the intrinsic and extrinsic pathways by which prothrombin activator (prothrombinase) is formed.

INTRINSIC MECHANISM. In spontaneous coagulation (intrinsic) as studied in vitro, plasma Factors XII, XI, X, IX, VIII and V interact with each other and platelets, in the presence of ionized calcium, to produce the activator of prothrombin. A deficiency of any one of these factors will cause either a delay in the formation of activator or a decrease in the amount of activator formed, or both, and will result in a delay and a decrease in the conversion of prothrombin to thrombin, and thus a delay in the conversion of fibrinogen to fibrin and in clot formation. The exact role of each of the coagulation factors in the complex reaction is not known, but considerable information has accumulated from studies on blood and plasma from patients with congenital deficiencies of a single coagulation factor and from partially purified preparations of coagulation factors derived from serum and plasma. For many years it has been recognized that blood or plasma exposed to foreign surfaces, such as glass, clots more rapidly than when exposed to nonwettable surfaces such as silicon-coated glass or plastics. It is now evident that this acceleration effect of surface is mediated entirely, or at least in great part, through activation of Factor XII, the Hageman factor. Calcium is not necessary for this reaction.[36-41]

Although Factor XII is necessary for coagulation to proceed normally in vitro, its role in hemostasis is questionable, because patients with a marked deficiency of this factor, exhibiting prolonged clotting times, do not bleed excessively even when subjected to surgery. That Factor XII may play some role in hemostasis is suggested by the fact that it is activated by collagen. Activated XII (XIIa) interacts with Factor XI (PTA) in a reaction which is not calcium-dependent to form an activation- or contact-product, presumably activated XI (XIa). In the widely-held "cascade" or "waterfall" concept

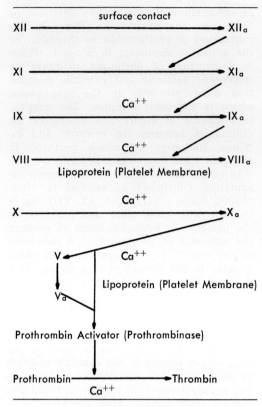

FIG. 27-4. First and second phases of coagulation: intrinsic mechanism. Subscript "a" indicates activated Factor.

of coagulation this is the first of a series of reactions in which protein clotting factors interact with each other in a step-wise manner, one factor acting as an enzyme and the other as a substrate (see Fig. 27-4). Thus activated, Factor XII acts as an enzyme in activating Factor XI which exists in its inactive form in plasma. Activated XI in turn

activates Factor IX. Ionized calcium is necessary for this reaction to take place, as it is for all the following reactions in the formation of prothrombin activator. Activated Factor IX activates Factor VIII. Not only is Ca^{++} essential for this reaction to take place but a lipoprotein derived from platelet membrane is also necessary for optimal activation. The lipid portion of this co-factor is a phospholipid. It has been shown that phosphatidyl ethanolamine and phosphatidyl serine which are present in platelet membranes can substitute in vitro studies for the platelet lipoprotein. It is postulated that activated Factor VIII then activates Factor X. A reaction then follows between activated X and Factor V in which calcium and phospholipid (lipoprotein derived from platelets) take part and the activator of prothrombin or prothrombinase is formed. This enzyme in turn splits the prothrombin molecule, the active portion of which, thrombin, is a proteolytic enzyme for which fibrinogen is a substrate.

Recent data indicates that certain modifications of this concept are probably in order. The evidence now available suggests that Factor X is activated by a complex of activated IX, VIII, Ca^{++} and phospholipid and not by VIIIa. Both Factors IX and VIII must be present for activation of X as indicated in Figure 27-5. Whether VIII is first activated or whether either the native or the activated form of VIII may function in this reaction is not known. The phospholipid apparently provides a surface to which IXa and VIII can adhere and form a complex and are so oriented in the presence of calcium that Factor X can be activated. A similar complex, it appears, is also formed between phospholipid, activated X, V, and calcium, which is the activator of prothrombin.

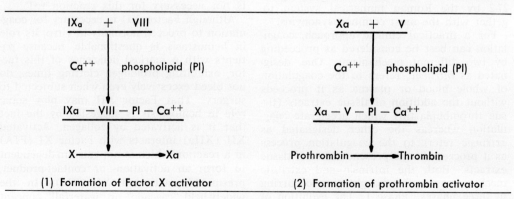

FIG. 27-5.

Exactly what role activation of Factor V plays in this reaction is not clear.

When blood clots in vitro there is a latent period during which the blood remains fluid and there is no conversion of prothrombin to thrombin. Once a small amount of prothrombin activator is formed, thrombin begins to appear at a slow rate and visible clotting begins. If the conversion of prothrombin to thrombin is followed, it is found to proceed very slowly at first and then to accelerate until conversion proceeds at a very rapid rate. This has been referred to as the autocatalytic nature of thrombin formation. Since the hemostatic effectiveness of coagulation depends more upon the velocity of thrombin evolution than its final yield, considerable attention has been focused on the autocatalytic reaction and various mechanisms have been postulated to explain this phenomenon. As outlined in Figure 27-4 the formation of prothrombin activator is a time-consuming process. At first only small amounts of prothrombinase are formed, which will slowly convert prothrombin to thrombin, but as the reaction proceeds, more and more of this prothrombin activator is formed. The accumulation of activator obviously will increase the velocity of thrombin formation from prothrombin. The development of prothrombinase activity also does not proceed at a steady rate, but it first develops slowly and then there is a period of a rapid acceleration of its formation, which also might be referred to as autocatalytic. Since the development of prothrombinase activity is dependent upon a chain of reactions, one catalyzing another, the velocity of each reaction would increase as the product of the preceding reaction increased. This would lead, of course, to an increasing velocity of prothrombinase production. In addition, there is also evidence that end products of certain reactions in coagulation can accelerate preceding reactions. Thus, there is evidence that minute amounts of thrombin activate Factor V (increase activity 3 to 5 fold) and that an increase in Factor V activity occurs early in the clotting of whole blood, before there is any evidence of fibrin formation or decrease in prothrombin content as determined by the available procedures.[50,51] Activation of Factor V by thrombin or other intermediary products may accelerate production of prothrombinase, and in turn, of thrombin. This activated Factor V in humans is more labile and the activity

disappears fairly rapidly. Thrombin also has been shown to cause clumping of platelets in plasma and to induce viscous metamorphosis and platelet lysis, thus making available more platelet factor 3, which in turn results in a more rapid and greater evolution of prothrombinase activity.[29,52,53,54] Evidence also indicates that trace amounts of thrombin activate Factor VIII (AHF), and by this means accelerate coagulation.[55] This occurs only at the stage of coagulation where minute amounts of thrombin are available, for higher activities of thrombin destroy Factor VIII. Factor VII activity is also increased in the early phase of coagulation before conversion of prothrombin to thrombin. How this is brought about is not known, since it is now generally agreed that Factor VII does not play a role in the intrinsic pathway of coagulation, but that it is essential for rapid coagulation of blood by tissue thromboplastin. An increase in Factor VII activity will accelerate coagulation induced by tissue thromboplastin, and this may be of importance in hemostasis.[56,57]

EXTRINSIC MECHANISM. As illustrated in Figure 27-3 certain of the plasma coagulation factors (XII, XI, IX and VIII) essential in the intrinsic mechanism of prothrombinase formation, are not necessary in the extrinsic pathway in which tissue thromboplastin is present in excess or optimal concentration. Factors V and X are necessary in both pathways for rapid prothrombinase formation and Factor VII plays a role only in the extrinsic pathway.[3,56-58] Tissue thromboplastin, Factors V, VII and X interact in the presence of ionized calcium to form a potent prothrombin activator.

The active component of tissue thromboplastin in this reaction is also a lipoprotein but it differs functionally and structurally from platelet lipoprotein. The sequence of events in the formation of the extrinsic prothrombin activator is not known but it appears that there is an initial reaction between the lipoprotein, Ca^{++}, and Factor VII with the formation of a complex which then activates Factor X. As in the intrinsic mechanism, for the formation of a potent prothrombin, activator V is also necessary. Whether or not a complex of VIIa- Xa-V-Ca-lipoprotein forms and is the prothrombin-activator is not clear. The extrinsic pathway for blood coagulation is that involved in the commonly used prothrombin time. It should be emphasized at this point that the prothrombin time is dependent not only upon the prothrombin level of the plasma but also upon the level of Factors V, VII, IX and fibrinogen.

PROTHROMBIN AND THROMBIN. From studies on purified preparations, the molecular weight of prothrombin has been estimated to be from 62,000 to 70,000 and that of thrombin to be about 30-32,000.[60] Thrombin is a proteolytic enzyme whose primary substrate is fibrinogen, but it also acts on Factors V and VIII, first activating them and then destroying their activity. In addition, it activates Factor XIII. It acts upon fibrinogen by splitting off two polypeptides (fibrinopeptides A and B) by hydrolysis of arginylglycyl linkages. Two A and two B peptides are liberated and one fibrin monomer formed from each molecule of fibrinogen. The fibrin monomers undergo polymerization by means of hydrogen bonding to form fibrin clots which are soluble in 5 molar area or 1 per cent monochloracetic acid. The polymerization depends on conditions such as pH and ionic strength but not on the presence of thrombin. Calcium is not essential for the action of thrombin on fibrinogen or for polymerization but it does affect the rate of these reactions.

FIBRIN-STABILIZING FACTOR. In the presence of calcium, thrombin converts the fibrin-stabilizing factor (Factor XIII) to its active form, a transglutaminase (XIIIa). This enzyme converts the soluble fibrin clot into an insoluble one by a transamidation reaction. Subjects with severe deficiencies of Factor XIII have a bleeding diathesis.

COAGULATION FACTORS IN SERUM. During coagulation of normal blood considerable changes occur in the various clotting factors so that the coagulant activity of plasma and serum are very different. Fibrinogen, of course, is converted to fibrin and is not present in serum. Most of the prothrombin is converted to thrombin and only small amounts remain in serum (0 to 10%). The thrombin formed is neutralized by the antithrombin in plasma and serum so that only tracer amounts persist for any length of time in serum Factors V and VIII, which are activated during clotting, are unstable in their activated state and little if any of their activity persists in serum. Factors VII and IX are also activated, but are relatively stable in this form, so that serum exhibits higher VII and X activity than plasma. Although some Factor X is activated in spontaneous clotting there is little if any difference found in the X activity between serum

and plasma. When blood clots in glass, Factors XII and XI are partially activated and in this state may adhere to surfaces so that the serum may show a loss of their activity. In addition, activated XI is neutralized by a plasma factor so that little activated XI remains in serum. Factor XIII activity of serum is considerably less than that of plasma.

CLOT RETRACTION. A minimal system for clot retraction must contain fibrinogen, intact platelets, thrombin, and magnesium or calcium, all reacting in a solution of appropriate pH and ionic strength. Glucose will enhance the retraction but is not essential with fresh normal platelets. When platelets are stored in vitro, their clot-retracting activity decreases and the loss of activity more or less parallels the loss of platelet ATP. Platelets that have been disrupted or have been repeatedly washed also lose their clot-retracting activity. Removal of calcium and magnesium completely inhibits retraction; inhibition thus caused can be reversed by the addition of either or both of these cations. Platelets have a high content of ATP and during the early phase of retraction there is increased glycolysis and increased ATP production resulting in a rise in ATP concentration. As clot retraction proceeds ATP decreases. Thrombosthenin, the contractile platelet protein, has actomyosin-like ATPase activity, and exhibits physical changes following the addition of ATP in the presence of calcium or magnesium, the same conditions necessary for clot retraction. It is presumed, therefore, that thrombosthenin participates in the retraction process, but must retain specific steric relationship in the cell, because disrupted platelets do not support clot retraction.

INHIBITORS OF COAGULATION. One of the most provocative and as yet unsolved questions concerning coagulation is how the fluidity of the blood is maintained in vivo. No matter how carefully blood is withdrawn and handled, and no matter in what type of container it is stored, if maintained at 37°C it will clot within minutes to several hours. Blood within a carefully isolated vascular segment will show small fibrin clots within 20 to 30 minutes although complete clotting-out of the fibrin may take longer than 8 hours.[67] These findings plus the short in vivo half-life of many of the coagulation factors (Factor VIII 6 to 12 hours, Factor VII 3 to 6 hours, Factor IX 20 to 24 hours, fibrinogen 4 to 5 days, platelets 3 to 4 days)

In the conditions transmitted through a *recessive sex-linked gene abnormality*, for example classical hemophilia and Factor IX deficiency, the disease is seen almost exclusively in males, and the female carriers are usually not symptomatic. The synthesis of Factors VIII and IX depend upon the presence of a gene located in the X chromosome which has no counterpart in the Y chromosome. A hemophilic male inherits an X chromosome from his carrier mother which has the abnormal allele, and from his normal father a normal Y chromosome. Half the male offspring of a union between a normal male and carrier female will inherit the normal X chromosome from the carrier mother and will be normal, and half will inherit the abnormal X chromosome and be hemophiliacs. Half the daughters will be carriers and half will be normal. A hemophilic male married to a normal female will have all normal sons, since they inherit their X chromosome from their mother, but all his daughters will be carriers, since they must inherit his abnormal X chromosome. The union of a female carrier with a hemophiliac male would be expected to produce a true hemophilic female (inheriting an abnormal X chromosome from each parent), a carrier female (abnormal X chromosome from the father and normal X chromosome from the mother), a normal male, and a hemophilic male. The occurrence of true female hemophilia is rare in humans[77] and it may well be that the inheritance of two such abnormal genes may be lethal to the fetus. However, by selective breeding and transfusion therapy Brinkhous and coworkers have been able to produce female hemophiliac dogs by mating carrier females with hemophiliac males. The bleeding manifestations in the females were similar to those seen in the males.[78]

If the average normal level of plasma antihemophilic factor is taken as 100 per cent, the levels among the normal male population are found to vary from about 70 to 150 per cent. Normal females are also found to have levels ranging from 70 to 150 per cent despite the fact that they have two normal X chromosomes and the male only one X chromosome. The antihemophilic factor level in female carriers tends to run lower than that of the normal female or male, varying from 20 to 130 per cent[79,80] with an average of about 60 per cent. It is not clear why the normal female with two X chromosomes and therefore two genes for antihemophilic factor has the same plasma level of this factor as males who have only one X chromosome and therefore only one such gene, whereas the female carrier of hemophilia with one normal gene and one abnormal allele tends to have a lower level than the male. The low level in the female carrier may be due to some modifying genes or it may be due to the production of an inhibitor controlled by the abnormal gene. The Factor VIII levels in both the normal and carrier female in relation to what is present in the normal male could also be explained if only one X chromosome is functional in the female and the other, forming the chromatin body seen on microscopy, is inactive; or the part of the chromosome containing the hemophilic or Factor VIII gene is inactive. Assuming that the X chromosome of a cell slated to be the active one is selected purely by chance, then the levels of Factor VIII found in the plasma of normal and carrier females would be expected. Similar findings for the levels of Factor IX (PTC) in normal females and in carriers have also been reported.[81,82]

In those conditions in which the hereditary pattern is characteristic of recessive or partially *recessive autosomal transmission*, severe hemorrhagic manifestations occur only in the presence of two abnormal genes. The carrier can be either male or female and may have a slight to moderate depression of the level of the coagulation factor in question which may or may not be associated with a mild bleeding tendency. Variation in the carrier state may be due to the variability of the recessiveness or penetrance of the abnormal gene. In these disorders the appearance of the homozygous individual, which would necessarily mean inheriting one abnormal gene from each parent, is frequently associated with consanguinity in the preceding generation. A carrier male or female married to a normal individual can transmit the carrier state to one half of the progeny, whether male or female. All the children of a male or female homozygous for the abnormal gene married to a normal individual will be carriers. Both the parents of a homozygous individual must either be carriers (heterozygous) or one must be a carrier and the other homozygous for the abnormality. There is fairly good evidence that the hereditary deficiencies of Factors XII,[83] XI,[84] X,[85] VII,[86] and V[87] fall into this group. The evidence for hereditary deficiency of prothrombin and fibrinogen belonging to this group is not as good.

In the pattern of *dominant inheritance,* only one abnormal autosomal gene occurring in either sex is necessary for the abnormality to manifest itself. In all probability the homozygous state for the abnormal dominant gene is not compatible with survival of the fetus. The abnormality is transmitted to half the male and female children by the single parent who is heterozygous for the abnormal gene. None of the single congenital coagulation deficien-

cies are inherited by this mode of transmission. In von Willebrand's disease, in which there is a mild Factor VIII deficiency and some vascular abnormality, inheritance appears to be of this type. Since in this syndrome the transmission is not sex linked, it is evident that Factor VIII (antihemophilic factor) synthesis is affected by more than the one gene on the X chromosome. Synthesis must also be affected by a gene on an autosomal chromosome. It would also appear that in this condition one is dealing with a double heterozygosity for a domi-

TABLE 27-4. CLASSIFICATION OF HEMORRHAGIC DISEASES

I. DEFECTIVE COAGULATION—DERANGEMENT IN PLASMA CONSTITUENTS

FIRST PHASE DEFECTS: DEFECTIVE THROMBOPLASTIN FORMATION

Deficiencies of plasma factors involved in intrinsic thromboplastin formation only:
  Factor VIII deficiency
    1. Congenital-hereditary (Classical hemophilia)
    2. Acquired: intravascular coagulation

  Factor IX deficiency
    1. Congenital-hereditary (Christmas disease)
    2. Acquired: vitamin K deficiency, drugs of coumarin and phenylindanedione types, hepatocellular disease, obstructive jaundice, neonatal

  Factor XI (PTA) deficiency
    1. Congenital-hereditary
    2. Acquired: hepatocellular disease, neonatal

Deficiencies of plasma factors involved in both intrinsic and extrinsic thromboplastin formation:
  Factor V deficiency (pseudohypoprothrombinemia)
    1. Congenital-hereditary (parahemophilia)
    2. Acquired: severe hepatocellular disease, severe sepsis, intravascular fibrinolysis or coagulation

  Factor X deficiency (pseudohypoprothrombinemia)
    1. Congenital-hereditary
    2. Acquired: vitamin K deficiency, drugs of coumarin and phenylindanedione type, hepatocellular disease and obstructive jaundice, neonatal

Deficiencies of plasma factors involved in extrinsic thromboplastin formation only:
  Factor VII deficiency (pseudohypoprothrombinemia)
    1. Congenital-hereditary
    2. Acquired: vitamin K deficiency, drugs of coumarin and phenylindanedione type, hepatocellular disease and obstructive jaundice, neonatal

Circulating anticoagulants inhibiting thromboplastin formation:
  Inhibitors of specific coagulation factors
    1. Antifactor VIII
    2. Antifactor IX
    3. Antifactor V
    4. Others

  Nonspecific inhibitors
    1. Acquired: dysproteinemias (hyperglobulinemia, macroglobulinemia, cryoglobulinemia, multiple myeloma, lupus erythematosus)
    2. Drugs (heparin, protamine, polybrene)

SECOND PHASE DEFECTS: DEFECTIVE THROMBIN FORMATION

Factor II (Prothrombin) deficiency
    1. Congenital (hypoprothrombinemia)
    2. Acquired: vitamin K deficiency, drugs of coumarin and phenylindanedione type, hepatocellular disease, and obstructive jaundice, neonatal

TABLE 27-4. CLASSIFICATION OF HEMORRHAGIC DISEASES (*Continued*)

DEFECTIVE COAGULATION—DERANGEMENT IN PLASMA CONSTITUENTS (*Continued*)

Thromboplastin inhibitors
1. Acquired: dysproteinemias (hyperglobulinemia, macroglobulinemia, cryoglobulinemia, multiple myeloma, lupus erythematosus)
2. Drugs: heparin and protamine

THIRD PHASE DEFECTS: DEFECTIVE FIBRIN FORMATION

Hypofibrinogenemia (Factor I deficiency)
Congenital-hereditary
Acquired
1. Decreased production: liver disease, polycythemia vera
2. Increased utilization: intravascular coagulation with defibrination (complication of pregnancy: premature separation of the placenta, intrauterine retention of a dead fetus, amniotic fluid embolism, septic abortion; carcinoma of prostate and stomach; pulmonary and cardiac surgery).
3. Increased destruction: increased fibrinolytic activity (complications of pregnancy as mentioned above: carcinoma of prostate, liver disease, polycythemia vera, leukemia, shock, anoxia, severe exertion, pulmonary and cardiac surgery, secondary to fibrinolytic therapy —streptokinase, plasmin).

Inhibition of thrombin-fibrinogen interaction:
1. Increased antithrombin activity: dysproteinemias, liver disease, products of fibrinogenolysis and fibrinolysis.
2. Drugs: heparin

Circulating anticoagulants directed against fibrinogen

II. DEFECTIVE COAGULATION PLUS VASCULAR ABNORMALITIES

THROMBOCYTOPENIC PURPURA

Megakaryocytic thrombocytopenia:
Conditions in which the life-span of platelets is predominantly reduced
Conditions in which an immune mechanism probably plays a role
1. Idiopathic thrombocytopenia (Werlhof's disease), acute and chronic primary thrombocytopenia
2. Sensitivity to drugs (Sedormid, Phenobarbital, Quinine, Quinidine, Sulfonamides, Penicillin, Chlortrimeton, Benadryl, Antazoline, Thiouracil, Propylthiouracil, organic arsenical compounds, Amidopyrine, Salicylates, Chlorothiazide compounds, Digitoxin, Chlorpropamide, DDT)
3. Infections, (Viral or probably viral: measles, rubella, chicken pox, mumps, cytomegalic inclusion disease, infectious hepatitis, infectious mononucleosis, upper respiratory tract viral infections; bacterial: particularly streptococcal infection but can occur in any bacterial infection; rickettsial: typhus)
4. Thrombotic thrombocytopenia purpura
5. Systemic lupus erythematosus
6. In association with auto-immune hemolytic anemia (Evans syndrome)
7. In lymphoproliferative diseases (chronic lymphatic leukemia, lymphosarcoma)
8. Neonatal thrombocytopenia (In babies born of mothers with idiopathic thrombocytopenia; in erythroblastosis, secondary to isoantibodies formed in the mother to the infant's platelets)

Conditions in which the platelets are sequestered, destroyed or utilized excessively
1. Splenomegaly with hypersplenism (Gaucher's disease, sarcoidosis, tuberculosis, congestive splenomegaly, myeloid metaplasia, lymphosarcoma, amyloidosis)
2. Congenital hemangiomatosis
3. Massive hemorrhage with replacement of blood loss by transfusion of platelet-poor blood
4. Intravascular coagulation

Conditions in which production of platelets is predominantly reduced (megakaryocytes present)
1. Nutritional deficiencies (Vitamin B_{12}, folic acid, ? vitamin C, Kwashiorkor)
2. Infiltration of marrow with abnormal cells (leukemia, metastatic carcinoma, multiple myeloma)
3. Splenomegaly of any cause, particularly congestive splenomegaly
4. Renal failure with severe azotemia
5. Lack of thrombopoetin

TABLE 27-4. CLASSIFICATION OF HEMORRHAGIC DISEASES (*Continued*)

DEFECTIVE COAGULATION PLUS VASCULAR ABNORMALITIES (*Continued*)
Pathogenesis of thrombocytopenia unknown
1. Congenital thrombocytopenia with eczema
2. Onyalai
3. Paroxysmal nocturnal hemoglobinuria

Amegakaryocytic thrombocytopenia:
1. Congenital-hereditary conditions (congenital hypoplastic anemia, Fanconi's anemia, congenital thrombocytopenia with other congenital abnormalities)
2. Aplastic anemia with thymoma
3. Idiopathic aplastic anemia
4. Secondary to drugs, chemicals, or ionizing radiation (nitrogen mustard and related components; antimetabolites such as folic acid antagonists, 6 mercaptopurine; organic solvents such as benzene; arsenicals; gold; mercury; antityroid drugs such as thiouracil; anti-convulsants such as Mesantoin and Tridione; insecticides such as DDT and chlordane; antibiotics such as chloramphenicol and less commonly the tetracyclines; carbutamide; barbiturates; promazines; meprobamate; Pyribenzamine; hair dyes; x-radiation, P32, etc.)
5. Displacement by other cells as in acute leukemia, chronic leukemia, multiple myeloma, myelofibrosis with and without myeloid metaplasia.

QUALITATIVE PLATELET ABNORMALITY PLUS (?) VASCULAR ABNORMALITY:
1. Hereditary hemorrhagic thrombasthenia (Glanzman's disease, thrombocytopathic purpura with impaired clot retraction)
2. Familial thrombocytopathic purpura due to deficiency in platelet factor 3
3. Acquired platelet factor 3 defect or other abnormality of platelets:
   Uremia
   Polycythemia vera
   Myeloid metaplasia
   Primary hemorrhagic thrombocytosis

VASCULAR ABNORMALITY (? DEFICIENCY OF A PLASMA FACTOR) PLUS A PLASMA COAGULATION DEFECT:
1. Vascular hemophilia, von Willebrand's disease, pseudohemophilia: vascular abnormality plus Factor VIII deficiency.
2. Vascular abnormality plus plasma deficiency of coagulation Factors other than VIII (IX, XI, etc.).

III. VASCULAR ABNORMALITIES

HEREDITARY
Hereditary hemorrhagic telangectasia (Rendu-Weber-Osler disease)

ACQUIRED
Vitamin C deficiency—scurvy
Anaphylactoid purpura
1. Idiopathic (Henoch-Schönlein purpura)
2. Secondary to drugs, chemicals and infections (purpura fulminans, Shwartzman reaction)
Probable vascular abnormality: Shamberg's disease, Majocchi's disease.
Purpura associated with hypertension, atherosclerosis, diabetes mellitus, and infections.

IV. CONNECTIVE TISSUE ABNORMALITIES
(VASCULAR AND EXTRAVASCULAR ABNORMALITIES)

HEREDITARY
Ehlers-Danlos syndrome
Osteogenesis imperfecta
Pseudoxanthoma elasticum

ACQUIRED
Pulmonary hemosiderosis

V. PATHOGENESIS UNCERTAIN

Purpura senilis, purpura in Cushing's disease and with corticosteroid therapy, auto-erythrocyte sensitization, auto-DNA sensitization, and other as yet unsolved hemorrhagic disorders which cannot at present be categorized.

nant autosomal gene, one affecting Factor VIII synthesis and another affecting the vasculature.[88] Also typical of this type of dominant inheritance is hereditary hemorrhagic telangiectasia. It is evident from clinical observations in this condition that there is considerable variation in the severity of the syndrome and the distribution of lesions from patient to patient,[71] indicating the variable penetrance of the dominant gene or a number of alleles.

HEMORRHAGIC DISEASES

The clinical and laboratory manifestations of pathologic bleeding depend largely upon which component or components of the hemostatic mechanisms are deranged. The classification of hemorrhagic diseases that occurs in Table 27-4 is intended solely as a guide and is based upon present knowledge of the defects underlying the various disorders. An attempt has been made to classify according to whether the disturbance is of the coagulation mechanism, the vasculature, the supporting tissue, or any combination of these, and as far as possible upon the pathogenesis of these disturbances. While considerable progress has been made in elucidating the pathogenesis of many hemorrhagic states, there are still areas of ignorance and controversy, consequently, certain categories in the classification may be questioned. However, any such classification should be considered flexible and should be altered as new information becomes available so that it remains a useful guide to the differential diagnosis of pathologic bleeding.

CONGENITAL HEREDITARY PLASMA COAGULATION DEFECTS

Hemophilia

Hemophilia was first recognized as a distinct clinical entity in 1803 by Otto,[89] who delineated the conditions governing its transmission. It is now well established, as described above, that hemophilia is transmitted as a sex-linked recessive characteristic, although approximately one third of the cases fail to give a positive family history. It is thought that sporadic cases do arise as a result of mutation of the controlling gene on the X chromosome. It is undoubtedly the occurrence of mutations that maintains the incidence of hemophilia, otherwise one would have anticipated that the incidence would have steadily declined to the point of disappearance of the disease, since relatively few of the males with hemophilia have children. It is of interest that the clinical severity of the disease and of the coagulation defect is approximately the same for all the members of a given family or pedigree. Severe, moderate, and mild cases (see below) do occur, and it has been suggested that such variation may be due to the fact that there are several alleles of the hemophilia gene[90] which result in different degrees of deficiency of the antihemophilic factor. It is also evident from the studies on patients with a vascular defect and varying degrees of antihemophilic factor deficiency that at least one gene on an autosomal chromosome has an effect upon the production of this factor. The true incidence of hemophilia is not known and in the countries where it has been most extensively studied (United States, England, Sweden, France, Switzerland, etc.) the estimated incidence varies from 1 in 10,000 to 20,000, to 1 in 100,000. Hemophilia has been reported in the negroid and mongoloid as well as in the caucasian races.

Hemophilia is due to a deficiency or qualitative abnormality of a single plasma protein, Factor VIII. This protein has been partially purified by a variety of techniques from normal human and animal plasma and has been found to correct the coagulation defect of hemophilia in vitro and in vivo.[91-93] Purification has not progressed to the point at which the protein can be accurately characterized. Although at one time Tocantins[94] and others held that the abnormality in hemophilic blood was due to an excess of a lipid inhibitor, it is now generally accepted that inhibitors are present only in those hemophilics who have developed resistance to the corrective effects of normal plasma or Factor VIII concentrates, and that the inhibitor is an antibody directed against Factor VIII.

That a vascular factor may also play a role in hemophilic bleeding is suggested by the findings that although the Factor VIII plasma level in a given hemophilic shows no significant variations, the ease with which hemorrhage develops varies considerably, from periods of complete freedom even with appreciable trauma, to periods in which only mild trauma will elicit major hemorrhage, or bleeding appears to start spontaneously, frequently at multiple sites. It has also been noted that capillary fragility may be increased at such times. Nevertheless, hemorrhage can be controlled even at such periods, if the circulating Factor VIII level is raised to 30 per cent of normal or above by the administration of plasma or of Factor VIII concentrates. Usually the severity of the clinical manifestations parallels the degree of Factor VIII deficiency. In severe hemophilia, hemorrhagic manifestations are frequent, occurring with minor trauma or spontaneously, the clotting time is markedly prolonged, usually greater than 45 minutes, prothrombin consumption is poor, and the Factor VIII level is less than 1 per cent. In those classified as moderate, the hemorrhagic manifestations are usually less extensive, rarely appear to be spontaneous but occur after mild to moderate trauma, the clotting times vary from normal to prolonged, the prothrombin consumption is almost always impaired, and the Factor VIII level ranges from 1 to 5 per cent of normal. In mild hemophilia, hemorrhage does not occur spontaneously, the abnormal hemostasis usually manifests itself as excessive bleeding only after moderate to severe trauma, the clotting times are almost always in the normal ranges, prothrombin consumption is usually normal, and the Factor VIII level ranges from 5 to 25 per cent of normal.

Clinical Manifestations. Episodic and persistent bleeding from or into various parts of the body constitutes the outstanding clinical feature of hemophilia. Certain areas of the body are particularly susceptible, notably the joints, the subcutaneous tissues, the muscles, and the mucous membranes of the mouth, the nose and the genitourinary tract. Chronic, crippling damage to joints from many repeated episodes of hemorrhage is particularly characteristic of hemophilia.[95-97] Curiously, intracranial bleeding is not as frequent as one might anticipate, probably because the brain is well protected against trauma. Petechiae are not characteristic, but may appear at times at the height of or preceding a bleeding episode. Usually the bleeding follows injury, which frequently is trivial. Sometimes it appears spontaneously, but there is always the possibility that the precipitating trauma may have passed unnoticed. Usually the bleeding is of the persistent oozing type, lasting for days or weeks, although it occasionally may be massive and accompanied by shock.

Hemophilia may be manifest at birth, for the defect is demonstrable in cord blood and occasionally the infant bleeds from injuries sustained at childbirth. Bleeding from the umbilical stump is unusual. The disease may first become evident because of severe bleeding at the time of circumcision although surprisingly some undergo this procedure without difficulty. Hemorrhagic episodes are uncommon during infancy, probably because the infant is not so liable to trauma. However, once the child begins moving around, and particularly when he begins to creep and try to walk, thus subjecting himself to trauma, "unexplained" hematomas may appear and may reach large proportions. Hemorrhagic manifestations are usually most severe during childhood and adolescence when it is difficult to restrict the affected child's activities, since he cannot readily appreciate or accept his abnormalities. If the hemophilic, as he matures, can learn to accept his limitations and if he can adjust his activities accordingly, hemorrhagic episodes are usually less frequent and less severe.

Hemarthrosis generally involves the knees, the elbows, the ankles, the hips and the shoulders, joints which are most subject to trauma. At first, the joint is stiff and painful, but as bleeding continues, it becomes swollen, warm to the touch, and when the capsule is distended, exquisitely tender. There is usually no discoloration around the joint except when subcutaneous ecchymosis is present due to the original trauma. The muscles crossing the joint may be in protective spasm. Bleeding is usually self-limited, arrest of the hemorrhage resulting largely from tamponade. When bleeding stops, the blood within the joint is gradually absorbed and mobility is slowly regained. However, damage to the joint occurs as a result of atrophic changes induced by high intra-articular pressure from the tamponaded blood and by disturbance in blood supply to the joint structure. Once a joint has been the site of hemarthrosis it is more likely to bleed again and with repeated hemorrhage permanent joint deformities occur. Vascular hyperplasia of the synovia and thickening of capsular and pericapsular tissue may develop, resulting eventually in scarring and contracture. The synovial tissues become impregnated with iron and thickened, the cartilages become thin and are invaded by hyperplastic synovial and subsynovial tissues. Cysts form in the subchondral bone due to the destruction of bone by vascular connective tissue. Bony proliferation, lipping, contractures and eventually ankylosis may occur. In children the epiphysial areas may become involved leading to premature closure of the epiphysis and eventual shortening of the bone. Each episode of hemarthrosis imposes an additional burden on both involved and uninvolved parts of the skeletal system. Locomotion becomes difficult, balance is impaired, other joints are subjected to unusual strain, and the likelihood of a new "spontaneous" or traumatic incident is enhanced. The clinical, pathologic and roentgenographic features of hemophilic arthropathy have been extensively reviewed.[95-97]

Intramuscular bleeding may also appear to occur spontaneously or following minor trauma particularly that which causes sudden tension or twisting of a muscle. Crippling often results from destruction of muscle, replacement by fibrous tissue, and subsequent contracture. Bleeding frequently continues until it is stopped by the effect of tamponade and this may result in embarrassment of blood supply to an extremity with subsequent contractures (Volkman's contracture) or gangrene. Paralysis may be produced by pressure on nerve trunks, such as the branches of the femoral plexus. Bleeding retroperitoneally into the psoas muscles may produce symptoms simulating acute appendicitis. Hemorrhage into muscular areas such as the chest wall, the buttock, the neck or the thigh may dissect widely as may retroperitoneal bleeding, resulting in a marked fall in circulating blood volume and shock, or encroachment on such structures as airways, esophagus, and ureters. With the accumulation of blood in muscular areas or in joints, the problem frequently arises whether one should relieve tension by aspiration. This poses a difficult problem to resolve because of the important role tamponade plays in the hemostatic mechanism, especially when clotting is deranged. Each case must be considered individually, but usually aspiration should not be attempted unless a sufficient quantity of plasma or of a potent Factor VIII preparation is available for adequate therapy (i.e., to maintain a Factor VIII level between 20 and 30 per cent of normal) for a period of several days to a week, depending upon the lesion. Hemorrhage into muscle may also result in the formation of cysts which can grow to such size that they become incapacitating.

Bleeding from the mucous membranes is one of the most common and serious hemorrhagic manifestations of hemophilia. The most trivial trauma (e.g. a cut tongue, loss or extraction of deciduous teeth, or trauma from ingestion of a relatively sharp object) can induce persistent oozing which may prove fatal despite all therapeutic measures when the bleeding point is not readily accessible, since the effect of tamponade is not operative in such bleeding. Epistaxis is very common in children. Melena, hematemesis and hematuria occur in about 30 per cent of the cases, are apt to recur and may last from days to weeks. There may be associated local manifestations such as distention, abdominal pain and increased peristalsis, or in case of genitourinary hemorrhage, symptoms of renal colic.

Bleeding into the nervous system probably occurs more frequently than is generally described. Besides hematomas in soft tissues that may compress or damage peripheral nerves, epidural, subdural, subarachnoid hemorrhage or focal bleeding into the central nervous system may occur. Signs and symptoms will depend upon the location and extent of such hemorrhage, and permanent damage of the central nervous system may occur.

LABORATORY. The laboratory abnormalities are confined to alterations of the clotting mechanism of the blood except that bleeding may cause melena, hematuria, anemia, etc. As indicated above, the capillary fragility (tourniquet test) and bleeding times are usually normal. All test procedures which measure the formation of plasma thromboplastin or prothrombinase by the intrinsic mechanism or the overall coagulation via the intrinsic mechanism will be abnormal if the deficiency of Factor VIII is great enough. The tests commonly employed which will reveal this first phase defect are the clotting time, recalcification time, partial thromboplastin time, prothrombin consumption and thromboplastin generation. Each of these tests has a different sensitivity to deficiency of Factor VIII. Thus, although a *prolonged clotting time* is generally considered one of the classical findings in hemophilia, it is a rather insensitive test for Factor VIII deficiency, for it is significantly prolonged only when the Factor VIII level is less than 1 to 2 per cent of normal. It is therefore not surprising that severe hemorrhagic manifestations may occur in a hemophilic with a normal clotting time. The *plasma recalcification time* is somewhat more sensitive

TABLE 27-5. CHARACTERISTIC LABORATORY FINDINGS IN HEMORRHAGIC DISORDERS

DISORDER	CAPILLARY FRAGILITY	BLEEDING TIME	CLOTTING TIME	PROTH.* TIME	PTT†	PROTH. CONSUMP.	TGT‡	STYPVEN TIME	THROMBIN TIME	COAGULATION CORRECTED BY NORMAL			
										PLASMA	ADSORBED PLASMA	SERUM	ADSORBED SERUM
XII Deficiency	Normal	Normal	Long	Normal	Long	Decreased	Abnormal	Normal	Normal	Yes	Yes	Yes	Yes
XI(PTA) Deficiency	Normal	Normal	Long	Normal	Long	Decreased	Abnormal	Normal	Normal	Yes	Yes	Yes	Yes
X(Stuart) Deficiency	Normal	Normal	Long	Long	Long	Decreased	Abnormal	Long	Normal	Yes	No	Yes	No
IX(PTC) Deficiency	Normal	Normal	Long	Normal	Long	Decreased	Abnormal	Normal	Normal	Yes	No	Yes	No
VIII Deficiency Classical Hemophilia	Normal	Normal	Long	Normal	Long	Decreased	Abnormal	Normal	Normal	Yes	Yes	No	No
VII Deficiency	Normal	Normal	Normal	Long	Normal	Normal	Normal	Normal	Normal	Yes	No	Yes	No
V Deficiency	Normal	Variable	Normal-Long	Long	Long	Decreased	Abnormal	Long	Normal	Yes	Yes	No	No
II (Prothrombin) Deficiency	Normal	Normal	?	Long	?	—	? Abnormal	Long	Normal	Yes	No	No	No
I Deficiency (Afibrinogenemia)	Normal	Normal-?Prolong.	Long-Infinite	Long-Infinite	Long-Infinite	Normal	Normal	Long-Infinite	Long-Infinite	Yes	Yes	No	No
Thrombocytopenia	Increased	Prolonged	Normal-Long	Normal	Normal	Decreased	Normal	Normal	Normal	No	No	No	No
von Willebrand Syndrome	Increased-Normal	Prolonged	Normal-Long	Normal	Long	Normal-Decreased	Abnormal	Normal	Normal	Yes	Yes	No	No
Anaphylactoid Purpura	Normal; Occ. Increased	Normal	Normal	Normal	Normal	Normal	Normal	Normal	Normal	—	—	—	—
Fibrinolysis	Normal-Increased	Normal-Prolonged	Normal-Long	Long	Long	Decreased	Abnormal	Normal-Long	Long	Variable			

* Proth. = Prothrombin
† PTT = Partial Prothrombin Time
‡ TGT = Thromboplastin Generation Test

upon the plasma levels of the affected coagulation factors is similar to that of vitamin K-deficiency. Factor VII appears to be the most sensitive and its plasma level falls after coumarin administration before there are significant changes in the levels of the other factors. However, there have been conflicting reports concerning the rate at which the concentration of each of these factors decreases and the extent to which each decreases with the same drug and with different coumarin drugs.[4,131,132] The discrepancies in these reports reflect both the individual variability of the subjects studied and differences in techniques used to determine plasma levels of these factors. It is generally agreed that Factor VII falls more rapidly than any of the other factors, and that prothrombin itself falls more slowly than the other factors, and usually does not decrease to the same extent as Factors VII and X. There is considerable difference of opinion as to how rapidly, and to what extent Factors IX and X fall. In my own experience with the usual therapeutic doses of Dicumarol and Warfarin, Factor IX falls to levels of 20 to 40 per cent within 48 to 72 hours and usually remains at this level with continued therapy. Factor X falls at about the same time and usually reaches levels of 10 to 20 per cent. Factor VII reaches levels of 10 to 20 per cent in 24 to 48 hours, whereas prothrombin usually does not fall below levels of 30 per cent, which is reached on the fourth to fifth day. With prolonged coumarin therapy, although the prothrombin time may not change significantly, the levels of the different coagulation factors may vary considerably and this may account for unexpected bleeding. With excessive doses of anticoagulant and in severe vitamin K-deficiencies all factors may fall to very low levels (0 to 10%).

Hematuria, melena, epistaxis, and easy bruising are the early hemorrhagic manifestations of the hemostatic defect caused by vitamin K-deficiency or coumarin administration. These manifestations may occur when the prothrombin time is 2 to 3 times as long as normal, a prolongation which is considered to be in the therapeutic range for anticoagulant therapy. With more profound alteration in coagulation there may be spontaneous ecchymosis, hematomas, severe gastrointestinal bleeding, bleeding into the central nervous system, hemarthrosis, prolonged bleeding after trauma or menorrhagia. The most charac-

teristic laboratory finding is *prolongation of the prothrombin time.* Since Factor VII is the first coagulation factor to fall, the *prothrombin time is prolonged before alteration of any tests which depend upon the intrinsic clotting mechanism.* With depression of prothrombin, Factors IX and X, the partial thromboplastin time and thromboplastin generation test become abnormal. Whole blood clotting times and recalcification times also become prolonged when these deficiencies are great enough, but these tests are less sensitive than the partial thromboplastin time and thromboplastin generation. The bleeding time is usually normal. However, when there is marked depression of the clotting factors, it becomes prolonged. Whether the prolonged bleeding time is due to the coagulation defect or to an effect upon the vasculature or platelets is not known. Recently it has been demonstrated that platelet adhesiveness is decreased in Dicumarol therapy,[133] and loss of adhesiveness may delay the formation of the platelet plug.

HEMORRHAGIC DISEASE OF THE NEWBORN also represents a deficiency of the vitamin K-dependent coagulation factors. The normal newborn infant, although exhibiting no hemorrhagic diathesis, does have coagulation deficiencies when compared to the adult. At birth prothrombin and Factors VIII, IX and X are only about 30 to 60 per cent of the normal adult levels.[4,134] Factors XI[135] and XII[2] are also reduced, whereas Factor V[136] is elevated. During the first two to three days of life there is normally a further fall in prothrombin and in Factors VII, IX and X and the plasma levels may fall to 10 to 20 per cent of normal. The levels then rise to their original values in about one week, and without supplementary vitamin K it may take 6 to 10 weeks before they reach normal adult levels. There is still some question whether or not vitamin K can accelerate this secondary rise, although there is evidence that the administration of the vitamin will accelerate the recovery from the low values reached on the second or third day. In premature infants even lower plasma levels of these factors are encountered, and vitamin K administration does not accelerate their rise towards normal. The failure of the premature infant to respond to vitamin K and the initial drop in coagulation factors in both the premature and the full term infant are probably due to incomplete development of the enzyme systems necessary for the synthesis of these proteins as well as due to low vitamin K levels in the liver. The higher plasma levels initially seen probably represent passage of these factors from the mother's plasma through the placenta to the infant's circulation. Hemorrhagic disease of the newborn represents an exaggeration of these abnormalities of the clotting mechanism ordinarily found in the asymptomatic newborn. Why these severe defects occur in some newborns is not clear. Certainly they occur when the mother is normal and it is still not certain that administration of vitamin K to the mother prior to delivery will prevent their occurrence.

Symptoms usually appear suddenly upon the second or third day after delivery, at the time when the newborn usually exhibits the greatest alteration in coagulation. However, they may occur at the time of birth. Bleeding is usually not massive but is characterized by persistent oozing from the stump of the umbilical cord, and from mucosal surfaces. Hemoptysis, hematemesis, melena, hematuria, vaginal bleeding and ecchymosis are common. Fatal hemorrhage into the central nervous system, the adrenals, the kidneys, and the liver may occur. The coagulation findings are those described in vitamin K-deficiency or coumarin administration. Unless associated with severe liver disease, the hemorrhagic manifestations and the coagulation defects respond within a matter of hours to vitamin K.

It should be pointed out that administration of *water-soluble vitamin K analogues* (menadione bisulfate, Synkayvite, Hykinone) may cause a *hemolytic anemia* in the infant with resulting kernicterus when given either to the mother shortly before delivery or to the infant. They should therefore be avoided in treating infants. The sensitivity of the infant's red cells to these drugs is due to the low content of glucose-6-phosphate dehydrogenase of these cells. The naturally occurring fat-soluble vitamin K_1 or K_1 oxide does not seem to have this hemolytic effect and probably the newer aqueous colloidal solutions of K_1 (Aqua Mephyton) do not. Therefore, these are the drugs of choice in infants, but overdosage should be avoided. In vitamin K-deficiency in the adult, whether due to malabsorption or dietary deficiency, the water-soluble vitamin K preparations are effective, but they appear to have little or no effect in counteracting the action of Dicumarol and related drugs. Vitamin K_1 and vitamin K_1 oxide intravenously or orally and Aqua Mephyton intravenously or intramuscularly will have a corrective effect within 2 to 3 hours and usually will raise the vitamin K-dependent clotting factors to safe levels within 4 to 12 hours. When very large doses of these preparations are used the patient may become resistant for a considerable period to the action of the coumarinlike drugs.

Deficiencies Associated With Liver Disease. Obstruction of the common duct, or cholangitis which is not associated with extensive parenchymatous liver disease but causes biliary stasis, results in poor absorption of vitamin K and of deficiency of the vitamin K-dependent clotting factors only. Such deficiencies respond to vitamin K administration. Extensive hepatocellular disease may also result in a marked deficiency of these clotting factors because there is inability to utilize vitamin K. However, other clotting factors may also be depressed, depending upon the severity of liver impairment. Factor V[74] and Factor XI[76] are frequently decreased and less frequently fibrinogen may be decreased. A progressive fall in Factor V is an ominous prognostic sign and a rise in Factor V frequently heralds the recovery phase of severe hepatitis. Occasionally, increased fibrinolytic activity is evident, but this usually is rather mild and not persistent. Not infrequently in viral hepatitis and more frequently in cirrhosis of the liver there may be an associated thrombocytopenia. Although the cause of this thrombocytopenia is not known, it apparently is not due directly to any alteration of liver function, but is related in cirrhosis to the associated congestive splenomegaly and in viral hepatitis to some extrahepatic effect of or reaction to the virus. A qualitative change in the platelets (a decrease in platelet factor 3 activity) has been reported in cirrhosis but this has not been confirmed. In addition to the depression of coagulation factors, a circulating anticoagulant or inhibitor may be present which interferes with the thrombin-fibrinogen reaction and may also interfere with thromboplastin generation.[137] In parenchymal liver disease, in contrast to biliary obstruction, there is little or no improvement of the coagulation defects after the administration of vitamin K.

Circulating Anticoagulants. Circulating anticoagulants may be defined as "abnormal endogenous components of blood which inhibit the coagulation of normal blood."[138] In general they may be divided into two groups, one group in which the inhibitor is directed against a specific coagulation factor and appears to destroy the activity of this factor; and a second group in which the inhibitor blocks or interferes with one of the reactions of coagulation but is not directed against a specific coagulation factor. Anticoagulants have been described against every clotting factor and against several of the recognized intermediary steps of coagulation. In addition, there are numerous case reports in which a circulating anticoagulant has been demonstrated, but its mode of action not identified. The hemorrhagic manifestations which are seen depend upon the level of the circulating anticoagulant and to some extent the nature of the anticoagulant. Inhibitors which are directed against a single specific clotting factor produce the type of bleeding seen in hereditary deficiencies of these factors.

ANTICOAGULANTS DIRECTED AGAINST A SPECIFIC CLOTTING FACTOR. Perhaps the most frequently encountered acquired anticoagulant is that directed against the antihemophilic factor. This type has been observed in four groups of patients: (1) patients with classical hemophilia; (2) women who develop a bleeding disorder resembling hemophilia within a year postpartum; (3) middle aged or elderly men and women with no history of hemophilia or any other hemorrhagic diathesis and in whom no other disease process can be found; and (4) middle aged or elderly men and women with no previous history of a hemorrhagic tendency but who have some other pathologic process. In this last group the anticoagulant has appeared after penicillin reactions, in the course of lupus erythematosus, rheumatoid arthritis, tuberculous adenopathy, and various dysproteinemias. The anticoagulants in these various groups of patients cannot be distinguished by their action or physiochemical characteristics.

The incidence of circulating anticoagulant in classical hemophilia has in various reports ranged from 0 to 21%. The true incidence is probably between 5 to 10%. Although the occurrence of this type of anticoagulant is almost entirely in the severe hemophilic, it has been reported in mild hemophilics also. The mechanism of the development of this type of anticoagulant is not known, but it is seen almost always in patients who have had repeated transfusions and therefore it has been considered by many as a result of such therapy. In favor of this concept is the observation that the titer of anticoagulant activity in a number of cases rose after transfusion and gradually decreased when transfusion therapy was withheld. These findings of course suggest that the anticoagulant activity is exerted by an antibody directed against Factor VIII, which can perhaps be considered a foreign protein to the hemophilic person. It has now been definitely established that these inhibitors are immunoglobulins and in almost all cases studied they have been identified as 7S (IgG) immunoglobulins.

The severity of the hemorrhagic manifestations usually does not increase or change in character with development of an inhibitor in the hemophilic. However, *transfusion becomes ineffective*, since it no longer corrects the clotting defect. In vitro it can also be demonstrated that the amounts of normal plasma which are usually sufficient to correct the clotting defect in classical hemophilia have little or no corrective effect upon clotting and recalcification times, prothrombin consumption, partial thromboplastin times and thromboplastin generation tests. When the inhibitor activity is sufficiently high, the patient's blood will inhibit the clotting of normal blood. Incubation of the patient's plasma with normal plasma destroys the Factor VIII activity of the latter. All coagulation factors other than Factor VIII are present in the patient's plasma at normal levels. Prothrombin times and thrombin times remain normal. If the anticoagulant is present in high titer when severe hemorrhage occurs, the usual transfusion therapy is ineffective and in order to get even transient restoration of hemostasis, it may be necessary to use exchange transfusions or very large amounts of Factor VIII-rich plasma fractions. Corticosteroids and ACTH are of questionable value even in large doses. The titer of inhibitor may gradually drop over the course of months or years and the patient again becomes responsive to transfusion therapy but in many instances the titer rises following such therapy.

Although the Factor VIII inhibitor which appears in nonhemophilics has the same physiochemical characteristics there is considerable variation in the clinical course. If women who develop such an inhibitor following pregnancy survive the initial hemorrhagic episode, the inhibitor gradually disappears. It does not seem to be increased by transfusion therapy and in at least one instance it did not recur following a subsequent pregnancy.[138] The anticoagulant which makes its appearance following a penicillin reaction also may not be increased in titer by transfusion therapy and usually disappears within the relatively short time of three to six months. In some previously normal individuals and in patients with a chronic disease process, the level of the inhibitor may remain elevated with little variation for months and years, whereas in other persons there may be significant improvement, with disappearance of the inhibitor.

The incidence of the development of an inhibitor in patients with Factor IX deficiency is probably about the same as that in classical hemophilia, however in these individuals the anticoagulant is directed against Factor IX. All the other coagulation factors are normal. The inhibitor again appears to be related to transfusion therapy since the titer rises after transfusion and gradually decreases when transfusions are withheld.[138,143] It is of interest that it is rare to find this type of inhibitor appearing in patients without pre-existing Factor IX deficiency, which is in contrast to the inhibitor of Factor VIII.

Anticoagulants directed against Factors V, VII, XI and fibrinogen have been reported but these are extremely rare and in most instances have occurred in patients with a pre-existing deficiency of the factor against which the anticoagulant is directed. The hemorrhagic manifestations are those seen in the corresponding deficiency state.

ANTICOAGULANTS DIRECTED AGAINST A REACTION IN COAGULATION. Of the inhibitors which appear to be directed at a reaction in coagulation rather than against a specific factor, an *inhibitor of thromboplastin or prothrombinase* is the most common. This occurs most frequently in disseminated lupus erythematosus but is also seen in other collagen diseases and occasionally in patients with abnormal plasma proteins (macroglobulin, cryoglobulin, and hypergammaglobulinemia). The hemorrhagic manifestations are usually mild, but ecchymosis, hematuria, bleeding from mucous membranes and menorrhagia have been reported. The most characteristic laboratory finding is a prolonged prothrombin time, particularly with diluted thromboplastin, in the presence of normal levels of all known clotting factors. In most cases the clotting time is only slightly to moderately prolonged, but the recalcification time of platelet-poor plasma is markedly prolonged.[138,144,145] The exact nature or mechanism of action of this type of anticoagulant is not known. Some patients with systemic lupus have in addition a significant decrease of prothrombin without other evidence of liver disease.

An anticoagulant which *inhibits the action of thrombin on fibrinogen* has been reported in liver disease and in patients with either hypergammaglobulinemia or abnormal plasma proteins as seen in multiple myeloma. The characteristic finding is a prolonged thrombin time which can be shortened by the addition of calcium or protamine in concentration greater than that needed to neutralize heparin.[138,146,147] This inhibitory activity has been referred to as antithrombin V. The mechanism of action is not known. As discussed above, the products of fibrinolysis also produce prolonged thrombin times and although this is frequently referred to as an antithrombin VI, the inhibition is against the polymerization of fibrin rather than the action of thrombin.

Although a number of reports have appeared describing *heparinlike* anticoagulants, it is doubtful that any of these cases, with the exception of one, represent true hyperheparinemia.[138,148] Since heparin is known to interfere with all three phases of coagulation, the characteristic findings should include prolonged clotting times, prothrombin times, and thrombin times. The clotting abnormality should be corrected both in vivo and in vitro by protamine, toluidine blue, or polybrene. However, in interpreting the results, it must be borne in mind that protamine in concentrations higher than that necessary to neutralize heparin will shorten the thrombin time of normal blood or of blood with nonheparin inhibitors of the thrombin-fibrinogen reaction as well as that of heparinized blood.

THROMBOCYTOPENIA

Thrombocytopenia is probably the most common cause of pathologic bleeding encountered by the physician. The characteristic hemorrhagic manifestations are a reflection of the unique role of platelets in hemostasis, particularly in relation to the small blood vessels. The platelets, by a mechanism that is not understood, contribute to the maintenance of the integrity and strength of these vessels. Platelets are also involved in the first response to injury of a vessel, that is platelet massing at the site of injury followed by formation of the platelet plug, which by itself is sufficient to control bleeding from small arterioles and capillaries. It is therefore not surprising that the most characteristic hemorrhagic lesions in thrombocytopenia are petechiae, which are due to rupture of or bleeding from the smallest arterioles or the arterial end of the capillary loop. Although the platelets also play a very important role in coagulation, large ecchymoses, hematomas and hemarthroses, so common in coagulation deficiencies, are usually not present except in the most severe cases. Two classical findings in thrombocytopenia, increased capillary fragility and prolonged bleeding time, are manifestations of the loss of platelet function in small blood vessels, and are usually not present in coagulation deficiency states.

In general, no matter what the etiology of the thrombocytopenia, the hemorrhagic manifestations are the same. Petechiae may be widely distributed but are most apt to occur in dependent areas, in areas overlying bony structures and in the mucous membranes of the mouth. These lesions are usually not palpable nor do they have an associated erythema as is noted in anaphylactoid purpura. Bleeding from mucous membranes is very frequent (epistaxis, gingival bleeding, bleeding into the gastrointestinal tract, and hematuria), although massive hemorrhage rarely occurs. In women there is usually a history of prolonged and profuse menses. Ecchymoses may occur without obvious trauma and prolonged and excessive bleeding from abrasions or minor lacerations is generally noted. In severe cases hemorrhagic blisters frequently appear on the mucous membranes of the lips, the mouth, the tongue, the nose and the pharynx. Intracranial bleeding is not common (particularly in children) and is most apt to occur in patients with associated aplastic anemia and acute leukemia. The typical laboratory findings are a prolonged bleeding time, increased capillary fragility, normal clotting time, poor prothrombin consumption and poor clot retraction. However, since all the plasma clotting factors are usually normal, there is normal partial thromboplastin time, prothrombin time and thrombin time. The diagnosis of thrombocytopenic purpura rests upon demonstrating a decreased number of platelets in the peripheral blood. Bleeding and derangement in coagulation rarely occurs until the platelets fall below 75,000 per cubic mm. Below this level there is no strict correlation between the severity of the clinical picture and the platelet level, although in general the lower the platelet count, the more severe the bleeding tendency. This suggests that other factors beside the number of platelets must play a role in the pathogenesis of purpuric bleeding. In some types of thrombocytopenia there may well be vascular damage due to antibody-antigen reaction or by abnormal proteins. There is also evidence that there may be qualitative differences in platelets in thrombocytopenia which could account, at least in part, for the clinical variability.[149]

Thrombocytopenia can occur in a large variety of conditions, many of which appear to have little in common except a decrease in the number of circulating platelets. Since the prognosis and therapy are often dependent upon the pathogenesis of the thrombocytopenia or at least upon the associated pathologic process, it is of importance for the physician to investigate the pathogenesis thoroughly. Any meaningful classification of the conditions which may be associated with or produce thrombocytopenia is limited by our inadequate knowledge of the mechanisms involved. However, a logical approach can be made by starting with the simple concept that the numerical level of circulating platelets will depend upon the rate of production of platelets versus the rate of destruction of platelets. Since the megakaryocytes of the bone marrow are the primary site for the production of circulating platelets, the initial consideration is the status of the megakaryocytes in the bone marrow. This can be determined from bone marrow aspiration or biopsy. Thrombocytopenic states can thus be classified into two major groups: (1) amegakaryocytic, and (2) megakaryocytic. In addition, the marrow may show abnormalities which point to a definitive diagnosis which may or may not have been suspected, such as leukemia, metastatic carcinoma, myeloma, Gaucher's disease, folic acid or vitamin B_{12} deficiency, etc.

Amegakaryocytic Thrombocytopenia. In amegakaryocytic thrombocytopenia decreased production of platelets is the major cause of the thrombocytopenia, although increased destruction of platelets may play a minor role. The hypoplasia of the megakaryocytes may be congenital or acquired, the latter being much more frequent.

The *congenital variety* may show a marked reduction of megakaryocytes without disturbance of other bone marrow elements. This type is sometimes associated with absence of the radii.[150] More frequently there is also hypoplasia of the myeloid and erythroid elements and sometimes this type is also associated with other congenital abnormalities (Fanconi syndrome).[151] It is of particular importance to differentiate the amegakaryocytic from the megakaryocytic type in infants since the prognosis and treatment are significantly different.

The *acquired form* is most frequently due to replacement of the marrow tissue with abnormal cells (leukemia, myeloma, etc.) with crowding out of the normal elements or to a generalized hypoplasia of the bone marrow secondary to chemicals, medications, or irradiation. The agents which have been reported to induce such changes are listed in Table 27-4. The sensitivity of individuals to these agents varies considerably. In some persons the same chemicals and drugs may produce thrombocytopenia by a different mechanism, that is, by peripheral destruction of the platelets, without hypoplasia. This will be discussed later. Idiopathic aplastic anemia with hypoplasia of the marrow is almost always associated with thrombocytopenia. Not infrequently in aplastic anemia it is the hemorrhagic complications which cause death.

Megakaryocytic Thrombocytopenia. The megakaryocytic type of thrombocytopenia may result from a variety of pathogenic mechanisms but they all cause the thrombocytopenia either by decreasing production of platelets or by increasing their peripheral destruction or both. A classification of megakaryocytic thrombocytopenia on this basis certainly has more logic and is more useful than the older classification of idiopathic and secondary or symptomatic thrombocytopenia. Cohen *et al.*[23] have proposed such a classification based on the life span of platelets determined by the Cr^{51} labeling technique. From their studies they divided cases of thrombocytopenia into three broad groups: (1) those that had a normal platelet survival and reduced production; (2) those with predominantly decreased production but with some decrease in life span; and (3) those in which shortened survival predominated but decreased production might be present. Since the division between the first and second groups and the second and third groups may be somewhat arbitrary, it is perhaps more useful clinically to divide the thrombocytopenias into two groups depending on whether the major factor is shortened survival or decreased production.

FACTORS REGULATING NUMBER OF CIRCULATING PLATELETS

Little is actually known concerning the normal regulatory mechanism determining the number of circulating platelets. Evidence indicates that many factors are involved.

Plasma Factor. Shulman *et al.*[19] have described a plasma factor which promotes megakaryocytic maturation and platelet production in an orderly and sequential manner. Lack of this factor can be responsible for thrombocytopenia in the presence of megakaryocytes in the bone marrow. This factor is apparently distinct from erythropoietin and has been referred to as thrombopoietin. A lack of this factor has so far been described in only one case and studies indicate that it is present in normal or excessive levels in the plasma of patients with so-called idiopathic thrombocytopenia and in patients with thrombocytosis.

Folic acid deficiency and vitamin B_{12} deficiencies are frequently associated with thrombocytopenia. Megakaryocytes are either somewhat decreased or normal in number in the marrow. Cohen and Gardner[23] have found normal survival of platelets in such patients, indicating that folic acid and B_{12} are essential for normal production. Treatment with folic acid or B_{12} will result in restoration of platelet levels to normal. Vitamin C has also been implicated in platelet production, particularly in relation to folic acid metabolism.[152]

Hormones seem to have an effect upon platelet levels which is probably related to platelet production rather than destruction. In normal women there is usually a slight to moderate fall in circulating platelets during the last two weeks of the menstrual cycle and a rapid return to normal after the onset of menses.[153] Whether or not this is related to changes in the levels of estrogens, progesterone or FSH is not known. A few cases of cyclic thrombocytopenia occurring in women at the time of the menses have been reported.[154,155] Corticosteroids and ACTH may also produce an increase in platelets when administered to patients without thrombocytopenia. What role they play in the normal regulatory mechanism is not known.

The role of the spleen still remains an enigma. An old observation that has been confirmed countless times is that following splenectomy for reasons other than thrombocytopenia, the platelet count rises above normal levels and remains elevated for weeks to months or even for years. This may also occur after splenectomy for "idiopathic" thrombocytopenia, and it is not unusual to find the platelets rising to levels three to five times normal within a week to ten days after splenectomy, and the patient, who but a few days before was having serious hemorrhagic manifestations, now suffers from thromboembolic phenomena. Although any surgical procedure may be followed by a moderate increase in circulating platelets, persistence of thrombocytosis for more than a few days occurs only after splenectomy. The effect of splenectomy can be interpreted as evidence either that the spleen has an inhibitory effect upon platelet production or that the spleen removes platelets from the peripheral blood by a process similar to its action in regard to red cells. Thrombocytopenia might therefore result from an increase in splenic activity regardless of which of these interpretations is correct. Studies indicate that under certain circumstances the spleen, at least when enlarged, does have an inhibitory effect upon platelet production. In rats fed methyl cellulose splenomegaly is induced and thrombocytopenia occurs. It has been shown that under these circumstances there is no change in the life span of the platelets, indicating a reduced production as the cause of the thrombocytopenia. In such animals, splenectomy results in a thrombocytosis even greater than that seen in splenectomized normal animals.[156] Cohen and Gardner[23] have found that in thrombocytopenia associated with congestive splenomegaly caused by portal hypertension the platelet survival time is only slightly reduced, whereas production is significantly reduced. Thus the thrombocytopenia would appear to be due in large part to a decrease in platelet production, possibly caused by a humoral factor produced in the chronically congested spleen. Relief of portal hypertension by portacaval shunt without splenectomy is almost always followed by a rise in the platelet count.[157] The role of

the spleen in platelet survival in normal persons is far from clear. Controversy still exists as to whether most platelets are removed from the blood stream by the spleen as they become senescent, as suggested by some platelet survival data,[20,22,25] or are utilized in a random manner in hemostasis as is suggested by the curvilinear survival curves reported by others.[21,23,24] That thrombocytopenia may result from increased utilization of platelets in intravascular coagulation has been demonstrated in animals and also is evident in certain clinical syndromes. It has also been shown that excessive platelet loss, as produced by plateletphoresis in animals[158] or by severe hemorrhage in man treated with a large volume of bank blood containing nonviable platelets,[159] will result in thrombocytopenia when the capacity of the bone marrow to produce platelets is exceeded, and that such thrombocytopenia may persist for three to four days after platelet loss stops and then the platelet count begins to rise. It is therefore evident that continued sequestration or destruction of platelets, by whatever means, can induce a severe thrombocytopenia and can also result in secondary decrease in platelet production due to bone marrow exhaustion. The thrombocytopenia which occurs in patients with giant hemangiomas is thought to be due to sequestration and destruction of the platelets within the abnormal vessels. Destruction of platelets results from intravascular coagulation within the hemangioma. In such cases splenectomy, corticosteroids and ACTH are ineffective and only a decrease in size of the hemangioma by surgery, radiation or spontaneous regression results in a rise in the number of circulating platelets.[160] In many seemingly unrelated thrombocytopenias it has been suggested that increased sequestration or destruction of platelets occurs in the spleen[161] with splenomegaly such as is seen in Gaucher's disease, sarcoid, lymphoproliferative syndromes, tuberculosis, etc. It has been postulated that hyperplasia or abnormality of the reticuloendothelial system causes an increase in this activity of the spleen, and that in "idiopathic" thrombocytopenia it occurs for some unknown reason. More recent developments would indicate that when increased destruction of platelets takes place in any of these conditions there may be more than one mechanism, and that a similar mechanism may be operative in different pathologic processes. Evidence has accumulated to indicate that thrombocytopenia may be of immunological origin in many of these cases and that the spleen may play a role both in production of platelet antibodies and in clearing the blood of platelets which have been coated with an antibody.

Immunologic origin of thrombocytopenia has been definitely proved in certain types of thrombocytopenia and there is suggestive and controversial evidence in others. In drug-induced megakaryocytic thrombocytopenia (Sedormid, quinine, quinidine, etc.) it has been demonstrated that an antibody exists in the plasma which in the presence of the offending drug and platelets will fix complement and lyse platelets, and when complement is not present will agglutinate platelets in vitro. The evidence indicates that the drug acts as a hapten-forming complex with a plasma protein to which the body reacts with the formation of an antibody. When the drug is added to the platelet-rich plasma or enters the blood stream of a sensitized individual a hapten-antibody complex is formed between the drug and the antibody which is non-specifically adsorbed onto the platelet surface. Complement is fixed to the platelet in this reaction. Adsorption of the complex alters the platelet so that it is lysed or removed from the circulation. In *in vitro* studies it has been demonstrated that the hapten-antibody complex is adsorbed onto normal platelets as well as onto platelets obtained from the sensitized subject. When the offending drug is given to a sensitized person with circulating antibody there is a marked fall in circulating platelets within an hour, indicating a peripheral destruction of platelets.[162,163] Recovery usually follows in these cases within one week following removal of the responsible agent.

It has long been known that blood platelets are isoantigenic. Serum antibodies which react with platelets have been demonstrated in patients who have received multiple blood transfusions and in multiparous women.[164,165,167] Plasma or blood from these individuals can produce acute thrombocytopenia in appropriate recipients. The demonstration of isoantibodies by the usual immunologic techniques (agglutination, antihuman globulin consumption, indirect Coombs, and complement fixation) in patients receiving multiple transfusions is rather low (3 per cent to 14 per cent, probably because these techniques are relatively insensitive. Recent studies on platelet survival by the Cr^{51} labeling technique after repeated transfusions of platelets into normal recipients indicate a much higher incidence of platelet antibody formation, as demonstrated by decreased survival times.[167,23] Such shortened survival times are found in the absence of positive results with the usual immunologic tests. How many platelet groups actually exist still remains controversial. At least two major antigen systems have been identified and probably more exist.[168] It has been definitely established that neonatal thrombocytopenic purpura, which occurs in otherwise normal children of healthy mothers, can be caused by maternal antibodies formed against fetal platelets.

Shulman[166] *et al.* have also presented evidence that an isoantibody provoked by mismatched platelet transfusion may destroy platelets in the sensitized individual. The mechanism suggested is that foreign platelet antigen survives in vivo longer than the period of antibody induction and that antibody, complexed with foreign antigen, is adsorbed by autologous platelets making them more susceptibile to processes of in vivo sequestration. It is also possible that antigen-antibody complexes in which the antigen is not related to platelets may induce thrombocytopenia since it has been demonstrated that adsorption of such complexes by platelets is a common immunologic phenomenon.[169] At present there is no definite evidence to indicate that this mechanism is involved in thrombocytopenic purpura.

In many thrombocytopenic states an immunologic process is suspected as the underlying mechanism. Supportive evidence for such a mechanism in "idiopathic" thrombocytopenia has been the demonstration that plasma from a fairly high percentage of such cases (40 per cent to 70 per cent) when transfused into a normal individual will induce thrombocytopenia in the recipient within the course of an hour or two.[164] Such reactions may also occur from plasma of patients with thrombocytopenia in the course of systemic lupus erythematosus and lymphatic leukemia. The spleen is not essential for the production of thrombocytopenia under these circumstances, but the evidence indicates that it is one of the areas of sequestration and destruction of the platelets in the recipient. The data that have been reported on the presence of platelet antibodies in the serum or plasma of patients with thrombocytopenia other than that due to drug sensitivity or in patients who have had multiple transfusions have been confusing and contradictory.

Harrington[170] and Tullis[171] using different techniques have reported positive tests for circulating antiplatelet antibodies in 50 to 60 per cent of patients with idiopathic thrombocytopenic purpura (ITP). However, as pointed out by Cohen et al.,[23] these two techniques frequently give conflicting results in a given patient and are often negative in cases of idiopathic thrombocytopenia in which platelet life span is markedly reduced. Others[172] have not been able to demonstrate platelet antibodies in ITP by immunologic techniques. Despite these rather disappointing results of immunologic techniques to demonstrate conclusively presence of platelet antibodies, the concept of an immunologic mechanism as the cause of thrombocytopenia in megakaryocytic thrombocytopenia with increased platelet destruction has continued to gain popularity. More recently Karpatkin et al.[170a] have reported a technique for identification of antibodies against platelets in patients with ITP. This work has as yet not been confirmed by others.

IDIOPATHIC THROMBOCYTOPENIA

At the present time this term refers to a thrombocytopenia which cannot be attributed to or associated with some other disease process. Characteristically, the marrow contains adequate or increased numbers of megakaryocytes, the spleen is not palpable, and the patient's symptoms are limited to manifestations of the bleeding tendency. Idiopathic thrombocytopenic purpura as defined above undoubtedly encompasses more than one disease entity or etiology. Although the platelet survival time is very short in most such cases, some cases have been shown to have normal platelet survival time,[23,164] indicating different mechanisms (decreased production) for the thrombocytopenia in patients who appear similar clinically. The thrombocytopenia-producing agent is not present in the plasma of all cases. Thrombocytopenia indistinguishable clinically from the idiopathic type may be the first manifestation of systemic lupus erythematosus.[174] The thrombocytopenia which occurs following measles, rubella, mumps, chickenpox, or infectious mononucleosis is very similar to the so-called acute form of idiopathic thrombocytopenia in the abruptness of onset, sex distribution, and the limited duration of

a few weeks or months. Since many cases of "acute idiopathic" thrombocytopenia do occur after upper respiratory infections, particularly in children, it is questionable whether or not there is any significant difference between such cases and those that occur after known viral infections. In all of these instances the thrombocytopenia may be secondary to sensitization of the platelets to sequestration by the absorption of antigen-antibody complexes to the platelet surface.

Clinically two types of idiopathic thrombocytopenic purpura are recognized, the acute and chronic forms. The *acute* form is characterized by an abrupt onset without previous history of a bleeding tendency, equal sex distribution, greater frequency in children and young adults, and spontaneous recovery in a few weeks to six months. When thrombocytopenia persists for longer than six months, the case is usually classified as chronic. However, the usual *chronic* type is characterized by a more gradual onset of hemorrhagic manifestations so that the patient may have a history of easy bruising, excessive bleeding after dental extraction, or menorrhagia dating back for several months or years before the appearance of purpura. This form is characterized by remission and exacerbation. The remissions are rarely complete, the platelet counts returning to 50 to 60 per cent of normal, which is usually sufficient to correct the hemostatic defect, and the relapses vary in severity. In contrast to the acute form, the chronic form occurs more commonly in females (3:2 to 3:1) and in adults. The distinction between acute and chronic is not always evident at the time a patient is first seen, since a chronic case may start out acutely and a relapse in a chronic case may give as severe hemorrhagic manifestations as those seen in the acute forms. The response of both the acute and the chronic forms to various types of therapy is not predictable from the clinical course. Although the acute form usually goes into complete remission spontaneously, a remission may be induced much sooner with corticosteroids or splenectomy. However, both of these forms of therapy may fail. In the chronic form response to corticosteroid therapy and splenectomy is also variable, and in a certain percentage of cases (this varies in the different series reported from 10 to 30 per cent), relapse occurs after an initial response to splenectomy or corticosteroids. Patients who fail to respond to steroids may respond to splenectomy and the reverse may also occur. The variability of the clinical course, and the varied response to therapy in ITP are further indications that this is *not a single disease entity, and that there is more than one pathogenic mechanism.* Although ITP is frequently referred to as autoimmuned thrombocytopenia, it should be pointed out that at the present time there is no substantiating evidence for this concept, since the evidence for platelet antibodies in any of these cases, as discussed above is still controversial. The occurrence of thrombocytopenia in other diseases considered as autoimmuned, such as systemic lupus erythematosus and autoimmuned hemolytic anemia, does lend weight to this concept as one cause of ITP.

It should be pointed out that *neonatal thrombocytopenia* occurs in about half the newborn infants of mothers who have idiopathic thrombocytopenic purpura or who have had a remission subsequent to splenectomy; whereas it does not occur if the mother has had a spontaneous remission.[164,175] Hemorrhagic phenomena are most pronounced in the first few days of life and then decrease as the platelet count usually starts rising, however it may not reach normal levels for two to three months.

Thrombotic Thrombocytopenic Purpura

This syndrome, first described by Moschcowitz,[176] is characterized by the triad of thrombocytopenia, hemolytic anemia, and transient bizarre neurologic signs and symptoms. The majority of cases have an abrupt onset and a rapid downhill course, death occurring within one to six weeks. Only recently have a few chronic cases been reported. The purpuric manifestations are the same as those of any severe thrombocytopenia. The bone marrow has many megakaryocytes, and platelet survival is probably very short. The cause of the short platelet life span is obscure. It is probably not due to the utilization of the platelets in the multiple small vessel thrombi seen in this disease, as was originally postulated. These thrombi appear to be composed primarily of fibrin with little platelet material as determined by immunofluorescent technique.[177] The initial lesion is in all probability a vascular one involving the small arterioles and is characterized by a proliferation of the vascular endothelium and an infiltration of the vascular wall with a homogeneous acidophilic fibrinoid material, with little or no inflammatory reaction. The thrombi are thought to occur secondary to the vascular lesion, since they are found in relation to changes in the vessel, whereas vascular lesions can be seen in the absence of thrombosis.[178] The purpuric manifestations are due to the thrombocytopenia. However, the neurologic abnormalities are usually due to the occlusive vascular lesions in the brain rather than to hemorrhage into the brain. So far no platelet antibodies have been identified, nor has a thrombocytopenia-producing factor been identified in the plasma of such patients.

The anemia seen in this disease is moderate to severe and is characterized by normochromic normocytic red cells, increase in reticulocytes, increase in serum bilirubin, shortened life span of the red cells, and in most cases a negative Coombs test. The bone marrow in addition to having numerous megakaryocytes, shows erythroid hyperplasia. The cause of the hemolysis is not known.

The etiology of the complex syndrome remains unknown. It has been suggested that thrombotic thrombocytopenia may represent (1) an autoimmuned process involving platelets, red cells and vascular endothelium; (2) a Shwartzman-like phenomenon in the human; (3) a hypersensitivity reaction to an infectious agent or drug; (4) a variation of systemic lupus erythematosus.

Qualitative Platelet Abnormalities

Qualitative abnormalities of platelets occur both on a congenital and an acquired basis and may be associated with hemorrhagic manifestations. Considerable confusion has arisen, particularly concerning the congenital variety, because of the indiscriminate nomenclature used in the literature and because of a multitude of new techniques for testing platelet aggregation, adhesiveness, and PF3 "release". However, the qualitative platelet disorders can be divided into two major groups: Thrombasthenia, and Thrombocytopathy or "Thrombopathia".

Thrombasthenia, first described by Glanzmann, is a hereditary platelet disorder characterized by poor to absent clot retraction. The hemorrhagic manifestations are easy bruising, excessive bleeding after surgical procedures, epistaxis, menorrhagia, and bleeding gums. The bleeding time is prolonged. Blood clotting other than impaired clot retraction is normal. The platelets appear normal by light microscopy and are present in normal numbers in the peripheral blood. There appears to be a defect in the platelet membrane so that it does not respond to external stimuli that ordinarily produce important changes in normal platelets. Although these platelets do adhere normally to collagen and connective tissue and under this stimulus release serotonin and ADP normally, they do not respond by aggregation to this released ADP or to added ADP. Nor do they aggregate to agents that operate through the ADP mechanism such as thrombin, epinephrine and serotonin. This failure to respond to aggregating agents may be the basis of the impaired hemostasis. Following exposure to connective tissue or thrombin, platelet factor 3 is available in normal or somewhat reduced amounts but not sufficiently decreased to significantly interfere with the development of prothrombin activator. These platelets fail to adhere normally to glass. Their thrombosthenin content seems to be normal. The platelet fibrinogen content has been reported as reduced, although the plasma fibrinogen is normal. Whether or not the low platelet fibrinogen is related to the poor clot retraction and the failure of ADP-induced aggregation remains to be determined. Reduced levels of enzymes in the glycolytic pathway have been reported in some patients. Such abnormalities would result in decreased production of ATP, thus interfering with the energy necessary for clot retraction. However, these enzyme deficiencies are not present in all patients studied.

Thrombopathia may well refer to a conglomerate of inherited or acquired platelet abnormalities. However, at this time, one can characterize the abnormality as follows: the patients present with a mild bleeding disorder manifested by spontaneous or easy bruising, mild epistaxis, and a variable history of excessive bleeding following surgery. The bleeding time is prolonged, clot retraction is normal, the platelet count is normal, and the platelets appear morphologically normal by light microscopy. Platelet adhesion to connective tissue or collagen is normal to impaired, but the characteristic reaction is failure of release of ADP under these conditions or under the stimulation of thrombin and epinephrine. This results in impaired aggregation by these agents. The platelets aggregate normally with ADP. After exposure to collagen and other agents such as kaolin, platelet factor 3 is not released or made available normally. This may be asso-

ciated with decreased formation of prothrombin activator during coagulation leading to poor prothrombin consumption. Platelet adhesiveness to glass may or may not be impaired. The above findings are similar to those encountered in patients who have ingested aspirin. They are seen in persons with family histories suggesting a hereditary background but are also seen in patients without such history and in patients with other disease processes such as cirrhosis or uremia, and in some patients with myeloproliferative syndromes (polycythemia vera, myeloid metaplasia with myelosclerosis, primary thrombocythemia). Although there have been reports of a hemorrhagic disorder due to defective platelet factor 3, it is more likely that most of the patients reported would fall into the group described above in which there is no true abnormality of the platelet factor 3, but rather a failure for it to be made available during the hemostatic and coagulation reactions.

The Wiskott-Aldrich syndrome, a rare disease of sex-linked inheritance, is characterized by a triad of eczema, thrombocytopenia and repeated infections. It is associated with immunologic deficiencies. The thrombocytopenia appears to be due to a shortened life span of the platelets, probably because of an intracorpuscular defect. Platelets from patients with this disease have a metabolic defect and fail to aggregate in the presence of collagen, ADP and epinephrine.[209]

VASCULAR ABNORMALITY PLUS A PLASMA COAGULATION DEFECT

A unique disorder called von Willebrand's disease is characterized by a "dual" or "hybrid" hemostatic defect: there is Factor VIII deficiency, but with normal, not with prolonged clotting time as in hemophilia; also in contrast to hemophilia there is prolonged bleeding time, suggesting that there is abnormality in the vascular or platelet phases of hemostasis. The condition is inherited as an autosomal dominant trait, but the genetic mode of transmission of the dual defect is unknown.

In 1926 von Willebrand described a hereditary bleeding disorder prevalent among both the male and female inhabitants of the Aland Island.[182] The characteristic finding was a prolonged bleeding time and a normal clotting time. The symptoms varied considerably from case to case and were similar to, but milder than, those of classical hemophilia. Hemarthrosis was much less common and joint deformities did not occur. Severe bleeding after operative procedures, menorrhagia, and bleeding at parturition were prominent features. In this first description of the syndrome it was referred to as pseudohemophilia, but later it was referred to in the literature as von Willebrand's disease. With improvement in methodology and advancement of our knowledge of hemostasis, the hemostatic defect in this syndrome has been considerably clarified but not completely worked out. After the initial report Jurgen and von Willebrand[183] concluded from further studies that the bleeding tendency was due to a qualitative defect of the platelets. Macfarlane[12] and others, however, believed that the bleeding tendency was due to a vascular abnormality in which the capillaries reacted abnormally to injury. Bizarre and tortuous capillary loops were also described.

In 1953 Alexander and Goldstein[184] reported low antihemophilic factor in two patients with prolonged bleeding times, normal platelets and irregular and distorted nail bed capillaries. Deficiency of Factor VIII was soon reported in many other patients considered to fall into this syndrome, and finally re-examination of the Aland Island patients revealed that they also had a deficiency of Factor VIII.[185] The Swedish group in addition reported that there was a factor in plasma which could correct the prolonged bleeding time. Fractionation of normal plasma revealed that this factor was not Factor VIII or fibrinogen although it was concentrated in Fraction I. Further studies revealed that this factor was present in at least normal levels in the plasma of patients with classical hemophilia. (To date it has not been possible to purify this factor to the extent that its physicochemical characteristics can be determined. It is, however, believed to be a protein.) Nilsson et al.[185] were able to correct the prolonged bleeding time without significantly increasing the Factor VIII level of the patient's blood by use of hemophilic plasma, or they could correct the Factor VIII level to normal without correcting the bleeding time by the use of certain purified Factor VIII fractions from normal blood. Cornu et al.[186] have confirmed these findings. From such data and studies on platelet adhesiveness it has been postulated that this plasma protein may play a role in platelet adhesion or massing at the site of vascular injury. Biggs,[187] however, found in four

patients that the bleeding time was never reduced to normal with the materials she used (fresh frozen plasma, several Factor VIII-rich plasma fractions, serum, and fibrinogen fractions). Although reduction in bleeding did occur in some instances it was of brief duration and the control of traumatic bleeding appeared to be correlated with the increase in Factor VIII levels rather than with the correction of the bleeding time.

All platelet studies are normal except for adhesion to glass. That is, there is normal adhesion to and aggregation by connective tissue, and normal release of ADP, serotonin and PF3. Aggregation by ADP, thrombin and epinephrine is normal. Adhesion to glass is reported to be abnormal but corrected by the addition of normal plasma.

Of interest in this syndrome is the finding that Factor VIII levels not only vary greatly from patient to patient but may vary significantly from one time to another in a given individual, which is distinctly different from what is found in classical hemophilia. In addition, exercise and the administration of adrenalin produce a much greater rise in the plasma Factor VIII activity than in the hemophilic. The effect of transfusion therapy upon the plasma Factor VIII levels is also significantly different in these two groups. In classical hemophilia the rise in plasma Factor VIII activity in response to transfusion reaches its peak immediately after completion of transfusion, the increase in activity is directly related to the total Factor VIII in the transfused material, and fall-off of activity begins immediately, with a half-life variously estimated as 10 to 20 hours. In contrast in the von Willebrand group the peak of Factor VIII activity occurs from several to 24 hours after completion of tranfusion. The rise in activity is greater than that expected from the total amount of Factor VIII administered. It has also been found that serum devoid of Factor VIII activity[187] and hemophilic plasma[186] will induce a delayed rise in Factor VIII which is equivalent to that produced by normal plasma. The fall-off rate is slower than that seen in hemophilia.

From these findings, it appears that the Factor VIII deficiency in von Willebrand's syndrome is not due to an inability to produce Factor VIII but rather to the *absence or deficiency of a stimulating factor* for Factor VIII production. The concept is compatible with the difference in the inheritance pattern between hemophilia and von Willebrand's disease, the former exhibiting a sex-linked recessive pattern and the latter an autosomal dominant pattern.

At the present time most investigators define von Willebrand's disease as a hemorrhagic disease characterized by a prolonged bleeding time, low Factor VIII plasma levels, and normal platelets both in quality and quantity. Bizarre and tortuous capillary loops may or may not be present. The bleeding time may vary from slightly above normal to markedly prolonged, and Factor VIII levels may vary from low normal to one to two per cent of normal. In general, the Factor VIII levels are not as low as those found in moderate to severe classical hemophilics. In the untreated patient there is no correlation between the decrease in Factor VIII and the prolongation of the bleeding time, and some cases which undoubtedly belong to this syndrome have been reported in whom the bleeding time was prolonged but the Factor VIII level was within the normal range. In all probability the reverse findings may also occur. Whether or not there is a decrease in a plasma protein which has no function in coagulation, but which plays some role in vascular integrity or platelet function remains to be clarified.

The variability of the clinical findings and symptoms and the conflicting reports in the literature concerning the nature of the hemostatic defect have led to the use of a number of terms in the literature, in addition to von Willebrand's disease, to refer to this syndrome: pseudohemophilia, pseudohemophilia B, angiohemophilia, and vascular hemophilia. It is still not clear what the relationship is between von Willebrand's disease as defined above and certain cases described in the literature. Cases have been reported in which abnormal platelet morphology or a decrease in platelet factor 3 was found in addition to prolongation of the bleeding time with or without reduction of Factor VIII or increased capillary fragility.[188] Cases have also been reported in which the prolonged bleeding time was associated with a decrease in Factor IX or XI rather than VIII.

HEREDITARY VASCULAR ABNORMALITIES

Hereditary hemorrhagic telangiectasia (Rendu-Osler-Weber disease) is a vascular disorder in which sporadic pathologic bleeding arises from localized, discrete vascular lesions which are usually widely distributed. This clinical entity, first recognized by Rendu

in 1896,[189] was more clearly delineated by Osler in 1901[190] and somewhat later by Weber.[191]

This vascular abnormality is transmitted as an autosomal dominant trait so that either parent if affected may transmit it to half the progeny both male and female. It is probable that the homozygous form of hereditary hemorrhagic telangiectasia is lethal. The vascular lesions, which may occur in any organ or tissue of the body, tend to be particularly prominent in the skin and mucous membranes. They are rarely evident in infancy or early childhood but usually tend to appear during the 2nd to 5th decade. In most affected individuals new lesions continue to appear throughout life, but lesions may also disappear over a period of months to years leaving no visible vascular abnormality.[7] The lesions in the skin and mucous membranes are of three types: macules, spiders, and nodules. The macule is the most common and earliest type and usually is a pin-point, red to purple spot which is not elevated and may even be depressed. The spider superficially resembles the vascular spider of cirrhosis but in contrast to the latter it usually does not blanch completely with pressure. This type of lesion does not make its appearance before the more characteristic macules. The nodules are red, or violaceous to purple lesions which may reach 5 to 8 mm. in diameter and are elevated above the surrounding skin. These too are usually a late manifestation. The vascular lesions may be distributed over the entire skin but are notable for their frequency on the palmar surface of the fingers and the hands, the fingernails, the lips, the ears, the face, the lower portion of the arms and the toes. The trunk and the abdomen are less often affected. As concerns pathologic bleeding, the more serious lesions are those in the mucous membranes of the nose, tongue, pharynx, larynx, trachea, bronchi, gastrointestinal tract, and the genitourinary tract. The basic histologic defect in the vascular lesions is the failure of muscle and connective tissue to develop properly in the wall of the vessel. The lesions consist of dilated small vessels (arterioles, capillaries, and venules) with walls that may be nothing more than a layer of endothelial cells with little or no muscular or elastic elements. Atrophy of the skin or mucous membranes overlying these lesions occurs, thus reducing the mechanical protection ordinarily afforded. The involved vessels fail to contract normally when traumatized.[12] The frequent hemorrhages result only from the vascular lesions, the hemostatic mechanism in unaffected vessels is normal and there is no coagulation or platelet abnormality. Accordingly, the clotting time, platelet count, bleeding time, tourniquet test, etc. are all normal.

Hemorrhage often begins spontaneously. Epistaxis is most common, frequently precipitated by sneezing or blowing the nose. Gastrointestinal hemorrhage is fairly frequent and is probably the most serious, since it is not possible to apply local measures to stop the bleeding. Hemoptysis is not unusual and may be fatal. It arises from the vascular lesions of the bronchi rather than from the arteriovenous fistulae. In the classical case, the triad of a familial background, episodic bleeding, and obvious multiple telangiectasia make diagnosis relatively simple. However, in some instances diagnosis may be difficult, particularly when lesions are not apparent and no family history of bleeding is elicited. Hemorrhage may be frequent and severe, often originating repeatedly in the same location, and may induce profound anemia. Since more and more lesions appear with advancing years, the frequency of hemorrhagic episodes usually increases with age. Lesions occurring in certain organs may complicate the picture. Pulmonary arteriovenous fistulae may occur. Such lesions are usually found only in adults and when they occur are very frequently multiple.[7] They may, of course, result in cyanosis, polycythemia, clubbing of the fingers, and heart failure. Vascular lesions may occur in all organs including the brain, the spleen, and the liver. In the liver and spleen these lesions may expand into cavernous hemangiomas.[192] Aneurysms of systemic arteries, such as the splenic and mesenteric arteries, have been reported.[7] It has also been reported that a specific form of cirrhosis of the liver may be associated with this disease.[7] As would be expected from consideration of the underlying pathology, effective therapy consists in local application of pressure when the angioma is accessible, followed by its extirpation surgically or by electrocautery. Systemic therapy has little to offer other than treatment of iron deficiency anemia when it is present. Estrogens[193] which have been reported as helpful are in general of little use.

Angiokeratoma Corporis Diffusum (Fabrey's Syndrome). Although this syndrome is not associated with pathologic bleeding, it is mentioned here because the vascular lesions which occur may be mistaken for petechiae or the lesions of hereditary hemorrhagic telangiectasia. However, careful examination of the lesions and their distribution usually is sufficient to distinguish them. It is sex-linked, occurring almost entirely in males. In Fabrey's syndrome the lesions vary in size from barely visible to 2 to 4 mm. in diameter. The small ones are flat and the larger ones are elevated slightly above the surface of the skin. They range in color from deep red to black. The smaller ones are usually the lightest in color and can be partially blanched by pressure. Since thrombosis may occur in a given lesion, it may closely resemble a petechial lesion, however, there are always lesions present which will blanch and which do not disappear in a few days as petechiae do. The lesions usually appear in clusters, and in contrast to hereditary telangiectasia, the most prominent clusters are between the level of the umbilicus and the knees, and in particular over hips, iliac crests, genitalia, lumbosacral area, buttocks, and around the umbilicus. The palms and soles are rarely involved and lesions on the face, scalp and ears have not been reported. The lesions may appear on mucous membranes of the mouth and pharynx, but rarely if ever on the dorsum of the tongue. The diffuse disease process involves many organs. The renal lesion is usually the most serious one and uremia in most cases supervenes by the 4th or 5th decade. Premature cerebral vascular and coronary artery disease resulting in strokes and myocardial infarctions are prominent manifestations. Superficial corneal opacities are common and varicosities of the retinal veins. From histologic studies it was suspected for some time that this process was a "lipid storage" disorder. Recent investigations reveal that there is an accumulation of a glycolipid ceramidetrihexoside due to the deficiency of the enzyme (ceramidetrihexosidase) which is necessary for its metabolic degradation.[193] The condition is hereditary and appears to be transmitted as a sex-linked recessive trait. However, it has been reported in females, but this is thought to represent a function of penetrance of the gene. There is no abnormality in hemostasis or coagulation. An excellent review on the subject by Wise *et al.* has been published.[194]

ACQUIRED VASCULAR ABNORMALITIES

Vitamin C Deficiency (Scurvy). Ascorbic acid deficiency causes a defect in intercellular collagenous cement substance which in turn results in increased permeability and fragility of the small blood vessels (arterioles, capillaries, and venules). Although this effect upon the vasculature is undoubtedly the principal cause of the hemorrhagic tendency of scurvy, it may not be the only factor. In some cases thrombocytopenia may also occur and may contribute to the hemorrhagic diathesis.[4,152] It is thought that the thrombocytopenia is due to decreased production of platelets. Qualitative platelet changes of questionable significance have also been described in patients with scurvy[195] and findings in scorbutic guinea pigs indicate that a coagulation defect (decreased Factors XI and XII) might play a role in bleeding. The coagulation defects have not as yet been demonstrated in humans.

Hemorrhagic manifestations consist of follicular and perifollicular purpura, ecchymoses, large subcutaneous extravasations of blood, and oozing from the gums. The gum bleeding is frequently associated with peridontal sepsis, loosening of the teeth, and gum retraction. In infants subperiosteal bleeding and petechiae are outstanding features. The subperiosteal bleeding causes severe pain made worse by movement. Since the hemorrhages occur most frequently at the lower end of the femur and the upper end of the humerus, the child refuses to move his limbs and tends to lie absolutely still with his legs flexed and widely abducted.

Usually the only test of hemostasis which is abnormal is the tourniquet test, which is often strikingly positive. The bleeding time and all coagulation tests are most often normal. If thrombocytopenia is present, a prolonged bleeding time, poor prothrombin consumption and poor clot retraction may occur. However, it is rare that the thrombocytopenia is of a severe enough degree to produce such changes. Both the increased vascular fragility and the thrombocytopenia are corrected within a few days by the administration of ascorbic acid (200 to 300 mg. daily).

Anaphylactoid Purpura. Anaphylactoid, allergic or Henoch-Schönlein purpura is a generalized disturbance of the small blood vessels in which purpura is but one of a wide variety of manifestations. Because of the widespread involvement of the small vessels, signs and symptoms referable to many organs (skin, mucous membranes, joints, gastrointestinal tract, urinary tract, central nervous system and heart) may be present. The characteristic vascular lesion is an angiitis of the arterioles and capillaries in which there is perivascular cuffing with varying numbers of polymorphonuclear, lymphocytic, histiocytic and eosinophilic cells. There may be swelling and proliferation of the endothelial cells which at times may be so marked as to occlude the vessel. The vascular wall may be necrotic and collagen fibers in the areas of intensive cellular reaction may be distorted and stain abnormally. In the areas of purpura extravasated erythrocytes are seen about the affected vessels. In the dermis and the mucous membranes there may be evidence of edema. The early renal lesions have many similarities to those of disseminated lupus erythematosus[197] whereas the older lesions are difficult to differentiate from subacute or chronic glomerulonephritis.[198]

The etiology of the syndrome is unknown. Osler was probably the first to attribute its pathogenesis to an anaphylactic or allergic mechanism because of its similarity to serum sickness. Although the concept has fallen out of favor from time to time, advances made in the study of the relations of the immune mechanism to disease states suggest that this syndrome is a result of an immune reaction involving blood vessels. Certain clinical and pathologic aspects of Henoch-Schönlein purpura give support to this theory. The joint manifestations and some of the skin lesions (urticaria, edema, erythema) are similar to those seen in serum sickness and known allergic reactions. Some cases with classical clinical and pathologic findings have been shown to be due to reactions to specific foods and drugs. In such cases recovery occurs when the offending agent is withdrawn and reappears when it is again given to the patient. Among the offending agents reported are milk, chocolate, wheat, beans, penicillin, barbiturates, quinine, chlorothiazide, salicylates, and influenza vaccine.[8,198,199] About 70 to 90 per cent of cases follow an upper respiratory infection occurring one to three weeks before onset of purpura.[198,200] In only about 25 to 30 per cent is the preceding infection due to beta hemolytic streptococci as determined by culture or antistreptolysin titers, in contrast to the infections more regularly preceding rheumatic fever and glomerulonephritis. None the less, the high incidence of recent upper respiratory infections is impressive. It is of course possible that antibodies formed in response to an infection might cross-react with vascular tissue, thus producing a generalized vascular lesion, but a more likely explanation in view of experimental findings in animals, is that soluble antigen-antibody complexes of various types produce the injury to blood vessels. Dixon et al.[201] caused vascular lesions in the kidney of rabbits by repeated injection of antigen (foreign protein), and the critical factor determining whether or not an animal would develop renal disease was the amount of antibody the animal formed. Vascular lesions have also been produced in animals by intravenous administration of a number of antigen-antibody complexes made soluble by the presence of excess antigen.[202] It is possible therefore that the lesions in this disease process are caused by "immunologic pathogens" which are without immunologic specificity for vascular tissue. Although Henoch-Schönlein purpura has been referred to as an "autoimmuned" disease, and lesions have been produced in animals which are similar to those seen in the human by the administration of heterologous antivascular serum, there has been no convincing demonstration of circulating antibodies in the serum of patients against any antigen in blood vessels or of tissue-localizing antibody in the vessel of patients as determined by fluorescent techniques.[203]

The onset and course of the disease is quite variable. It may begin with fever, headache and anorexia, or purpura, arthralgia, abdominal pain or hematuria may be the first manifestation. Although it occurs commonly in children under the age of eight, it may occur at any age. The sexes are probably affected equally since in some series males were found to predominate, whereas in others it occurred more frequently in females.[198] Each episode usually lasts no more than a few weeks, but recurrent attacks occur in about 50 per cent of the cases.

Hemorrhage in Henoch-Schönlein purpura is rarely severe enough to endanger life. There is no generalized breakdown of the hemostatic mechanism, and bleeding occurs only at the site of vascular damage. There is no alteration in the coagulation mechanism and platelets are usually qualitatively and quantitatively normal. Occasional cases with an associated thrombocytopenia have been described. The tourniquet test is usually negative and the bleeding time normal.

Skin involvement has been reported in almost all cases, probably because without it the diagnosis is rarely if ever made. A wide variety of lesions occur which may or may not be hemorrhagic. The rash is often urticarial at first and is then replaced by a red macular or maculopapular lesion. These lesions, which can occur without the preceding urticaria, may remain small and discrete but usually they enlarge and often become confluent. Hemorrhages occurring in these lesions give the characteristic purpura of the disease. Frequently, hemorrhage occurs early in the formation of the lesion so that the underlying erythema is not apparent. In such instances the purpura may be confused with that of thrombocytopenia, although certain characteristics help differentiate it. The purpuric lesions are usually larger and more confluent than those seen in thrombocytopenia and small round petechiae are uncommon. The distribution is also different, since in allergic purpura the purpura is most prominent over the lower extremities and buttocks and may be limited to these areas; however, the arms, face and rarely the lower trunk may become involved. The lesions are more prominent on the extensor surfaces of the extremities and in the joint areas. Other skin lesions such as blebs, bullae, and erythema nodosa may appear. Localized areas of edema, particularly on the hands, the feet, and around the face, the eyes, the neck, the lips and the penis are often present.

Joint symptoms are a very common manifestation. The joints most frequently affected are the ankles and the knees. Joint pains often seem excessively severe, out of proportion to the objective evidence. The involved joint is usually slightly to moderately swollen and tender, but rarely red or warm. Roentgenographic examination reveals periarticular soft tissue swelling without any change in the joint space. Joint involvement is usually transient and not migratory, but may recur during the course of the illness and does not respond well to salicylates.

Gastrointestinal symptoms consist of colicky abdominal pain, vomiting, melena and hematemesis. The abdominal pain is the most common symptom and is thought to be due to edema and/or bleeding into the intestinal wall. Intussusception is the most serious gastrointestinal complication and occurs most often in children under the age of eight.

In about 40 to 60 per cent of the cases there is evidence of renal involvement as indicated by hematuria, proteinuria, or elevation of blood urea. In most cases there is complete recovery, but in about 20 to 25 per cent of cases some abnormality of renal function persists for years, and in a small percentage it progresses to renal failure and death.[198]

Involvement of the central nervous system may result in transient attacks of paresis, epileptiform convulsions, chorea, and subarachnoid bleeding.

PURPURA PROBABLY DUE TO AN ACQUIRED VASCULAR DISORDER

This group is composed of syndromes characterized by mild hemorrhagic skin lesions associated with other vascular abnormalities and pigmentary disorders.

Shamberg's Disease (progressive pigmentary dermatitis) is characterized by appearance of reddish pin-head-sized lesions on the lower extremities. These coalesce to form larger irregular-shaped lesions which gradually fade and become brown to yellow in color. Histologically there is a proliferation of capillaries and of endothelial cells and some vessels become dilated, allowing diapedesis of red cells. The brownish color which develops is in part due to accumulation of hemosiderin in phagocytes in the skin. *Majocchi's disease (purpura annularis telangiectodes)* is characterized by purpuric and pigmented macules and rings which do not fade on pressure and which usually begin in the lower extremities but subsequently involve the arms and trunk. Telangiectasia may occur. Histologically the lesions reveal atrophy of the epidermis, perivascular inflammatory reaction of small vessels with polymorphonuclear and lymphocytic cells, and thickening of the vascular wall with occlusion occurring in some vessels. The etiology of these two conditions is not known nor is their relationship to each other or to syndromes such as Henoch-Schönlein purpura clear. There are several other similar conditions described in the dermatologic literature. However, all of these are rare, and none are associated with any severe bleeding or a generalized disturbance of the hemostatic mechanism.

DISEASES OF CONNECTIVE TISSUE WITH HEMORRHAGE PROBABLY DUE TO VASCULAR DEFECTS AND ABNORMALITY OF SUPPORTING TISSUE

There are a number of syndromes which appear to be hereditary disorders of connective tissue or collagen in which hemorrhagic manifestations are common.[204] In these cases the abnormal bleeding tendency is thought to be due to a vascular defect which may be enhanced by a defect of the supporting tissue.

Ehlers-Danlos syndrome is a hereditary disorder of both sexes which is inherited as a simple dominant trait. It is characterized by hyperelasticity of the skin, hyperextensibility of the joints, increased fragility of the skin and blood vessels, dislocation of the lens and increased incidence of dissecting aneurysm of the aorta. Hemorrhagic manifestations are easy bruising, petechiae, epistaxis, bleeding from the gums, hematuria, melena, menorrhagia and excessive bleeding after surgical procedures. In most cases the only test of the hemostatic mechanism which is abnormal is the tourniquet test. Occasionally the bleeding time is slightly prolonged and in scattered cases mild thrombocytopenia, qualitative defect of platelets, or low Factor IX has been reported. These defects have usually been rather mild and ordinarily would not be expected to cause any serious defect in hemostasis. In all probability the bleeding tendency is due to the abnormal formation of elastic tissue in the blood vessels and surrounding tissue.

Osteogenesis imperfecta is thought to be a hereditary disorder of collagen formation and may be associated with hemorrhagic manifestations such as ecchymosis, hematoma, melena, subconjunctival hemorrhages, etc. The bleeding tendency is assumed to be due to a vascular defect caused by abnormal collagen formation. However, qualitative abnormalities of platelets (decreased platelet factor 3 activity) has recently been reported in this syndrome. Whether or not this platelet defect is always present and is responsible for the hemorrhagic diathesis has not been determined.

Pseudoxanthoma elasticum may be associated with bleeding from virtually any organ. The cause remains obscure. As yet, no abnormality in coagulation has been reported. The pathologic abnormality (which is a hereditary one, although its hereditary pattern is as yet not certain) appears to be a defect of either the elastic tissue or collagen. The small and medium-sized arteries may show degenerative changes in the elastic membrane, and capillaries and small veins may be widely dilated. These vascular changes may well be responsible for the bleeding tendency.

Pulmonary hemosiderosis[205] is characterized by recurrent, subacute episodes of pulmonary hemorrhage and progressive pulmonary insufficiency. About 80 per cent of the cases occur in children and the remainder in young adults. The onset is often insidious. The pulmonary bleeding may be mild, giving rise only to blood-tinged sputum. However, at some time during the course of the disease frank hemoptysis usually occurs. Dyspnea and cough are almost always present and become much more pronounced during episodes of bleeding, at which time cyanosis also becomes prominent. With recurrent pulmonary hemorrhages, pulmonary symptoms increase and become more persistent. Pulmonary fibrosis progresses and cor pulmonale may occur eventually, giving rise to signs of right-sided heart failure. Frequently a moderate to severe anemia develops due to iron deficiency, for although there is a great deal of iron in the pulmonary tissue, it is not available for hemoglobin synthesis. The accumulation of iron in the lung results in the appearance of hemosiderin-laden histiocytes in the sputum, an important diagnostic finding. The hemorrhagic tendency is confined to the lungs. All coagulation studies are normal, and there is no evidence of any platelet or generalized vascular disorder.

The etiology of this syndrome is obscure. There is no evidence of an increased familial incidence. It is classified here in the group of connective tissue disorders because the characteristic pathologic findings have been considered to be a degeneration of the alveolar, interstitial and vascular elastic fibers. However, these changes are now thought to be secondary to the hemosiderin deposited in the lung from repeated bleeding. Three postulations have been advanced: (1) A defective vasomotor control of the pulmonary vessels gives rise to pulmonary hypertension with subsequent diapedesis of red cells. (2) An auto-immuned process or some immunologic reaction affects the pulmonary vessels leading to hemorrhage. (3) This disease represents primarily an abnormality of alveolar epithelial growth and function which critically affects the mechanical stability of the alveolar capillaries. As yet none of these theories have been substantiated. The relation between this syndrome and *Goodpasture's syndrome* (pulmonary hemorrhage and extensive glomerular disease) also is obscure.

PURPURA AND BLEEDING OF OBSCURE ETIOLOGY

Autoerythrocyte Sensitization. In 1955 Gardner and Diamond first described a peculiar chronic recurrent purpura which occurred in women.[206] It usually first makes its appearance shortly after an injury or surgical procedure. The lesions arise spontaneously or following minor trauma and are most frequently limited to the extremities. Characteristically, the patient first notes a tingling or painful sensation and within a few minutes an urticarial or erythematous skin lesion appears. Within minutes or hours the area becomes ecchymotic and painful. The ecchymosis area may be ringed by an area of erythema. After a week or two the ecchymosis disappears. At irregular intervals new lesions appear. Associated with such episodes left upper quadrant pain similar to that of a splenic infarct, or melena, hematuria, hemiparesis or hemiplegia may occur. Gardner and Diamond demonstrated that these lesions could be induced by intradermal administration of the patient's own red cell stroma, but not by plasma, white cells or hemoglobin, and postulated autoerythrocyte sensitization as the mechanism producing the purpura. Histamine has also been shown to produce the lesions in such patients. Most of the affected persons have rather severe emotional disturbances. Agle and Ratnoff[207] have emphasized this and have reviewed the relationship of emotional disturbance and hemorrhagic phenomena. Although no definite conclusion can be drawn, the author suggest a trial of psychiatric therapy for treatment of patients with this type of purpura.

A somewhat similar condition has been reported in which the purpuric lesions appear to be due to *autosensitization to deoxyribonucleic acid.*[208,209] The lesions begin as erythematous swelling which increases in size over a period of a few hours, after which ecchymosis replaces the erythema. Chloroquin is effective in treatment.

Polycythemia Vera. That thromboembolic phenomena occur in polycythemia vera is not surprising in view of the increased viscosity of the blood, the resulting decrease in velocity of blood flow, and the thrombocytosis which is frequently present. However, the cause of the hemorrhagic diathesis, which is often present even when there is evidence of intravascular coagulation, is for the most part obscure. Increased fibrinolytic activity, marked hypofibrinogenemia, or severe liver damage with resulting decrease in coagulation factors produced in the liver can account for bleeding in an occasional case. In the remainder a variety of mechanisms have been suggested. Because of the increased red cell mass and high hematocrit, the level of plasma coagulation factors per volume of whole blood is reduced even though the plasma levels may be normal. However, studies do not indicate that such reduction is usually sufficient to account for hemorrhage, and in addition the hemorrhagic tendency remains even after reduction of red cell mass and hematocrit to normal levels by venesection. It is possible that the clot formed is inadequate because of the increased number of red cells or because of some qualitative abnormality in the fibrin clot which is suggested by the abnormally high red cell fallout observed in vitro. The increased fallout may occur even when the hematocrit and platelet levels have been reduced to normal by therapy. Decreased platelet 3 activity has been reported but is rarely if ever of sufficient degree to account for bleeding. It has also been postulated that there is a vascular defect perhaps caused by prolonged over-distention of the vascular tree by the increased blood volume, which results in the loss of vascular response to injury.

Hemorrhagic Thrombocythemia. As might be anticipated, intravascular thrombosis is one of the complications of thrombocytosis. However, a hemorrhagic diathesis, which is characterized by easy bruising and excessive bleeding following trauma or surgery, also occurs.[210] The mechanism by which thrombocythemia leads to bleeding has been the subject of much speculation, but there is little to support any of the suggested theories. The underlying cause of the thrombocytosis, (whether polycythemia vera, myeloid metaplasia, chronic granulocytic leukemia, or idiopathic) does not seem to be a determining factor in whether or not a bleeding tendency is present. Although in patients with bleeding there seems to be a relationship between the level of the platelet count and the tendency to bleed, other patients with equally high counts have no bleeding tendency. It has been suggested that the bleeding is due to: (1) A defect in platelet factor 3, which has been demonstrated in some patients. (This defect, however, is not always present nor does it ever seem severe enough to be the cause of bleeding.) (2) A vascular defect which may or may not be related to the thrombocythemia (There usually is no evidence by the tests available of a defect in vascular integrity.) (3) A defect in plasma coagulation factors. (Such a defect may be present because there frequently is involvement of the liver by the underlying disease process; however, it rarely is severe enough to account for the bleeding.) (4) The anticoagulant effect of excessive platelets, a phenomenon which can be demonstrated in vitro. (In the majority of cases the platelet elevation does not appear to be of sufficient magnitude to cause this coagulation defect.)

The most recent investigations suggest that there is a platelet defect in thrombocythemia which is similar to that described under thrombopathia. Although the platelets adhere normally to collagen and connective tissue there is an abnormality in the release phenomenon of ADP and serotonin and platelet factor 3.

HEMORRHAGIC MANIFESTATION IN ASSOCIATION WITH PLASMA PROTEIN ABNORMALITIES

Hyperglobulinemic purpura is a clinical entity first reported by Waldenström in 1943. It is characterized by episodic purpura and an increase in serum gamma globulin.[211,212] The increased gamma globulin is of the 7S type and, unlike myeloma globulin, migrates as a broad band on paper electrophoresis. This syndrome has been observed most frequently in middle-aged women but has been reported in males. The condition usually begins insidiously with occasional attacks of purpura over the distal lower extremities but over the course of years the attacks become more frequent and more extensive, involving the entire lower extremity and occasionally the trunk. The purpura usually occurs after prolonged standing or exercise and may be heralded by burning or stinging and may be preceded or accompanied by edema of the legs, pain in the knees or ankles, and low grade fever. Most often no underlying disease can be found, but it has been described in patients with sarcoid, lupus erythematosus, Sjögren's syndrome and Mikulicz's disease. The bleeding tendency is limited to the skin. The purpuric lesions consist of small petechiae or ecchymoses ranging from a few mm. to 2 cm. in diameter. The rash gradually fades over a week or two and at first disappears without a trace, but after repeated bouts, persistent pigmentation develops. The purpura is not associated with any significant disturbance of blood coagulation. All the usual coagulation tests are normal and although in some cases a mild thrombocytopenia or a moderate decrease in platelet factor 3 activity has been reported it is unlikely that such changes play any role in the purpura. The bleeding time is normal and the tourniquet test is normal in most cases. Pathologic examination reveals a vasculitis which is limited to the areas of the purpuric lesion. Vessels in normal-appearing skin either from the lower extremities or elsewhere seem histologically normal. The early pathologic changes are found in the capillaries and small arterioles and consist of perivascular edema, and infiltration with leukocytes, plasma cells and histiocytes. Proliferation of the endothelial cells also occurs and may completely occlude the vessel. Later changes consist of fibrinoid degeneration of the collagen fibers and loss of elastic fibers. The purpura obviously is secondary to the vascular lesion. However, the etiology of these lesions and role of the hypergammaglobulinemia remains obscure. There is no good evidence to implicate antibodies against the vascular wall or sensitization to altered gamma globulin. However, immunologic mechanisms cannot be excluded for as discussed in the previous section on Henoch-Schönlein purpura, studies have demonstrated the vascular toxicity of soluble antigen-antibody complexes; such a mechanism has not been ruled out in this condition. It is of interest that it has been reported that thioguanine therapy resulted in marked improvement in two patients with hyperglobulinemic purpura without significantly altering the plasma proteins by the parameters used.[213]

Hyperglobulinemia Associated With Multiple Myeloma. In multiple myeloma a bleeding tendency characterized by ecchymoses, petechiae, epistaxis, gingival bleeding, hematemesis, and excessive bleeding at surgery is commonly encountered. The pathogenesis of the hemorrhagic diathesis varies from patient to patient. In some it is due to thrombocytopenia, and in a rare case increased fibrinolysis is the cause. However, in most cases the pathogenesis is not so clear cut. In some instances the abnormal protein may delay clotting by acting as an inhibitor of the action of thrombin or fibrinogen or of the polymerization of fibrin the protein is ever responsible for bleeding is not clear. In other cases no explanation for bleeding has been found.

Cryoglobulinemia. Cryoglobulins are proteins which precipitate or gel when whole blood or plasma is cooled, and at body temperature increase the viscosity of the blood if present in high enough concentrations. They may have the molecular weight of normal gamma globulin, or may be macroglobulins. In most cases there is an underlying disease process such as multiple myeloma, lymphoproliferative disease, Hodgkin's disease or lupus erythematosus, but an essential or idiopathic variety has also been reported. There is considerable variation not only in the level of these proteins from one case to another but also in their physical properties. In some cases lowering the temperature of the blood just a few degrees below body temperature results in gel formation or precipitation whereas in others this does not take place unless the temperature is dropped considerably below room temperature. Symptoms vary depending upon the concentration and physical properties of the protein. Slowing of the circulation is caused by the increased viscosity of the blood, and as the temperature drops there may be complete cessation of the flow of blood in the small vessels. The circulatory alterations result in cyanosis, particularly of the exposed portions of the body, and may cause Raynaud's phenomenon. Complete obstruction of vessels may lead to injury of the vessel with thrombosis and/or hemorrhage. Ecchymosis, epistaxis, melena, retinal hemorrhage, and excessive bleeding after trauma or surgery have been reported. The mechanism of the bleeding is not clear. However, several abnormalities in coagulation have been noted: prolonged prothrombin times, decreased prothrombin and Factor VII and V levels, increased clotting and partial thromboplastin times may occur. Many of these findings are probably caused by interference by the abnormal protein in the clotting process. It has also been postulated that these proteins may form complexes with certain of the coagulation factors and thus make them unavailable. They also may interfere with the thrombin-fibrinogen reaction and clot retraction. The clots that are formed are friable, and this may contribute to the defect in hemostasis. Coating of the platelets with these proteins, particularly if they are macroglobulins, may interfere with platelet function and in particular with release of platelet factor 3.

Macroglobulinemia. Normally about 2 to 5 per cent of the plasma proteins have a molecular weight of 1,000,000 or more. Occasionally the concentration of these macroglobulins is high. Such an increase may be associated with some underlying disease process such as cirrhosis, lymphoproliferative diseases, myeloma or lupus, but in other instances it appears to be part of a distinct syndrome referred to as Waldenström's macroglobulinemia.[214,215] In this syndrome there are many peculiar cells in the bone marrow, and at times in the spleen and lymph nodes which have features of both lymphocytes and plasma cells and may represent some transition form between the lymphocyte and plasma cell. It is believed that these cells produce the macroglobulin. Subjects with high levels of macroglobulin may have a severe hemorrhagic diathesis characterized by bleeding from mucous membranes, particularly of the gums and nose. These mucosal surfaces frequently show persistent oozing which is difficult to control. Minor surgery may be complicated by severe and persistent hemorrhage. Bleeding into the skin and subcutaneous tissues (petechiae and ecchymoses) occur much less commonly as does bleeding into the eye, the central nervous system and the gastrointestinal tract. Typically the bleeding time is prolonged and the tourniquet test is normal. Coagulation studies have produced a remarkable variety of findings. The clotting time of whole blood may be prolonged, particularly if carried out in siliconized tubes. Subnormal prothrombin, Factor V and VII levels have been reported as well as inhibitors directed against thromboplastin formation, the action of thrombin on fibrinogen, or the polymerization of fibrin. Prothrombin consumption may be markedly decreased during coagulation. In some patients thrombocytopenia does occur, but it is usually not of a severe enough degree to produce prolonged bleeding times or poor prothrombin consumption. It has been reported that at least in some patients poor prothrombin consumption can be due to a lack of release of platelet factor 3. Although the platelets of the patients reported contained normal amounts of this factor, it appeared that macroglobulin on the surface of the platelets seemed to inhibit the release of factor 3. The macroglobulin in these patients was also shown to coat red cells and white cells.[216] Despite all these reports there are cases in which none of these abnormalities appear to adequately explain the bleeding tendency. It has been postulated that the macroglobulins in some way impair the function of the small vessels. That the macroglobulins are in some way directly responsible for the hemorrhagic diathesis would appear to be substantiated by the decrease in the bleeding tendency following reduction of the level of macroglobulin by plasmapheresis.[217]

SUMMARY

Pathologic bleeding occurs when there is impairment of the hemostatic mechanism, in which extravascular, vascular, and intravascular factors all play a role. Study of the various components involved has helped to clarify the pathogenesis and explain the clinical manifestations of many hemorrhagic disorders. In this chapter an attempt has been made to summarize our present knowledge of the hemostatic mechanism and to indicate how it is altered in various hemorrhagic states. Although our present knowledge is far from complete, it does permit a rational approach to the study, diagnosis, and treatment of pathologic bleeding.

REFERENCES

1. Quick, A. J. Hemorrhagic Diseases and Thrombosis, ed. 2, Philadelphia, Lea & Febiger, 1966.
2. Ratnoff, O. D.: Bleeding Syndromes, A Clinical Manual, Springfield, Ill., Thomas, 1960.
3. Biggs, R., and Macfarlane, R. G.: Human Blood Coagulation and Its Disorders, ed. 3, Oxford, Blackwell Scientific Publ., 1962.
4. Owen, C. A., Bowie, E. J. W., Didiaheim, P. and Thompson, J. H.: The Diagnosis of Bleeding Disorders, Boston, Little, Brown, 1969.
5. Poller, L., Ed.: Recent Advances in Blood Coagulation, Boston, Little, Brown, 1969.
6. Marcus, A. J. and Zucker, M. B.: The Physiology of Blood Platelets, New York, Grune and Stratton, 1965.
7. Bean, W. B.: Vascular Spiders, and Related Lesions of Skin, Springfield, Ill., Thomas, 1958.
8. Marcus, A. J.: Platelet function, New Eng. J. Med. 280:1213, 1969.
9. Biggs, R. and Macfarlane, R. G.: Treatment of Hemophilia and Other Coagulation Disorders, Philadelphia, F. A. Davis Co., 1966.
10. Hardaway, R. M.: Syndromes of Disseminated Intravascular Coagulation, Springfield, Charles C Thomas, 1966.
11. Tocantins, L. M.: The mechanisms of hemostasis, Ann. Surg. 125:292, 1947.
12. Macfarlane, R. G.: Critical review: the Mechanisms of hemostasis, Quart. J. Med. 34:1, 1941.
13. Kramár, J.: The determination and evaluation of capillary resistance—a review of methodology, Blood 20:83, 1962.

14. Chambers, R., and Zweifack, B. W.: Vaso-motion in the hemodynamics of the blood capillary circulation, Ann. N. Y. Acad. Sci. 49:549, 1948.

15. Weiner, M., and Udenfriend, S.: Relationship of platelet serotonin to disturbances of clotting and hemostasis, Circulation 15:353, 1957.

16. Nilsson, I. M., Blömback, M., and Blömback, B.: von Willebrand's disease in Sweden: its pathogenesis and treatment, Acta med. scandinav. 164:263, 1959.

17. Duke, W. W.: The relation of blood platelets to hemorrhagic disease, J.A.M.A. 55:1185, 1910.

18. Ivy, A. C., Shapiro, B. F., and Melnick, P.: The bleeding tendency in jaundice, Surg. Gynec. Obstet. 60:781, 1935.

19. Shulman, I., Pierce, M., Lukens, A., and Currimbhog, Z.: Studies on thrombopoiesis. I. A factor in normal human plasma required for platelet production; chronic thrombocytopenia due to its deficiency, Blood 16:943, 1960.

20. Harker, L. A.: The kinetics of thrombopoiesis, J. Clin. Invest. 47:458, 1968.

21. Adelson, E., Rheingold, J. J., and Crosby, W. H.: Studies of platelet survival by in vivo tagging with P^{32}, J. Lab. Clin. Med. 50:570, 1957.

22. Leeksma, C. H. W., and Cohen, J. A.: Demonstration of the life span of human blood platelets using labeled diisopropylfluorophosphate, J. Clin. Invest. 35:964, 1956.

23. Cohen, P., and Gardner, F. H.: Reclassification of thrombocytopenia by Cr^{51} labeling method for measuring platelet life span, New Eng. J. Med. 234:1294, 1350, 1961.

24. Aster, R. H.: Pooling of platelets in the spleen: Role in the pathogenesis of hypersplenic thrombocytopenia, J. Clin. Invest. 45:645, 1966.

25. Baldini, M., Costea, N., and Dameshek, W.: The viability of stored human platelets, Blood 16:1669, 1961.

26. Roskam, J., Hughes, J., Bounameaux, Y., and Salmon, J.: The part played by platelets in the formation of an efficient hemostatic plug, Throm. et Diath. Hem. 3:510, 1959.

27. Lüscher, E. F.: Blood platelets—there relationship to the blood clotting system and to hemostasis, Vox. Sang. 5:259, 1960.

28. Berman, J. B., and Fulton, G. P.: Platelets in the Peripheral Circulation, in Blood Platelets, International Symposium, Johnson, S. A., Monto, R. W., Rebuck, J. W., and Horn, R. C. eds. Boston, Little, Brown, 1961.

29. Zucker, M. B., and Borrelli, J.: Viscous metamorphysis, clot retraction and other morphologic alterations of blood platelets, J. Appl. Physiol. 14:575, 1959.

30. Mason, R. G., Hocutt, E. J., Wagner, R. H., and Brinkhous, K. M.: Evolution and decay of platelet-agglutinating activity in normal and pathological human plasma, J. Lab. Clin. Med. 59:645, 1962.

31. Marcus, A. J., and Spaet, T. H.: Platelet phosphatides: their separation, identification and clotting activity, J. Clin. Invest. 37:1836, 1958.

32. Troop, S. B., Reed, C. F., Marinetti, G. V., and Swisher, S. N.: Thromboplastic factors in platelets and red blood cells: observations on their chemical nature and function in in vitro coagulation, J. Clin. Invest. 39:342, 1960.

33. Salmon, J., and Bounameaux, V.: Etude des Antigens Plaquettes et en particulier du Fibrinogène, Thromb. Diath. Hem. 2:93, 1958.

34. Bounameaux, Y.: L'Accolement des Plaquette aux Fibres Sous-endothéliales, Compt. Rend. Soc. Biol. 153:865, 1959.

35. Bettex-Galland, M., and Lüscher, E. F.: Extraction of an actomyosin-like protein from human platelets, Nature 184:276, 1959.

36. Ratnoff, O. D., and Colopy, J. E.: A familial hemorrhagic trait associated with a deficiency of a clot promoting fraction of plasma, J. Clin. Invest. 34:602, 1955.

37. Ratnoff, O. D., and Rosenblum, J. M.: Role of Hageman factor in the initiation of clotting by glass, Amer. J. Med. 25:160, 1958.

38. Ratnoff, O. D., Davie, E. W., and Mallett, D. L.: Studies on the action of Hageman factor: evidence that activated Hageman factor in turn activates plasma thromboplastin antecedent, J. Clin. Invest. 40:803, 1961.

39. Davie, E. W. and Ratnoff, O. D.: Waterfall sequence for intrinsic blood clotting, Science 145:1310, 1964.

40. Macfarlane, R. G.: An enzyme cascade in the blood clotting mechanism and its function as a biochemical amplifier, Nature 202:498, 1964.

41. Soulier, J. P., and Prou-Wartelle, O.: New data on Hageman factor and plasma thromboplastin antecedent. The role of contact in the initial phase of blood coagulation, Brit. J. Hemat. 6:88, 1960.

42. Rosenthal, R. L., Dreskin, O. H., and Rosenthal, N.: New hemophilia-like disease caused by deficiency of a third thromboplastin factor, Proc. Soc. Exp. Biol. Med. 82:171, 1953.

43. Rosenthal, R. L.: Plasma thromboplastin antecedent (P.T.A.) deficiency in man; clinical, coagulation, hereditary, and therapeutic aspects, J. Clin. Invest. 33:961, 1954.

44. Bergsagel, D. E., and Hougie, C.: Intermediate stages of the formation of blood thromboplastin, Brit. J. Hemat. 2:113, 1956.

45. Hougie, C.: The role of Factor V in the formation of blood thromboplastin, J. Lab. Clin. Med. 50:61, 1957.

46. Osterud, B. and Rapoport, S.: Synthesis of intrinsic Factor X activator. Inhibition of the function of formed activator with antibodies to Factor VIII and IX, Biochemistry 9:1854, 1970.

47. Fisch, U., and Duckert, F.: Some aspects of kinetics of the first stages of blood thromboplastin formation, Throm. Diath. Haem. 3:98, 1959.

48. Yin, E. T., and Duckert, F.: The formation of intermediate product I in a purified system. The role of Factor IX or of its precursor and of a Hageman-PTA fraction, Thromb. Diath. Haem. 6:224, 1961.

49. Horowitz, H. I., and Spaet, T. H.: Generation of coagulation product I and its interaction with platelets and phospholipids, J. Appl. Physiol. 16:112, 1961.

50. Barton, P. G., Jackson, C. M. and Hanahan, D. J.: Relationship between Factor V and activated X in generation of prothrombinase, Nature 214:923, 1967.

51. Lewis, J. H., Didisheim, P., Ferguson, J. H., and Hattori, K.: Changes occurring during coagulation in glass. I. Normal human blood, Thromb. Diath. Haem. 4:1, 1959.

52. Quick, A. J., Shanberge, J. N., and Stefanini, M.: The role of platelets in the coagulation of blood, Amer. J. Med. Sci. 217:198, 1949.

53. Alexander, B., Goldstein, R., Rich, L., LeBolloc'h, A. G., Diamond, L. K., and Borges, W.: Congenital afibrinogenemia: a study of some basic aspects of coagulation, Blood 9:843, 1954.

54. Mason, R. G., Hocutt, E. J., Wagner, R. H., and Brinkhous, K. M.: Evolution and decay of platelet-agglutinating activity in normal and pathologic human plasmas, J. Lab. Clin. Med. 59:645, 1962.

55. Rapaport, S. I., Schiffman, S., Patch, M. J., and Ames, S. B.: Rapid clotting in the presence of activation product plus traces of thrombin, Proc. IX Congress Int. Society of Hemat. 1962.

56. Goldstein, R., and Alexander, B.: Coagulation factors concerned with thromboplastin generation, Fed. Proc. 14:219, 1955.

57. ———: Further studies on proconvertin deficiency and the role of proconvertin, in Hemophilia and Hemophiloid Diseases, p. 93, Brinkhous, K. M., ed. Chapel Hill, U. North Carolina Press, 1957.

58. Hougie, C., Barrow, E. M., and Graham, J. B.: Stuart clotting defect. Segregation of hereditary hemorrhagic state from heterogeneous groups heretofore called "stable factor" (SPCA, proconvertin, Factor VII) deficiency, J. Clin. Invest. 36:485, 1957.

59. Nemerson, Y.: Characteristics and lipid requirements of coagulant proteins extracted from lung and brain: The specificity of the protein component of tissue factor, J. Clin. Invest. 48:322–331, 1969.

60. Seegers, W. H., Levine, W. G., and Shepard, R. S.: Further studies on the purificaction of thrombin, Can. J. Biochem. Physiol. 36:603, 1958.

61. Seegers, W. H., Ed.: Blood Clotting Enzymology, New York, Academic Press, 1967.

62. Gladner, J. A., Folk, J. E., Laki, K., and Carroll, W.: Thrombin-induced formation of cofibrin I. Isolation, purification and characterization of co-fibrin, J. Biol. Chem. 234:62, 1959.

63. Scheraga, H. A.: Thrombin and its interaction with fibrinogen, Ann. N. Y. Acad. Sci. 75:189, 1958.

64. Gross, R.: Metabolic Aspects of Normal and Pathological Platelets, p. 407, in Blood Platelets, Boston, Little, Brown, 1961.

65. Lorand, L., and Jacobsen, A.: Studies on the polymerization of fibrin, The role of the globulin: fibrin-stabilizing factor, J. Biol. Chem. 230-421, 1958.

66. Duckert, F., Jung, E., and Shmerling, D. H.: A hitherto undescribed congenital hemorrhagic diathesis probably due to fibrin stabilizing factor deficiency, Thromb. Diath. Haem. 5:179, 1960.

67. Wessler, S.: Studies in intravascular coagulation. I. Coagulation changes in isolated venous segments, J. Clin. Invest. 31:1011, 1952.

68. Fell, C., Ivanovic, N., Johnson, S. A., and Seegers, W. H.: Differentiation of plasma antithrombin activities, Proc. Soc. Exp. Biol. Med. 85:199, 1954.

69. Wessler, S., Ward, K., and Ho, C.: Studies in intravascular coagulation. III. The pathogenesis of serum-induced venous thrombosis, J. Clin. Invest. 34:647, 1955.

70. Spaet, T. H., Horowitz, H. L., Zucker-Franklin, D., Cintron, J., and Biezenski, J. J.: Reticuloendothelial clearance of blood thromboplastin by rats, Blood 17:196, 1961.

71. Sherry, S.: Fibrinolysis, Ann. Rev. Med. 19:247, 1968.

72. Niewiarowski, S., Kowalski, E., and Stachurska, J.: Influence of fibrinogen derived antithrombin (antithrombin VI) on the blood coagulation, Acta. Biochem. 6:45, 1959.

73. Fletcher, A. P., Alkjaersig, N., and Sherry, S.: Pathogenesis of the coagulation defect developing during pathological plasma proteolytic (fibrinolytic states. I. The significance of fibrinogen proteolysis and circulating breakdown products, J. Clin. Invest. 41:896, 1962.

74. Finkbiner, R. B., McGovern, J. J., Goldstein, R., and Bunker, J. P.: Coagulation defects in liver disease and response to transfusion during surgery, Amer. J. Med. 26:199, 1959.

75. Dodds, W. J.: Storage, release, and synthesis of coagulation factors in isolated perfused organs, Amer. J. Physiol. 217:879–883, 1969.

76. Rapaport, S. I.: Plasma thromboplastin antecedent levels in patients receiving coumarin anticoagulants and in patients with Laennec's cirrhosis, Proc. Soc. Exp. Biol. Med. 108:115, 1961.

77. Mersky, C.: Hemophilia occurring in the human female, Proc. Int. Soc. Hemat. p. 441, 1950.

78. Brinkhous, K. M., and Graham, J.: Hemophilia in the female dog, Science 111:723, 1950.

79. Nilsson, I. M., Blömback, M., Thelin, A., and Von Francken, I.: Carriers of hemophilia A: a laboratory study, Acta Med. scand. 165:357, 1959.

80. Rapaport, S. I., Patch, J. M., and Moore, F. J.: Anti-hemophilic globulin levels in car-

riers of hemophilia A, J. Clin. Invest. 39:1619, 1960.

81. Barrow, E. M., Bulloch, W. R., and Graham, J. B.: A study of the carrier state for PTC deficiency utilizing a new assay procedure, J. Lab. Clin. Med. 55:936, 1960.

82. Didisheim, P., and Vandervoort, L. E.: Detection of carriers for Factor IX (PTC) deficiency, Blood. 20:150, 1962.

83. McCain, K. F., Chernoff, A. I., Graham, J. B.: Establishment of the inheritance of Hageman defect as an autosomal recessive trait. Hemophilia and other hemorrhagic states, p. 179, Chapel Hill, U. North Carolina Press. 1959.

84. Rapaport, S. I., Proctor, R. R., Patch, M. J., and Yettra, M.: The mode of inheritance of PTA deficiency: evidence for the existence of major PTA deficiency and minor PTA deficiency, Blood. 18:149, 1961.

85. Graham, J. B., Barrow, E. M., and Hougie, C.: Stuart clotting defect: genetic aspects of a "new" hemorrhagic state, J. Clin. Invest. 36:497, 1957.

86. Denson, K. W. E., Lurie, A., DeCataldo, F. and Mannucci, P. M.: The Factor X defect: Recognition of abnormal forms of Factor X, Brit. J. Hemat. 18:317, 1970.

87. Friedman, I. A., Quick, A. J., Higgens, F., Hussey, C. V., and Hickey, M. E.: Hereditary labile factor (Factor V) deficiency, J.A.M.A. 175:116, 1961.

88. Graham, J. B.: The inheritance of "vascular hemophilia" a new and interesting problem in human genetics, J. Med. Educ. 34:385, 1959.

89. Otto, J. C.: An account of hemorrhagic disposition existing in certain families, Med. Reposit. 61:1803.

90. Graham, J. B., McLendon, W. W., and Brinkhous, K. M.: Mild Hemophilia, an allelic form of the disease, Amer. J. Med. Sci. 225:46, 1953.

91. Wagner, R. H., Richardson, B. A., and Brinkhous, K. M.: A study of the separation of fibrinogen and antihemophilic factor in canine, porcine and human plasmas, Thromb. Diath. Haem. 1:1, 1957.

92. Blömback, M.: Purification of antihemophilic globulin. I. Some studies on the stability of the antihemophilic globulin activity in fractions I-0, and a method for its partial separation from fibrinogen, Arkiv. F. Kemi. 12:387, 1958.

93. Bidwell, E.: The purification of antihemophilic globulin from animal plasma, Brit. J. Haemat. 1:386, 1955.

94. Tocantins, L. M.: Hemophilic syndromes and hemophilia, Blood. 9:281, 1954.

95. DePalma, A. F., and Colter, J.: Hemophilic arthropathy, Clin. Arthrop. 8:163, 1956.

96. Ivins, J. C.: Bone and Joint Complications of Hemophilia, p. 225, in Hemophilia and Hemophilioid Diseases. Chapel Hill, U. North Carolina Press, 1959.

97. Jordan, H. H.: Hemophilic Arthropathies, Springfield, Ill., Thomas, 1958.

98. Nye, S. W., Graham, J. B., and Brinkhous, K. M.: The partial thromboplastin time as a screening test for the detection of latent bleeders, Amer. J. Med. Sci. 243:279, 1962.

99. Aggeler, P. M., White, S. G., Glendenning, M. B., Page, E. W., Leake, T. B., and Bates, G.: Plasma thromboplastin component (PTC) deficiency, a new disease resembling hemophilia, Proc. Soc. Exper. Biol. Med. 79:692, 1952.

100. Biggs, R., Douglas, A. S., Macfarlane, R. G., Dacie, J. V., Pitney, W. R., Merskey, C., and O'Brien, J. R.: Christmas disease, a condition previously mistaken for hemophilia; Brit. Med. J. 2:1378, 1952.

101. Aggeler, P. M., White, S. G., and Spaet, T. H.: Deuterohemophilia. Plasma thromboplastin component (PTC) deficiency, Christmas disease, hemophilia B, Blood 9:246, 1954.

102. Rapaport, S. I., Shiffman, S., Patch, M. J., and Ware, A. G.: A simple specific one-stage assay for plasma thromboplastin antecedent activity, J. Lab. Clin. Med. 57:771, 1961.

103. Rosenthal, R. L.: The Present States of Plasma Thromboplastin Antecedent Deficiency, p. 116, in Hemophilia and Hemophilioid Diseases. Brinkhous, K., ed. Chapel Hill, U. of North Carolina Press, 1957.

104. Alexander, B., Goldstein, R., Landwehr, G., and Cook, C. D.: Congenital SPCA deficiency: a hitherto unrecognized coagulation defect with hemorrhage rectified by serum and serum fractions, J. Clin. Invest. 30:596, 1951.

105. Owren, P. A.: Parahemophilia: hemorrhagic diathesis due to absence of a previously unknown clotting factor, Lancet 1:446, 1947.

106. Alexander, B., and Goldstein, R.: Parahemophilia in three siblings (Owren's disease), Amer. J. Med. 13:255, 1952.

107. Shapiro, S. S., Martinez, J. and Holborn, R. R.: Congenital dysprothrombinemia: a structural disorder of human prothrombin, J. Clin. Invest. 48:2251, 1969.

108. Borchgrevink, C. F., Egeberg, O., Pool, J. G., Skulason, T., Stormorken, H., and Waller, B.: A study of a case of congenital hypoprothrombinemia, Brit. J. Hemat. 5:284, 1959.

109. Pool, J. G., Desai, R., and Kropatkin, M.: Severe congenital hypoprothrombinemia in a Negro boy, Thromb. Diath. Haem. 7:235, 1962.

110. Gitlin, D., and Borges, W. H.: Studies on the metabolism of fibrinogen in 2 patients with congenital afibrinogenemia, Blood 8:679, 1953.

111. Frick, P. G., and McQuarrie, I.: Congenital afibrinogenemia, Pediatrics 13:44, 1954.

112. Jackson, D. P. and Beck, E. A.: Inherited abnormal fibrinogens, in Brinkhous, K. (ed.) Hemophilia and New Hemorrhagic States, Chapel Hill, U. of North Carolina Press, 1969.

113. Sherry, S., Lindmeyer, R. I., Fletcher, A. P., and Alkjaersig, N.: Studies on enhanced fibrinolytic activity in man, J. Clin. Invest. 38:810, 1959.

114. Tagnon, H. J., Levenson, S. M., Davidson, C. S., and Taylor, F. H. L.: The occurrence of fibrinolysis in shock, with observation on the prothrombin time and the plasma fibrinogen during hemorrhagic shock, Amer. J. Med. Sci. 211:88, 1946.

115. Sawyer, W. A., Fletcher, A. P., Alkjaersig, N., and Sherry, S.: Studies on the thrombolytic activity of human plasma, J. Clin. Invest. 39:426, 1960.

116. Ratnoff, O. D., Pritchard, J. A., and Copley, J. E.: Hemorrhagic states during pregnancy, New Eng. J. Med. 254:63, 1955.

117. Weiner, A. E., Reid, D. E., and Roby, C. C.: Incoagulable blood in severe premature separation of the placenta. A method of management, Amer. J. Obstet. Gynec. 66:475, 1953.

118. Pritchard, J. A., and Wright, M. R.: Pathogenesis of hypofibrinogenemia in placental abruption, New Eng. J. Med. 261:218, 1959.

119. Schneider, C. L.: Fibrin embolism (disseminated intravascular coagulation) with defibrination as one of the end results during placenta abruptio, Surg., Gynec. Obstet. 92:27, 1951.

120. Gollub, S., Ulin, A., Paxson, N. F., Winchell, H. S., O'Riordan, J., Black, M., and Ambrus, J. L.: Obstetrical hemorrhage in criminal abortion and abruptia placentae, J. Lab. Clin. Med. 53:765, 1959.

121. Reid, D. E., Weiner, A. E., and Roby, C. C.: Intravascular clotting and afibrinogenemia: the presumptive lethal factors in the syndrome of amniotic fluid embolism, Amer. J. Obstet. Gynec. 66:465, 1953.

122. Albrechtsen, O., Storm, O., and Troll, D.: Fibrinolytic activity in circulating blood following amniotic fluid infusion, Acta Hemat. 14:309, 1955.

123. Pritchard, J. A., and Ratnoff, O. D.: Studies of fibrinogen and other hemostatic factors in women with intrauterine death and delayed delivery, Surg., Gynec. Obstet. 101:467, 1955.

124. Jackson, D. P., Hartman, R. C., and Busby, T.: Fibrinogenopenia complicating pregnancy: clinical and laboratory studies, Obstet. Gynec. 5:223, 1955.

125. Chalnot, P., Michon, P., and Lochard, M.: Afibrinémie Mortelle à L'occasion d'une Intervention Endothoracique, Rev. Hemt. 7:27, 1952.

126. von Kaulla, K. N., and Swan, H.: Clotting deviations in man during cardiac by-pass: fibrinolysis and circulating anticoagulant, J. Thoracic Surg. 30:519, 1958.

127. Pisciotta, A. V., and Schulz, E. J.: Fibrinolytic purpura in acute leukemia, Amer. J. Med. 19:824, 1955.

128. Sirridge, M. S., Bowman, K. S., and Garber, P. E.: Fibrinolysis and changes in fibrinogen in multiple myeloma, Arch. Int. Med. 101:630, 1958.

129. Mersky, C., Johnson, A. J., Kleiner, G. J. and Wohl, H.: The defibrination syndrome: Clinical features and laboratory diagnosis, Brit. J. Hemat. 13:528, 1967.

130. Tagnon, H. J., Schulman, P., Whitmore, W. F., and Levine, L. A.: Prostatic fibrinolysis: study of a case illustrating role in hemorrhagic diathesis of cancer of the prostate, Amer. J. Med. 15:875, 1953.

131. Bachmann, F., Duckert, F., and Koller, F.: The Stuart-Prower factor assay and its clinical significance, Thromb. Diath. Haem. 2:24, 1958.

132. Owren, P. A.: Control of anticoagulant therapy, Arch. Int. Med. 111:249, 1963.

133. Murphy, E. A., and Mustard, J. F.: Dicumarol therapy and platelet turnover, Circ. Res. 9:402, 1962.

134. Aballe, A. J., Banus, V. L., de Lamerens, S., and Rosengvaig, S.: Coagulation studies in the newborn period. Alterations of thromboplastin generation and effects of vitamin K in full-term and premature infants, Amer. J. Dis. Child. 94:589, 1957; III. Hemorrhagic disease of the newborn, Amer. J. Child 97:524, 1959; IV. Deficiency of Stuart-Prower factor as a part of the clotting defect of the newborn, Amer. J. Dis. Child. 97:549, 1959.

135. Hilgartner, M. W.: Personal communication.

136. Fresh, J. W., Ferguson, J. H., Stamey, C., Morgan, F. M., and Lewis, J. H.: Blood prothrombin, proconvertin, and proacceleran in normal infancy. Questionable relationship to vitamin K, Pediatrics 19:241, 1957.

137. Shanberge, J. N., and Regan, E. E.: The thromboplastin generation heparin tolerance test (TGHTT) in hypocoagulable states, Fed. Proceed. 19:3, 1960.

138. Margolius, A., Jr., Jackson, D. P., and Ratnoff, O. D.: Circulating anticoagulants: a study of 40 cases and a review of the literature, Medicine 40:145, 1961.

139. Lewis, J. H., Ferguson, J. H., Fresh, J. W., and Zucker, M. B.: Primary hemorrhagic diseases, J. Lab. Clin. Med. 49:211, 1957.

140. Biggs, R., and Bidwell, E.: A method for the study of antihemophilic globulin inhibition with reference to six cases, Brit. J. Hemat. 5:379, 1959.

141. Breckenridge, R. T., and Ratnoff, O. D.: Studies of the nature of the circulating anticoagulant directed against antihemophilic factor: with notes on an assay for antihemophilic factor, Blood 20:137, 1963.

142. Feinstein, D., Chang, M., Kasper, C. K., and Rapoport, S. I.: Hemophilia A: Polymorphism detectable by a Factor VIII antibody, Science 163:1071, 1969.

143. Goldstein, R., Gelfand, M., Sanders, M., and Rosen, R.: Anticoagulant appearing in

plasma thromboplastin component (PTC) deficiency, J. Clin. Invest. 35-707, 1956.

144. Conley, C. L., and Hartman, R. C.: A hemorrhagic disorder caused by circulating anticoagulant in patients with disseminated lupus erythmatosus, J. Clin. Invest. 31:621, 1952.

145. Lee, S. L., and Sanders, M.: A disorder of blood coagulation in systemic lupus erythematosus, J. Clin. Invest. 34:1814, 1955.

146. Frick, P. G.: Inhibition of the conversion of fibrinogen to fibrin by abnormal proteins in multiple myeloma, Amer. J. Clin. Path. 25: 1263, 1955.

147. Wayne, L., Goldsmith, R. E., Glueck, H. I., and Berry, H. K.: Abnormal calcium binding associated with hyperglobulinemia, clotting defects, and osteoporosis: a study of this relationship, J. Lab. Clin. Med. 54:958, 1959.

148. Heni, F., and Krauss, I.: Angeborene Familiare Gerinnungsstorung durch Heparintige Hemmkorper, Klin. Wschr. 34:747, 1956.

149. Czernobilsky, H., and Alexander, B.: Some Qualitative Aspects of Platelet Function in Normal, Thrombocytopenic and Thrombocytopathic States, p. 565, in Blood Platelets, Henry Ford Hospital International Symposium, Boston, Little, Brown, 1961.

150. Emery, J. L., Gordon, R. R., Rendle-Short, J., Varadi, S., and Warrack, A. J. N.: Congenital amegakaryocytic thrombocytopenia with congenital deformities and leukemoid blood picture in newborn, Blood 12:567, 1957.

151. Reinhold, J. D. L., Neumark, H., Lightwood, R., and Carter, C. O.: Familial hypoplastic anemia with congenital abnormalities (Fanconi's syndrome), Blood 7:915, 1952.

152. Cox, E. V., Meynell, M. J., Cooke, W. T., and Gaddie, R.: Scurvy and anemia, Amer. J. Med. 32:240, 1962.

153. Pohle, F. J.: Blood platelet counts in relation to menstrual cycle in normal women, Amer. J. Med. Sci. 197:40, 1939.

154. Pepper, H., Liebowitz, D., and Linsay, S.: Cyclical thrombocytopenic purpura related to the menstrual cycle, Arch. Path. 61:1, 1956.

155. Minot, G. R.: Purpura hemorrhagica with lymphocytosis. An acute type and an intermittent type, Amer. J. Med. Sci. 192:445, 1936.

156. Hjort, P., and Paputchis, H.: Platelet life span in normal, splenectomized and hypersplenic rats, Blood 15:45, 1960.

157. Ekman, C.: Portal hypertension, diagnosis and surgical treatment, Acta Chir. scandinav. Supp. 222:1, 1957.

158. Craddock, C. G., Jr., Adams, W. S., Perry, S., and Lawrence, J. S.: Dynamics of platelet production as studied by depletion techniques in normal and irradiated dogs, J. Lab. Clin. Med. 45:906, 1955.

159. Jackson, D. P., Krevans, J. R., and Conley, C. L.: Mechanism of the thrombocytopenia that follows multiple whole blood transfusions, Trans. Ass. Amer. Physicians 69:155, 1956.

160. Sutherland, D. A., and Clark, H.: Hemangioma associated with thrombocytopenia. Report of a case and review of the literature, Amer. J. Med. 33:150, 1962.

161. Wright, C. S., Doan, C. A., Bouroncle, B. A., and Zollinger, R. M.: Direct splenic arterial and venous blood studies in hypersplenic syndromes before and after epinephrine, Blood 6:195, 1951.

162. Ackroyd, J. B.: Pathogenesis of thrombocytopenic purpura due to hypersensitivity to Sedormid, Clin. Sci. 7:249, 1949.

163. Shulman, R. R.: Immunoreactions involving platelets. I. A steric and kinetic model for formation of a complex from a human antibody, quinidine as a haptene, and platelets: and for fixation of complement by the complex, J. Exp. Med. 107:665, 1958.

164. Harrington, W. J., Sprague, C. C., Minnich, V., Moore, C. V., Aulvin, R. C., and Dubach, R.: Immunologic mechanisms in idiopathic and neonatal thrombocytopenic purpura, Ann. Int. Med. 38:433, 1953.

165. Dausset, J., Colin, M., and Colombani, J.: Immune platelet iso-antibodies. Vox. Sang. 5:4, 1960.

166. Shulman, R., Aster, R. H., Leitner, A., and Hiller, M. C.: Immunoreactions involving platelets. V. Post-transfusion purpura due to a complement-fixing antibody against a genetically controlled platelet antigen. A proposed mechanism for thrombocytopenia and its relevance in "autoimmunity", J. Clin. Invest. 40:1597, 1961.

167. Baldini, M., Costea, N., and Ebbe, S.: Studies in Antigenic Structure of Blood Platelets, p. 378, Proc. VIII Cong. Europ. Soc. Hemat. 1961. Basel and New York, S. Karger, 1962.

168. Shulman, R., Aster, R. H., Pearson, H. A., and Hiller, M. C.: Immunoreactions involving platelets. VI. Reactions of maternal isoantibodies responsible for neonatal purpura. Differentiation of a second platelet antigen system, J. Clin. Invest. 41:1059, 1962.

169. Miescher, P., and Cooper, N.: The fixation of soluble antigen-antibody-complexes upon thrombocytes, Vox. Sang. 5:138, 1960.

170. Harrington, W. J., and Arimura, G.: Immune Reactions of Platelets, p. 659, in Blood Platelets, Henry Ford Hospital International Symposium, Boston, Little, Brown, 1961.

170a. Karpatkin, S. and Siskind, G.: In vitro detection of platelet antibody in patients with ITP and systemic lupus erythematosus, Blood 33:795, 1969.

171. Tullis, J. L.: Identification and significance of platelet antibodies. New Eng. J. Med. 255:541, 1956.

172. Corn, M., and Upshaw, J. D., Jr.: Evaluation of platelet antibodies in idiopathic thrombocytopenic purpura, Arch. Int. Med. 109:117, 1962.

173. Jackson, D. P., Schmid, H. J., Zieve, P. D., Levin, J., and Conley, C. L.: Nature of a platelet-agglutinating factor in serum of pa-

tients with idiopathic thrombocytopenic purpura, J. Clin. Invest. 42:383, 1963.

174. Rabinowitz, Y., and Dameshek, W.: Systemic lupus erythematosus after "idiopathic" thrombocytopenic purpura: a review, Ann. Int. Med. 52:1, 1960.

175. Epstein, R. D., Lozner, E. L., Coffey, T. S., and Davidson, C. S.: Congenital thrombocytopenic purpura. Purpura hemorrhagica in pregnancy and in the newborn, Amer. J. Med. 9:44, 1950.

176. Moschcowitz, E.: An acute pleiochromic anemia with hyaline thrombosis of the terminal arterioles and capillaries, Arch. Int. Med. 36:89, 1925.

177. Craig, J. M., and Gitlin, D.: The nature of the hyaline thrombi in thrombotic thrombocytopenic purpura, Amer. J. Path. 33:251, 1957.

178. Orbsin, J. L.: Morphology of thrombotic thrombocytopenic purpura with demonstration of aneurysms, Amer. J. Path. 28:129, 1952.

179. Glanzmann, E.: Hereditare Hammorrhagische thrombasthenie. Ein Beitrag zur Pathologia der blutplattchen, J. Kinderheills 88:113, 1918.

180. Weiss, H. J.: Platelet aggregation, adhesion and adenosine diphosphatate release in thrombopathia (platelet factor 3 deficiency): Comparison with Glanzman's thrombasthemia and von Willebrand's disease, Amer. J. Med. 43:570, 1967.

181. Ulutin, O. N.: The Qualitative Platelet Diseases, p. 553, in Blood Platelets, Henry Ford Hospital International Symposium, Boston, Little, Brown, 1961.

182. von Willebrand, E. A.: Hereditare Pseudohemofili, Finska, Lab.-sallsk. hande. 68:87, 1926.

183. von Willebrand, E. A., and Jurgens, R. I.: Ueber eine neue Bluterkrankheit, die konstitutionelle Thrombopathie, Klin. Wschr. 12:414, 1933.

184. Alexander, B., and Goldstein, R.: Dual hemostatic defect in pseudohemophilia, J. Clin. Invest. 32:551, 1953.

185. Nilsson, I. M., Blömback, M., Jorpes, E., Blömback, B., and Johansson, S. A.: von Willebrand's disease and its correction with human plasma fraction I-O, Acta Med. scand. 159:179, 1957.

186. Horowitz, H. I. and O'Leary, D.: von Willebrand's disease: A critical evaluation of diagnostic criteria, N.Y. State J. Med. 65:2236, 1965.

187. Biggs, R., and Matthews, J. M.: The treatment of hemorrhage in von Willebrand's disease and the blood level of Factor VIII (AHG), Brit. J. Hemat. 9:203, 1963.

188. Baccuglia, G., and Neel, J. V.: Congenital vascular defect associated with platelet abnormality and antihemophilic factor activity, Blood, 15:807, 1960.

189. Rendu, M.: Epistaxis répétees chex un Sujet Sufferant Pour Angiomes Cutanés et Muquex, Bull. Mem. Soc. Med. Hosp. Paris 13:731, 1896.

190. Osler, W.: On a familial form of recurring epistaxis associated with multiple telangiectases of the skin and mucous membrane, Bull. Johns Hopkins Hosp. 12:333, 1901.

191. Weber, F. P.: A case of multiple hereditary developmental angiomata (telangiectasis) of the skin and mucous membrane associated with recurring hemorrhages, Lancet 2:160, 1907.

192. Bird, R. M., and Jaques, W. E.: Vascular lesion of hereditary hemorrhagic telangiectasia, New Eng. J. Med. 260:597, 1960.

193. Brady, R. O., Gal, A. E., Bradley, R. M., Martensen, E., Warshaw, A. L. and Laster, L.: Enzymatic defect in Fabry's disease, New Eng. J. Med. 276:1163, 1967.

194. Wise, D., Wallace, H. J., and Jellinek, E. H.: Angiokeratoma corporis diffusum, a clinical study of eight affected cases, Quart. J. Med. 31:177, 1962.

195. Cetingil, A. I., Ulutin, O. N., and Karaca, M.: A platelet defect in a case of scurvy, Brit. J. Hemat. 4:350, 1958.

196. Flute, P. T., and Howard, A. M.: Blood coagulation in scorbutic pigs: a defect in acceleration by glass contact, Brit. J. Hemat. 5:421, 1959.

197. Vernier, R. L., Farquhar, M. G., Brunson, J. G., and Good, R. A.: Chronic renal disease in children, J. Dis. Child. 96:306, 1958.

198. Allen, D. M., Diamond, L. K., and Howell, D. A.: Anaphylactoid purpura in children (Schönlein-Henoch syndrome) review and a follow-up of the renal complications, J. Dis. Child. 99:833, 1960.

199. Ackroyd, J. F.: Allergic purpura including purpura due to foods, drugs and infections, Amer. J. Med. 14:605, 1953.

200. Bywaters, E. G. L., Isdole, I., and Kempton, J. J.: Schönlein-Henoch purpura, Quart. J. Med. 26:161, 1957.

201. Dixon, F. J., Feldman, J. D., and Vasquez, J. J.: Experimental glomerulonephritis. The pathogenesis of a laboratory model resembling the spectrum of human glomerulonephritis, J. Exp. Med. 113:899, 1961.

202. Benacerrai, B., Patter, J. L., McCluskey, R. T., and Miller, F.: The pathologic effects of intravenously administered soluble antigen-antibody complexes. II. Acute glomerulonephritis in rats, J. Exp. Med. 111:195, 1960.

203. Cruichshank, B.: The role of auto-antibodies in anaphylactoid purpura, Immunology 2:123, 1959.

204. McKusick, V.: Heritable Disorders of Connective Tissue, ed. 3, St. Louis, Mosby, 1966.

205. Soergel, K. H., and Sommers, S. C.: Idiopathic pulmonary hemosiderosis and related syndromes, Amer. J. Med. 32:499, 1962.

206. Gardner, F. H., and Diamond, L. K.: Autoerythrocyte sensitization: a form of purpura producing painful bruising following auto-

sensitization to red cells in certain women, Blood, 10:675, 1955.

207. Agle, D. P., and Ratnoff, O. D.: Purpura as a psychosomatic entity, Arch. Int. Med. 109:89, 1962.

208. Levin, M. B., and Pinkus, H.: Autosensitivity to desoxyribonucleic acid (DNA) report of a case with inflammatory skin lesions controlled by chloroquin. New Eng. J. Med. 264:533, 1961.

209. Kuramoto, A., Steiner, M., and Baldini, M. G.: Lack of platelet response to stimulation in the Wiskott-Aldrich syndrome, New Eng. J. Med. 282:475, 1970.

210. Gunz, F. W.: Hemorrhagic thrombocythemia. A critical review, Blood 15:706, 1960.

211. Strauss, W. G.: Purpura hyperglobulinemia of Waldenström: report of a case and review of literature, New Eng. J. Med. 260:857, 1959.

212. Goetz, R. W., and Good, R. A.: Benign hyperglobulinemic purpura. Relation to Mikulicz's disease, Sicca syndrome and epidermolysis bullosa dystrophica, Arch. Dermat. 83, 26, 1961.

213. Weiss, H. J., Demis, D. J., Elgart, M. L., Crawford, S. B., and Crosby, W. H.: Treatment of two cases of hyperglobulinemic purpura with thioguanine, New Eng. J. Med. 268:753, 1963.

214. Rosen, F. S.: The macroglobulins, New Eng. J. Med. 267:491, 1962.

215. Ritzman, S. E., Thurm, R. H., Truax, W. E., and Levin, W. C.: The syndrome of macroglobulinemia. Review of the literature and a report of two cases of macroglobulinemia, Arch. Int. Med. 105:939, 1960.

216. Pachter, M. R., Johnson, S. A., Neblett, T. R., and Truant, J. P.: Bleeding, platelets, and macroglobulins, Amer. J. Clin. Path. 31:467, 1959.

217. Schwab, P. J., and Fahey, J. L.: Treatment of Waldenström's macroglobulinemia by plasmapheresis, New Eng. J. Med. 263:574, 1960.

28

Anemia, Weakness and Pallor

EDWARD H. REINHARD

Definition of Anemia

Introduction

**Pathophysiology of the Symptoms
and Signs of Anemia**
  Weakness and Fatigue
  Apathy and Lassitude
  Pallor and Other Skin Changes
  Cardiovascular Symptoms and Signs
  Gastrointestinal Symptoms and Signs
  Genitourinary Symptoms and Signs
  Neurological Symptoms and Signs
  Fever
  Splenomegaly, Hepatomegaly and
    Lymph Node Enlargement
  Jaundice

Pathologic Physiology of the Anemias
  Structure and Physiologic Function of
    the Normal Human Erythrocyte
  Classification of the Anemias
  Iron-Deficiency Anemias
  Vitamin B-12 and Folate Deficiency
    Anemias
  Hemolytic Anemias
  Other Types of Anemia

Definition. Anemia refers to a reduction of the oxygen-carrying capacity of the blood below normal values due to an abnormality in the quantity or quality of the red blood cells. In the great majority of cases, anemia involves a reduction below normal in the number of erythrocytes, the quantity of hemoglobin, and the volume of packed erythrocytes per 100 ml. of blood. However, only one or two of these values may be reduced in certain types of anemia. For example, in microcytic, hypochromic anemia due to iron deficiency, the total number of erythrocytes per 100 ml. of blood may be within the normal range, but the hemoglobin value (and hence the oxygen-carrying capacity of the blood) is below normal. Indeed, in certain conditions such as methemoglobinemia and carboxyhemoglobinemia, the patient may be functionally anemic even though the red blood cell count, the hemoglobin value, and the hematocrit reading are all normal. In these disorders, there is adequate hemoglobin present in the blood, but it is in a chemical form, which will not transport oxygen. At the other extreme, it is possible for the erythrocyte count, the hemoglobin concentration, and the hematocrit value all to be reduced below normal without the patient being anemic. Overhydration due to excessive intravenous administration of fluids is an example of this; the physiological abnormality is an increase in the plasma volume, with resultant hemodilution producing an apparent but not a real "anemia." This reduces the oxygen-carrying capacity of each 100 ml. of blood, and may even result in tissue anoxia, but the fundamental abnormality does not involve the production or the survival of the red blood cells or hemoglobin.

It is extremely important to emphasize that the normal ranges of variation of the erythrocyte count, the hemoglobin value, and the hematocrit are considerably greater than is generally appreciated, and normal ranges vary with age and sex as illustrated in Figure 28-1.[1,2] In adults, the normal range of hemoglobin values is approximately 14 to 18 Gm./100 ml. for men and 12 to 16 Gm./100 ml. for women. When a patient's hemoglobin level is in the uncertain area between normal and abnormal, it is very helpful to secure previous values obtained over a period of years if such records are available; only in this way can one determine whether a specific value is normal for a given patient. Nothing in medicine is more futile than trying to raise a "low normal" hemoglobin or hematocrit value to *average* normal levels by the administration of "shotgun" hematinics.

INTRODUCTION

Deficiency in the oxygen-carrying capacity of blood often results in disturbances in the function of many organs and tissues, and these disturbances may lead to a wide variety of symptoms. The complaints vary from patient to patient, as well as with the rapidity of development of the anemia and with its severity. In general, anemia of slow and insidious onset is surprisingly well-tolerated by young, otherwise healthy individuals, and there may be no symptoms whatever until the hemoglobin value and the hematocrit fall to levels below 50 per cent of normal, or even lower. Under these circumstances, the individual may first seek medical attention, not because he has any complaints, but because friends have commented upon his pale appearance. In contrast, when anemia is of rapid onset, dyspnea and palpitation may occur when the hemoglobin and hematocrit values are considerably above 50 per cent of normal; when the blood loss is sudden or very severe, shock may ensue.

Anemia itself may cause certain signs and symptoms, but other *unrelated diseases* often play an important part in determining the degree of anemia required to precipitate the symptoms, or even the nature of the specific symptoms in a given patient. For example, a patient with arteriosclerosis of a coronary artery which has resulted in some narrowing of the coronary lumen may not have chest pain, but the subsequent development of anemia may result in sufficient myocardial ischemia to produce angina pectoris. The extent to which the coronary artery is narrowed will determine the severity of the anemia which must develop before angina occurs.

A second group of signs and symptoms are caused by the effect of the anemia on *various organs*. Reference has already been made to the fact that anemia may precipitate angina. Under similar circumstances, the sudden onset of a sufficiently severe anemia may be the immediate precipitating cause of myocardial infarction, cerebral in-

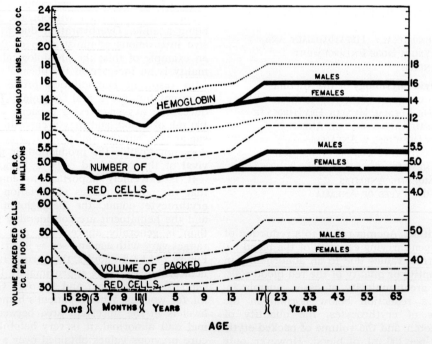

FIG. 28-1. Normal curve for hemoglobin, red blood cells, and volumes of packed red cells, from birth to old age. The mean values are heavily outlined. The range of variation is indicated by dotted lines for hemoglobin, interrupted lines for red blood cell count, and dotted interrupted lines for volume of packed red cells. The scales for hemoglobin, red blood cell count, and volume of packed red cells are similar, and therefore the relative changes in these three values are apparent on inspection. The scale for age, however, is progressively altered. (Courtesy of Dr. Maxwell Wintrobe[1,2])

farction, or the infarction of almost any viscus. Severe anemia can certainly precipitate congestive heart failure. Anemia may cause impairment of renal function or aggravate pre-existing renal disease without producing actual infarction. Conversely, in severe renal failure with uremia due to any cause, anemia may develop as a *result* of the renal failure. Anemia may contribute to the development of congestive heart failure as a result of several different pathophysiological mechanisms.

A third group of signs and symptoms are caused by disorders *etiologically associated* with the anemia, rather than being caused by the anemia itself. In pernicious anemia, the vitamin B-12 deficiency results in anemia but also gives rise to soreness of the tongue, numbness and tingling of the extremities, and diarrhea. Jaundice and splenomegaly may first attract attention before anemia is evident in hereditary spherocytosis.

The pathophysiology of the symptoms and signs occurring in association with various types of anemia will be discussed below. Under each symptom or sign, emphasis will be placed on whether the clinical manifestation is due to the anemia per se, to the underlying deficiency or disease responsible for the anemia, or to aggravation by the anemia of some totally unrelated disorder.

PATHOPHYSIOLOGY OF THE SYMPTOMS AND SIGNS OF ANEMIA

Weakness and Fatigue. There is a widely held misconception that anemia is the commonest cause of weakness and fatigue; this is definitely not true. As is pointed out earlier in this chapter, many patients have moderately severe anemia without any weakness or fatigue whatever, and, conversely, weakness and fatigue, which probably constitute the most common of all complaints in late 20th century America, may be due to a tremendous variety of causes, prominent among which are boredom, depression, anxiety, and other psychophysiological abnormalities. This subject is discussed in Chapter 29. Although an adult with moderately severe anemia may not complain of weakness or fatigue at rest, exercise tolerance is often lowered. In children, however, even severe anemia may be asociated with very little decrease in exercise tolerance.[3]

Apathy and Lassitude. Although anemia is not the most common cause of apathy, lassitude, and fatigue, these symptoms do occur in association with moderate to severe anemia. Their pathogenesis is not clear. However, no close correlation exists between these symptoms and the degree of anemia, and it would seem that psychosomatic mechanisms contribute, in some cases, to the development of these complaints. The anemic patient sometimes shows a lack of interest in his surroundings, and diminished enthusiasm for his work. It has been suggested that neurotic symptoms and even psychoses may be triggered or aggravated by chronic anemia.[4]

PALLOR AND OTHER SKIN CHANGES

Pallor refers to an abnormally pale appearance of the patient. Although pallor may be manifest on examining the skin, this can be misleading, since there is wide normal variability in skin color because of individual differences in the size and depth below the surface of the small skin blood vessels. Thus, some individuals with normal blood counts may appear pale, whereas others with similar blood values may appear plethoric. Hence, a change in skin color may be more important than the absolute shade. There is less normal variation in the color of *mucous membranes*, and hence one can estimate the degree of anemia more accurately by examining the conjunctivae, mouth, pharynx, and lips. The color of the *fingernail bed* is also more reliable than skin color in estimating anemia. It is common practice to inspect the hands for pallor. As the hemoglobin level drops, the palms become pale first, but the creases in the palms become pale only with severe anemia. Inspection of the palms, although a more reliable index of anemia than examination of other parts of the skin, is valid only if the hands are warm and held at the level of the heart. Cold hands may appear pale because of vasoconstriction.

A light lemon-yellow tint to the skin is characteristic of severe untreated pernicious anemia (mild bilirubinemia plus pallor). The severe anemia resulting from acute hemorrhage gives rise to a very white waxy appearance of the skin. With more chronic blood loss, the skin color is sallow. Pallor is often severe in leukemia, and it has been stated the the skin may have a grayish tint.

In severe aortic regurgitation, the patient may appear pale although there is no anemia, whereas in mitral stenosis and mitral regurgitation, there is a redness of the facies that may mask an existing anemia. These changes result from the relative blood supply to blood vessels near the skin surface.

In certain types of anemia, the skin may become dry and shrivelled. In pernicious anemia graying of the hair often occurs early, and most pernicious anemia patients have blue eyes.

Chronic ulcers around the ankles occur in association with various blood dyscrasias, but particularly in sickle-cell anemia and other hemolytic anemias.[5,6] The leg ulcers in sickle-cell anemia are probably due to a combination of factors. Occlusion of small vessels and the anemia, per se, lower the oxygen tension in areas where the circulation is normally sluggish. The lowered oxygen tension then further aggravates the situation by causing an increase in the viscosity of the sickle-cell blood.

CARDIOVASCULAR SYMPTOMS AND SIGNS

Most otherwise healthy patients who have mild or moderate anemia have no cardiorespiratory symptoms at rest, although they may have diminished exercise tolerance. As the anemia becomes more severe, exercise tolerance progressively decreases, until finally *dyspnea, tachycardia,* and *palpitation* may be present even at rest. Factors that determine the degree of anemia required to produce these symptoms include the age of the patient and the status of the cardiovascular system.[7]

The cardiac output is usually normal in patients with mild anemia, but as the anemia becomes more severe, cardiac output increases. This is a reflex phenomenon mediated via the sympathetic nervous system and may be thought of as an attempt to compensate for the decreased oxygen-carrying capacity of the blood. Once the anemia becomes sufficiently marked to produce increased cardiac output, relatively small further decreases in the hemoglobin and hematocrit produce comparatively large increases in the cardiac output.[8] The increase in cardiac output is brought about by an increase in the heart rate and an augmentation of the stroke volume. However, the distribution of the blood to the various organs resulting from this increased cardiac output is not uniform, and variations in the degree of constriction of the small blood vessels operate to bring about a proportionately greater distribution of blood to organs that are more sensitive to oxygen deprivation, with less blood going to organs that can tolerate oxygen deprivation better. For example, in severe anemia, the blood flow to the hands and

TABLE 28-1. PATHOPHYSIOLOGY OF CARDIOVASCULAR SIGNS AND SYMPTOMS THAT MAY BE CAUSED BY ANEMIA

THE FOLLOWING ARE INCREASED	GIVING RISE TO THE FOLLOWING CLINICAL FINDINGS
Heart rate	Fast pulse, palpitation
Stroke volume	Increased arterial pulsation (e.g., throbbing carotids), increased pulse pressure, capillary pulsations in fingertips, cardiac murmurs
Velocity of blood flow	Shortened circulation time, cardiac murmurs
Cardiac work	Increase in heart size; may lead to angina and congestive heart failure
Pulmonary ventilation	Tachypnea, dyspnea
Residual air volume and minute ventilation	Detected by pulmonary function studies

THE FOLLOWING ARE DECREASED	GIVING RISE TO THE FOLLOWING CLINICAL FINDINGS
Blood viscosity	Contributes slightly to increased circulation time (primarily due to increased stroke volume and heart rate)
Peripheral resistance	Contributes to increased circulation time
Total blood volume (decreased in *acute* blood loss)	Signs and symptoms of hypovolemia
A-V oxygen difference	— — —
Vital capacity, respiratory reserve volume, and complemental air volume	Increased respiratory rate, dyspnea
Renal blood flow	Azotemia, edema

NOT ALTERED
Central venous pressure and intracardiac pressure (right atrial pressure may at times be elevated)
Blood pressure

kidneys may be greatly decreased,[9] and it has been suggested that the relatively small renal blood flow is an important factor leading to the development of *edema*.[10]

The increase in the cardiac output resulting from moderate to severe anemia involves increased cardiac work, and, as would be anticipated, prolonged anemia may result in *cardiac hypertrophy*, usually of moderate degree. If the increased cardiac output is insufficient to compensate for the reduced oxygen-carrying capacity of the blood, the heart muscle, like other tissues, suffers from hypoxia; angina pectoris and congestive heart failure may ensue.

Slowly developing anemia does not give rise to changes in either the systemic or pulmonary blood pressure. The cardiac output and the velocity of blood flow are increased without any increase in blood pressure as a result of lowered peripheral vascular resistance.[11]

The increased velocity of blood flow in anemic patients tends to diminish tissue oxygenation, as is evidenced by the decreased arteriovenous oxygen difference. However, in anemic patients there is a compensatory decrease in the affinity of hemoglobin for oxygen, manifested by a shift of the oxygen dissociation curve to the right, which enables tissues to extract oxygen more efficiently.[12]

The lungs of patients with anemia show no anatomical alteration, and pulmonary function may be normal. However, with increasing anemia, as the cardiovascular abnormalities develop, the rate and depth of respiration increase, and the patient may become aware of dyspnea (at first only on mild exertion, but later, with very severe anemia, there may be dyspnea even at rest). These symptoms correlate with a decrease in the vital capacity, the respiratory reserve volume, and the complemental air volume.[13] The minute ventilation and the residual air volume are increased.[14]

On the basis of the preceding considerations, it is apparent that, as increasing anemia develops, certain physiologic adjustments in cardiovascular and pulmonary function occur and give rise to specific physical signs as outlined in Table 28-1.

Cardiac murmurs are common in association with severe anemia. Murmurs caused by blood abnormalities are called *hemic murmurs*. They occur most commonly at the apex, but almost as frequently at the pulmonic area[15]; in some cases, the murmur may be audible over the whole precordium, but it tends, in these circumstances, to be loudest in the apical or pulmonic areas. The functional murmur of anemia is almost always systolic in time; rarely, however, diastolic murmurs are heard in patients with severe chronic anemia but without organic heart disease.[16] The diastolic murmur may be mid-diastolic or presystolic, and may be heard best at the apex, thus simulating the murmur of mitral stenosis.[16,17] In sickle-cell anemia, particularly, the murmurs may be indistinguishable from those of organic valvular disease.

The classical systolic murmur heard in association with moderate to severe anemia has been attributed to the increased quantity and speed of flow of blood of low viscosity passing through a pulmonic valve, which is relatively stenotic (i.e., the lumen is "normal" but inadequate to allow the increased amount of blood to pass through without producing eddy currents); this has been referred to as a "systolic flow murmur." Another mechanism of production of systolic murmurs in anemic patients is ventricular enlargement with dilatation of the atrioventricular rings, resulting in functional mitral or tricuspid regurgitation.[18] The rare diastolic murmurs heard in association with very severe anemia have been attributed to greatly increased blood flow, producing a relative stenosis of the mitral or tricuspid valves. Both the systolic and diastolic murmurs tend to disappear when the anemia is relieved, and are accentuated when the anemia becomes worse.

Bruits are sometimes heard bilaterally over the carotid arteries in the neck in association with severe anemia, and in the absence of any disease of the arteries.[19] A continuous humming sound of venous origin can be heard also in some anemic patients on auscultation over the jugular vein; this has been referred to as the "bruit de diable." Again, these bruits and hums are thought to be due to the production of swirling of the blood and eddy currents resulting from the increased rate of flow of the blood of low viscosity through the blood vessels.

Electrocardiographic Changes. Mild anemia, unaccompanied by organic heart disease, does not produce any electrocardiographic abnormalities. However, in one study[20] 11 of 100 patients with severe anemia due to various causes had electrocardiographic changes that did not appear to be due to associated cardiac disease or hypokalemia. The most common abnormalities are S-T segment depression and flattening, or depression of the T waves.[15,20] These changes are presumably attributable to hypoxia of the myocardium. Similar changes have been observed with anemia resulting from acute blood loss.[21] Other changes including low voltage of the QRS complexes and prolongation of the P-R interval, have been noted occasionally. The electrocardiographic findings usually return to normal when the anemia is corrected.[22]

Sickle-Cell Anemia. The cardiovascular disturbances that are observed in association with sickle-cell anemia deserve special mention. Homozygous sickle-cell disease is one of the few disorders in which the anemia is consistently severe enough so that in nearly every case cardiac symptoms develop sooner or later. Furthermore, sickle-cell anemia is often accompanied by a thin body build, an immature appearance in relation to the patient's age, aching pains in the joints and elsewhere, loud cardiac murmurs, and other symptoms and signs, which may lead to an incorrect diagnosis of acute rheumatic fever, rheumatic or congenital heart disease, or subacute bacterial endocarditis. In addition, vascular thrombi in the pulmonary arteries and a reactive arteritis occur in association with sickle-cell anemia.[23] This multiple occlusion of small pulmonary arteries may be so extensive that pulmonary hypertension develops, eventually leading to cor pulmonale.[24,25]

Congestive Heart Failure. Dyspnea on exertion, palpitation, tachycardia, cardiomegaly, and edema are all common in severe chronic anemia; these findings may be incorrectly interpreted as indicating congestive heart failure. The diagnosis of cardiac decompensation is justified only if the patient also has orthopnea, râles in the lungs, distended neck veins, and an increased venous pressure.

When frank congestive heart failure does develop in an anemic patient, the possibility of some type of underlying organic heart disease always should be considered. There may be unsuspected coronary artery disease, or a murmur, which was considered to be hemic in origin, may actually be due to rheumatic valvulitis. However, severe anemia itself may occasionally result in heart failure in the absence of organic heart disease.[26] With increasingly severe anemia, compensatory physiologic adjustments (discussed in an earlier section) may fail to maintain the circulation, and finally decompensation occurs.

It has been shown that anemic patients have a significantly lower arterial oxygen tension and a considerably higher alveolar-arterial oxygen tension gradient than do normal subjects.[27] Anemia, per se, should not adversely affect the attainment of equilibrium between the oxygen tension in the alveolar air and that in the pulmonary capillary bed. Evidence has been presented that the increased alveolar-pulmonary artery oxygen tension gradient that is observed in anemic subjects is due to admixture with venous blood, possibly through such channels as thebesian veins, and bronchial veins that connect with pulmonary veins; or it might result from blood flow through imperfectly aerated regions of the lung.[27] Carbon dioxide transport is also affected in anemic subjects, in whom there is a deficiency in carbonic anhydrase.[28] This enzyme deficit, together with the decreased availability of hemoglobin for carbon dioxide transport, results in a decreased ability to absorb carbon dioxide from the tissues and release it in the lungs.

By expanding available hemodynamic compensatory mechanisms, the anemic individual at rest is able to manage the delivery of oxygen and the transport of CO_2 in relatively adequate fashion. During vigorous exercise, however, despite maximal utilization of all available hemodynamic adjustments, the supply of oxygen delivered to cells is sharply limited and the release of CO_2 from cells and its transportation also is curtailed.[29] If the hemoglobin level falls progressively, exercise tolerance steadily diminishes, and eventually the compensatory mechanisms are unable to maintain an adequate circulation even at rest and cardiac failure results.

Myocardial Infarction. A patient with fairly marked arteriosclerosis of the coronary arteries may be able to maintain reasonably normal circulatory dynamics for a considerable period of time. Such a patient tends to have reduced exercise tolerance, but he may be asymptomatic with limited activity. However, the sudden development of an acute blood loss anemia, or even acute hemolytic anemia, may lower the oxygen tension in the myocardium below the critical level with resultant myocardial infarction. In this situation, the sudden development of anemia is an important contributory cause, but not the primary cause, of the myocardial infarction. Anemia per se probably never causes myocardial infarction in patients with perfectly normal hearts, as a progressively falling hemoglobin value in such patients would result in death due to cerebral anoxia and perhaps shock before myocardial infarction would develop.

GASTROINTESTINAL SYMPTOMS

A great variety of gastrointestinal symptoms occur commonly in conditions characterized by anemia. These symptoms may be directly due to the anemia, they may be the result of a deficiency state, which simultaneously affects the hematopoietic organs and the gastrointestinal tract, or they may even aggravate the anemia by interfering with proper nutrition. The symptoms include sore mouth, a sore tongue, dysphagia, anorexia, abdominal distention and flatulence, nausea, vomiting, diarrhea, or constipation.

Almost any part of the digestive system may be involved. Recurring episodes of glossitis are common in untreated pernicious anemia. During these episodes, the patient may complain of marked soreness or actual pain in the tongue. The tongue appears beefy red either over its whole dorsum or in a patchy distribution. Occasionally, vesicles or small white ulcers simulating aphthous stomatitis may appear. Rarely, the patient may complain of burning of the entire mouth and pharynx and even pain on swallowing. The glossitis tends to subside spontaneously even in the absence of treatment, only to recur again. With the passage of time the epithelium of the tongue becomes smooth and slick and, upon examination with a magnifying glass, it is seen to be devoid of papillae. These atrophic changes develop even in patients who have never had any soreness of the tongue. When adequate therapy is given, there is usually partial restoration of the papillae.[30]

The essential lesion of pernicious anemia is absence of secretion of *intrinsic factor* by the gastric mucosa, associated with an obvious *atrophy of the gastric mucosa*. There is considerable evidence that immune mechanisms play a part in the pathogenesis of the gastric lesions.[31] About 90 per cent of patients with pernicious anemia possess serum antibodies that react specifically with the parietal cells of the gastric fundus. These antibodies fix complement and are directed against microsomal antigens in the parietal cells. More than half of all patients with pernicious anemia also have antibodies against microsomal antigens of thyroid acinar cells and, conversely, approximately one-third of patients with Hashimoto's thyroiditis and myxedema have antibodies against gastric parietal cell constituents.[32]

Iron also plays an important role in maintaining the integrity of epithelial tissues, as evidenced by the characteristic abnormalities in the nails associated with iron deficiency.[33] Cheilosis and glossitis are common in association with chronic iron deficiency anemia, and these manifestations are said to be relieved by iron therapy even when the patients remain on a poor diet.[34] Dysphagia, which is the outstanding symptom in the Plummer-Vinson's syndrome, has also been attributed to iron deficiency.[35] However, cheilosis, glossitis, and dysphagia have been found to be rare in East Africans with severe iron deficiency.[36] It has been suggested that the chronic fatigue and other symptoms which accompany iron deficiency states might be due to a deficiency of iron-containing enzymes,[37] but this has not been definitely established.

Ulcerated and necrotic lesions may be seen in the mouth and pharynx in association with agranulocytosis and aplastic anemia, and similar lesions are seen in mouth, rectum, and vagina in patients with acute leukemia. Lowered resistance to infection would seem to be the primary cause of such evidences of diseased epithelium. Examination of such lesions at necropsy usually shows acute and chronic inflammation, necrosis, and infiltration with leukemic cells.

GENITOURINARY SYMPTOMS

Menstrual disturbances are common in association with anemia. The most common disturbance is amenorrhea, but menorrhagia also occurs and may be severe. Anemia in the male may lead to loss of libido. The pathogenesis of these symptoms has not been defined.

Slight *proteinuria* is not uncommon in various types of anemia. *Polyuria* may occur, and *hyposthenuria* has been reported, particularly in association with sickle-cell anemia. Moderate *azotemia* may develop in severe anemias.

The pathogenesis of the reduced renal function has been elucidated only partially. It has been shown that the effective renal blood flow is markedly reduced in chronic anemia,[38] presumably as a result of constriction of afferent and efferent glomerular arterioles. As mentioned earlier, this constriction of renal arterioles diverts blood to other organs more sensitive to oxygen deprivation and may be thought of as an advantageous compensatory mechanism, but it certainly contributes to the development of azotemia in very severe anemic states or in patients who have underlying renal disease. Tubular excretion of Diodrast is also significantly reduced in chronic anemia.

Edema is common in association with severe anemia, even in the absence of demonstrable organic renal disease or congestive heart failure. Factors that contribute to the development of edema include reduced renal blood flow, hypoproteinemia, and decreased tissue oxygen tension, which results in increased capillary permeability.[39] Direct studies of water retention in association with various types of anemia have shown that water retention following salt administration is directly related to the degree of anemia, except in pernicious anemia. Salt loading did not result in water retention in untreated pernicious anemia.[40]

NEUROLOGICAL SYMPTOMS

Headache (often pounding in character), a tendency to fainting, dimness of vision, tinnitis, vertigo, irritability, restlessness, inability to concentrate, and drowsiness are all common in association with severe anemia. Presumably, these symptoms are due to hypoxia of the nervous system, and thus are attributable to the anemia itself.

Papilledema in association with blood loss anemia has been reported.[41] Retinal hemorrhages are seen frequently in patients with leukemia, aplastic anemia, and pernicious anemia. Thrombocytopenia and a hemorrhagic diathesis occur in all of these conditions and these abnormalities, plus the direct effect of anemia on capillary permeability,[39] account for the hemorrhages. The retinal hemorrhages may be of almost any type,[42] but flame-shaped and punctate hemorrhages are the most common in the author's experience.

The neurological manifestations of pernicious anemia are not due to the anemia per se, since they may appear in the absence of significant anemia. Indeed, paresthesia may be the first clinical manifestation of pernicious anemia. Vitamin B-12 is essential to the maintenance of normal nervous tissue metabolism, and vitamin B-12 deficiency due to any cause may lead to degeneration of the dorsal and lateral columns of the spinal cord, and even to degenerative changes in the peripheral nerves and in the brain itself. These degenerative changes are thought to be due to defective RNA synthesis, which occurs particulary in the long axons of nerve cells in the spinal cord.[43]

Symptoms referable to the nervous system occurred in from 70 to 95 per cent of cases of pernicious anemia, according to reports published prior to 1935[44,45,46]; in 25 per cent of cases, the neurological manifestations occurred prior to the development of recognized anemia. Since effective therapy and much better diagnostic tests for pernicious anemia have come into general use, the frequency of severe neurological manifestations has markedly decreased.[47] In recent years, instances of serious neurological manifestations have occurred in patients having the pathophysiologic defects of true pernicious anemia, but who have been taking multivitamin capsules containing sufficient folic acid to prevent the anemia at the time when they developed vitamin B-12 deficiency.[48]

The earliest neurological symptoms of pernicious anemia are numbness and tingling in the extremities and difficulty in walking. The earliest physical signs are first, loss of vibratory sense, and, next, loss of position sense in the distal extremities. There may be loss of touch sensation, but pain and temperature sensation usually remain intact. Ataxia, Romberg's sign, decreased or increased deep tendon reflexes, pathological toe signs, muscle flaccidity or spasticity, and sphincter paralysis may occur as the degenerative process in the spinal cord progresses. Visual disturbances and optic atrophy occasionally occur. Peripheral nerve degeneration occurs, as well as the typical spinal cord lesions[49,50]; the former may be responsible for the numbness as well as the rare instance of stocking hypesthesia and hyperesthesia of the soles of the feet.

Paresthesias also occur in association with chronic iron-deficiency anemia. Numerous neurologic manifestations occur in association with sickle-cell anemia,[51] including headache, convulsions, drowsiness, stupor, coma, aphasia, hemiplegia, stiff neck, nystagmus, pupillary changes, blindness, cranial nerve palsies, and paresthesias. It is likely that these manifestations are due to impairment of circulation to the nervous system, resulting from sickling of the red blood cells and the increased viscosity of such blood.

FEVER

Low-grade fever is not uncommon in association with severe anemia. In some cases, the fever is undoubtedly not due to the anemia per se, but rather to the underlying disease that caused the anemia or to an associated condition. For example, aplastic anemia and chronic lymphocytic leukemia, even when accompanied by severe anemia, rarely cause fever unless there is an associated infection. On the other hand, fever is extremely common in all types of acute leukemia.[52] High fever occasionally occurs in chronic granulocytic leukemia in the absence of infection, and the fever may subside promptly when the white blood cell count is lowered to normal by appropriate therapy.[53] The incidence of fever in chronic granulocytic leukemia is much lower than in the acute leukemias.

The pathogenesis of the fever of the acute leukemias and chronic granulocytic leukemia is unknown, but it is interesting to speculate that it might be related to the development of antibodies against the foreign (i.e. malignant) leukocytes in the patient's blood, bone marrow, and tissues. It has been shown that severe febrile reactions following blood transfusion are common in patients who have received a large number of transfusions, and in such patients, antibodies against the donor leukocytes have been demonstrated.[54,55] That these antibodies against the foreign leukocytes are responsible for the febrile reactions is strongly supported by the fact that the chills and fever can be prevented by the administration of blood from which most of the leukocytes have been removed.[56] Furthermore, in one large series, complete leukoagglutinins could be found in the serum of 58 per cent of patients who had posttransfusion chills and fever, and such leukoagglutinins were present in only 9 per cent of patients who had no reactions following transfusion.[57] If the repeated transfusion of foreign leukocytes can give rise to the production of antibodies against these leukocytes, which then react with antigens in the same type of foreign leukocytes on subsequent transfusion with resultant fever, it seems reasonable to speculate that similar mechanisms might operate in the patient with acute leukemia or chronic granulocytic leukemia where the antigenic make-up of the malignant cells might be foreign to the host, and where large numbers of cells are being constantly broken down. In addition to this hypothetical mechanism, it is clearly established that the basal metabolic rate and, hence, the body's heat production, are significantly increased in the acute leukemias and in most cases of chronic granulocytic leukemia. This undoubtedly contributes to the fever. The increased basal metabolic rate is thought to be due to the

increased rate of proliferation and enhanced oxygen consumption of the leukemic cells. The hypermetabolism is not related to increased thyroid activity.

Fever also occurs in association with acute hemolytic anemias. Rapid blood destruction due to a single episode of acute hemolytic anemia, or to a hemolytic crisis occurring during the course of a chronic hemolytic anemia, may be accompanied by symptoms suggesting an acute infection such as malaise, headache, severe aching pain in the back, extremities, or abdomen, and, also, chills and fever. In extreme cases, prostration and shock may develop. Under such circumstances there is a rapid destruction of red blood cells which results in a reduction in the total blood volume,[58] and the breakdown products of the red blood cells are rapidly removed by the body tissues. It seems likely that these varied symptoms, including the fever, are somehow related to the rapid lysis of the erythrocytes and the subsequent metabolism of the breakdown products.

SPLENOMEGALY, HEPATOMEGALY AND LYMPH NODE ENLARGEMENT

These physical signs are not due to anemia per se, but are often encountered in disorders characterized by anemia. The spleen, the liver, and the lymph nodes are commonly enlarged, firm, and nontender in the leukemias and malignant lymphomas; the enlargement is usually due to direct involvement of these organs by the neoplastic cells. Splenomegaly is an essential feature of chronic congestive splenomegaly (Banti's syndrome). In this syndrome, the liver may or may not be enlarged; there is usually an associated leukopenia and thrombocytopenia. Splenomegaly also occurs frequently in pernicious anemia and in association with many types of hemolytic anemia. In sickle-cell anemia, the spleen is enlarged early in life, but later undergoes multiple infarctions, fibrosis, and shrinkage, so that at autopsy it often weighs less than 50 Gm.[59] Splenomegaly persisting into adult life is common in many other hemoglobinopathies, including thalassemia. If an adult patient has significant splenomegaly and sickle cells are seen in the blood smear, the most likely diagnosis is that the patient is simultaneously heterozygous for HgS and another abnormal hemoglobin (often HgC), or thalassemia. Splenomegaly, often marked, occurs in as many as two-thirds of such cases.[60] In iron deficiency anemia, enlargement of both the liver and spleen may occur. The incidence of spleno- megaly in this type of anemia is a matter of considerable dispute. According to one often-quoted report published in 1933,[61] the spleen was palpable in approximately one- third of cases of hypochromic anemia occur- ring in adults. In the author's experience, the incidence of a palpable spleen in asso- ciation with iron deficiency anemia is less than 5 per cent; this could be related to the fact that iron deficiency anemia is now diag- nosed and treated much earlier than was the case in 1933.

Localized bone tenderness not related to trauma and not accompanied by spontane- ous bone pain, is an important physical sign that often indicates acute leukemia. This sign is most readily elicited by moderate pressure over the sternum. It is present less commonly in patients with chronic leu- kemia and multiple myeloma, and only rarely in patients with myelophthisic anemia due to metastatic cancer invading the bone marrow.

JAUNDICE

When jaundice occurs in association with anemia, it may be either due to a hemolytic process, in which case there is an increased production of bilirubin, or to an obstructive process, in which case there is usually dis- ease of the liver (either due to the underly- ing disease causing the anemia or to some secondary hepatic disturbance) which inter- feres with bile drainage.

Hemolytic anemia is characterized by: (1) various laboratory findings that are charac- teristic of increased red blood cell destruc- tion and, (2) laboratory findings that are related to the compensatory increase in erythrocyte production which almost always accompanies significant hemolysis. The in- creased red blood cell destruction results in an increased production of bilirubin, which is present in the serum primarily in the form of unconjugated (indirect reacting) bilirubin. Most of this passes through the liver cells and is excreted in the bile as conjugated bilirubin, which is then converted in the intestine by bacterial organisms into uro- bilinogen. There is, therefore, an elevated urobilinogen content in the feces, but bili- rubinuria is not usually observed, because unconjugated bilirubin is not excreted by the kidneys. In severe hemolytic anemia, small amounts of conjugated bilirubin may be present in the urine.[62] In addition, the blood smear may show changes in the red blood cells which are characteristic of a par- ticular type of hemolytic anemia. Thus, in hereditary spherocytic anemia, large num- bers of spherocytes are present; in heredi- tary hemolytic ovalocytosis, many of the erythrocytes have an elliptical shape; in sickle-cell anemia, sickle cells are seen; in thalassemia, target cells are prominent; and in microangiopathic hemolytic anemia, many bizarrely shaped red blood cells, including burr cells, helmet cells, schistocytes, and crenated cells are seen.[63]

The laboratory findings indicative of a compensatory increase in red blood cell pro- duction include an elevation of the reticulo- cyte count above the normal range (some- times to levels greater than 50 per cent), the appearance of nucleated red blood cells, chiefly normoblasts, in the peripheral blood, and an increase in the erythroid to myeloid cell ratio on bone marrow examination. In severe hemolytic anemias, there may be many more nucleated red blood cells than there are myeloid cells, in contrast to the normal E:M ratio of 1:3 or 1:4.

The jaundice seen in association with non- hemolytic anemia is of the obstructive type, and may be due to many different mecha- nisms. The anemia may be secondary to primary liver disease, such as cirrhosis of the liver. Or, the liver may be secondarily involved by the disease causing the anemia, such as infiltration with leukemic cells, car- cinoma cells, or Hodgkin's tissue. Hodgkin's disease is an outstanding example of a dis- order in which jaundice may occur as a re- sult of many different mechanisms. In one autopsy study of 57 jaundiced patients with Hodgkin's disease, the cause of the jaundice was liver invasion by Hodgkin's tissue in 70.2 per cent, hemolytic anemia in 5.2 per cent, extrahepatic bile duct obstruction by Hodgkin's tumor (lymph nodes) in 3.5 per cent, hepatitis in 3.5 per cent, choledocho- lithiasis in 1.8 per cent, hepatic cirrhosis in 1.8 per cent and unexplained in 14 per cent.[64]

Another general category of obstructive or hepatocellular jaundice associated with ane- mia includes those cases in which the jaun- dice is secondary to the therapy for the anemia (serum hepatitis following blood transfusion), or to treatment for the under- lying disease (cholestatic jaundice due to testosterone therapy for certain types of re- fractory anemia and myelofibrosis, or to 6-mercaptopurine therapy for leukemia, etc.). In all of these cases, the laboratory findings are characteristic of obstructive jaundice of either intrahepatic or extrahepatic type (see Ch. 24). Laboratory changes indicative of a compensatory increase in red blood cell production usually are not present.

PATHOLOGIC PHYSIOLOGY OF THE ANEMIAS

STRUCTURE AND PHYSIOLOGIC FUNCTION OF NORMAL HUMAN RED BLOOD CELLS

The normal mammalian erythrocyte is a biconcave disc (with a slightly depressed central portion) which is flexible and elastic. In the dog, it has been shown to fold up into a cup-shaped form with a hollow center as the cell flows into small capillaries.[65] The outer portion of the red blood cell functions as a membrane, the composition of which may not be homogeneous. Evidence has been presented indicating that there is a higher concentration of cholesterol around the periphery of the biconcave red cell than elsewhere on the cell membrane,[66] and it has been suggested that differences in surface tension resulting from this variation in cholesterol concentration may be responsible for the unique biconcave discoid shape of the cell. When excess water diffuses into the mature erythrocyte, it becomes smaller in its maximum diameter and spheroidal in shape. About 65 per cent of the red blood cell is water, 34 per cent is hemoglobin, and the remaining approximately 1 per cent consists of stroma, glucose, electrolytes, vitamins, enzymes, and other substances.

The function of the erythrocyte is oxygen transport. Oxygen combines with the hemoglobin molecule as the red corpuscle passes through the lung capillaries, and oxygen is then released in the tissues in accordance with the oxyhemoglobin dissociation curve. The hemoglobin in the red corpuscle also acts as a buffer in carbon dioxide transport. Carbon dioxide exists within cells chiefly joined with sodium as sodium bicarbonate, and this base loses its sodium to the hemoglobin molecule, thus allowing CO_2 to diffuse out of the cell. The shape of the mammalian red blood cell provides a maximum surface area for efficient gas diffusion. It is remarkable that the red blood cell loses its nucleus before entering into its phase of greatest physiological function.

The earliest recognizable red blood cell precursor in the bone marrow undergoes approximately three mitotic divisions over a period of three or four days in the process of developing into a reticulocyte. In the human adult, during this developmental period, heme and 2 alpha globin and 2 beta globin polypeptide chains are synthesized within the cell and united to form hemoglobin. It is thought that 10 to 15 per cent of the developing red blood cells in the bone marrow of normal healthy persons disintegrate without ever reaching maturity. In pernicious anemia and certain other anemias, the degree of "ineffective erythropoiesis" is much greater; this hemolysis of immature cells in the marrow contributes to the lemon-yellow color characteristic of these disorders (mild bilirubinemia plus pallor).

Many red blood cells, at the time of their delivery into the peripheral blood, are at the reticulocyte stage of development, but some of the cells lose their reticular substance prior to release. Under conditions of greatly increased erythropoiesis, the release of reticulocytes is accelerated, and the percentage of reticulocytes in the peripheral blood roughly parallels the rate of red blood cell production. Normoblasts may also appear in the peripheral blood, and some of the red blood cells may stain basophilic with Wright's stain (a dark bluish tinge to the cytoplasm) as a result of retained RNA.

The life-span in the circulation of a normal red blood cell is approximately 120 days. Thus, 1/120 or 0.8 per cent of the total red blood cell mass is broken down and must be replaced each day. As erythrocytes age, the concentration of certain vital enzymes, including glucose-6-phosphate dehydrogenase, decreases and other changes occur leading to senescence. About 90 per cent of the senescent cells are broken down and phagocytized in the reticuloendothelial system, and the other 10 per cent hemolyze intravascularly.

In animals, the production of polycythemia by hypertransfusion results in cessation of red blood cell production by the bone marrow, and, conversely, lowering the red blood cell mass below normal by phlebotomy results in a prompt resumption of erythropoiesis.[67] The same mechanism that brings about these changes is constantly brought into play in maintaining the red blood cell mass within normal limits under physiological conditions. When the red blood cell mass falls below normal, as well as in various other conditions causing an inbalance between oxygen supply and demand, *erythropoietin* is produced by the kidneys, apparently in the glomeruli[68] and perhaps in the juxtaglomerular cells. There is some

TABLE 28-2. Morphologic, Etiologic and Clinical Classification of Anemias
(Modified from Wintrobe, M. M.: Clinical Hematology, ed. 6
pp. 466–467, Lea and Febiger, Philadelphia.)

Morphologic Type	Etiologic Type or Mechanism Causing Anemia	Clinical Condition or Syndrome
Macrocytic $\left(\begin{array}{c} \text{M.C.V.} > \\ 94 \text{ cu. } \mu \\ \text{M.C.Hb.C.} \\ \text{normal} \end{array} \right)$	1. Vitamin B-12 or folate deficiency (megaloblastic anemias)	(a) Pernicious anemia (b) Malabsorption syndromes (c) Post-gastrectomy (total) (d) Nutritional macrocytic anemias (e) Due to antimetabolite therapy (f) Miscellaneous: megaloblastic anemias of infancy and of pregnancy, fish tape worm, etc.
	2. Macrocytosis due to reticulocytosis (reticulocytes are larger than mature rbc)	(a) Hemolytic anemias (b) Following acute hemorrhage
	3. Exact mechanism unknown	(a) Severe chronic liver disease (b) Hypothyroidism (may be normocytic)
Normocytic, normochromic $\left(\begin{array}{c} \text{M.C.V.} \\ 80\text{-}94 \text{ cu. } \mu \\ \text{M.C.Hb.C.} \\ > 30 \text{ percent} \end{array} \right)$	1. Sudden blood loss	(a) Hemorrhage from any cause (rbc may be macrocytic at time of peak reticulocytosis)
	2. Hemolytic anemias due to intracorpuscular defects	(a) Hemoglobinopathies including sickle-cell anemia, hereditary spherocytosis, paroxysmal hemoglobinuria, enzyme deficiency anemias, and other congenital nonspherocytic hemolytic anemias, etc.
	Extracorpuscular defects	(a) Hemolytic anemias due to immunoglobulins including isoagglutinins, cold, warm, and blocking antibodies (b) Hemolytic anemias due to chemical, physical, vegetable and animal agents, and infectious organisms (c) "Symptomatic" hemolytic anemias

	3. Depression of blood formation (excluding vitamin B-12 and folate deficiencies)	(a) Primary "refractory anemias"
		  1. Hypoplastic anemia of unknown cause
		  2. Due to agents that regularly produce marrow hypoplasia: ionizing radiation, alkylating agents, etc.
		  3. Due to agents that produce marrow hypoplasia in occasional individuals: antibiotics, anticonvulsants, many other drugs

[*Anemia is usually normocytic and normochromic, but may be normocytic and hypochromic, or, rarely, microcytic] ← see		(b) Anemias associated with chronic infections, chronic inflammatory diseases,* renal failure, malignant neoplasms (c) Myelophthisic anemias due to involvement of marrow by cancer cells, leukemia, fibrous tissue or bone (myelofibrosis, myelosclerosis) (d) Anemia associated with endocrine deficiencies (thyroid, adrenal, testicular, or anterior pituitary deficiency)

TABLE 28-2. Morphologic, Etiologic and Clinical Classification of Anemias (*Cont.*)

Type Morphologic	Etiologic Type or Mechanism Causing Anemia	Clinical Condition or Syndrome
Microcytic, hypochromic $\left(\begin{array}{c} \text{M.C.V.} < \\ 80 \text{ cu. } \mu \\ \text{M.C.Hb.C.} \\ < 30 \text{ percent} \end{array}\right)$	1. Iron deficiency	In adults, is most commonly due to chronic bleeding (chronic blood loss) In infants, most commonly due to iron deficient diet Other causes include defective absorption; excessive demands for iron (during rapid growth, repeated pregnancies); combinations of all factors mentioned above
	2. Copper, pyridoxine?	Rare anemias in infants responsive to copper and iron; rare anemias partially responsive to vitamin B-6
	3. Genetic anomaly	Thalassemia major
	4. Unknown	Sideroblastic refractory anemia

experimental evidence that tissues other than the kidneys may at times produce an erythropoietic substance in response to hypoxia.[69] Erythropoietin is thought to be a glycoprotein of high molecular weight which acts primarily at the stem cell level to initiate erythropoiesis in the bone marrow. It has been claimed that erythropoietin also stimulates hemoglobin synthesis and promotes the release of marrow reticulocytes.[70]

The methods of assaying erythropoietin are relatively crude, and usually the minute amount presumed to be present in normal plasma is too small to be detected. As would be expected, increased amounts of erythropoietin can be demonstrated in the plasma in blood loss anemia, in individuals with cyanosis due to congenital heart disease with associated secondary polycythemia, and in some patients with anemia due to leukemia. Erythropoietic activity has also been detected in the fluid from renal cysts and in extracts of tumors (particularly renal tumors) removed from patients with polycythemia presumed to be secondary to these lesions. Assayable levels of erythropoietin are usually *not* found in the serum of patients with polycythemia vera or hemolytic anemias. *High* levels of erythropoietin are found in association with hypoplastic anemia, presumably because the kidneys secrete normal or increased amounts of the substance, but because of the absence of erythropoietic tissue, it is not utilized.

Classification of the Anemias

The anemias may be classified on the basis of etiologic, morphologic, or clinical criteria. Etiologic factors would seem to be the most basic criteria for classification, but such a classification presents difficulties in that the anemia associated with certain specific diseases may involve several different etiological mechanisms. For example, the anemia associated with uremia involves defective erythropoiesis, but the red blood cell survival time may also be significantly shortened; the anemia of chronic blood loss involves the actual loss of blood which must be replaced, but iron deficiency develops and affects hemoglobin synthesis. The morphologic classification is based on the mean red blood corpuscle volume (M.C.V.) and the mean corpuscular hemoglobin concentration (M.C.Hb.C.). This classification has the great advantage that, once a careful red blood cell count, hemoglobin determination, and hematocrit level have been obtained, the M.C.V. and M.C.Hb.C. can be quickly calculated, and an immediate classification is available which considerably reduces the diagnostic possibilities and provides guidance in planning further diagnostic studies. Obviously, if the calculated M.C.V. and M.C.Hb.C. are inaccurate, the classification may be grossly misleading. Another shortcoming of this classification is that macrocytosis due to one disease, for example, pernicious anemia, may be masked by an-

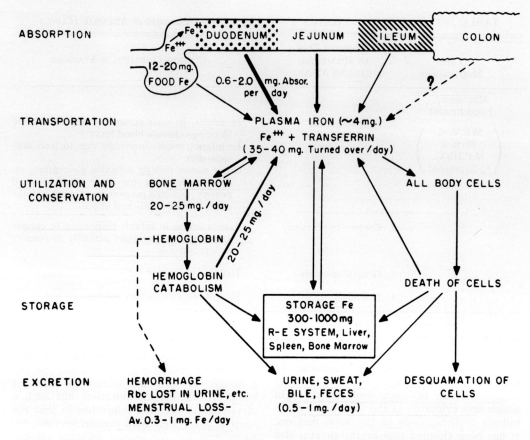

Fig. 28-2. Schematic outline of iron metabolism in the human adult. (Courtesy of Dr. C. V. Moore *in* Beeson and McDermott (eds.): Cecil-Loeb Textbook of Medicine, ed. 12, Philadelphia, Saunders, 1967)

other disorder, such as iron deficiency due to blood loss from an associated gastric carcinoma. The physician can avoid this pitfall by a careful examination of the blood smear, which, in this case, would reveal the presence of both macrocytic erythrocytes and hypochromic, microcytic cells.

A combined morphologic, etiologic and clinical classification is presented in Table 28-2. The reader must remember that a given patient may have anemia due to more than one etiological mechanism, so that morphologic characteristics may be impure. The table is not complete; several rare and relatively unimportant types of anemia have been excluded deliberately for the sake of conciseness.

The remainder of this chapter will be devoted to a consideration of the pathologic physiology of the more important types of anemia based on the etiological diagnoses (see column 2 of Table 28-2). Although it is listed last in the table, iron deficiency anemia will be discussed first because of its paramount importance.

IRON-DEFICIENCY ANEMIA

Iron deficiency is probably the most common cause of anemia in nontropical countries, and it usually responds readily to oral iron therapy. An understanding of the mechanism of production of the iron deficiency is crucial, since only by removing or correcting the underlying cause of the anemia can the patient be restored permanently to good health.

In chronic iron-deficiency anemia, the red blood cells are microcytic and hypochromic, the leukocyte level is normal or slightly reduced, and the platelet count is usually normal but may be increased. The serum bilirubin is normal or reduced, and the fecal urobilinogen is reduced. The serum iron level is below normal (i.e., less than 40 mcg.

per 100 ml.), the plasma iron-binding capacity is elevated, and transferrin, the iron-binding protein, is less than 15 per cent saturated. Bone marrow slides stained with special iron stains show a decrease in siderotic granules (hemosiderin) in the normoblasts and RE cells.

In recent years, extensive erythrokinetic studies utilizing radioiron have vastly increased knowledge concerning iron metabolism.[71,72,73] Some of the more important features are presented schematically in Figure 28-2. Food iron, present mostly in the ferric state, is reduced in the stomach and upper intestine to the ferrous form. Absorption is most efficient in the duodenum, and decreases progressively as food moves caudally. The intestine plays an important role in adjusting the amount of iron that is absorbed; it varies in accordance with the needs of the body. A current concept is that the amount of iron stored as ferritin in the columnar epithelial cells of the small intestine regulates the amount of iron absorption. When there is little or no ferritin in the mucosal cells, iron is rapidly transported across the cells and delivered into the capillaries. In the normal state, the mucosal cell contains iron (as ferritin) supplied from the body stores, and this minimizes transport of iron from the gut to the capillaries. In iron overload states, sufficient ferritin is present in the cells to inhibit transfer of iron from the gut to the capillaries. The ferritin in a mucosal cell is lost into the gut when the cell sloughs on reaching senescence.[74] Hence, iron absorption is enhanced in iron-deficiency states, it is minimal when the serum iron is normal, and it is markedly reduced in iron overload states. Other factors that decrease iron absorption include depressed erythropoiesis from any cause; clay-eating and diets high in phytates and phosphates, which bind iron in insoluble forms; gastrectomy, steatorrhea, and chronic diarrhea.

Iron is transported in the blood bound to transferrin (the "iron-binding protein") which is a beta$_1$ globulin. The total amount of transferrin, or total iron-binding capacity (T.I.B.C.), of normal adults is usually between 300 and 360 mcg. per 100 ml., with an extreme normal range of 250 to 400 mcg. per cent. Normally, about one-third of the transferrin is bound to iron. The total amount of iron in the body of an adult male is 3 to 5 Gm., of which approximately 55 per cent is in hemoglobin, 25 per cent in storage depots, 15 per cent in myoglobin, and the re-

mainder in tissue (cytochrome) enzymes. Only the hemoglobin iron and the storage iron are available for synthesis of new hemoglobin.

There is a striking conservation of iron by the body. The amount of iron lost from the healthy human body via desquamated skin and intestinal mucosa, sweat, urine, and bile is between 0.5 and 1 mg. per day. There are 12 to 20 mg. of iron in the normal adult diet in the United States (or about 6 mg./1000 calories) of which approximately 5 to 10 per cent is absorbed. If one averages these figures, the mean amount of iron absorbed per day is about 1.2 mg., only slightly more than the normal daily loss. Normal menstrual blood loss varies from 25 to 60 ml., or about 10 to 30 mg. of iron per period, which, if distributed over the entire month, would amount to between 0.35 and 1 mg. per day. Pregnancy places a further heavy, but variable, strain on the ability of the mother to maintain iron balance. Iron is required for the fetus, for the milk if the baby is nursed, and 30 to 170 mg. are lost in the placenta and cord as well as an estimated 90 to 310 mg. loss via hemorrhage at the time of delivery. It has been estimated that 9 months of pregnancy plus 6 months of lactation would increase the total iron loss for this period by an average of 1 to 2.5 mg. per day over and above basal losses.

From these data it is apparent that in adult males there is a modest favorable iron balance, whereas in infants and females during the menstrual and reproductive years, the balance is very precarious indeed. The ability of the intestinal mucosal cells to transport more iron into the blood stream when the serum iron begins to fall prevents hypochromic microcytic anemia from developing more often than it does. However, any protracted excessive menstrual blood loss can be expected to exhaust the iron stores eventually.

The time required for hypochromic microcytic anemia to develop is dependent on the amount and duration of blood loss and on the adequacy of iron stores in the body. Reserve iron is stored primarily in RE cells, mainly in the liver, spleen, and bone marrow. The total iron in storage depots is less in women than in men, and averages about 300 to 1000 mg. This is readily available, and equals the normal iron loss over a period of one to five years, which explains the long delay required for hypochromic microcytic anemia to develop when iron loss due to bleeding is only slightly in excess of iron absorption.

The most common causes of iron-deficiency anemia are excessive menstrual bleeding and chronic gastrointestinal hemorrhage. If excessive menstrual bleeding and multiple pregnancies can be excluded, and careful questioning fails to uncover any history of known blood loss, a gastrointestinal neoplasm or other source of chronic occult gastrointestinal blood loss should be considered. Innumerable lesions other than tumors can cause occult, as well as frank chronic blood loss from the gastrointestinal tract, including esophageal varices, peptic ulcer, hiatus hernia, diverticulosis, intestinal parasitic infestation, regional enteritis, ulcerative colitis, and hemorrhoids.

Less common causes of iron deficiency anemia are *improper diet* (including diets low in iron content and diets that contain substances that interfere with iron absorption), and *impaired absorption* due to gastrointestinal disease. In order for iron deficiency to develop because of a low iron content in the diet, the diet must be grossly deficient and very low in animal protein. The constant eating of clay, particularly by women and children, is common among economically deprived people. Clay reduces iron absorption by chelating the metal, or precipitating it as insoluble compounds in the gut. Reference has already been made to the effects of phytates and phosphates (in cereals) in converting iron into insoluble compounds.

Gastrointestinal disorders that interfere with iron absorption include sprue (adults), celiac disease (children), steatorrhea, chronic diarrhea from any cause, total or partial gastrectomy, and atrophic gastritis with achlorhydria. Mechanisms contributing to the reduced iron absorption include specific abnormalities of the gastrointestinal mucosa which are associated with reduced iron absorption (celiac disease, nontropical sprue, and atrophic gastritis), absence of gastric acid, which interferes with absorption of iron from some foods but not others (atrophic gastritis with achlorhydria), increased amounts of fat in the stool (steatorrhea), and shortened transit time, allowing less time for absorption (chronic diarrhea).

MACROCYTIC ANEMIAS

There are two major types of macrocytic anemias: (1) those characterized by the presence of increased numbers of immature but otherwise presumably normal red blood cells in the peripheral blood due to any one of a variety of nonspecific causes (sometimes referred to as the *nonmegaloblastic macrocytic anemias*), and (2) those anemias specifically due to deficiency of vitamin B-12 or folate (or both), which results in a qualitative abnormality in erythrocyte development (*the megaloblastic anemias*). This term derives from the fact that the earliest recognizable red blood cell in the bone marrow in these anemias is the megaloblast, an abnormal cell, the further maturation of which produces abnormally large mature red blood cells.

The nonmegaloblastic macrocytic anemias constitute a heterogeneous group. Any condition that causes marked reticulocytosis may result in macrocytosis, since reticulocytes are larger than mature erythrocytes. The M.C.V. is very rarely above 110 cu. μ in this situation. This group of anemias includes certain types of hemolytic anemia of obscure etiology, the postacute hemorrhage state when reticulocytosis may show a transient sharp rise, and sickle-cell anemia. The red blood cells in sickle-cell anemia are usually normocytic and may even be microcytic, but they occasionally may be macrocytic when the anemia is very severe. The size of the red corpuscles in this disease varies with oxygen saturation; treatment of such blood with carbon dioxide results in a substantial increase in the volume of packed red blood cells.[75] It should be emphasized that the mean corpuscular volume is normal in most cases of hemolytic anemia, in spite of elevated reticulocyte counts.

In one series of 132 cases of various types of *liver disease*, the incidence of macrocytic anemia was 32.6 per cent, normocytic anemia 30.3 per cent, microcytic anemia (usually due to chronic blood loss) 14.4 per cent, and there was no anemia in 22.7 per cent of the patients.[76] Macrocytic anemia was most common in association with severe long-standing liver disease, particularly cirrhosis, and was not found in acute hepatic necrosis. The pathogenesis of the anemia of chronic liver disease is very complex and involves shortening of the red blood cell survival time, impaired red cell production as measured by radioiron incorporation studies,[77] sequestration and destruction of erythrocytes in the spleen,[78] and, in some cases, bleeding from esophageal varices. The cirrhotic liver has a decreased ability to store folic acid.[79] Lastly, it has been shown that, in anemic folate-deficient patients, alcohol suppresses the erythropoietic response to minute doses of folate in the range of the minimal daily requirement.[80] Vitamin B-12 deficiency *does not* appear to play a significant role, even though the vitamin B-12 level is occasionally below normal in chronic liver disease, and impaired absorption or impaired hepatic deposition of labeled vitamin B-12 is common.[81] The degree to which these multiple factors operate on a given patient presumably determines the type of anemia manifested at a given time.

In *hypothyroidism*, also, the associated anemia may be macrocytic, normocytic, or even microcytic, and it is sometimes difficult to determine whether the anemia is due to the primary disease or an associated condition, such as iron deficiency. However, hypothyroidism per se does produce anemia; anemia develops regularly after total thyroid ablation in both animals[82] and man.[83] The red blood cells are larger than normal, the marrow is sometimes hypoplastic, and the reduction in the total red blood cell mass may be greater than is apparent because the plasma volume as well as the total blood volume is reduced. The pathogenesis of the anemia is uncertain, but it seems clear that thyroid hormone has an influence on erythropoiesis, because the red blood cell survival time is normal. Thyroid therapy alone will correct the anemia of severe hypothyroidism, although the response is very slow; the blood values rarely return to normal in less than 3 months, and complete correction sometimes requires 6 to 9 months.

The megaloblastic anemias constitute the most common group of macrocytic anemias; their recognition is extremely important, since they usually can be treated very effectively. The megaloblastic anemias are characterized by slowly progressive anemia, leukopenia, and thrombocytopenia, the presence of abnormal megaloblastic erythroid precursors in the bone marrow, the frequent association of neurological and mucous membrane lesions affecting the mouth, tongue, and stomach, and in the great majority of cases the hematological manifestations are corrected and the neurological and oral abnormalities are ameliorated by either vitamin B-12 or folate therapy.

The pathologic physiology of the megaloblastic anemias has been studied intensely in recent years. There is a great deal of evidence, based on ferro-kinetic studies utilizing radioactive iron, that in this group of ane-mias there is much greater iron utilization by the bone marrow than can be accounted for by the number of labeled red blood cells which are delivered to the circulation.[84] This phenomenon has been referred to as "ineffective erythropoiesis." It is now established that this ineffective erythropoiesis is due to deficiency, either absolute or relative, of vitamin B-12 or folate, or to an abnormal metabolism of these vitamins. The vitamin deficiency may be the result of *impaired absorption* (pernicious anemia, sprue, following total gastrectomy, etc.), *increased requirements* (certain cases of hemolytic anemia, and possibly myelofibrosis[85] and hemochromatosis[86]), or *interference with folic acid metabolism* (patients receiving folic acid antagonists such as amethopterin, antimetabolites such as 6-mercaptopurine or 5-fluorouracil, or anticonvulsants such as diphenylhydantoin sodium, primidone, and possibly certain barbital derivatives).

The basic derangement resulting from vitamin B-12 or folate deficiency is disordered synthesis of deoxyribonucleic acid (DNA). The biochemical derangement has been summarized clearly in recent reviews.[87,88] These two vitamins play an essential role in the formation of deoxyribosyl precursors of DNA. When inadequate amounts of deoxyribosyl precursors are synthesized in proliferating cells which are preparing for division, the cells are unable to replicate their full complement of DNA during the DNA synthetic phase of the cell division cycle. The synthetic phase is thus prolonged, and cells accumulate in midcycle with a content of DNA greater than that of a normal somatic cell but less than twice the normal amount that would be required for two cells produced by mitosis. Those cells that finally reach the phase of mitosis often show minor chromosomal abnormalities, but actual mitotic arrest is not prominent. However, during each subsequent synthetic phase, the risk of a lethal delay in DNA replication increases. In contrast to the impaired synthesis of DNA, RNA synthesis is not significantly disturbed in most megaloblastic anemias, and the RNA content of the cytoplasm may be very high. Consequently, there is little or no impairment of hemoglobin synthesis. As a result of these biochemical changes, the red blood cell precursors in the marrow develop bizarre nonhomogeneous chromatin patterns, enlarged deformed nuclei, and, eventually, marked karyorrhexis and karyolysis. During the prolonged synthetic phase of cell division hemoglobin continues to accumulate in spite of the arrested maturation of the nucleus. This results in large cells with immature-appearing nuclei and old-appearing orthochromatic or eosinophilic cytoplasm. Many of the erythroblasts are permanently arrested during one of their several cycles of cell division, and these cells eventually lyse within the marrow. This accounts for the observed greater radioiron utilization by the bone marrow than can be accounted for by the number of labeled erythrocytes which are delivered to the circulation, as well as by the slight hyperbilirubinemia that occurs in these anemias. As a result of this intramedullary red blood cell lysis, there is increased erythrophagocytosis, larger amounts of hemosiderin can be demonstrated by appropriate stains, and the serum lactic dehydrogenase level is elevated. The erythroblasts that do survive are abnormal in appearance, and the characteristic macrocytosis of the red blood cells in the peripheral blood may be in part due to omission of one of the cell divisions, with resultant release of some cells having up to twice the normal cell volume. From these considerations, it is apparent that the major defect in the megaloblastic anemias is a profound disturbance in erythropoiesis. However, not only is there intramedullary hemolysis of abnormal red cell precursors, but the erythrocytes that are delivered into the circulation have a shortened survival time, many being sequestered prematurely in the spleen.

The maturation of the granular leukocytes and the megakaryocytes is similarly affected by the derangement in DNA synthesis in vitamin B-12 and folate deficiency states. In pernicious anemia, the morphologic changes in the leukocytes often precede marked changes in the red cells. The characteristic abnormalities include leukopenia due to neutropenia, an increased size of many of the polymorphonuclear leukocytes, hypersegmentation of the nucleus with as many as 8 to 10 lobes, some of which may be abnormal in shape, the appearance of rare metamyelocytes and myelocytes in the peripheral blood, and abnormally large band forms, metamyelocytes, and myelocytes in the bone marrow and occasionally in the blood. The platelet count is also reduced, and giant platelets and bizarre-shaped platelets appear. The megakaryocytes may also appear abnormal. The biochemical derangement is not confined to the blood cells, but also affects epithelial cells. Giant cells may be seen in

scrapings of the mucosa of the mouth and vagina and are also present in the stomach mucosa. The nervous system is likewise affected; the most characteristic lesion is *degeneration of the posterolateral columns in the spinal cord*, with resultant absent reflexes, disturbed position and vibratory sense, and difficulty in walking, but peripheral nerve degeneration also occurs which may produce numbness.[89]

Specific Diseases Characterized by Megaloblastic Anemia. The varied mechanisms that may interfere with vitamin B-12 or folate absorption or utilization have already been discussed. In this section we will discuss in somewhat more detail the two most important diseases that give rise to megaloblastic anemia in temperate climates, pernicious anemia and malabsorption syndromes. In tropical countries pernicious anemia is rare, and nutritional megaloblastic anemias are common.

Pernicious anemia is a disease characterized by atrophy of the mucous membrane in the fundus of the stomach, usually with absence of the parietal and chief cells, as a result of which inadequate amounts of intrinsic factor are secreted. Intrinsic factor is a glycoprotein substance secreted by the parietal and/or chief cells which preferentially binds vitamin B-12 and is essential to its later absorption in the lower ileum. The gastric lesion is almost always associated with achlorhydria. Both genetic and environmental factors may be involved in the production of the basic lesion (gastric atrophy). One out of every five patients with this disease gives a family history of pernicious anemia. The disease appears to be more common in individuals of northern European descent, and it affects primarily blue-eyed individuals with a short broad face with the eyes set far apart, with large ears and a tendency to develop early greying of the hair. The frequency of blood group A in patients with pernicious anemia and in their normal relatives is higher than in the general population. The family incidence of juvenile pernicious anemia is much more striking than is the case with the adult disease, and it has been suggested that the juvenile form of the disease may represent the homozygous inheritance of the disease from heterozygous parents, in one or the other of which the disease may not be clinically expressed.[90,91] The mode of inheritance has not been established, but the evidence is consistent with the concept that a single dominant autosomal gene determines the basic gastric mucosal defect[92] (which, however, may not alone be sufficient to produce clinically manifest pernicious anemia). In recent years, evidence has accumulated which suggests strongly that *immunological mechanisms* play a part in the pathogenesis of the gastric lesion. Antibodies which react specifically against gastric parietal cells have been shown to be present in the sera of 80 to 90 per cent of patients with pernicious anemia.[93] These antibodies are complement-fixing, precipitating antibodies, which are directed against microsomal antigens in the parietal cells; they are not species specific. Similar antibodies have been detected in the sera of 36 per cent of nonanemic relatives of patients with pernicious anemia. Almost 50 per cent of patients with pernicious anemia also have antibodies against thyroid microsomal antigens; conversely, many patients with Hashimoto's thyroiditis (and less frequently, other types of thyroid disease), have antibodies against gastric parietal cells. The significance of these antibodies is difficult to determine, because they are also present in the serum of most patients with chronic gastritis and in 5 to 10 per cent of apparently healthy people. Serum antibodies directed specifically against human intrinsic factor are also present in more than 50 per cent of patients with pernicious anemia.[94] These antibodies block the enhancing effect of intrinsic factor on vitamin B-12 absorption. Unlike antibodies against parietal cells, these antibodies are almost specific for pernicious anemia, since they are very rarely demonstrable in any other condition. These data have led to the presently popular hypothesis that: (1) gastric atrophy is controlled by inheritance through a dominant gene; (2) affected individuals react by forming antibodies against either parietal cell antigens, or against intrinsic factor (in response to repeated presumed episodes of minor damage or trauma to the gastric mucosa); and (3) the antibodies then effectively either prevent intrinsic factor production or block its function of enhancing vitamin B-12 absorption. Antibody assays in juvenile pernicious anemia have been essentially negative,[95] which suggests that this possibly homozygous form of the disease involves a congenital inability of the parietal cells to synthesize intrinsic factor.

Nontropical sprue (adult celiac disease, gluten enteropathy) is one of the more important disorders in which megaloblastic anemia may develop on the basis of folate deficiency; sprue will be discussed as a prototype of a group of disorders of the gastrointestinal tract characterized by a malabsorption defect and accompanied by megaloblastic anemia. In this group also are certain nutritional macrocytic anemias, and some surgical and mechanical disorders of the gastrointestinal tract, including resection of considerable segments of small intestine, intestinal strictures, gastrocolic fistulas, diverticuli, and "blind loops." It must be emphasized that the megaloblastic anemia that sometimes develops in these disorders usually is due to a combination of *folate and vitamin B-12 deficiency.* However, malabsorption of vitamin B-12 *alone* may occur. When blind loops, diverticuli, strictures or other causes of intestinal stasis are present, an overgrowth of intestinal bacteria in the involved segment of intestine may result in competitive utilization of vitamin B-12 by the organisms, so that the intestinal contents reaching the lower ileum where B-12 is absorbed are devoid of this vitamin. There is an intimate relationship between the metabolism of folate and vitamin B-12, and deficiency of one affects the need for the other. This interrelationship is most clearly exemplified by pernicious anemia, in which the basic defect is clearly failure of absorption of vitamin B-12; however, oral folate administration will produce a temporary and often incomplete hematologic remission, although it in no way alleviates the neurological lesion, and may actually accentuate it by further lowering the serum vitamin B-12 level.

Nontropical sprue is a syndrome characterized clinically by malabsorption of many nutrients and pathologically by a striking atrophy of the villi of the small intestine. Many, but not all, patients with this syndrome respond dramatically when foods containing wheat, barley, and rye flour are excluded from the diet. The specific agent responsible for the disorder resides in the protein (gluten) fraction of the flour. The mechanism by which *gluten* produces the anatomical and physiological lesions responsible for the malabsorption is not known, but the two prevalent theories are (1) that immune mechanisms are involved or (2) that the basic fault is an enzymatic defect in the epithelium. There is no convincing support for either of these hypotheses, but an inheritable factor does appear to be involved.

Folic acid is only one of many important nutrients which is inadequately absorbed. The malabsorption is caused by the villous atrophy of the small intestine and is aggravated by the diarrhea.

The term folic acid includes several related compounds, of which the simplest to show physiological activity is pteroylglutamic acid. Vegetables and liver are particularly rich in "folic acid" and the normal balanced diet contains at least 10 times the minimal daily requirement of the vitamin. Following absorption, folic acid is reduced by the action of specific liver enzymes to tetrahydrofolic acid, various derivatives of which constitute the active forms of the vitamin. The primary function of the active derivatives, such as tetrahydrofolate, is in the transfer of one carbon (C_1) groups. Folic acid is thereby involved in the biosynthesis of purines, thymidine, and, ultimately of DNA and RNA. Specifically, in the presence of pyridoxal, tetrahydrofolic acid catalyzes the transfer of the B carbon of serine to homocysteine forming methionine. In this reaction, an important intermediate, N^5, N^{10}-methylene-tetrahydrofolate is formed, and this, in the presence of thymidylate synthetase, catalyzes the methylation and subsequent conversion of deoxyuridylate to thymidylate, an essential precursor of DNA synthesis. The failure of this metabolic pathway is presumably the basic defect responsible for the megaloblastic changes that occur in "folic acid deficiency."[96] Tetrahydrofolate and its derivatives are intimately involved in synthetic reactions in which vitamin B-12 is also involved, and a deficiency of one of these vitamins may lead to an overutilization or some other abnormality in the metabolism of the other. It is thus not surprising that folic acid deficiency may result in hematologic and gastrointestinal abnormalities that are indistinguishable from those of pernicious anemia.

HEMOLYTIC ANEMIAS

All of the hemolytic anemias are characterized by more rapid than normal destruction and disappearance of red blood cells from the circulation; the basic laboratory finding that documents this phenomenon is shortening of the life-span of the red cells as measured by the rate of disappearance from the blood of cells that have been tagged with radioactive chromium (Cr^{51}). This procedure may be the only laboratory test that will detect a mild degree of hemolysis not otherwise manifested (because slight to moderate increase in the rate of red blood cell destruction often does not cause hyperbilirubinemia, and is compensated for by increased erythrocyte production in the bone marrow). The laboratory procedures that are helpful in the diagnosis of more severe degrees of anemia have been discussed in Chapter 24, on Jaundice. If liver function is normal, considerably increased amounts of bilirubin can be excreted rapidly into the bile, and hemolytic anemia, not accompanied by clinical icterus, may still be brisk enough to produce reticulocytosis and an increase in the erythroid to myeloid ratio in the bone marrow.

Hemolytic anemia may be due to many different causes. The hemolytic anemias can be divided conveniently into two groups, (1) those due to a defect in the red corpuscle itself, and (2) those primarily due to extracorpuscular factors (see classification in Table 28-2). There is overlapping between these two groups because extracorpuscular hemolytic mechanisms and serum factors sometimes act on defective red cells, and, conversely, hemolysis primarily due to a defect in the red blood cell may be aggravated or influenced by extracorpuscular mechanisms.

The remainder of this section will be devoted to a brief discussion of the pathogenesis of some of the more important types of hemolytic anemia.

Hemolytic Anemias Due to Intracorpuscular Defects

The fact that a given hemolytic anemia is primarily due to a defect of the red blood cells rather than to serum factors can be established conclusively by cross transfusion experiments. If red blood cells from the patient tagged with radiochromium disappear rapidly when transfused into normal recipients, and normal erythrocytes survive for a normal period of time when transfused into the patient, it is apparent that the primary defect is in the cells rather than the serum of the patient. However, extracorpuscular factors may play an important secondary role in such a patient. For example, in hereditary spherocytosis, the primary abnormality is an inherited defect of the red cells, but these abnormal cells may be able to survive normally after the spleen is removed, whereas they are rapidly destroyed on passing through the unique circulation of the normal spleen. Other similar examples will be given later.

Sickle-Cell Anemia. "Sickling" of the red blood cells is a phenomenon that occurs as a direct result of the presence in the red cells of an abnormal hemoglobin referred to as sickle (or S) hemoglobin. The cells under certain conditions assume abnormal shapes, appearing in profile like sickles, crescents, or oat grains. This is a hereditary disease of Negroes in which the presence of S-hemoglobin in the erythrocytes is genetically controlled as an autosomal intermediate. About 7 per cent of the Negroes in the United States harbor this gene, which may be transmitted by either parent. Thirty-nine out of every 40 of those persons having the gene have the heterozygous form of the disease (sickle-cell trait), which is an asymptomatic disorder unaccompanied by significant anemia. There is no anemia in persons carrying only the "trait," because sickling does not occur in these individuals in vivo unless there is an associated condition causing *hypoxia* (such as chronic pulmonary insufficiency or high altitude flying). One out of 40 of those harboring the gene have the homozygous state (sickle-cell anemia), a serious disease characterized by in vivo sickling with severe continuous hemolytic anemia and multiple symptoms. Most (76 to 100 per cent) of the hemoglobin in the erythrocytes of patients with sickle-cell anemia is S-hemoglobin, and the remainder is fetal hemoglobin. In the sickle-cell trait, 22 to 45 per cent of the hemoglobin is S-hemoglobin, the remainder being normal (A) hemoglobin.

Across Central Africa there is a very high incidence of sickle-cell trait, ranging up to 46 per cent of the population among the pygmoids in East Africa.[97] Thus, sickle-cell trait in Africa is far more common than among American Negroes. This has been attributed to the fact that sickle-cell hemoglobin is a relatively unfavorable substrate for the metabolism of malaria organisms, and patients with the sickle-cell trait therefore have this advantage in natural selection in areas of high malarial incidence.[98] This may mean that in Africa, where malaria is common and severe, that the mortality from malaria is higher among those without the sickle-cell gene, so more survivors live to transmit the hereditary trait.

Sickle-cell hemoglobin has the characteristic property of forming birefringent, highly anisomeric units[99] (referred to as tactoids) within the cell in a manner analogous to crystallization; the abnormal shape assumed by the red blood cells is directly related to this "crystallization" of the hemoglobin. Conditions that favor crystallization are (1) a high percentage of S-hemoglobin in the cells; (2) a low oxygen tension, either due to factors affecting the entire body such as a low atmospheric pressure, or local causes such as stasis; and (3) a low pH, such as occurs normally in the renal medulla and in the pulmonary arterioles. As the percentage of sickled cells increases, the viscosity of the blood increases markedly, further aggravating stasis. The lesions that are produced and the resultant symptoms are thought to be related to multiple vascular occlusions, local tissue hypoxia, and infarction. The typical course of events can thus be envisaged as follows. Hypoxia from any cause (general or local) results in increased numbers of sickle cells forming in areas of stasis or low pH; these may block the terminal capillaries and venules leading to still further stasis, local anoxia, and a decrease in pH. This vicious cycle may progress until significant infarction occurs. In turn, multiple vascular occlusions with or without actual tissue infarction presumably account for the autosplenectomy, the leg ulcers, the aseptic necrosis of the head of the femur and of the humerus, hematuria, priapism, the bone and joint pains of sickle-cell crisis, the abdominal pains simulating acute abdominal conditions, and the neurological manifestations.

Other clinical manifestations, such as jaundice, cholelithiasis, stunted growth, cardiac complications, and symptoms referable to the anemia are the direct results of the hemolytic process. This, in turn, is probably due to the increased mechanical fragility of the bizarre-shaped red cells, which have been shown to have a markedly shortened life-span.

Thalassemia. Another very important hemoglobinopathy is thalassemia. This is also a genetically determined (probably recessive) disease, which exists in a heterozygous state (thalassemia minor) and in a homozygous state (thalassemia major, Cooley's anemia). The genetic mechanisms involved in the thalassemia syndromes are exceedingly complex, and combinations of the thalassemia defect with other abnormal hemoglobins are relatively common, as is also true of sickle-cell disease. Thalassemia is characterized by unusually thin erythrocytes, aniso- and poikilocytosis, microcytosis, stippled cells, and target cells. When the anemia is severe, large numbers of nucleated red blood cells appear in the circulation. The exact nature of the basic biochemical abnormality in the synthesis of hemoglobin in the thalassemic disorders is unknown, but there is strong evidence that there is a defect in the synthesis of individual polypeptide chains. As a result, normal hemoglobin (HgA) is decreased, and fetal hemoglobin and HgA_2 synthesis are increased. It now appears that there are two varieties of thalassemia, one involving defective β-chain synthesis (the common form) and another involving α-chain synthesis. Unlike the other hemoglobinopathies, thalassemia does not involve the production of a truly abnormal hemoglobin.

Many other abnormal hemoglobin syndromes have been described in recent years. Most of these hemoglobinopathies may occur in combination with the sickle cell or the thalassemia defect, giving impure syndromes.

Hereditary spherocytosis is a genetic disorder of the red blood cell transmitted by either parent as a Mendelian dominant in which the erythrocytes assume a spherical shape, which results in *increased osmotic fragility*. Hemolysis is continuous, but hemolytic exacerbations accompanied by vomiting, tachycardia, abdominal pain, and fever may occur periodically and apparently spontaneously. Acute aplastic crises also occur during which there is leukopenia, thrombocytopenia, reticulocytopenia, aplasia of the bone marrow, and disappearance of jaundice and urobilinuria (apparently due to unexplained sudden depression of hematopoiesis and cessation of hemolysis).[100] It has been suggested that the genetically determined physiological defect in this disorder is an abnormal permeability of the red blood cell membrane for sodium ions which favors absorption of water and swelling of the cell. As sodium and water enter the cells, potassium is lost. There is a decrease in the lipid content of the membrane of these cells, and the physiological abnormality may be caused by physiochemical alterations in the cell surface related to the loss of membrane lipids.[101]

Splenectomy almost invariably corrects the anemia of hereditary spherocytosis. Spherocytes washed out of the spleen after its removal show *greatly increased osmotic fragility* compared to cells removed from the peripheral blood of the same patient. When spherocytes are incubated in vitro (a situation probably comparable to the trapping of erythrocytes for significant periods of time in the sinusoids of the intact spleen), there is a marked decrease of all lipid and possibly certain protein components in the red cell membrane. The addition of glucose to the blood being incubated markedly reduces potassium loss and decreases the abnormal osmotic fragility by retarding adenosine triphosphate depletion in the cells. Red cells sequestered in the spleen probably have inadequate access to glucose. Thus, trapping and stagnation of the spherocytes in the splenic sinusoids may aggravate the surface membrane defect believed to be responsible for the increased permeability which, in turn, is ultimately responsible for swelling and rupture of the cells.

Hemolytic anemias due to genetically determined deficiencies of enzymes in erythrocytes may be classified into two groups: (1) those deficiencies in enzymes or cofactors related to the pentose phosphate pathway, and (2) those related to the Embden-Meyerhof pathway of glycolysis.

Glucose-6-phosphate dehydrogenase (G-6-PD) deficiency is by far the most important of the deficiencies related to the pentose phosphate pathway. This group of genetic disorders, carried on the X chromosome, occurs in about 13 per cent of American Negroes; enzyme levels are 10 to 15 per cent of normal in homozygous males and homozygous females, heterozygous females usually showing much higher levels. In normal and affected individuals the activity of G-6-PD steadily decreases as the cells age, older cells thus being more susceptible to hemolysis. Ordinarily, these patients have a mild hemolytic state readily compensated for by increased erythropoiesis. However, a large number of drugs which can function in the red cells as oxidant compounds will initiate overt hemolysis in these patients. These drugs include primaquine, pamaquine, sulfonamides, nitrofurans, phenacetin, para-aminosalicylic acid, and certain vitamin K derivatives. G-6-PD is involved in the regeneration of nicotinamide adenine dinucleotide phosphate (NADPH), and this, in turn, is required for the reduction of oxidized glutathione to reduced glutathione. It is this pathway that provides the reductive capacity of the cell. The oxidant drugs increase the demands on this pathway, and when it is defective, as occurs in G-6-PD deficiency, oxidative denaturation of hemoglobin and constituents of the erythrocyte membrane is favored with resultant hemolysis. Certain illnesses, particularly bacterial infections (especially pneumonia), viral infections, and metabolic disturbances (particularly diabetic ketoacidosis) also precipitate hemolysis in these patients. In one series of 102 patients with erythrocyte G-6-PD deficiency, acute hemolytic episodes occurred more frequently in association with such illnesses alone than with drug therapy alone.[102] The combination of an infection or metabolic disturbance such as diabetic ketoacidosis with oxidant drug therapy provides the optimum conditions for hemolysis.

The incidence of erythrocyte G-6-PD deficiency is much lower in Caucasions than in Negroes. A screening survey on 10,000 consecutive male donors in the Presbyterian Hospital (New York) blood bank revealed an incidence of only 0.9 per cent in Caucasian males, as contrasted with 13 per cent in Negro males.[102] However, when the deficiency does occur in Caucasians, the disease tends to be more severe, because the enzyme levels are much lower, and *chronic hemolytic anemia may result.*

Red blood cell enzyme defects involving almost all of the enzymes of the Embden-Meyerhof pathway have now been described. These are relatively rare disorders; pyruvate kinase deficiency is by far the most common defect. The pentose phosphate shunt provides a reducing mechanism, which protects erythrocytes from the oxidant effects of drugs and certain diseases, whereas the Embden-Meyerhof pathway involves the conversion of glucose to lactate through a series of phosphorylated intermediates with the production of energy in the form of two moles of ATP for each mole of glucose consumed. This energy is essential for maintaining the normal cation concentration and balance of the red blood cells, as well as for other vital cell functions. These differences help explain why enzymatic defects in the Embden-Meyerhof glycolytic pathway result in *persistent chronic anemia,* whereas deficiencies in the pentose phosphate shunt are generally associated with anemias *only when oxidant drugs are given or the patient has certain illnesses.*

Paroxysmal nocturnal hemoglobinuria is a relatively rare disorder in which chronic hemolytic anemia occurs as a result of an *acquired* erythrocyte defect. There is associated hemoglobinemia, which is accentuated during sleep, and this results at times in the passage of dark urine when the patient first awakens. There are two populations of cells in the blood of patients with PNH, one short-lived and the other longer-lived; the short-lived cells are younger cells (reticulocytes being particularly susceptible to hemolysis).[103] The nature of the red cell defect is unknown. Acetylcholinesterase activity in the membrane of these erythrocytes is decreased[104] and electron microscopy studies reveal abnormalities including surface pitting,[105] but these changes may result from, rather than be the cause of, the membrane defect. A valuable screening test for PNH (*the sucrose water test*) is performed by incubating 1 volume of blood in 9 volumes of a 10 per cent solution of sucrose in water; a red color in the supernatant fluid following centrifugation indicating hemolysis constitutes a positive test. When normal erythrocytes are incubated with serum diluted in sucrose solutions, they become coated with complement. A positive sucrose water test is thought to result from the increased sensitivity of PNH cells to complement components.[106] The diagnosis is established by the acid hemolysis test (*Ham's test*); hemolysis of the patient's red blood cells in slightly acidified normal human serum constitutes a positive test. All known components of human complement, as well as calcium and magnesium, must be present in the serum for hemolysis of these cells to occur. Hemosiderinuria occurs in all cases of this disease and may result in the development of a secondary iron deficiency. Thrombotic complications are common, presumably because of the release of thromboplastic substances from the PNH cells.[107] The PNH defect has developed in the erythrocytes of some patients following what appeared to be drug-induced hypoplastic anemia, and the suggestion has been made that in some cases the abnormal PNH cells derive from a mutant clone of precursors following the injury to the marrow cells which resulted in hypoplasia.

Hemolytic anemias due to extracorpuscular defects include those due to immune mechanisms, those due to chemical, physical, vegetable, and animal agents and infectious organisms, and those secondary to other diseases (the so-called "symptomatic hemolytic anemias").

The "auto-immune" hemolytic anemias are characterized by the presence on the patient's red blood cells (and often free in the serum) of globulins, which render the cells susceptible to hemolysis. The most common type of "auto-immune" hemolytic anemia is associated with warm gamma globulins (i.e., those that react with red blood cells at body temperature). These are incomplete antibodies, and their presence can be detected readily by the Coombs test. Coombs serum is prepared from the serum of rabbits that have been immunized against human globulins. This serum does not affect normal erythrocytes but, under proper conditions, causes the agglutination of sensitized red blood cells, which are coated with "antibody" globulin (a positive direct Coombs test). A positive indirect Coombs test indicates the presence of incomplete antibody globulins free in the serum. The serum to be tested is incubated with appropriate normal cells; the cells are then washed free of serum, and Coombs serum is added. Agglutination indicates that incomplete antibody globulins in the test serum become fixed to the normal cells, which are then agglutinated by the antiglobulin rabbit serum. In general, a positive indirect Coombs test indicates that there is more antibody present than the patient's red cells can adsorb. Warm antibodies adsorbed to erythrocytes are usually present in large amounts, and give a positive reaction (agglutination) with high dilutions of Coombs serum; but the antibodies in the serum, if found at all, are present in much lower titers, and they are more readily demonstrated when trypsinized cells are used. The Coombs antiglobulin test may also be positive when cold agglutinins are present, but it is usually very weakly positive; hemolysins, by contrast, are rare in warm antibody disorders, and common in association with cold agglutinins.

It seems clear that a positive direct Coombs test is indicative of adsorbed antibodies on the erythrocytes in patients with Rh sensitization, and in some cases of sensitivity reactions to drugs. In idiopathic acquired hemolytic anemia, on the other hand, it is not certain that a positive Coombs reaction indicates "autosensitization" of the red cells. It is possible that in these cases the avidity of the adsorbed globulin for the red blood cells may be due to the formation of abnormal globulins that may have nothing to do with auto-immune mechanisms.

There are three different mechanisms that may be involved in the induction of a direct positive Coombs test in drug-induced anemias: (1) the haptene type, associated with high dose penicillin therapy, resulting in a positive antigamma globulin Coombs test, (2) the "innocent bystander" reaction, seen after quinine administration, associated with an anticomplement Coombs test, and (3) the

alpha-methyl-dopa type, in which the anti-gamma-G Coombs test is positive, but the drug need not be present in the test system.[108] The most important example of the *haptene type* of drug induced Coombs positive hemolytic anemia is seen in rare patients, who have received large doses of penicillin, usually more than 20,000,000 units per day for several weeks. In these patients, the positive direct Coombs test is of the gamma G type. The hemolytic anemia may persist for several weeks after the drug is discontinued. Antipenicillin antibody is present in the serum and can be eluted from the patient's red blood cells. These antibodies react only with penicillin coated erythrocytes and not with normal cells. The *"innocent bystander"* reaction occurs in association with the administration of quinine, quinidine, stibophen, and probably aminopyrine. The incidence of this reaction is low, but when it does occur, thrombocytopenia and leukopenia, as well as hemolytic anemia or any combination of these, may occur. The direct positive Coombs reaction is of the complement type. The cell that is injured is dependent on the type of antibody, at least when quinine is the offending drug. The antibody that causes red blood cell injury is a 19 S gamma M globulin, whereas the antibody that causes platelet injury is a 7 S gamma G globulin. The antibody that is involved is directed against the drug, and the drug-antibody complex then becomes attached to the red blood cells, white blood cells, or platelets, which serve as innocent bystanders. Complement is then fixed to the cell surface, with resultant cell injury, that ultimately leads to lysis of the cells. The *alpha-methyl-dopa* (Aldomet) type of reaction presents several unusual features. About 20 per cent of patients treated for hypertension with Aldomet develop a positive direct Coombs test of the gamma-G type[109]; however, only a small percentage of these patients develop a hemolytic anemia. This phenomenon is dose dependent, and usually occurs after the ingestion of more than 500 mg. of the drug per day for at least 4 to 6 months. Although many patients develop a positive Coombs test without evidence of a hemolytic process, when anemia does occur it is reversible; cessation of drug administration is followed by cessation of hemolysis.[110] The antibody involved in these cases is not directed against the drug, but rather against red cell antigens, usually of the Rh system.[110] The

TABLE 28-3. FREQUENCY OF "AUTOANTIBODIES" IN ACQUIRED HEMOLYTIC ANEMIA*

I. Warm type (75 per cent of total)
A. Idiopathic 58%
B. Secondary: (1) Chronic lymphocytic leukemia 6%
(2) Malignant lymphomas 4%
(3) Disseminated lupus .. 4%
(4) Other 3%

II. Cold type (25 per cent of total)
A. Idiopathic 12%
(1) Atypical pneumonia .. 7%
(2) Malignant lymphoma. 4%
(3) Other 2%

* Dacie, J. V.: The Hemolytic Anemias: Congenital and Acquired. Part II: The Autoimmune Hemolytic Anemias. New York, Grune and Stratton, 1962.

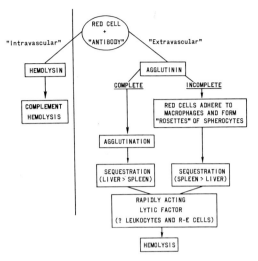

FIG. 28-3. Postulated sequence of events resulting in increased erythrocyte destruction in hemolytic anemias. (Courtesy of Dr. W. B. Castle, modified by Dr. Castle from table *in* Sodeman and Sodeman (eds.): Pathologic Physiology, ed. 4, Philaphia, Saunders, 1967, p. 800)

Coombs test is positive in the absence of any drug in the test system. The importance of obtaining a detailed drug history from patients with a Coombs-positive hemolytic anemia cannot be overemphasized.

Approximately three-fourths of patients with non-drug-induced Coombs-positive hemolytic anemias have warm-type "antibodies," and one-fourth have cold "antibodies." The relative frequency of cases that are idiopathic and cases that are secondary to specific diseases has been reported as shown in Table 28-3.[111]

It has been demonstrated by slit lamp microscopy of the scleral conjunctiva in patients with acquired autoimmune hemolytic anemia that in vivo aggregation of red cells occurs as evidenced by granularity of the flowing blood, and this phenomenon correlates with the severity of the hemolytic process.[112] The antibodies apparently do not injure the red blood cells directly. Fibrinogen seems to enhance the agglutination of erythrocytes coated with antibody and this, in turn, increases mechanical filtration of red cell aggregates.[113] Globulin-coated red blood cells are sequestered and removed from the circulation by the reticuloendothelial system. If the erythrocytes are coated with complete antibodies, such as those of the ABO system which fix complement and cause agglutination in saline, the cells are sequestered throughout the RE system. However, the red cells coated with incomplete warm antibodies, such as those associated with idiopathic acquired Coombs-positive hemolytic anemia, are removed primarily in the spleen. When the hemolytic process is very severe or prolonged, the liver removes more erythrocytes than the spleen, and the bone marrow also removes cells when the liver and spleen are overloaded.[114] Splenectomy diminishes hemolysis significantly, at least temporarily, in about 50 per cent of patients with Coombs-positive hemolytic anemia both because the spleen is one source of antibody production and because it also filters out weakly agglutinated erythrocytes. Steroid therapy is very effective both because steroids presumably decrease antibody production, and also because they decrease the adhesion of sensitized cells to blood vessel walls. The latter effect diminishes red cell trapping in the liver and spleen.

The sequence of events resulting in increased erythrocyte destruction is summarized diagrammatically in Fig. 28-3. *Hemolysins* are complete antibodies against red blood cell components which activate the C_1 component of complement to a substance having esterase activity. Electron photomicrographs of sheep red blood cells treated with Forsman antibody and guinea pig complement have shown that this activated component of complement produces innumerable holes in the erythrocyte membrane through which hemoglobin escapes.[115] This type of red blood cell destruction occurs intravascularly.

ber of complex synthetic organic compounds used in preserving and processing foods, in cosmetics, in clothing (dyes, synthetic processors), in innumerable industrial and agricultural processes, about the home (paint removers, paints, adhesives, insecticides), and perhaps even air pollutants in heavily industrialized areas. It is probable that at least some cases of *"idiopathic"* bone marrow failure are, in fact, due to unidentified exposure to such compounds.

The pathogenesis of the bone marrow failure due to drugs and chemicals which regularly produce marrow injury in sufficient dosage is uncertain. Benzene may be considered as the prototype of this group of compounds. Anemia is the most common blood abnormality observed in exposed workers, thrombocytopenia and leukopenia being next in frequency. The anemia is primarily due to decreased erythrocyte production, but the earliest effect may be increased red blood cell destruction. In normal rabbits, extirpation of portions of the bone marrow is followed by an orderly sequence of events characterized first by the appearance of sheets of primitive reticular cells and bone trabeculae; then fat cells appear, and finally recognizable hematopoietic cells appear. Similar studies in benzene-poisoned animals showed that the extirpated marrow was replaced by primitive reticular cells, but no further regeneration beyond this point occurred, suggesting that benzene inhibits cell division and maturation beyond the primitive reticular cell level.[121] Benzene poisoning in humans may be associated early with a regenerative blood picture and even a leukemoid reaction, and the bone marrow may be hypercellular, whereas the ultimate effect of heavy exposure is invariably marrow aplasia. This suggests that idiopathic bone marrow failure, or bone marrow failure due to drugs and other chemicals, may pass through a series of stages characterized early by normal cellularity or hypercellularity of the bone marrow, which later is succeeded by hypoplasia and then by more or less complete disappearance of cells from the marrow. If this hypothesis is correct, the degree of hypocellularity would be a function of the dose and duration of the exposure to the myelotoxic drug.

The pathogenesis of the bone marrow failure that follows ingestion of those drugs that only occasionally or very rarely produce marrow toxicity is unknown. Chloramphenicol may be taken as a prototype for this group. Approximately 1 out of 60,000 patients taking chloramphenicol develops fatal aplastic anemia.[122] Studies have shown that about half of patients receiving chloramphenicol develop slight anemia, neutropenia, and thrombocytopenia, the reticulocyte count falls, and the serum iron level rises.[123,124] Vacuolization of the nucleus and the cytoplasm of the blood cell precursors in the bone marrow is common between the 11th and 14th day after initial exposure to the drug. However, these toxic effects are reversible[125] and probably have nothing to do with the development of aplastic anemia. It has been suggested that the pathogenesis of the aplastic anemia, when it does develop, may be related to a biochemical defect involving some essential metabolic pathway.

Anemia of Chronic Infection, Chronic Inflammatory Disorders, and Malignant Neoplastic Diseases. Normocytic, normochromic anemia, usually mild, is common in association with chronic infections, chronic inflammatory diseases, and cancer. Anemia has been observed in two-thirds of cases of subacute bacterial endocarditis,[126] and it is common also in association with tuberculosis, brucellosis, bronchiectasis, lung abscess, and empyema. Anemia is common also in patients with rheumatoid arthritis and active rheumatic fever. Many different pathogenic mechanisms play a part in the production of anemia in association with malignant neoplastic diseases. Cancers of the gastrointestinal tract often result in iron-deficiency anemia due to chronic blood loss, but they may also interfere with appetite and absorption and give rise to macrocytic anemia.[127] Certain cancers, particularly those of the prostate, tend to metastasize widely to bone marrow, thus causing myelophthisic anemia. When these specific mechanisms are eliminated, there remains a form of anemia seen in association with many different types of cancers which is similar to the anemia of chronic infection and chronic inflammation.

This type of anemia (due to infection, inflammation, or cancer) is characterized by a rapid disappearance of radioiron from the plasma, a normal or slightly increased plasma iron turnover rate, normal or slightly increased iron utilization for hemoglobin synthesis, and an increase in the fraction of red blood cells renewed daily.[128] Thus, erythropoiesis is normal or slightly increased. The rate of red blood cell destruction is also increased, as evidenced by a shortened red blood cell survival time[129] and an increase in the fraction of erythrocytes renewed daily. The survival of red blood cells from patients with these disorders in normal recipients is normal, and the survival of normal red blood cells in the circulation of patients with rheumatoid arthritis is shortened, thus indicating that the *hemolytic process* must be due to *a serum factor.*[129] The nature of this extracorpuscular factor is unknown.

It has been shown that the *release of iron* from the stores in the reticuloendothelial tissues is defective in association with infections,[130] rheumatoid arthritis,[131] and cancers.[132] The low serum iron and the decrease in marrow sideroblasts seen in all of these conditions is thought to be attributable to the defective mobilization of iron from the RE system, and this, in turn, results in inhibition of erythropoiesis. The anemia, then, is due to (1) a minor decrease in red cell survival time in a patient (2) whose bone marrow is not able to respond in a normal fashion because of unavailability of iron, in spite of plentiful iron stores.

Certain bacteria may produce *hemolysins,* and some infections are associated with the production of cold agglutinins or cold hemolysins. In these circumstances, much more severe anemia may occur than is seen in the usual chronic infection.

Anemia of Chronic Renal Disease. Chronic renal disease accompanied by azotemia sooner or later inevitably results in anemia. In general, the severity of the anemia correlates well with the level of the blood urea nitrogen. The blood smear may show stippling, moderate anisocytosis, and poikilocytosis, and occasional normoblasts may be seen. The anemia is usually normocytic and normochromic, but may be slightly microcytic or hypochromic.

Anemia with azotemia results from (1) decreased erythropoiesis and (2) increased hemolysis.

Curiously, the marrow remains normally cellular, and no significant decrease in the erythroid to myeloid ratio can be detected, even though the reticulocyte count is depressed and ferrokinetic studies consistently show depressed erythropoiesis. The cause of the decreased erythropoiesis is unknown. Since the kidney is the major organ of erythropoietin production, it is logical to suppose that *decreased erythropoietin production* might be a factor in the pathogenesis of the anemia. Methods of assaying the plasma

levels of the substance are so crude that it is extremely difficult to measure the amount in normal plasma, much less in conditions where erythropoietin is decreased.

The red blood cell survival time is decreased, particularly in severe long-standing uremia, and this is because of unknown extracorpuscular plasma factors. When hemolysis is relatively severe, reticulocytosis may occur, but the marrow is totally unable to compensate for the increased rate of red blood cell destruction by sufficiently accelerated red blood cell production.

Myelophthisic Anemia. The term myelophthisic implies wasting of the marrow, but in actual practice the term is used to include those conditions in which anemia is associated with invasion or involvement of the bone marrow by some space-occupying lesion, such as carcinoma cells (particularly prostate, breast, lung, adrenal, and thyroid cancer), lymphomatous tissue, including Hodgkin's disease, leukemia, multiple myeloma, multiple granulomatous lesions due to tuberculosis or diffuse fungus infections, fibrous tissue (myelofibrosis), or xanthomatous cells. In these conditions the leukocyte level may be depressed or elevated, and moderate thrombocytopenia is not uncommon. Normoblasts and young granulocytic cells (metamyelocytes and myelocytes) are usually seen in the peripheral blood. The pathogenesis of these changes is obscure, but it does not seem to be a simple "crowding out" of the marrow by the abnormal cells or tissue. Ferrokinetic studies have revealed normal or slightly increased erythropoiesis, and the red blood cell survival time is significantly shortened.[133] Anemia develops because erythropoiesis does not increase sufficiently to compensate for the degree of hemolysis, but the mechanism for these phenomena and the explanation for the appearance of immature red blood cells and granular leukocytes in the peripheral blood is unknown.

Anemia Associated with Endocrine Dysfunctions. Anemia occurs in association with myxedema, adrenal cortical insufficiency, and hypopituitarism. The anemia of hypothyroidism is usually normocytic, but may be macrocytic. Impaired absorption of vitamin B-12 with or without impaired intrinsic factor activity has been observed in hypothyroidism.[134] Furthermore, there is an increased incidence of true pernicious anemia in patients with myxedema. Hypothyroidism per se, however, also causes anemia, since total ablation of the thyroid regularly produces mild anemia, which responds slowly, but eventually completely, to thyroid therapy. Hypoplasia of the bone marrow is sometimes observed in myxedema.[135] The mechanism by which thyroid hormone influences erythropoiesis is unknown. In Addison's disease (chronic adrenocortical insufficiency), there is usually normocytic anemia, which appears to be mild, but the total red blood cell mass is decreased more than is apparent because the blood volume is markedly reduced. Anterior pituitary failure also results in anemia, which may be accompanied by leukopenia.[136] Again, the mechanism by which these hormones affect blood cell equilibrium is unknown.

REFERENCES

1. Wintrobe, M. M.: Blood of normal men and women, Bull. Hopkins Hosp., 53:118, 1933.
2. Wintrobe, M. M.: The Erythrocyte, in Clinical Hematology, ed. 6, Ch. 2, p. 91, Philadelphia, Lea & Febiger, 1967.
3. Parsons, C. G., and Wright, F. H.: Circulatory function in the anemias of children, Amer. J. Dis. Child. 57:15, 1939.
4. Romano, J., and Evans, J. W.: Symptomatic psychosis in a case of secondary anemia, Arch. Neurol. Psychiat. 39:1294, 1938.
5. Pascher, F., and Keen, R.: Chronic ulcers of the leg associated with blood dyscrasias, Arch. Derm. Syph. 66:478, 1952.
6. Taylor, E. S.: Chronic ulcer of the leg associated with congenital hemolytic jaundice, J.A.M.A. 112:1574, 1939.
7. Wintrobe, M. M.: The cardiovascular system in anemia, Blood 1:121, 1946.
8. Brannon, E. S., Merrill, A. J., Warren, J. V., and Stead, E. A., Jr.: The cardiac output in patients with chronic anemia as measured by the technique of right atrial catheterization, J. Clin. Invest. 24:332, 1945.
9. Bradley, S. E., and Bradley, G. P.: Renal function during chronic anemia in man, Blood 2:192, 1947.
10. Whitaker, W.: Some effects of severe chronic anemia on the circulatory system, Quart. J. Med. 25:175, 1956.
11. Bäckman, H.: Circulatory studies in slowly developing anemias, Scand. J. Clin. Lab. Invest. (supp. 57) vol. 13, 1961.
12. Pickering, G. W., and Wayne, E. J.: Observations on angina pectoris and intermittent claudication in anemia, Clin. Sci. 1:305, 1933.
13. Blumgart, H. L., and Altschule, M. D.: Clinical significance of cardiac and respiratory adjustments in chronic anemia, Blood 3:329, 1948.
14. Rankin, J., McNeill, R. S., and Forster, R. E.: The effect of anemia on the alveolar-capillary

exchange of carbon dioxide in man, J. Clin. Invest. 40:1323, 1961.
15. Hunter, A.: The heart in anaemia, Quart. J. Med. 15:107, 1946.
16. Goldstein, B., and Boas, E. P.: Functional diastolic murmurs and cardiac enlargement in severe anemias, Arch. Intern. Med. 39:226, 1927.
17. Gunewardene, H. O.: The cardiac complications of ankylostoma infection with special reference to a presystolic murmur occurring in these cases, J. Trop. Med. Hyg. 36:49, 1933.
18. Friedberg, C. K.: Diseases of the Heart, ed. 3, p. 1683, Philadelphia, Saunders, 1966.
19. Wales, R. T., and Martin, E. A.: Arterial bruits in anaemia, Brit. Med. J. 2:1444, 1963.
20. Gonzáles-de-Cossía, A., Sanchez-Medal, L., and Smyth, J. F.: Electrocardiographic modifications in anemia, Amer. Heart J. 67:166, 1964.
21. Scherf, D., and Klotz, S. D.: Electrocardiographic changes after acute loss of blood, Ann. Intern. Med. 20:438, 1944.
22. Christ, C.: Experimentelle kohlenoxydvergiftung, herzmuskelnekrosen und electrokardiogramm, Beitr. Path. Anat. 94:111, 1934.
23. Steinberg, B.: Sickle-cell anemia, Arch. Path. 9:876, 1930.
24. Yater, W. M., and Hansmann, G. H.: Sickle-cell anemia: a new cause of cor pulmonale, Amer. J. Med. Sci. 191:474, 1936.
25. Winsor, T., and Burch, G. E.: The electrocardiogram and cardiac state in active sickle-cell anemia, Amer. Heart. J. 29:685, 1945.
26. Friedberg, C. K.: Diseases of the Heart, ed. 3, p. 1684, Philadelphia, Saunders, 1966.
27. Ryan, J. M., and Hickam, J. B.: The alveolar-arterial oxygen pressure gradient in anemia, J. Clin. Invest. 31:188, 1952.
28. Blumgart, H. L., and Altschule, M. D.: Clinical significance of cardiac and respiratory adjustments in chronic anemia, Blood 3:329, 1948.
29. Sproule, B. J., Mitchell, J. H., and Miller, W. F.: Cardiopulmonary physiological responses to heavy exercise in patients with anemia, J. Clin. Invest. 39:378, 1960.
30. Oatway, W. H., and Middleton, W. S.: Correlation of lingual changes with other clinical data, Arch. Intern. Med. 49:860, 1932.
31. Fisher, J. M., and Taylor, K. B.: A comparison of autoimmune phenomena in pernicious anemia and chronic atrophic gastritis, New Eng. J. Med. 272:499, 1965.
32. Doniach, D., and Raitt, I. M.: An evaluation of gastric and thyroid autoimmunity in relation to hematologic disorders, Seminars Hemat. 1:313, 1964.
33. Waldenström, J.: Iron and epithelium. Some clinical observations. I. Regeneration of the epithelium, Acta Med. Scand. (supp. 90) p. 380, 1937.
34. Darby, W. J.: The oral manifestations of iron deficiency, J.A.M.A. 130:830, 1946.

35. Waldenström, J., and Kjellberg, S. R.: The roentgenological diagnosis of sideropenic dysphagia (Plummer-Vinson's syndrome), Acta Radiol. 20:618, 1939.

36. Jacobs, A.: Epithelial changes in anemic East Africans, Brit. Med. J. 1:1711, 1963.

37. Beutler, E., Larsh, S. E., and Guruey, C. W.: Iron therapy in chronically fatigued non-anemic women: a double blind study, Ann. Intern. Med. 52:378, 1960.

38. Bradley, S. E., and Bradley, G. P.: Renal function during chronic anemia in man, Blood 2:192, 1947.

39. Földi, M., Korányi, A., and Szabo, G.: Über die Entstehung anämischer Ödeme, Acta Med. Scand. 129:486, 1948.

40. Strauss, M. B., and Fox, H. J.: Anemia and water retention, Amer. J. Med. Sci. 200:454, 1940.

41. Schwaber, J. R., and Blumberg, A. G.: Papilledema associated with blood loss anemia, Ann. Intern. Med. 55:1004, 1961.

42. Marshall, R. A.: A review of lesions in the optic fundus in various diseases of the blood, Blood 14:882, 1959.

43. Nieweg, H. O., Farber, J. G., deVries, J. A., and Kroese, W. F. S.: The relationship of vitamin B-12 and folic acid in megaloblastic anemias, J. Lab. Clin. Med. 44:118, 1954.

44. Goldhamer, S. M., Bethel, F. H., Isaacs, R., and Sturgis, C. C.: Occurrence and treatment of neurologic changes in pernicious anemia, J.A.M.A. 103:1663, 1934.

45. Grinker, R. R., and Kandel, E.: Pernicious anemia: results of treatment of neurologic complications, Arch. Intern. Med. 54:851, 1934.

46. Smithburn, K. C., and Zerfas, L. G.: The neural symptoms and signs in pernicious anemia, Arch. Neurol. Psychiat. 25:1110, 1931.

47. Davidson, S.: Clinical picture of pernicious anemia prior to introduction of liver therapy in 1926 and in Edinburgh subsequent to 1944, Brit. Med. J. 1:241, 1957.

48. Ellison, A. B. C.: Pernicious anemia masked by multivitamins containing folic acid, J.A.M.A. 173:240, 1960.

49. Greenfield, J. G., and Carmichael, E. A.: The peripheral nerves in cases of subacute combined degeneration of the cord, Brain 58:483, 1935.

50. Van der Scheer, W. M., and Koek, H. C.: Peripheral nerve lesions in cases of pernicious anemia, Acta Psychiat. Neurol. 13:61, 1938.

51. Baird, R. L., Weiss, D. L., Ferguson, A. D., French, J. H., and Scott, R. B.: Studies in sickle-cell anemia. XXI. Clinico-pathological aspects of neurological manifestations, Pediatrics 34:92, 1964.

52. Silver, R. T., Utz, J. P., Frei, E., III, and McCullough, N. B.: Fever, infection and host resistance in acute leukemia, Amer. J. Med. 24:25, 1928.

53. Wintrobe, M. M.: Clinical manifestations of leukemia, in Clinical Hematology, ed. 6, Ch. 19, p. 1006, Philadelphia, Lea and Febiger, 1967.

54. Brittingham, T. E., and Chaplin, H., Jr.: Febrile transfusion reactions caused by sensitivity to donor leukocytes and platelets, J.A.M.A. 165:819, 1957.

55. Payne, R., and Rolfs, M. R.: Further observations on leukoagglutinin transfusion reactions, Amer. J. Med. 29:449, 1960.

56. Chaplin, H., Jr., Brittingham, T. E., and Cassell, M.: Methods of preparation of suspensions of buffy coat-poor red blood cells for transfusion, Amer. J. Clin. Path. 31:373, 1959; Transfusion 2:216, 1962.

57. Jenson, K. G.: The significance of leukoagglutinins for the development of transfusion reactions, Danish Med. Bull. 9:198, 1962.

58. Fox, C. L., Jr., and Ottenberg, R.: Acute hemolytic anemia from the sulfonamides, J. Clin. Invest. 20:593, 1941.

59. Diggs, L. W.: Siderofibrosis of the spleen in sickle-cell anemia, J.A.M.A. 104:538, 1935.

60. River, G. L., Robbins, A. B., and Schwartz, S. O.: S-C hemoglobin, Blood 18:385, 1961.

61. Wintrobe, M. M., and Beebe, R. T.: Idiopathic hypochromic anemia, Medicine 12:187, 1933.

62. Tisdale, W. A., Klatskin, G., and Kinsella, E. D.: The significance of the direct-reacting fraction of serum bilirubin in hemolytic jaundice, Amer. J. Med. 26:214, 1959.

63. Brian, M. C., Dacie, J. V., and Hourihane, D. O'B.: Microangiopathic hemolytic anemia, Brit. J. Haemat. 8:358, 1962.

64. Levitan, R., Diamond, H. D., and Craver, L. F.: Jaundice in Hodgkin's disease, Amer. J. Med. 30:99, 1961.

65. Guest, M. M., Bond, T. P., Cooper, R. G., and Derrick, J. R.: Red blood cells: change in shape in capillaries, Science 142:1319, 1963.

66. Murphy, J. R.: Erythrocyte metabolism. VI. Cell shape and the location of cholesterol in the erythrocyte membrane, J. Lab. Clin. Med. 65:756, 1965.

67. Gurney, C. W., and Pan, C.: Studies on erythropoiesis in experimental polycythemia, Proc. Soc. Exp. Biol. Med. 98:789, 1958.

68. Fisher, J. W., Taylor, G., and Porteous, D. D.: Localization of erythropoietin in glomeruli of sheep kidney by fluorescent antibody technique, Nature 205:611, 1965; Proc. Soc. Exp. Biol. Med. 122:1015, 1966.

69. Erslev, A.: Humoral regulation of red blood cell production, Blood 8:349, 1953; ibid., 9:1055, 1954; ibid., 10:616 and 954, 1955; ibid., 14:386, 1959; ibid., 24:331, 1964; Medicine 43:661, 1964.

70. Gallagher, N. I., McCarthy, J. M., and Lange, R. D.: Erythropoietin production in uremic rabbits, J. Lab. Clin. Med. 57:281, 1961.

71. Bentler, E., Fairbanks, V. F., and Fahey, J. L.: Clinical Disorders of Iron Metabolism; New York, Grune & Stratton, 1963.

72. Beveridge, B. R., Bannerman, R. M., Evanson, J. M., and Witts, L. J.: Hypochromic anemia: a retrospective study and follow-up of 378 in-patients, Quart. J. Med. 34:145, 1965.

73. Moore, C. V.: Iron Metabolism and Nutrition, Harvey Lect., Ser. 55, p. 67, 1961; International Symposium on Iron Metabolism, p. 241, Berlin, Springer-Verlag, 1964; Series Hematologica 6:1, 1965.

74. Crosby, W. H.: The control of iron balance by the intestinal mucosa, Blood 22:441, 1963.

75. Winsor, T., and Burch, G. E.: Diagnostic physio-chemical blood tests in sickle-cell anemia, Amer. J. Med. Sci. 207:152, 1944.

76. Wintrobe, M. M.: The relation of disease of the liver to anemia, Arch. Intern. Med. 57:289, 1936.

77. Kimber, C., Deller, D. J., Ibbotson, R. N., and Lander, H.: The mechanism of anemia in chronic liver disease, Quart. J. Med. 34:33, 1965.

78. Jandl, J. H.: The anemia of liver disease: observations on its mechanism, J. Clin. Invest. 34:390, 1955.

79. Cherrick, G. R., Baker, H., Frank, O., and Leevy, C. M.: Observations on hepatic avidity for folate in Laennec's cirrhosis, J. Lab. Clin. Med. 66:446, 1965.

80. Sullivan, L. W., and Herbert, V.: Suppression of hematopoiesis by ethanol, J. Clin. Invest. 43:2048, 1964.

81. Kimber, C. L., Deller, D. J., and Lander, H.: Megaloblastic and transitional megaloblastic anemia associated with chronic liver disease, Amer. J. Med. 38:707, 1965.

82. Kunde, M. M., Green, M. F., and Burns, G.: Blood changes in experimental hypo- and hyper-thyroidism (rabbit), Amer. J. Physiol. 99:469, 1931–1932.

83. Stein, B., and Altshule, M.D.: Hematologic studies in hypothyroidism following total thyroidectomy, J. Clin. Invest. 15:633, 1936.

84. Finch, C. A., Coleman, D. H., Motulsky, A. G., Donohue, D. M., and Reiff, R. H.: Erythrokinetics in pernicious anemia, Blood 11:807, 1956.

85. Forshaw, J., Horwood, L., and Weatherall, D. J.: Folic acid deficiency and megaloblastic erythropoiesis in myelofibrosis, Brit. Med. J. 1:671, 1964.

86. Frick, P. G., and Brunner, H. E.: Megaloblastäre forsäuremangel—anämie bei hämochromatose, Deutsche Med. Wschr. 89:161, 1964.

87. Johns, D. G., and Bertino, J. R.: Folates and megalo-blastic anemia, a review, Clin. Pharmacol. Ther. 6:372, 1965.

88. Jandl, J. H.: Section on megaloblastic anemias in Beeson and McDermott, (eds.): Cecil and Loeb, Textbook of Medicine, Philadelphia, Saunders, 1967.

89. Van der Scheer, W. M., and Kolk, H. C.: Peripheral nerve lesions in cases of pernicious anemia, Acta Psychiat. Neurol. 13:61, 1938.

90. Lambert, H. P., Prankerd, T. A. J., and Smellie, J. M.: Pernicious anemia in childhood, Quart. J. Med. 30:71, 1961.

91. Waters, A. H., and Murphy, M. E. B.: Familial juvenile pernicious anemia: a study of the hereditary basis of pernicious anemia, Brit. J. Haemat. 9:1, 1963.

92. McIntyre, P. A., Harn, R., Conley, E. L., and Glass, B.: Genetic factors in predisposition to pernicious anemia, Bull. Hopkins Hosp. 104:309, 1959.

93. Jeffries, G. H., and Sleisenger, M. H.: Studies of parietal cell antibody in pernicious anemia, J. Clin. Invest. 44:2021, 1965; 45:803, 1966.

94. Taylor, K. B., Roitt, I. M., Doniach, D., Couchman, K. G., and Shapland, C.: Autoimmune phenomena in pernicious anemia: gastric antibodies, Brit. Med. J. 2:1347, 1962.

95. Dimson, S. B.: Juvenile pernicious anemia, Arch. Dis. Child. 41:216, 1966.

96. Johns, D. G., and Bertino, J. R.: Folates and megaloblastic anemia: a review, Clin. Pharmacol. Ther. 6:372, 1965.

97. Raper, A. B.: Sickle-cell disease in Africa and America—a comparison, J. Trop. Med. Hyg. 53:49, 1950.

98. Allison, A. C.: Protection afforded by sickle-cell trait against subtertian malarial infection, Brit. Med. J. 1:290, 1954.

99. Pauling, L., Itano, H. A., Singer, S. J., and Wills, I. C.: Sickle-cell anemia, a molecular disease, Science 110:543, 1949; J. Biol. Chem. 187:221, 1950.

100. Owren, P. A.: Congenital hemolytic jaundice. The pathogenesis of the "hemolytic crisis," Blood 3:231, 1948.

101. Jacob, H. S., and Jandl, J. H.: Increased cell membrane permeability in the pathogenesis of hereditary spherocytosis, J. Clin. Invest. 43:1704, 1964; Amer. J. Med. 41:734, 1966.

102. Burka, E. R., Weaver, Z., III, and Marks, P. A.: Clinical spectrum of hemolytic anemia associated with glucose-6-phosphate dehydrogenase deficiency, Ann. Intern. Med. 64:817, 1966.

103. Kan, S. Y., and Gardner, F. H.: Life span of reticulocytes in paroxysmal nocturnal hemoglobinuria, Blood 25:759, 1965.

104. Auditore, J. V., and Hartmann, R. C.: Paroxysmal nocturnal hemoglobinuria. II. Erythrocyte acetyl cholinesterase defect, Amer. J. Med. 27:401, 1959.

105. Lewis, S. M., Danon, D., and Marikovsky, Y.: Electron microscope studies of the red cell in paroxysmal nocturnal hemoglobinuria, Brit. J. Haemat. 11:689, 1965.

106. Hartmann, R. C., and Jenkins, D. E., Jr.: The sugar-water test for paroxysmal nocturnal hemoglobinuria, New Eng. J. Med. 275:155, 1966.

107. McKellar, M., and Dacie, J. V.: Thromboplastic activity of the plasma in paroxysmal nocturnal hemoglobinuria, Brit. J. Haemat. 4:404, 1958.

108. Craft, J. D., *et al*.: Coombs test positivity induced by drugs. Mechanisms of immunologic reactions and red cell destruction, Ann. Intern. Med. 68:176, 1968.

109. Carstairs, K. C., Breckenridge, A., Dollery, C. T., and Worlledge, S. M.: Incidence of a positive direct Coombs test in patients on α-methyl dopa, Lancet 2:133 and 135, 1966.

110. Worlledge, S. M., Carstairs, K. C., and Dacie, J. V.: Autoimmune hemolytic anemia association with α-methyl dopa therapy, Lancet 2:135, 1966.

111. Dacie, J. V.: The Hemolytic Anemias: Congenital and Acquired. Part II: The Autoimmune Hemolytic Anemias, New York, Grune & Stratton, 1962.

112. Wasastjerna, C., Dameshek, W., and Kominos, Z. D.: Direct observations of intravascular agglutination of red cells in acquired autoimmune hemolytic anemia, J. Lab. Clin. Med. 43:98, 1954.

113. Jandl, J. H., Simmons, R. L., and Castle, W. B.: Red cell filtration and the pathogenesis of certain hemolytic anemias, Blood 18:133, 1961.

114. Jandl, J. H.: Mechanisms of antibody-induced red cell destruction, Series Hematologia 9:35, 1965.

115. Borsos, T., Dourmaskin, R. R., and Humphrey, J. H.: Lesions in erythrocyte membranes caused by immune hemolysis, Nature 202:251, 1964.

116. LoBuglio, A. F., Cotran, R. S., and Jandl, J. H.: Red cells coated with immunoglobulin G: binding and sphering by mononuclear cells in man, Science 158:1582, 1967.

117. Wintrobe, M. M.: Hemolytic anemias, *in* Clinical Hematology, ed. 6, Ch. 12, p. 606, Philadelphia, Lea and Febiger, 1967.

118. Young, L. E.: Section on Extracorpuscular hemolytic agents and mechanisms, from chapter on Diseases of the Blood, *in* Beeson and McDermott (eds.): Cecil and Loeb Textbook of Medicine, ed. 12, p. 1034, Philadelphia, Saunders, 1967.

119. Brain, M. C., Dacie, J. V., and Hourihane, D. O'B.: Microangiopathic hemolytic anemia, Brit. J. Haemat. 8:358, 1962.

120. Bull, B. S., Rubenberg, M. L., Dacie, J. V., and Brain, M. C.: Red blood cell fragmentation in microangiopathic hemolytic anemia: in-vitro studies, Lancet 2: 1123, 1967.

121. Steinberg, B.: Bone marrow regeneration in experimental benzine intoxication, Blood 4:550, 1949.

122. Smick, K. M., Condit, P. K., Proctor, R. L., and Sutcher, V.: Fatal aplastic anemia, J. Chron. Dis. 17:899, 1964.

123. Saidi, P., Wallerstein, R. O., and Aggeler, P. M.: Effect of chloramphenicol on erythropoiesis, J. Lab. Clin. Med. 57:247, 1961.

124. Gussoff, B. D., and Lee, S. L.: Chloramphenicol-induced hematopoietic depression: A controlled comparison with tetracycline, Amer. J. Med. Sci. 251:8, 1966.

125. Scott, J. L., Finegold, S. M., Belkin, G. A., and Lawrence, J. S.: A controlled double blind study of the hematologic toxicity of chloramphenicol, New Eng. J. Med. 272:1137, 1965.

126. Middleton, W. S., and Burke, M.: Streptococcus viridans endocarditis lenta, Amer. J. Med. Sci. 198:301, 1939.

127. Morgensen, E.: The anemia of gastric cancer, Folia Haemat. 56:206, 1936.

128. Cartwright, G. W.: The anemia of chronic disorders, Seminars in Hematology, 3:351, 1961.

129. Freireich, E. J., Ross, J. F., Bayles, T. B., Emerson, C. P., and Finch, S. C.: Radioactive iron metabolism and erythrocyte survival studies of the mechanism of anemia associated with rheumatoid arthritis, J. Clin. Invest. 36:1043, 1957.

130. Haurani, F. I., Green, D., and Young, K.: Iron absorption in hypoferremia, Amer. J. Med. Sci. 249:537, 1965.

131. Haurani, F. I., Burke, W., and Martinez, E. J.: Defective re-utilization of iron in the anemia of inflammation, J. Lab. Clin. Med. 65:560, 1965.

132. Haurani, F. I., Young, K., and Tocantins, L. M.: Re-utilization of iron in anemia complicating malignant neoplasms, Blood 22:73, 1963.

133. Hyman, G. A.: Anemia in malignant neoplastic disease, J. Chronic Dis. 16:645, 1963.

134. Tudhope, G. R., and Wilson, G. M.: Anaemia in hypothyroidism, Quart. J. Med. 29:513, 1960; Lancet 1:703, 1962.

135. Jones, R. M.: Human sternal marrow in hyperthyroid and myxedematous states, Amer. J. Med. Sci. 200:211, 1940.

136. Daughaday, W. H., Williams, R. H., and Daland, G. A.: The effect of endocrinopathies on the blood, Blood 3:1342, 1948.

137. Bunn, H. F., and Jandl, J. H.: Control of hemoglobin function within the red cell, New Eng. J. Med. 282:1414, 1970.

29

Nervousness and Fatigue

GEORGE L. ENGEL

INTRODUCTION

Nervousness and fatigue are terms used by patients to indicate certain common and nonspecific symptoms that characterize many types of illness, physical and emotional. **Nervousness** refers to a feeling of tension, arousal, and uncertainty; **fatigue** to a feeling of weakness, depletion, and exhaustion. The common denominator of *nervousness* is a sense of actual or threatened loss of control over mind or body, associated with feelings of alarm and vulnerability. The common denominator of *fatigue* is a feeling of inability to mobilize energy to carry on, associated with a desire to rest and sleep. Patients complaining of nervousness often complain of fatigue as well.

Nervousness and fatigue are nonspecific psychological accompaniments of the activity of the two major neurobiological emergency systems, **flight-fight**[1] and **conservation-withdrawal**.[2,3,64] The *flight-fight* system readies the organism to meet threats by warning of dangers and mobilizing neuroendocrine and other physiological mechanisms to prepare the body for action and possible injury. The reaction ceases as soon as effective action or the possibility of a solution is realized. The *conservation-withdrawal* system protects against exhaustion by warning of the possibility of energy depletion and initiating processes to conserve supplies, including reduction of activity and heightening of the stimulus threshold. The reaction dissipates after rest or sleep, as energy supplies are replenished, or when the warning of energy depletion proves to be unfounded. The conservation-withdrawal reaction protects against overstress, and hence replaces the flight-fight response when the latter proves ineffective.

From the psychological perspective, *nervousness* encompasses mainly the affects of fear, anxiety, and anger, along with a high degree of arousal. Such affects reflect the feeling that available mental mechanisms are inadequate to cope with anticipated circumstances, which consequently are perceived as threatening. With *fear* the danger is seen as real and external, and the desire is to escape and avoid injury. With *anxiety* the danger is obscure and omnipresent. The orientation is to anticipate injury and to be prepared for escape or attack; hence, the high level of arousal. Anger is an intense feeling that someone or something must be acted upon to destroy it as a threat or to force it to comply or provide a needed or wanted gratification. When the feelings of anxiety, fear, or anger are not recognized as such, the resulting tension usually is referred to as *nervousness*. Fatigue, on the other hand, has a closer affinity with depression, the affects of giving up (helplessness and hopelessness), and apathy.[4] These reflect the feeling that one is no longer able or interested enough to engage in the activity necessary to achieve gratification. They may be evoked by a sense of bodily incapacity, psychological failure, or environmental deprivation.

BIOLOGY OF NERVOUSNESS AND FATIGUE

NEURAL ORGANIZATION OF THE FLIGHT-FIGHT AND CONSERVATION-WITHDRAWAL SYSTEMS

The central nervous system is organized so that sensory information, from the body as well as the environment, is coded into signals capable of eliciting meaningful patterns of response. This processing of sensory input is accomplished simultaneously by several interconnected analyzer-integrator systems, which differ in phylogenetic age and in the degree of crudeness or refinement with which the sensory pattern is dealt.[5] The emergency biological defense systems of flight-fight and conservation-withdrawal are mediated through the more primordial analyzer-integrator-effector circuits represented in the limbic system, the hypothalamus, and the reticular formation of the brainstem and midbrain. This circuit also regulates the stability of the internal milieu, mediates the preformed behavioral and physiological response patterns required for such activities as foraging, feeding, and mating, and provides the neural basis for the elaboration and expression of emotions.[5,6] By virtue of direct neocortical connections with the frontal and temporal cortex and indirect connections through the reticular systems, the limbic system is receptive to input from the older as well as from the more recently developed neural organizations. Hence, it can respond to at least three different levels of input: (1) changes in the physicochemical properties of the blood as sensed by chemoreceptor neurons in the reticular formation and hypothalamus; (2) sensory signals transmitted along afferent pathways from within the body and from the environment; and (3) sensory information based on memory, experience, and the symbols of the personal and cultural milieu, transmitted through neocortical connections.[7] The reticular formation, through its excitatory and inhibitory functions, can both facilitate the flow of sensory information from the various sense receptors and screen out irrelevant or excessive input.[8,9]

The existence of direct and indirect neocortical connections with the limbic system-midbrain circuit and the hypothalamus provides the mechanisms whereby behavior can be organized in terms of long-term goals, opportunities, and dangers. These are represented in the form of the memory traces of past successes and failures. In this way, behavior in response to internal (bodily) and environmental changes is based on available mental or motor patterns, which have been effective in the past.

In effect, past experience enables the animal to predict how successfully any particular behavioral pattern will control the environment or assure gratification of needs. As long as analysis of sensory input confirms the availability of an effective behavioral response, the animal can function efficiently and with confidence of the outcome. But the moment sensory input is analyzed as incongruent with available behavioral responses, predictability fails and the stability of the system is jeopardized. At this juncture the emergency systems are likely to be activated, first as arousal, then as flight-fight, and finally as conservation-withdrawal if no resolution has been achieved and exhaustion threatens. The reticular formation plays an especially important role in regulating the levels of arousal and inhibition characteristic of these states.[8,9]

The extensive activation of the nervous system and the development of emergency responses when an animal has no available behavior to control its environment can be illustrated by the free operant avoidance conditioning situation.[10] When placed for the first time in a conditioning box, the animal initially displays alerting and orienting behavior, examining the new setting for sensory information congruent with past experience. This arousal behavior is accompanied by widespread cortical and subcortical responses, as recorded from implanted electrodes, which disappear as soon as the animal becomes adjusted to its new surroundings. Upon the introduction of a new stimulus, such as a regularly appearing 10 per second flickering light, arousal behavior is again elicited, and synchronous 10 per second activity appears in many areas of the brain, reflecting the dissemination of the sensory information to many different analyzer-integrator currents. But as the animal again becomes accustomed to the new stimulus, he no longer responds to it, and the synchronous 10 per second response becomes largely limited to the visual system. If now the periodic light becomes a warning for an electric shock, which will follow regularly after a fixed interval, the animal displays, upon each occasion, marked agitation and a desperate effort to escape the anticipated shock. Such behavior exemplifies the flight-fight reaction and includes searching, running, hiding, trembling, cowering, vocalizing, and at times pilo-erection, urination, and defecation. At the same time, recordings from implanted electrodes reveal widespread responses throughout the nervous system, reflecting both the extensive dissemination of the sensory input in the form of synchronous responses, as well as activation of many different circuits. However, if in the course of such behavior some act, such as depressing a lever, is associated with failure of the shock to follow the light, the animal is likely to repeat the act to verify the reliability of this association. In this way he discovers a new behavioral response with which he can again predictably control his environment. At this point the flight-fight response is replaced by an efficient instrumental act and the animal is able to resume his ordinary activity, assured of no shock as long as he depresses the lever. At the same time the generalized excitability of the cortex and of the neural structures mediating the emergency response disappears, and responses synchronous with the light persist only in the visual system, amygdala, and anterior ventral nucleus of the thalamus, areas presumably concerned with attention to the stimulus of execution of the learned response.

The same situation can also be used to illustrate the *transition* from the **flight-fight response** to the **withdrawal response.** Animals placed in a situation in which no effective response is possible or in which a previously effective response, such as lever pressing, is no longer available or effective, at first again become strikingly agitated. But ultimately many give up, becoming quiet, inactive, hypotonic, poorly responsive, sometimes dozing or sleeping for long periods of time.[11,12,13]

The two emergency defense systems are separately represented in the nervous system in what Hess has designated as (1) the **ergotropic** and (2) the **trophotropic** zones of the diencephalon and mesencephalon.[14] The ergotropic system, in a broad sense, discharges over the *sympathetic outflow* and *neuroendocrine systems*, the trophotropic over the *parasympathetic outflow.* The ergotropic system is concerned with the mobilization and utilization of energy, the trophotropic with local defense mechanisms and conservation of energy. The *ergotropic system* is thus *dynamogenic*, whereas the *trophotropic* protects against overstress. Ergotropic activity facilitates alertness and preparation for action, whereas trophotropic activity lowers responsiveness and facilitates drowsiness and sleep.

Ordinarily ergotropic and trophotropic reactions do not occur at the same time.[15] They are reciprocally related, responsiveness of one system declining progressively with increasing activity of the antagonistic system. However, under the influence of increasingly strong stimuli and in states of heightened central excitability, parasympathetic and sympathetic discharges may both occur (viz., urination and defecation during the flight-fight response). Under such conditions, the trophotropic system may ultimately become dominant, with the result that noxious stimuli, which previously elicited ergotropic (sympathetic) responses, may now elicit trophotropic reactions, including drowsiness and sleep. Apparently a feedback mechanism exists between the neocortex and the reticular formation so that excessive cortical excitation induces corticofugal impulses that inhibit the reticular formation. This provides the homeostatic control whereby the excitation of the ergotropic system is effectively limited, a first step in the conservation-withdrawal reaction protecting the organism from exhaustion. This relationship is demonstrated behaviorally in the transition from the active behavior of the flight-fight reaction to the inactivity of the conservation-withdrawal response when no escape or solution is possible.

PHYSIOLOGY OF FLIGHT-FIGHT AND NERVOUSNESS

The physiologic processes of the flight-fight (ergotropic) reactions vary according to the degree to which organized activity is possible. As illustrated by the avoidance conditioning experiments, this may range from a state of general arousal and alarm, during which no effective action is available, to one in which the animal vigilantly maintains readiness to institute a specific behavior to avoid trauma, whether it be literally to flee or to fight or merely to perform an instrumental act, as lever pressing. In general, the physiological reactions of flight-fight serve to *anticipate* needs rather than being *responses* to actual body changes. Hence, the system is most sensitive to psychological influences, and the physiological changes are most pronounced in situations of greatest uncertainty.[16]

According to Mason, the widespread **hormonal changes** associated with arousal and the flight-fight reaction may be classified into two groups.[16,38] One shows a monophasic response curve, hormone production increasing during the reaction and returning to the baseline during the recovery period. The second shows a biphasic pattern, decreasing during the reaction and increasing during recovery. **The first group** includes ACTH,[17] corticosteroids (17-OHCS),[18] epinephrine, norepinephrine,[19,20] antidiuretic hormone,[21] aldosterone,[22] thyroid,[23,24] and growth hormone (GH).[25] **The second group** includes insulin,[26] estrogens,[27] testosterone,[28] and the androgenic metabolites.[29] The hormonal responses are prompt—within minutes for some —except for thyroid hormone, which may not become elevated until several days have elapsed and may remain elevated until well into the recovery period. The hormone responses are also sustained throughout the period of reaction, except for epinephrine, which is usually most elevated early. The rebound during the recovery period may last a week or more. Most thoroughly studied has been the pituitary-adrenal cortical system, which is regulated through the limbic system via amygdala-hippocampal interactions.[17,30,31] Elevations in 17-OHCS correlate very closely with the degree of arousal and emotional distress in both man and animals. Levels fall as effective coping mechanisms develop and comfort and tranquillity return, sometimes even in the face of unrealistic or psychotic ideation. Patients facing surgery or diagnostic procedures,[32,44] parents of mortally ill children,[33] men in combat,[34,35] and psychotic patients[36,37] may show normal 17-OHCS levels as long as they manage to perceive their situations as not disturbing or threatening. The moment such defenses become ineffective and distress is felt, 17-OHCS levels rise.

Mason points out that the first subgroup have mainly "**catabolic**" effects on energy metabolism, the second "**anabolic**."[38] For example, fuel sources are increased by the glycogenolytic effect of epinephrine and free fatty acid releasing effects of epinephrine and norepinephrine.[39,40] The adrenal steroids promote hyperglycemia, facilitate free fatty acid release,[41] support muscular work capacity,[42] and increase the capacity of cells to produce energy anaerobically, a critical factor for strenuous muscular work.[43] GH accelerates triglyceride breakdown and fatty acid release.[45] Thyroxine increases rates of oxidation and potentiates some of the catabolic effects of epinephrine.[46,47] On the other hand, insulin promotes glycogenesis and lipogenesis and stimulates protein synthesis[47,48]; testosterone and related androgens promote protein synthesis, and both estrogens and androgens may potentiate some effects of insulin on carbohydrate metabolism.[49,50] All of these events appear to be oriented toward the common end of efficient mobilization of energy resources during flight-fight and replenishment of depleted stores afterward.

The antidiuretic and aldosterone responses are probably related to conservation of water and electrolytes for the temperature regulation and muscular activity required of the animal preparing for action.[21,22]

Other effects of these hormone changes may have to do with preparation for injury. These include the effects of epinephrine on blood coagulation and the role of adrenal steroids in preventing the capillary damage associated with excessive sympathetic activity.[51]

The catecholamines and the adrenal steroids may also play a role in the functioning of the central nervous system. Epinephrine contributes to the central excitation of the neocortex and of the ergotropic system as a whole.[52] Norepinephrine exists in high concentrations in the hypothalamus and parts of the limbic system.[53] Its accumulation or release in these sites appears to play an important role in mediating alertness and vigilance. ACTH and the adrenal steroids have significant effects on the development of conditioned responses.[54,55,83]

Prominent during flight-fight are the circulatory and respiratory preparations for muscular activity. During periods of greatest unpredictability the circulatory changes are largely mediated through the diffuse effects of epinephrine and include an increase in cardiac output and in rate of vigor of the heart beat; enhanced blood flow to the heart, skeletal muscles, and brain; and rise in systolic and slight fall in diastolic blood pressure.[56,57] As more organized behavior develops, norepinephrine secretion at sympathetic nerve endings dominates in the regulation of regional circulatory adjustments.[92] Thus, appropriate cardiac adjustment is regulated by reflex sympathetic control, while blood flow to striated muscle, heart, and brain is assured by sympathetically mediated (norepinephrine) vasoconstriction in less essential areas, such as the gastrointestinal tract, kidneys, skin, and those muscles necessary for the behavioral response. If heat production is excessive, cutaneous vasoconstriction is replaced by vasodilation and sweating. Cholinergic sympathetic activity yields local vasodilation in muscles and sweating of palms and soles.[58]

Respiration is typically accentuated during preparation for activity, often leading to significant hyperventilation and hypocapnia. The consequent reduction in plasma pH increases the capacity of the blood to buffer acid metabolites of muscular activity and prolongs breathholding time, a crucial factor for the use of the torso for a sustained effort.[59]

PHYSIOLOGY OF CONSERVATION-WITHDRAWAL AND FATIGUE

As a signal for the need to replenish or conserve energy, fatigue is intimately related to the waking-sleep cycle and activity of the trophotropic system.[14,60] This fatigue normally develops in a cyclical fashion in relation to the circadian rhythm, as well as in response to any situation centrally interpreted as a threat of exhaustion. This ranges from a psychological judgment that further effort is fruitless (a feeling of fatigue) to a physiologic feedback that further effort is impossible (actual exhaustion). Fatigue, of course, may be felt long before exhaustion develops, and performance, mental or physical, can be sustained or resumed in spite of the feeling of fatigue. Further, training may raise the threshold for fatigue by enhancing performance capability both physiologically and psychologically. In general, the development of fatigue is delayed as long as there is expectation or hope of success and hastened as soon as the prospects dim. In this way, fruitless expenditure of energy is minimized.

Exhaustion of energy at the cellular level determines the absolute limit of performance. Presumably multiple feedback mechanisms exist whereby the neural regulating system receives information indicating the imminence of such a state, whether brought about by work or by some interference with energy-yielding chemical reactions resulting from disease processes. As yet, little is known about these mechanisms.

Nor is there much information concerning the physiological correlates of the *feeling of fatigue* per se or of more extreme conditions of giving up. In general, there is a dampening of physiologic and metabolic processes required for active engagement with the environment and a shift toward metabolic adaptations geared to anabolic processes and the use of endogenous sources of substrate. Many of the changes are similar to those observed during sleep.[61,62] All sympathetic and some parasympathetic activities are inhibited.[57] There is a decrease in motor activity and muscle tone, the latter involving reduced activity of the gamma system[57]; general reduction in the activity of the cardiovascular system, including slower heart rate, lower blood pressure, and probably reduced cardiac output[57]; reduced sensitivity of the respiratory center to CO_2, with rise in CO_2, fall in pH, and decrease in ventilation[57,63]; diminished secretion, motor activity, and blood flow of the stomach[65,66] and intestinal tract[67]; decrease in the state of arousal[14,57,64]; fall to baseline or below of levels of epinephrine, norepinephrine, ACTH, and 17-OHCS[33,37,38] and GH.[25,44] With the more chronic conservation-withdrawal response, there may also be weight loss and, in children, failure to grow and develop.[64,69,70,71]

CLINICAL MANIFESTATIONS OF NERVOUSNESS AND FATIGUE

NERVOUSNESS

The clinical manifestations of nervousness are comprised of various combinations of the affects of anxiety, fear, and anger, along with somatic expressions of activity of the flight-fight system.

The most common form of nervousness involves predominantly the affects of **anxiety** and **fear**. The patient experiencing *anxiety* may describe himself as tense, upset, shaky, jittery, worried, anxious, scared, or on edge. He has a sense of uneasiness, foreboding, apprehension, sometimes for no evident reason, sometimes associated with some definite concern (fear). Sleep is poor and often disturbed by frightening dreams. He may speak of weakness, fatigue, giddiness, quivering inside, "butterflies in the stomach," blurred vision, and difficulty concentrating. His voice may be high-pitched and tremulous, and there may be an irregular tremor of the lips and outstretched hands. He may complain of weakness, breathlessness, flushing, cold hands and feet, palpitations, rapid heart action, and skipped beats. Heart rate fluctuates widely, often from 70 to 140 or faster over short periods of time, and may show unusual acceleration upon standing (orthostatic tachycardia) or after hyperventilation or the Valsalva maneuver; yet it usually slows during sleep. There may be frequent premature supraventricular contractions. Blood pressure is labile, usually with some systolic elevation and widened pulse pressure. Hands and feet typically are cold and wet with perspiration. Breathing is sometimes irregular, with frequent sighing. Appetite is generally decreased, but some patients overeat to overcome the feeling of tension, and hence gain weight; more show a modest weight loss. Occasional patients also have irregular, mild diarrhea, usually with peristaltic rushes and without blood or significant mucus. There may be transient frequency of urination and occasionally nocturia and polyuria due to excessive water drinking.

Among some patients the complaint of nervousness reflects a struggle to control **anger,** often mixed with anxiety as well. Feeling their anger to be excessive, inappropriate, or hazardous, they try to hide it and sometimes succeed even to the extent of denying anger to themselves. As a consequence, they often feel tense, irritable, "ready to fly off the handle," "tight as a drum," "ready to explode," or "blow my top." The struggle to contain anger is usually revealed in the patient's manner as well as language, which may be replete with imagery of violence even when anger is denied; things "explode," "crash," or "burst." Sleep may be disturbed by dreams of violence. The patient tends to hold himself rigidly, the brow furrowed, the lips pinched tightly, the jaws clamped together, and the fists clenched. Such chronic muscle tension may result in band-like, bitemporal, or fronto-occipital headaches and aches in the back of the neck, the shoulders, and upper back. There may be flushing or blanching of the face, slight tachycardia and elevation of systolic and diastolic blood pressures, occasionally reaching hypertensive levels. Extremities are warm and dry unless anxiety is also present.

People working under pressure may also feel nervous as a consequence of sustained arousal. They use such terms as "keyed up," "excited," "wound up," "pressured," "tense," "worried," or "irritable." Impatient, in a hurry, moving and speaking rapidly, unable to relax, and constantly concerned that the job will not be done, their sleep is disturbed and insufficient, their eating irregular. Physical findings are less pronounced in this group.

FATIGUE

Exemplified by such terms as weary, "all in," tired, worn out, listless, no pep, and no more interest, fatigue is marked by a feeling of insufficient energy to carry on and a strong desire to stop, rest, or sleep.

At least three components may be involved. It may be felt as lassitude, or tiredness, as is typical after a full day's activity, relief from which is sought through sleep. It may be felt as muscular, as occurs upon physical exertion, which may be relieved simply by resting. Or it may be mental, as develops with sustained emotional and intellectual effort or lack of stimulation, which may be relieved by relaxation or diversion. Motivation plays a powerful role, for the length of time one may persevere at a task without fatigue depends very much on interest and determination. Pleasure and satisfaction raise the threshold for fatigue, disinterest and discomfort lower it.

It is difficult to associate any physical findings with fatigue per se, especially when it reflects major underlying disease. In general the patient tends to appear worn, wan, lethargic, slowed down, and lacking in verve and energy. The face sags, the body slumps, and the voice may be dull and toneless. There are no specific circulatory or respiratory changes.

DIFFERENTIAL DIAGNOSIS OF NERVOUSNESS AND FATIGUE

NERVOUSNESS

Most patients complaining of nervousness are suffering from emotional disturbances of some sort. In a few, the nervous symptoms are the result of abnormalities involving the neural or endocrine systems mediating the flight-fight reaction. The diagnostic problem involves first differentiating between these two major categories and then delineating the various entities that comprise each.

Occasional patients use the term nervousness loosely to refer to such complaints as intention tremor, ataxia, chorea, epilepsy, and the loss of emotional control of pseudobulbar palsy. Such conditions are easily identified and are not considered here.

Psychological Disturbances

Transient situational disturbances are the most frequent explanation for nervousness. Sometimes the patient is quite aware of the problem that is disturbing him; more often he has dismissed it from his mind but not resolved it. In either case he is facing some situation, which evokes apprehension or anger or places him under pressure, but he feels unsure or powerless how to cope with it. The resulting uncertainty induces the symptoms of nervousness and leads the patient to seek medical attention. Because of the prominence of physical symptoms, some individuals actually believe themselves to be suffering from a physical illness. The task for the physician is to recognize the psychological nature of the complaint and elucidate its basis. Usually he can gain some understanding, and often appreciably help the patient, simply by encouraging him to describe his life situation around the time of symptom onset. An accepting and understanding manner generates confidence and often enables the patient to acknowledge or recall what had triggered his feelings. Virtually any type of life change or conflict may be responsible and ordinarily the symptoms subside when the external situation is resolved. If not, one must consider some other explanation.

Among hospitalized patients, circumstances surrounding clinical study and care may be important in provoking such nervous reactions. Patients may become anxious or angry anticipating diagnostic procedures or surgery, particularly if they have not been adequately prepared emotionally, have previously had unpleasant experiences, or lack confidence in the physician. The symptoms or distress of a patient in a nearby bed or an ill-considered remark by a staff member may be upsetting. Uncertainty on the part of the doctor about the diagnosis, obvious disagreement among the physicians as to management, and failure to communicate with the patient are potent determiners of anxiety and sometimes anger, especially among patients with complex or obscure illnesses. Not to be overlooked are worries about affairs and relationships outside the hospital. In general, providing the patient with an opportunity freely to discuss his concerns often resolves the issue and is more efficacious than the use of tranquilizing drugs. Indeed the common practice of immediately sedating an upset patient rather than first letting him talk about what concerns him can only be condemned.

The somatic changes of physical illness may secondarily induce fear or anxiety, which often persists until medical help arrives or some rational explanation is provided. Certain physical derangements have an especially high potential for generating anxiety, notably difficulty in breathing, sudden paralysis, bleeding, loss of vision, and inability to speak. *Delirium*, the result of cerebral metabolic insufficiency, may be accompanied by profound anxiety. The anxiety is easily understandable as the patient's reaction to his difficulty in memory, orientation, and in comprehending what is going on about him.[72]

Some symptoms, especially pain or paralysis, may be frustrating and provoke anger in some patients.

Sometimes the nervousness results from a more personal response to a relatively minor symptom. For example, a patient may become unduly agitated about a slight cough, his concern really being related to his father's death from a lung ailment or his own earlier bout with tuberculosis. If such concerns represent realistic anxiety rather than neurotic preoccupation or hypochondriasis, they will readily be relieved by reassurance.

Neurotic reactions differ from the acute situational disturbances by virtue of the more pervasive and enduring quality of the nervousness and its less obvious association with the environmental conditions. The nervousness generally reflects the anxiety, often mixed with depression, which marks the failure or inadequacy of psychologic defenses. Some patients are chronically anxious; they continually feel apprehensive, uncertain, and fearful, about others as well as themselves. Many are profoundly disabled by their physical symptoms, which reflect a more or less chronic flight-fight response, often no longer related to the original psychological problems; the physical symptoms themselves generate more anxiety in a never-ending vicious cycle. Other patients externalize the fear in the form of a phobia, which enables them to reduce their discomfort by avoiding the phobic situation. Common phobias concern being alone, darkness, crowds, confining spaces, heights, and animals. Fears of dirt, contamination, germs, or poisons are more difficult to control. The **obsessive-compulsive neurotic** person attempts to do so with the aid of complex rituals, but rarely with much success; hence, anxiety symptoms are promi-

TABLE 29-1. COMPARISON OF HYPERTHYROIDISM AND PSYCHOGENIC NERVOUSNESS

	HYPERTHYROIDISM	PSYCHOGENIC NERVOUSNESS
Appetite	Usually increased	Usually decreased
Food intake	Increased	Decreased or increased
Weight	Loss	Loss or gain
Sweating	Generalized	Hands and feet
Skin temperature	Warm	Variable, usually cool
Flushing	Generalized, persistent	Blush area, intermittent
Temperature complaints	Persistent heat intolerance	More often feel cold, sometimes with hot flashes
Hands and feet	Warm and moist	Cold and moist
Heart rate	Persistent sinus tachycardia, awake and asleep; atrial fibrillation occasionally	Variable tachycardia, normal during sleep
Blood pressure	Widened pulse pressure, diastolic pressure low	Widened pulse pressure, systolic pressure high
Generalized weakness and fatigue	Persistent	Variable
Muscle weakness	Proximal muscle groups; may be wasting	No objective evidence
Tremor	Fine, rapid, persistent	Coarse, slower, variable
Thyroid enlargement	Usually demonstrable	Absent
Exophthalmos and eye signs	Present	Lid retraction may be present

nent. Hypochondriacal concerns are peculiarly distressing and show no response to reassurance.

Psychotic reactions may be associated with periods of diffuse anxiety or may be ushered in by panic. Such patients may believe themselves to be the intended victim of an attack or organized plot, hallucinate menacing voices or terrifying visions, imagine they are being controlled by radio waves, or fear they are undergoing some bodily changes. In general the psychotic person appears intense, disorganized, detached, or distractible and the examiner may find it difficult to maintain contact with him or to follow the sense of what he is saying. His language may be bizarre, stilted, or excessively concrete. There may be peculiar gestures, mannerisms, or facial expressions, and emotional expression may be inappropriate. The longer the patient is allowed to talk and the less direction he is given, the more evident will become the psychotic nature of his disturbance.

Delirium tremens, a withdrawal reaction in chronic alcoholism, is marked by severe anxiety, with confusion, visual hallucinations, and fear of attack, usually coming on 3 or 4 days after discontinuing alcohol. It is commonly heralded by insomnia and rapidly mounting nervousness. The patient shows hyperkinesis, coarse tremor, startle, stare, and often marked tachycardia and sweating, and sometimes circulatory collapse.

ABNORMALITIES INVOLVING THE FLIGHT-FIGHT (ERGOTROPIC) SYSTEM

In these conditions, abnormalities affecting the function of components of the system mediating flight-fight may be responsible for nervousness, either by producing some of the physiological changes of or by lowering the threshold for a flight-fight reaction.

Hyperthyroidism. Nervousness is a prominent feature of hyperthyroidism, not only because the disease commonly develops in a setting of emotional disturbance,[23] but also because the synergistic action of the excess thyroid hormone accentuates the physiological effects of catecholamines centrally as well as peripherally.[73,74] Hence, hyperthyroid patients may have both a lower threshold for anxiety and an enhanced physiologic responsivity.

The clinical differentiation between hyperthyroidism and nervousness of other origin rests on demonstrating the more specific metabolic and mesodermal effects of thyroid hormones. The hypermetabolism and the consequent need to dissipate heat result in generalized sweating and peripheral vasodilation, even in the presence of intense anxiety. Hence the cold, wet hands and feet of the anxious patient are virtually never encountered in hyperthyroidism, especially under the bed covers. The hyperthyroid patient typically casts aside his covers, even on a cool day; the anxious patient, although restless, is more likely to remain covered.

Table 29-1 summarizes the salient clinical differences between the two conditions.

Pheochromocytomas produce symptoms that resemble the effects of an intravenous infusion of the catecholamines, and hence may duplicate some of the physiological manifestations of the acute anxiety attack. Adrenal medullary tumors generally secrete both epinephrine and norepinephrine, whereas extra-adrenal paraganglion tumors secrete predominantly norepinephrine. However, in contrast to the anxiety attack, physiological symptoms predominate in pheochromocytoma attacks, whereas feelings of anxiety, if they develop at all, come later. This is consistent with the experimental observation that the administration of the catechols produces the physiological, but not necessarily the psychological phenomena of anxiety.[91] With pheochromocytoma, physiological symptoms are likely to be quite dramatic. They include profuse sweating, severe palpitation, pronounced throbbing in the neck, pounding headache, dyspnea, choking, anterior chest pain, nausea, vomiting, abdominal cramps, and dysuria. Attacks come on abruptly, usually last minutes up to an hour, but may occasionally last hours, leading to "epinephrine shock."[75] During the attack, the patient appears quite ill, drenched with sweat, tremulous, with cold blanched face and extremities, dilated pupils and severe tachycardia and hypertension. When pronounced feelings of apprehension accompany the attack, the physician may be misled into ascribing it to psychological causes, especially when the attack has been precipitated by an emotional upset, as occasionally occurs.[75]

Between attacks, the patient may feel quite well, which would be unusual for a patient experiencing recurring anxiety attacks.

Hyperkinetic Heart Syndrome (Hyperdynamic B-Adrenergic Circulatory State)[76,77,78] defines a clinical syndrome characterized by a chronically overactive circulatory state, thought to be due to increased responsiveness of B-adrenergic receptors, and characterized by disturbing palpitations, chest discomfort, rapid heart action, and in many cases variable hypertension. Symptoms are most pronounced at times of great anxiety or following exercise, are markedly intensified by infusion of a B-adrenergic stimulator (isoproterenol), and are relieved by a B-adrenergic blockading agent (propranolol). Such pharmacologic responses are not found among individuals with anxiety alone.[78] The syndrome likely includes patients who in the past were referred to as "neurocirculatory asthenia."

Ictal anxiety, a rare manifestation of **epilepsy,** usually originating from the temporal lobe, is characterized by pronounced feelings of anxiety, at times approaching terror, that come on and cease abruptly, usually in seconds, or a minute or two at the most.[79,80] This sudden on-and-off character differentiates ictal from ordinary anxiety attacks, which may begin abruptly, but last longer and taper off more slowly. The attack may include terrifying ideas or images, such as being attacked from behind, which recur in a stereotyped manner. Sometimes a grand mal seizure or a more complex psychomotor spell follows. During the attack the patient may suddenly cease activity and stare with a look of terror on his face. The pupils may be widely dilated and the lids retracted. As the attack ends, he may momentarily appear confused or surprised. Any type of temporal lobe lesion, including neoplasm, may be responsible.

Hypoglycemia, regardless of etiology, may occasionally be responsible for episodes of nervousness. Falling blood sugar characteristically induces a sympathetic response, with epinephrine and norepinephrine secretion and the accompanying physiologic effects, notably tremulousness, tachycardia, sweating, weakness, and feelings of apprehension.[81] Such symptoms are more pronounced with milder degrees of hypoglycemia, especially when the rate of fall is rapid, whereas confusion and coma characterize more severe hypoglycemia (below 30 mg. per cent). The distinguishing features are the relation of the attacks to the fasting state, the profuse, generalized sweating, the progression to confusion and coma, and the prompt relief of all symptoms upon administration of carbohydrate.

Drugs, especially those that produce arousal or act on the sympathetic nervous system, may be responsible for feelings of nervousness when used in excessive quantities. Important among them are caffeine, sympathicomimetic drugs, atropine, the amphetamines, the monoamine oxidase inhibitors, tricyclic antidepressants, thyroid hormone, adrenal steroids, and ACTH. The amphetamines are adrenergic agents and probably directly stimulate the ergotropic system. The monoamine oxidase inhibitors interfere with the destruction of norepinephrine,[53] whereas the tricyclic antidepressants may potentiate the effects of norepinephrine in the central nervous system.[82] ACTH and the steroids also have central effects.[83]

Patients discontinuing *barbiturates* and other sedative drugs after prolonged usage may become tense, sleepless, irritable, and anxious during the *withdrawal* period. Occasionally a convulsion occurs. Marked agitation accompanies withdrawal from *heroin* and related addictive drugs.

FATIGUE

Fatigue may be considered a symptom when it becomes the occasion for complaint, as when one becomes fatigued with less effort or at unusual times of the day; or when rest is no longer recuperative or diversion as distracting. Fatigue is probably the most prevalent symptom of illness, physical as well as mental, and is often its first indication. Like normal fatigue, symptomatic fatigue may be general, muscular, mental, or any combination of these. When the muscular component is prominent the patient speaks more of weakness; when the mental component dominates, he reports more loss of interest and energy. Many patients take so for granted the fatigue that ordinarily accompanies an illness that they may not even mention it unless asked. Hence, when fatigue is stressed as a symptom, either it is very pronounced, a decided departure from normal, or lack of vigor or energy has important psychological meaning for that person. For example, the emotionally healthy

aging person expects his strength and vigor to decline with advancing age. Hence *a complaint* of fatigue by an older person usually indicates some physical or psychological disturbance and should not be dismissed as simply a reflection of aging.

Denial of fatigue may be as important as complaint of fatigue. Some patients respond to gradually developing fatigue by reducing their activity, thereby eliminating the symptom. The physician may then discover the fatigue only in the course of inquiring into the patient's activities and work habits. Thus he may learn that the patient has reduced his golf game from 18 to 9 holes, applied for a sitting-down job, or started taking an afternoon nap. As a general rule, the patient who tries to minimize his fatigue in this manner is more likely suffering from an organic than a psychological disorder; he is avoiding facing the alarming implications of the symptom.

There are no reliable figures as to the prevalence of physical as compared to psychological causes of fatigue. Certainly in many instances both are operating. Clinical experience suggests that the majority of patients who present with chronic fatigue and no other localizing manifestations are suffering primarily from psychological disturbances.[84] But psychological influences also commonly contribute to the fatigue of patients with chronic physical disease. Accordingly, both psychological and physical factors must always be evaluated.

Psychological Disorders

Symptomatic fatigue of psychic origin is most related to overstress, deprivation, and giving up. Thus, fatigue is common in persons who are exposed to excessive noise, heat, vibration, and other physical factors as well as in persons involved in recurring, chronic, and unresolved conflict. It is all pervasive with chronic pain and typically punctuates the sustained vigilance, anxiety, or controlled anger which give rise to nervousness. Fatigue is a prominent symptom among patients suffering the emotional deprivation of a loss, and even more so among those who psychically give up.[4,85] In terms of clinical syndromes, fatigue may characterize any neurotic or psychotic illness and is a dominant symptom in all forms of depression, as well as during grief.[86]

All of these situations are marked by a relative lack of emotional gratification. Conflict involves increased psychic work coupled with the frustration of little reward. Here the fatigue reflects the wish to be relieved of the necessity to continue the struggle, as well as a feeling of imminent exhaustion. It may disappear dramatically the moment the conflict is resolved. Deprivation, whether real or fantasied, constitutes a situation in which gratification appears to be no longer adequate or available. Under such conditions, the person may not only feel depleted, he may also give up trying to achieve gratification. Both carry the implication of a risk of exhaustion, in the biological sense, and evoke a warning to conserve energy. The feeling of fatigue serves this function.

Anxiety, anger, chronic conflict. The association of fatigue with anxiety, anger, and chronic tension has already been discussed (see Nervousness). Some patients who are struggling to control aggression do not manifest nervousness so much as a general inhibition, which may be felt as fatigue.[87] Paradoxically, such fatigue may be relieved by calisthenics or sports, which allow for muscular discharge or socially acceptable competition. These patients often are not aware of their aggressive inclinations, viewing themselves as exceptionally peaceful and kindhearted. They may develop fatigue when aggressive fantasies are stimulated, as when watching scenes of violence on television or being in a situation of actual conflict. Some are constantly fatigued. Headache or other pains, based on conversion or chronic muscle tension, commonly accompany the fatigue (see Chap. 30 on Conversion Symptoms).

Sometimes patients plunge into frenetic activity to avoid facing emotional problems or to overcome a loss. The excessive expenditure of energy, inadequate sleep and nutrition, and the enervating effect of the underlying conflicts combine to produce fatigue, sometimes culminating in exhaustion or collapse.

Depressive reactions characteristically are dominated by various expressions of fatigue, including weakness, tiredness, drowsiness, lack of energy, loss of interest, apathy, discouragement, a sense of weight or heaviness, and a general feeling that it is no longer worthwhile to exert oneself. The adjective, depressive, as used here, refers to a wide range of reaction patterns, including the mood swings of everyday life, normal and pathological grief and loss reactions, and the major affective disorders (neurotic depressive reaction, psychotic depressive reaction,

involutional melancholia, and manic-depressive illness).

In a broad sense, the depressive reactions all occur in response to a real, threatened, or fantasied loss of sources of emotional gratification, be it a loved person, home, job, status, strength, physical attractiveness, or even ideals or goals. Such losses may include illness, death, marriage, graduation, military service or any other real or threatened separation from a loved person; or they may involve any life change, including chronic illness or disability, which requires one to give up or modify relationships or way of living. Especially important are the crises of middle and later life. Men may become concerned about failure to achieve goals in work, family, or social relations; women about fading attractiveness, loss of childbearing capacity, and decline in the importance of their maternal functions. The fading of life goals reduces motivation and incurs a feeling of futility, often experienced primarily as fatigue. Often the frustrated hopes of the parent are projected onto the child, whose failure to fulfill his parent's expectations shatters the parent's illusion and precipitates a depressive reaction. A sense of loss may also stem from intrapsychic and interpersonal conflict, in the course of which one feels alienated from one's sources of emotional gratification; this defines a fantasied loss. Whatever the determinants, some type of depressive reaction ensues when the person feels he has no adequate means to overcome his own feelings of loss and no means to regain the missing gratification. Under such circumstances, feelings of sadness, loneliness, guilt, shame, helplessness, or hopelessness dominate, at times also intermingled with anxiety or anger. There may also be concomitant psychophysiological disturbances, which reflect activation of both the conservation-withdrawal (trophotropic) and flight-fight (ergotropic) systems as the person alternately feels overwhelmed by the loss and struggles to overcome it. Fatigue reflects activity of the conservation-withdrawal pattern.

Grief is the normal response to a *permanent loss*.[86,88] It involves an initial period, lasting weeks to months, during which the predominant feeling is a painful awareness of the loss, marked by sadness, loneliness, at times mixed with varying degrees of bitterness, resentment, or guilt. Fatigue may be overwhelming during this first phase. The grieving person feels inclined to disengage from the activities or pleasures of life, which he can no longer enjoy. After an active process of mourning, in the course of which the expectation of real gratification from the lost object is little by little given up and replaced by gratifying memories, the mourner re-establishes his links with life. The major work of mourning often occupies one year or more and is completed during the second year as the mourner relives the first anniversaries of meaningful occasions previously shared with the deceased, as birthdays or holidays. Many grieving patients do not associate their weakness or fatigue with their grief, and hence seek medical attention.

Some patients, especially those with ambivalent feelings toward the deceased, do not cry or feel the usual sense of loss at the time of a death. Instead they develop fatigue, often with anorexia, aches and pains, and insomnia, sometimes at the time of the loss, sometimes after an interval of several months. They are usually aware of and disturbed about their *failure to grieve* and inability to cry. Occasionally a psychotic depression follows after an interval of a few months.

There are also patients who grieve for years (**unresolved grief**), especially when they had been extremely dependent on the deceased person or have no prospects of a replacement. They typically develop symptoms, especially fatigue, on anniversaries or other occasions when the person would have played an important role were he still alive. Among many, the sense of deprivation is so pervasive that they feel chronically fatigued. Characteristically, the patient is unable to speak of his loss without crying or feeling sad. Crying spells are common, especially when alone.

It is important to appreciate that such depressive reactions, including grief, also constitute settings in which physical illness may develop.[4,85] Hence, the physician must be careful not to overlook an underlying organic disease.

Depressive neurosis defines the illness of a group of patients, usually with long-standing neurotic difficulties and conflict, who readily respond with feelings of discouragement and helplessness even to minor rebuffs or demands. Basically they are extremely dependent and clinging people who have not achieved the maturity of adulthood. They feel themselves to be weak, inadequate, and incompetent, and indeed often behave as such. They lack initiative and enthusiasm

and are extremely sensitive to losses and to changes in their supporting environment. Fatigue is a prominent symptom.

Psychotic depressive reactions, involutional melancholia, and *manic-depressive illness (depressed)* all designate major depressive illnesses, marked by a severely depressed mood; mental and motor retardation, often mixed with severe agitation; and anorexia, weight loss, constipation, and insomnia with early morning awakening. These patients have a profoundly pessimistic outlook and are burdened with intense and unrealistic feelings of guilt and shame, which may take the form of hallucinations or delusions, including ideas of internal organs rotting or drying up. **Manic-depressive illness** is characterized by recurring episodes of depression or alternating cycles of mania and depression, often without obvious precipitating factors. **Psychotic depressive reactions** have no regular cycle and usually are precipitated by some psychological stress. When occurring for the first time in the menopausal period, the illness may be designated **involutional melancholia.** All of these disorders carry a high risk of *suicide.* It is clinically important to note that these disorders may be ushered in by a period of *fatigue* which may last for weeks or longer before the more profound depressive mood becomes obvious. Associated manifestations of worry, loss of interest, self-deprecation, constipation, decline in appetite, and poor sleep may accurately forewarn of an impending major depression, especially if such episodes have occurred in the past.

Conversion. Fatigue may be a conversion symptom, commonly representing an identification with another person with a chronic illness marked by weakness and fatigue. It is closely related to the conversion symptoms of weakness and paralysis and may have the same symbolic meanings (Chap. 30).

Organic brain syndromes, especially those of gradual development, as the arteriosclerotic and senile dementias, are typically characterized by fatigue, sometimes appearing well before the distinctive cognitive defects are appreciated. Such fatigue partly reflects the increased effort required to carry on mental operations previously performed with ease. The victim of a chronic organic brain syndrome (dementia) has a lessened capability to comprehend and retrieve new information and relate it to old information, as revealed in the greater effort required for such mental tasks as simple arithmetic, and his poor memory, narrowing range of attention, and lessened ability to think abstractly. The patient who is becoming demented commonly exhibits decreased interest and activity and a tendency to doze or sleep more. Dementia is an important cause of fatigue in the aging person.

Physical Disorders

Some degree of fatigue is an accompaniment of most active diseases. It is likely to be a prominent symptom in conditions that affect primarily the metabolic support of the body as a whole or interfere with neuromuscular function in particular, as well as in slowly developing diseases, which have not yet given rise to specific symptoms. Most patients, however, do not complain only or predominantly of fatigue, but readily reveal the tell-tale evidences of the underlying disease. Hence, this discussion only calls attention to some of the disorders that should be considered among patients whose main complaint is fatigue.

The **endocrine disorders** in their early stages commonly present primarily as problems in fatigue. The patient with developing **adrenal insufficiency** is often aware of a decline in strength and vigor for weeks or months before any of the other manifestations appear. Notable is a tendency for the fatigue and weakness to increase strikingly in the presence of a minor infection or other stress. The sense of fatigue is usually quite pervasive and is little alleviated by rest and sleep. The **hypothyroid** patient usually has such a gradual decline in his vigor that he is often unaware of the change until the disease is well-developed. Drowsiness and a tendency to sleep more are characteristic responses. The combination of fatigue, somnolence, and cold intolerance of gradual and progressive development over months to years suggests the diagnosis. The fatigue of **hypopituitarism** is related to target gland insufficiency, secondary to inadequate production of gonadotropic, adrenocorticotropic, and thyrotropic hormones. Hypogonadism is the most common manifestation of hypopituitarism and usually precedes the other endocrine deficiencies, by months and sometimes by years. Injury, infection or anesthesia may bring out the latent adrenal insufficiency, often in the form of an abrupt and marked increase in fatigue. The various forms of **hypogonadism,** other than those secondary to pituitary failure, are not ordinarily associated with fatigue, contrary to popular belief; the fatigue observed in older persons with declining gonadal function is complex in origin and no doubt has an important psychic component. The weakness and fatigue of **hyperparathyroidism** is mainly due to hypercalcemia, as is that sometimes seen in the hypercalcemia of sarcoidosis, hypervitaminosis D, milk alkali syndrome, and various neoplasms with and without bone metastases. These symptoms are probably related to the role of the calcium ion in muscle function, and hence commonly are experienced as muscle weakness. When the serum ionized calcium level is high enough to induce weakness and fatigue, there is usually also constipation, vomiting, and sometimes pruritus.

Diabetes mellitus may be ushered in by a period of fatigue, the other symptoms being less prominent or less stressed by the patient. Sometimes such a complaint may reflect a depressive reaction, a common setting of onset for diabetes.[89]

The relationship of **nutritional deficiency** to fatigue is quite evident in cases of obvious dietary insufficiency or starvation.[90,92] Indeed, conservation-withdrawal activity, expressed as fatigue and a tendency to reduce activity, is a predictable biological response to the curtailed energy production. With starvation, depletion of energy resources ultimately becomes the limiting factor determining strength and fatigability. The nutritional deficiency may be total, or it may involve specific food elements, notably protein, thiamine, riboflavin, niacin, and ascorbic acid, leading to specific deficiency syndromes. Ordinarily the evidences of nutritional deficiency, such as weight loss, edema, or the signs of specific vitamin lack, are already evident when fatigue becomes the major symptom. Actually, the role of lesser degrees of nutritional lack in producing fatigue is difficult to evaluate, because many situations in which nutritional deficiency develops also involve some major psychological stress as well. The capacity to tolerate a severe degree of chronic starvation and weight loss without fatigue is vividly demonstrated in the syndrome of **anorexia nervosa,** in which the body weight may fall to 50 per cent of normal, and still the patient may remain astonishingly active.

Chronic anemia may be responsible for fatigue, but is unlikely to be the only factor when the hematocrit is above 30. The marked fatigue of **pernicious anemia** is clearly not dependent on the oxygen-carrying capacity of the blood, because it responds dramatically within a few days to the administration of vitamin B-12, well before any rise in hematocrit. Prominent fatigue with moderate anemia should suggest the possibilities of chronic infection, neoplasia, nutritional deficiency, systemic lupus erythematosus, some other occult organic disorder, or a psychological disorder.

Derangements in electrolyte or water balance, including hyponatremia, as may occur consequent to excessive sweating or too vigorous diuresis; **dehydration; hypokalemia** and **hyperkalemia; alkalosis** and **acidosis** all may be associated with marked fatigue. Electrolyte disturbances have general metabolic consequences. Because of the role of potassium in muscle contraction, the fatigue occurring with hypokalemia and hyperkalemia, either of which may be associated with intracellular potassium deficit, is likely to involve muscle weakness. **Aldosteronism** and **renal tubular acidosis** are two conditions in which weakness and fatigue may be the only manifestations of hypokalemia.

Occasionally fatigue is the first symptom of **renal insufficiency** and **uremia.** Usually considerable anemia is also involved.

A remarkable degree of fatigue characteristically accompanies **hepatitis,** and often persists for weeks after the laboratory evidence of active liver disease has cleared. It typically is exacerbated by physical exertion, following which there may be a mild reactivation of the hepatopathy, as evidenced by elevation of serum transaminase activity. The occasional case of **anicteric hepatitis** is especially likely to present as fatigue of obscure origin. Fatigue is a common manifestation of **hepatic insufficiency.**

Chronic heart disease, involving low cardiac output and inadequate tissue oxygenation, is marked by moderate to severe fatigue and weakness. Patients whose physical activity has already been restricted because of some disability, such as arthritis, peripheral vascular disease, or severe angina, may experience fatigue rather than dyspnea with advancing heart failure. Drowsiness and fatigue are common among patients with **chronic pulmonary insufficiency,** especially when there is CO_2 retention. Fatigue may precede by weeks or months the manifestations of right heart failure in cases of **primary pulmonary hypertension.**

Various **drugs** and **toxic chemicals** may be responsible for fatigue. The intake of tranquilizers and sedatives over an extended period of time is an extremely common cause of fatigue and one which is readily overlooked. The drug is usually prescribed for some form of nervousness and the patient expects to achieve a feeling of relaxation and well-being; instead he develops torpor, drowsiness, and fatigue, the basis for which is not appreciated by the physician. Because fatigue may be a symptom of toxic or other reactions to many different drugs, the medications taken by the patient with obscure fatigue should always be carefully reviewed. Similarly must be considered exposure to toxic chemicals, such as carbon monoxide, substances producing methemoglobinemia or sulphemoglobinemia, heavy toxic metals, and various organic compounds. The fatigue of the heavy consumer of alcohol is complex, involving toxic, nutritional, hepatic, and psychological factors.

Neuromuscular defects. *The myopathies* are marked by weakness, which may be generalized or involve specific muscle groups. Patients with such disorders have no difficulty in identifying the muscular system as the site of the symptom, and readily differentiate muscle weakness from the more general symptoms of fatigue. The weakness is directly related to use of the muscle. In *myasthenia gravis* there is very rapid exhaustion of muscle strength upon use but recovery with rest. Ptosis and diplopia are common early symptoms. Various forms of *primary myopathy* are characterized by weakness and wasting, predominantly of the proximal and limb girdle muscles. The *myopathy* of *occult malignant disease* and *hyperthyroidism* are also characterized by proximal weakness, as well as pronounced fatigue. *Neurological disease* involving motor function is typically associated with fatigue.

An important cause of fatigue which is often overlooked is *overload based on some physical disability.* The most common example is massive *obesity,* where the fatigue is largely a product of the work involved in moving the heavy body about. Even a modest weight reduction may have a salutory effect. In obese patients with the so-called *Pickwickian syndrome* (reduced vital ventilatory capacity), hypoventilation with CO_2 retention and somnolence are additional factors. Patients accustomed to being active who become crippled as the result of such conditions as arthritis, paraplegia, hemiparesis, or amputations, may suffer intensely from fatigue as they struggle to overcome their disabilities.

Fatigue may be an early symptom of some *occult disease* process, as *neoplasia, lymphoma, leukemia, tuberculosis, subacute bacterial endocarditis, chronic pyelonephritis,* or *chronic brucellosis;* the last is an unlikely diagnosis in the absence of a history of an acute attack.

Constitutional

In addition to these specific conditions, attention must also be drawn to the person with no particular physical or psychological disorder whose entire life has been marked by low energy and easy fatigability. Some with such life-long fatigue do occasionally prove to be the victims of some obscure myopathy, endocrine problem, or nutritional deficit in infancy, but for most only the vague and unsatisfactory interpretation of a "constitutional" factor can be invoked. Such persons appear to be peculiarly ill-equipped to cope with environmental stresses and are likely to have long and imperfect convalescences even from relatively minor illnesses.

FATIGUE AS A COMPLICATION IN ORGANIC DISEASE

When fatigue persists or develops despite apparently effective treatment of or convalescence from a 'physical disorder, other explanations must be considered. The patient may be experiencing some concern about the implications of his illness, the reactions of other patients, his relationship with his physician, problems at home, or the prospects of returning—or not returning—to full activity. To any of these he may respond in a **depressive** fashion. Less common are **untoward reactions to treatment,** such as hypokalemia with overvigorous diuresis, or the beginning toxic effect of some medication. Overuse of sedatives may produce iatrogenic fatigue. How fatiguing some modern diagnostic procedures are for some patients may be underestimated, as may be the difficulty some patients have in getting adequate rest on a busy hospital floor. Unexpected complications or recurrent disease must also be kept in mind.

DIFFERENTIATION BETWEEN FATIGUE OF PSYCHIC AND PHYSICAL ORIGINS

Psychological factors always play a role in fatigue, regardless of its origin. Hence, the practical problem is to distinguish those instances in which physical factors are significantly involved from those in which they are not. The problem is made especially complex by virtue of the fact that certain types of depressive reactions, especially those characterized by feelings of giving up, appear to predispose to the development of a wide variety of organic illnesses.[4,85] Hence, patients whose fatigue is *primarily* a reflection of a depressive reaction may have an *organic disease as well,* which may also be contributing to the fatigue in its own right. The patient who develops leukemia in the setting of loss is a typical example.[95] Accordingly, the discovery that fatigue has developed in a setting of psychological upset by no means proves that the syndrome itself is psychological in nature. Whether there is a physical illness will have to be investigated by careful interview and examination designed to uncover possible clues indicating an organic process. Since most patients whose fatigue is based on physical determinants sooner or later develop other symptoms or signs, it often suffices to keep them under observation for a period before embarking on an extensive—and expensive—laboratory work-up. Fatigue not of physical origin usually shows considerable variability, the patient being "exhausted" under one circumstance and full of energy on another, perhaps only a few minutes later. Psychotically depressed patients feel most fatigued when they get up in the morning and gradually improve as the day wears on; the reverse sequence is the rule when physical factors are responsible. Patients with physical fatigue are more likely to show at least some restoration after a good rest or sleep, whereas depressed or anxious patients commonly feel as fatigued or even more fatigued when they get up. When organic factors are responsible for muscle fatigue there is generally a clear relationship between muscle use and its rapid fatigue. The extent of muscle weakness demonstrable at the bedside after a brief period of use is usually greater than it was before use. When weakness is of psychological origin, it is less readily demonstrable and less likely to show a decrement upon brief testing.

As mentioned earlier, patients who appear or are described as weak and tired, and yet deny fatigue or weakness, are almost certain to be suffering from an organic, not a psychological disturbance.

REFERENCES

1. Cannon, W. B.: Bodily Changes in Pain, Hunger, Fear, and Rage, New York, Appleton, 1929.
2. Engel, G. L.: Psychological Development in Health and Disease, Ch. XXXIII, Philadelphia, Saunders, 1962.
3. ———: Clinical observation. The neglected basic method of medicine, J.A.M.A. 192:849, 1965.
4. Schmale, A. H.: Relationship of separation and depression to disease. I. A report on a hospitalized medical population, Psychosom. Med. 20:259, 1958.
5. MacLean, P. D.: The limbic system with respect to self-preservation and the preservation of the species, J. Nerv. Ment. Dis. 127:1, 1958.
6. Papez, J. W.: A proposed mechanism of emotion, A.M.A. Arch. Neurol. Psychiat. 38:725, 1937.
7. Nauta, W. J. H.: Central nervous system organization and the endocrine motor system, in Nalbandov, A. V. (ed.): Advances in Neuroendocrinology, p. 5, Urbana, Univ. of Ill. Press, 1963.
8. Hernandez-Peon, R.: Reticular mechanisms of sensory control, in Rosenblith, W. A. (ed.): Sensory Communication, p. 497, New York, Wiley, 1961.
9. ———: Psychiatric implications of neurophysiological research, Bull. Menninger Clin. 28:165, 1964.
10. John, E. R., and Killam, K. F.: Electrophysiological correlates of avoidance conditioning in the cat, J. Pharmacol. Exp. Ther. 125:252, 1959.
11. Richter, C.: On the phenomenon of sudden death in animals and man, Psychosom. Med. 19:191, 1957.
12. Maier, S. F., Seligman, M. E. P., and Solomon, R. L.: Pavlovian fear conditioning and learned helplessness, in B. A. Campbell (ed.): Punishment, New York, Appleton-Century-Crofts, 1968.
13. Stroebel, C. F.: The importance of biological clocks in mental health, Mental Health Program Reports, 2:323, 1968; PHS Publ., 1743.
14. Hess, W. R.: The Functional Organization of the Diencephalon, New York, Grune and Stratton, 1957.
15. Gellhorn, E.: Physiological analysis of ergotropic and tropotrophic imbalances, in Principles of Autonomic-Somatic Integrations, Ch. II, pp. 40–70, Minneapolis, Univ. of Minn. Press, 1967.
16. Mason, J. W.: Organization of psychoendocrine mechanisms, Psychosom. Med. 30:565, 1968.
17. ———: A review of psychoendocrine research on the pituitary-adrenal cortical system, Psychosom. Med. 30:576, 1968.
18. ———: Plasma and urinary 17-OHCS responses to 72-hr. avoidance sessions in the monkey, Psychosom. Med. 30:608, 1968.
19. ———: A review of psychoendocrine research on the sympathetic adrenal medullary system, Psychosom. Med. 30:631, 1968.
20. Mason, J. W., Tolson, W. W., Brady, J. V., Tolliver, G. A., and Gilmore, L. I.: Urinary epinephrine and norepinephrine responses to 72-hr. avoidance sessions in the monkey, Psychosom. Med. 30:654, 1968.
21. Mirsky, I. A.: Secretion of antidiuretic hormone in response to noxious stimuli, Arch. Neurol. Psychiat. 73:135, 1955.
22. Mason, J. W., Jones, J. A., Ricketts, P. T., Brady, J. V., and Tolliver, G. A.: Urinary aldosterone and urine volume responses to 72-hr. avoidance sessions in monkeys, Psychosom. Med. 30:733, 1968.
23. Mason, J. W.: A review of psychoendocrine research in the pituitary-thyroid system, Psychosom. Med. 30:666, 1968.
24. Mason, J. W., Mougey, E. H., Brady, J. V., and Tolliver, G. A.: Thyroid (plasma butanol-extractable iodine) response to 72-hr. avoidance sessions in the monkey, Psychosom. Med. 30:682, 1968.
25. Mason, J. W., Wool, M., Wherry, F. E., Pennington, L. L., Brady, J. V., and Beer, B.: Plasma growth hormone response to avoidance sessions in the monkey, Psychosom. Med. 30:774, 1968.
26. Mason, J. W., Wherry, F. E., Brady, J. V., Beer, B., Pennington, L. L., and Goodman, A. C.: Plasma insulin response to avoidance sessions in the monkey, Psychosom. Med. 30:746, 1968.
27. Mason, J. W., Taylor, E. D., Brady, J. V., and Tolliver, G. A.: Urinary estrone, estradiol, and estriol responses to 72-hr. avoidance sessions in monkeys, Psychosom. Med. 30:696, 1968.
28. Mason, J. W., Kenion, C. C., Collins, D. R., Mougey, E. H., Jones, J. A., Driver, G. C., Brady, J. V., and Beer, B.: Urinary testosterone response to 72-hr. avoidance sessions in the monkey, Psychosom. Med. 30:721, 1968.
29. Mason, J. W., Tolson, W. W., Robinson, J. A., Brady, J. V., Tolliver, G. A., and Johnson, T. A.: Urinary androsterone, etiocholanolone, and dehydroepiandrosterone responses in 72-hr. avoidance sessions in monkeys, Psychosom. Med. 30:710, 1968.
30. Mason, J. W.: Plasma 17-hydroxycorticosteroid levels during electrical stimulation of the amygdaloid complex in conscious monkeys, Amer. J. Physiol. 196:44, 1959.
31. Mason, J. W., Nauta, W. J. H., Brady, J. V., Robinson, J. A., and Sachar, E. J.: The role of limbic system structures in the regulation of ACTH secretion, Acta Neuroveg. 23:4, 1961.
32. Price, D. B., Thaler, M., and Mason, J. W.: Preoperative emotional states and adrenal cortical activity, A.M.A. Arch. Neurol. Psychiat. 77:646, 1957.

33. Wolff, C. T., Friedman, S. B., Hofer, M. A., and Mason, J. W.: Relationship between psychological defences and mean urinary 17-OHCS excretion rates. I. A predictive study of parents of fatally ill children, Psychosom. Med. 26:576, 1964.

34. Bourne, P. G., Rose, R. M., and Mason, J. W.: Urinary 17-OHCS levels. Data on seven helicopter ambulance medics in combat, Arch. Gen. Psychiat. 17:104, 1967.

35. ———: 17-OHCS levels in combat, Arch. Gen. Psychiat. 19:135, 1968.

36. Sachar, E. J., Harmatz, J., Bergen, H., and Cohler, J.: Corticosteroid responses to milieu therapy of chronic schizophrenics, Arch. Gen. Psychiat. 15:310, 1966.

37. Sachar, E. J., MacKenzie, J. M., Binstock, V. A., and Mack, J. E.: Corticosteroid responses to psychotherapy of depressions. I. Evaluations during confrontation of loss, Arch. Gen. Psychiat. 16:461, 1967.

38. Mason, J. W.: Organization of multiple endocrine responses to avoidance in the monkey, Psychosom. Med. 30:774, 1968.

39. Ellis, S.: The metabolic effects of epinephrine and related amines, Pharmacol. Rev. 8:485, 1956.

40. Hagen, J. H., and Hagen, P. B.: Actions of adrenalin and noradrenalin on metabolic systems, in Litwack, G., and Kritchevsky, D. (eds.): Actions of Hormones on Molecular Processes, p. 268, New York, Wiley, 1964.

41. Fajans, S. S.: Some metabolic actions of corticosteroids, Metabolism 10:951, 1961.

42. Ingle, D. J.: Metabolic effects of adrenal steroids, in Gordon, E. S. (ed.): A Symposium on Steroid Hormones, p. 150, Madison, Univ. of Wisconsin Press, 1950.

43. Grossfield, H.: Actions of adrenal cortical steroids on cultured cells, Endocrinology 65:777, 1959.

44. Greene, W. A., Conron, G., Schalch, D. S., and Schreiner, G.: Psychological correlates of growth hormone and adrenal secretory responses in patients undergoing cardiac catheterization, Psychosom. Med. 31, 1969.

45. Randle, P. J.: Endocrine control of metabolism, Ann. Rev. Physiol. 25:291, 1960.

46. Hoch, F. L.: Biochemical actions of thyroid hormones, Physiol. Rev. 42:605, 1962.

47. Tepperman, J.: Metabolic and Endocrine Physiology, Chicago, Year Book Pub., 1968.

48. Krahl, M. E.: The Action of Insulin on Cells, New York, Academic Press, 1961.

49. McKerns, K. W., and Bell, P. H.: The mechanism of action of estrogenic hormones on metabolism, Recent Progr. Hormone Res. 16:97, 1960.

50. Talaat, M., Habib, Y. A., and Habib, M.: The effect of testosterone on the carbohydrate metabolism in normal subjects, Arch. Int. Pharmacodyn. 111:215, 1957.

51. Ramey, E. R., and Goldstein, M. S.: The adrenal cortex and the sympathetic nervous system, Physiol. Rev. 37:155, 1957.

52. Bonvallet, M., Dell, P., and Hubel, G.: Sympathetic tonus and electrical activity of the cortex, EEG Clin. Neurophysiol. 6:119, 1954.

53. Kety, S. S.: Psychoendocrine systems and emotion: biological aspects, in Glass, D. C. (ed.): Neurophysiology and Emotion, p. 103, New York, Rockefeller Univ. Press, 1967.

54. Mirsky, I. A., Miller, R., and Stein, M.: The influence of ACTH on the avoidance conditioned reflex in monkeys, Psychosom. Med. 15:574, 1953.

55. Lissak, K., and Endroczi, E.: Neuroendocrine interrelationships and behavioral processes, in Bajusz, E., and Jasmin, G. (eds.): Major Problems in Neuroendocrinology, p. 1, Baltimore, Williams & Wilkins, 1964.

56. Kelly, D. H. W., and Walter, C. J. S.: The relationship between clinical diagnoses and anxiety, assessed by forearm blood flow and other measurements, Brit. J. Psychiat. 114:611, 1968.

57. Gellhorn, E.: Principles of Autonomic-Somatic Integrations, Minneapolis, Univ. of Minn. Press, 1967.

58. Uvnas, B.: Sympathetic vasodilator system and blood flow, Physiol. Rev. (supp. 4) 40:69, 1960.

59. Ferris, E. B., Engel, G. L., Stevens, C. D., and Webb, J. B.: Voluntary breathholding. III. The relation of the maximum time of breathholding to the O_2 and CO_2 tensions of arterial blood, J. Clin. Invest. 25:734, 1946.

60. Richter, C. P.: Biological Clocks in Medicine and Psychiatry, Springfield, Ill., Thomas, 1965.

61. Kleitman, N.: Sleep and Wakefulness, Chicago, Univ. of Chicago Press, 1963.

62. Bulow, K.: Respiration and wakefulness in man, Acta Physiol. Scand. supp. 209, vol. 59, 1963.

63. Dudley, D. L., Martin, C. J., and Holmes, T. H.: Psychophysiologic studies of pulmonary ventilation, Psychosom. Med. 26:645, 1964.

64. Engel, G. L., and Reichsmann, F.: Spontaneous and experimentally induced depressions in an infant with a gastric fistula, J. Amer. Psychoanal. Ass. 4:428, 1956.

65. Wolf, S., and Wolff, H. G.: Human Gastric Function, New York, Oxford Univ. Press, 1943.

66. Engel, G. L., Reichsmann, F., and Segal, H. L.: A study of an infant with gastric fistula. I. Behavior and the rate of total acid secretion, Psychosom. Med. 18:374, 1956.

67. Grace, W. J., Wolf, S., and Wolff, H. G.: The Human Colon, New York, Hoeber, 1951.

68. Mason, J. W.: Psychoendocrine approaches in stress research, in Symposium on Medical Aspects of Stress in the Military Climate, p. 375, Washington, D. C., Walter Reed Army Institute of Research, 1964.

69. Spitz, R. A.: Hospitalism, Psychoanal. Stud. Child, 1:53, 1945.

70. Patton, R. G., and Gardner, L. I.: Growth Failure in Maternal Deprivation, Springfield, Ill., Charles Thomas, 1963.

71. Powell, G. F., Brasel, J. A., and Blizzard, R. M.: Emotional deprivation and growth retardation simulating idiopathic hypopituitarism, New Eng. J. Med. 276:1271, 1967.

72. Engel, G. L., and Romano, J.: Delirium, a syndrome of cerebral insufficiency, J. Chronic Dis. 9:260, 1959.

73. Harrison, T. S.: Adrenal medullary and thyroid relationships, Physiol. Rev. 44:161, 1964.

74. Ramey, E. R.: Relation of the thyroid to the autonomic nervous system, in Levine, R. (ed.): Endocrines and the Central Nervous System, Res. Publ. Ass. Res. Nerv. Ment. Dis. 43:309, 1966.

75. Engel, F. L., Mencher, W. H., and Engel, G. L.: "Epinephrine shock" as a manifestation of pheochromocytoma of the adrenal medulla, Amer. J. Med. Sci. 204:649, 1942.

76. Gorlin, R.: The hyperkinetic heart syndrome, J.A.M.A. 182:823, 1962.

77. Brill, I. C.: Sinus tachycardia, Arch. Intern. Med. 115:674, 1965.

78. Frohlich, E. D., Tarazi, R. C., and Dustan, H. P.: Hyperdynamic beta-adrenergic circulatory state, Arch. Intern. Med. 123:1, 1969.

79. Penfield, W., and Jasper, H.: Epilepsy and the Functional Anatomy of the Brain, Boston, Little, Brown, 1954.

80. Daly, D.: Ictal affect, Amer. J. Psychiat. 115:97, 1958.

81. Sussman, K. E., Crout, J. R., and Marble, A.: Failure of warning in insulin-induced hypoglycemia, Diabetes 12:38, 1963.

82. Schildkraut, J. J., and Kety, S. S.: Biogenic amines and emotion, Science 156:21, 1967.

83. Weiss, J. M., McEwen, B. S., Teresa, M., Silva, A., and Kalkut, M. F.: Pituitary influences on fear responding, Science 163:197, 1969.

84. Allan, F. N.: Differential diagnoses of weakness and fatigue, New Eng. J. Med. 231:414, 1944.

85. Engel, G. L.: A life setting conducive to illness. The giving up—given up complex, Ann. Intern. Med. 69:293, 1968.

86. Lindemann, E.: Symptomatology and management of acute grief, Amer. J. Psychiat. 101:141, 1944.

87. Shands, H. C., and Finesinger, J. E.: A note on the significance of fatigue, Psychosom. Med. 14:309, 1952.

88. Engel, G. L.: Psychological Development in Health and Disease, Ch. 26, Philadelphia, Saunders, 1962.

89. Hinkle, L. E., and Wolf, S.: A summary of experimental evidence relating life stress to diabetes, J. Mount Sinai Hosp. N. Y. 19:537, 1952.

90. Keys, A., and Brozek, J.: The Biology of Human Starvation, Minneapolis, Univ. of Minn. Press, 1950.

91. Schachter, S., and Singer, J.: Cognitive, social, and physiological determinants of emotional state, Psychol. Rev. 69:379, 1962.

92. Schiele, B., and Brozek, J.: Experimental neuroses resulting from semistarvation in man, Psychosom. Med. 10:31, 1948.

93. von Euler, U. S.: Some aspects of the role of noradrenaline and adrenaline in circulation, Amer. Heart J. 54:469, 1958.

94. Mason, D. T.: The autonomic nervous system and regulation of cardiovascular performance, Anesthesiology 29:670, 1968.

95. Greene, W. A., Young, L. E., and Swisher, S. N.: Psychological factors and reticuloendothelial disease, Psychosom. Med. 18:284, 1956.

30

Conversion Symptoms

GEORGE L. ENGEL

INTRODUCTION

Psychosomatic symptoms have received, quite properly, much attention in recent years. Both patient and physician may be well aware, for example, that under conditions of emotional upset patients may develop headaches or back pain; or nausea, vomiting, and epigastric distress; or palpitation, sweating, and muscle tension. Such symptoms may be brought about by a variety of mechanisms. Sometimes the symptoms reflect psychophysiological changes that accompany affects, as the nervousness, tremulousness, palpitation, and sweating of anxiety; or the fatigue, weakness, and anorexia of the depressive affects (Chapter 29—Nervousness and Fatigue). Sometimes they are the result of organic disorders precipitated or exacerbated by emotional disturbances, such as peptic ulcer, angina pectoris, or migraine. But very commonly such symptoms are the result of *conversion*, a psychic mechanism whereby an idea, fantasy, or wish *is expressed* in bodily rather than verbal terms and *is experienced* by the patient as a physical rather than a mental symptom. The

prevalence of conversion as a mechanism of symptom formation and the variety of bodily systems that may be implicated are so great that conversion has been called the great imitator of organic disease (Table 30-1). In 1873 Sir James Paget proposed the term "nervous mimicry."[1]

Known to the ancients, conversion symptoms have been ascribed to many different mechanisms, perhaps the most influential being "wandering of the uterus"; hence, the term *hysteria* and the erroneous assumption that these mechanisms are peculiar to females.[2,3] Appreciation of a psychological origin began in the early 19th century, whereas modern understanding was ushered in by Breuer and Freud's classic, *Studies on Hysteria* in 1895.[4] Freud was the first to propose the concept of conversion to explain the somatic symptoms of hysteria, but subsequent writers have shown that conversion symptoms are by no means restricted to patients diagnosed as having the medical condition now called hysteria.[5,6]

DEFINITIONS

In ordinary clinical usage, the term *symptoms* refers to what the patient experiences and reports as manifestations of illness. Thus, symptoms are subjective (psychological) in the sense that the patient can report only that of which he is aware. From the patient's point of view, symptoms either are considered as *bodily* (*physical*) in origin, meaning they are interpreted as arising from some disturbance in the body, such as nausea, pain, shortness of breath, or paralysis; or they are considered as *mental* (*psychological*) in origin, meaning they are perceived as reflecting some disturbance in psychological functioning, such as anxiety, obsessions, fears, or memory loss.

Conversion symptoms originate in the mind but are experienced as bodily (physical) in origin. They derive from stored mental representations (memories) of bodily activities or functioning which are utilized to express symbolically unconscious wishes or impulses as a means of coping with a psychological conflict. Hence, the conversion symptom is completely intrapsychic in nature. In contrast, *symptoms of organic origin* derive from awareness of *actual changes taking place in the body.* To illustrate, shortness of breath as a conversion symptom originates from the memory of some past respiratory experience, which is being used to express symbolically some fantasy, as, for example, that of being smothered or of smothering someone else. Here the fantasy of smothering reactivates a memory of feeling unable to breathe and leads to the sensation (symptom) of breathlessness and the response of hyperventilation. Shortness of breath as a symptom of congestive heart failure, in contrast, originates from an awareness of the actual increased effort of breathing required to achieve ventilation in the face of pulmonary congestion. Here the afferent input to the respiratory center is primary, whereas the sensation of being unable to breathe gives rise to the idea of "breathlessness" or "smothering."

Conversion refers to the intrapsychic processes whereby an unacceptable idea or fantasy is experienced and expressed symbolically as (converted to) a bodily sensation or feeling. *Conversion symptoms* include the fantasied bodily sensations as well as behavioral or physiological reactions that occur in response to the sensation, e.g., the sensation of nausea may lead to vomiting, a feeling of weakness may be displayed as paralysis. *Conversion complications* are biochemical or physiological processes inappropriately set in motion by conversion symptoms. For example, nausea and vomiting as conversion symptoms may lead to metabolic alkalosis; shortness of breath and hyperventilation to respiratory alkalosis. The resulting symptoms of alkalosis, namely, lightheadedness, paresthesias, or tetany, are organic in origin, not psychogenic; they have no psychologic meaning and in no way express symbolically the fantasy underlying the conversion vomiting or hyperventilation. A list of conversion complications is found in Table 30-2.

INCIDENCE AND PREVALENCE

No accurate figures on the incidence or prevalence of conversion symptoms are available. Ljungberg estimates the prevalence of "hysterical reactions" in the general population of Sweden as 5 per cent, whereas Farley gives a figures of 39 per cent in a consecutive series of 100 post-partum women. Pa-

tients with conversion symptoms consult all varieties of medical specialists, but rarely psychiatrists, since they consider their complaints to have a physical origin. Hence, psychiatric confirmation of diagnosis is infrequent, and prevalence figures are unreliable. Working as both internist and psychiatrist, it is the impression of this writer that as many as 20 to 25 per cent of patients admitted to a general medical service have manifested conversion symptoms at some time in their lives. Such symptoms are two or three times as common among women as among men, and may first appear at as early an age as seven or eight years. They may range from transient, minor symptoms to major and often disabling symptoms, which constitute the illness for which the patient seeks help. Although more frequent among hysterics, they may occur with any personality type, as well as in the course of any organic or psychiatric illness. The belief that conversion symptoms are more common or are even restricted to the uneducated, unsophisticated, or to members of culturally more primitive groups is not supported by clinical observation; rather, such persons are more likely to display dramatic or bizarre conversion syndromes, sometimes based on primitive or religious notions. However, more sophisticated patients nowadays manifest symptoms more consonant with prevailing notions of physical illness. On the other hand, certain social situations are conducive to epidemics of conversion symptoms, as when groups are swept by intense emotions. Fainting of teenagers in the crowd listening to the singing idol of the day, or hyperventilation attacks among students in a girls' school upon the rumor of the pregnancy of a class member, are typical of such epidemics.[9]

CONVERSION SYMPTOMATOLOGY

The great variety of conversion symptoms is illustrated in Table 30-1, conversion complications in Table 30-2. Most patients present with multiple symptoms in the form of syndromes resembling organic disease.

MECHANISMS (PATHOPSYCHOLOGY)

How Can Bodily Symptoms Originate from an Idea or Fantasy?

At first glance, it is difficult to grasp how such physical symptoms as pain, nausea, blindness, or paralysis may, in fact, be expressing ideas or fantasies rather than be the result of some bodily change. Yet it is not unusual for some body activity to be used to express ideas. Gesture and panto-mime are the most familiar. In the well-known game of charades, the performer may express the notion that something is invis-ible or should not be seen by closing his eyes or acting blind. Everyday language, particu-larly metaphors, contains many instances of ideas being expressed in body terms, such as "It took my breath away," "I'm fed up," "I can't bear it." The person who speaks metaphorically of "keeping anger in," of something being "rammed down my throat," or "falling by the wayside," clearly is using body imagery to express himself.[10] Such ex-pressions remind us that before the infant becomes capable of expressing his feelings and wishes in words, he uses his body. Fur-ther, his first knowledge of his surroundings is formed out of his own bodily reactions and sensations in response to the environ-ment.[11] The metaphor, "I can't swallow that," no doubt, has roots in the recollection in bodily terms of an earlier period when everything was examined by putting it in the mouth. The distinction between good and bad in terms of what is taken into the mouth and what is rejected is one of the infant's earliest cognitive generalizations. It con-tinues to be exhibited in adulthood by pinch-ing the lips tightly together to express rejec-tion, even though nothing literally is to be taken into the mouth.

The dream is the most common mental activity in which wishes, fantasies, and ideas are expressed predominantly in nonverbal terms as visual imagery, body sensations, and even physical symptoms. As Freud has shown, the content of the dream reflects the dreamer's continuing preoccupation in sleep with the problems of his waking life.[12] Cut off in sleep from the reality of the external environment and deprived of the possibility of action, the dreamer falls back on more archaic modes of thinking characteristic of the unconscious mental processes of the pre-verbal period of childhood. Aside from its patent illogic, the dream is marked by the tendency to express complex fantasies or ideas in symbolic forms derived from earlier body experiences and sensations. Especially relevant to the problem of con-version are dreams in which one is sick or disabled or is suffering such symptoms as blindness, weakness, paralysis, dyspnea, or pain. Analysis of such dreams reveals that sometimes the symptom is a direct symbolic expression in its own right; e.g., blindness symbolizes the wish to see something for-

bidden or the failure to recognize or face something. At other times it derives from memories of a symptom that the dreamer himself had once before experienced and/or that he had observed or imagined some other person to suffer. Thus, shortness of breath or a sensation of suffocation in a dream may rise from a childhood memory of being pleasurably smothered by mother's embrace or from the recollection of a pant-ing athlete at the moment of triumph, the symptom thereby expressing, symbolically, a regressive wish to be reunited with the mother or to be like the triumphant athlete; or it may originate from memories of a childhood attack of croup or of a parent's asthmatic attack, symbolically expressing the wishes or concerns that marked that original experience.

The occurrence of symptoms in dreams is commonplace, and the reader will have no difficulty recalling, from his own dreams, how real such symptoms may seem at the time. This demonstrates that the capability to express ideas or wishes symbolically through the modality of a bodily symptom is a normal mental phenomenon. What needs to be considered now is how this may come about in the waking state.

PSYCHIC REQUIREMENTS FOR CONVERSION

Conversion symptoms characteristically develop under conditions of deprivation or frustration, and constitute a regressive way both of gratifying an unfulfilled need and of relating to others. The choice of the particu-lar symptom is based on its suitability to represent symbolically the particular wish or fantasy that is incapable of being fulfilled.[13] In this regard, the mechanism underlying conversion symptoms has much in common with that responsible for the form taken by the dream.[12] In both instances, the frustra-tion encourages regressing to earlier modal-ities of expression and relating, as substi-tute modes of gratification. This in turn mobilizes buried (unconscious) wishes or fantasies, which cannot be permitted access to consciousness except in a disguised form. In the dream, the unrecognizable symbolic representation of the fantasy permits the dreamer to "enjoy" his dream and sleep peacefully; should the disguise be threat-ened, the dream becomes unpleasant and the dreamer may awaken. With the conversion symptom, the patient's conviction that he is suffering from a physical disorder similarly keeps him from recognizing the unacceptable fantasy symbolically represented by the symptom. The following is an example.

A man that is involved in a conflict with his partners dreams that he is playing golf with four or five men. They all have golf clubs and are hitting the ball skillfully. He has only a broomstick, and is hitting at a pile of leaves, when he suddenly realizes that he has been beating a squirrel cowering underneath. He awakens feeling anxious. Later in the day, shortly before he is to meet with his partners, he develops a severe aching pain over his back and shoulders and is obliged to go home. This was a conversion symptom.

The dream clearly expressed the patient's feeling of inferiority to his partners, and in only a thinly disguised manner his rage toward them, displaced to the helpless squirrel. The conversion backache symbolically expressed the same aggressive fantasy, now turned on himself as punishment. The patient, however, was conscious only of a physical discomfort, which obliged him to leave work, and thereby incidentally to avoid a confrontation with his partners. In their eyes, as in his own, his pain identified him as sick and entitled to the privileges of the sick role.

As the example indicates, the conversion symptom develops in relation to the internal (intrapsychic) conflict that is mobilized by the frustrating or threatening life situation. The emergence of a wish or fantasy toward which the person himself feels strong disapproval is met by repression, preventing it from becoming conscious. The ensuing conversion symptom has four aims: (1) *to permit expression* of the forbidden wish (although in a disguised form) recognizable neither by the patient nor by the person toward whom it is intended; (2) *to impose punishment* through suffering and disability for entertaining, even unconsciously, such a wish, and thereby to atone for guilt; (3) *to remove the patient* from the threatening or disturbing life situation; and (4) *to provide a new mode of relating,* namely, the sick role, which is sanctioned by society. Thus, the conversion symptom is a compromise solution, and as such serves an adaptive function for the patient. The symptom is the lesser of two evils, because, if successful, the patient enjoys it as a substitute gratification, while he is protected from the anxiety, guilt, shame, or helplessness, which otherwise would have been engendered by the frustrat-

ing life situation and the unacceptable fantasies ("primary gain"). At the same time, he achieves a "secondary gain" by virtue of his sick role.

The effectiveness of this adaptation is measured by the presence or absence of unpleasant affects or of other disturbances. The patient for whom a conversion symptom is serving its purpose best is likely to manifest little anxiety or depression and to be relatively indifferent to the symptom ("la belle indifference"), although he is required to act like a patient in order to fulfill the sick role. When the conversion symptom is not effectively defending against the emergence of the threatening fantasy, he shows more evident suffering from the symptoms, is more insistent in the demand for help, and may be manifestly anxious or depressed as well.

A "successful" conversion symptom is illustrated in the case of a 45-year old bachelor farmer with bilateral ptosis and blepharospasm, the sudden development of which dramatically prevented him from shooting a bull tethered to a fencepost. From that point on he was unable to raise his lids. Although he was no longer able to care for the farm, he exhibited surprisingly little concern, considering how disabling the symptom was. Only after a year of persistent urging from his family did he consent to consult a physician. The symptom, it turned out, had developed on the anniversary of the death of his father, an irascible, alcoholic widower who owned the farm and for whom the son worked. Dominated and abused by the father, he had never succeeded in emancipating himself. On the day of the father's death, the son was horrified to come upon his body lying dead in a pool of blood (from a massive hematemesis), his eyes wide open and staring. The son became nauseated, vomited, and then fled in horror. Thereafter, he had many frightening dreams of the father staring at him accusingly, and he upbraided himself for not having at least lowered the lids of the dead man. The decision one year later to slaughter the bull, his father's prize possession, was an impulsive one, for which he could give no adequate explanation. With the development of the conversion symptom, the frightening dreams ceased and his depression ameliorated. However, when the examining physician forcibly elevated his lids, the patient became acutely anxious, broke out in a cold sweat and fainted (vasodepressor syncope). As he was losing consciousness he had hallucinations in which there were eyes staring at him.

DETERMINANTS OF THE CHOICE OF A CONVERSION SYMPTOM

The raw materials for a conversion symptom are body sensations experienced in the past, that is, the memories of body sensations. Thus, any body parts or functions that can give rise to sensations or have cerebral representation can be implicated in the development of a conversion symptom.[14,45] Thus, contractions of the stomach giving rise to cramps may contribute to a memory trace later utilizable for conversion, whereas increased secretion of gastric acid, a silent physiological process, cannot.

Whether or not such memories can be utilized for conversion depends on whether they have or can contribute to the formation of cognitive structures; that is, ideas, wishes, or fantasies. If so, they are then available to represent the wish or fantasy when it cannot be entertained or expressed in words. A patient's choice of a particular conversion symptom, e.g., a sticking pain in the right cheek, a feeling of being unable to breathe, or blurred vision, thus depends on his individual, often idiosyncratic, past cognitive experience of the underlying sensation.

A woman experienced pains in her arms after her second baby was stillborn. She rationalized that the baby might be better off dead, since perhaps it had been damaged by her toxemia, yet blamed herself for the death. But in speaking of how much she missed the baby, she said, "My arms just ached to hold her."

Some sensations common to infancy and early childhood have a high potential for conversion use by virtue of constituting preverbal body experiences contributing to language formation. This already has been discussed in respect to the use of metaphors and other body imagery for expression. Other sensory experiences qualify for conversion utilization by virtue of being chronologically associated with strong feelings. Such experiences may include not only actual sensations originating from one's own body, but also sensations induced by imagining how someone else feels.

A woman whose conversion manifestations consisted of shaking chills (without fever) and pain in her face, "as if it had been scraped along the ground," had been involved in an auto accident when 11 years old. In the darkness she was thrown into a snow pile where she shivered unnoted for what seemed an interminable period; her mother was dragged along the pavement by the car, her face scraped and bloodied. The patient remembered her hospitalization as the only time in her life when her mother was affectionate to her. The conversion symptoms developed when her marriage, which her mother had strongly disapproved of, was breaking up.

The sensation of being cold and shivering expressed symbolically her yearning for her mother's affection, whereas the face pain symbolized her rage toward the mother who was so frustrating. We can imagine that the little girl took some grim satisfaction in her mother's injury, only to feel guilty when her mother was so kind to her.

The phenomenon of taking on another's symptom, as just illustrated, exemplifies an important determinant of symptom choice. Moved by strong feelings of guilt toward another person, a patient may impose upon himself the same symptoms that he imagined the other person to suffer. In so doing, he follows the primitive *law of the talion*, "an eye for eye, a tooth for tooth." In effect, he responds to the other's symptoms as if he were responsible for them, and must therefore suffer in kind. This is a primitive form of thinking, characteristic of unconscious mental activity.

Ordinarily, the probability of a particular body experience being utilized for conversion is reinforced by numerous associations over years. Thus, a single symptom may effectively condense and express simultaneously a number of different motifs, another typical characteristic of unconscious mental activity. Hidden in such associations are numerous gratifying fantasies or experiences of the past, sometimes quite remote from the conflict immediately underlying the symptom.

Attacks of breathlessness and hyperventilation in a woman had as their immediate determinant the stertorous breathing of her comatose dying mother-in-law at whose bedside she sat for five days. In the background of her childhood, however, were memories and fantasies of (1) the heavy breathing of her father when he was angry at her or quarreling with her mother; (2) the sounds of breathing of her parents engaged in sexual intercourse in the bedroom next to hers; (3) holding her breath so that she could better hear what was going on in the next room, only to become frightened that she might not be able to take another breath; (4) feeling suffocated as she was held by her father while being anesthetized for a minor surgical procedure; and (5) pleasant early childhood memories of inhaling the fragrance of her mother's bosom, later replaced by a fear that the mother might suffocate her. Through all these associations the sensation of breathlessness and the hyperventilation successfully expressed many different childhood fantasies of love and hate, as well as those immediately linked with her ambivalent feelings about her mother-in-law.

The various examples of conversion cited thus far also serve to emphasize the extent to which human relationships are involved in determining which body sensations become the representatives of the repressed wish or fantasy. Just as the original body experiences somehow were implicated in the sharing of feelings with the other person, so too the conversion symptom also is meant to communicate a message and elicit a response from those for whom the repressed wish or fantasy is intended. It is both a disguised communication and a technique of relating. Indeed, to the patient, it often appears to be the only satisfactory way of relating and expressing himself. Hence, the patient conspicuously displays his symptom even when the symptom itself is of no great concern to him. Accordingly, conversion symptoms are usually more pronounced when the patient is with persons significant to him. Although patients with symptoms of organic origin may feel ashamed of or frightened by them, this is virtually never the case with a conversion symptom. For some patients, relating through conversion manifestations may become a way of life, long after the responsible conflict has ceased to be an active issue.

MECHANISMS OF CONVERSION COMPLICATIONS[14]

In the conversion process, a physical sensation from memory used to represent an idea is endowed with the quality of current reality. A conversion complication may result if the neural systems concerned with homeostasis respond by initiating physiological reactions, as though the remembered sensations were indeed real. For example, if the conversion sensation is feeling unable to breathe, the response is to increase ventilation. So imperative may such a message be, that negative feedback transmitted through chemoreceptors *is ignored*, and CO_2 is blown off to the point of respiratory alkalosis. Similarly, a conversion involving a fantasy of injury may initiate

physiological responses to injury at the site implicated in the fantasy. This process is mediated through a neurosecretory mechanism involving antidromic activity along afferent nerves, with the secretion at the nerve terminals of polypeptides of the kinin group.[15,16] In some instances local lesions, including ecchymoses, allergic dermatitis, and urticaria, may develop at such sites, presumably by virtue of interaction with other pre-existing pathogenic factors.[17,18,19] It is conceivable that the stigmata of certain religious mystics may be explained by such a mechanism.[20,21] In such cases, conversion is responsible for the location and time of onset of the lesion, not for its pathological nature or its subsequent course.[14]

CLINICAL DIAGNOSIS

In most cases, the diagnosis of conversion can be established on the first examination. To do so calls for understanding of the mechanism of conversion, familiarity with the diagnostic criteria, and a style of interviewing that yields the relevant psychological data. The diagnosis cannot be based merely on the exclusion of organic disease, especially since many conversion patients have coexisting organic disease (the conversion presenting as an additional symptom or as an exaggeration of the organic symptom).[22] More often than not, the problem is to establish which symptom is based on conversion and which on an organic process.

INTERVIEW TECHNIQUE

Since conversion symptoms are common and readily confused with organic symptoms, the physician should approach every patient with this possibility in mind. This is best accomplished by always utilizing an interview style that elicits social and psychological data concurrently with the physical symptomatology. Actually, such an approach is economical and efficient in the evaluation of any illness, because it insures fuller understanding of those personal, family, and social circumstances which are most relevant to the understanding of the illness and the care of the patient. The details of such an interview approach are presented elsewhere[23] (see also Chapter 1, The Study of Symptoms).

In considering conversion, the interview technique must take into account the fact that, although conversion symptoms are triggered by some circumstance of the patient's life, the patient is *unaware* of the association. This precludes direct questioning as a means of discovering such relationships. The patient who insists that he is not aware of anything upsetting him, unless it be the symptom itself, is being quite honest, for the conversion serves the function of protecting him from the distress that he would otherwise experience were he to face his conflicts directly. Accordingly, the responsibility to recognize the connection between life events and symptoms rests solely on the physician, who listens for associations, spontaneously brought up, although not recognized by the patient. This requires that every new area being investigated be initiated with open-ended, nondirective questions, so that the patient is induced to respond in his own words and to provide his own associations. More specific questions are then developed on the basis of the information so obtained. For example, the open-ended query "Tell me what the problem has been?" enables the patient to respond in his own way, while the interviewer notes what is of main concern to the patient and how he spontaneously relates elements of his illness and his life. The patient is then invited to elaborate on whatever detail of the story the interviewer deems pertinent, e.g., "Tell me more about the pain," following which he explores with more specific questions what the patient has related, until the particular subject has been fully characterized. Each area is investigated in this manner until all the details have been clarified and the full history has been obtained.

In order to uncover relationships between life events and symptoms, both must be explored simultaneously, not as independent categories. This is accomplished by inquiring carefully into all the circumstances surrounding the onset of the symptom, as well as indicating interest each time the patient makes reference to his life circumstances. For example, when the patient passingly mentions his work, his wife, or his neighbors; or that he was home asleep, on the job, on vacation, or expecting a visit from his mother-in-law when the symptoms began, the interviewer promptly inquires about the item brought up, "What is your work?" or "What were you doing at that point?" or "Who was with you?" Sometimes merely an echoing question will suffice, "Your wife?" "Your mother-in-law?" This approach is based on the principle that a patient is more likely to elaborate on personal matters when he, rather than the physician, introduces the subject. For many patients, a formal inquiry

into "social history" or "family history" seems irrelevant, if not intrusive. Further, the relevance of the life circumstance to the symptom is more readily clarified when both are considered in the context in which the patient introduced the theme. Often the patient with a conversion betrays the connection through his choice of words, gestures, or slips of the tongue. On other occasions, the sequence of the symptom occurring immediately after or on an anniversary of a life event provides the clues. The interviewer takes care not to reveal to the patient that he suspects a connection, for this may only block further associations. Hence the physician does not dwell on the personal data beyond what the patient seems willing to discuss, returning to a continuation of the account of symptoms when the patient shows signs of reticence.

DIAGNOSTIC CRITERIA

Ideally, the diagnosis of conversion would require elucidation of the unconscious meaning of the symptom, clarification of the intrapsychic conflict for which it is an attempted solution, and disappearance of the symptoms upon resolution of the conflict. In practice, the suspicions of the physician are usually first aroused by certain unusual features of the symptom, and by how the patient reports his illness. These constitute *suggestive criteria*, and justify exploration for the *confirmatory criteria:*

Suggestive Criteria

1) The Manner in Which the Symptom is Reported. Because of the psychological value of the symptom to the patient, his manner of reporting is ambivalent. On the one hand, he is likely to display suffering and disability, sometimes in a dramatic manner, while on the other hand he subtly betrays attachment to, and even pleasure in, the symptom. Hence, a conversion etiology may be suspected when the patient appears relaxed, even smiling, as he describes a distressing symptom; when he appears unconcerned about the effect on his life of such disabling symptoms as blindness or paralysis ("la belle indifference"); when he gratuitously insists that the symptom *must* have an organic origin; or when he emphasizes his own ability to tolerate the suffering, while describing the terrible effect it is having on his family. The language used in describing a conversion symptom may be rich in imagery, often conveying the hidden psychological meaning.

For example, a man reported a sudden severe pain in his back. "I was just starting to sit down when I got this shot in the back. Boy I come up quick, just bang! Felt like something going through a hole, like a pencil." The pain lasted only a second. A few days earlier he had attempted to rape the wife of an acquaintance, but was interrupted before he could complete the act. He fled from the back door imagining that the husband was pursuing him with a gun. The pain occurred when he heard a radio report that the assailant had been identified. The patient's choice of words neatly condensed the imagery of both the sexual attack and being shot.

Because of the central role of repression in the mechanism of conversion, patients are likely to be vague and imprecise in describing a conversion symptom and the circumstances surrounding its development; this may contrast with their ability to describe the details of a symptom of organic origin. In effect, the repression encompasses not only the pathogenic conflict, but associated events as well. Accordingly, one may find patients with otherwise good memories for dates and events unable to remember the details of even striking events that happen to be associated with the development of the conversion symptom.

2) Inconsistency with Somatic Processes. The form of the conversion symptom is determined by the psychological needs it is intended to meet, not by the anatomical or physiological properties of the body part involved. Hence, the possibility of conversion should be entertained whenever the symptom does not make sense in anatomical or physiological terms (e.g., inability to perceive vibration over one-half of the sternum; or a pain that radiates from the occiput to the groin); when expected physical signs or laboratory findings are absent (e.g., normal vital signs, color, and EEG during syncope or active corneal reflex with hemianesthesia of the face); when the clinical characteristics or course are inconsistent (e.g., intermittent amblyopia with mild nonprogressive exophthalmos or dyspnea and precordial pain, unaffected by exertion).

3) Hysterical Personality Features. Susceptibility to conversion symptoms is not limited to any particular personality type, but is decidedly greater among patients with hysterical traits. Hence, conversion as the explanation of symptoms must always be kept in mind with patients who demonstrate the following characteristics of hysteria:

(a) *Colorful and dramatic expression, language and appearance.* The hysteric needs to attract attention to himself and to affect others. He does so by his manner of dress and grooming and by being charming, entertaining, winsome, appealing, and sometimes frankly provocative or seductive. The style of behavior is characteristically exaggerated, whether it be as the shy innocent little girl, the teasing, seductive woman, the charming, flamboyant man-about-town or the inhibited, timid young man. So too is the manner of presenting the history, which is commonly dramatic and self-centered. At times, the theatrical appearance of the patient permits the diagnosis to be made almost at a glance.

(b) *Role playing.* An unusual ability to put himself in the place of others and to play their roles makes the hysteric a born actor and mimic, and he readily shifts from one role to another as the occasion demands. This chameleon-like quality contributes to the impression of the hysteric being dramatic, colorful, charming, entertaining, and, above all, unpredictable. Thus, such a person may in a few moments change from the apparently desperately ill patient to the charming hostess who puts the physician at his ease, only to resume the wan, languid look of illness as soon as the doctor focuses on the symptoms.

(c) *Use of body language and expression.* The hysteric characteristically makes much use of his body for expression. His language is replete with metaphorical body references. His descriptions are supplemented by demonstrations, sometimes startlingly dramatic.

A mother, for example, describing her child's attack of croup, not only began to speak in a high-pitched, whining tone of voice, but also sighed, gasped, choked, clutched her throat, and rolled her eyes about, dramatically re-enacting the little boy's attack, while at the same time exhibiting her own helplessness, fear, and anger. Her conversion manifestation was choking and hyperventilation.

(d) *Demanding dependency.* Hysterical people are hungry for attention, admiration, and support, and hence are quick to solicit an emotional involvement with the physician. They have an intuitive ability to sense what will be most appealing to the doctor, but their basic self-centeredness (narcissism) proves difficult to gratify, and ultimately frustrating to both. Physicians often eventually become impatient, while the patient typically responds by becoming even more manipulative, demanding, angry, and finally changes doctors. This sequence of first overvaluation and then disillusionment with each doctor is sufficiently typical as to have diagnostic value. A similar sequence often characterizes other relationships as well.

(e) *Suggestibility.* These patients are highly suggestible and readily take on the symptoms of others, whether it be a family member or the patient in the next bed. In groups with strong emotional ties this may assume epidemic proportions.[9] The physician may unwittingly suggest new symptoms or modify old ones simply by implying that he expects a symptom to be present, or by appearing especially interested in a particular symptom. The open-ended interview approach, by not revealing what the doctor has in mind, minimizes such distortions.

(f) *Manifest sexual problems.* Hysterical women, although commonly attractive and seductive, usually are, in fact, frigid, anesthetic, or dyspareunic; they may be shy, inhibited, and fearful of sexual activity, or they may be promiscuous. Hysterical men may be colorful and flamboyant or shy and inhibited, often with an active fantasy life, but a relatively ineffectual sexual life. Marital relations are likely to be unstable, with separations, divorces, and extramarital relations common.

(g) *Previous history of multiple conversion symptoms.* Many hysterical patients experience their first conversion symptoms in adolescence, and repeated symptoms thereafter. Purtell has identified a group of chronic hysterical patients who present a dramatic or complicated medical history beginning before age 35 and marked by as many as 25 conversion symptoms persisting over a period of years.[24,25] They go from doctor to doctor, and by mid-life usually have been subjected to many diagnostic and surgical procedures, occasionally with transient relief of a symptom, but more often with unexpected complications, persistence of old symptoms, or the appearance of a new symptom. Usually these symptoms are reported in traditional medical terms, e.g., "pleurisy," "kidney stones," or "gall bladder attacks," and hence their conversion origin is likely to be overlooked by the physician who does not carefully review the symptomatology. Abdominal pain of conversion origin is so frequently misdiagnosed as appendicitis in young women that the history of an appendectomy performed between the ages of 14 to 22 always should be carefully investigated.[26,27]

(h) *Psychiatric symptoms.* Hysterical patients are also prone to phobias, dissociative states, fugues, and amnesia. Episodes of depression are common, as are suicide gestures with drug overdosage or wrist slashing (often revealed by scars). Excessive dependence on medication is common.

Confirmatory Criteria

Any of the foregoing criteria only *suggest* the diagnosis of conversion. All are equally compatible with an organic diagnosis as well. To make a certain diagnosis, *all* of the following *confirmatory criteria* must be fulfilled. If some, but not all, of the confirmatory criteria are met, conversion may be regarded as a probable diagnosis, but additional study will be required.

1) Precipitation of Symptoms by Psychological Stress. This is a necessary but hardly sufficient criterion, because any illness, organic as well as psychological, may develop in a setting of psychological stress.[28,29,46] However, the patient with a conversion illness is typically oblivious to any connection between his life situation and the symptoms, whereas an organically ill patient often suggests a relationship himself. In fact, a patient's insistence on a psychic origin for a somatic symptom strongly favors an organic rather than a conversion etiology.

Many stressful circumstances may induce conversion symptoms. In general, the more blatantly hysterical the individual, the more subtle may be the stimulus precipitating the conversion symptom; for example, merely a faintly suggestive remark may provoke conversion syncope in an inhibited hysterical girl struggling with sexual fantasies. The more usual settings include real or threatened losses and separations, acute grief, interpersonal conflicts, and sexual threats or temptations, to which the individual responds with a sense of frustration and helplessness. Such feelings may be fleeting or prolonged, but disappear, and often are forgotten when the conversion symptom develops. Because the patient does not consciously connect the situation with the symptom, the interviewer must carefully note dates and the sequence of events. Especially important are symptoms developing on the anniversary of significant events.

The farmer cited earlier, who developed blepharospasm and ptosis on the first anniversary of his father's death, is a case in point.

This information emerged not when he was describing his symptom, but when he was telling how he had acquired his farm; the coincidence with the anniversary had not occurred to him.

Quite often the psychological stress of a physical illness provides the setting for a conversion symptom, especially among patients facing surgical or diagnostic procedures or patients with chronic disease, puzzling or undiagnosed illness, or illnesses of uncertain prognosis. These are all situations in which a patient is likely to feel helpless and frightened, extremely dependent upon his physician, and vulnerable to vivid fantasy.

A patient recovering from a very severe myocardial infarction developed a hyperventilation attack on the day of discharge; a woman facing cystoscopy found herself unable to void; a diabetic who saw a fellow patient with an amputation in his doctor's waiting room developed pain and numbness in his foot when his doctor went on vacation.

Such conversion symptoms are usually short-lived if the physician recognizes their origin and responds to the patient's underlying concerns; they may become quite intractable if approached as evidence of organic illness.

2) Demonstration of the Determinants of the Symptom Choice. This is the most valuable diagnostic criterion. There are four possible determinants of the choice of the symptom, any one or combination of which may be implicated.

(a) *Body language.* The conversion manifestation may be selected by virtue of its capability to express in body terms the unconscious fantasy and the punishment, as a pain in the chest being a "heartache," a paralyzed hand representing an inhibition of a wish to masturbate or to strike someone, or morning nausea indicating a wish to be pregnant. However, the mere fact that a symptom can be so translated is not sufficient to establish its relevancy; it is also necessary to produce supporting evidence. The patient with chest pain must have related the term "heartache" to a real situation in his life; the man with the paralyzed hand must reveal some basis for a wish to masturbate or hit someone; and the woman with morning nausea must betray some evident concern about pregnancy. Further, the patient *remains unaware* of the real meaning of the symptom. When a patient volunteers that perhaps he is paralyzed because

he wanted to hit someone, either that is not the real basis for the conversion, or the symptom has an organic etiology.

(b) *A physical symptom previously experienced by the patient.* Past illnesses must be carefully explored, not only as to details of the symptoms, but even more importantly in respect to the surrounding circumstances. Illness experiences, especially those of childhood, which involved a great deal of secondary gratification or were used to manipulate or control others, are especially likely to provide the basis for future conversion symptoms. Such replication of symptoms of an earlier illness then becomes the means of recreating a more gratifying life situation and averting current frustrations. A familiar example is the recurrence of chest pain in the convalescing coronary patient.[32]

(c) *Symptoms observed in someone else.* This is a common determinant of symptom choice. It involves identification with another person with whom the patient is or has been in conflict or in relationship to whom he is currently suffering frustration. The discovery of the connection with the other person's symptom usually comes about in the course of eliciting information about the illnesses of family members and others. Here the *patient's idea* of what the other person's symptoms were like is more important than the actual diagnosis. Sometimes patients ascribe symptoms to the other person that are not ordinarily part of the alleged illness. For example, the victim of acute pulmonary edema may have been perceived as suffering pain in his chest; the pain of myocardial infarction may be assigned to the region of the nipple. Sometimes one manifestation dominates in the patient's mind, as exemplified in the staring eyes of the dead father serving as the basis for the conversion blepharospasm of the farmer described earlier. The more closely the patient's description of the other person's symptoms corresponds to his own, the more likely it is that they are the model for a conversion. Careful attention to dates and sequences is necessary to establish that the patient's symptom did indeed develop *after* he learned of the other person's symptom. The relationship with the person whose symptom provided the model for the conversion usually is a close but ambivalent one. He is usually a family member or close friend, but may also be someone who merely resembles or can represent the more important person, as a fellow employee or the patient in the next bed.

A woman with autoerythrocyte sensitization developed a severely painful ecchymosis on her lower right thigh; one week earlier, she saw a neighbor youth bleeding from a gunshot wound in the same location. To her mind, he had a close resemblance to her brother.[21] The location and timing of the lesion was determined by conversion mechanisms; the lesion was a conversion complication.

Identity of location is an important diagnostic requirement, but sometimes patients will claim inability to recall the exact location of the other person's symptom. It may then be noted that, while protesting ignorance, the patient is at the same time unwittingly indicating the location of his own symptom.

A woman who mentioned in passing that her father had lost an eye in a shooting accident could not remember which eye, yet while trying to recall unconsciously placed her finger to her left eye, the site of symptoms ultimately proven to be due to conversion (pain, blurring of vision, and twitching of the lids.)

(d) *Symptoms wished on someone else.* The curses of everyday language, e.g., "drop dead," "I wish he'd break his neck," may be translated into conversion symptoms when they evoke conflict and guilt. Thus, a person may faint or develop a pain in the neck rather than entertain, much less utter, the terrible (for him) thought. Here the wish is felt as equivalent to the deed, and the patient inflicts the curse upon himself rather than upon his intended victim. Often the wish is more personal, such as the infertile woman, envious of her sister's pregnancy, who developed as a conversion symptom lower abdominal cramps rather than persist in her secret wish that the sister abort. Sometimes the symptom is based on an actual incident earlier in life.

A middle-aged unmarried woman developed a "sticking pain" in her left cheek soon after her roommate of many years got married. They had been "like sisters." As a child she had, in a fit of anger, thrown an open safety pin, which lodged in her sister's left cheek. She never again permitted herself to feel angry, even when she felt deserted by her roommate.

3) **Primary and Secondary Gains.** *The primary gain* refers to the effectiveness of the conversion symptom in providing a satisfac-

tory symbolic expression for the repressed wishes, and thereby the averting underlying frustration. It is measured by the degree to which the conversion mechanism appears to be protecting the patient from the emotional distress that accompanied (or would accompany) the open conflict. Thus, the primary gain may be considered maximal when the patient is free of anxiety or depression and has little or no concern about the symptom. The serene woman with paralyzed legs, "resigned to God's will," who says she has come to the doctor only because of the insistence of the family, exemplifies an extreme degree of effectiveness of the conversion. *Secondary gain* refers to the advantages conferred on the patient by the illness itself. Any illness provides some gain for most patients, but the patient with a conversion symptom seeks to extract as much advantage as he can. He deliberately uses his symptom to influence and manipulate others, to gain their sympathy and attention, and to avoid certain responsibilities. For him the sick role is a desirable one. Although he may protest his determination to be rid of the symptom, the discerning physician will detect a resistance to any approach that might reveal the underlying psychological problems.

COMMON CONVERSION SYMPTOMS

Most patients present a number of conversion manifestations, sometimes in the form of complex syndromes, sometimes as apparently unrelated symptoms. Only occasionally is the conversion monosymptomatic. Combinations of symptoms commonly simulate familiar illness patterns. The monographs by Breuer and Freud, and by Abse provide excellent descriptions of conversion syndromes.[3,4]

Pain[30,31]

Pain is the conversion symptom seen most commonly today. It may involve any part of the body, the head, back, and abdomen being the most frequent. Pain in the abdomen and face is more common among women, in the back and heart region among men. Conversion pain may occur in conjunction with other conversion symptoms, as dyspnea or nausea, or may confuse the picture of an organic disease.

The choice of pain rather than of some other conversion symptom rests mainly on the relation of pain to aggression and punishment (see Chapter 3). Hence, conversion pain syndromes occur most commonly among persons who are struggling with

TABLE 30-1. CONVERSION SYMPTOMS

MOTOR SYSTEM

Generalized weakness (pseudomyasthenia gravis), fatigue
Paralysis or weakness of extremities
Muscle spasms, stiffness, contractures, pseudo-contractures, torticollis, camptocormia (bent back), writer's cramp
Abnormal movements, tics, tremors, localized seizures
Gait disturbances, astasia-abasia
Aphonia, dysphonia
Occular fixation, ptosis, blepharospasm, blinking

SENSORY SYSTEMS

Pain, aching, pressure, burning, fullness, hollowness, pruritus
Anesthesia, hypesthesia, dysesthesia, hyperesthesia
Sensations of dizziness, swaying, falling
Sensations of coldness, localized or generalized
Sensations of warmth, localized or generalized
Blindness, amblyopia, clouding of vision, tubular vision, scotomata, monocular diplopia, polyplopia
Deafness
Loss of taste, bitter taste, burning tongue

LEVEL OF CONSCIOUSNESS

Fugue, amnesia
Stupor, coma
Convulsions, seizures
Syncope
Dizziness, lightheadedness, faintness, giddiness
Sleepiness, narcolepsy, somnambulism

RESPIRATORY SYSTEM

Cough, tickle, hoarseness

Dyspnea, choking, suffocation, smothering, inability to breathe, hyperventilation
Sighing, yawning
Wheezing
Breath holding
Pain in chest, upper, or lower respiratory passages

CARDIOVASCULAR SYSTEM

"Pain in the heart"
Palpitations
Dyspnea, orthopnea

GASTROINTESTINAL SYSTEM

Sensations of dryness, burning, "acid" in mouth or throat
Anorexia
Bulimia
Thirst, polydipsia
Dysphagia, lump in the throat (globus)
Nongaseous abdominal distention, bloating
Pain, burning, fullness, and other abdominal sensations
Diarrhea, frequent bowel movements, tenesmus, constipation
Anorectal sensations—fullness, burning, pruritus ani

URINARY SYSTEM

Retention, incontinence, urgency, frequency, dysuria, pain

GENITAL SYSTEM

Anesthesia, parasthesias, pain, pruritus, fullness, and other sensations
Dyspareunia, vaginismus
Pseudocyesis

---

underlying feelings of aggression and guilt which they attempt to deal with through the atonement of self-inflicted pain. Unacceptable angry feelings directed toward a deceased person, for example, may be symbolically represented by pain, the site of which often is based on a pain that the deceased had suffered. In this way, expression of aggression is averted, and feelings of guilt are assuaged.

Certain individuals are excessively prone to suffer pain, especially conversion pain.[30] Such "pain-prone" persons are dominated by conflicts around issues of aggression, guilt, self-punishment, and atonement. Typically, they have a history of repeated painful disorders, accidents, injuries, or operations, usually with uncertain diagnoses and indifferent treatment results. Often, no sooner is one pain problem resolved when another de-

velops. The pain is commonly described with vivid imagery, portraying injury, torture, and mutilation ("like being stabbed with a red-hot poker"; "like a bullet going through me"; "like my flesh is being torn"). Some patients parade their suffering; others display the patient resignation of martyrs. In their backgrounds is often a history of violence and brutality; parents who fought, cruel punishments, an abusive alcoholic father, or alternation between angry and recriminating, and cold and distant relationships. Occasionally, they report a childhood marked by uninterrupted love, peace, and serenity; a picture actually too good to be true.

The pain-prone women characteristically emphasize hardships, difficulties, defeats, and humiliations, but paradoxically they appear to have solicited such situations rather than to have sought to avoid or overcome them.[30]

They report bad marriages to abusive inconsiderate husbands, mistreatment by neighbors or employers, dirty, demeaning jobs, and just plain "bad luck." Actually their bitter lives are reported with a certain relish, suggesting masochism, and curiously an inverse relationship often exists between the occurrence of pain and the difficulties of the life situation. When life is treating them badly, they are pain free; when they have a success or prospect of relief, pain develops and denies them of its enjoyment. Evidently, when the environment does not impose sufficient suffering to appease guilt, they inflict punishment upon themselves in the form of the pain.

Pain-prone men are less masochistic and more sadistic in their orientation.[31] They struggle with intense hostility, sometimes of homicidal character, which they attempt to control by relative isolation from others or by involvement in dangerous, often solitary activities, as hunting, fast driving, and scuba diving. Such men are decidedly accident-prone. They show a delicate balance between pain and acts of aggression; pain inhibits agressive activity, whereas controlled aggressive behavior with a high risk of self-injury sometimes relieves the pain. A less severe and usually socially better adjusted group appear mainly as hypermasculine individuals who place a great premium on strength, courage, daring, and endurance. They fear being weak or passive and may greatly over-estimate their own potential. The pain syndrome often develops when they suffer a defeat or loss or are thrust into a position of too great responsibility. An accident on the job may be the final step precipitating the chronic pain, permitting the patient to rationalize his defeat and subsequent inactivity. Some industrial compensation cases fall into this group. Among middle-aged men, pain in the heart region (pseudoangina) is a particularly common form, perhaps fostered by the notion that the heart attack is the price of success and overwork.[32]

Hyperventilation Syndrome[33,34]

A common conversion manifestation, hyperventilation may also be a concomitant of anxiety (Chapter 29). Most patients are unaware of overbreathing, instead reporting the symptoms of hypocapnia and respiratory alkalosis, namely, lightheadedness, dizziness, buzzing in the head, numbness and tingling of the lips and fingertips, and rarely tetany. Commonly, they also complain of choking sensations, suffocation, or inability to take in a deep breath. Although dizzy and lightheaded, they rarely faint. Patients with the hyperventilation syndrome sigh frequently, especially when sensitive topics are being explored in the interview. They are prone to use imagery of breathing as, "It took my breath away," "I just gasped when . . .," and to display inspiratory and expiratory exclamations, such as "Oh!," "Ah." The symptoms may be reproduced by having the patient overbreathe for one minute, preferably with no explanation at the end of the examination. Although most persons easily tolerate the hypocapnic symptoms induced by two to three minutes of overbreathing, the patient with the hyperventilation syndrome is highly sensitive and often cannot persevere beyond 30 seconds without experiencing severe symptoms identical with the spontaneous attacks. To avoid suggestion, the patient should be asked "What did you feel?" or "Have you ever felt like this before?" rather than "Was it like your symptoms?"

Syncope, Stupor, and Coma[34,35]

Conversion syncope, sometimes called hysterical syncope, is more common among women than men. Typically the faint occurs in the presence of others, the patient sliding or slumping to the ground, rarely suffering any injury. Unconsciousness may last from seconds to minutes and often is not complete, the patient reporting voices as from a great distance. During the faint there are no changes in vital signs, color, or sweating, unless the patient is also hyperventilating, as may occasionally occur. The lids may flutter and the patient may moan, mutter, or move about. A sharp command may terminate the attack. Sometimes the examiner may provoke a faint by having the patient hyperventilate or by a strong suggestion that a particular manipulation, e.g., massaging the neck, will induce an attack. At times, the periods of unconsciousness last long enough to be classified as *stupors* or *comas*. Such episodes may be ushered in by a period of sleepiness or confusion and may last days at at a time. Usually the patient can be aroused to cooperate in eating or toileting, although he appears dazed and confused. The episode may terminate abruptly, the patient claiming amnesia for the period. The electroencephalogram (EEG) obtained while the patient is unconscious is always normal. In all types of syncope and coma involving some interference with cerebral metabolism, the EEG is abnormal, usually slow, during the period of unconsciousness.[34,36]

Convulsions

In contrast to the stereotyped sequence of grand mal epilepsy, the conversion (hysterical) convulsion is marked by an unpredictable course, with clutching, grasping, pulling, struggling, tearing at the clothes, rolling from side to side, bizarre postures and expressions, and sometimes blatantly coital movements. Tongue biting and incontinence are infrequent. Consciousness may not be completely lost, the patient sometimes being able to report details of the seizure. Corneal, pupillary, and deep reflexes are present, and attempts to open the eye are resisted. Postictal confusion and somnolence are unusual.

A normal EEG *during* or the first minute or so following the seizure strongly favors conversion. Since some epileptic patients may also have conversion convulsions, an abnormal interseizure EEG does not rule out conversion.

Paralysis

Conversion paralysis may be limited to the movement of only one joint, a finding virtually unknown with a neurological disorder. When the patient attempts to move the paralyzed limb he may contract the antagonistic muscles as well as the prime movers; this may be detected by placing the finger on the tendon of the antagonistic muscle while the patient attempts to move the limb. With spasticity of conversion origin the rigidity increases as the examiner intensifies his effort to move the limb; the resistance of organic spasticity is overcome by increased pressure.

Conversion paralysis is paralysis en masse and is usually more pronounced peripherally; lower motor neuron paralysis generally involves individual muscles, while upper motor neuron paralysis is more pronounced proximally. The leg of a patient with conversion paralysis is dragged when walking, that with an upper motor neuron lesion is circumducted. Lower facial paresis and homonymous hemanopia may accompany organic, but not conversion, hemiparesis.

When a supine patient attempts to raise his paralyzed leg, he will not make use of the leverage available from the nonparalyzed leg if the paralysis is on a conversion basis; on the other hand, he will use the paretic limb to help raise the good leg. The opposite prevails in the case of organic paralysis; the good leg is used for leverage while the paralyzed leg is not. This may be tested by placing the hand under each heel in succession and noting whether the patient presses down when asked to raise the other leg. One may also observe whether or not the paralyzed limb lifts off from the bed as the patient attempts to raise himself to the sitting position with his arms folded and his legs separated; with conversion the affected leg will remain firmly on the bed.

Weakness and Fatigue (Pseudomyasthenia Gravis)[37]

Conversion myasthenia differs from myasthenia gravis in that weakness occurs throughout the waking hours, is unrelieved by rest or sleep, and is not directly related to severity of exercise or the muscle group used. The weakness may be intensified under unusual circumstances, such as eating or during a headache. Inconsistencies of muscle strength are apparent when tested neurologically and functionally, e.g., during position holding, deep knee bends, or stair climbing. True ptosis does not occur, although a profound sense of tiredness may be expressed as "I couldn't hold my eyes open." Symptoms usually persist chronically over a period of years, and are not progressive.

Gait Disturbances

In the conversion syndrome of *astasia-abasia* the patient is able to move his legs normally when lying down, and yet is unable to stand and walk. Conversion gait disturbances are characterized by awkward postures and modes of progression which require complex muscular coordination to prevent falling.

Cutaneous Sensory Disturbances

Conversion hemisensory disturbance commonly involves the entire half of the body, including head and face, more often left than right, the line of demarcation being exactly at the midline. Usually all modalities of sensation are involved, leading to the physiologically illogical finding of absent or diminished vibratory sensation over half of the sternum or skull. Patchy sensory disturbances, hypesthetic or hyperesthetic,

TABLE 30-2. CONVERSION COMPLICATIONS

CONVERSION SYMPTOM	CONVERSION COMPLICATIONS
1. Paralysis	Muscle atrophy, contracture
2. Spasms	Contractures
3. Localized cutaneous pain, burning, dysesthesia	Localized flushing, swelling, purpura, vesicles, or dermatoses
4. Dyspnea, choking, smothering suffocation, panting (hyperventilation)	Respiratory alkalosis, with secondary symptoms (lightheadedness, paresthesias, tetany)
5. Anorexia, nausea, vomiting, dysphagia	Weight loss, inanition, electrolyte or nutritional deficiencies, alkalosis
6. Bulimia	Weight gain, obesity
7. Thirst	Polyuria, nocturia

which vary from day to day and are inconsistent with patterns of innervation, are likely to be of conversion origin. The margins of sensory loss in conversion are usually sharp, not graded as with nerve lesions, with which levels also differ for touch and pin prick.

Blindness and Amblyopia

The sudden onset of total blindness as a conversion symptom may be verbalized as "Why have the lights been turned off?", when the patient should know that normally some vision is retained, even in the dark. A blink reflex may be provoked by a sudden faint. Conversion *amblyopia* is suggested when the patient hesitates as much over the 20/200 level as over the subsequent lines of the Snellen chart. Visual field testing on the tangent screen may reveal no enlargement of the field as the distance from the screen is increased (tubular vision). Further, the conversion visual field typically is circular, with no normal temporal enlargement, and is the same size whether obtained by a 5-mm. object or a large sheet of white paper. With conversion visual problems, the subject may be able to see better through one color lens than another.

Anorexia, Nausea, Vomiting

Conversion anorexia is likely to be expressed as distaste for food or dislike of eating rather than as lack of appetite. Anorexia, nausea, or vomiting may be provoked by certain foods and not by others, especially foods conducive to fantasy, as fluid egg white, scum on milk, or raw meat. Such symptoms may occur before or after eating, on the sight of food, or only in certain settings or with certain people. A good appetite may abruptly be replaced by nausea at mealtime, only to return as soon as the meal is over. Commonly, food is taken into the mouth gingerly, in small morsels, and delayed in the forepart of the mouth, the act of swallowing threatening to evoke a gag. Vomiting, unless it occurs soon after a meal, is likely to consist only of mucus or a small amount of bile-stained gastric juice, but it can be copious enough to lead to alkalosis and electrolyte imbalance. Morning nausea, gagging, and vomiting may indicate unconscious pregnancy fantasies in men as well as women; similar symptoms occurring at night may reflect an unconscious wish for and rejection of an oral sexual experience. The rejection of any repugnant idea may be expressed by anorexia, nausea, or vomiting.

Dysphagia

Conversion dysphagia is typically intermittent, nonprogressive, and referred to the throat or high in the esophagus as a sensation of sticking. When observed eating, the patient may be noted to pucker his face and act as if it is difficult to move the bolus into the esophagus. The symbolic meaning of the food is more important than its consistency, some solid foods being swallowed with ease; some soft or liquid foods producing discomfort.

Globus Hystericus

This is a feeling of a lump felt in the lower part of the neck or behind the upper part of the sternum, comparable to that experienced during crying ("choked up"). It more often occurs between meals. Not only does it usually not interfere with swallowing, it may be relieved by drinking something. The symptom is intermittent in character, usually recurring over a period of years, and never progressing. Schatzki believes the sensation to arise as a physiological response to frequent swallowing without adequate saliva formation, suggesting as the basis an underlying unconscious wish to swallow.[38]

Dysphonia and Aphonia

Dysphonia presents as whispering or a high-pitched expiratory or inspiratory stridor, aphonia as a complete inability to utter any word at all. There is sometimes an accompanying sensation of tightness in the throat or chest. A normal voice may unexpectedly reappear when the patient is startled or during sleep. The vocal cords move properly, approximate accurately, and are free of lesions. Conflicts about speaking or revealing secrets are prominent.[39,40]

Nongaseous Abdominal Bloating[41]

This syndrome occurs almost exclusively among hysterical women with intense longings to be pregnant. The marked abdominal protuberance is brought about by simultaneously relaxing the abdominal musculature and thrusting the lumbar spine forward, often so much so that the hand may easily be passed beneath the spine of the reclining patient. Though seemingly well-relaxed, the patient is unable to make her abdomen flatten by conscious effort, but the protuberance sometimes can be reduced by turning the patient on her side and quickly and forcibly bringing the knees up to the chest. The enlargement may develop within a few minutes, but more often reaches a peak only by the end of the day and disappears during sleep.

Pruritus Vulvae and Ani[42]

A conversion origin may be suspected when there is evidence of sexual frustration and conflict, as among widows, spinsters, and wives of impotent husbands. Scratching may be a substitute for masturbation. Commonly there is perineal or perianal factitious injury from scratching, with mild infection, lichenification, and other secondary changes, often misinterpreted as the primary cause. Conversion pruritus ani is more common among men, and often represents an unconscious homosexual fantasy; such men often show paranoid features as well.

Urgency, Frequency, and Retention

These symptoms commonly are associated with unconscious sexual or pregnancy fantasies. The urge to urinate may be intense and entirely unrelieved by emptying the bladder, yet the patient may not report nocturia. Urinary findings are minimal, considering the intensity of the symptoms. Retention may be total, with enormous distention of the bladder requiring catheterization for relief. The urethral meatus ordinarily appears normal, with the sphincter firmly closed. Evidence of superficial irritation may prove to be secondary to trauma inflicted by the patient.

DIFFERENTIATION FROM OTHER PSYCHOSOMATIC SYMPTOMS

Psychophysiologic Symptoms

Psychological symptoms result when psychologic defense and coping mechanisms, including conversion, are ineffective or fail. Under such conditions, more primitive neurobiological systems of defense and adaptation are invoked, involving mainly autonomic neuroendocrine outflow systems. These include mechanisms to prepare the organism for flight, struggle, and defense against injury (the flight-fight pattern, the ergotropic system) or for conservation of resources and insulation against trauma (the conservation-withdrawal pattern, the trophotropic system). See Chapter 29, Nervousness and Fatigue, for further discussion of psychosomatic symptoms.

The failure of mental mechanisms to maintain adjustment is experienced by the patient in terms of unpleasant affects, such as anxiety, fear, anger, sadness, helplessness, or hopelessness, whereas the activation of the biological systems involves such demonstrable physiological changes as tachycardia, sweating, vasoconstriction, or hyperperistalsis. The patient's awareness of such physiological processes results in such symptoms as palpitation, sweating, cold hands and feet, diarrhea, or fatigue. In this respect, although remotely induced by psychological processes, the psychophysiological symptom itself is of organic origin, deriving as it does from the patient's awareness of actual bodily changes. In contrast to the conversion symptom, it has no primary symbolic meaning and serves no psychological function.

The basic difference of psychophysiologic symptoms and signs from conversion is perhaps best highlighted by the clinical observation that, when the conversion mechanism is *failing* in its adaptive function, the patient may become anxious or depressed and manifest psychophysiologic changes and symptoms; conversely, the development of a conversion symptom may *terminate* such symptoms. The farmer with conversion ptosis and blepharospasm, mentioned earlier, who became acutely anxious and fainted when his lids were held open, illustrated this inverse relationship.

Hypochondriacal Symptoms

The hypochondriacal patient appears to be unusually aware of even the most trivial physical sensation and to ascribe to it grave consequences. Minor aches and pains, intestinal gas, borborygmi, cough, flushing, sweating, premature ventricular contractions, indeed virtually any perceptible physiological change may become the object of intense concern; so too may the discovery of a minor skin blemish, a palpable lymph node, or a visible arterial pulsation. The patient's concerns generally are couched in terms of fear of some serious or fatal disease. No amount of reassurance, no matter how soundly based, gives more than transient relief. Further, any suggestion that the feared disease may indeed be present intensifies the patient's concern. This contrasts to the behavior of the patient with a conversion symptom, who does not view his symptom with such intense alarm and indeed may even seem relieved when an organic diagnosis is proposed. Resignation to suffering, as is sometimes encountered with conversion symptoms, is never associated with the hypochondriacal symptom. Most confusion arises from the hysterical patient with chronic conversion symptoms whose efforts to gain the attention of the physician are misinterpreted as genuine hypochondriacal concern. Some hypochondriacal patients are basically schizophrenic and their somatic symptoms are delusional in character.

Somatic Delusions

Somatic delusions are psychotic manifestations and may be observed in patients with schizophrenia, paranoid states, psychotic depression and delirium, dementia, or drug-induced psychoses. Although also originating in the mind, they differ from conversion symptoms by virtue of their palpably bizarre character. Thus, patients may believe internal organs are shriveling up or disappearing, the nose is misshapen or enlarged, the genitals are deformed or missing, a foreign object is in the rectum, abdominal cavity, uterus, or gullet, insects are crawling under the skin, or an extremity is enlarged or shrunken. Although most such patients present no difficulty in diagnosis, an occasional patient whose delusions have been challenged in the past succeeds in couching the complaint in terms that suggest conversion or an organic process. However, when encouraged to elaborate, the patient who may have first defined his symptom as "pain" will eventually introduce the bizarre features that establish the delusional quality of the symptom.

Malingering

Physicians often are quick to accuse patients with conversion symptoms of malingering. In actuality, malingering, the conscious simulation of disease, is rare in the general practice of medicine. Most cases occur in settings in which there is an immediate and usually obvious gain to be achieved by being sick, as in penal institutions, the military, or when litigation is involved. Some unscrupulous individuals simulate for dishonest purposes, but they ordinarily avoid medical contacts lest they be unmasked. Children and some immature adults may make clumsy, amateurish efforts to play sick in order to avoid a difficult situation, but these are easily identified by virtue of the naïvete of their notions of illness. Among children, such malingering may hide a school phobia. More difficult to identify as malingering are patients who seek to prolong convalescence by simulating continuing symptoms of an illness, or who are receiving compensation, or facing a lawsuit.

The ability to malinger successfully requires intellectual knowledge of and familiarity with disease pictures. Hence, successful malingerers are commonly drawn from among nurses, aides, attendants, x-ray technicians, members of the medical corps of the armed services, and occasionally persons who have previously been hospitalized for extended periods. An important group is drug addicts, who simulate pain to secure narcotics; the telltale marks of previous injections usually betray them.

The determinants of malingering are complex. Prominent are intense needs to be taken care of and/or to suffer. Some merely act out the symptoms of disease, whereas others fake fever by heating the thermometer, or bleeding by putting blood in sputum or urine. Some go so far as to injure themselves by inducing bruising or abscesses, introducing foreign bodies, or taking such drugs as digitalis, coumadin, atropine, insulin, or thyroid hormones. The distribution of self-inflicted lesions is ordinarily limited by the patient's reach and handedness. Such self-destructive behavior may carry over into everyday life in the form of accident-proneness and masochistic relationships in which they are physically abused.

The so-called *"Munchausen syndrome"* refers to a group of psychiatric illnesses manifested by chronic factitious symptomatology.[42,43] The diagnostic features include (1) the dramatic presentation of medical complaints, suggesting a major emergency; (2) factitious evidence of disease; (3) evidence of many previous hospital experiences, particularly laparotomy scars and cranial burr holes; (4) eager submission to painful diagnostic and therapeutic procedures; (5) pathological lying and false elaboration of the symptoms that intrigue the listener (pseudologia fantastica); (6) a history of signing out of hospital against medical advice and wandering from hospital to hospital across the country ("hospital hoboes"); and (7) aggressive, unruly, truculent behavior. Like the imposter, these patients know they are acting, but they cannot stop; their bizarre behavior has become a way of life.

The differentiation between malingering and conversion is at times difficult. In general, the malingerer is aloof, suspicious, hostile, secretive, unfriendly, and more concerned about his symptom; the patient with conversion is more dependent, appealing, clinging, and although clearly acting out the sick role, shows less than the expected concern about the symptom. Because the skillful malingerer applies his intellectual knowledge of the disease in the simulation, the end result is more likely to resemble the real thing. Careful observation, especially when the patient is unaware that he is being observed, often will reveal that the patient is not as disabled as he claims. Unlike the patient with a conversion, the malingerer must work to maintain his ruse. Hence, he cannot always resist the temptation to relax the deception, especially when he believes himself to be alone. Amelioration of symptoms with the establishment of an effective relationship with the physician is more characteristic of conversion than malingering. Indeed the malingerer, because he is consciously involved in a deception, is unlikely to relate well. The malingerer may be reluctant to cooperate in diagnostic procedures which unmask him; the conversion patient is eager for confirmation of an organic explanation for his symptom.

Deliberate deception of patients by physicians, as with the use of placebos or sterile hypos, is of little diagnostic value and indeed may irrevocably damage the relationship with the patient. It is a far better method for the physician to try to understand the psychological reason for the symptom, whether it be based on conversion or on conscious simulation.

REFERENCES

1. Paget, J.: Nervous mimicry (Lancet, 1873), *in* Paget, J., Clinical Lectures and Essays, New York, Appleton & Co., 1875.
2. Veith, I.: Hysteria. The History of a Disease, Chicago, Univ. of Chicago Press, 1965.
3. Abse, D. W.: Hysteria and Related Mental Disorders, Baltimore, Williams & Wilkins, 1966.
4. Freud, S.: Studies on hysteria (with Breuer, J.) 1893: Freud S., standard ed., Vol. II, p. 5, London, Hogarth Press, 1955.
5. Freud, S.: Fragment of analysis of a case of hysteria (1905): Freud, S., standard ed., Vol. 7, p. 3, London, Hogarth Press, 1954.
6. Rangell, L.: The nature of conversion, J. Amer. Psychoanal. Ass. 7:632, 1959.
7. Ljungberg, L.: Hysteria. A clinical prognostic, and genetic study, Acta Psychiat. Neurol. Scand. (supp. 112) Vol. 32, 1957.
8. Farley, J., Woodruff, R. A., and Guze, S. B.: The prevalence of hysteria and conversion symptoms, Brit. J. Psychiat. 114:1121, 1968.
9. Knight, J. A., Friedman, T. I., and Sulianti, J.: Epidemic hysteria: A field study, Amer. J. Public Health 55:858, 1965.
10. Sharpe, E. F.: Psychophysical problems revealed in language: An examination of metaphor, Int. J. Psychoanal. 21:201, 1940.
11. Piaget, J.: Six Psychological Studies, New York, Random House, 1967.
12. Freud, S.: The Interpretation of Dreams (1900): Freud, S., standard ed., Vol. 9, London, Hogarth Press, 1953.
13. Fenichel, O.: Conversion, *in* The Psychoanalytic Theory of Neurosis, Ch. XII, New York, W. W. Norton, 1945.
14. Engel, G. L.: A reconsideration of the role of conversion in somatic disease, Compr. Psychiat. 9:316, 1968.
15. Chapman, L. F., Ramos, A. O., Goodell, H., and Wolff, H. G.: Neurohumoral features of afferent fibers in man, their role in vasodilation, inflammation, and pain, Arch. Neurol. 4:617, 1961.
16. Chapman, L. F., Ramos, A. O., Goodell, H., and Wolff, H. G.: Evidence for kinin formation resulting from neural activity evoked by noxious stimulation, Ann. N. Y. Acad. Sci. 104:258, 1963.
17. Barchilon, J., and Engel, G. L.: Dermatitis: An

hysterical conversion symptom in a young woman, Psychosom. Med. 14:295, 1952.

18. Seitz, P. F. D.: Symbolism and organ choice in conversion reactions, Psychosom. Med. 13: 254, 1951.

19. Seitz, P. F. D.: Experiments in the substitution of symptoms by hypnosis, Psychosom. Med. 15:405, 1953.

20. Lifschutz, J. E.: Hysterical stigmatization, Amer. J. Psychiat. 114:527, 1957.

21. Ratnoff, O. D., and Agle, D. P.: Psychogenic purpura: A re-evaluation of the syndrome of autoerythrocyte sensitization, Medicine 47: 475, 1968.

22. McKegney, F. P.: The incidence and characteristics of patients with conversion reactions. I. A general hospital consultation service sample, Amer. J. Psychiat. 124:542, 1967.

23. Morgan, W. L., and Engel, G. L.: The approach to the medical interview, in The Clinical Approach to the Patient, Ch. III, Philadelphia, W. B. Saunders, 1969.

24. Purtell, J. J., Robbins, E., and Cohen, M. E.: Observations on clinical aspects of hysteria. A quantitative study of 50 hysterical patients and 156 control subjects, J.A.M.A. 146:902, 1951.

25. Perley, M., and Guze, S. B.: Hysteria—the stability and usefulness of clinical criteria. A quantitative study based on a follow-up period of six to eight years in 39 patients. New Eng. J. Med. 266:421, 1962.

26. Hardy, H. E.: A notable source of error in the diagnosis of appendicitis, Brit. Med. J. 2:1028, 1962.

27. Barraclough, B. M.: Appendicectomy in women, J. Psychosom. Res. 12:231, 1968.

28. Schmale, A. H.: Relationship of separation and depression to disease, Psychosom. Med. 20:259, 1958.

29. Engel, G. L.: A life setting conducive to illness: The giving-up—given-up complex, Ann. Intern. Med. 69:293, 1968.

30. Engel, G. L.: "Psychogenic" pain and the pain-prone patient, Amer. J. Med. 26:899, 1959.

31. Tinling, D. C., and Klein, R. F.: Psychogenic pain and aggression. The syndrome of the solitary hunter, Psychosom. Med. 28:738, 1966.

32. Engel, G. L.: Pseudoangina, Amer. Heart J. 59:325, 1960.

33. Engel, G. L., Ferris E. B., and Logan, M.: Hyperventilation: Analysis of clinical symptomatology, Ann. Intern. Med. 27:683, 1947.

34. Engel, G. L.: Fainting, ed. 2, Springfield, Ill., Thomas, 1962.

35. Romano, J., and Engel, G. L.: Studies of syncope. III. Differentiation between vasodepressor and hysterical fainting, Psychosom. Med. 7:3, 1945.

36. Engel, G. L., and Romano, J.: Delirium, a syndrome of cerebral insufficiency, J. Chronic Dis. 9:260, 1959.

37. Fullerton, D. T., and Munsat, T. L.: Pseudomyasthenia gravis: A conversion reaction, J. Nerv. Dis. 142:78, 1966.

38. Schatzki, R.: Globus hysteria (globus sensation), New Eng. J. Med. 270:676, 1964.

39. Tyrer, J. H., Emerson, B. T., and Murphy, K. J.: Hysterical laryngeal spasm and the production of paroxysmal arterial hypertension, Quart. J. Med. 28:315, 1959.

40. Barton, R. T.: The whispering syndrome of hysterical dysphonia, Ann. Otol. 69:156, 1960.

41. Alvarez, W. C.: Hysterical type of nongaseous abdominal bloating, Arch. Intern. Med. 84:217, 1949.

42. Rosenbaum, M.: Psychosomatic factors in pruritus, Psychosom. Med. 7:52, 1945.

43. Bursten, B.: On Munchausen's syndrome, Arch. Gen. Psychiat. 13:261, 1965.

44. Spiro, H. R.: Chronic factitious illness, Munchausen's syndrome, Arch. Gen. Psychiat. 18:569, 1968.

45. Engel, G. L., and Schmale, A. H.: Psychoanalytic theory of somatic disorder: Conversion, specificity, and the disease onset situation, J. Amer. Psychoanal. Ass. 15:344, 1967.

46. Adamson, G. D., and Schmale, A. H.: Object loss, giving up, and the onset of psychiatric disease, Psychosom. Med. 27:557, 1965.

31

Coma and Convulsion

JAMES L. O'LEARY and WILLIAM M. LANDAU

INTRODUCTION

Coma and convulsion, outstanding symptoms of cerebral disorder, occupy the extremes of an excitability gradient that extends from a zone of hypoexcitability at one end of the normal range to one of hyperexcitability at the other. Coma can develop as the state of neural excitability enters either of these end-zones. Suspension of consciousness can occur either during a generalized epileptic attack (hyperexcitability) or when trauma, anoxia, infection, systemic metabolic disturbance, toxin, poison, or drug markedly depresses neural functioning (hypoexcitability).

We digress to discuss certain rudiments of neurophysiology. The human brain contains some ten billion nerve cells arranged in an intricate communication net roughly analogous to a telephone system or a computer, but infinitely more intricate than either. Each single cell component functions both as a receiver-transmitter (cell body and dendrites) and as a conductor (axon). The axon terminals of one nerve cell are applied to the cell body or dendrites of others to produce circuits of varying complexity. Information is propagated along axons as variations in the spacing between a quick succession of *all-or-none* impulses. At the synapses the digital all-or-none information carried by axons is transformed into an analogical *graded* process. Two basic kinds of information are thus transmitted—excitatory and inhibitory. Naturally, it is the excitatory processes upon which the nervous system depends chiefly for its operations, the inhibitory either preventing overaction or slowing or stopping action in progress. The richness of the interconnections between neurons makes for ready distribution of coded information through the neural net. However, inhibitory controls restrict normal activity to purposive channels. Under conditions of *exalted excitability* (i.e., epileptic states) distribution of information is far too permissive, particularly when inhibitory brakes are also ineffective. In such circumstances, a few neurons discharging at frequencies up to 800 per second (a speed not uncommon at the site of epileptogenic lesions) may transmit impulses that rapidly infiltrate neighboring neurons poised on the threshold of discharge, drawing them into the orbit of excessive firing from a small start. Thus, a convulsion may avalanche across wide areas of the cerebral gray matter.

The depressed functioning of the *hypoexcitable state* is occasioned by elevation of the synaptic threshold and subnormal responsiveness of the membrane that invests the nerve cell, the former being one specific expression of the properties of the latter.

Upon the relative reactivity of the membrane depend the important functions of synaptic transfer and impulse propagation: impaired excitability of the membrane greatly slows the operations of the system as a whole. Such slowing may cause abnormal scarcity of circulating impulses within the neural net and abolition of all but the most vital activities. Thus unconsciousness results.

The state of hyperexcitability, a prelude to convulsion, is manifested by low resistance at the synaptic bridges and a high tide of irritability. The latter leads to the discharge of spurts of impulses of excessive length and astonishingly high frequency. This has the effect of overloading the system with a jam of circulating signals, and, through resultant overaction, suspending the logistics of normal functioning. Besides interrupting consciousness, the impulses discharge outward through avenues of diminished synaptic resistance, massively invading the nerve routes leading to skeletal muscle and producing the overt signs of convulsion. Since the nervous system depends largely upon energy sources transported via the blood supply, the time is relatively brief during which the chaotic overaction of convulsion can be maintained. As a result, more likely than not, a convulsion will terminate with the brain in a depressed state. Thus, during and after a generalized seizure, the accompanying unconsciousness can occur for two reasons that appear in succession, the first that of overactivity associated with the convulsion proper, and the second (postictal parasomnia) with terminal underactivity.

By unconsciousness we mean a void of consciousness. The range of consciousness extends from the alert wakefulness (vigilance) of the expectant mind, through clouding (obtundity) and stupor, to precoma and coma. Any loss implies the prior existence of a state of *normal consciousness*, the introspective yardstick that the experienced observer uses to estimate the severity of the loss. It is the definition of normal consciousness which is most difficult. Its meanings are obscured in a haze of metaphysics, and Brain[1] has pointed out that to different savants it can mean six things: forms of behavior by which we distinguish the unconscious from the conscious individual; psychological terms used to describe conscious states such as sensory and perceptual experiences; consciousness as related to the activity of the nervous system; role of consciousness in the biological functions of the living organism; the logical terms that can be applied to conscious experience; and the metaphysical status of consciousness. The notion of distinguishing between *content of consciousness* and the *state of awareness* in which it exists is also prevalent, the phrase *spontaneity of consciousness* being used for the latter. Sartre,[2] for example, alludes to consciousness as a pure spontaneity, "confronting the world of things which is sheer inertness." James[3] challenged its very foundations in an essay, "Does Consciousness Exist?"

HISTORICAL RÉSUMÉ

Efforts to comprehend how body and mental states conjoin go back some 2,400 years. Viewed in retrospect they signify man's most prolonged struggle to comprehend his own nature. One lesson taught is that speculations based upon erroneous structural and physiologic information can long persist as a habit of thinking even though challenged occasionally during the passage of centuries. The ancients certainly knew something of the brain, recognizing at the least that the ventricles contained fluid, because in several instances hydraulic terms were applied to brain parts that adjoined ventricular channels, such as pons, aqueduct, and valve. Thus the erroneous view that the ventricles contain a "pneuma" (air, gas, or vapor) arose as speculation after a fair start had already been made in the right direction. The error resulted from sheer laziness to observe, reliance being placed instead upon the transmission of book knowledge. Such speculation continued to be accepted as fact until near our own time when Magendie (1825) proved the fluid content of the brain ventricles in freshly dead bodies.

Aristotle viewed the seat of animal spirits as existing in the heart. However, Hippocrates formed a more correct opinion of the importance of the brain to mental states. Erasistratus, a student of Aristotle, taught also that animal spirits derive from the head. Plato recognized three mental faculties, of which the rational was related to the brain. Most of the ancients, including Galen, believed that the ventricles received a pneuma through nasal passages and sphenoid bone, and that this mixed in the ventricles with vital spirits brought upwards from the heart by the arteries. The animal spirits there produced were supposed to be transmitted downward through the ventricles to be distributed over the nerves.

Galen also conceived of the brain as having movements of diastole and systole. In the former he supposed that it receives air and vital spirits into the ventricles, and in the latter distributes animal spirits via the nerves. Later, it was denied that animal spirits were formed in the ventricles, and taught instead that they were generated in the substance of the brain, since dissections showed that nothing macroscopic could pass inward through channels in sphenoid and ethmoid bones. Nevertheless, the view long persisted that the ventricles had an excretory function, dispelling to the outside effete material that arises as a waste product during nutrition of the brain.

The modern era began with the phrenologists who, in addition to fathering an outlandish theory of brain localization related to cranial protuberances, were masters of brain dissection. Their rivals of the more orthodox school were forced to seek corresponding proficiency as dissectors, and thus emphasis turned inevitably to re-establishing the science of observation. Prochaska,[4] for example, supported the view (based on dissection) that the nerves of sensation and of motion met and communicated in the medulla oblongata, giving rise there to a "seat of the sensorial consciousness." Later (about 1850) that seat was moved forward to the thalamus, where we leave it to take up work of our own time which also appears to support a thalamic center for consciousness.

Theoretical considerations arising out of the modern studies dominate today's thinking upon the subject, and are in opposition to the view that the whole brain acting together performs the function of consciousness. This dichotomy of thinking was recognized long before the present epoch, and is stated clearly in the following quotation from Richerland[5]:

> The existence of a centre, to which all the sensations are carried, and from which all motions spring, is necessary to the unity of a thinking being, and to the harmony of the intellectual functions. But is this seat of the principle of motion and of sensation circumscribed within the narrow limits of a mathematical point? or rather should it not be considered as diffused over the whole brain?

For these purposes, consciousness is definable as a generalized product of the functioning of the waking brain, and is only recognizable through introspection. It is divisible into a state (or states) of awareness and a changing mental content to which we attend. The content includes items of both primary and subsidiary import and is evident either in present perception or (after recall) in the memory of past events. Phylogenetically, its origin is said to lie in feeling.

Coma, deriving from the Greek *koma* meaning deep sleep, designates a state of unconsciousness from which the subject cannot be aroused. The state of impaired consciousness which gradually develops into coma leads through obtundation (a state of drowsiness, indifference, and apathy in which the threshold of arousal is significantly increased), through stupor (requiring vigorous, sometimes continuous, stimulation to maintain arousal), to deep coma in which both the psychological and motor responses to stimulation are lost. Pupillary reactions, ocular motility, and abnormalities of respiration are valuable guides to the etiology of coma and, if structurally caused by a brain stem lesion, lead to the probable site of severe impairment. Irreversible coma is the sign of a permanently nonfunctioning brain.[54]

The advent of heart transplants has led to a re-evaluation of the criteria for irreversible coma, and a comprehensive definition has been provided by an ad hoc committee of the Harvard Medical School appointed to examine the criteria of brain death.[54] Those arrived upon include: (1) total unawareness to externally applied stimuli and inner need and complete unresponsiveness; (2) no movements or breathing; (3) no reflexes; (4) a flat or isoelectric electroencephalogram with the presumptions that the personnel conducting the recording were competent, the sensitivity of the equipment adequate, and the apparatus operating normally. For (4), they recommend the use of one channel for EEG and another for a noncephalic lead to pick up extraneously derived artifacts and identify them.

NEURAL BASIS OF CONSCIOUSNESS

CONTRIBUTION OF STUDIES UPON SLEEP

The vagueness of our concept of consciousness was alluded to previously, as was the behavioral significance of *awareness* or *vigilance* as expressions of the state, if not the content, of mind. Any stimulus that usurps the attention of animal or man simultaneously produces vigilance and "activates" the scalp- (or brain-) recorded electroencephalogram (EEG); that is, it converts the usual spontaneous rhythm of the waking brain into an irregular tracing of low voltage in which no remainder of usual activity is evident. From that change we deduce the importance of the sensory paths to the cortex in the maintenance of awareness. Sensory monotony, or deprivation, has the opposite effect, lending itself to sleep.

In animals, a brain stem severance at the mesodiencephalic junction, which permanently deprives the cerebral cortex of a sensory inflow, leads to perpetual slumber along with the ocular and EEG manifestations of sleep.[6] Analysis of the phenomena of normal sleep in animals and man has aided importantly in the neurologic appraisal of consciousness and unconsciousness. It is recognized, of course, that in sleep the mental operations of animal and man most closely approach equivalence. Hereafter we examine sleep as a prelude to matters that concern the pathological suspension of consciousness.

The notion of a sleep center did not originate with von Economo,[7] the German neurologist who is credited with describing the form of encephalitis called sleeping sickness, but he gave it a strong impetus by concluding that a *wakefulness center* exists in the hypothalamic wall of the third ventricle because the destructive lesions of encephalitis center there. He also described a *sleep center* situated just ahead of that area, verging upon the preoptic region. Lesions at the latter site were characterized by wakefulness (asomnia) and von Economo theorized that it produced sleep by inhibition of the remainder of the brain. Between them, these half-centers were presumed to establish the diurnal sleeping-waking cycle. Later, W. R. Hess,[8] stimulating a corresponding region of the ventralmost thalamus with slowly repetitive electrical pulses of long duration, also produced sleep. He, too, proposed a more posteromedially situated wakefulness center.

Bremer[6] is credited with replacing this older static view of a sleep center with the more dynamic one that sleep is due to an interruption of a continuous stream of afferent impulses which flows past the mesodiencephalic junction upwards and outwards to cerebral cortex. He believed the lemnisci to be the channels of flow, whereas later workers describe instead a collateral path (derived from the lemnisci) which filters more gradually through the in-lying brain stem tegmentum to connect at the level of the center median thalamic nucleus with a a diffuse thalamocortical system, to be described next.

Bremer showed that severance of the brain stem at the mesodiencephalic junction produced a state closely akin to sleep, and replaced usual waking frequencies of the EEG with diffusely slow (delta) activity interrupted by spindles closely similar to those recorded in human EEG sleep tracings. Dempsey and Morison[9] proved the origin in the mid-line thalamus of a fiber system which distributes diffusely to the cortex. Through repetitive electrical stimulation at the thalamic source they produced generalized wave sequences (recruiting response) in the cortex which closely resemble the spontaneously repetitive spindles of light sleep. Later, Moruzzi and Magoun[10] showed that rapidly repetitive stimulation in the brain stem tegmentum can convert the sleep type EEG with spindles (such as is produced during barbiturate anesthesia) to the low voltage desynchronized tracing characteristic of a just awakened alert animal. Tonic drive feeding into the diffuse thalamocortical system of Dempsey and Morison[9] is presumed responsible for maintenance of the waking state. When the tonic drive is interrupted sleep intervenes. Thus the origin of the term *reticular activating system* used by the followers of Moruzzi and Magoun.

For a long time, deepest sleep was associated with very slow delta EEG activity and spindles as observed by Bremer in his animals with brain stem transection. It came as a surprise, therefore, when a still deeper stage of sleep was recognized in the cat (Dement,[11] Jouvet[12]). It was dubbed *paradoxical sleep* because the EEG closely resembles that of the awake, alert animal. Nevertheless, if the cat is stimulated during paradoxical sleep it only reverts to the stage of sleep with slow waves and spindles, not to full awakening. It is known that the nervous system is peculiarly sensitive to auditory arousal. Thus it is not surprising that responses of single tegmental neurones to auditory clicks are reduced during usual deep sleep and are practically absent during paradoxical sleep. However, in curious contrast is the fact that the spontaneous activity of the same neurone is greatest during paradoxical sleep.[13] It has been shown recently that usual sleep with slow waves and spindles depends upon the integrity of cerebral mechanisms, whereas paradoxical sleep requires the operation of rhombencephalic mechanisms. The latter also has been called archisleep, suggesting a more archaic origin than has telecephalic sleep.

Out of modern studies upon sleep and activation has come a renewed interest in a mesodiencephalic center of consciousness. Penfield[14] theorizes that the highest level of integration in the brain of man, "to which all the sensations are carried and from which all motions spring," is situated in the mesodiencephalic region.[5] Penfield incorporates into his hypothesis much of the evidence just presented and other data based upon evaluation of the unconscious state associated with brain lesions in man. Walshe[15] has reviewed the Penfield evidence critically and with enviable lucidity. His easily accessible account should be read by everyone interested in the problems of mind and brain.

Unconsciousness in Brain Stem Lesions in Man

Much has been learned of the site of origin of comatose states from study of patients with lesions of the brain stem or the superstructure. One important source has been observations upon anencephalic and hydrocephalic monsters.[16,17]

It appears that such mesodiencephalic subjects sleep and wake, react to hunger, loud sounds, and crude visual stimuli by movement of eyes, eyelids, and facial muscles. Such an infant may see and hear, taste and smell, reject the unpalatable and accept such food as it likes, utter sounds, show displeasure when hungry and pleasure when sung to. He may also perform crude limb movements spontaneously. All this can perhaps be described collectively as rudimentary awareness, or indeed as crude consciousness, if we could somehow make ourselves aware of its content.

Cairns[18] analyzed the effect upon consciousness of lesions at lower and upper brain stem levels, the latter, of course, including involvement of thalamic centers. He found that a disturbance of the medulla or the pons can produce sudden loss of consciousness, ordinarily with associated disturbance of breathing and circulation. The question arises as to whether anoxia resulting from the cardiorespiratory deficit might not be the cause of coma in lower brain stem lesions. However, in some instances, loss of consciousness has been shown to precede the drop in blood pressure and respiratory change. Howell[19] analyzed the case histories of six patients who showed foraminal impaction of the brain stem at postmortem. He found the most common feature of this syndrome to be the hydrocephalic attack, consisting in its mildest form of a brief *agonizing headache* (often lasting only a minute or two) with or without transitory confusion, deafness, or amaurosis. Inconstant features were bilateral cranial nerve palsies (involving nerves seven to ten inclusively), neck rigidity and sustained hydrocephalus developing insidiously. Between attacks patients were found to be alert, in contrast to the global impairment of consciousness seen with upper brain stem compressions. In fact, Howell states that global impairment is no part of this syndrome, and that with medullary compression a patient alert one moment may be dead the next. When coma occurred it lasted a minute in one case, several hours in three others, with possible upper brain stem compression as well.

Two main varieties of loss of consciousness occur in upper brain stem and thalamic lesions, one intermittent and the other continuous.[18] The former is exemplified by petit mal epilepsy, the latter by coma with decerebrate rigidity, coma with hyperthermia, hypersomnia, and akinetic mutism. In hypersomnia, persistent unconsciousness may resemble sleep, with quiet breathing, muscular relaxation, and loss of the expression that characterizes the waking state. The patient can be aroused temporarily, and the EEG is of the sleep type with diffuse delta activity, as is also true with other kinds of unconsciousness. In akinetic mutism the eyes may follow the observer about, but the patient is otherwise unresponsive.

Because of their acute development, the signs of coma associated with downward pressure from supratentorial mass lesions may be significantly more dramatic. Two possible sequences of brain stem dysfunction may accompany such conditions.[20] In one, the signs of uncal herniation occur, including third nerve involvement and lateral midbrain compression. The other reflects bilateral diencephalic impairment, Cheyne-Stokes respiration, "doll's head" (oculocephalic) eye movements, and bilateral motor involvement.

Howell,[19] whose study upon brain stem and foraminal impaction already has been mentioned, examined some 150 cases of upper brain stem compression. He reports that the main features of the syndrome are sufficiently constant for it to be distinguished from other conditions causing coma. Increased headache, vomiting, and stiffness of neck develop at the onset. The most constant feature is a global impairment of all mental functions progressing rapidly or slowly, from lethargy to a semicomatose state. Patients in his series might die before they became fully comatose, and thus death could only be attributed to coma when severe aspiration or hypostatic pneumonia developed. Bradycardia occurred less frequently than tachycardia. Hyperpyrexia was common. In rapidly developing compression, sudden respiratory arrest might be seen, and this could follow a phase of slow, shallow, grunting respiration. Loss of pupillary light reflex was very constant, although it might not be observed until compression is far advanced. Dilation of the pupil is usual, but the pupils may remain small or even contracted. Decerebrate rigidity is common, and it is exceptional not to detect extensor spasm of the limbs in response to painful stimulation at some stage of the illness.

Plum and Posner[55] view abnormalities of pupils, respiration, and the oculocephalic and oculovestibular reflexes as having important localizing value in brain stem lesions. It is the combinations between them which produce the important syndromes recognized by neurologists and ophthalmologists as pointing to the probable site of disorder. In progressive involvement extending rostrocaudally, one combination of deficit may replace another indicative of the descent of the impairment. Associated cranial nerve deficits may confirm the site of the pathology.

Among respiratory abnormalities Cheyne-Stokes respiration occurs most frequently in association with alterations lying deep in the cerebral hemispheres. Central neurogenic hyperventilation (sustained, regular, rapid, and deep hyperpnea) occurs in certain patients with involvement of the brain stem tegmentum having lesions situated between lower mid-brain and lower pons. Apneustic breathing (inspiratory cramp) is indicative of damage to the respiratory controls situated at mid- or caudal pontine levels. Ataxic breathing may at times be confused with Cheyne-Stokes respiration. It retains its burst rhythmicity, but is completely irregular within the bursts.

Mention of a few of the more common pupillary abnormalities will illustrate their localizing value.[55] In mid-brain damage, nuclear lesions may interrupt both sympathetic and parasympathetic ocular circuits leaving the pupil in midposition and fixed to all stimuli. Pontine lesions produce bilaterally small pupils, and lateral medullary lesions an ipsilateral Horner's syndrome with slight ptosis.

In examining ocular motility, chief reliance is placed upon the state of the eyes at rest and upon components of oculocephalic and oculovestibular reflexes, the former produced by brisk rotation of the head from side to side and up and down, the latter by caloric (ice water) stimulation. In light coma the oculocephalic reflexes can be demonstrated consistently, and caloric stimulation produces tonic lateral deviation. With greater cortical depression, which leaves brain stem mechanisms relatively intact, both reflexes become very brisk. There are two principal intrinsic deficits in optic motility having localizing value. One, a conjugate gaze paralysis, points to the pontine tegmentum; the other, paralysis of adduction called internuclear ophthalmoplegia, is a disconjugate gaze paralysis due to involvement of the median longitudinal fasciculus between the vestibular and III nerve nuclei.

"Drop attacks"[56] occasionally signal a susceptibility to transient brain stem ischemia. The attack occurs while the subject is standing or walking, and comes on abruptly without warning. It is produced by a transient loss of strength in the lower extremities, and characteristically there is no alteration of consciousness; vision, hearing, and speech remain intact.

Ingvar and Lundberg[21] recorded EEG and ventricular fluid pressure (VFP) simultaneously in patients showing increased intracranial pressure associated with brain tumor. Paroxysmal variations in the VFP were observed in the form of large, suddenly appearing plateau waves with peaks of 100 mm. Hg and rhythmically recurring VFP variations showing a frequency of 1 to 2 per minute. It is important to note that high plateau waves can be accompanied by loss of consciousness and tonic-clonic movements. Only subtle EEG changes are found to accompany plateau waves. The onset of such a wave can be accompanied by the arousal type of EEG change; its termination with hyperventilation shows an increase in slow activity. However, despite the loss of consciousness and obvious tonic-clonic movements, no convulsive activity appears in the electroencephalogram. They conclude that the convulsive phenomena observed resulted from brain stem seizures.

The evidence from organic lesions of brain stem and thalamus points to the consciousness inherent in this region as being essentially a *crude consciousness*. This leaves the cerebral cortex essential for the manifestation of higher levels of consciousness, even though a healthy cerebral cortex cannot of itself maintain the conscious state. Massive bifrontal lesions in man, for example, have been shown not to disturb crude consciousness, but instead to impair will, initiative, foresight, and judgment.[18]

ABNORMAL STATES OF CONSCIOUSNESS AND THEIR ETIOLOGIES

Figure 31-1 presents a scheme of the relationships of the waking state to normal sleep and to coma of a variety of etiologies as taken up in the ensuing account.

In a 1933 survey of patients who entered Boston City Hospital in coma, alcohol was held responsible for 50 per cent, trauma for 13 per cent, and cerebrovascular disorders for 10 per cent.[22-24] Other causes, each accounting for 3 per cent or fewer patients, were poisoning, epilepsy, diabetes, meningitis, pneumonia, cardiac decompensation, exsanguination, CNS syphilis, uremia, and eclampsia. Those causes in which prompt diagnosis and emergency treatment are imperative were diabetes, hyperinsulinism,

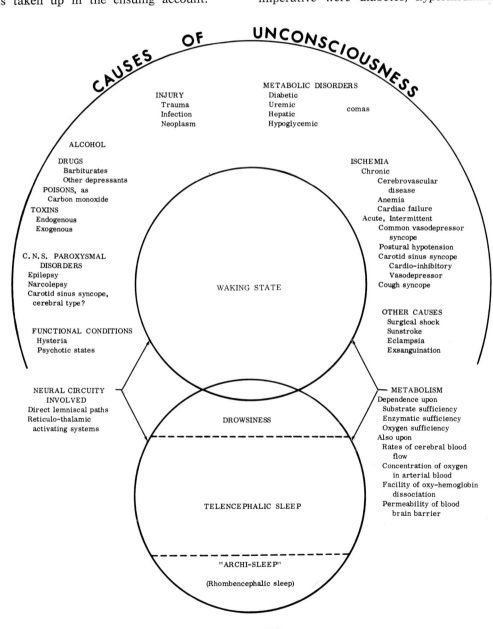

FIGURE 31-1.

TABLE 31-1. PHYSICAL CHANGES HELPFUL IN THE DIAGNOSIS OF COMA AND THE
CONDITIONS IN WHICH THEY OCCUR*

Odor of breath
   Alcohol ....alcoholism
   Acetone ....diabetes, uremia
   Illuminating gas ..carbon monoxide poisoning

Color of skin and mucous membranes
   Hyperemic ....alcoholism
   Cherry red ....carbon monoxide poisoning
   Cyanosis ....cardiac decompensation,
                          pneumonia
   Pallor ....hemorrhage, pernicious anemia
   Jaundice ....cholemia

Local signs of injury ....trauma, burns,
         hemorrhage, epilepsy, erysipelas

Temperature
   Increased ....pneumonia, meningitis,
                       encephalitis
   Decreased ....carbon monoxide poisoning,
                        diabetes
Pulse
   Rapid ....diabetes, pneumonia,
                 meningitis, eclampsia
   Irregular ....cardiac decompensation
   Slow ....Stokes-Adams disease

Respiration
   Kussmaul ....diabetes
   Increased ....pneumonia

Hemiplegia ....cerebral vascular lesions

Observation of convulsions ....epilepsy, cerebral
      vascular lesions, central nervous
          system syphilis, alcoholism
Vomiting ....cerebral hemorrhage,
                     poisoning
Stiffness of the neck ....meningitis, cerebral
                 vascular lesions
Kernig's leg sign positive ...meningitis, cerebral
                 vascular lesions
Chest signs
   Consolidation ....pneumonia
   Fluid ....empyema, ruptured aortic
                     aneurysm
Pulmonary congestion ....ascites, enlarged
        liver, distended neck veins,
          cardiac decompensation

Distention and spasticity of
   the abdomen ......ruptured esophageal varix,
       carcinomatous erosion of the
       gastrointestinal tract, ruptured
       ectopic pregnancy, miliary
           tuberculosis
Muscular twitchings ....uremia
Abdominal tumor ....eclampsia
Bulging fontanels ....meningitis
Soft eyeballs ....diabetes
Wounds or scars on the tongue ....epilepsy
Vaginal examination abnormal .....pelvic malig-
      nancy, ruptured ectopic pregnancy
Blood pressure
   Increased ....cerebral vascular lesions,
               uremia, eclampsia
   Decreased ....trauma

* Courtesy of Solomon and Aring: J.A.M.A. 105:7.

poisoning, traumatic shock, exsanguination, subdural hematoma, brain tumor, abscess, meningitis, and eclampsia. History was of immediate importance in 60 per cent of cases, and ambulance drivers were instructed to bring in a relative, or other witness whenever possible to facilitate obtaining a history. Depth of coma, state of reflexes and pupils were not found to be of great diagnostic importance, although of course neurological signs ordinarily depended upon the depth of the coma. Tables 31-1 and 31-2, from Solomon and Aring,[22] provide excellent summaries of physical and laboratory observations helpful in the differential diagnosis of coma and of the conditions in which it occurs.

Hereafter we outline the salient features of a variety of conditions which cause coma. The discussion is necessarily far from complete.

HEAD TRAUMA

The best possible history and neurologic appraisal are always obtained. For future reference Symonds[25] advises us to distinguish between patients who are never unconscious, those unconscious but a few moments, and those who exhibit prolonged periods of unconsciousness. Patients with cerebral contusion may show focal neurologic signs. Those with severe head injury (as in automobile accidents) who come to postmortem often show severe laceration of the orbital surfaces of the frontal lobes and the tips of the temporal lobes.[26] In middle meningeal hemorrhage (epidural hematoma) a brief interval of unconsciousness following the accident may be succeeded by lucidity, and several hours later a rapidly deepening coma may develop. Subdural hematoma may be acute or chronic. In the latter instance gradually

TABLE 31-2. LABORATORY OBSERVATIONS
HELPFUL IN THE DIAGNOSIS OF COMA AND
THE CONDITIONS IN WHICH THEY OCCUR*

Lumbar puncture: spinal fluid
Pressure
    Increased ....cerebral vascular
        lesions, meningitis trauma,
        central nervous system syphilis
    Decreased ....diabetes
Bloody fluid ....cerebral vascular
        lesions, trauma
Purulent fluid ....meningitis
Organisms by smear and culture ...meningitis
Sugar
    Low ....meningitis
    High ....diabetes
Protein high ....meningitis; central
        nervous system syphilis
Spinal fluid Wassermann positive ..central nervous system syphilis
        vous system syphilis
Blood examination
Sugar
    High ....diabetes
    Low ....insulin shock
Nonprotein nitrogen high ....uremia
Wassermann test positive .....central nervous
        system syphilis
Low red blood count,
    abnormal smear ....pernicious
        anemia, leukemia
Culture positive ....pneumonia,
        meningitis, septicemia
Spectroscopy ....carbon monoxide
        poisoning, methemoglobinemia

Urine examination
Sugar ....diabetes
Gross albuminuria ....eclampsia,
        uremia, cardiac
        decompensation
Gastric lavage
Examination of gastric contents .....poisoning

Roentgenogram
Skull ....fracture across middle
        meningeal artery in
        extradural hemorrhage
Lungs ....pneumonia, empyema,
        miliary tuberculosis
Heart ....cardiac decompensation

Electrocardiogram ....heart block,
        cardiac decompensation

* Courtesy of Solomon and Aring: J.A.M.A., 105:7.

increasing coma and progressive paralysis may develop even when there is no history of an accident. In all cases of head injury, proved or suspected, a careful watch should be made for signs of increased intracranial pressure (as estimated from repeated re-cordings of blood pressure), respiration, and pulse. Roentgenograms are important as early as the condition of the patient will permit. An excellent brief survey of post-traumatic epilepsy is available.[27]

In prolonged unconsciousness due to head injury with brain stem impairment, it is important not to discuss prognosis in the presence of the patient, for such cases may recover and remember what went on about them.

NEOPLASM AND BRAIN ABSCESS

Either neoplasm or abscess may cause coma with or without paralysis. The history is that of progressive neurologic deficit of variable duration. Important historical data concern headache, vomiting, convulsion, paralysis, or incoordination with failing vision or personality change in the background. Papilledema is an important sign. In possible abscess inquiry should be made about past lung, ear, or sinus disease with or without operative intervention. A history of skull fracture also may be important. In tumor, suddenly developing coma may result either from secondary hemorrhage or tentorial or foramen magnum herniation due to increased pressure.

MENINGITIS AND ENCEPHALITIS

In meningitis severe headache may develop, acutely followed by loss of consciousness. The important diagnostic signs are nuchal rigidity, and Kernig and Brudzinski signs. Dissociation in ocular movements, pupillary abnormalities, convulsion, and focal neurologic signs may be seen. Tuberculous meningitis is gradual in onset and isolated cranial nerves may be affected.

There are several types of encephalitis, any of which may show hypersomnia as an acute symptom. However, lethargic encephalitis is outstanding for producing hypersomnia. Demyelinating encephalitides are associated with vaccinia, smallpox, measles, and antirabies treatment. Dissociated eye movements may feature viral encephalitis. Diagnosis of specific viral etiology may be sought through neutralization and complement-fixation tests. These may be done on successive serum samples obtained during the course of the illness, seeking a rise in titer.[28] Hemagglutination of cells is used in the case of arthropod viruses. It may be possible to isolate virus from the spinal fluid.

"Slow viruses" recently have been recognized as opening new vistas of explanation for some of the less protracted dementias of man which may eventuate in comas. In such virus infections, evidence of disease may not appear until months or years after the virus enters the body. Kuru, a familial degenerative disease of the nervous system occurring in the Highlands of New Guinea, evidently has been transmitted to chimpanzees, and transmission from chimpanzee to chimpanzee also was effected, with shortening of the incubation period.[57] Brain biopsy material from a patient having Creutzfeldt-Jakob disease with severe status spongiosus also has been inoculated into the chimpanzee; after 13 months the animal developed a clinical course remarkably similar to that of the patient and died. Neuropathological findings were also very similar.[58]

CEREBROVASCULAR DISEASE

Coma may occur at the onset of cerebral hemorrhage, but often it develops gradually. It is uncommon with cerebral thrombosis. Associated hemiplegia is frequent. Sudden loss of consciousness in cerebral hemorrhage is due to massive explosive injury to the cerebrum and to accompanying neural shock. Cerebral embolism shows a sudden onset, but loss of consciousness is far less likely than with cerebral hemorrhage. Subarachnoid hemorrhage is distinguished by sudden onset of intense headache, often following exertion. Coma may come on more gradually. The pulse may be slowed, and meningeal signs are observed. Coma also may develop in hypertensive encephalopathy, either with or without convulsions; there is usually a history of severe hypertension.

When vascular lesions involve the lesser brain stem vessels, as the branches of the vertebrobasilar system, localizing signs and symptoms commonly occur without loss of consciousness unless the lesion is hemorrhagic. However, symptoms of attacks of vertebrobasilar and carotid insufficiency may appear as the prodrome of a massive cerebral thrombosis with unconsciousness. For that reason we list below principal symptoms of the two main types of insufficiency drawn from a USPHS cerebrovascular survey report:[29]

Vertebrobasilar Insufficiency
Dizziness
Diplopia
Blurred vision
Blindness
Pupillary change
Memory lapses
Confused behavior
Unilateral or bilateral numbness
Unilateral or bilateral weakness
Dysarthria
Dysphagia
Impaired hearing
Numbness of face
Staggering gait
Hiccuping

Carotid System Insufficiency
Unilateral weakness or numbness
Dysphasia
Confusion
Ipsilateral monocular blindness
Homonymous field defects
Headache
Possibly focal epileptic seizures

Recently Ingvar et al.[59] had the opportunity to examine hemispheric blood flow in a man of 60 who had suffered an acute vascular lesion of the brain stem from which he remained unconscious and unresponsive over an eight-month period. The EEG was depressed, showing a low voltage delta pattern. Contrast media injection of the left internal carotid showed some tortuosity of the carotid syphon; otherwise the cerebral arterial pattern was normal. Circulation time across the cerebral capillary bed was six seconds, and air study revealed only moderate cerebral atrophy. In spite of these findings, hemispheric blood flow as determined by krypton 85 showed an average flow of about one-quarter of the normal, and cerebral oxygen consumption which was reduced proportionately. A biopsy of frontal cortex presented normal findings with no evidence of neuron loss or gliosis. The case illustrates the marked reduction of cerebral metabolism and circulation which can occur after a lesion of the upper brain stem with permanent coma.

Obrist et al.[60] present statistical results open to a somewhat different interpretation. They examined the relation between EEG and cerebral blood flow and metabolism in 26 white males ranging in age from 65 to 81, comprising a healthy community group. These were compared with 26 white males, 67 to 84, of a psychiatric group. The results lend credence to the view that slow activity in the senescent electroencephalogram (as in the psychiatric group) is associated with reduction in cerebral blood flow and oxygen consumption. The healthy group failed to show any relationship between EEG characteristics and cerebral circulation or metabolism, whereas the psychiatric patients yielded statistically significant correlations between EEG frequency measurements and both circulatory variables. The indicated result of this study would appear to place dependence in the relationship between resting EEG and cerebral metabolic function in elderly people upon the existence of pathological processes.

BRAIN METABOLISM AND METABOLIC COMA

Under normal conditions, the brain derives most of its energy from the oxidation of glucose. It can metabolize other substrates, but they would provide poor substitutes because the blood-brain barrier prevents them from entering the brain in sufficient quantity to maintain a normal metabolic rate.[55] Each 100 Gm. of brain takes up 5.5 mg. of glucose per minute, and all but about 15 per cent of this substrate is used in combustion with oxygen to form CO_2 and energy as ATP. Only one-third is so metabolized rapidly, the rest being incorporated into amino acids, proteins, and lipids. A continuous supply of oxygen also is required. Without it some glucose evidently can still be metabolized to lactic acid with some energy provided; but this minor source could not fulfill the requirements of the adult human brain for more than a few seconds.

The adult brain (which comprises only 2 per cent of total body mass) utilizes 20 per cent of the total oxygen and 65 per cent of the total glucose consumed by the body, and requires 15 to 20 per cent of the total blood circulation per minute to deliver the high requirements for oxygen and glucose. Thus, when supplies of one or both are cut off, neural function fails with disastrous rapidity.[30] It has been estimated that the cerebral blood flow of a recumbent normal man is 750 ml. per minute. At any moment the blood circulating through the brain contains 7 ml. of oxygen, an amount sufficient to supply its needs for less than ten seconds. However, under conditions of reduced systemic blood pressure, as little as 32 ml. of blood per minute per 100 Gm. of brain can maintain consciousness—a little over half the usual supply. In experiments of Rossen, Kabat, and Anderson,[31] in which the human brain was deprived of oxygen by sudden and complete arrest of cerebral circulation,

consciousness was lost in six seconds. Restoration within 100 seconds was followed by rapid return of consciousness without objective evidence of brain injury.

When evaluating metabolic coma, the state of consciousness, respiration, pupillary reactions, eye movements, and biochemical blood data are important in distinguishing metabolic from (1) structural brain disease and (2) psychogenic unresponsiveness. Plum and Posner[55] point out important distinguishing criteria. The state of consciousness is particularly important in the subtle manifestations that can be detected as a warning signal in disease conditions known to feature coma as a complication. Hyper- or hypoventilation with coma may have different meanings depending upon whether one or the other is a response to primary respiratory stimulation or a compensation therefor. Thus, in defining acidosis or alkalosis, biochemical data become of paramount importance. In deep coma, the state of the pupils is very important in distinguishing between metabolic and structural conditions. Preserved pupillary light reflexes together with caloric unresponsiveness and either decerebrate rigidity or motor flaccidity suggest metabolic coma. Early in coma the eye movements are of roving character, later in deep coma they are directed forwards. In light coma the response of the eyes to cold caloric stimulation may still produce conjugate deviation toward the stimulated side, whereas minimal if any response is elicited in deep coma.

Diabetic coma usually is attributed to the gradual accumulation of aceto-acetic and beta-hydroxybutyric acids in the blood. However, Fazekas and Bessman[32] note that in diabetic coma cerebral oxygen consumption is greatly depressed, although cerebral blood flow, vascular resistance, and oxygen delivery may be normal and glucose supply far greater than normal. They attribute the condition to inhibition of cerebral enzymatic activity, adding that they find no support for the contention that diabetic coma is due to the accumulation of ketone bodies, or to changes in water or electrolyte metabolism. Others point to the difficulty in assigning a primary enzymatic cause. Plum and Posner,[55] in addition to discussing the more common diabetic acidosis with ketonemia, describe a lactic acidosis occurring especially in those diabetics treated with oral hypoglycemic agents. In the latter, ketonemia is lacking.

Hypoglycemic Coma. Arteriovenous oxygen differences in the brain are related closely to the blood sugar level, and intense hypogylcemia causes severe impairment in oxygen uptake by the brain. The almost sole dependence of the brain upon the constant delivery of glucose makes it particularly vulnerable to hypoglycemic states. Although it has other causes, hypoglycemic coma not uncommonly presents in those with a history of insulin treatment for diabetes. It may present as a delirium, as a coma with accompanying facets of brain stem dysfunction, as a strokelike illness, or as an epileptic attack with postical coma. Whereas the neurological deficits incurred may be reversible, the longer the hypoglycemia lasts, the more likely is irreversible neuronal loss.

Uremic coma is due to the accumulation of noxious substances as a result of impaired excretory and detoxifying mechanisms as well as to disturbances in water and electrolyte metabolism.[32] Laboratory determinations do not delineate clearly the cause of the coma, since the renal failure in which it occurs is accompanied by complex biochemical changes and the azotemia varies in those with equally serious symptoms.[55] The best hypothesis is the existence of a toxin of small molecular size.

Hepatic Coma. Depth of hepatic coma appears to be related to blood ammonia level. Ammonia is produced in the intestine by bacterial action and conveyed to the liver by the portal vein. In the presence of either liver failure or extensive collateral circulation such as develops in hepatic cirrhosis, ammonia accumulates in the blood in increasing amounts.[33] The slowing of the EEG correlates well with the extent of neurologic and mental disturbance. Reduction of dietary protein and administration of neomycin for gut sterilization may improve the character of the EEG. Increasing protein intake or administering methionine or ammonium chloride causes the EEG to deteriorate.[34] When the liver is unable to eliminate the ammonia, either because it is bypassed or diseased, coma or death may ensue.

Clinically, full coma rarely develops suddenly unless there has been overwhelming liver damage or massive gastrointestinal hemorrhage. Blood ammonia is almost always elevated above 50 μGm. per 100 ml., and nearly all patients have respiratory alkalosis.[61] Hume et al.[62] recently have described treatment by colectomy which can reduce blood ammonia levels and normalize the EEG, paralleling improvement in clinical status.

Pulmonary Disease. Profound hypoventilation can develop because of lung failure and lead to serious CO_2 retention along with the hypoxemia and acidosis, which aggravate the situation. The neurological symptomatology to be observed correlates well with CO_2 acidosis of spinal fluid, and perhaps with intracellular acidosis as well (Posner, Swanson, and Plum[63]). Such patients hypoventilate and can become cyanotic. Where there is obstructive emphysema as well, the patients wheeze, gasp, or puff.[55] Headache is a common feature of the symptomatology, and this can be accompanied by slowly developing drowsiness, stupor, or coma. The pupils are often small, reactive to light, and the ocular movements are normal. If papilledema occurs, it reflects increased intracranial pressure. Seizures are rare; myoclonus is common.

Endocrine Conditions. Coma can occur with myxedema with an onset that is rapid or subacute. Hypothermia and other evidences of severe prolonged hypometabolism should be evident (hair loss, thick, dry skin, etc.). Diagnosis can be confirmed by tests of thyroid function.

Coma also may develop in addisionian crises. Such patients may have flaccid weakness with hypoactive or absent tendon reflexes, resulting presumably from hyperkalemia. Generalized convulsions also may occur, attributable perhaps to hyponatremia and water intoxication.

Electrolyte Disturbances. Lesser variations in either the potassium or the sodium level of plasma are said not to affect the brain wave tracing.[35] However, in hypokalemia with familial periodic paralysis, the EEG has been reported to be normal in some instances and disordered in others. Severe sodium depletion also has been said to slow the EEG and produce sleepiness leading to coma.[36] Calcium deficit leads to convulsions and also produces EEG slowing. Excessive hydration in combination with sodium depletion can lead to convulsions and also slows the EEG or transforms it into a convulsive pattern. Impaired consciousness also can result. Uncomplicated acidosis does not produce an unusual EEG effect, although that occasioned by inhalation of CO_2 brings about some increase in background fast activity and lowers the voltage of the EEG. Temporary alkalosis, as produced by hyperventilation, slows the EEG trace and produces amplitude build-up, especially in the frontal leads. More prolonged alkalosis (from vomiting, for example) occasions clouding of consciousness and produces runs of high-voltage, rhythmic, slow activity.[35]

SYNCOPAL ATTACKS

Syncopal Attacks. The pathophysiology of fainting (syncope) is discussed in Chapter 33, and is correlated with the many clinical conditions in which it may occur.

Pathophysiologic factors in the various kinds of faints have been systematized by Engel,[37] who classifies them under broad categories of peripheral circulatory inadequacy, cardiac arrhythmias, and respiratory or pulmonary disorders. Such brief periods of unconsciousness can be brought about in one of three ways: by cerebral ischemia, localized or generalized; by change in composition of the blood; by reflex cerebral dysfunction.[38]

Ischemia is the most important of these, and the site most vulnerable is believed to be the upper brain stem, a locus already discussed with respect to brain lesions, which are prone to cause suddenly developing unconsciousness in the experimental animal or man. With prompt restoration of blood supply such lost consciousness is readily reversible. The EEG is a very sensitive indicator of anoxia, and the rapidity with which a slow delta pattern replaces usual background activity during an attack is intimately related to the abruptness of onset of unconsciousness. If ventricular standstill occurs (as may happen in Adams-Stokes attacks), brain wave slowing can be closely related to alterations in pulse and blood pressure. Under these circumstances the pulseless period that precedes the onset of unconsciousness may be variable, extending from a few to ten or more seconds.

Vasodepressor syncope[37] is the most common form of fainting, and can be precipitated by fear, anxiety, pain, or injury. It practically never occurs except in the erect posture, and symptoms usually are relieved by lying down. At the onset of an attack pulse and blood pressure may be somewhat elevated, blood pressure falling thereafter, systolic more rapidly than diastolic. Ordinarily recovery is rapid. Slowing of the EEG has been observed as consciousness is lost. An important factor is said to be the shunting of blood from brain to muscle by vaso-

dilation mediated through the cholinergic vasodilator system.

Postural hypotension can develop in several ways, the common denominator being the repeated occurrence of fainting upon a rise from bed. Limited capacity for postural adjustment is important, and micturition or postmicturition syncope occurring in the middle-aged man who arises from a deep sleep to hurry to the bathroom may have this precipitating base. In chronic orthostatic hypotension, the classical form of postural hypotension, blood pressure falls rapidly upon assumption of the erect posture. Both systolic and diastolic pressures fall, but there is little or no pulse alteration.[37] Consciousness also is lost rapidly, and is restored rapidly upon correction of the precipitating postural change. Diffuse disease of the autonomic nervous system is often held responsible.

Micturition syncope long has been believed to be due to a combination of orthostatic tension and the reflex action of a distended bladder. Recently, Tudor[64] has concluded that the syndrome results from a cerebral hypoxia due to reflex cardioinhibitory and vasodepressor mechanisms triggered by emptying of the bladder.

Adams-Stokes syndrome is the most widely known of the episodic syncopal attacks that occur in cardiac conditions. Such instances are divisible into two categories, one associated with permanent complete heart block and slow pulse (Adams-Stokes syndrome) and the other rising from reflex and/or metabolic factors with or without structural changes.[37] In Adams-Stokes syndrome, the attacks of syncope are believed to be due to decrease in cerebral blood flow resulting from ventricular standstill, tachycardia, or fibrillation. The duration of asystole may be long, and convulsion caused by cerebral hypoxia may occur. High-voltage, slow EEG activity occurs during asystole, and if the standstill persists the tracing may flatten out. Among the instances that arise in individuals with reflex and/or metabolic factors are those with transient and paroxysmal heart block. Afferents of vagal reflexes arising from the upper gastrointeric tract, respiratory tract, mediastinum, and external auditory canal may contribute to causation, as may afferent paths arising in eye or nasopharynx and carried in trigeminal and glossopharyngeal nerves.[37] Increased activity of the vagus nerves resulting from such heightened afferent impulses may cause sinoatrial standstill or atrioventricular block. This is true especially if associated with metabolic or organic changes affecting the mechanisms controlling origin and conduction of the stimulus to the heart beat. Reflex cardiac standstill and syncope can result in patients with intense paroxysmal pain in the glosso-pharyngeal distribution (glossopharyngeal neuralgia).

Carotid Sinus Hypersensitivity. Syncope associated with hypersensitivity of the caro-tid sinus also utilizes an afferent arm, which passes over a branch of the glossopharyn-geal nerve. In this disorder the specific nerve endings in the carotid sinus may be the major source of activation, but summate with overly sensitive afferents from other sources, which augment vagal outflow. Sig-nificantly more persons show carotid sinus hypersensitivity to massage than ever show spontaneous fainting of this origin. Engel[37] advocates demonstration of identity between induced (by massage) and spontaneous faints, differentiation between massage of the sinus and of the carotid below it, and abolition of the hypersensitivity by atropine as criteria for establishing the carotid sinus as the source of troubles. He points out that the sinus region in such cases usually is exquisitely sen-sitive to stimulation. Besides prolonged asys-tole, there is a vasodepressor type of response in which fall of blood pressure is independent of change of heart rate. According to Wayne[38] this is abolished by epinephrine administra-tion only.

A cerebral type of carotid sinus syncope also is described in which fainting is not re-lated to change in blood pressure or pulse and is uninfluenced by either atropine or ephed-rine.[39] Gurdjian et al.[40] believe this form to be misinterpreted and to result instead from partial or complete occlusion involving com-ponents of the contralateral arterial supply. They believe, of course, that a carotid sinus inhibitory reflex may be associated with the ischemic response. Engel has contraverted this evidence using the criteria set forth above. He has found that the cerebral type of carotid sinus reflex may be elicited by very gentle and brief nonocclusive stimulation of the sinus. Reese, Green, and Elliott[41] have re-ported a case in which the features of the cerebral type of hypersensitivity were ob-served and yet panarteriography failed to show significant disease of the cervical arteries.

Respiratory and Pulmonary. Among forms of syncope associated with respiratory and pulmonary disorders, two are selected for brief mention, cough syncope and Pickwickian syndrome.

Cough syncope is prone to occur in robust middle-aged men. Severe cough from any cause, may, if sufficiently strenuous and repe-titious, cause loss of consciousness. The faint is caused by rapidly repeated inspiration, in-complete expiration, and rapidly repeated very forceful expiratory effort against a closed glottis. Increased intrathoracic pres-sure results, which obstructs the return of blood from the cranium.

In Pickwickian syndrome the association of obesity with hypersomnolence, hypoventila-tion, and polycythemia occurs, and in this instance attention is directed to somnolence instead of to syncope. Drachman and Gum-nit[42] showed by intensive investigation of a single case that oxygen lack was the predom-inant factor in driving the subject's respira-tion and in awakening her from the somno-lent state that she might fall into.

Alcohol, Drugs, and Poisons. Alcohol is by far the most frequent cause of hospital admis-sions for coma. The signs and symptoms of *acute alcoholism* are too well-known to need emphasis here. For medicolegal purposes the concentrations of alcohol in blood, urine, sa-liva, or exhaled air can be determined. As in other kinds of unconsciousness, brain rhythms are slowed by alcohol, the degree of slowing being roughly related to the severity of intoxication.

About 20 per cent of hospital admissions for acute drug intoxication are for *barbitu-rate* poisoning. When the subject is dis-covered in acute poisoning, deep sleep or coma is characteristic. Cyanosis may be prominent and Cheyne-Stokes respiration may occur. The involvement of superficial and deep reflexes relates to the degree of central depression, and toe signs may be obtained. Pupils tend to be somewhat constricted, although they may dilate late in the course of the poisoning. The EEG shows the high-voltage slow delta activ-ity that is a general characteristic of brain activity in comatose patients. Identification can be made of barbiturates in the stomach contents, blood, and urine. For treatment, Plum and Swanson[43] believe that there is no substitute for the direct physiological treat-ment of depressed respiration or circulation; the use of analeptic drugs in their hands pro-vided little additional help. The immediate dangers to the patient admitted in a comatose state generally are respiratory. The airway must be cleared scrupulously and one must insure adequate intake of oxygen. Circulatory treatment should include starting venoclysis at the time of admission to provide an immediate route if plasma expanders or vasopressor drugs become necessary.

Opium, morphine and other opium derivatives should also be remembered as possible causes of coma. Diacetylmorphine (heroin) is 5 times as potent as morphine and is especially apt to cause addiction. It is not an official drug in the United States and its importation into or manufacture in this country is prohibited by law. Not uncommonly *salicylate* poisoning may occur (especially in children) and need consideration in differential diagnosis.

Among the poisonous gases causing coma *carbon monoxide* is important,[44] most often from automobile exhaust or from gases used in the home or produced in industry. Skin, lips and nail beds may be a cherry-red color, pupils dilated, temperature subnormal, and respirations irregular, rapid or shallow. Blood chemistry studies for carbon monoxide and for methemoglobin may be diagnostic.

Dinitro-ortho-cresol, a weed killer, should be considered where poisoning is suspected, as should pesticides which are DFP congeners. The latter inactivate cholinesterases.

HYSTERIA

Considered as a cause of unconsciousness, hysteria usually occurs in females with chronic multiple system complaints, often starting at adolescence. By age 30, such women frequently have had several surgical operations. When periods of unconsciousness are of brief duration they may have been preceded by difficulty in breathing at a time of emotional stress with subsequent hyperventilation and respiratory alkalosis (with numbness, muscle cramps, etc.).

CONVULSIVE DISORDERS

The convulsion, describable for the generalized attack as a violent involuntary contraction (tonic, then clonic) or series of massive contractions of the voluntary musculature, gives the arresting appearance to the epileptic event. However, it needs to be understood that there is no single kind of epileptic event. The seizure, as one is often referred to descriptively, may involve only brief episodes of staring, as in the *petit mal* or "absence" attack of childhood. It may be *myoclonic,* consisting of quick, contractile muscle bursts, which may be single or repetitive. *Akinetic seizures* present brief losses of muscle tone

instead of contractions and may resemble the "drop attacks" described previously. There are also a variety of *partial seizures,* which point to a focal origin within the cerebral hemispheres and relate to the pattern of cerebral localization. Of these, *jacksonian seizures* develop in an orderly march, commencing with a signal contraction in a local area of the musculature and sometimes progressing to a full-fledged generalized convulsion. Finally, there are *focal seizures,* which present with automatisms or even a complex sequence of automatisms such as is ordinarily referred to as a *psychomotor attack.* The common denominator for all of these kinds of attack is the occurrence of paroxysmal electrical disturbances of unique form and high voltage in the encephalogram. They are the sign of excessive synchronization in neuronal discharge such as occasions a seizure. Repetitive-spike and spike-and-wave discharges are the principal kinds. They and others are depicted in the EEG classification presented in Fig. 31-2. In generalized seizures of any consequence, an associated interval of *unconsciousness* is invariable, and stupor or sleep may extend the coma into the postictal period.

ANALYTIC VALUE OF BRAIN WAVES
AND CLASSIFICATION

The electroencephalogram is the most important adjunct we have to the clinical appraisal of convulsive states. In general, we believe that refractoriness to anticonvulsant drugs correlates positively with excessive, persistent disorders of brain rhythm. Certain types of seizures known to respond effectively to one medication but not to another often can be identified from unique characteristics of a disordered EEG, when other bases of clinical appraisal leave the issue in doubt. Examples are the 3 per second generalized spike-wave EEG of petit mal epilepsy and the asynchronous spikes that arise from a background of suppression (called hypsarrhythmia). In the latter condition, steroids may provide the base for successful treatment of a severely incapacitated infant.

In adults, when an aura or signal symptom (Fig. 31-2) points to a focal seizure originating at a particular site upon one side of the brain, the electroencephalogram may confirm the supposition in an interseizure interval by producing evidence of an associated spike or slow wave focus. Finally, if generalized seizure first occurs in middle adult life, the EEG may yield the first evidence localizing a brain tumor. For these reasons it is profitable to consider EEG rhythms and their classification as a prelude to discussion of the pathophysiology of seizure.

Background Activity. The first recordings of spontaneous brain rhythms in animals were obtained long before the electronic era produced a technology capable of coping with the clinical aspects of electrical recording. Berger is credited with the first indubitable records of brain activity in man. His clinical success activated a universal interest in brain recording. At the start, Adrian and Buy-

EEG CLASSIFICATIONS

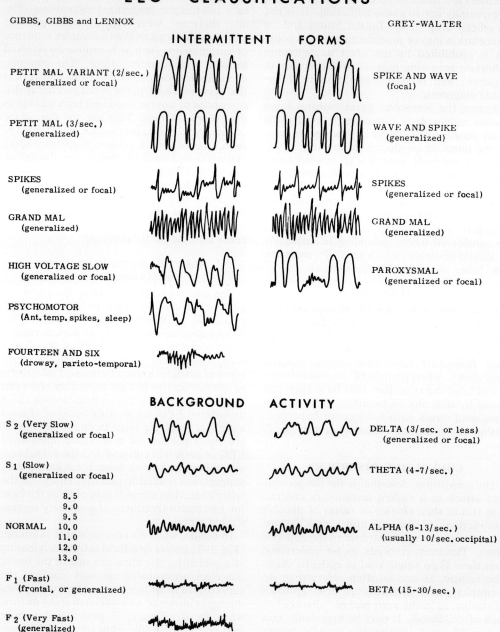

GIBBS, GIBBS and LENNOX   GREY-WALTER

INTERMITTENT   FORMS

PETIT MAL VARIANT (2/sec.)
(generalized or focal)   SPIKE AND WAVE
                                                                 (focal)

PETIT MAL (3/sec.)
(generalized)   WAVE AND SPIKE
                                                                 (generalized)

SPIKES
(generalized or focal)   SPIKES
                                                                 (generalized or focal)

GRAND MAL
(generalized)   GRAND MAL
                                                                 (generalized)

HIGH VOLTAGE SLOW
(generalized or focal)   PAROXYSMAL
                                                                 (generalized or focal)

PSYCHOMOTOR
(Ant. temp. spikes, sleep)

FOURTEEN AND SIX
(drowsy, parieto-temporal)

BACKGROUND   ACTIVITY

S₂ (Very Slow)
(generalized or focal)   DELTA (3/sec. or less)
                                                                 (generalized or focal)

S₁ (Slow)
(generalized or focal)   THETA (4-7/sec.)

                    8.5
                    9.0
                    9.5
NORMAL   10.0   ALPHA (8-13/sec.)
                   11.0   (usually 10/sec. occipital)
                   12.0
                   13.0

F₁ (Fast)
(frontal, or generalized)   BETA (15-30/sec.)

F₂ (Very Fast)
(generalized)

FIGURE 31-2.

tendijk[45] were able to show that the isolated brain stem of the goldfish gives forth a rhythm that has the same frequency as the movement of the gills in the intact fish. Ever since, spontaneous rhythms have been accepted as another manifestation of the essential rhythmicity that sustains many of life's processes. Adrian also confirmed Berger's interpretation of the 10 per second adult alpha rhythm, which is recorded from the parieto-occipital scalp area in the relaxed subject, who has his eyes closed. A variety of other electrical manifestations of the activity of the human brain also can be recorded through scalp electrodes, differences appearing in individuals awake and asleep, and at different stages of life from infancy to old age. At birth the electroencephalogram shows only low, slow waves of 4 per second or lower frequency. For the first year of life, these slow patterns increase in amplitude and are then replaced by intermediate slow frequencies at 4 to 7 per second. Finally (in a small percentage of infants beginning as early as the tenth month) the precursor of the adult alpha rhythm in turn replaces the intermediate frequencies as the principal background pattern of the human electroencephalogram. In old age, metabolic letdown again introduces slow activity into the normal tracing, and the ravages of cerebrovascular disease can markedly hasten this process. As with animals, rhythm at 1 per second characterizes the human brain asleep, and it is also the principal pattern associated with pathologic loss of consciousness for whatever reason. This rhythm (called delta and assigned limits of 1 to 4 per second) also appears focally as a pathological process over sites of cerebral infarct, contusion, abscess, or tumor.

Intermittent Forms Characteristic of Convulsive States. In addition to the spontaneous background activity described in the above, intermittent wave patterns also occur. Often these show a voltage 4 to 20 times greater than that of the background activity. They signify abnormally synchronized electrical disturbances of unique wave form, which has a very high correlation with seizure state, and can be recorded in interseizure traces. Such intermittent forms can occur as single wave complexes, or repeat the identical wave shape continuously over intervals extending from seconds to minutes. When diffusely recorded from scalp (that is, showing no localization), they are presumed to signify a generalized cortical disturbance projected from a limited

central source situated at the mesodiencephalic origin of the diffuse thalamic projection system. Grand and petit mal seizure discharges of the usual idiopathic variety belong in this category, and Penfield and Jasper[46] would list them as *centrencephalic seizures.* In the case of repetitive spike-wave disturbance, it is important that brief runs lasting four to six seconds can occur without either a petit mal seizure or lapse of consciousness intervening. Such are called *subclinical or electrical seizures.* When closely repetitive large spikes occur at 12 to 24 per second they correlate with grand mal seizures and complete loss of consciousness. Such are difficult to record during an attack because electrodes are easily torn off. However, very adequate records have been obtained by use of immobilizing drugs. There are also other unique intermittent wave forms, such as single spikes or spike waves, which appear focally over an underlying epileptogenic focus of the brain. Such indicators of the site of a focal seizure often may be recorded in the interseizure period. Thus, they are a valuable asset to the electroencephalographer, because he does not have to depend upon recording a seizure. Presumably when a seizure spreads widely from such a focus, these spikes become a confluent series that spreads as an avalanche to the remotest areas of the brain, producing generalized seizure manifestations.

It is important to understand that EEG classifications developed simultaneously in several different parts of the world. Those of Gibbs, Gibbs, and Lennox[47] and Grey-Walter[48] are in most common use (Fig. 31-2). They agree in general principles, but differ in detail of subclassification of both background and intermittent forms. In interpretation one must understand that even in the absence of the intermittent types of activity which have a high correlation with convulsive state, the degree of departure of background activity from the expected normal for age also has use in establishing an unknown electroencephalogram as obtained from a subject with a convulsive disorder. Thus, the S-2 (very slow) pattern of the adult electroencephalogram[47] occurs 20 times as frequently in epileptics as it does with normal controls. By contrast, a mildly slow tracing occurs only twice as often.

During sleep, several unique intermittent (convulsive) features can appear which are not evident in the waking state. Outstanding among these are the anterior temporal spikes, which derive from the tips of the temporal lobes in psychomotor epilepsy. Another such pattern is the "14 and 6" pattern of the drowsy state. This is most easily recorded from the temporoparietal areas in monopolar records, and is believed by some authorities to correlate highly with behavior disorder, abdominal epilepsy, etc. However, these relations have not been established firmly.

BROAD SPECTRUM OF
CONVULSIVE DISORDER

Convulsions are of common occurrence, appearing, for example, in one of two hundred draftees and in a significantly higher incidence of still younger individuals. Attacks are far more diversified than can be encompassed under the combined symptoms of loss of consciousness and massive generalized spasm. The term *epilepsy* also includes a variety of focal seizure patterns in which consciousness is either not lost at all or (at most) is altered, and those others which show fleeting but complete interruption of consciousness attended by a minimum of rhythmic movement. Features common to all attacks are episodic occurrence, brief duration, and coincidence in the EEG of the unique wave forms mentioned in the last section. Such are the inseparable accompaniments of the epileptic attack, and their occurrence as brief interludes of the interseizure EEG trace caused Gibbs, Gibbs, and Lennox[47] to refer to epilepsy as a *paroxysmal cerebral dysrhythmia*. There may be instances in which seizure develops without concomitant scalp-recorded EEG change. However, if it does, its site of origin is either at a considerable distance from the scalp leads through which it might be recorded or else it is so exquisitely small as not to spread to even a nearby electrode. Undoubtedly, both circumstances arise rarely.

The causes of epileptic attacks are multiple and can be systematized in a number of ways. One classification sets generalized against focal attacks. The origin of a focal attack is ascribed to one discrete area of the brain, and the sequence of development of the seizure somehow exemplifies the function attributed to parts through which it spreads. Focal seizures are usually symptomatic of an organic brain lesion and fall into the group called *symptomatic epilepsy*. Thus, only secondarily do they signify a pathophysiologic process. By contrast, generalized seizures of the kind referred to as *idiopathic* (or by Penfield as centrencephalic) represent a primary pathophysiologic process arising through some predisposition, genetically determined or otherwise. It is important to remember that instances of symptomatic epilepsy are not infrequent among generalized seizures. The perinatal period particularly abounds in contributory causes. Among them are changes in the uterine environment such as predispose to congenital malformations (as viral or bacterial infections of the mother), kernicterus, anoxia, and mechanical birth trauma. Encephalitis and meningitis occurring in the postnatal period also take a significant toll, and postnatal trauma is the precipitating cause in some instances. In later life, the residuals of CNS infectious processes, cerebrovascular disease, and neoplasm precipitate the condition. Thus the relative proportion of the remainder of generalized seizures attributable to *genetic predisposition* remains moot. Lennox[49] estimated that in a group of 2,000 epileptics a family history was obtained in about 20 per cent. However, the same writer has pointed out the similarity in detail of spike and wave discharges as they occur in uniovular twins. As in other disorders of paroxysmal recurrence, heredity and environment are not mutually exclusive determinants, but interact considerably.

GENERALIZED SEIZURES

We restrict the term generalized to seizures in which there is an interruption of consciousness, however fleeting, and in which the EEG discharge appears simultaneously or successively from leads over the two hemispheres.

Grand Mal. Onset is usually sudden and may be ushered in by an expulsion of air through a partially closed glottis, giving rise to an epileptic cry. Ordinarily the convulsion is of the tonic-clonic type. Loss of control of bladder or bowels and biting of the tongue are common. During and immediately following a seizure, the pupils may be fixed and positive toe signs may be found. Postictal drowsiness or automatism can occur and last for several hours. Although repetitive spike activity of the type called grand mal is the most common seizure finding, tracings from young children may show a high amplitude, synchronized slow pattern instead.

Petit Mal. A momentary stare or blank look (indicative of a suspension of consciousness) is the minimal finding, and not unusually such lapses occur for some time before being discovered by teacher or parent. The episodes may be called spells, blackouts, trances, daydreaming, even thinking, by distracted parents. They are of abrupt onset and ending, often occur very frequently, and are of brief duration. However, *petit mal status* may occur. Status attacks consist of longer lapses from consciousness, sometimes lasting for many seconds or even several minutes, without a fall or convulsion. Gibbs and Gibbs[50] detected a history of status in approximately one-quarter of their petit mal cases. The diagnosis can be established by detection of the classical 3 per second spike and wave pattern in the electroencephalogram. When such sequences are more than a few seconds long they invariably are accompanied by a typical lapse. Hyperventilation producing alkalosis, ingestion of a large amount of alkali, hydration, anoxia, hypoglycemia, or emotional disturbance may precipitate attacks. Facial twitches and jerks of the limbs may accompany a lapse, individual twitches correlating in time with the spikes of the spike-wave pattern. Sometimes there also are minor automatisms such as licking the lips or shuffling the feet. The subject remains erect if standing.

Other seizure types related to petit mal by the similar occurrence of generalized spike and wave activity are myoclonic attacks, ranging from small jerks to mass spasms, and falling spells sometimes called *akinetic epilepsy*.

Psychomotor Seizures. There is confusion between authorities as to the exact limits of psychomotor seizure phenomena and terminology for and site of origin of the seizures. Attacks with which they may be confused are automatisms of frontal or temporal origin,[45] uncinate attacks, and psychic equivalents of temporal lobe origin (as *déjà vu* and *déjà pensée*). It would appear that a nuclear pattern of automatism can attach to a variety of reported psychic experiences, including those of fear, rage, and the dream state. We are concerned, however, with the pattern of attack associated with anterior temporal spikes in the sleep electroencephalogram. That is best described by Gibbs and Gibbs.[50] For hours or days before a seizure the patient may be irritable. A seizure commences with a wild look, an inappropriate phrase, or a peculiar gesture. The movements during an attack may appear to be purposeful, but are poorly co-ordinated. To a degree they are automatic and repetitive. They may consist of simple acts like lip smacking, hand wringing, or clutching or plucking at objects. In some cases they consist in more elaborate posturing or movements which have the appearance of being purposive, such as undressing or sweeping with a broom. Content of speech is commonly affected, and may be rambling or tangential. Inability to recollect events points toward a sufficient suspension or diversion of the stream of consciousness to mark the seizures as generalized. EEG traces that we have recorded during such seizures also show bilateral disorder, even though interseizure spiking during sleep may be principally unilateral.

FOCAL SEIZURES

It is the sensory aura or the motor signal symptom (Fig. 31-3) which lends distinctive character to a focal seizure. In the case of the *jacksonian motor seizures* there are three predominant foci in the motor cortex: for movements of thumb and the index finger, the angle of the mouth, and the hallux (great toe). All such attacks spread from these parts in an ordered march of convulsion, which as a rule corresponds fairly closely with the localization of motor control in the cortex.[50] However, the march need not invariably follow the points indicated upon the familiar charts of cerebral localization. A jacksonian motor seizure, of course, may spread from an exquisitely localized source, such as the thumb or hallux, and become generalized. Other seizures with more massive signal symptoms derive from other areas of the frontal lobe. For example, the *frontal adversive seizure*, combining head and eye turning toward the opposite side, derives from the premotor territory. The *supplemental motor seizure*, which is initiated by the assumption of a posture in which the contralateral arm is raised and the head turned toward the arm,[51] derives from frontal marginal cortex extending posteriorly to the paracentral lobule and inferiorly to the cingulate gyrus.

Seizures of *sensory* origin present a variety of auras, each suggestive of a site of origin in one of the major sensory receiving areas of the cortex. Among them are auditory, visual, olfactory (uncinate), and sensory jacksonian types (Fig. 31-3). The last is the sensory replica of the motor jacksonian seizure with march, arising instead in the general sensory cortex just behind the major central sulcus, which divides the frontal from the parietal lobes. Spread of

the disturbance from any one of these may eventuate in a generalized motor seizure. Other focal seizure types are the masticatory and the aphasic (of which speech arrest is one kind), arising, respectively, from temporal and frontal regions of the brain.

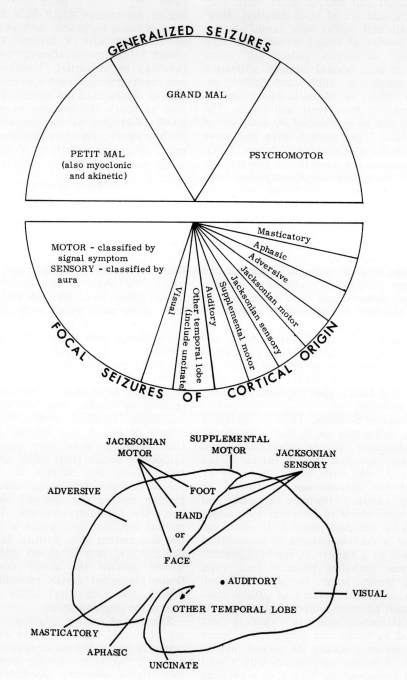

FIGURE 31-3.

Evaluation of the epileptic significance of episodic psychic aberrations rests upon uncertain ground unless indisputable neurologic concomitants occur. Such seizures pass through an intervening shadowland into mental experiences that would only engage the attention of a psychiatrist.

On occasion, sensory stimuli are known to precipitate seizures; instances of such activation by touch, pain, smell, noise, and music have been recorded. *Reading epilepsy* is a special variety of the latter,[52] about 20 cases having been reported to date. Seizures occur during reading precipitated by intermittent brief involuntary movements of the jaw. Several types of EEG abnormalities have been observed in such cases.

NARCOLEPSY

In cases in which narcolepsy occurs with all of its commonly related symptoms, recurrent attacks of sleepiness are associated with cataplexy (attacks of tonelessness), "sleep paralysis," and hallucinatory phenomena. The etiology of the disturbance is unknown, but it is believed to center in the sleep areas of the hypothalamus, if such exist. Sleep attacks may occur without warning many times a day. Ordinarily they happen when the subject is sitting quietly in a chair or lying in bed. The attack occurs without warning and may last up to half an hour. Normal persons experience a fragment of a cataplectic episode every time their "knees become weak" through fear. Laughter, anger, fright, or surprise can bring on an attack. Besides the tonelessness of the somatic musculature, the voice may grow weak and the eyelids droop. After about a minute, recovery occurs. "Sleep paralysis" is a corresponding state of tonelessness that occurs when the subject is falling asleep or awakening. Frightening hallucinations also occur in some narcoleptics.

Rechtschaffen *et al.*[65] examined the nocturnal sleep and eye movements of narcoleptics as compared with those of normal persons. Seven of the nine narcoleptics showed a distinctive phenomenon unknown in pathological conditions or in normal persons. They presented "stage I" rapid eye movement periods at sleep onset rather than approximately 90 minutes thereafter, as normal subjects do. The authors suggested that the narcoleptic is susceptible to precocious triggering of the pontine reticular substance.

SUMMARY

The chapter commences with a review of the pathophysiology of coma and convulsion. Sleep is used to illustrate a normal, reversible kind of unconsciousness that has its pathologic counterpart in lesions that destroy the rostral brain stem tegmentum. Coma also may result from a sufficient general depression of brain metabolism. The brain is almost entirely dependent for its energy upon the delivery of oxygen and glucose across the blood-brain barrier. For example, at any moment the blood circulating through the brain carries only enough oxygen to sustain functioning for a matter of ten seconds. Even a brief failure of delivery of these important energy sources through ischemia (for example in common vasodepressor syncope, or in an Adams-Stokes attack) can produce a corresponding suspension of consciousness. Disordered systemic metabolism may produce a more prolonged, although a less drastic effect upon the brain than does arrest of circulation. Uremia, diabetes, hypoglycemia, and liver disease can produce coma through interference with the delivery of glucose, or by suppression by toxins of the cerebral enzymatic activity necessary to convert glucose and oxygen to energy.

Coma also accompanies generalized seizures. In fact, a brief suspension of consciousness is the outstanding symptom in one type of generalized seizure called petit mal. In another type (grand mal), loss of consciousness is of longer duration and accompanied by massive tonic-clonic spasm of the somatic musculature. In a third type, a diversion of the stream of consciousness occurs, coupled with an episode of automatism (psychomotor). Electroencephalograms of these three principal types have distinguishing characteristics that are very useful diagnostically.

A variety of focal seizures also occur. These arise at a spot of cortical damage that results from invasion by neoplasm, anoxia, or scarring due to injury. The seizure process is the same as in the generalized seizure, and the focal attack may spread to produce one. It is the sensory aura or the motor signal symptom which lends a distinctive character to a focal seizure, pointing to the site of origin in the plan of cerebral localization. Seizures of sensory origin present a variety of auras, each suggestive of a site of origin in one of the major sensory receiving areas of the cortex. Among these seizures are auditory, visual, olfactory, and sensory jacksonian types. Focal motor seizures commence in the motor cortex ahead of the central sulcus as jacksonian motor seizures with signal symptoms in thumb and index, hallux, or side of mouth. Other types of focal motor seizure are "adversive" and "supplemental motor," which arise from other areas of the frontal lobe. In all instances, it is important to discover the etiology of a focal seizure, because it may be caused by a surgically remediable condition.

REFERENCES

1. Brain, R.: The physiological basis of consciousness, Brain 81:426, 1958.
2. Sartre, J. P.: Imagination. A psychological critique, Williams, F. (transl.), Ann Arbor, Univ. of Mich. Press, 1962.
3. James, W.: A Pluralistic Universe, New York, Longmans, Green & Co., 1932.
4. Prochaska, G.: Dissertation on the Functions of the Nervous System, Laycock, T. (ed. and transl.), London, Sydenham Society, 1851.
5. Richerland, A.: Elements of Physiology, de Lys, G. J. M. (transl.), Philadelphia, Dobson & Son, 1813.
6. Bremer, F.: Cerveau isolé et physiologie du sommeil, Compte Rend. Biol., Paris, 118:1235, 1935.
7. von Economo, C. J.: Sleep as a problem of localization, J. Nerv. Ment. Dis. 71:249, 1930.
8. Hess, W. R.: The Functional Organization of the Diencephalon, New York, Grune & Stratton, 1957.
9. Dempsey, E. W., and Morison, R. S.: The production of rhythmically recurrent cortical potentials after localized thalamic stimulation, Amer. J. Physiol. 135:293, 1942.
10. Moruzzi, G., and Magoun, H. W.: Brain stem reticular formation and activation of EEG, Electroenceph. Clin. Neurophysiol. 1:455, 1949.
11. Dement, W.: The occurrence of low voltage, fast, electroencephalogram patterns during behavioral sleep in the cat, Electroenceph. Clin. Neurophysiol. 10:291, 1958.
12. Jouvet, M.: Telencephalic and rhombencephalic sleep in the cat, in Wolstenholme, G. E. W., and O'Connor, M. (eds.): The Nature of Sleep, a Ciba Symposium, Boston, Little, Brown, 1960.
13. Huttenlocher, P. H.: Evoked and spontaneous activity in single units of medial brain stem during natural sleep and waking, J. Neurophysiol. 24:451, 1961.
14. Penfield, W.: Centrencephalic integrating system, Brain 81:231, 1958.
15. Walshe, F. M. R.: The brain stem conceived as the "highest level" of function in the nervous system; with particular reference to the

16. Puetsch, P., Guilly, P., Fischgold, H., and Bounes, G.: Un cas d'anencephalie hydrocephalique, Rev. Neurol. 79:117, 1947.
17. Nielsen, J. M., and Sedgwick, R. P.: Instincts and emotions in an anencephalic monster, J. Nerv. Ment. Dis. 110:387, 1949.
18. Cairns, H.: Disturbances of consciousness with lesions of the brain stem and diencephalon, Brain 74:109, 1952.
19. Howell, D. C.: Upper brain stem compression and foraminal impaction with intracranial space-occupying lesions and brain swelling, Brain 82:525, 1959.
20. McNealy, D. E., and Plum, F.: Brain stem dysfunction with supratentorial mass lesions, Arch. Neurol. 7:10, 1962.
21. Ingvar, D. H., and Lundberg, N.: Paroxysmal symptoms in intracranial hypertension, studied with ventricular fluid pressure recording and electroencephalography, Brain 84:446, 1961.
22. Solomon, P., and Aring, C. D.: The causes of coma in patients entering a general hospital, Amer. J. Med. Sci. 188:805, 1934.
23. ———: The differential diagnosis in patients entering the hospital in coma, J.A.M.A. 105:7, 1935.
24. ———: A routine diagnostic procedure for the patient who enters the hospital in coma, Amer. J. Med. Sci. 191:357, 1936.
25. Symonds, C. P.: Concussion and contusion of the brain and their sequelae, in Brock, S., (ed.): Injuries of the Skull, Brain and Spinal Cord, ed. 4, Baltimore, Williams & Wilkins, 1960.
26. Courville, C. B.: Pathology of the Central Nervous System, Mountain View, Calif., Pacific Press Pub. Ass., 1937.
27. Walker, A. E.: Posttraumatic Epilepsy, Springfield, Ill., Thomas, 1949.
28. Robbins, F. C.: The clinical and laboratory diagnosis of viral infections of the central nervous system, in Fields, W. S., and Blattner, R. J. (eds.): Viral Encephalitis, Springfield, Ill., Thomas, 1958.
29. Survey Report: Cerebrovascular Study Group, Institute of Neurological Diseases and Blindness, National Institutes of Health, Bethesda, Md. and St. Louis, Mo., revised ed. Bardgett Printing & Publishing Co., 1965.
30. Tower, D. B.: Neurochemistry, Report of an Extramural Survey and Program Committee, Neurological & Allied Sciences, U.S. Public Health Service, Bethesda, Md. and St. Louis, Mo., Bardgett Printing & Publishing Co., 1960.
31. Rossen, R., Kabat, H., and Anderson, J. P.: Acute arrest of cerebral circulation in man, Arch. Neurol. Psychiat. 50:510, 1943.
32. Fazekas, J. F., and Bessman, A. M.: Coma mechanisms, Amer. J. Med. 15:804, 1953.
33. McLagen, N. F.: The biochemistry of coma,

automatic apparatus of Carpenter (1850) and to the "centrencephalic integrating system" of Penfield, Brain 80:510, 1957.

in Biochemical Aspects of Neurological Disorders, Oxford, Blackwell Scientific Pub., 1959.

34. Parsons-Smith, B. G., Summerskill, W. H. J., Dawson, A. M., and Sherlock, S.: The electroencephalogram in liver disease, Lancet 2:867, 1957.

35. Kiloh, L. G., and Osselton, J. W.: Clinical Electroencephalography, London, Butterworths, 1961.

36. Moyer, C. A.: Fluid Balance, Chicago, Year Book, 1953; Personal communication.

37. Engel, G. L.: Fainting, Springfield, Ill., Thomas, 1962.

38. Wayne, H. H.: Syncope, Amer. J. Med. 30:418, 1961.

39. Weiss, S., and Baker, J. P.: The carotid sinus reflex in health and disease. Its role in the causation of fainting and convulsions, Medicine 12:297, 1933.

40. Gurdjian, E. S., Webster, J. E., Hardy, W. G., and Lindner, D. W.: Nonexistence of the so-called cerebral form of carotid sinus syncope. Neurology 8:818, 1958.

41. Reese, C. L., Green, J. B., and Elliott, F. A.: The cerebral form of carotid sinus hypersensitivity, Neurology 12:492, 1962.

42. Drachman, D. B., and Gumnit, R. J.: Periodic alteration of consciousness in the "Pickwickian" syndrome, Arch. Neurol. 6:471, 1962.

43. Plum, F., and Swanson, A. G.: Barbiturate poisoning treated by physiological methods with observations on effects of betamethylglutarimide and electrical stimulation, J.A.M.A. 163:827, 1957.

44. Polson, C. J. and Tattersall, R. N.: Advances in clinical toxicology, Practitioner 187:549, 1961.

45. Adrian, E. D., and Buytendijk, F. J.: Potential changes in the isolated brain stem of the goldfish, J. Physiol. 71:121, 1931.

46. Penfield, W., and Jasper, H.: Epilepsy and Functional Anatomy of the Brain, Boston, Little, Brown, 1954.

47. Gibbs, F. A., Gibbs, E. L., and Lennox, W. G.: Electroencephalographic classification of epileptic patients and control subjects, Arch. Neurol. Psychiat. 50:111, 1943.

48. Grey-Walter, W.: Normal rhythms—their development, distribution and significance, *in* Electroencephalography, a Symposium on its Various Aspects, London, MacDonald, 1950.

49. Lennox, W. G.: Epilepsy and Related Disorders, vol. 1, Boston, Little, Brown, 1960.

50. Gibbs, F. A., and Gibbs, E. L.: Atlas of Electroencephalography, vol. 2, Cambridge, Mass., Addison-Wesley, 1952.

51. Walshe, F. M. R.: On the mode of representation of movements in the motor cortex with special reference to "convulsions beginning unilaterally," Brain 66:104, 1943.

52. Ajmone Marsan, C. and Ralston, B. R.: The Epileptic Seizure: Its Functional Morphology and Diagnostic Significance, Springfield, Ill., Thomas, 1957.

53. Bickford, R. G., Whelan, J. L., Klass, D. W., and Corbin, K. B.: Reading epilepsy: clinical and electroencephalographic studies on a new syndrome, Trans. Amer. Neurol. Ass., pp. 100–102, 1956.

54. Ad Hoc Committee, Harvard Medical School, Report to examine the definition of brain death, J.A.M.A., 205:337, Aug. 5, 1968.

55. Plum, F., and Posner, J. B.: Diagnosis of Stupor and Coma, Contemporary Neurology Series, Philadelphia, Davis & Co., 1966.

56. Kubala, M. J., and Millikan, C. H.: Diagnosis, pathogenesis and treatment of "drop attack," Arch. Neurol. 11:107, 1964.

57. Gajdusek, D. C., Gibbs, C. J., Jr., and Alpers, M.: Transmission and passage of experimental Kuru to chimpanzees, Science 155:212, 1968.

58. Gibbs, C. J., Gajdusek, D. C., Asher, D. M., Alpers, M. P., Beck, E., Daniel, P. M., and Matthews, W. B.: Creutzfeldt-Jakob Disease (Spongiform encephalopathy): Transmission to the chimpanzee, Science 161:388, 1968.

59. Ingvar, D. H., Haggendal, E., Nilsson, N. J., Sourander, P., Wickbom, I., and Lassen, N. A.: Cerebral circulation and metabolism in a comatose patient, Arch. Neurol. 11:13, 1964.

60. Obrist, W. D., Sokoloff, L., Lassen, N. A., Lane, M. H., Butler, R. N., and Feinberg, I.: Relation of EEG to cerebral blood flow and metabolism in old age, Electroenceph. Clin. Neurophysiol. 15:610, 1963.

61. Plum, F.: Metabolic encephalopathies *in* Conn, H. F., Clohecy, R. J., and Conn, R. B. (eds.): Current Diagnosis, Philadelphia, Saunders, 1966.

62. Hume, H. A., Erb, W. H., Stevens, L. W., and Hallahan, J. D.: Treatment of hepatic encephalopathy by surgical exclusion of the colon, J.A.M.A. 196:593, 1966.

63. Poser, J. B., Swanson, A. G., and Plum, F.: Acid-base balance in cerebrospinal fluid, Arch. Neurol. 12:479, 1965.

64. Tudor, I.: Sincopa la mictiune, Neurologia (Bucur.) 11:229, 1966.

65. Rechtschaffen, A., Wolpert, E. A., Dement, W. C., Mitchell, S. A., and Fisher, C.: Nocturnal sleep of narcoleptics, Electroenceph. Clin. Neurophysiol. 15:599, 1963.

32

Disturbances of Movement

WILLIAM M. LANDAU and JAMES L. O'LEARY

Because the distribution of activity in the neuromuscular system is appraised readily by visual inspection, manipulation, and palpation, both in spontaneous behavior and reflex activation, clinical observation alone has proved to be a remarkably successful analytic method. By 1900 most of the major disorders mentioned in this chapter were well-described, and in many cases correlated with neuropathologic findings. Most of the groundwork had been laid during the time that Cajal and Sherrington were developing our modern concepts of the neuron doctrine, the synapse, the reflex, and the final common path. In fact, many of the important early studies in neuroanatomy were derived from clinical material. In physiology, as Walshe has pointed out, the experiments demonstrating the electrical excitability of the motor cortex in animals were based upon the clinical observations and inferences of Hughlings Jackson.

The fact that Jackson's early studies upon the natural experiments of disease proved accurate and valid warrants more than an historical footnote, because the integrative theory of nervous functioning which he developed remains important. These ideas are the philosophical premises of most modern thinking and investigation in neurology (not of the motor system alone) and, although not often admitted, of experimental neurophysiology and psychology as well.

Here, as a framework for discussion of the pathophysiology of movement, we have space only to assert principles. For a better understanding of their derivation, the interested reader is referred to Walshe's review,[1] and thence to some of the classical studies upon the subject.

Disturbances of muscle activity may result from the following:

1. Primary muscle disorders
2. General body conditions affecting muscles
3. Disorders affecting the neuromuscular junction
4. Peripheral nerve disorders
5. Central nervous system disorders
6. General body conditions, which may affect the peripheral nerves, the central nervous system, or both.

Symptoms may be due solely to the absence of function following a destructive lesion, as when, for example, a muscle is completely paralyzed by transection of its motor nerve. In contrast, a discharging lesion is one in which diseased elements are abnormally active, as when the anterior horn cells fire spontaneously in fasciculation, or the motor cortex, in convulsion.

There are both negative and positive results of central nervous system lesions. The negative aspect of a lesion in the motor cortex may be the loss of skilled movement, whereas a positive aspect would be the organization of remaining neural tissue into activity patterns that produce simpler, less variably adaptive movements and hyperactive reflexes. This also is called release of function. It is inferred that neural connections that become hyperactive are normally controlled and regulated by the regions damaged. Whether or not this regulation includes direct inhibition is seldom clear.

Jackson emphasizes the view that both normal and injured nervous systems perform adaptive functions as an integrated whole. This does not mean that functional analysis is impossible, or that all regions are equipotential. It means rather that behavioral function can be analyzed best in terms of levels of complexity. The nervous system clearly is not like a system of electrical relays, the higher triggering the lower. Rather it is the ultimate organ of adaptation: its flexibility and variability of response are functions of the available multiplicity of connections. Jackson put it most simply: "the more gray matter, the more movements."

This leads to his concept of levels of neural integration. The lowest level of representation of movement in Jackson's language is the anterior horn cell and the local segmental reflex connections. This stump of the nervous system is capable of mediating stereotyped protective and ambulatory movements. A higher level of adaptive response in organized behavior is possible when the organism has available brain stem and motor cortical connections. The highest level of behavior is available with the complete nervous system.

A specific example of the levels of CNS dysfunction may be presented for the tongue. If the motor nerve is damaged, there is complete paralysis. If the pyramidal tract and brain stem connections are damaged, the motoneuron and the muscle remain intact, and can be activated in some reflexes, but most complex organized movement is not possible. If the motor cortex is relatively spared, the tongue may move quite well in complex movements of swallowing and purposeful movements of the tongue upon command. But if the region around the left Sylvian fissure is damaged, the patient will be aphasic and still unable to use the tongue in the most complex movements of speech.

Many movement disorders have several aspects of malfunction. Thus, their arbitrary assignment in the classification that follows is only for convenience of presentation.

IMPAIRED MOVEMENT

Muscular Dystrophy

The primary symptom of muscle disease is the weakness in the movements of affected muscles. Clinical definition depends upon the distribution and the course of impairment. Distortions of movement may result from compensatory efforts to overcome weakness.

There are several varieties of progressive muscular dystrophy.[2,3] The majority have their onset early in life, with progression slowly over a period of years, and with impairment of the proximal musculature early and most severely. The most common type is inherited as a sex-linked recessive. It probably occurs only in boys, begins during the first few years of life, and leads to severe disability before maturity. The early symptoms are difficulty in climbing stairs and in arising from the recumbent position. Observation of this performance shows that the patient uses his hands to climb up the furniture or his own extremities in order to overcome the weakness of his trunk and pelvic girdle muscles. There is usually a swayback posture. The gait is waddling because of gluteal weakness. Stretch reflexes and response to direct muscle percussion are decreased. The calf muscles are prominently spared early in the course of the disease and may be enlarged by increased size of muscle fibers. However, true "pseudohypertrophy" due to fatty infiltration, with or without weakness, is rare.

Other varieties may affect either sex, may be inherited as dominant or recessive characters, usually start in the later first to third decades, progress less rapidly, and may affect primarily the face and shoulder girdles or both limb girdles. There are rare families afflicted with dystrophy of distal limb muscles. Hereditary extraocular muscle dystrophy presents symptoms in adult life.

The most common cause of distal myopathy in early adult life is myotonic dystrophy. In addition to slowly progressive involvement of the forearms and legs, along with the diagnostic myotonic phenomenon (see below), there are prominent atrophy of the sternomastoid and facial muscles, baldness, early lenticular cataract, gonadal atrophy, and other endocrine hypofunction.

The hypotonic, floppy infant is a complex diagnostic problem.[3,4] Many such patients suffer from diffuse brain damage, either congenital or progressive, and generally are severely retarded. When such processes are excluded, the most common disease of floppy babies is infantile motoneuron disease (Werdnig-Hoffman). Also progressive is an infantile variety of progressive muscular dystrophy. Recent muscle biopsy studies using electronmicroscopy and histochemical techniques have defined several varieties of rare genetically determined myopathies associated with clinical pictures of nonprogressive or very slowly progressive weakness and hypotrophy. Infantile varieties of polyneuritis, polymyositis, and myasthenia gravis also may occur.

POLYMYOSITIS

This is one of the collagen diseases. When there is associated skin or gastrointestinal involvement, it is called dermatomyositis. The disease may develop at any age but appears most commonly in adult life and then is often associated with a malignant neoplasm. Symmetrical muscle wasting and weakness, usually in a proximal distribution, develop over periods of weeks to years. Muscle tenderness and pain may occur but are relatively uncommon. The clinical and even the biopsy findings may be quite similar to those of hereditary dystrophy, and only the age of onset, the clinical course, and the absence of family history may be distinctive.[5] Since many cases respond well to steroid therapy, clinical distinction is of practical importance. The EMG often shows fibrillation potentials and small motor units. Several serum enzymes also may be increased. Rare causes of localized or diffuse myositis are sarcoidosis and trichinosis.

METABOLIC MYOPATHIES

Rarely, myopathy is related to endocrine malfunction. Weakness usually is diffuse, but sometimes is more prominent proximally or distally.

Hyperthyroid myopathy may be proximal or general. Fasciculation, bulbar weakness, and eye muscle involvement may occur along with wasting. Thus there may be confusion with motoneuron disease or with myasthenia gravis; indeed, the latter also may be present. Hyperthyroidism is char-

acterized by weakness, sometimes muscle enlargement, and a unique slowed relaxation due to abnormality of the contractile mechanism. This may be clinically evident in the tendon jerks. A proximal or diffuse weakness and wasting has been reported with hyperparathyroidism.

A proximal or generalized myopathy may occur in Cushing's syndrome, spontaneous or induced. Myopathy in Addison's disease is associated with joint contractures thought related to primary affection of facial tissue.

Hyperinsulinism may produce a distal, or less often proximal muscle impairment. Evidence for both primary myopathy and neuropathy has been recorded. There is controversy concerning the occurrence of a primary myopathy in diabetes mellitus.

Congenital deficiency of muscle phosphorylase (McArdle) results in inability to metabolize muscle glycogen. The patient suffers painful muscle cramping leading to muscle contracture and weakness when he attempts to exercise beyond a minimum rate. These patients also may have myoglobinuria following excessive exercise. Muscle wasting is not conspicuous. When the syndrome occurs in middle age or beyond, there is a significantly increased incidence of associated malignant disease, especially carcinoma of the lung. In this and several other enzymatic disturbances which prevent normal glycogen degradation (glycogenoses), a useful screening test is the absence of normal elevation of lactate in venous blood derived from ischemically exercised muscle.[45] The specific defect then may be defined by biochemical and histochemical studies of biopsy material.

PERIODIC PARALYSIS

Normal muscle membrane resting potential is determined primarily by the relative concentrations of K^+ inside and outside the cell. The resting membrane is relatively impermeable to Na^+ and the K^+ concentration gradient is maintained by a metabolically active pump which extrudes Na^+. The K^+ thus diffuses inward to maintain ionic equilibrium; there is evidence that potassium is actively pumped inward also by linkage with the sodium pump mechanism.

Secretion of acetylcholine at the endplate results there in a drastically increased membrane conductance for both Na^+ and K^+. The propagated action potential is then sustained by a transient regenerative and explosive increase in Na^+ conductance and inward flux, resulting in a transient reversal of membrane potential. With inactivation, the restoration of Na+ impermeability, rapid diffusion of K+ out of the cell, accelerated by a transient increase in K+ conductance, returns the membrane to the resting level. The sarcolemmal conducted action potential is thought to extend into the muscle fibre via the transverse tubule system, resulting in the activation of a process involving Ca+ release which causes the actin and myosin protein fibrils to slide together and thus shorten the muscle. There is evidence that depression of resting potential augments the ionic pump maintenance mechanism. Combined microelectrode, biochemical, and metabolic studies are beginning to explore the possible disturbances of these complex processes that may occasion the symptoms of the conditions under consideration here.

Periodic paralysis is a recurrent acute familial syndrome of severe weakness leading to paralysis which comes on over a period of minutes to hours. Each episode lasts a few hours to a day or more. The originally described periodic paralysis is usually associated with hypokalemia during attacks that may be reversed by potassium therapy. The paralysis is characteristically ascending and tends to spare the respiratory muscles.

Attacks of familial periodic paralysis occur during exercise or following a rest, often at night, and may be provoked by the administration of glucose or insulin, or both, and sometimes by adrenalin. An association is suggested between the movement of glucose into cells and the movement of K+, and a related effect on Na+ conductance or an effect on K+ and Na+ transport. Microcystic lesions are seen within muscle fibers during attacks. Especially among Japanese, the condition may be associated with hyperthyroidism and may be cured by treatment of the latter. A unique feature is the electrical inexcitability of both motor nerves and muscles during an attack. Muscle membrane potentials have been shown to be normal at this time. Potassium therapy may help.

When diabetes mellitus is treated vigorously with insulin, especially when high insulin doses are used in the treatment of diabetic acidosis, extracellular K enters cells with glucose; serum K, initially high, may fall to subnormal levels and muscle weakness may become a striking symptom.

Subnormal K in extracellular fluids is associated with muscular weakness or paralysis in many conditions other than the rare "familial periodic paralysis." These include the following: (1) High K loss via the renal route from any cause: (a) rapid, heavy or prolonged diuresis; (b) potassium-losing nephropathies (renal tubular acidosis, etc.); (c) steroid hormone effects with renal K loss and Na retention: Cushing's syndrome, hyperaldosteronism, hyperadrenocorticism, steroid therapy. (2) High K loss via the gastrointestinal route: vomiting, diarrheal diseases, excessive catharsis.

Paradoxically, a periodic weakness may also occur with intoxication. Chapter 35 discusses potassium metabolism.

Studies have not yet explained how or why both hypokalemia and hyperkalemia are associated with muscle paralysis. Gamstorp has described a familial periodic paralysis associated with hyperkalemia or normokalemia. Attacks usually follow shortly upon exercise, and yet sometimes may be "worked off" by resuming activity. They may be provoked by potassium administration and often may be prevented by K+ retaining diuretics. Muscle fibers are significantly depolarized during attacks.[46]

Paramyotonia congenita is an hereditary disease related to myotonia in which symptoms of stiffness and paralysis are provoked by exposure to cold or occur spontaneously. Several authors think that this is essentially the same as Gamstorp's disease.

A subacute syndrome of generalized weakness may be due to **poisoning** of the neural portion of the muscle endplate by botulinus toxin. The toxin secreted by some species of ticks produces progressive paralysis by poisoning of the motor neuron fiber. Removing the tick reverses the paralysis.

MYASTHENIA

Myasthenia gravis is the archetype of disease at the muscle end-plate. Classically, this has been considered to be a disorder of neuromyal transmission, analogous to poisoning by competitive acetylcholine blocking agents like curare. Because individual muscles vary in their degree of clinical and pharmacologic impairment, it has been postulated that there is a localized defect in acetylcholine metabolism or in the end-plate membrane with curarelike poisoning by a metabolic product like choline.[6,7]

The *neuromuscular junction* consists of the motor end-plate and the terminal fibers of the motor nerves that penetrate it. The nerve fibers and muscle membrane are not in direct contact, but are separated by a small gap. Present belief is that a neurohumoral agent, presumably *acetylcholine*, transmits the impulse from nerve to muscle.

The acetylcholine is supposed to be released from the nerve terminals, and it is believed that its action is to depolarize and establish the true end-plate potential; the impulse is propagated along the sarcolemmal membrane as the muscle action spike potential, which in turn initiates muscular contraction.

The acetylcholine survives only a few milliseconds. It is destroyed rapidly by the enzyme cholinesterase, which is normally present at the end-plate.

The essential pathophysiology of myasthenia gravis is still an enigma, but it seems definitely to be a disorder of neuromuscular transmission. Anticholinesterase drugs combine directly with cholinesterase and prevent it from destroying acetylcholine. Carefully adjusted individualized doses improve muscle strength for hours, and medication given several times daily often provides fairly satisfactory maintenance therapy. The drugs employed provoke parasympathomimetic effects, in addition to the effects discussed at the cerebrospinal neuromuscular junctions. They vary in intensity and duration of action and include neostigmine (Prostigmin), pyridostigmine (Mestinon), ambenonium (Mytelase), and edrophonium (Tensilon).

The most impressive evidence for a humoral agent is the occurrence of transient neonatal myasthenia in the offspring of affected mothers. Increasing evidence has developed that the long-known association of myasthenia with thymus disease implicates an autoallergic mechanism involving the contractile substance of muscle.[9] Such a phenomenon may relate to the neonatal disease, but embarrassingly for such a theory, autoantibodies conspicuously do not fix to end-plate structures.

More recent physiological studies[8,47,48] localize the conduction defect to the presynaptic neural elements, which histological examinations show to be characteristically different from the normal. Normal sensitivity of the end-plate muscle membrane to applied acetylcholine and related drugs negates the hypothesis of curariform action. Normal excitability cycle behavior with nerve stimulation, and normal frequency and reactivity of miniature end-plate potentials (MEPPs) indicate that the mechanism of extrusion of acetylcholine vesicles also is intact. However, the amplitude of myasthenic MEPPs is significantly depressed, and the characteristically prolonged increased block following strong sustained contraction in patients is simulated by the pharmacological model of hemicholinium, which interferes with the formation of acetylcholine. Thus, it is inferred that the functional defect resides in defective formation and packaging of acetylcholine, or possibly in the synthesis of a similar but physiologically inactive substance.

The hallmark of the clinical picture is fatigability, particularly affecting the extraocular and bulbar muscles, limb muscles being involved in the more severe generalized cases. Symptoms of diplopia or dysarthria are typically worse later in the day. Stretch reflexes are intact although sometimes fatigable, and muscle wasting occurs only rarely in severely affected muscles. Characteristically there are spontaneous exacerbations and remissions. Severe generalized weakness with respiratory paralysis is called myasthenic crisis. Diagnosis is established by symptomatic improvement with administration of Tensilon or Prostigmin, which block the cholinesterase enzyme at the end-plate. Prostigmin and related drugs have therapeutic value because the enzyme normally competes for acetylcholine molecules with binding sites on the muscle end-plate membrane; more acetylcholine released by nerve terminals is therefore available to produce muscle depolarization and consequent action potential and contraction.

A myasthenic syndrome (Lambert-Eaton),[10] usually but not always associated with carcinoma, especially "oat-cell" lung cancer, presents with weakness and fatigability which affect limb musculature more prominently than cranial nerves. A characteristic feature demonstrated by motor nerve stimulation at rapid rates (20 to 40 per second) is a dramatically increased response to successive volleys. At low frequencies (3 per second), transmission may be increasingly blocked as is seen typically in myasthenia gravis. The augmentation phenomenon of the myasthenic syndrome may be apparent clinically as increasing strength of persistent voluntary grasp and by a striking though transient postexercise facilitation of strength. Microelectrode studies indicate normal amplitude of MEPPs, but a deficiency in the ability of nerve endings to eject acetylcholine.[49] Along with anticholinesterase drugs, guanidine has specific therapeutic value in augmenting transmitter ejection, perhaps in relation to the sensitivity of the nerve endings to Ca^{++} and Mg^{++} concentrations. The fact that neomycin and botulinus toxin polypeptides also interfere with transmitter release suggests that some cancer cells may secrete a similar substance.

A slight degree of neuromuscular block also may occur in motor neuron disease, somehow related to disturbed function of the diseased neurons.

PERIPHERAL NEUROPATHY

The basic motor symptom of peripheral nerve disease is weakness. Following section of nerve the motor axons become electrically inexcitable in a few days and undergo wallerian degeneration. The muscle fibers supplied by the nerve undergo atrophy, and gross muscle atrophy may be apparent in two to three weeks. Affected muscles are flaccid, and although stretch reflexes are absent, myotatic response to direct muscle percussion may be increased. Sensory impairment and distortion of sensation are appropriate to the superficial distribution of mixed motor and sensory nerves.

If the gross nerve structure remains intact, or after surgical anastomosis when the nerve is severed, the central motor axons grow out toward the denervated muscles at a rate of 1 to 3 mm. a day. If reinnervation occurs, the muscle mass may be restored to a varying degree. Functional recovery may be diminished if some nerve axons grow back into muscles other than those originally supplied.

Acute contusion of a nerve may produce a physiologic block for a period of days to weeks without degeneration of the distal axons. The distal axons remain electrically excitable, there is no significant muscle wasting, and recovery is usually excellent. Even when a lesion in continuity is severe enough to produce degeneration of the distal axons, the recovery is usually better than that following surgical anastomosis because the nerve sheath relationships that guide axon growth are better preserved.

Chronic trauma may be produced by compression in several entrapment syndromes, the most common of which is carpal tunnel compression of the median nerve. In addition to symptoms of pain and sensory loss or distortion, there may be weakness and wasting in the muscles of the thenar eminence. In many cases there is a significant delay of conduction of nerve impulses under the compressed region when the motor nerve is stimulated electrically.[11] This test is of diagnostic value; the physiologic explanation of delay is uncertain, but it is probably due to inactivation of one cr more nodes of Ranvier.

Other commonly vulnerable loci are the peroneal nerve at the fibula (as affected in habitual leg crossing), the ulnar nerve at the elbow, and the brachial plexus at the first rib. Spinal roots are commonly compressed by herniated intervertebral disks near the intervertebral foramina. The anatomic distribution of muscle involvement defines the level at which a population of motoneurons is affected. Mononeuropathies are particularly prone to occur with trivial mechanical insult when there is systemic disturbance, such as alcoholism, malnutrition, or diabetes.

Multiple mononeuritis may occur in diabetes, polyarteritis nodosa, and other conditions. The more common polyneuritis is a syndrome of diffuse involvement of those motor and sensory axons which extend farthest from their cell bodies. Thus, weakness, wasting, loss of stretch reflexes, and proprioception usually are most marked in a diffuse distal pattern, particularly in the legs and the feet. The time course of neuropathies may vary from months and weeks in metabolic disturbances to an acute or subacute picture in toxic, porphyric, or postinfectious polyneuritis, lupus erythematosus, etc.

Predominant motor impairment is particularly characteristic of porphyric and chronic lead intoxication neuropathies. The earliest symptoms of subacute combined system disease, like pernicious anemia related to B_{12} deficiency, indicate mixed sensory and motor peripheral nerve impairment. Central involvment also affects the dorsal column spinal projection of sensory neurons, pyramidal tracts, optic nerves, and even general cerebral functions.

ANTERIOR HORN CELL DISEASE

Amyotrophic lateral sclerosis is a disease of adults in which there is a progressive degeneration of anterior horn cells in the spinal cord, along with the homologous cranial motor neurons, excepting those to the extraocular muscles. In addition, there is an ascending degeneration of pryamidal tract fibers, the symptoms of which overlap those of the lower motor neuron process. Thus, instead of the decreased stretch reflexes that might be expected with the muscle wasting and weakness of motoneuron damage, there are paradoxically increased stretch reflexes (as long as some motoneurons survive) and often extensor plantar responses (see below). Hyperirritable surviving motoneurons fire spontaneously, resulting in muscle fasciculation. The clinical picture is defined by the diffuse craniospinal involvement. An infantile variety of anterior horn cell disease (Werdnig-Hoffman) is not associated with corticospinal tract involvement.

UPPER MOTOR NEURON SYNDROME

This expression generally is used in reference to the corticospinal tract, for this is the largest single efferent internuncial pathway. Polemical controversy about which effects of upper motor neuron lesions are pyramidal, and which, if any, are exclusively extrapyramidal, is tending toward resolution by recent physiological studies in monkeys. Predominant effects of pyramidal lesions upon fine movements may be attributed to the finding that the most potent motor cortex projections, long known (as in the Penfield homunculus pictures) to be directed to distal extremity muscles, are mediated by direct corticomotoneuronal synaptic connections, whereas proximal and axial musculature are reached only indirectly by interneuronal relays.[50] But the pyramidal tract is not the only important effector pathway arising from motor cortex, since grossly somatotopic movements still may be elicited by stimulation of the motor cortex after section of the medullary pyramids in the baboon.[51] In other experiments, a significant repertory of fine limb movements which survives pyramid section is seriously impaired by the additional destruction of the lateral brain stem and cord extrapyramidal tracts in the same animals, whereas axial and proximal limb movement are impaired only by medial extrapyramidal tract lesions.[52] Naturally occurring lesions in man are practically never limited to the pyramidal tract. However, it may be that the upper motor neuron syndrome should be attributed to destruction of the most direct paucisynaptic pathways to motor neurons, most of which are carried in the corticospinal tract.

Spinal shock is a condition of severe reflex depression in the distal spinal cord following acute transection. This lasts for several weeks in man, with gradual recovery of both nociceptive and stretch reflexes. The former, although they are polysynaptic, recover first, and may be present in depressed form immediately after the lesion is made. At this time, the two-neuron stretch reflex is severely depressed. Yet the same motoneurons *can* be excited by electrical stimulation of stretch receptor nerve fibers (H reflex). This suggests that depression occurs at the stretch

receptor end-organs, which are less sensitive because of temporarily decreased activity in the fusimotor (gamma efferent) system.[12]

The shock phenomenon seems to be reasonably explicable on the basis of the sudden diminution of synaptic barrage at both interneuron and motoneuron synapses. The recovery of reflexes not only to the normal level, but to the hyperactive state, has not been explained satisfactorily. It has been suggested that postsynaptic membranes, thus partially denervated, become hyperexcitable to the transmitter substance from surviving presynaptic terminals.[13] Another explanation for the development of increased reflexes over a long period of time is that dorsal root neurons develop additional collateral branches, which increase the number of synaptic connections in the reflex pathway.[14] The suggestion that hyperreflexia is due to increased fusimotor tone has not been confirmed.[15,53]

A transient period of hyporeflexia with flaccid paralysis also occurs with massive lesions of the upper motor neuron in a cerebral hemisphere. This is thought to be homologous to spinal shock, but less severe and prolonged because of the larger proportion of surviving efferent connections.

The classical model of chronic upper neuron lesion is the condition evolving from a lesion of the internal capsule. If the lesion develops slowly, the hyperreflexic state evolves continuously without the initial depressed phase of acute lesions. The paralysis is characterized by being most severe in the fine dexterous movements of the extremities. Thus, finger movement is more impaired than forearm, and forearm more than shoulder. Muscle strength is usually reduced, but severe disability may be present even with good strength of individual muscles because the repertoire of performance is greatly limited. Thus the hemiplegic patient may be limited to a movement including flexion of the fingers, the wrist, and the elbow, and protraction and elevation of the arm regardless of which movement of the fingers he is attempting to perform.

Long ago Beevor[16] showed that trunk muscles may be functionally weak for postural maintenance in one position in space and quite strong in another. Thus, with a right hemispheral lesion the sitting patient falls to the left, and the *right* paraspinal muscles are weak in the effort to sit up straight. The same muscles are quite strong in abducting from the upright position toward the right.

Conversely, the *left* trunk muscles are strong in adduction from right to mid-line and weak in continuation of the movement to abduction from mid-line toward the left. Beevor concluded that the motor cortex is concerned primarily in contralateral *movements,* not simply related to contralateral muscles in the fashion of marionette strings.

After an acute capsular lesion, the phasic stretch reflexes (tendon jerks) on the affected side are slightly decreased or normally active for several days. They then become more and more hyperactive. When the hyperactivity becomes extreme, a steady stretch stimulus applied to the muscle will result in four to seven rhythmic contractions per second, each followed by a silent period, and the renewed stretch response. This is clonus. Increased resistance to passive limb movement manifests spasticity (see below).

Associated with the development of hyperactive reflexes is a functional recovery of behavioral movement conditioned by proprioceptive stimuli. If movement evolves toward complete recovery, there is also return of the stretch reflexes toward the normal level and, according to Twitchell,[17] the grasp reflex may appear transiently as evidence of the facilitatory influence of contactual stimuli.

The plantar reflex elicited by nociceptive stimulation of the lateral planta normally produces a reflex withdrawal of the foot from the stimulus. The prime movement is plantar flexion of the hallux, along with dorsiflexion of the ankle and irregular flexion at the hip and the knee. When the upper motoneuron is damaged, this reflex becomes hyperactive in a very special way: the extensor hallucis longus, which is silent in the normal plantar reflex, becomes by reflex irradiation a synergic cocontractor of the neighboring ankle dorsiflexors, tibialis anticus, and extensor digitorum longus. As a result, the hallux *dorsiflexes* even though there is active contraction of the hallux flexors. This is the *extensor toe sign of Babinski* (Fig. 32-1).[18]

The pathologic reflex usually has a lower threshold for response than the normal; increased excitability also is indicated by the spatial irradiation of the afferent arc, so that stimuli applied elsewhere on the extremity than the lateral planta may be effective. On the efferent side, the extensor reflex tends to recruit a more vigorous generalized limb muscle synergy than does the normal flexor pattern.

The plantar reflex has great clinical value because it often becomes abnormal early in

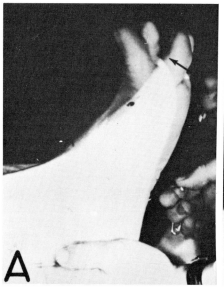 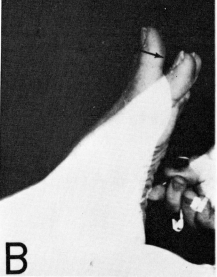

Fig. 32-1. Extensor plantar reflex (Babinski sign). (A) Superposed motion picture frames showing dorsiflexion of the hallux along with dorsiflexion of the foot. (B) Same subject after block of the peroneal nerve, which paralyzes foot and toe dorsiflexors. The prime movement of hallux plantar flexion is apparent. In *A* this movement is overcome by the stronger contraction of extensor hallucis longus.

TABLE 32-1. CONDITIONS CAUSING MUSCULAR WEAKNESS

DISEASE	DISTRIBUTION	ATROPHY	FASCICULATION	TENDON JERKS	TONE	DIRECT MYOTATIC RESPONSE	PLANTAR REFLEX	ASSOCIATED SENSORY LOSS
Myopathy	Usually proximal	Usual except hypertrophic calves	None	Decreased	Decreased	Decreased	Normal	None
Myasthenia gravis	Eye and throat, variable in limbs	Rare	None	Normal or fatigable	Normal	Normal	Normal	None
Periodic paralysis	Ascending	None	None	Absent	None	None	None	None
Root or nerve disease	In root or nerve innervation	Present	Rarely evident	Decreased	Decreased	Increased or normal	Normal or depressed	Often in nerve or root distribution
Lower motor neuron syndrome	Usually distal; can be generalized	Prominent	Present	Decreased	Normal or decreased	Increased or normal	Normal or depressed	None
Upper motor neuron syndrome (chronic)	Movements of distal parts more affected	Minimal, if any	None	Increased	Spasticity	Normal	Extensor	Sometimes as a result of other cerebral damage
Parkinsonism	Generalized hypokinesia	None	None	Normal	Rigidity; often cog-wheeling	Normal	Normal	None
Cerebellar disease	Ataxia, most prominent in limbs. Weakness is mild	None	None	Normal (pendular)	Hypotonic	Normal	Normal	None

the course of disease before other signs or symptoms of pyramidal tract damage are apparent. Extensor toe signs may occur in transient conditions of cortical depression and coma.

In progressive paraparesis due to spinal cord disease, hyperreflexia in the extensor muscles is more prominent; the resting posture is one of extension. With progression, this commonly evolves into paraplegia in flexion in which the lower extremities tend to remain flexed at the hip, the knee, and the ankle. This is also the end stage of the phasic hyperactive flexion reflex or flexor spasm, an exaggerated plantar reflex. The paraplegic limb may respond with vigorous transient flexion to a slight movement of the bed sheets, to the stimulation of trophic skin lesions, or (apparently) spontaneously. Since, it has been possible to maintain patients with complete cord transection for an indefinite period of time, it has been found that some remain in extension most of the time, and some in flexion, without significant relationship to the level of the cord lesion. Flexor spasms may occur in either circumstance. There is no clear understanding why some patients with complete section assume one posture and others another.

A transient upper motor neuron paralysis (Todd) may be associated with the period immediately following a focal convulsive seizure. Although it has usually been assumed that this represents postconvulsive fatigue and decreased tonic activity in the appropriate motor cortex, critical analysis indicates that there also may be an element of active inhibition.[19]

Highest level paralysis occurs with cortical lesions in the motor region and is called apraxia. Here the patient may have preserved the capacity to use muscles in complex co-ordination for automatic or associated movements and yet be unable to perform a skilled act purposefully, as using a key, a fountain pen, or a comb. The grasp reflex and instinctive grasp reactions generally are correlated with frontal or diffuse cortical lesions.

DISTORTIONS OF MOVEMENT AND POSTURE

SPASTICITY*

The tendon jerk is the most sensitive measure of stretch reflex excitability, because the synchronous activation of muscle spindle stretch receptors results in temporal summation at the spinal cord. Spasticity is evident when the reflex synapses are so sensitive that even asynchronous afferent impulses, ineffective in a normal subject, result in muscle contraction.[53] Thus, when excitability is high, even slow passive extension of a muscle will result in reflex contraction that increases in intensity as the stretch increases, and then suddenly gives way (lengthening reaction). This whole reaction is the *clasp-knife phenomenon which, by definition, is clinical spasticity*. The release of the clasp-knife tension is attributed to the auto-inhibitory action of high tension on the muscle tendon (Golgi) stretch receptors.

Between a stage of increased tendon jerks and that of fully developed spasticity, varying degrees of incremental-decremental plastic resistance to passive movement may be observed. In human subjects, these tend to be variable and are often difficult to distinguish from poor co-operation. True spasticity *never* occurs except in association with hyperactive phasic stretch reflexes. In spite of the reflex hyperexcitability, spastic muscles are flaccid and electrically silent when the limb is positioned so that there is no passive muscle stretch.

Although such terms as spastic hemiparesis are in common usage, the disturbance of movement is more the result of loss of control (negative effect) than it is a manifestation of increased stretch reflexes (positive release effect). To be sure, in hemiparesis, the flexed posture of the upper extremity and the extended posture of the lower one reflect the effect of stretch reflexes. But the shoulder-arm synergy of the upper extremity and the coarse circumducting movement of the lower extremity in walking, accomplished largely with the proximal musculature, are essentially the same regardless of the degree of hyperreflexia. The tendency of the extremities to cross in the gait of upper neuron paraparesis does indicate a disability due to exaggeration of the stretch reflex in the thigh adductors.

*The terms flaccid and spastic are confusing because they denote different methods of observation. *Muscle tone is determined by evaluating the resistance to passive stretch.* In normal relaxed subjects this resistance is slight but significant as compared with the hypotonia of severe neuropathy, myopathy, or cerebellar disease. Hypertonia in spasticity, as well as in some other conditions, is due to muscle contraction *induced* by the act of passive muscle lengthening. *Flaccidity is an observation of visual inspection and palpation of the muscle at rest;* this term properly contrasts with contraction. Thus, a muscle affected by tetanus toxin or parkinsonism will show activity at rest by inspection and palpation, which also can be shown by passive joint movement.

Decerebrate rigidity in animals was originally defined by Sherrington as a state of hyperactivity of antigravity (extensor) stretch reflexes in all limbs resulting from midbrain transection. The homologous condition of hyper-reflexia in man with lesions of the corticospinal tract (probably, parallel descending pathways, too) is called spasticity; spasticity and decerebrate rigidity are physiologically synonymous.

There is much misunderstanding of the pathophysiology of decerebrate rigidity or decerebrate posturing in man. A widely held view among clinicians is that brainstem transection in man produces a *steady state of marked extensor posture* of the lower extremities, with associated extension and hyper-pronation of the upper extremities. This is contrasted with a putative condition of decorticate rigidity, attributed to upper motoneuron lesion at a forebrain level and manifested by similar lower extremity posture with flexion of the upper extremity.

Clinical studies and the results of animal experiments indicate that "decerebrate posture" is *a transient state* evoked by a strong noxious stimulus or by a central pathological process (hypoxia or compression) that could produce direct brainstem irritation.

New experiments with monkeys (M. Feldman, in press) indicate that complete transection of the primate midbrain produces a flaccid animal with increased tendon jerks. "Decerebrate posturing" can be produced by noxious stimulation, neck extension, or transient hypoxia. Related clinical studies affirm the view that spontaneous evolution of "decerebrate posturing" indicates an active irritative process of the central nervous system. The concept of a diagnostically significant decorticate posture is unsupported by the clinical and experimental studies.

PARKINSONIAN RIGIDITY

The pathologic basis of this syndrome is still controversial, although many authors believe that lesions in the substantia nigra are the most significant ones. There are also lesions of the basal ganglia, particularly the pallidum, and Denny-Brown emphasizes the damage to corticopallidal and striopallidal fibers.[20] There are two major aspects to the clinical syndrome: (1) constant innervated contraction of most of the musculature at rest, and (2) generalized weakness and difficulty in starting movements (hypokinesia). The abnormal resting tone sometimes may

be relaxed by careful positioning of limbs, but it is practically always present in the waking state and is much exaggerated by emotional stress or attention. Although the generalized rigidity seriously interferes with motor activity, fine movements of the fingers may be relatively well-preserved as compared with the syndrome of the upper motoneuron. Afflicted patients move slowly with stooped posture, short steps, and lack of associated movements in the upper extremities.

Passive movement at affected joints reveals a continuous resistance throughout the excursion tested. Most often this rigidity has a rhythmic phasic quality (*cogwheeling*), which is clearly related to the tremor (*paralysis agitans*) that many patients have. Rigidity is partially sustained by proprioceptive reflex drive, since desensitization of muscle stretch receptors by anesthetic block of fusimotor fibers can abolish the hypertonicity.[21] An abnormality of fusimotor tone is unlikely. Although there is controversy about the relationship between rigidity and tremor, we think it most probable that tremor represents a reciprocal organization at the spinal level of the increased tonic neural drive from above, somehow released by the primary lesions.[54] (See Tremor, below.)

Most useful drugs for parkinsonian rigidity and tremor are related either to antihistamines (Benadryl), or to the belladonna alkaloids; their mechanism of action never has been clear. The syndrome may occur in manganese poisoning and as a toxic effect of the therapeutic use of reserpine and phenothiazine drugs (rarely with permanent effect). Occasionally such agents produce instead a choreic picture. These observations have suggested localized differences in neural transmission mechanisms in the affected regions of the forebrain.

Biogenic amines are decreased in affected substantia nigra and striatum of parkinsonian brains, a finding that was presumed to reflect the destruction of neurons containing the amines. However, administration of large doses of a presumed transmitter substance precursor, dihydroxyphenylalanine (DOPA, the L form of which is the active agent), may produce dramatic improvement of symptoms, including hypokinesia.[55] Interesting neurological side-effects may include psychological changes and choreic movements. Whether the therapeutic effect has any relationship to the pathological cell changes remains to be seen.

MYOTONIA

This is a hereditary disturbance of muscle excitability and structure in which individual fibers are hyperirritable and may fire repetitively and produce prolonged contraction in response to physiologic activation by motoneurons, or mechanical stimulation by percussion.[22] In addition, myotonic muscle continues to contract throughout the flow of threshold stimulation by direct electrical current, instead of firing only when the cathodal current is turned on, as in normal muscle. Electromyographic (EMG) recording indicates that individual muscle fibers may even go into high frequency activity without any apparent triggering stimulus. Intracellular recording has shown spontaneous oscillations of membrane potential similar to those seen in experimentally hypersensitive membranes like that of hypocalcemic nerve.[23] Involuntary muscle contraction after a handgrasp or percussion may last 10 to 30 seconds. Associated with this hindrance to normal movement, there may be innervated contraction of both the primarily affected and associated muscle (after-spasm). Myotonia may be produced in normal animals and man by the administration of desmosterol, which presumably becomes structurally incorporated into the muscle membrane so that its excitability characteristics are changed.[56]

In *myotonia congenita*, the stiffness of the proximal muscles of the lower extremities results in an unusual stiff gait, resembling that associated with hip joint disease. The myotonic phenomenon usually improves with exercise (warming-up) and may be helped to some degree by quinine or procaine amide therapy.

In *dystrophia myotonica* a similar myotonia is seen in adults. The gait is disturbed by myotonia; moreover weakness and atrophy of the quadriceps and the dorsiflexors of the feet are striking and further interfere with walking. There is also often wasting and myotonia of the facial muscles, the sternomastoids, and the muscles of the forearm. Most patients with this condition are unaware of the muscle stiffness and come to medical attention because of the distal muscle wasting and weakness.

ATAXIA

Irregular failure of co-ordination in purposeful movement generally is attributed to disease of the cerebellum or its tracts. Except for their temporal course, the symptoms are qualitatively indistinguishable, whether lesions are confined to the tracts of the cerebellar peduncles, as in hereditary degenerations; to the cortex, as in degeneration due to distant carcinoma or other toxic effect (e.g., excessive Dilantin medication); to single focal lesions, such as tumor or infarction; or to scattered lesions of cerebellum and its brain stem tracts, as in multiple sclerosis.

Limbs affected by cerebellar lesions have some degree of hypotonia and weakness, and difficulty in maintaining a stable position against gravity. When the hand is directed toward a target, the movement tends to be decomposed into oscillations toward either side of the target with a crescendo increase of amplitude, finally arrested to greater or less degree when the target is reached. This is called intention tremor. Similar dysfunction in respiratory and bulbar musculature produces explosive, scanning, dysarthric speech.

Stretch reflexes are normal in amplitude, but the hypotonic state may be seen in pendulous oscillations following the initial contraction. This is particularly evident for the knee jerk.

Although Sherrington defined the cerebellum as the head ganglion of the proprioceptive system, more recent studies have shown that afferent pathways from skin, ear, and eye also project to the cerebellum. Patients with cerebellar lesions have no sensory loss and the function of these projections is unknown.

Walshe[24] has emphasized that cerebellar symptoms are not present when there is superposed affliction of the cerebrospinal pathways, and this also has been shown when a pyramidal tract lesion is superposed on a cerebellar lesion in monkeys.[25] In the monkey, improvement is reported following lesions of the pallidum, and in man, following contralateral thalamic lesions.[26] Thus, the cerebellum is implicated in motor behavior in relation to forebrain projection rather than directly in organization at the spinal level. The theory that cerebellar symptoms are due to fusimotor hypotonia has not been confirmed.[21] Some current theories of the mechanism of cerebellar symptoms reduce to the absurd position that the function of the normal cerebellum is to prevent cerebellar ataxia. No more satisfactory explanation has been brought forward.

There is some degree of somatotopic localization of the cerebellum, in that midline lesions of the vermis tend to be related to instability and ataxia of the trunk, whereas lesions of the medial anterior lobe produce predominance of lower extremity symptoms, and the upper extremities may be involved by more lateral posterior lesions. If the dentate nucleus is spared, large ablations of neocerebellum may produce very little disability. Because the major cerebellar afferent paths and its efferent tract in the superior peduncle as far as the midbrain are uncrossed, unilateral cerebellar lesions produce ipsilateral ataxia.

Behavior resembling cerebellar symptomatology also may occur in other conditions. The fact that frontal lobe tumors may simulate contralateral cerebellar lesions has not been explained satisfactorily. The fact that ablation of the frontal lobe does not produce such symptoms has led to the argument that the phenomenon is due to distortion of brain stem structures by the mass of the tumor. Occasionally, a cerebral lesion that affects both precentral and parietal regions, associated with loss of position and localization sense, may also result in ataxia, whether the eyes are open or not.

Severe proprioceptive loss, such as occurs most typically with degeneration of large nerve fibers in dorsal roots and dorsal columns in tabes dorsalis (due to syphilis), may result in a movement ataxia, which is exaggerated when visuomotor control is subtracted by closing the eyes (Romberg sign). Other signs of dorsal root affection include shooting pains and absent muscle stretch reflexes. Occasionally, too, the weakness associated with neuropathy affecting the motor nerves, or even with debilitating systemic disease, may simulate true ataxia.

DYSTONIA

This term, indicating disordered muscle tone, usually is used more specifically to define conditions like *dystonia musculorum deformans*, in which there are severe tonic distortions of posture and movement most conspicuously affecting truncal, neck, and proximal limb musculature. Jung and Hassler[27] have called the dystonic syndrome proximal athetosis. Denny-Brown[20] uses the term in a more literal and general sense as a relatively fixed attitude, emphasizing early distortions of limb movement as the disease develops. Degenerative lesions seem to be primarily but not exclusively in the putamen along with thalamic and cortical involvement. Dystonic rigidity may be the major finding in some patients with Huntington's chorea, in which the most impressive degeneration is in the caudate nucleus. The pathophysiology of dystonia is poorly defined. Denny-Brown believes that this released activity is a common feature of the advanced stages of the other basal ganglia conditions, and that it represents released contactual reflexes.

Probably the increased motor neuron activity level represents a release effected at an internuncial level of spinal cord or brain stem, as in parkinsonism, rather than at the final common path, as in spasticity.[57]

ATHETOSIS

Denny-Brown has defined this term in relation to its literal meaning of lack of fixation or stability of position, but it is used generally to define a condition with bizarre, wormlike distortions of movement, particularly affecting the hands, distal limb segments, and face. When quiet, there is no resistance to passive movement in affected extremities. The abnormal movements are usually irregular and tend to be stereotyped, e.g., hyperextension of the fingers with hyperflexion at the wrists. Lesions affect the putamen predominantly. Denny-Brown believes that the instability represents the competition for expression of an approach reaction to cutaneous stimulation released by lesions of the precentral cerebral system, with avoidance reaction released by lesions of the parietal lobe system. Usually the symptoms are present from birth, although rarely the condition develops progressively. Athetosis often is associated with the spontaneous movements of chorea.

Tabetic athetosis is associated with severe loss of proprioceptive sense due to dorsal root and dorsal column disease. Irregular small movements of the distal extremities, particularly the fingers, are observed during posture maintenance, and sometimes at rest. It has been suggested that the phenomenon represents denervation sensitization of motoneurons.[28]

SPONTANEOUS MOVEMENT

FIBRILLATION

Spontaneous, often rhythmic, contractions of individual muscle fibers constitute fibrillation.[29,30] Since normal muscle fibers are less than one-tenth of a millimeter in diameter, and atrophied fibers even smaller, it is obvious that these contractions are not usually visible. Occasionally fine vermicular movements can be seen when the affected muscle is in the tongue or underlies thin skin over portions of the hand. Elsewhere they are detected by EMG as brief (1 msec.), low voltage potentials uninfluenced by voluntary effort.

The most common cause of fibrillation is separation of muscle fibers from their motoneuron, whether the lesion occurs at cord, root, or peripheral nerve. The orphaned muscle fibers undergo progressive atrophy for a month or more during which there are also progressive physiologic changes. Instead of the normal localized sensitivity to acetylcholine at the end-plate, the fiber becomes equally sensitive over its entire surface.[31] There also are changes in the electrical characteristics of the membrane, so that adaptation to a continuous stimulating electric current does not occur. Whereas normal muscle fibers will contract only at the make of a continuous threshold current, denervated fibers will fire repetitively throughout the flow of current and at lower threshold. There is also an increase in mechanical excitability; fibrillations are stirred up readily by movement of an EMG recording needle electrode. They are diminished by cooling. Although they may persist for many years after nerve section, they may not be present if there is excessive fibrosis. When motor axons grow back into a denervated muscle and begin to form effective contact, threshold for electrical stimulation rises and fibrillation disappears before spontaneous innervated movement occurs.

Increased muscle fiber irritability and frank persistent fibrillation are seen sometimes in primary myopathies, particularly those that develop very rapidly, such as polymyositis.[32] The diffuse inflammatory reaction may produce direct changes in muscle membrane irritability and also may effectively produce denervation by the destruction of muscle fiber segments between motor end-plates and surviving segments. Fibrillations are observed quite rarely in muscular dystrophy. Disappearance of previously observed fibrillations in polymyositis may serve as a measure of therapeutic clinical improvement.

FASCICULATION

Fasciculation is defined as the spontaneous isolated contraction of individual motor units. The muscle fibers supplied by a single motoneuron produce a brief twitch of a muscle fascicle, the size being larger in large muscles. Normal motor units in limb muscles may include many hundreds of muscle fibers, whereas those of the extraocular muscles contain only a few. Fasciculations usually occur irregularly at slow frequencies ranging from once every several seconds to two or three a second.

Fasciculations are most notorious as a sign of diffuse motoneuron disease in amyotrophic lateral sclerosis. Curiously, these patients practically never complain of fasciculation and come to medical attention because of muscle weakness. By EMG the fasciculation units in this disease are often several-fold larger and more polyphasic than normal.[33] This seems to be because surviving motoneurons put out collateral axon branches to reinnervate orphaned muscle fibers. The hyperexcitability of the motoneuron in this condition extends beyond the cell body, because fasciculations have been observed to persist when the motor nerve is blocked or even severed. This hyperirritability, plus that related to newly growing axonal sprouts, may explain why muscle percussion is a useful technic for bringing out latent fasciculation.

Fasciculations also occur with other varieties of spinal cord disease. They may be seen associated with the early inflammatory reaction of poliomyelitis, or chronically, when the cord is damaged by neoplasm, compression, or scar.

Benign fasciculation commonly is seen in normal subjects, often when they are tense and anxious or overfatigued. Neurologists in a medical school are accustomed to visits from medical students who become concerned about themselves after hearing a lecture about amyotrophic lateral sclerosis. In middle age and beyond, benign fasciculations of the calf muscles are common. Benign twitches are not intrinsically different from those seen with motoneuron disease, except that the giant, more irregularly shaped fasciculation potentials are not seen in the EMG. Nor are there muscle fibrillations, atrophy, or weakness.

Nerve root compression may give rise to localized fasciculation more often, it seems, than does peripheral nerve compression. These fasciculations may be single, or they may be brief tetani of two to several action potentials at a rate of 60 to 100 per second. These fasciculations may appear more prolonged to visual inspection than do the usual single twitches.

Myokymia is a benign condition of unknown mechanism in which the patient may complain of spontaneous muscle twitching which characteristically occurs in the multiple high frequency pattern.[34] This symptom is usually present in the calf muscles, but it may be generalized.

The involuntary muscle contraction of shivering looks like, and is by definition, fasciculation, although the discharge rate is faster. Thus it is important that the patient be examined for pathologic fasciculation in a warm environment. Fasciculations often are seen with electrolyte disturbance in toxic states like uremia. Contraction fasciculation is purposeful movement in muscles reduced to a very few motor units by the decimation of disease.

SPASM

This is a marked, if not violent, contraction of a muscle or group of muscles which is often but not always painful. The most common variety is common muscle cramp. It may occur in normal subjects when a muscle is contracted maximally, especially if it is in the shortened position, as when the triceps surae is strongly contracted with the foot plantar-flexed. Once the cramp is set up, it cannot be stopped by relaxation, but may be resolved by massage and passive extension. The EMG during cramp shows high frequencies of unit discharge, several times the 20 to 30 per second seen in normal movement.[35] Cramp may occur more readily after excessive exercise, and in patients with peripheral vascular disease, and those with motoneuron disease. Its mechanism is not known.

The spasm of tetany occurs predominantly in the distal extremities (carpopedal spasm), with the characteristic flexion of fingers and hands and flexion of toes with inversion of feet. It is due to low concentration of ionized calcium in the serum. Low blood calcium may be caused by hypoparathyroidism, in which characteristic tetany develops spontaneously. Hyperventilation from any cause may produce respiratory alkalosis, with resultant lowering of Ca^{++} concentration and associated tetany, even when the total serum calcium is normal. Excitability of isolated nerve fibers is increased in a medium containing subnormal Ca^{++} concentration. Synaptic responsiveness of neuron somata likewise is exaggerated and may be manifest clinically as convulsions.

The diagnosis of tetany may be suggested by revealing latent tetany (when it is not overtly present). Increased mechanical irritability is shown by twitching of facial muscles evoked by tapping the cheek over the facial nerve (Chvostek's sign). Irritability is exaggerated by the metabolic effects of ischemia, as shown by carpal spasm following occlusion of forearm circulation by a cuff (Trousseau's sign).

Tetany in hypoparathyroidism follows primary elevation of serum phosphorus, with consequent fall in Ca^{++}. Renal disease (glomerular insufficiency) may produce similar hyperphosphatemia and hypocalcemia with tetany, as may excessive phosphorus ingestion. Other possible causes of symptomatic hypocalcemia include: low calcium intake; high intestinal calcium loss (vitamin D deficiency, sprue, diarrhea); high urinary loss of calcium (essential hypercalciuria, renal tubular acidosis).

Tetanus toxin may provoke localized sustained muscle contraction, in the beginning only as a prolongation of normal movement, later as sustained contraction. Such a condition may last for many days. Systemic spread of the toxin early affects the muscles of mastication and produces trismus. In addition to the increased neuromuscular excitability, there may be similar effects within the spinal cord attributable to block of synaptic inhibition of motor neurons.

A condition of unknown etiology with some clinical similarity to tetanus, consists of persistent involuntary muscle contraction, (the "stiff-man" syndrome). The mechanism of the often dramatic improvement with Valium administration is also unknown. An even rarer similar condition, in which the disturbance has been localized to irritability of motor axons, responds remarkably to Dilantin.[58]

Postdenervation muscle spasm most commonly affects the facial musculature after nerve regeneration from Bell's palsy. Here there may be background activity of single motor units in the multiple fasciculation pattern of myokymia along with intermittent high frequency bursts of one or more units associated with the clinical spasm. Here, as in nerve root compression, one suspects a primary hyperirritable state in the proximal portion of the motor axon.

Generalized recurrent muscle spasm may be seen with many varieties of diffuse neuronal irritation, such as virus infection (rabies), strychnine poisoning, and various subacute degenerative neuronal diseases.

TREMOR

This term implies a relatively continuous state during which individual muscle contraction varies in a rhythmic pattern. Parkinsonian tremor (paralysis agitans) is characteristically a tremor of rest. There is a regular contraction at 4 to 7 per second which is most prominent in the upper extremities, producing the characteristic pill-rolling movement in the hand with spread to involve proximal muscles. Less often tremor may involve the lower extremities and the facial muscles. During active movement, the silent periods between motor unit bursts may be filled in by contraction of the same and other motor units as the tremor becomes less evident or disappears, only to reappear as the limb comes to a new resting position.[36] However, sometimes this filling-in does not occur, and movement may be produced by increased amplitude of tremor bursts. In most cases there is reciprocal relaxation of antagonistic muscles, but there may be "overflow" contraction in the antagonists, which is obviously a handicap to movement. Thus, muscle contraction may occur in agonists and antagonists without gross movement. Cogwheel rigidity observed with passive movement in parkinsonian patients reflects a basic tremor, whether or not visually apparent. Tremor frequency may increase during active movement, and may vary spontaneously, or even independently in antagonistic muscles.

As noted previously, we believe that resting tremor is essentially a segmental phenomenon of reciprocal reaction to a tonic efferent discharge released by forebrain lesions.[54] The rhythm and reciprocal relationships are like those of clonus released by corticospinal tract damage. Unlike clonus, the stretch reflexes are not increased, but stretch receptor function is essential for the maintenance of both conditions, since both are stopped by local anesthetic block of fusimotor fibers and consequent desensitization of muscle spindles, or by dorsal root section.[21] Shivering provides a useful physiologic model, because the involuntary hypothalamic discharge produced by cooling leads first to diffuse muscle contraction and thence to alternating reciprocal clonus.[37] Liberson[38] has shown that, when the median nerve is stimulated electrically in a patient with parkinsonian tremor, the tremor rhythm in that hand is reset so that the next burst after the shock comes at the same interval as that between preceding and succeeding spontaneous bursts. This resetting hardly could occur if the tremor pattern were established elsewhere than in the segmental level concerned. Moreover, although tremor may be affected by stimulation of various deep brain structures, no gross ganglionic tremor rhythms have been recorded from them. Tremor rhythm has been detected in single neurons of thalamic nucleus ventralis lateralis, but there is no basis for believing that this represents other than the normal afferent activity triggered by the tremor itself.[59]

Denny-Brown[20] has observed in some patients with hepatolenticular disease the evolution of less regular athetosis into regular tremor. He believes that tremor, like athetosis, represents antagonistic movement patterns released by deranged forebrain mechanisms. He also believes that tremor primarily relates to lesions of the inner globus pallidus. However, concerning neuropathologic findings in parkinsonism, it is fair to say that there is no widely accepted correlation of symptoms with specific lesions. It is certain that parkinsonian symptoms may be associated with various degrees and distributions of pathologic findings among several basal forebrain structures.

Parkinson himself observed that resting tremor disappears in the limbs affected by hemiplegia, only to return if there is sufficient recovery of voluntary movement. Thus, it may be presumed that some pyramidal tract tonic activity is necessary for the maintenance of the abnormal movement. Indeed, Bucy[39] suggests that therapeutic lesions aimed at the globus pallidus or thalamus to relieve tremor do so by inadvertent damage to the internal capsule. Lesions in the thalamus seem more likely to produce good results. Whatever the mechanism, it is not specific to resting tremor, because symptoms of dystonia, chorea, essential tremor, and ataxic intention tremor also are said to be improved by the same lesion.[40-43] When the underlying disease process is progressive, relief of symptoms by brain lesions is usually transient.

Purdon-Martin[26,44] believes that the pallidum is released to excessive activity by lesions of the substantia nigra, that the pallidum is the major efferent path of the basal forebrain neuronal complex, and that this explains why lesions of the pallidum may be helpful.

Although some workers have reported occasional monkeys with ventral midbrain lesions that allegedly simulate parkinsonian resting tremor, the results are inconstant and difficult to relate anatomically to the human condition. Thus, there is no convenient experimental model. The ventralis lateralis nucleus of the thalamus, which seems to be the most effective target for therapeutic lesions, is a site of convergence of pathways ascending from the cerebellum and basal ganglia to the motor cortex.[60] Obviously, neural activity leading to behavioral movement must descend from the cortex by both pyramidal and extrapyramidal routes, and probably from other brain structures as well. Carman's concepts[60] of initiation of movement by "precortical motor activity," "state of balance" of motor pathways, an origin of tremor rhythm in the thalamus, "imbalance or deficiency in the total input," a special central control of the fusimotor system, or the provision to cortex of "inappropriate information" from the thalamus, are unsupported by or are contradictory to facts, or else they are so vague that they have no operational significance that is subject to test. The paradoxical relative preservation of voluntary movement as abnormal movement is suppressed by thalamic lesions remains a tantalizing problem.

Senile tremor may be related to the parkinsonian variety. Head tremor is conspicuous and the hand tremor may be exaggerated by movement. It is seldom disabling and rigidity is not significant. Essential or heredofamilial tremor usually becomes evident in adolescence. There is a regular alternating tremor of the outstretched hands, usually somewhat faster than that of parkinsonism, and not present at rest. The tremor may be exaggerated during movement, diminishing at termination. Patients afflicted with this condition often can do remarkably fine work in spite of the tremor during limb transit. The condition usually is not progressive and there is no rigidity. Pathologic and physiologic bases are unknown. Flapping or wing-beating tremor of the outstretched hands in hepatolenticular degeneration (Wilson's disease, due to toxic accumulation of copper in liver and brain as a result of a genetic metabolic disorder) is slower than parkinsonian tremor, is less prominent or absent at rest, but has both clinical and pathological features related to parkinsonism and athetosis. The lesions are most prominent in the putamen.

A "liver flap," first described in other varieties of severe liver disease, is called asterixis. It also has been seen in other severe metabolic disorders, renal or pulmonary. Affected patients have clinical and EEG evidence of diffuse encephalopathy. Irregular lapses of muscle contraction shown by EMG are manifest clinically as an irregular 4 to 10 per second "metabolic" tremor or by sudden lapse of posture in the outstretched hands when the silences are prolonged (asterixis).[61] The symptom seems to indicate a limited capacity of the toxic brain to maintain a steady state of motor outflow.

Tremor attributed to midbrain lesions has features related to both the parkinsonian and cerebellar syndromes.[20] The resting tremor tends to be variable and includes pronation and supination of the forearm and protraction of the shoulder. With movement, the tremor may resemble the intention pattern of cerebellar disease.

The tremor of hyperthyroidism is irregular, rapid, and fine; it is maintained by tonic contraction of active muscles. It is not easily confused with those due to neurologic lesions. The tremor of anxiety states may be similar or more coarse, but it is faster than parkinsonian tremor, and usually does not show the parkinsonian alternation in antagonists. The tremulousness seen in various chronic alcoholic conditions is manifest during movement, is irregular, unsteady, and slow, but not ataxic in the usual sense. It is probably related to asterixis.

CHOREA

The name of this symptom is derived from the Greek word for dance. Involuntary movements at rest are irregular, jerky, and highly varied; a finger or hand may twitch or flick in any direction. Often minor movements are covered up by the patient's concealing them beneath some quasi-purposeful movement like scratching. Irregular twitching movements of the tongue, the face, and the lower extremities are usual. In advanced cases the movements involve whole extremities, and the patient may be bedridden.

Symptomatic relief may be obtained from reserpine and phenothiazine derivatives, which can produce the parkinsonian syndrome. Other sedatives also may be helpful.

In hereditary chorea (Huntington) there is progressive degeneration of the striatum, particularly the caudate nucleus, but degeneration is also more widespread. Muscle tone and the ability to move purposefully between abnormal movements are normal, as are the reflexes. Denny-Brown emphasizes a continual flow of motion in chorea, but this is not present in early cases. He proposes that choreic movement, like athetosis, is a manifestation of conflicting movement biases triggered by sensory input, and released by the striatal lesions. Others propose damage to an inhibitory system with consequent release of abnormal function. The possibility of a discharging lesion is not excluded.

In rheumatic chorea (Sydenham) the pathologic findings that have been described are quite diffuse and nonspecific. Possibly the choreic symptoms are due to anoxia related to rheumatic arteritis. Some authors believe that the movements of this disease can be distinguished from Huntington's chorea. Chorea or parkinsonism may result from carbon monoxide poisoning.

Chorea sometimes develops in the older age group without a family history. The lesions are thought to be similar to those of the hereditary variety. Hemichorea may occur following a vascular lesion in the internal capsule region. As the patient recovers from hemiparesis, the permanent lesion of the striatum manifests itself in the abnormal movements.

BALLISM

This symptom is usually present unilaterally following a contralateral lesion in or near the subthalamic nucleus of Luys.[26,44] Affected extremities undergo extreme flinging movements with such vigorous involvement of proximal muscles that the patient may injure other portions of his body or head. There may be slight weakness. Purposeful movement can be carried out between the abnormal ones. Whether these movements differ more than in degree from those of Huntington's chorea has been debated. Denny-Brown emphasizes the rotatory movements in ballism, together with internal rotation at elbow and wrist.[20] This syndrome can be reproduced by experimental lesions in the monkey, and as in man, it can be relieved by secondary lesions in the pallidum or thalamus. Such movements also are diminished by motor cortex or pyramidal tract lesions.[25] Again, the symptoms are explained as a manifestation of released inhibitory control.

OCULOGYRIC CRISES

These are involuntary tonic upward movements of the eye which may last minutes to hours. The patient may be able to look downward briefly, but the abnormal movement soon overcomes his effort. The condition is seen in postencephalitic parkinsonism and also in the parkinsonian syndrome due to phenothiazine drugs. It is presumably due to a disorder of upper brain stem function. Some varieties of torticollis and tic may also relate to undefined brain stem and basal ganglia lesions. The majority of these disorders are believed to be psychogenic, but they are notoriously resistant to psychiatric treatment.

PALATAL MYOCLONUS

This is a regular rhythmic elevation of the palate at a frequency of 1 to 2 per second, persisting even during sleep in many cases. Concomitant synchronous or asychronous movements may occur in facial, extraocular, and respiratory muscles. Lesions of various etiologies have been associated, but always in the brain stem region bounded by the inferior olivary nucleus, dentate nucleus, and red nucleus. The mechanism is unknown.

CLONIC CONVULSIVE MOVEMENTS

Focal motor seizures most often affect the thumb and fingers, the great toe, or the perioral region, presumably because the motor cortex has powerful direct corticomotoneuronal connections to these distal muscles.[50] The strong muscle contractions are brief tetani, rhythmic or irregular, and are impossible to control by effort. The movements are produced by sudden bursts of high frequency discharge into the pyramidal tract. In general, such seizures connote abnormal discharge in the motor cortex rather than in subcortical regions. Clonic jerks may sometimes build up into tonic prolonged contractions, usually with spread to other areas (jacksonian seizure).

Short rhythmic bursts of muscle jerks (myoclonus), at the brain wave rhythm of 2 to 3 per second, may involve whole limbs or parts of limbs in children with convulsive disorder. Such myoclonic seizures occur with diffuse neuronal disease at any age.

SUMMARY

Disturbances of function of striated muscle are related to disease of muscle, the motoneurons, the spinal cord, or the brain.

Varieties of dysfunction include weakness, distortions of posture, movement, and co-ordination, abnormal reflexes, distortions of muscle tone, and spontaneous movements. Pathophysiologic analysis must include consideration of the function of uninjured tissue when normal structures are destroyed or become pathologically overactive. In many areas, pathophysiologic understanding lags far behind clinicopathologic correlation.

REFERENCES

1. Walshe, F. M. R.: Contributions of John Hughlings Jackson to Neurology. A brief introduction to his teachings, Arch. Neurol. 5:119, 1961.
2. Walton, J. N., and Nattrass, F. J.: On the classification, natural history and treatment of the myopathies, Brain 77:169, 1954.
3. Adams, R. D., Denny-Brown, D. E., and Pearson, C. M.: Diseases of Muscle. A Study in Pathology, ed. 2, New York, Hoeber-Harper, 1962.
4. Greenfield, J. G., Cornman, T., and Shy, G. M.: The prognostic value of the muscle biopsy in the "floppy infant," Brain, 81:461, 1958.
5. Greenfield, J. G., Shy, G. M., Alvord, E. C., and Berg, L.: An Atlas of Muscle Pathology in Neuromuscular Diseases, London, Livingstone, 1957.
6. Grob, D., Johns, R. J., and Harvey, A. M.: Studies in neuromuscular function. IV. Stimulating and depressant effects of acetylcholine and choline in patients with myasthenia gravis and their relationship to the defect in neuromuscular transmission, Bull. Hopkins Hosp., 99:153, 1956.
7. Churchill-Davidson, H. C., and Richardson, A. T.: Neuromuscular transmission in myasthenia gravis, J. Physiol. 122:252, 1953.
8. Dahlback, O., Elmqvist, D., Johns, T. R., Radner, S., and Thesleff, S.: An electrophysiologic study of the neuromuscular junction in myasthenia gravis, J. Physiol. 156:336, 1961.
9. Strauss, A. J. L., Seegal, B. C., Hsu, K. C. Burkholder, P. M., Nastuk, W. L., and Osserman, K. E.: Immunofluorescence demonstration of muscle binding complement-fixing globulin fraction in myasthenia gravis, Proc. Soc. Exp. Biol. Med. 105:184, 1960.
10. Eaton, L. M., and Lambert, E. H.: Electromyography and electric stimulation of nerves in diseases of motor unit. Observations on myasthenic syndrome associated with malignant tumors, J.A.M.A. 163:1117, 1957.
11. Lambert, E. H.: Clinical Examinations in Neurology, Ch. 15, Philadelphia, Saunders, 1957.
12. Weaver, R. A., Landau, W. M., and Higgins, J.: Fusimotor function: II. Evidence of fusimotor depression in human spinal shock, Arch. Neurol. 9:127, 1963.
13. Teasdall, R. D., and Stavraky, G. W.: Responses of deafferented spinal neurons to cortico-spinal impulses, J. Neurophysiol. 16:367, 1953.
14. McCouch, G. P., Austin, G. M., Liu, C. M., and Liu, C. Y.: Sprouting as a cause of spasticity, J. Neurophysiol. 21:205, 1958.
15. Meltzer, G. E., Hunt, R. S., and Landau, W. M.: Fusimotor function: III. The spastic monkey, Arch. Neurol. 9:133, 1963.
16. Beevor, C.: Remarks on paralysis of the movements of the trunk in hemiplegia, and the muscles which are affected, Brit. Med. J. 1:881, 1909.
17. Twitchell, T. E.: The restoration of motor function following hemiplegia in man, Brain 74:443, 1951.
18. Landau, W. M., and Clare, M. H.: The plantar reflex in man, with special reference to some conditions where the extensor response is unexpectedly absent, Brain 82:321, 1959.
19. Efron, R.: Post-epileptic paralysis: Theoretical critique and report of a case, Brain 84:381, 1961.
20. Denny-Brown, D. E.: The Basal Ganglia and their Relation to Disorders of Movement, London, Oxford, 1962.
21. Landau, W. M., Weaver, R. A., and Hornbein, T. F.: Fusimotor nerve function in man: differential nerve block studies in normal subjects and in spasticity and rigidity, Arch. Neurol. 3:10, 1960.
22. Landau, W. M.: The essential mechanism in myotonia. An electromyographic study, Neurology 2:369, 1952.
23. Norris, F. H., Jr.: Unstable membrane potential in human myotonic muscle, Electroenceph. Clin. Neurophysiol. 14:197, 1962.
24. Walshe, F. M. R.: The significance of the voluntary element in the genesis of cerebellar ataxy, Brain 50:377, 1927.
25. Carpenter, M. B.: Brainstem and infratentorial neuraxis in experimental dyskinesia, Arch. Neurol. 5:504, 1961.
26. Martin, J. P.: Further remarks on the functions of the basal ganglia, Lancet 1:1362, 1960.
27. Jung, R., and Hassler, R.: The extrapyramidal motor system, in Handbook of Physiology, vol. 2, sec. 1, Ch. 35, p. 863, Washington, American Physiological Society, 1960.
28. Moldaver, J.: Contribution a l'étude de la regulation réflexe des movements, Arch. Int. Med. Exp. 11:405, 1936.
29. Denny-Brown, D., and Pennybacker, J.: Fibrillation and fasciculation in voluntary muscle, Brain 61:311, 1938.
30. Landau, W. M.: Synchronization of potentials and response to direct current stimulation in denervated mammalian muscle, Electroenceph. Clin. Neurophysiol. 3:169, 1951.

31. Thesleff, S.: Effects of motor innervation on the chemical sensitivity of skeletal muscle, Physiol. Rev. 40:734, 1960.
32. Lambert, E. H., Sayre, G. P., and Eaton, L. M.: Electrical activity of muscle in polymyositis, Tran. Amer. Neurol. Ass. 79:64, 1954.
33. Erminio, F., Buchthal, F., and Rosenfalck, P.: Motor unit territory and muscle fibre concentration in paresis due to peripheral nerve injury and anterior horn cell involvement, Neurology 9:657, 1957.
34. Denny-Brown, D., and Foley, J. M.: Myokymia and the benign fasciculation of muscular cramps, Trans. Ass. Amer. Physicians 61:88, 1948.
35. Norris, F. H., Jr., Gasteiger, E. L., and Chatfield, P. O.: An electromyographic study of induced and spontaneous muscle cramps, Electroenceph. Clin. Neurophysiol. 9:139, 1957.
36. Bishop, G. H., Clare, M. H., and Price, J., Patterns of tremor in normal and pathological conditions, J. Appl. Physiol. 1:123, 1948.
37. Denny-Brown, D., Gaylord, J. B., and Uprus, V.: Note on the nature of the motor discharge in shivering, Brain 58:233, 1935.
38. Liberson, W. T.: Monosynaptic reflexes and their clinical significance, Electroenceph. Clin. Neurophysiol. [Suppl.] 22:79, 1962.
39. Bucy, P. C.: The cortico-spinal tract and tremor, in Pathogenesis and Treatment of Parkinsonism, p. 271, Springfield, Ill., Thomas, 1958.
40. Cooper, I. S.: Neurosurgical Alleviation of Parkinsonism, Springfield, Ill., Thomas, 1956.
41. ——: Neurosurgical alleviation of intention tremor of multiple sclerosis and cerebellar disease, New Eng. J. Med. 263:441, 1960.
42. ——: Heredofamiliar tremor abolition by chemothalamectomy, Arch. Neurol. 7:129, 1962.
43. ——: Dystonia reversal by operation on basal ganglia, Arch. Neurol. 7:132, 1962.
44. Martin, J. P.: Remarks on the function of the basal ganglia, Lancet 1:999, 1959.
45. Salter, R. H.: The muscle glycogenoses, Lancet 1:1301, 1968.
46. Brooks, J. E.: Hyperkalemic periodic paralysis. Intracellular electromyographic studies, Arch. Neurol. 20:13, 1969.
47. Thesleff, S.: Acetylcholine utilization in myasthenia gravis, Ann. N. Y. Acad. Sci. Art. 1, 135:195, 1966.
48. Desmedt, J. E.: Presynaptic mechanisms in myasthenia gravis, Ann. N. Y. Acad. Sci. Art. 1, 135:209, 1966.
49. Elmqvist, D., and Lambert, E. H.: Neuromuscular transmission in patient with the myasthenic syndrome sometimes associated with bronchogenic carcinoma, Proc. Mayo Clin. 43: 689, 1968.
50. Phillips, C. G.: Corticomotoneuronal organization. Projection from the arm area of the baboon's motor cortex, Arch. Neurol. 17: 188, 1967.
51. Lewis, R., and Brindley, G. S.: The extrapyramidal motor map, Brain 88:397, 1965.
52. Lawrence, D. G., and Kuypers, G. J. M.: The functional organization of the motor system in the monkey. II. The effects of lesions of the descending brain-stem pathways, Brain 91:15, 1968.
53. Landau, W. M., and Clare, M. H.: Fusimotor function. Part VI. H reflex, tendon jerk, and reinforcement in hemiplegia, Arch. Neurol. 10:26, 1964.
54. Landau, W. M., Struppler, A., and Mehls, O.: A comparative electromyographic study of the reactions to passive movement in parkinsonism and in normal subjects, Neurology 16:34, 1966.
55. Cotzias, G. C., Van Woert, M. H., and Schiffer, L. M.: Aromatic amino acids and modification of parkinsonism, New Eng. J. Med. 276:374, 1967.
56. Winer, N., Martt, J. M., Somers, J. E., Wolcott, L., Dale, H. E., and Burns, T. W.: Induced myotonia in man and goat, J. Lab. Clin. Med. 66:758, 1965.
57. Landau, W. M., and Clare, M. H.: Pathophysiology of the tonic innervation phenomenon in the foot, Arch. Neurol. 15:252, 1966.
58. Wallis, W. E., Van Poznak, A., and Plum, F.: Generalized muscular stiffness, fasciculations, and myokymia of peripheral nerve origin, Arch. Neurol. 22:430, 1970.
59. Jasper, H. H., and Bertrand, G.: Thalamic units involved in somatic sensation and voluntary and involuntary movements in man, in Purpura, D. P., and Yahr, M. D. (eds.): The Thalamus, pp. 364–390, New York and London, Columbia University Press, 1966.
60. Carman, J. B.: Anatomic basis of surgical treatment of Parkinson's disease, New Eng. J. Med. 279:919, 1968.
61. Leavitt, S., and Tyler, H. R.: Studies in asterixis, Arch. Neurol. 10:360, 1964.

33

Fainting (Syncope)

EUGENE A. STEAD, JR.

Pathogenesis

Fainting from Arteriolar Dilatation
    COMMON FAINT (VASODEPRESSOR SYNCOPE)
    CAROTID SINUS DEPRESSOR REFLEX
    DISEASE OF THE SYMPATHETIC NERVOUS
    SYSTEM (POSTURAL HYPOTENSION)

Fainting: Main Causes
    A SHARP FALL IN CARDIAC OUTPUT
        WITHOUT CARDIAC STANDSTILL
    VENTRICULAR STANDSTILL (ADAMS-STOKES
        ATTACKS)
    COUGH; WITH OBSTRUCTIVE EMPHYSEMA
        AND TRACHEAL OR LARYNGEAL
        OBSTRUCTION
    EXTERNAL COMPRESSION OF THE THORAX
        WITH GLOTTIS CLOSED
    CEREBRAL ANOXEMIA IN TETRALOGY OF
        FALLOT
    EXTRACRANIAL OBSTRUCTION OF THE
        CEREBRAL VESSELS
    OBSTRUCTION OF MITRAL VALVE BY BALL
        THROMBUS OR TUMOR
    EMBOLUS LODGING IN A CEREBRAL ARTERY
    HYPERVENTILATION
    ANOXEMIA
    HYPOGLYCEMIA
    HYSTERIA

Less Well-Understood Causes
    HEART DISEASE
    PLEURAL SHOCK
    REMOVAL OF FLUID FROM BLADDER OR BODY
        CAVITIES
    MICTURITION

Diagnostic Approach
    HISTORY: ESPECIALLY SUGGESTIVE FEATURES
    PHYSICAL EXAMINATION AND SPECIAL TESTS

DEFINITION

Fainting and syncope are terms commonly used interchangeably to describe a transient loss of consciousness caused by reversible disturbances in cerebral function from (1) transient ischemia, (2) change in composition of blood perfusing the brain, and (3) changes in the pattern of central nervous system activity by stimuli entering the central nervous system.[1] Loss of consciousness accompanied by the clinical or electroencephalographic features of epilepsy is excluded.

PATHOGENESIS

The words *fainting* and *syncope* imply brief loss of consciousness and suggest that the fundamental disturbance must be quickly reversible. Fainting must be distinguished from more prolonged, less quickly reversible losses of consciousness, which are discussed in Chapter 31. The most common cause of syncope is a sudden decrease in the blood supply to the higher nerve centers, i.e., the centers of *consciousness*. For a discussion of these centers, see Chapter 31.

Among the physiologic disturbances that may cause a decrease in the blood supply to the brain are (1) peripheral arteriolar vasodilatation, (2) failure of normal peripheral vasoconstrictor activity, (3) sharp fall in cardiac output from heart disease or from a decrease in blood volume, (4) constriction of cerebral vessels as CO_2 is lost by hyperventilation, (5) occlusion or narrowing of internal carotid or other arteries to the brain, (6) ventricular asystole and (7) obstruction in the heart by myxoma. The first four disturbances rarely produce unconsciousness when the patient is in the horizontal position.

Less frequent in the pathogenesis of true syncope are reflex effects upon the cerebral centers of consciousness. Whether these act directly on the nervous system, or indirectly, by local changes in blood supply, remains to be determined.

Changes in the constituents of the blood caused by chemical or metabolic derangements may be associated with syncope and may predispose the involved person to its occurrence. These disorders include hypoxia, alkalosis, acidosis, hypoglycemia, etc. Such conditions are more apt to be implicated in the causation of other types of unconscious states; they are less frequent as etiological factors in syncope.

FAINTING FROM ARTERIOLAR DILATATION

THE COMMON FAINT
(VASODEPRESSOR SYNCOPE)

The benign faint, produced by such stimuli as bad news, the sight of blood, hypodermic injection or venipuncture, commonly occurs while the subject is standing or sitting. The signs and the symptoms of the faint result from reflex activity from a variety of sensory stimuli. The afferent impulses producing the faint may arise from the emotional content of thought, or from any sensory nerve endings. Whether or not a subject faints from a given stimulus depends to a great degree upon the amount of anxiety mobilized in him by the stimulus. The intensity of the stimulus and the organ stimulated are less important.

In a few subjects a given stimulus will cause fainting no matter how often it is repeated. More commonly, the same stimulus causes less and less reaction each time. Many persons faint at the time of their first venipuncture, but never have any reaction to subsequent ones.

Clinical Picture. The clinical picture of the common faint is well-known. The patient, in the erect or sitting position, complains of a feeling of warmth in his neck and face; he becomes deathly pale and beads of sweat appear on his forehead. Yawning, belching, nausea, increased peristalsis of the gut, dilatation of the pupils, coldness of the hands and the feet, and profound weakness are noted. The heart rate is usually increased and the pulse pressure is narrowed. The radial pulse becomes weak and may be imperceptible, although the femoral and the carotid pulses remain full. When the mean arterial pressure approaches the level of 25 mm. of Hg, the heart rate slows and high-voltage synchronous slow waves appear in the electroencephalogram. Hyperventilation occurs frequently. By as yet undetermined mechanisms, the cerebral vascular resistance is decreased more than the resistance in the remainder of the systemic arterial bed.[2] If the subject is standing, he becomes uncon-

scious. When he is placed in the horizontal position, consciousness returns quickly. Occasionally there may be a short period of disorientation. The arterial pressure usually rises immediately when the patient is placed in the recumbent position, but at times it remains depressed for minutes or hours. Pallor, nausea, weakness, and sweating frequently persist for a few minutes to two hours; occasionally they persist for 24 hours. If the patient stands up before recovery is complete, a precipitous fall in arterial pressure with syncope may again occur. If the subject remains upright after loss of consciousness, clonic movements of the hands and the legs are not infrequent.

In many instances, all of the phenomena usually preceding and following the loss of consciousness occur, although the patient remains conscious. To these signs and symptoms, which frequently but not necessarily terminate in syncope, the term *fainting reaction* has been applied.[3]

The fainting reaction without loss of consciousness is seen frequently in patients who are in the horizontal position when an appropriate stimulus occurs. In blood-donor centers, an occasional person loses consciousness in the recumbent position. In some of these instances, convulsions with tonic and clonic phases and urinary incontinence occur in persons who never have had seizures before.

The circulatory dynamics during the fainting reaction induced in blood donors by venesection have been studied intensively during the last few years.[4,5] The reaction is reflex in nature and may occur before anything is done to the donor. It may occur before the needle is inserted, after the venipuncture but before any blood is drawn, or it may occur during or shortly after the venesection. The sharp fall in arterial pressure, the feeble radial pulse, and the intense pallor suggest a sudden marked fall in cardiac output. Studies of the cardiac output indicate that the fall does not occur simultaneously with the fainting reaction. The sudden fall in arterial pressure without a corresponding fall in cardiac output indicates a great decrease in peripheral resistance, as would be expected with widespread arteriolar dilatation. Studies of the blood flow in the forearm demonstrate *an increase in blood flow to the muscles* in spite of the low arterial pressure and the decrease in blood flow in the skin.[4] Vasoconstriction in the skin with vasodilatation in the muscles is not an unusual response. Epinephrine reduces the blood flow to the skin and increases it in the muscles.

The mechanism of the loss of consciousness in patients in the upright position during a precipitous fall in arterial pressure is understood easily. The arterial pressure reaches such a low level that it is insufficient to maintain the blood flow to the head against the force of gravity. Complete unconsciousness is always accompanied by high-voltage slow waves in the electroencephalogram. When the patient is placed in the recumbent position, the arterial pressure is sufficient to restore the cerebral circulation and consciousness returns.

Detailed observations have not been made on persons who have lost consciousness while in the recumbent position. It is not known whether the entire reaction represents a more profound degree of arteriolar dilatation with a drop in arterial pressure to such a low level that the circulation cannot be maintained even with the head level with the heart, or whether some other factor such as reflex ventricular asystole occurs in these severe reactions.

The demonstration that the *cardiac output is well-maintained in the fainting reaction* accounts for the fact that the fall in arterial pressure in this condition does not usually lead to serious complications. In spite of the appearance of the patient and the low arterial pressure, the over-all blood flow to the tissues remains relatively normal.

This reaction of generalized activity of the autonomic nervous system with a precipitous fall in blood pressure has been called *primary shock* or *acute circulatory collapse* when it has occurred in injured persons. It may occur with any type of injury. At times it complicates the circulatory failure produced by a small blood volume. In patients with broken bones or severe injuries, manipulation of the parts or movement of the patient may be followed by circulatory failure.

It is of interest to note that signs of stimulation of both the sympathetic and the parasympathetic systems are present in the person with the fainting reaction. From a theoretical point of view, the activity of the autonomic nervous system might result from the fall in arterial pressure, or the fall in arterial pressure might be one of the manifestations of an over-stimulated nervous system. In the first instance, the signs and the symptoms of the fainting reaction would result from the fall in arterial pressure; in the second, they would be part of the response to the afferent stimulus producing the fall in arterial pressure but not caused by the fall in pressure itself. The signs and the symptoms of the fainting reaction frequently occur without the fall in arterial pressure and may persist long after the pressure has returned to normal. They may not occur when the blood pressure falls profoundly in patients with postural hypotension. These observations suggest that the symptoms are not caused by the fall in arterial pressure, but are responses to the same stimulus as that producing the drop.

The relationship between the intensification of the fainting reaction and the upright position of the subject is of interest. After a patient has apparently recovered in the recumbent position, assumption of the upright position often causes a recurrence of the entire reaction. After venesection, blood donors frequently have no symptoms until they resume the standing position. Acute infections, chronic illnesses, acute or chronic blood loss, fever, high external temperature, dehydration, and ingestion of nitrites frequently are associated with fainting when the patient assumes the upright position. The upright position causes pooling of blood by gravity in the portions of the body below the heart, with a reduction of cardiac output because of a decrease in venous return to the heart and a progressive fall in arterial pressure. The upright position is a strong stimulus to increased activity of the autonomic nervous system and greatly increases the number of visceral afferent stimuli entering the nervous system. This combination of a decreased pressure head and increased nervous system activity results in a precipitous fall in arterial pressure, the final sharp break in pressure being caused by reflex arteriolar dilatation.

In at least one situation, fainting may be precipitated by lying down and relieved by standing up. The writer has made observations on two pregnant women near term who fainted if they were placed on their backs in the recumbent position. The clinical picture was that of reflex vasodepressor syncope. They were able to lie on their sides without difficulty.

CAROTID SINUS DEPRESSOR REFLEX

Pressure on the carotid sinus may rarely cause a striking fall in arterial pressure, with or without the other signs and symptoms of the fainting reaction, which cannot be accounted for by slowing of the heart rate.[6]

Fig. 33-1. Diagram of the cardio-vascular reflex mechanisms. Afferent vagal fibers are shown by broken lines; sinus nerve fibers by a dotted line; efferent fibers to the heart and to the blood vessels by a continuous line. The afferent fibers are represented as causing reciprocal effects upon the medullary centers. (Best, C. H., and Taylor, N. B.: The Physiological Basis of Medical Practice, ed. 8, Baltimore, Williams & Wilkins)

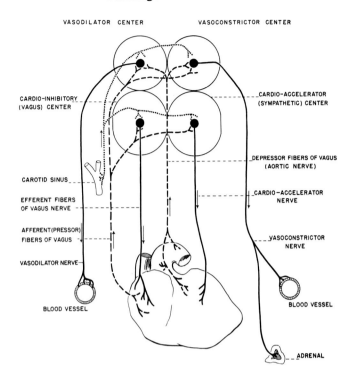

VASODILATOR CENTER   VASOCONSTRICTOR CENTER

CARDIO-INHIBITORY (VAGUS) CENTER

CARDIO-ACCELERATOR (SYMPATHETIC) CENTER

DEPRESSOR FIBERS OF VAGUS (AORTIC NERVE)

CAROTID SINUS

CARDIO-ACCELERATOR NERVE

EFFERENT FIBERS OF VAGUS NERVE

AFFERENT (PRESSOR) FIBERS OF VAGUS

VASOCONSTRICTOR NERVE

VASODILATOR NERVE

BLOOD VESSEL

BLOOD VESSEL

ADRENAL

Pressure on the carotid sinus may cause a precipitous fall in arterial pressure after cardiac slowing has been eliminated by atropinization. If the subject is upright, unconsciousness may occur. Epinephrine prevents the fall in arterial pressure when the carotid sinus is stimulated and syncope does not occur (Fig. 33-1).

DISEASE OF THE SYMPATHETIC NERVOUS SYSTEM (POSTURAL HYPOTENSION)

Syncope occurring only when the patient is in the upright position and without any of the unpleasant symptoms that are characteristic of the common faint, may be caused by postural hypotension.[7] In this condition, the arterial pressure is normal or elevated when the patient is horizontal, but falls precipitously upon standing. It is usually seen in middle-aged or elderly people, but may occur much earlier. Syncope is more likely to occur in the morning and often follows exercise. There are frequently signs and symptoms of disturbance in the central or peripheral nervous systems. Pupillary abnormalities, fixed heart rate, bladder disturbances, diarrhea, impotence, loss of sweating over a part of the body, loss of vasoconstriction and vasodilatation in the extremities when the body is cooled or

heated are seen frequently, either singularly or in any combination.

Postural hypotension is usually the result of a disease of the autonomic nervous system. It is seen most frequently in *diabetic neuropathy* and *tabes dorsalis*. In many instances, the etiology of the neurologic disease remains obscure. Postural hypotension also develops after extensive *bilateral sympathectomy* has been performed to relieve hypertension.

Persons with postural hypotension show either an abnormal fall in cardiac output upon standing with good arteriolar constriction, or an inability to vasoconstrict in response to a fall in arterial pressure, or a combination of the two. These abnormal responses reflect a state of circulatory incoordination dependent upon partial autonomic paralysis. No more than the usual amount of blood is pooled in the portions of the body below heart level. The response to the average amount pooled is abnormal, and does not maintain a normal arterial pressure. The fact that rapid infusion of albumin solution with the patient standing restores the arterial pressure to normal demonstrates the importance of the postural shift in blood volume. The ability of the heart to respond normally to a fall in arterial pressure, the ability of the veins to constrict in response to usual stimuli, and the ability of the arterioles to constrict when the cardiac output falls—all may be impaired in varying degrees. The lack of coordination in the circulation is caused by loss of function of the autonomic nervous system. This may be peripheral, as in the postural hypotension caused by sympathectomy; it may be in the spinal cord, as in patients with transverse myelitis; or it may be in the medulla or the hypothalamus.[8]

Postural hypotension resulting from disease of the sympathetic nervous system must be differentiated from the vasodepressor syncope precipitated by standing, which is common in persons with Addison's disease, with febrile illnesses, with blood loss, and with chronic wasting diseases. In these patients, the vasodepressor reaction, with the accompanying signs and symptoms of the fainting reaction, improve as the general condition of the patient improves. In the patient with postural hypotension caused by a disease of the autonomic nervous system, the fall in arterial pressure upon standing is not accompanied by other signs of stimulation of the autonomic nervous system, and the reaction persists regardless of the general condition.

FAINTING FROM A SHARP FALL IN CARDIAC OUTPUT WITHOUT CARDIAC STANDSTILL

Conditions causing a great decrease in cardiac output, such as a marked decrease in blood volume, acute pericardial tamponade, or massive myocardial infarction, may decrease the cardiac output to such a degree that the arterial pressure is greatly lowered, in spite of normal or increased arteriolar tone. When the drop in pressure is sufficient to decrease the circulation to the brain, syncope occurs. A pressure adequate to maintain the circulation to the brain with the subject in the horizontal position may be inadequate to overcome the force of gravity when the subject is upright.

In many illnesses, a decrease in venous tone leads to excessive venous pooling in the erect position. When inadequate filling of the heart is present, syncope follows.

In certain patients with diabetic neuropathy, a marked fall in arterial pressure occurs in spite of normal or excessive arteriolar constriction. The cardiac output is strikingly reduced and returns to normal when the blood volume is increased. Whether this represents a loss of venous tone common to many illnesses or whether it represents disease of the autonomic nerves supplying the veins remains to be determined.

Fainting at times occurs at the onset of an attack of paroxysmal tachycardia. The tachycardia may cause a sufficient fall in cardiac output to cause fainting on the basis of cerebral ischemia. Other mechanisms may be operative, however. Awareness of a disturbance in cardiac function may cause sufficient anxiety to precipitate an attack of vasodepressor syncope in an anxious subject. Comeau[9] described a patient with paroxysmal atrial fibrillation in whom attacks of syncope were caused by complete cardiac arrest between the cessation of normal rhythm and the establishment of atrial fibrillation. Carefully taken histories reveal that this is a common sequence of events in fainting associated with atrial tachycardia.

FAINTING FROM VENTRICULAR STANDSTILL (ADAMS-STOKES ATTACKS)

When the ventricles stop pumping blood for a few seconds, consciousness is lost. The effects of brief periods of acute arrest of the cerebral circulation in normal subjects have been reported by Rossen and his collaborators.[10] Arrest of the cerebral circulation was accomplished by means of a cervical pressure cuff (a constricting band about the subject's neck). These patients showed fixation of the eyes, tingling, constriction of the visual fields, loss of consciousness, and, immediately after restoration of blood flow, a brief, mild tonic and clonic seizure. The average time from arrest of the cerebral circulation to loss of consciousness was seven seconds. The corneal reflex may disappear in less than ten seconds. The investigators found that arrest of the circulation for 100 seconds may be followed by rapid recovery of consciousness and no objective evidence of injury.

Weiss and Baker[6] observed that, after complete arrest of the heart, syncope usually occurred in eight seconds, and occurred regularly within 12 seconds. Rossen, et al.[10] point out that the somewhat longer maintenance of consciousness following cardiac asystole than that following the use of the cervical cuff may be explained on the basis that arrest of the heart fails to arrest cerebral circulation as rapidly as does occlusion of the arteries supplying blood to the brain.

The ventricle may cease pumping blood as the result of (1) sinus standstill or heart block, and (2) ventricular fibrillation. Heart block may be caused either by abnormal reflex activity or by organic disease in the conduction system of the heart.

Stimulation of the efferent endings of the vagus causes ventricular asystole either by sinus standstill or auriculoventricular block. Pressure on the carotid sinus is frequently an effective afferent stimulus. Less frequently, pressure on the eyeball causes cardiac standstill. Stimulation of the pharynx, the esophagus, the duodenum, or the bronchi may produce the same effect. Less often, afferent stimuli from other areas may cause sinus standstill or atrioventricular block.

Patients with organic heart disease frequently have periods of ventricular asystole sufficient to produce syncope. These periods of cardiac standstill characteristically occur when the rhythm of the heart shifts from normal sinus rhythm or partial heart block to complete heart block. When the impulses from the atria are completely blocked, several seconds may elapse before a site of impulse formation becomes active in the ventricles. In some patients, however, with constant complete atrioventricular block, syncope will occur because of periods during which the idioventricular rhythm fails. The diagnosis of syncope due to heart block is easy if the patient has some evidence of block at the time he is seen. In certain patients, normal sinus rhythm will be present the majority of the time, and repeated observations must be made before characteristic abnormalities are detected and the diagnosis of heart block can be definitely established.

The symptoms caused by ventricular standstill are the same regardless of the cause of the standstill. The patient has none of the unpleasant symptoms of overactivity of the autonomic nervous system so characteristic of the common faint. He notices only blurring of vision and loss of consciousness. Upon inspection, slight pallor may be noted, followed by a flush as the ventricles begin to pump blood. If the period of asystole is prolonged, hyperventilation and convulsive movements follow. Recovery is usually prompt when the ventricles begin to contract.

In the writer's experience, patients with ventricular standstill from heart block because of disease of the conduction system often have attacks in their sleep, whereas patients with ventricular standstill from reflex activity do not. The intravenous injection of atropine will restore normal sinus rhythm if the block is caused by reflex activity.

Patients with serious heart disease may rarely have attacks of asystole caused by short periods of ventricular fibrillation.[11] Upon physical examination, no evidence of ventricular activity can be detected. The electrocardiogram shows the characteristic bizarre pattern of ventricular fibrillation. At times in patients with complete heart block the syncope is caused by ventricular fibrillation rather than ventricular standstill.

TUSSIVE FAINTING WITH OBSTRUCTIVE EMPHYSEMA, TRACHEAL, OR LARYNGEAL OBSTRUCTION

Patients who have uncontrolled violent attacks of coughing may lose consciousness if they are unable to collapse their lungs in a normal manner.[12] Hysterical closure of the glottis, obstructive emphysema, or tracheal obstruction, most commonly from aneurysm, may prevent normal collapse of the lungs. When strong pressure is exerted by the chest wall and diaphragms on noncollapsible lungs, a very high intrathoracic pressure results. This pressure is transmitted to the systemic arteries. The rise in pressure is buffered by the elastic qualities of the systemic arteries outside the thorax and the abdomen, and the increase in arterial pressure is less than the increase in intrathoracic and intra-abdominal pressures. The aorta and the large vessels within the thorax and abdomen are collapsed. The cerebrospinal pressure rises as blood is forced into the extradural venous plexus, and soft tissues are displaced inward through the vertebral foramina. This rise in cerebrospinal pressure is not buffered as is the arterial pressure, and the cerebrospinal pressure becomes equal to the intrathoracic pressure and greater than the arterial pressure, thus forcing blood from the cranium. In cough syncope, the circulation is interfered with at two levels: (1) at the capillary level in the brain, and (2) at the lung and heart level by direct compression.[13] Subjects who stretch vigorously with the glottis closed may occasionally faint.

FAINTING FROM EXTERNAL COMPRESSION OF THE THORAX WITH GLOTTIS CLOSED

Fainting may occur during external compression of the thorax, or upon release of the compression.[14] It is assumed that the thoracic compression interferes with the flow of blood through the lungs, causing a fall in cerebral blood flow and loss of consciousness. If syncope does not occur during the compression, it may occur when it is released. Upon removing the compression, the blood from the right heart fills the empty lungs. This may cause a temporary fall in the rate of filling of the left heart, and may result in a sharp fall in cardiac output. The importance of reflex changes as accessory or primary factors in this type of fainting has not been determined.

FAINTING FROM CEREBRAL ANOXEMIA IN TETRALOGY OF FALLOT

Patients with tetralogy of Fallot may become unconscious upon exertion. It has been shown that during exercise the oxygen content of the arterial blood becomes much lower than it is at rest.[15] The exercising muscles extract nearly all of the oxygen from the blood passing through them. This dark, unoxygenated blood enters the systemic arteries through the interventricular septal defect without passing through the lungs. The oxygen content of the arterial blood falls sharply, and the patient becomes unconscious because of cerebral anoxemia.

FAINTING FROM EXTRACRANIAL OBSTRUCTION OF THE CEREBRAL VESSELS

Atherosclerosis may cause various degrees of obstruction of all major vessels to the head and upper extremities as they leave the aorta.[16] The carotid and brachial pulses may be absent. If one vessel is partially open, a systolic and diastolic murmur will be present. A diastolic murmur over a partially occluded artery occurs only when the collateral circulation is greatly reduced. Upon standing, the patient may lose consciousness, not because the arterial pressure in the aorta falls, but because, in the presence of occlusive disease, the normal aortic pressure cannot perfuse the head against the increased force of gravity produced by the upright position.

In extracranial disease of the internal carotid arteries, syncope, intermittent paralysis, and transient blindness may occur. A systolic stenotic murmur frequently may be heard over the area of the carotid bifurcation, over the mastoid process, or over the eyeball. When one internal carotid is completely occluded, the murmur will be heard over the open vessel. No murmur on one side and a systolic and diastolic murmur over the opposite side is an ominous sign. It means that the collateral circulation from the carotid and vertebral arteries is severely impaired and that there is a large pressure gradient during systole and diastole. A loud systolic murmur at the bifurcation of the common carotid may indicate localized narrowing of the external rather than internal carotid artery.

When the subclavian vessel is occluded just proximal to the vertebral vessel, an interesting syndrome may develop. Vigorous exercise of the arm on the occluded side may cause weakness in the opposite side of the body. The sharp fall in peripheral resistance caused by the exercise of the arm reverses the direction of blood flow in the vertebral artery and blood is channeled from the circle of Willis into the exercising arm. This syndrome has been called the "vertebral steal."

Obstruction of the common carotid artery below the carotid sinus for 15 to 25 seconds may produce syncope or other neurological manifestations by decreasing the blood flow to the brain. This is more likely to occur if the opposite internal carotid artery is occluded by disease. Many of these patients will have sensitive carotid sinuses and will have sinus arrest, heart block, or a drop in arterial pressure if the carotid sinus is massaged. These reflex causes of cerebral ischemia must be separated from those produced by obstruction of the common carotid artery.[17]

FAINTING FROM OBSTRUCTION OF MITRAL VALVE BY BALL-VALVE THROMBUS OR TUMOR

Intermittent obstruction of the mitral valve by a myxoma or ball thrombus in the left atrium causes sudden loss of consciousness. Peripheral embolization is common in both conditions.

FAINTING FROM EMBOLUS LODGING IN A CEREBRAL ARTERY

Transient periods of unconsciousness without focal neurologic signs are occasionally seen in patients in whom small vessels are being occluded by emboli. In one patient with subacute bacterial endocarditis, these episodes recurred frequently over several days. Usually emboli produce focal neurologic signs rather than syncopal attacks.

FAINTING FROM HYPERVENTILATION

An increase in ventilation above that required by metabolic needs of the body results in alkalosis because of the loss of CO_2 from the body. Numbness and tingling of the mouth, the face, and the extremities, coldness of the extremities, feeling of light-headedness and confusion, and at times tetany, are characteristic symptoms. The overventilation may be voluntary or reflex in origin. Anxiety is the most common cause of involuntary hyperventilation, but stimuli from any sensory organ or nerve may be the cause.

The disturbance in the level of awareness results from changes in cerebral metabolism produced by alkalosis. The electroencephalogram shows slow large waves. Consciousness is usually not lost when the subject remains in the recumbent position, but when he is upright, a typical vasodepressor reaction may develop with a sudden fall in arterial pressure and loss of consciousness.

FAINTING FROM ANOXEMIA

Loss of consciousness may result from an inadequate supply of oxygen to the brain when the blood supply is adequate but the blood transport of oxygen is deficient. This may occur in anemia; thus persons with severe anemia are especially apt to faint whenever any of the other possible causes are added to this predisposing cause. Carbonmonoxide poisoning may lower the ability of the red cells to carry oxygen.

Inadequate oxygen concentration in the inspired air or interference with access of oxygen through the lungs to the blood may result in oxygen-want in the tissues. Since the cerebral centers are particularly sensitive to lack of oxygen, a tendency to syncope may be an early evidence of such a condition.

FAINTING FROM HYPOGLYCEMIA

The symptoms produced by a decrease in blood sugar are strikingly similar to those produced by anoxia. In both instances, cerebral metabolism is interfered with: in one case by oxygen lack, in the other by the lack of fuel to utilize the oxygen.

Hypoglycemia affects the function of both the autonomic and the central nervous systems. Weakness, sweating, flushing, pallor, and trembling are evidences of disturbance in the autonomic nervous system. Anxiety, difficulty in concentrating, lightheadedness, disorientation, amnesia, unconsciousness, or convulsions may result from disturbance in cerebral metabolism. Administration of glucose by vein results in prompt recovery.

The signs and the symptoms of hypoglycemia are most frequently seen in patients with diabetes who have received an overdose of insulin. Hypoglycemia occurs spontane-

ously in patients with insulin-secreting adenomas of the isles of Langerhans or with functional hyperactivity and hyperplasia of the islets. It is seen also in patients with adrenal cortical insufficiency, hypophyseal deficiency, and liver disease. Evidences of hypoglycemia may appear in some otherwise normal subjects a few hours after ingestion of a large carbohydrate meal. Profound heart failure is occasionally associated with severe hypoglycemia. In most instances this occurs in irreversible situations, but we have seen one patient with pericardial tamponade from purulent pericarditis in whom the recognition of the hypoglycemia was life-saving.

Sudden transient loss of consciousness without any other symptom has not, in the author's experience, been caused by hypoglycemia. Mental confusion, with abnormal behavior, occurring when no food has been ingested for several hours, with or without loss of consciousness, suggests hypoglycemia. Many apparently normal persons complain of weakness, tremor, and lightheadedness when the interval between meals is prolonged. Although in such instances the clinical symptoms suggest hypoglycemia, the blood sugar level is usually normal.

HYSTERICAL FAINTING

Certain patients seem to lose consciousness without any changes in the circulation or respiration. The differentiation between hysterical fainting and syncope associated with altered cerebral metabolism has been discussed by Romano and Engel.[19] Hysterical fainting tends to occur more often in women. Other hysterical manifestations are frequently present and the patient may manifest little concern about the repeated faints. The loss of consciousness, which usually occurs in the presence of other people, is abrupt and not preceded by premonitory symptoms of nausea, sweating, and pallor. There are no changes in the heart rate, the respiration, the arterial pressure, or the electroencephalogram. All types of syncope except hysterical syncope are accompanied by alteration in cerebral metabolism which can be demonstrated by changes in the electroencephalogram.

LESS WELL-UNDERSTOOD CAUSES OF FAINTING

Noncyanotic Heart Disease. Persons with heart disease and left ventricular failure are prone to syncope. The combination of angina pectoris, dyspnea, and syncope is not uncommon. Syncope occurs with unusual frequency in three obstructive lesions of the heart and the pulmonary circulation: aortic stenosis, isolated pulmonic stenosis, and primary pulmonary hypertension. The mechanism of the syncope has not been determined. Although one or more of the causes of syncope discussed previously may be operative, when the patient is examined after recovery the responses to motionless standing, carotid sinus pressure, and hyperventilation are normal.

Pleural Shock. Syncopal attacks have occurred on introduction of a needle into the pleural space. In rare instances, such syncope has proved fatal. In many instances, the faint has occurred while air was being introduced to produce a pneumothorax, but in some the reaction has occurred before the introduction of air. The reactions appear to be of two types: (1) vasodepressor syncope from stimulation of the pleura, and (2) air embolus from introducing air into the pulmonary veins. Air normally in the lungs may enter the pulmonary veins through a tear in the lung, or it may be injected directly into the pulmonary veins.

Fainting From Removing Fluid From Bladder or Body Cavities. Transient loss of consciousness and, rarely, even death have occurred after draining a distended bladder or after removing fluid from the pleural or the peritoneal cavities. When this has occurred with drainage of a distended bladder or after removal of a large quantity of ascitic fluid, the syncope has been attributed to the pooling of blood in the venous system as the result of the decrease in the pressure of the urine or fluid. This hypothesis has never been tested experimentally. The role of reflex responses in this type of reaction has not been investigated.

Micturition Syncope. During or immediately after micturition, syncope may occur. It usually happens in the night and is more common in males. The loss of consciousness is brief, and there is no postsyncopal confusion or weakness.[20,21]

DIAGNOSTIC APPROACH IN REFERENCE TO CHIEF COMPLAINT OF FAINTING

HISTORY

Diseases that Predispose to Vasodepressor Syncope. Hemorrhage, dehydration, or any condition that lowers the blood volume, febrile illnesses, chronic wasting diseases, and trauma are important. Pregnancy and high external temperatures must be considered. Determine the relation of the attacks to minor respiratory illnesses and fatigue, as these predispose to vasodepressor syncope.

Circumstances Attending the Fainting Attacks. Vasodepressor syncope is very common in situations that cause anxiety. Vasodepressor syncope, with its characteristic changes in brain metabolism demonstrated by altered electroencephalographic activity, must be differentiated from hysteria in which the metabolism of the brain is unaltered and the electroencephalogram unchanged.[2]

Relation to Posture. Syncope produced by vasodepressor reaction, by cardiac standstill from reflex causes, and by fall in arterial pressure from stimulation of the carotid sinus occurs only rarely when the patient is recumbent. Mental confusion from hyperventilation in the recumbent position is common, but loss of consciousness rarely occurs except when the patient sits or stands. The patient with postural hypotension never has any syncopal symptoms when recumbent. A person with sensitive carotid sinus reflex may have attacks varying from a feeling of lightheadedness to loss of consciousness upon turning the head sharply, particularly if he wears a tight collar.

Heart Rate and Nature of Pulse During Attack. A very slow heart rate with a strong radial pulse suggests heart block. A slow rate with a very weak radial pulse suggests vasodepressor syncope.

Relation of Loss of Consciousness to Exercise. Syncope in patients with postural hypotension and aortic stenosis frequently occurs during exercise.

Presence of Other Symptoms Typical of the Fainting Reaction. These are absent in patients with ventricular standstill and postural hypotension. They do not occur with hyperventilation unless this reaction is accompanied by vasodepressor syncope. They are present in vasodepressor syncope and hypoglycemia.

Duration of the Unconsciousness. Unconsciousness from syncope usually lasts only a few seconds *except in patients with aortic stenosis, left ventricular failure, hypoglycemia, and hysteria.* Patients with vasodepressor syncope characteristically have persistence of weakness, sweating, pallor, and nausea after recovering consciousness; those with ventricular asystole or postural hypotension have no residual symptoms. The somnolence and headache, which are so frequently seen after an epileptic seizure, are not often present after fainting.

Symptoms of Heart Disease. Syncope may accompany attacks of angina pectoris; syncope may occur with left ventricular failure.

Relation to Sleep. Ventricular standstill from disease of the conduction system may cause syncopal attacks during sleep. Seizures during sleep are common in patients with epilepsy.

Presence of Incontinence and Tonic and Clonic Movements. Rhythmic jerking movements of the upper and lower extremities commonly occur in persons who faint and do not fall to the floor. A tonic and clonic convulsion with incontinence is rare in vasodepressor syncope, but does occur. Convulsive seizures with incontinence and biting of the tongue strongly suggest the diagnosis of epilepsy.

Symptoms Produced by Hyperventilation. Was the attack accompanied by numbness, tingling, and coldness of the extremities? Did tetany develop? These are the characteristic symptoms of hyperventilation.

Relation to Meals. Patients with hypoglycemia may be found unconscious after sleeping through the night (prolonged fasting). After fasting they may develop abnormalities of behavior and amnesia, which are promptly relieved by food.

Occurrence of Abnormal Behavior and Amnesia. Transient loss of consciousness may be preceded or followed by peculiar behavior or amnesia, not only in hypoglycemia, but also in patients with "epileptic equivalents."

PHYSICAL EXAMINATION AND SPECIAL TESTS

1. Look for evidence of diseases considered in the section entitled HISTORY (above).

2. Listen for systolic murmurs of localized arterial stenosis over common carotids, at the carotid bifurcation, over the mastoid processes and over the eyeballs. Stenotic murmurs over the aorta, renal vessels, iliac, and femoral vessels are frequently present in patients with extracranial vascular occlusion.

3. Have the subject sit in chair; massage first the right and then the left carotid bulb. Note any change in color, heart rate, arterial pressure, level of awareness, or focal neurologic signs. Massage may cause a cholesterol or calcium embolus and should not be done if there is evidence of disease in the carotid system.

4. While the patient remains sitting, have him hyperventilate maximally for two minutes. Question him as to any similarity between his spontaneous attacks and the symptoms produced by hyperventilation.

5. Determine the arterial pressure and the pulse rate with the patient recumbent and after he has stood leaning against the wall for one minute.

6. Examine heart for evidence of block, both by auscultation and by the electrocardiograph. Look for the physical signs of aortic stenosis and insufficiency.

7. Monitor the heart by continuous electrocardiography.[18]

8. Look for evidence of diffuse neurologic damage. Postural hypotension may accompany tabes dorsalis, combined system disease, or diabetic peripheral neuritis.

9. Feel radial pulse and take arterial pressure while the patient coughs. Repeat during forced expiration against closed glottis.

10. Determine the blood sugar concentration in the fasting state.

11. Cerebral angiograms may be indicated.

12. If myxoma is suspected, angiocardiograms are needed.

SUMMARY

Fainting (syncope) implies a brief, quickly reversible loss of consciousness. It is usually caused by diminution suddenly occurring in the blood supply to the centers of consciousness in the brain. It may be of no clinical importance, or it may be the first symptom of occlusion of the extracranial circulation. Less frequently, syncope may result from changes in the constituents of the blood. Other causes include primary neurophysiologic disorders.

Fainting with unconsciousness lasting only a few seconds may occur in aortic stenosis or left ventricular failure. These two conditions and others, such as hypoglycemia and hysteria, however, are apt to produce longer lapses. Such longer periods of unconsciousness, with the pathogenic mechanisms involved, are discussed in Chapter 31.

It is important to recognize syncope and to find its cause, and also to be able to distinguish it from other unconscious states, since the choice of therapy depends upon such differential diagnosis, and proper therapy may prevent permanent impairment or death.

REFERENCES

1. Wayne, H. H.: Syncope. Physiological consideration and an analysis of the clinical characteristics in 510 patients, Amer. J. Med. 30:418, 1961.
2. Karp, H. R., Weissler, A. M., and Heyman, A.: Vasodepressor syncope: EEG and circulatory changes, Arch. Neurol. 5:94–101, 1961.
3. Engel, G. L.: Mechanisms of fainting, J. Mount Sinai Hosp. N.Y. 12:170–190, 1945.
4. Warren, J. V., Brannon, E. A., Stead, E. A., Jr., and Merrill, A. J.: Effect of venesection and pooling of blood in extremities on atrial pressure and cardiac output in normal subjects with observations on acute circulatory collapse in 3 instances, J. Clin. Invest. 24:337–344, 1945.
5. Barcroft, H., Edholm, O. G., McMichael, J., and Sharpey-Schafer, E. P.: Posthemorrhagic fainting; study by cardiac output and forearm flow, Lancet 1:489–490, 1944.
6. Weiss, S., and Baker, J. P.: Carotid sinus reflex in health and disease; its role in causation of fainting and convulsions, Medicine 12:297, 1933.
7. Bradbury, S., and Eggleston, C.: Postural hypotension, Amer. Heart J. 1:73–86, 1933.
8. Stead, E. A., Jr., and Ebert, R. V.: Postural hypotension; disease of sympathetic nervous system, Arch. Intern. Med. 67:546–562, 1941.
9. Comeau, W. J.: Mechanism for syncopal attacks associated with paroxysmal auricular fibrillation, New Eng. J. Med. 227:134–136, 1942.
10. Rossen, R., Kabat, H., and Anderson, J. P.: Acute arrest of cerebral circulation in man, Arch. Neurol. Psychiat. 51:510–528, 1943.
11. Levine, S. A.: Clinical Heart Disease, ed. 5, Philadelphia, Saunders, 1958.
12. McCann, W. S., Bruce, R. A., Lovejoy, F. W., Jr., Yu, P. N. G., Pearson, R., Engel, G., and Kelly, J.: Observations on a case of tussive syncope, Trans. Ass. Amer. Physicians 62:116, 1949.
13. McIntosh, H. D., Estes, E. H., and Warren, J. V.: Circulatory effects of cough; the mechanism of cough syncope, Clin. Res. Proc. 3:82, 1955.
14. Weiss, S.: The Oxford Medicine, vol. 2, Chicago, Oxford, 1943.
15. Blalock, A., and Taussig, H.: The surgical treatment of malformations of the heart in which there is pulmonary stenosis or pulmonary atresia, J.A.M.A. 128:189, 1945.
16. Conference on Vascular Diseases of the Brain, Neurology 11: no. 4, Pt. 2, pp. 1–176, 1961.
17. Gurdjian, E. S., Webster, J. E., Martin, F. A., and Hardy, W. G.: Observations on unilateral compression and palpation of the carotid bifurcation, J. Neurosurg. 14:160–170, 1957.
18. Ira, G. H., Floyd, W. L., and Orgain, E. S.: Syncope with complete heart block. Differentiation of real and simulated Adams-Stokes seizures by radiotelemetry, J.A.M.A. 188:707–710, 1964.
19. Romano, J., and Engel, G. L.: Studies of syncope; differentiation between vasodepressor and hysterical fainting, Psychosom. Med. 7:3–15, 1945.
20. Engel, G. L.: Fainting, Springfield, Ill., Thomas, 1962.
21. Tudor, I.: Sincopa la mictiune, Neurologia (Bucur.) 11:229, 1966.

34

Vertigo and Dizziness

H. H. HYLAND

DEFINITIONS

The word *vertigo* is used in medical practice to imply a symptom that has certain specific characteristics. However, this word is rarely used by patients; the layman refers to it as "dizziness" or "giddiness," two terms that are commonly used to describe a wide variety of sensations as well as vertigo.

Dictionaries include among the synonyms of *dizziness* "foolish" or "stupid" and of *giddiness* "insane" or "possessed by a god," showing that originally these words implied a mental as well as a physical disturbance of equilibrium. To some extent this conception still exists, and the words are used interchangeably by patients to describe many symptoms, such as feelings of mental confusion, a general sense of insecurity, swimming or spinning sensations within the head, lightheadedness with or without brief visual impairment, a feeling of unsteadiness on the feet, a subjective sensation of movement of the individual or of his surroundings, etc.

Analysis of these abnormal sensations makes it evident that they vary in their pathogenesis, since they include symptoms accompanying psychogenic disorders and syncope as well as disturbed vestibular function. Because vertigo comes within the meaning of dizziness and giddiness, it would avoid much confusion if physicians would confine their use of these words to the symptom of vertigo and to those sensations that, although not truly vertigo, are related to it.

The physician always should obtain a detailed description of the actual sensations that have been experienced by the patient in order to be sure whether or not vertigo exists. This may take time and patience because many people find difficulty in describing accurately abnormal sensations of this nature. Those symptoms that are clearly not vertigo or related to it must be evaluated in the light of the history and findings upon examination. The necessity of careful inquiry from the patient was stressed by Hughlings Jackson[1] years ago: "The term vertigo is often used somewhat loosely. I do not take the explanation giddiness from the patient's mouth always to mean true giddiness. We have to put down not his name for, but the description he gives of the sensation he calls giddiness."

Vertigo is derived from the Latin verb *vertere* meaning "to turn," so that by its derivation it implies a sensation of turning either of the body or its surroundings. However, it is agreed generally that the word should not be restricted to the sensation of rotation but should be used to describe a hallucination of movement in any plane. The observations of McNally and Stuart[2] give justification for not interpreting vertigo too narrowly, since they found that the descriptions given by patients following vertigo induced by caloric tests indicate a variety of other sensations as well as that of turning.

Vertigo has been defined concisely by Russell Brain[3] as "the consciousness of disordered orientation of the body in space." The essential symptoms are a *hallucination of movement either of the surroundings or of the person himself.* In the former, objects may seem to move in a rotary, horizontal, vertical, or oblique fashion. In the latter, the false feeling of movement may consist of sensations of the body spinning, falling, or being pushed in various directions. Sometimes the sensation is confined to the head, which is felt to be revolving, swaying, or rocking. Observation of the patient during an attack of vertigo may reveal no objective movement of his body, but if the vertigo is at all severe he will stagger and may even fall to the ground.

Symonds[4] has emphasized that following all attacks of true vertigo there is a sensation of unsteadiness of the legs, usually lasting some hours. Another sensation that may occur as a common accompaniment or independently is a general sense of uncertainty in equilibrium upon walking, sometimes with a vague sense of movement of the surroundings. The patient often relates it to movement, particularly of the head. Although not necessarily implying a hallucination of movement, these two symptoms are closely akin to vertigo since they are common and sometimes persistent complaints from patients with vestibular disorders. Their regular occurrence as the aftermath of an acute attack of vertigo is helpful in identifying atypical attacks in which the patient may fall, with little or no awareness of preceding vertigo.

It is not clear what determines whether the false sense of movement in vertigo will be related to the surroundings or to the patient himself. The former occurs more commonly than the latter. Brain[3] considers that, for consciousness, the orientation of the body in space is normally an orderly dynamic relation between the bodily schema and the schema of the external world. Vertigo is the state of consciousness that arises when this relation becomes disordered. He points out that electrical stimulation at the cortical level has shown that a hallucination of rotation, either of the body in one direction or the environment in the other direction, may be evoked from the same region.[5] This suggests to him that what is evoked primarily is the functional relation between the body schema and the schema of the external world, thus indicating relative movement between them. Which is felt to be moving and which is felt to be stationary probably depends upon the pre-existing background provided by the proprioceptors of the body. This could be determined by their past conditioning relative to movement.

ANATOMIC AND PHYSIOLOGIC CONSIDERATIONS

The maintenance of equilibrium depends upon the integration by the brain of various afferent stimuli from the periphery that operate (for the most part) without entering consciousness. These include afferent impulses from the retinae, the skin, and the labyrinths, together with proprioceptive impulses from the ocular muscles, the neck, the trunk, and the lower limbs. Vertigo is the false sense perception that develops in consciousness when a disturbance or imbalance occurs in these peripheral mechanisms or their central connections. The most important of the peripheral mechanisms in maintaining orientation in space are the labyrinths; the most severe and clearly defined vertigo occurs if their function is disturbed.

The inner ear or labyrinth lies embedded within the petrous portion of the temporal bone; it consists of two intercommunicating parts; the cochlea, having to do with hearing, is anterior, whereas the vestibule and semicircular canals, concerned with equilibrium, are posterior. All of the membranous vestibular structures lie within bony canals and are bathed in and protected by perilymph. They contain another fluid called endolymph, which has direct continuity with the cochlear portion of the inner ear via the ductus reuniens. The three semicircular canals, known as the anterior and posterior (vertical) and the lateral (horizontal), lie in planes approximately at right angles to one another. The cavities of the three canals open by both extremities into the wall of a small saclike structure known as the utricle, which in turn connects with a similar structure called the saccule, by way of the ductus endolymphaticus. The utricle and the saccule are situated in the ovoid bony chamber known as the vestibule. The saccule communicates with the cochlea through the cochlear duct. Part of the epithelium forming the walls of the utricle and saccule is specialized for sensory reception. These structures, called the *macula utriculi* and the *macula sacculi,* each consists of a plaque of sensitive hair cells covered by a layer of gelatinous material upon which is situated a mass of tiny crystals of calcium carbonate. The maculae, which lie in different planes in relation to each other, are known as the otolith organs, and impulses from them are transmitted by branches of the vestibular nerve (Fig. 34-1). The function of the saccule is not completely understood, but it is thought to be involved mainly in cochlear function and to have relatively little to do with the maintenance of posture. This neural mechanism may serve to record bony vibrations as distinct from vibrations through air. The appreciation of the sound of one's own voice therefore may depend upon saccular as well as upon cochlear function. The utricle appears, from experimental study, to be an organ of static sense influencing muscle tone and serving to maintain posture. It registers the position of the head in space and governs the statotonic reflexes, the righting reflexes, and the compensatory positions of the eyes. An additional function suggested for the otolith structures is that they are the receptor organs concerned with linear acceleration.[6]

A branch of the vestibular nerve passes to the ampulla of each semicircular canal, where it terminates in a receptor organ called the *crista*. This also consists of specialized epithelium (hair cells) imbedded in a gelatinous fluid material known as the cupula, which fits hermetically into the ampulla. The motion of the cupula caused by the movement of the endolymph stimulates the hair cells of the crista, bringing about the perception of motion. Thus the crista has to do with kinetic sense, in contrast to the utricle, and is responsible for the statokinetic reflexes, which are the compensatory movements of eyes and limbs brought about by movements of the head. The crista responds to changes in the velocity and in the direction of movement. The response is accomplished through the effect that movements of the head exert upon the endolymph in the particular canal, the plane of which is involved in the movement.

The sensory impulses from the cristae of the semicircular canals, along with those from the maculae of the utricle and the saccule, proceed by way of the vestibular nerve, which originates from the bipolar cells of the vestibular ganglion. It passes through the internal auditory meatus, as the median part of the eighth nerve, to the cerebellopontine angle, and then separates

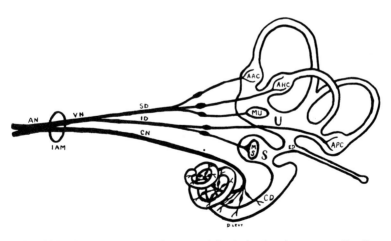

Fig. 34-1. Diagram of membranous labyrinth showing nerve distribution. AN, acoustic nerve; IAM, internal auditory meatus; VN, vestibular nerve; SD, superior division of vestibular nerve; ID, inferior division of vestibular nerve; CN, cochlear nerve; AAC, ampulla of anterior semicircular canal; AHC, ampulla of horizontal semicircular canal; APC, ampulla of posterior semicircular canal; U, utricle; MU, macula utriculi; S, saccule; MS, macula sacculi; CD, cochlear duct; ED, endolymphatic duct.

from the cochlear division upon entering the brain stem. Apart from some fibers passing directly to the cerebellum, the nerve terminates in four cellular masses constituting the vestibular nuclei, which extend from the pons to the upper part of the medulla, located in the floor and the lateral wall of the fourth ventricle.

From the vestibular nuclei, secondary tracts are given off to the cerebellum, the oculomotor nuclei, the spinal cord, and the cortex (Fig. 34-2). The fibers to the cerebellum, including those coming directly from the vestibular nerve and the secondary fibers from the vestibular nuclei, pass primarily into the flocculonodular lobe, according to Larsell and Dow.[7] This structure, consisting of the nodulus in the mid-line and paired lateral parts known as the flocculi, is situated in the postero-inferior part of the posterior lobe of the cerebellum. Secondarily, fibers pass to adjacent parts, which include the uvula, the lingula, and the fastigial or roof nuclei. It is possible that secondary vestibular fibers also reach other parts of the cerebellar cortex.[8] In addition to receiving only vestibular

fibers, the flocculonodular lobe sends efferent fibers only to the vestibular nuclei.[7] Therefore, the *flocculonodular mechanism* is entirely vestibular in function and is concerned with the maintenance of equilibrium. The uvula, lingula, and fastigial nuclei also send fibers to the vestibular nuclei.

Axons from the medial, spinal and superior vestibular nuclei go to form a large portion of the median longitudinal bundle of the same and opposite sides. This tract passes up the brain stem to the nuclei of the oculomotor, trochlear, and abducens nerves. Thus, each vestibular nucleus is able to influence ocular movement of both eyes. The tract passes downward to the nuclei of the spinal accessory nerve and to the anterior horn cells of the cervical portion of the spinal cord. Therefore, the median longitudinal bundle constitutes a pathway for the reflex control of movement of the head, the neck, and the eyes in response to vestibular stimulation. From the lateral vestibular nucleus (Deiters' nucleus) arises the vestibulospinal tract, which descends to the motor neurons of

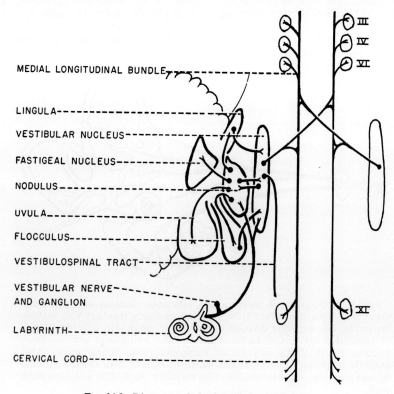

Fig. 34-2. Diagram of the vestibular pathways.

the spinal cord, conveying impulses concerned with the maintenance of tone and equilibrium. There is evidence that the reticular formation in the brain stem acts as a control mechanism, both inhibiting and facilitating motor responses initiated from the vestibular and proprioceptive end organs. Both the receptor-induced stimuli and modifying impulses from the cortex, autonomic nervous system, and cerebellum are received at the reticular substance and are modulated to produce a resulting balance.[9]

The course of the connections between the vestibular nuclei and the cortex is not definitely established as yet, but it is believed that the thalamus lies on the route.[10] Clinical and experimental evidence shows that certain parts of the cortex are capable of initiating vertigo and respond by increased activity to the stimulation of the labyrinth. As a result of observations on epileptics, including stimulation experiments on the exposed cortex, Penfield[11] considers that area 22 in the first temporal convolution is the end station of the vestibular tract, the auditory and the vestibular representations lying close together. With stimulation of this region, he found that the sensation of vertigo may occur as an aura of an induced seizure, or it may occur alone, or it may be associated with a humming sound (auditory vertiginous seizure). Penfield[12] has concluded from his studies that the pathway of vestibular sensory information makes a detour from the thalamus out to the cortex, where the vestibular area is next to the auditory area in the superior temporal convolution on both sides. From there, the pathway probably returns to the higher brain stem, where it enters the centrencephalic integrating system. He has found that removal of the superior temporal convolution on either side is not followed by any defect of vestibular function or auditory acuity. Foerster[5] induced severe vertigo by stimulation of the superior lip of the interparietal sulcus. His description of the result indicates that true vertigo with either a subjective or objective sensation of movement may occur. "The patient sees the objects before him moving towards the side of stimulation, or he has the sensation of turning towards the contralateral side," although objectively no movement of the head or trunk is observed. Foerster refers also to cases of epilepsy in which the lesions proved to be present in this anatomical loca-

tion, (area 5), which showed an aura of sudden vertigo. These various observations suggest that there are areas of cortex in the temporal and parietal regions which are concerned with the reception of vestibular impulses. These impulses provide conscious information about the position and movements of the head, and interference with them is likely to cause vertigo.

Vertigo that occurs with lesions involving the labyrinth may be accompanied by incoordination of movement and nystagmus as well as by certain visceral symptoms, including pallor, sweating, nausea and vomiting, and occasionally diarrhea. These visceral symptoms point to a spread of abnormal impulses from the vestibular nuclei to other centers, including the vagus nuclei. It has been suggested that there are connections, direct or indirect, between the vestibular nuclei and the vagus nuclei.[13] Incoordination of movement, including falling and past pointing, is the result of abnormal motor impulses transmitted to the skeletal muscles from the vestibular nuclei by way of the vestibulospinal tracts. The nystagmus that accompanies vertigo is caused by abnormal impulses transmitted from the vestibular nuclei to the oculomotor nuclei by way of the median longitudinal bundle. It has two components, a quick and a slow. The latter is the more important, being of vestibular origin, and is a reflex response resulting from abnormal stimulation of the semicircular canals. The direction of the slow component of the nystagmus, together with the falling and the past pointing, during an attack of labyrinthine vertigo, all are to the side of the more active labyrinth, whereas the quick component is directed toward the opposite side. Vertigo, together with the other signs of labyrinthine imbalance, can be produced physiologically by means of the *caloric and the rotation tests*, as well as by disease. When the caloric test is carried out with cold water on a normal subject the labyrinth on the tested side becomes the more active one. The direction of the vertigo is toward the opposite side, but the objective signs such as falling, past pointing, and the slow (vestibular) component of the nystagmus are to the side stimulated. When a subject is rotated with the head erect, the vertigo induced will be in the horizontal plane, that is, in the plane of the horizontal canals, its direction being opposite to his previous rotation and therefore opposite to the direction of the endolymph movement. The falling, past pointing, and the slow component of the nystagmus will be to the side corresponding to the direction in which he was rotated.

CLINICAL SIGNIFICANCE OF VERTIGO AND DIZZINESS

There will follow a consideration of various pathologic conditions in which vertigo and dizziness occur. The mechanism of production of these symptoms, their character with lesions in different anatomic sites, and the diagnostic features concerned will be discussed.

AURAL VERTIGO

Inflammatory. A common form of vertigo is that which is often called "viral labyrinthitis." It is acute in onset, benign in course, and occasionally occurs in small epidemics in a community.[14,15] The vertigo usually is induced or aggravated by movements of the head or change in posture. There is no deafness and rarely any tinnitus, although occasionally a transitory tinnitus has been noted. Vague sensations of fullness may be referred to an ear, and mild reduction in responses to caloric testing is occasionally found. Nausea, vomiting, and nystagmus may be present during acute episodes of vertigo. Recovery is usually gradual over a period of a few days or weeks and, although sometimes relapses occur, it is always ultimately complete. Diplopia with actual ocular muscle paresis has been found in some of the epidemic cases and this has led to the assumption that these patients may be suffering from a form of encephalitis, although the cerebrospinal fluid usually has been found normal. In some instances, where an increase in cells has been recorded, it is slight.[16] Sometimes the onset of the vertigo is preceded by a respiratory or other systemic infection, and hence it has been assumed to be due to an infectious agent, probably a virus. However, in many cases there is no evident infection and no premonitory malaise.

Dix and Hallpike[17] studied 100 cases similar to those described in the preceding paragraph except in regard to duration of the symptoms. They state that in their patients, recovery generally took place in the course of a few years. The patients presented with vertigo, usually, but not always paroxysmal, and were entirely free of cochlear signs or symptoms. Investigations showed that acute or quiescent focal infection, in the nose and throat particularly, was commonly present, and such infection is believed by the authors to play an important part in the pathogenesis. The caloric responses consistently were reduced. This was unilateral in 53 per cent and bilateral in 47 per cent. Since there was no evidence of involvement of the cochlear apparatus, the authors believe that the lesion is central to the labyrinth involving the vestibular nervous pathways up to and including the vestibular nuclei in the brain stem. They have called the condition "vestibular neuronitis." They consider it to be essentially benign and state that it responds well to treatment of focal infection when this is present. In a few cases they have observed the re-establishment of caloric responses with recovery from symptoms.

Hallpike[18] considers the nomenclature used in the various publications on epidemic labyrinthitis to be lax. The absence of any cochlear involvement in these cases makes a labyrinthine lesion very unlikely; yet the idea of such a lesion is incorporated in the name. Also, very few of the relevant publications include any satisfactory data upon the results of vestibular functional tests. He believes that if more attention is given to these tests and more careful terminology of the various members of this group of disorders is then used, vestibular neuronitis probably is the one that otologists and neurologists are most likely to encounter.

Cawthorne[16] regards the condition of vestibular neuronitis to be due to sudden failure of one vestibular end organ. He points out that the onset is sudden and severe and that the vertigo and nystagmus, which are intense at the onset, gradually diminish, so that after three weeks the nystagmus has disappeared and vertigo is likely to occur only on sudden movements of the head. This recovery is due to compensation within the central nervous system for the loss of one set of end organs. In his experience, the only physical sign is the absence or reduction of the normal response to caloric stimulation on one side. Although the lesion can be anywhere in the vestibular nerve from the end organ to the vestibular nuclei in the brain stem, he thinks it is quite possible that Scarpa's ganglion is the site.

Basser[19] has reported 17 cases of benign paroxysmal vertigo occurring sporadically in childhood. The disorder is purely vestibular, with the age of onset usually in the first four years of life, and the frequency of attacks showing considerable variation. The duration of an attack rarely exceeds a few minutes. The attacks come on abruptly, are very severe, and consist solely of vertigo. There are no precipitating factors and no significant infection was noted with the onset. The attacks cease spontaneously after a period varying from several months to six years. Caloric tests typically show moderate to severe reduction in response, unilateral or bilateral, which remains unchanged after cessation of the attacks. Basser regards the condition as a variety of vestibular neuronitis, but he points out that it differs significantly from this disorder as it has been described in adults. Differences include the uniformity and purely paroxysmal nature of the attacks, their brevity and recurrence at intervals, the absence of prolonged dysequilibrium or aggravation by head movement, and the absence of any evidence of infection at the onset.

Vertigo may develop in the presence of middle ear suppuration, indicating labyrinthine involvement. Another cause for the onset of attacks of vertigo in patients with long-standing middle-ear disease is the development of a cholesteatoma extending to involve the inner ear. Vertigo may appear also during certain specific febrile illnesses, notably mumps, indicating the complication of a neurolabyrinthitis. In the preceding disorders the vertigo is due to the resulting imbalance between the two labyrinths.

Noninflammatory. The condition of spontaneous aural vertigo was first recognized as being of labyrinthine origin by Meniere in 1861. Since that time it has been called Meniere's syndrome or Meniere's disease, the former term having been preferred because the etiology was unknown, and cases were considered to be due to a variety of causes. Numerous conditions have been suggested as playing a part in the etiology. These include abnormalities of fluid metabolism,[20] sodium retention in the body,[21] local alterations in capillary permeability resulting in local edema,[22] vasomotor disturbance in the inner ear,[23] angioneurotic crisis,[24] allergic responses of the inner ear,[25,26] stenosis of the eustachian tube,[27] hypothyroidism,[27-29] focal sepsis,[3,30] psychogenic disturbances,[31] etc. Autopsy studies had been lacking until some light was shed on the problem through the demonstration

of a pathologic condition common to a number of cases with Meniere's syndrome. In 1938, Hallpike and Cairns[32] found in two cases a marked dilatation of the endolymphatic system of the inner ear, suggesting the existence of increased endolymphatic pressure. Since that time other cases have been described, although the scarcity of pathologic material in this disease makes the number small. In 1945, Altman[33] collected 14 cases from the literature, in nine of which the involvement was unilateral. The cochlear duct was dilated in all, the saccule in most, the utricle in many, but the semicircular canals were dilated in none. No inflammatory changes were demonstrated, and it is assumed that the disorder is due to an overproduction or a diminished resorption of the endolymph, or to a combination of both. The cause of this condition of an obstructive distention of the endolymph system is unknown. It has been called *idiopathic hydrops of the labyrinth* to distinguish it from the hydrops associated with serous labyrinthitis, which shows more widespread degenerative change.

These pathologic observations have provided a basis for understanding the syndrome, but the fundamental etiology remains obscure and the explanation of the signs and symptoms is not entirely clear. Hallpike and Cairns[32] consider the attacks of vertigo to be due to a sudden rise of endolymphatic pressure with "rapidly initiated bouts of asphyxia" of the vestibular end organs. Lindsay[34] has described recent histopathologic studies with light microscopy. These have shown dilatations and herniations of the membranous labyrinth. The herniations have been found at the junction of canal ampullae with the utricle. This leads him to believe that variations in the frequency and severity of the attacks of vertigo, as well as the variable responses to vestibular tests, have a mechanical basis since the resulting distortions of the walls of the ampullae, as well as possible ruptures at these sites, are conditions subject to localized change during increase or decrease in the distention of the membranous labyrinth. Any shift in the wall of an ampulla, with its consequent effect on the cupula, could create an imbalance between its functional response and that of the ampulla in the same plane on the opposite side, thereby creating vertigo.

The syndrome consists of attacks of vertigo in an otherwise healthy adult, accompanied by deafness and tinnitus. The attacks occur spontaneously (bearing no relation to activity) at intervals that may vary from a few hours to several years. In most instances there is no warning before an attack, but sometimes there may be an increase in the intensity of the tinnitus and perhaps also of the deafness preceding the onset. In some cases cephalic sensations occur before an attack, such as sensations of fullness, pressure or stiffness in the back of the head, or in the region of the ear, which may last throughout the attack and persist for some time afterward. The attacks of vertigo characteristically come on abruptly, last usually a matter of minutes (rarely for an hour or more), and terminate abruptly. During the attack the patient is prostrated, desiring to remain motionless, with pallor, sweating and spontaneous nystagmus, either horizontal or rotatory. He is liable to be nauseated throughout, and commonly vomits repeatedly in the later stages of the attack. Recovery is usually rapid, although the patient is likely to have a sensation of unsteadiness upon standing lasting up to several hours, and abrupt movements of the head may result in brief vertiginous sensations. The nystagmus subsides with the cessation of vertigo or shortly afterward. Occasionally transitory loss of vision without unconsciousness may occur in an attack. Diplopia also has been described and attributed to skew deviation, a disorder of ocular posture emanating from the labyrinth.[3]

Loss of consciousness occasionally has been observed in severe attacks but it is not common. In such cases epilepsy always has to be excluded although the loss of consciousness may be due to vasovagal syncope resulting from the vasomotor disturbance, which accompanies severe vertigo. Rarely patients with long-standing Meniere's disease may develop epileptic attacks that seem to be a product of the labyrinthine disorder. The writer has had such a case under observation. This middle-aged man developed convulsive seizures eight years after the onset of perceptive deafness, tinnitus, and attacks of vertigo. The seizures were infrequent and took place without warning but on recovery of consciousness he experienced vertigo lasting 10 to 15 minutes. The interictal electroencephalogram was normal. The convulsive attacks ceased after a period of five years, coinciding with a spontaneous remission of the attacks of vertigo. The remission lasted for the next three years that he was under observation. During this time, he had no attacks of any kind. This case conforms with what has been called "vestibular epilepsy," i.e., a form of epilepsy in which seizures are provoked by excessive spontaneously arising discharge from the vestibular apparatus. Occasionally patients with Meniere's disease are subject to sudden brief attacks, without loss of consciousness, in which the limbs go limp and they fall. These attacks may occur with no accompanying vertigo, and they have been attributed to a disorder of the otolith organs ("the otolithic catastrophe" of Tumarkin).[35]

Subjective deafness, with or without tinnitus, commonly precedes the onset of attacks of vertigo, sometimes by many years. This is not surprising since the observed pathologic change appears to have its initial expression in the cochlear structures. It has been suggested that Meniere's disease may have loss of hearing as its only clinical symptom[36] but probably, if the patients survive long enough, attacks of vertigo will occur in the great majority. In a smaller number of patients the deafness and tinnitus appear at approximately the time of onset of the first attack of vertigo and in occasional instances they are not manifest for a considerable time after the attacks commence. The patient usually notices the deafness and tinnitus only in one ear at the start and often for a long time afterward. If these symptoms become bilateral they tend to preponderate on one side, being often relatively slight in the other ear. Cawthorne, Fitzgerald, and Hallpike[37] studied 50 cases of Meniere's disease finding objective impairment of cochlear function in all. They were able to show that this was bilateral in 86 per cent of the cases.

A characteristic feature of the deafness in this disease is its variability, particularly in the early stages when sudden changes are common. It is likely to be more marked at a time when attacks of vertigo are occurring, and it may lessen materially between attacks, suggesting that—in the early stages at least—a reversible factor must be present in its causation. It is a perceptive deafness showing either a uniform loss of hearing throughout the entire scale in the affected ear, or a predominant loss for low tones. Distortion of sounds (diplacusis) and hypersensitivity to loud sounds (subjective recruitment) occur, as well as the hearing loss, and may be very distressing to the patient. Lindsay[38] considers the auditory disturbances to be caused by the distortion of the saccule and the membrane of Reissner, associated with the hydrops, thus interfering with the sound transmission in the column of fluid in the cochlea.

The tinnitus likewise is usually more marked at the time when attacks of vertigo occur. It commonly consists of a high-pitched ringing or hissing sound with a low-pitched roaring or pounding, which is continuous even in the quiescent periods between attacks.[39] The tinnitus has been explained on the basis of irritation of the nerve endings by increased endolymph pressure, but the fact that section of the eighth nerve does not usually abolish the tinnitus makes it necessary to postulate a central factor in its causation, in some cases at least.

Tests for vestibular function in Meniere's disease reveal abnormal reactions in a large proportion of the cases if the tests are properly carried out. According to Altman,[33] there are abnormal caloric reactions in 90 per cent of the cases, with the majority showing a decrease in vestibular irritability on the affected side. Cawthorne,[40] who studied 400 cases, states that with the method of caloric testing used, he rarely failed to reveal a lack of balance between the two labyrinths, the most common finding being a depression of function on the side of the deafness. He points out that it affords almost the only and the most consistent physical sign of a vestibular disorder, and since each labyrinth is tested separately, it gives valuable information as to whether or not the disorder is limited to one labyrinth, a point of great importance if operative treatment is being considered. In contrast to what was found in testing cochlear functions, definite bilateral vestibular involvement was revealed in less than 5 per cent of these cases. Usually, but not always, the more affected labyrinth is on the side with the greater hearing loss. As in the case of the deafness, there may be considerable variation in the amount of labyrinthine response where tests are carried out at intervals and the latter usually parallels the deafness in degree.[39]

Between attacks the patient is characteristically well and free of symptoms, except deafness and tinnitus, which gradually become less variable and more severe over the years. In some cases the fear of attacks may lead to an anxiety state with resulting tension symptoms, which add materially to the disability. In Meniere's disease, as in other paroxysmal disorders, emotional maladjustments with morbid anxiety may aggravate and precipitate attacks of vertigo.

A feature of Meniere's disease which has not received the attention it merits is the frequent tendency to spontaneous remissions of the vertigo. Patients who have had many attacks of vertigo for months or years may experience periods of lessened frequency, whether they are receiving treatment or not. In about 50 per cent of long-standing cases, a history can be obtained of attacks having stopped spontaneously for months or years, although they tend to recur eventually.[41]

In this connection the observations of Picard[42] are of interest. He followed 37 patients with Meniere's disease treated only with placebos. Their previous attacks had existed for varying periods up to nine years, although some patients reported after the first attack. After 12 months' observation only 11 patients were continuing to have attacks, and after two years this number was reduced to five. He concludes that in 86 per cent of cases, Meniere's disease is self-limiting, and that in probably 70 per cent attacks will have ceased within a year. Although relapses may occur, they do not necessarily indicate a bad long-term prognosis.

It is important to consider this remitting character of the disease in evaluating any method of therapy. The removal of an abscessed tooth, eliminating a food from the diet, administering thyroid extract, inflating an eustachian tube, removing a plug of wax from the ear, etc., if carried out at the time a spontaneous remission is due to occur, may be considered of therapeutic value, and lead to false conceptions about causal relationship. The auditory symptoms are likely to continue and may progress during these periods of remission of the vertigo, indicating that, although a temporary balance may have developed in labyrinthine function, the underlying disorder is not quiescent.

Aural vertigo occasionally results from a vascular accident such as hemorrhage within the otic labyrinth, or perhaps more commonly thrombosis or embolism of the internal auditory artery. Such lesions cause explosive attacks of vertigo, usually accompanied by a high degree of permanent deafness.[43] It has been anatomically established that the internal auditory artery separates into branches, which supply the cochlea and the labyrinth, respectively, the branch to the labyrinth commonly being an end artery. Milliken et al.[44] have suggested that certain patients who have an instantaneous onset of severe vertigo associated with nausea and vomiting but no pain, tenderness, or hearing loss, nor any symptoms or signs of neuro-logical dysfunction, have suffered an occlu-sion of the labyrinthine division of the in-ternal auditory artery. Caloric studies in such patients reveal a dead labyrinth, and the total loss of function appears to be permanent. Vertigo and nystagmus are severe for weeks, with ultimate gradual recovery.

Acute unilateral obstruction of the eusta-chian tubes often is stated to be a cause of vertigo as well as conductive deafness, but the mechanism of the production of vertigo is not entirely clear. Usually it is attributed to an alteration of the pressure relationship that exists in the middle ears, since normally this is kept equal to the outside atmosphere by the passage of air through the eustachian tubes. Tubal catarrh may occur as a result of infection or in the presence of anedoids.

In aviation medicine the term "bara-trauma" has come into frequent use. It implies the middle-ear damage than can result from violent and tremendous pressure changes caused by climbing and power div-ing. Deafness and tinnitus are the most common symptoms, but vertigo may be an occasional accompaniment.

Vertigo and Dizziness With Lesions of the Eighth Nerve

Vertigo occurring in attacks and compar-able in severity to that of Meniere's disease is uncommon with lesions that are confined to the eighth nerve. The usual site of involve-ment of this nerve is in the cerebellopontine angle. Tumors, particularly acoustic neu-roma, are the most common lesions, but vascular anomalies, including aneurysms and abnormally distributed arteries undergoing arteriosclerotic change, occasionally may af-fect the eighth nerve directly. Chronic syphilitic pachymeningitis, arachnoiditis, and platybasia are uncommon causes. Vertigo, deafness, and tinnitus occasionally accom-pany the herpes oticus, facial palsy, and pain of the Ramsay Hunt syndrome. They are considered to be due to an associated neu-ritis of the eighth nerve.

Several statistical studies have been made on cases with verified lesions (mainly tumors of the eighth nerve) to estimate the fre-quency of vertigo.[4,41,45,46,47] Combined fig-ures from the various sources show that vertigo occurred in about 22 per cent of 293 verified cases. Thus, it is not common and when present, it is usually a late manifesta-tion accompanied by other neurologic signs

and symptoms which help to distinguish it from labyrinthine disease. Very rarely ver-tigo occurring in attacks may be the first or an early symptom in acoustic neuroma.[4,45,48] The inconstancy of true vertigo in lesions affecting the eighth nerve, and its tendency to appear as a late symptom if at all, sug-gest that when it occurs in cerebellopontine angle tumors it may be the result of involve-ment of the vestibular nuclei in the adjacent brain stem, either by the lesion directly or through changes resulting from internal hydrocephalus.

The rather surprising finding that lesions of the vestibular nerve itself rarely produce vertigo in any way comparable to what oc-curs with lesions of the end organ receives support from the observations of Dandy.[49] He sectioned the eighth nerve for labyrin-thine vertigo in three cases under local anes-thetic. In two there were no sensations when the nerve was being liberated or di-vided. The third patient experienced tran-sient vertigo when the nerve was being manipulated, but this stopped when it was divided. These observations provide a great contrast to the results from stimulation or sudden destruction of the labyrinth itself.

In the rare instances in which vertigo is an early symptom with tumors in the cerebello-pontine angle, there may be difficulty in dif-ferentiation from Meniere's disease, since unilateral perceptive deafness and tinnitus are likely to be present in both conditions. However, with a few exceptions, a careful neurologic examination is likely to show evi-dence of involvement of the fifth and pos-sibly the seventh cranial nerve, persistent nystagmus, and signs of cerebellar dysfunc-tion when tumor is the cause. A fluctuating tendency in the deafness and tinnitus, to-gether with the presence of loudness recruit-ment and diplacusis, which are attributed to disease of Corti's organ, favors Meniere's disease. The degree of impairment of ves-tibular function by caloric test is likely to be much greater with acoustic neuroma than is usually found in Meniere's disease. Al-though verified cases of acoustic neuroma have been recorded which are said to have shown good vestibular reactions on the af-fected side prior to operation, Dix and Hall-pike[48] found abnormal caloric responses in 100 per cent of their large series by use of the particular method of testing they employ.

Brief dizziness, consisting of sensations of unsteadiness in walking and uncertainty of equilibrium occurring upon change of posture, is much more common than true vertigo with tumors involving the eighth nerve. These symptoms are most prone to occur when signs of increased intracranial pressure are present, and it is possible that they are caused by edema and altered vascularity in the central vestibular pathways resulting from distention of the fourth ventricle associated with hydrocephalus.

Vertigo and Dizziness with Lesions in the Brain Stem

Lesions that involve the vestibular nuclei in the brain stem are likely to cause very severe vertigo comparable to that seen in labyrinthine disease. Atkinson[23] considers that only lesions in this situation will produce true objective vertigo other than those in the labyrinth itself. Lesions of the brain stem most prone to cause vertigo are those that occur acutely, such as *vascular accidents*.

Important vestibular pathways, including the large part of the vestibular nuclei situated in the pons, receive blood supply from the anterior inferior cerebellar arteries, and a thrombosis of one of these vessels or a hemorrhage arising from a pontine branch, would be expected to cause vertigo. Much more commonly, occlusion of a posterior inferior cerebellar artery occurs, giving rise to severe vertigo at the onset together with the other characteristic findings due to involvement of certain structures in the dorsolateral portion of the medulla. Both the posterior inferior cerebellar and the anterior inferior cerebellar arteries show considerable variation in their relative sizes and distributions, but ordinarily the major part of the descending vestibular nucleus is included in the distribution of the posterior inferior cerebellar artery.[50] The severity and duration of the vertigo with thrombosis or emblism affecting this vessel doubtless depend upon the degree and extent of the occlusion and the corresponding amount of damage to the vestibular structures in the upper medulla.

Vertigo may occur with acute exacerbations of *multiple sclerosis*, since plaques are not uncommonly situated in the brain stem —particularly in the pontine reticular substance. The vertigo in multiple sclerosis is often transitory, but sometimes it is very severe and protracted, accompanied by vomiting and lasting for days. Alpers[51] analyzed 156 cases, finding vertigo the first, or early, symptom in 26 and a late symptom in 11. He points out that when it occurs as an early

symptom, other findings characteristic of multiple sclerosis may be absent, rendering diagnosis difficult. However, careful inquiry in such cases will often reveal mild subjective symptoms accompanying the vertigo, like numbness on one side of the face or brief diplopia, which aid in their recognition.

Gradually developing lesions, such as *tumors*, situated in the brain stem occasionally give rise to vertigo, as a prominent and early symptom. Fifty-seven verified cases of tumor involving the brain stem were analyzed at the Toronto General Hospital[52] Vertigo occurring in spontaneous attacks or upon change of posture was an initial or very early symptom in eight patients. Two other patients had less specific dizziness as a presenting symptom. In eight of these cases the tumors arose primarily in the brain stem; the other two arose in the fourth ventricle. In Cairns' series of nine verified cases of brain-stem tumor, vertigo was present in two.[53] The reason vertigo does not occur more often with tumors in this situation is probably because slowly developing lesions enable adjustments to take place. Symonds[4] suggests that, when vertigo is a symptom of a brain-stem tumor, it is probably due to a phase of congestion or edema of rapid development. Episodes of vertigo accompanied by headache and visual disturbance upon movements of the head occasionally occur with tumors and cysts situated in the fourth ventricle (Brun's syndrome). Syringobulbia may very rarely cause severe and prolonged vertigo.

Symptoms of dysequilibrium upon change of posture, similar to those described with tumors of the eighth nerve, occur commonly with tumors in this region, particularly with those arising in the fourth ventricle. They are probably due to changes in the vestibular connections in the brain stem, caused by the tumor directly or as a result of the associated hydrocephalus.

The differentiation between vertigo originating in the brain stem and that of labyrinthine origin occasionally is difficult. If headaches and vomiting precede the onset of vertigo, a central cause must be suspected. The vertigo with brain-stem lesions has the same quality as labyrinthine vertigo but it is very sensitive to movements of the head which may precipitate or aggravate it. Both peripheral and central vertigo may be influenced by change in posture but, according to Denny-Brown,[54] this is more common with central lesions. In contrast to labyrinthine

sions affecting the vestibular structures in the brain stem. Harrison,[75] on the other hand, concludes from his studies that "serious, persistent dizziness following head injuries, not necessarily associated with skull fracture, is very frequently, particularly if it is of a rotational character, due to traumatic lesions of the otolithic apparatus." Caloric tests, using the technic described by Fitzgerald and Hallpike, showed abnormalities in most but not all of his cases. The diagnosis depends upon the demonstration of positional nystagmus with postural vertigo when the head is retracted and turned, first to one side and subsequently to the other, with the patient supine (as was described discussing brain-stem lesions). The nystagmus occurs in the one critical position, takes a few seconds to appear, lasts briefly, lessens with repetition of the test, and never changes direction. It has lateralizing value, since it usually beats towards the pathological ear when that ear is undermost.

Barber[76] found positional nystagmus with these characteristics in about 25 per cent of 165 patients exhibiting postural vertigo or dizziness following head injury. The frequency was nearly 50 per cent in 85 of the cases where longitudinal fracture of the temporal bone had occurred. There is good reason to believe that when the so-called "benign paroxysmal positional nystagmus," as described previously, is found after head injury, it is a result of a lesion in the vestibular end-organ,[18,55,75,77] probably involving the otoliths in many instances. However, the diagnostic and lateralizing significance of positional nystagmus has not been accepted uniformly,[78] and further pathological evidence is necessary before definite conclusions can be drawn.

The common "whiplash" injury sustained in automobile accidents occasionally is followed by postural vertigo. In some instances, this may be the result of damage to the vestibular end-organ, notably the utricle.[9] In those patients, however, in whom cervical muscle spasm, associated with persistent pain, exists, the vertigo is more likely the result of an interference with the tonic neck reflexes.[78] These reflexes are important in postural adjustments and are mediated through the dorsal roots of the upper cervical segments.

The mechanism of production of the less specific type of dizziness that follows cerebral trauma is not clearly understood, although its occurrence upon change of posture, like true vertigo after head injury, suggests a causal relationship. Most observers agree that two elements are involved in causing the dizziness: these are the *physical effect* of the injury on the structures inside the skull and the *psychogenic factors* arising out of the circumstances associated with the head injury. It is very difficult and, in many instances, impossible to be sure of the relative parts these play in a given case. However, the finding of positional nystagmus in a patient complaining of post-traumatic postural dizziness is positive evidence of organic disorder. This observation may be of great value in assessing cases involving litigation in which all other tests are negative.

The degree and persistence of this type of dizziness do not bear so clear a relationship to the severity of the head injury as does true vertigo. Its nature and close association with change of posture has given rise to speculation as to whether it could be due to a defect in vasomotor adjustment,[71,74,80] perhaps resulting from medullary concussion.[68,81] It seems possible that this may be an important factor in causing the dizziness as well as the headache in the first few months after head injury, but the available evidence is not conclusive.

When dizziness persists for many months or years after head injury it is usually accompanied by headaches and evidences of an anxiety state. Such patients often show no signs of structural damage from the trauma upon neurologic investigation. Inquiry frequently reveals evidence of nervous instability in the past history of the patient, with varying degrees of maladjustment, resentment arising from the circumstances of the injury or the compensation received, pending litigation, anxiety regarding future employment, etc. Although the foregoing factors are important in many cases with prolonged post-traumatic dizziness, there is not always a consistent relationship between the occurrence of the symptoms and the emotional disturbances. In addition, the incidence of prolonged dizziness is decidedly higher in patients with more severe head injuries.[70] Therefore, there is reason to believe that impairment of function, resulting from primary injury to some part of the vestibular mechanism from the peripheral end organ to the cortex, or secondary to post-traumatic vasomotor disturbance, is a fundamental basis of all post-traumatic dizziness; however, it seems probable that emotional factors, when present, may aggravate and prolong the symptoms.

Vertigo and Dizziness in Cardiovascular and Cerebrovascular Disease

In cardiovascular and blood diseases true vertigo is a rare complaint, but sensations described as dizziness related to change of posture or to sudden exertion occur more frequently. The sensations include unsteadiness, a swimming feeling, visual blurring, and lightheadedness, which are usually transitory and often immediately relieved by lying down. Among the conditions in which this type of dizziness may be a complaint are postural hypotension, severe anemia, aortic valvular disease (particularly aortic stenosis), Stokes-Adams syndrome, the carotid sinus syndrome, severe cardiac dysrhythmias and, rarely, coronary thrombosis. In these disorders it is likely that cerebral *anoxia* due to transitory ischemia is the usual cause of the symptoms, since they are allied more often to syncope than to vertigo. As a rule such patients experience no hallucination of movement of themselves or of objects, and nystagmus does not accompany the postural dizziness. In certain cases, however, there is degenerative disease of the cerebral arteries present as well. In this event the location of the latter may determine that the maximum anoxia resulting from the circulatory disorder is somewhere in the vestibular pathways, thus causing more specific vertiginous sensations.

Brief dizzy sensations, often of a vertiginous type, are a common complaint of the elderly, and usually prove to be a manifestation of cerebrovascular disease. They are induced or aggravated by change of posture, and less commonly by exertion, suggesting that they are due to imperfect vasomotor adjustment as a result of diseased blood vessels. It is movement and not position alone that is the provoking factor, so that the symptoms often can be lessened by changing posture slowly and also by avoiding excessive physical activity, which these patients soon learn to do.

Patients with hypertension sometimes complain of dizziness or vertigo but it is difficult to see how hypertension per se could cause these symptoms, unless possibly through sudden marked fluctuations occurring in the blood pressure. It is more probable that the symptoms are due to the underlying state of the blood vessels causing recurrent local circulatory insufficiency in some part of the vestibular system, perhaps the result of vasospasm associated with hypertensive vascular disease.

In cases where deafness is associated with the attacks of vertigo in hypertensive vascular disease, it can be inferred that the internal auditory artery is one of the vessels at fault.

Stenosis of the vertebral and basilar arteries may lead to intermittent vascular insufficiency with relative ischemia of the brain stem, causing periodic vertigo, which often is accompanied by other manifestations indicating interference with the basilar circulation. These include blurred vision, frank diplopia, obscuration of vision, tingling in the face, ataxia, weakness of the legs, and even loss of consciousness. The diagnosis is based on the periodic return of symptoms after intervals of time. A transient diminution of blood flow, causing symptoms of which vertigo is the most constant, may be brought about by such factors as fluctuations in blood pressure or recent dehydration associated with diarrhea. The vestibular nuclei far out in the pons are especially vulnerable under these circumstances because they are supplied by tenuous, long branches of the vertebral and basilar arteries. The parent vessels of the basilar arteries, the vertebral arteries, also are long, ascending through the foramina in the transverse processes of the upper six cervical vertebrae. They are extremely subject to congenital anomaly as well as to pressure from osteophyte formation, and they are particularly liable to atherosclerosis.[82] Apart from involvement of the vestibular nuclei in the brain stem in cases of stenosis of the vertebral-basilar system, there may be intermittent vascular insufficiency that affects the labyrinth directly and results from impaired blood flow through the internal auditory branches of the basilar. Attacks of vertigo due to this cause will not be accompanied by signs of brain-stem involvement.

Reversal of blood flow in a vertebral artery due to occlusion of the proximal portion of the subclavian, from which it arises, may cause episodic vertigo, often accompanied by other symptoms of brain-stem ischemia.[82] This condition, known as the *subclavian steal syndrome*, was described in 1961.[83] With total occlusion of the proximal portion of a subclavian, the more distal vertebral branch acts as a collateral to the arm by siphoning blood down the vessel from the other vertebral artery to the distal sub-clavian bed. The symptoms occur spontane-ously, or may be precipitated by neck move-ment or by exercise of the affected arm. A marked reduction of blood pressure in the arm, as compared with the opposite side, often with an audible supraclavicular bruit, aid in recognizing the condition, which can be confirmed by arteriography.

In addition to intermittent, spontaneous vertigo resulting from insufficiency of the vertebral-basilar arterial system as described previously, atherosclerotic individuals may suffer vertigo produced mainly by neck-turning in a right or left backward direction. Radiologic studies, after injections of opaque substances into the vertebral arteries of cadavers, have demonstrated narrowing of the lumen of the contralateral vertebral ar-tery, at the level of the joint between the atlas and the axis, upon rotational movements of the neck.[85] In normal individuals symp-toms do not occur because there is adequate circulation from the opposite side. However when the blood flow is impaired through atherosclerosis, perhaps accompanied by ob-struction from without due to cervical spon-dylosis and/or by a vascular anomaly with one vertebral artery being extremely small, then symptoms and signs are liable to occur with neck turning. Evidence that symptoms produced in this way are more common than is generally believed is obtained from the observations of Biemond,[86] who investigated a series of patients over 60 years of age with signs of arteriosclerosis. Twisting the neck in a right or left lateral direction resulted in the repeated appearance of a horizontal-rotatory type of nystagmus, as well as the frequent occurrence of pathologic plantar responses and a slight dysarthria.

Other conditions that will cause vertigo and nystagmus with turning movements or retraction of the head have to be differen-tiated from vertebral artery insufficiency, but this usually is not difficult. The syndrome may occur in primary labyrinthine disease but the lack of a history of previous *spon-taneous* attacks of vertigo and the absence of cochlear symptoms, together with normal caloric responses, usually enables this to be excluded. Little difficulty should be expe-rienced with so-called "benign paroxysmal positional nystagmus," which has been at-tributed to a lesion of the otolithic appa-ratus, traumatic, infective, or vascular. With this condition, the nystagmus and vertigo occur when the head is placed in a certain critical position and are not produced by neck movements per se. The patients are in a younger age group as a rule, and upon repetitive positional tests the nystagmic re-sponse becomes characteristically reduced, even to the point of abolition,[70] which is not the case with vertebral artery insufficiency. Abnormalities of the foramen magnum such as the Arnold-Chiari malformation as well as posterior fossa tumors, particularly mid-line cerebellar tumors, may cause vertigo and nystagmus upon retraction of the head which develop immediately and continue as long as the position is maintained. These lesions usually can be recognized readily by the accompanying neurologic signs, but Cawthorne and Hinchcliffe[87] have reported several cases of metastatic cerebellar tumor in which this central type of postural vertigo and positional nystagmus was the main find-ing, and it led to investigations that re-vealed the correct diagnosis. The occurrence of vertigo upon neck movement following cervical injury that has caused interfer-ence with the tonic neck reflexes has already been discussed. Such patients will have pain, muscle spasm, and possibly radiological findings in the cervical region, which help in identifying the condition.

VERTIGO DUE TO DRUGS

A toxic disturbance of the vestibular mecha-nism is a well-recognized complication from the administration of certain drugs. Vertigo sometimes accompanies the deafness and tinnitus which may occur when large doses of *quinine* or *salicylates* are administered. The association of deafness, tinnitus, and vertigo suggests that the site of the toxic effect is the peripheral cochlear and labyrinthine structures, with possible involvement of the eighth nerve also. The inhalation of *tobacco* smoke by susceptible individuals or *alco-holic* intoxication may cause vertigo, which is probably due to a toxic effect on the cen-tral vestibular mechanism. Toxic doses of certain anticonvulsant drugs, particularly Dilantin, occasionally cause vertigo although more commonly the symptoms consist sim-ply of ataxia, horizontal nystagmus, and dysarthria.

The otic complications of *streptomycin* therapy have received considerable atten-tion during the past 20 years since the introduction of the drug for the treatment of tuberculosis. Large doses and long administration are important factors in their occurrence. Symptoms become manifest between 30 and 35 days after beginning treatment,[88] and deafness and low-pitched tinnitus sometimes develop with the vertigo. If the drug is promptly discontinued complete recovery is likely to occur. Even if total loss of reactions on vestibular testing remains permanently, the patient usually recovers from any deafness that may have been present. In this event accessory balance mechanisms may compensate for the bilateral labyrinthine loss, although some constant unsteadiness of gait and posture may remain.[89] Such patients also may complain of inability to focus objects with the eyes when the head is in motion. Objects seem to dance or oscillate before the patient's eyes when he is walking or riding in a vehicle. These visual phenomena are due to the loss of the vestibulo-ocular reflexes, which influence the extra-ocular muscles in such a manner as to compensate for movements of the head. In addition to clinical studies, which have shown that streptomycin injures the vestibular nerve peripherally,[90] studies on experimental animals indicate that the localization of lesions after streptomycin is central as well as peripheral. The vestibular ganglion and Deiters' nucleus in the brain stem, together with the nerve, were found to show definite changes.[91]

More recently the drugs kanamycin and neomycin also have been shown to have ototoxic properties.[92,93]

PSYCHOGENIC DIZZINESS

Many patients who show in their histories and upon examination positive evidence of psychoneurosis give "dizziness" or "giddiness" as one of their symptoms. The complaint is often poorly described, and, when pressed, the patient may not be able to do more than reiterate "just a dizzy feeling." Sometimes it is described as "a feeling as if I am going to fall"; although the patient never falls and will usually admit that she never even staggers, yet it may keep her confined to the house for long periods. In such cases the sensation would seem to be a symbolic reflection of the inherent sense of insecurity caused by adjustment difficulties relating to the environment. The symptom is continuous, not coming in attacks, and may persist for weeks, months, or years. Brain[3] has suggested that it symbolizes the patient's fear of impending collapse—mental, moral, and physical.

Dizziness also may be a complaint in some psychotic patients, particularly in schizophrenia and depressive states. Inquiry shows that the word is used to indicate "thickheadedness" or an inability to think consecutively resulting from preoccupation or mental blocking.

Although dizziness is common in anxiety states, one must not assume that the dizziness is entirely a product of it. The converse may be true. Patients with paroxysmal vertigo are very prone to develop anxiety states as a result of their fear and apprehension about attacks, and in such cases a careful study of the patient may be necessary to evaluate correctly the symptoms. It should also be emphasized that the symptom of dizziness is not to be considered psychogenic because the patient's description does not indicate true vertigo. The complaint always should be interpreted in the light of the total findings, and other positive evidence must be found before concluding that it is a product of the mental state. Lord Brain[94] summarizes the matter very well when he says: (1) In all cases of giddiness, however great the psychological factor, investigate the labyrinth. (2) In all cases of giddiness, however great the organic factor, never forget the psychological reactions.

OCULAR VERTIGO AND MOTION SICKNESS

Ocular disorders are not a common cause of vertigo. Vertigo has been described as occurring at the onset of diplopia when an ocular muscle becomes suddenly paralyzed and is attributed to the faulty projection of the visual field of the affected eye. Looking down from heights and watching moving trains from a stationary platform causes vertiginous sensations in certain people due to the discrepancy between the visual perceptions and the proprioceptor impulses from elsewhere in the body.

It was formerly considered that in seasickness and certain other types of motion sickness the ocular factor was prominent in causing the vertigo. However, it is now generally believed that the disturbance is primarily vestibular in all forms of motion sickness, although the nature of the physiologic mechanisms at fault is still a matter of conjecture and theory. The condition has been attributed to excessive stimulation of the peripheral labyrinthine mechanism by the repetitive movement,[95] but the absence of spontaneous nystagmus in the various types of motion sickness has led to the opinion that the cause is excessive stimulation of the macula utriculi rather than the labyrinth. It is of interest that Bard and his associates[96] have cured car sickness in susceptible dogs by isolated removal of the nodulus of the cerebellum, thus apparently localizing a central pathway concerned in the disorder.

SUMMARY

Vertigo is a specific subjective sensation, consisting of a hallucination of movement of the individual or his surroundings. It may result from lesions affecting the vestibular pathways from the labyrinth to the cortex, but in its most developed form it is confined to lesions of the labyrinth or the vestibular structures in the brain stem.

Vertigo is encountered most commonly with labyrinthine disturbances, which may result from inflammatory, vascular, or toxic disorders or from the idiopathic hydrops of the labyrinth that accompanies Meniere's disease. The vertigo arising from disturbed function of the vestibular structures in the brain stem may be due to their direct involvement by vascular lesions or it may result from ischemia caused by impaired circulation in the basilar-vertebral arterial system. Plaques of multiple sclerosis, as well as neoplasms, also may involve the vestibular nuclei to produce vertigo. Persistent vertigo following cerebral trauma is the result of damage to the labyrinth or the vestibular nuclei. A particular type of postural vertigo after head injury, in which there is paroxysmal vertigo and nystagmus when the head is placed in certain critical positions, is believed to be due to a traumatic lesion of the otolithic apparatus. Intracranial expanding lesions not directly involving the brain stem may cause vertigo as a result of edema and changes in vascularity in the region of the vestibular nuclei associated with increased intracranial pressure. In subtentorial neoplasms there is likely to be the additional factor of distention of the fourth ventricle which accompanies hydrocephalus. Tumors and other lesions involving the eighth nerve may give rise to vertigo as an early symptom but not with anything like the consistency seen with disease of the labyrinth itself. Lesions strictly confined to the cerebellum give rise to a characteristic disturbance of equilibrium but there is no substantial evidence that vertigo results unless the brain stem is involved, directly or indirectly, as well. Destructive lesions of the forebrain rarely cause vertigo. When they do, it is a less severe and less clearly defined variety than that accompanying disorders of the labyrinth and the brain stem. Not infrequently, migraine and epilepsy are associated with vertigo. It may occur as the aura of an attack in either condition, and in migraine sometimes it may replace the headache or be present throughout the attack. In rare cases of chronic labyrinthine disease, epileptic seizures may develop which appear to be provoked by the excessive spontaneous discharge arising from the vestibular apparatus (vestibular epilepsy).

The complaints of "dizziness" and "giddiness" lack specific meaning. They are used to include not only vertigo and related sensations but also sensations pertaining to disturbed mental equilibrium and to syncope. Therefore, it is always necessary to obtain an *exact description* from the patient of what he feels in order to evaluate the symptom correctly.

A type of dizziness that may be associated with vertigo or occur alone is particularly important and probably has a basic mechanism similar to vertigo. It consists of sensations of unsteadiness in walking and uncertainty of equilibrium, often with a feeling of some sort of movement within the head, but it lacks the hallucination of movement of the individual or his surroundings that distinguishes vertigo. In cases of cerebral neoplasm, dizziness of this kind is a more common symptom than true vertigo. It is assumed to be due to changes affecting vestibular structures in the brain stem associated with increased intracranial pressure and it is particularly likely to occur with subtentorial tumors where obstruction and distention of the fourth ventricle are present. It occurs also as an aftermath of attacks of true vertigo, is frequently a symptom following head injury, and may be present in cerebral vascular disease, with or without hypertension. In these various conditions it is commonly brought on by change of posture. The symptoms described as dizziness which occasionally accompany certain cardiovascular diseases likewise may be induced by change of posture or by exertion, but for the most part their nature indicates a relationship to syncope, and they probably result from acute cerebral ischemia and anoxia.

It is evident that vertigo and dizziness

may be symptoms in a variety of pathologic conditions affecting the peripheral labyrinthine mechanism and the vestibular pathways in the brain. In order to localize the lesion correctly and to arrive at an accurate diagnosis of the cause of these symptoms, a carefully taken history and a thorough examination of the patient, medical and neurological, together with appropriate investigations of the auditory and vestibular functions, always are essential.

REFERENCES

1. Jackson, H.: Selected Writings, vol. 1, p. 309, London, Hodder & Stoughton, 1931.
2. McNally, W. J.: The physiology of the vestibular mechanism in relation to vertigo, Ann. Otol. 56:514, 1947.
3. Brain, W. R.: Vertigo: its neurological, otological, circulatory and surgical aspects, Brit. Med. J. 2:605, 1938.
4. Symonds, C. P.: The clinical significance of vertigo, Lancet 2:959, 1933.
5. Foerster, O.: The motor cortex in man in the light of Hughlings Jackson's doctrines, Brain 59:135, 1936.
6. Lindsay, J. R.: Postural vertigo and positional nystagmus, Ann. Otol. 60:1134, 1951.
7. Larsell, O., and Dow, R. S.: Cerebellum; new interpretation, Western J. Surg. 47:256, 1939.
8. Ransom, S. W., and Clark, S.: The Anatomy of the Nervous System, ed. 10, Philadelphia, Saunders, 1959.
9. Dolowitz, D. A.: Vertigo, Laryngoscope 75:805, 1965.
10. Kunkle, E. C.: Central causes of vertigo, J. S. Carolina Med. Ass. 50:161, 1954.
11. Penfield, W., and Erickson, T. C.: Epilepsy and Cerebral Localization, Springfield, Ill., Thomas, 1941.
12. Penfield, W.: Vestibular sensation and the cerebral cortex, Ann. Otol. 66:691, 1957.
13. Simonton, K. M.: The symptom of dizziness: its significance in general practice, Proc. Staff Meet. Mayo Clinic 16:465, 1941.
14. Burrowes, W. L.: Acute labyrinthitis, Brit. Med. J. 2:1182, 1952.
15. Leishman, A. W. O.: Acute labyrinthitis or epidemic vertigo, Lancet 1:228, 1955.
16. Cawthorne, T.: Vertigo, Proc. Roy. Soc. Med. 52:529, 1959.
17. Dix, M. R., and Hallpike, C. S.: The pathology, symptomatology and diagnosis of certain common disorders of the vestibular system, Proc. Roy. Soc. Med. 45:341, 1952.
18. Hallpike, C. S.: Vertigo of central origin, Proc. Roy. Soc. Med. 55:364, 1962.
19. Basser, L. S.: Benign paroxysmal vertigo of childhood, Brain 87:141, 1964.
20. Dedering, D.: Clinical and experimental examinations in patients suffering from MB Menieri including a study of the problem of bone conduction, Acta Otolaryng. (supp. x-xi), 1929.
21. Furstenberg, A. C., Lashmet, F. H., and Lathrop, F.: Ménière's symptom complex; medical treatment, Ann. Otol. 43:1035, 1934.
22. Shelden, C. H., and Horton, B. T.: Treatment of Ménière's disease with histamine administered intravenously, Proc. Staff Meet. Mayo Clinic 15:17, 1940.
23. Atkinson, M.: The dizzy patient, Eye, Ear, Nose, Throat Monthly 22:53, 1943.
24. Fischer, J. J.: Otologic aspects of vertigo, New Eng. J. Med. 241:142, 1949.
25. Harley, D.: Some observations on the fundamentals of allergy with special reference to its aural manifestations, J. Laryng. 62:1, 1948.
26. Lempert, J., et al.: A new theory for the correlation of pathology and symptomatology in Ménière's disease, Ann. Otol. 61:717, 1952.
27. Merica, F. W.: Vertigo due to obstruction of the eustachian tubes, J.A.M.A. 118:1282, 1942.
28. Athens, A. G.: Vertigo in hypothyroidism, Minnesota Med. 29:562, 1946.
29. Levy, I., and O'Leary, J. L.: Incidence of vertigo in neurological conditions, Ann. Otol. 56:557, 1947.
30. Wright, A. J.: Labyrinthine giddiness, its nature and treatment, Brit. Med. J. 1:668, 1938.
31. Fowler, E. P., and Zeckel, A.: Psychosomatic aspects of Ménière's disease, J.A.M.A. 148:1265, 1952.
32. Hallpike, C. S., and Cairns, H.: Observations on the pathology of Ménière's syndrome, J. Laryng. 53:625, 1938.
33. Altman, F.: Dizziness of peripheral vestibular origin, Laryngoscope 55:164, 1945.
34. Lindsay, J. R.: Pathology of vestibular disorders, Ann. Otol. 76:193, 1968.
35. Tumarkin, A.: The otolithic catastrophe, Brit. Med. J. 2:175, 1936.
36. Williams, H. L., Horton, B. T., and Day, L. A.: Endolymphatic hydrops without vertigo, Arch. Otolaryng. 51:557, 1950.
37. Cawthorne, T. E., Fitzgerald, G., and Hallpike, C. S.: Observations on the clinical features of "Ménière's" disease with especial reference to the results of the caloric tests, Brain 65:161, 1942.
38. Lindsay, J. R.: Labyrinthine dropsy and Ménière's disease, Arch. Otolaryng. 35:853, 1942.
39. Day, K. M.: Hydrops of labyrinth (Ménière's disease) diagnosis—results of labyrinth surgery, Laryngoscope 56:33, 1946.
40. Cawthorne, T.: Ménière's disease, Trans. Amer. Laryng. Rhinol. Otol. Soc., p. 352, 1946.
41. Hyland, H. H.: The diagnosis of Ménière's syndrome, Bull. Acad. Med., Toronto 19:8, 1945.

42. Picard, B. H.: The prognosis in Ménière's disease, Proc. Roy. Soc. Med. 60:968, 1967.
43. Furstenberg, A. C.: Symposium on vertigo, Ann. Otol. 56:576, 1946.
44. Milliken, C. H., Siekert, R. G., and Whisnant, J. P.: The syndrome of occlusion of the labyrinthine division of the internal auditory artery, Proc. Amer. Neurol. Ass. 1959.
45. McNally, W. J., and Stuart, E. A.: Vertigo from the standpoint of the otolaryngologist, Trans. Amer. Acad. Opthal. Otolaryng., p. 33, Nov.-Dec., 1941.
46. Cushing, H.: Tumors of the Nervus Acusticus and the Syndrome of the Cerebellopontile Angle, Philadelphia, Saunders, 1917.
47. Edwards, C. H., and Patterson, J. H.: The symptoms and signs of acoustic neurofibromata, Brain 74:144, 1951.
48. Dix, M. R., and Hallpike, C. S.: Discussion on acoustic neuroma, Proc. Roy. Soc. Med. 51:889, 1958.
49. Dandy, W. E.: Ménière's disease, its diagnosis and a method of treatment, Arch. Surg. 16:1127, 1928.
50. Alexander, L., and Suh, T. H.: Arterial supply of lateral parolivary area of medulla oblongata in man, Arch. Neurol. Psychiat. 38:1243, 1937.
51. Alpers, B. J.: Vertigo: its neurological features, Trans. Amer. Acad. Ophthal. Otolaryng., p. 38, Nov.-Dec., 1941.
52. Barnett, H. J., and Hyland, H. H.: Tumours involving the brain stem, Quart. J. Med. 83:265, 1952.
53. Cairns, H.: *Quoted by* Symonds (4).
54. Denny-Brown, D. E.: Neurologic aspects of vertigo, New Eng. J. Med. 241:144, 1949.
55. McCabe, B. F.: Clinical aspects of the differential diagnosis of end organ vertigo, Ann. Otol. 78:193, 1968.
56. Phillips, D. G.: Vertigo, New Zeal. Med. J. 45:219, 1946.
57. Fulton, J. F.: The William Withering Memorial Lectures, London, The Clarendon Press, Oxford, 1949.
58. Dow, R. S.: Effects of unilateral and bilateral labyrinthectomy in monkey, baboon and chimpanzee, Amer. J. Physiol. 121:392, 1938.
59. Spiegel, E. A., and Alexander, A.: Vertigo in brain tumors with special reference to the results of labyrinth examination, Ann. Otol. 45:979, 1936.
60. Abbott, W. D., and Kaump, D. H.: Subdural hematoma, Amer. J. Surg. 49:64, 1940.
61. Mollison, W. M., and Cloake, P.: Diagnosis and treatment of vertigo, Trans. Med. Soc. London 65:45, 1948.
62. Gowers, W. R.: Borderland of Epilepsy, Philadelphia, Blakiston, 1907.
63. Williams, D. J.: Vertigo, Proc. Roy. Soc. Med. 60:961, 1967.
64. Carmichael, E. A., Dix, M. R., Hallpike, C. S., and Hood, J. D.: Some further observations upon the effect of unilateral cerebral lesions on caloric and rotational nystagmus, Brain 84:571, 1961.
65. Behrman, S.: Vestibular epilepsy, Brain 78:471, 1955.
66. Bickerstaff, E. R.: Basilar artery migraine, Lancet 1:15, 1961.
67. Linthicum, F. H., and Rand, C. W.: Neuro-otological observations in concussion of the brain, Arch. Otolaryng. 13:785, 1931.
68. Russell, W. R.: Cerebral involvement in head injury, Brain 55:549, 1932.
69. Glaser, M. A.: The cause of dizziness in head injuries, Ann. Otol. 46:387, 1937.
70. Friedman, A. P., Brenner, C., and Denny-Brown, D.: Post-traumatic vertigo and dizziness, J. Neurosurg. 2:36, 1945.
71. Phillips, D. G.: Investigation of vestibular function after head injury, J. Neurol. Neurosurg. Psychiat. 8:79, 1945.
72. Osnato, M., and Gilberti, V.: Post-concussion neurosis—traumatic encephalitis, Arch. Neurol. Psychiat. 18:181, 1927.
73. Schuster, F. P.: Head injuries with ear symptoms, Southwest Med. 11:116, 1927.
74. Symonds, C. P., and Lewis, A.: Discussion on differential diagnosis and treatment of post-contusional states, Proc. Roy. Soc. Med. 35:601, 1942.
75. Harrison, M. S.: Notes on the clinical features and pathology of post-concussional vertigo with special reference to positional nystagmus, Brain 79:475, 1956.
76. Barber, H. O.: Dizziness and head injury, Canad. Med. Ass. J. 92:974, 1965.
77. Eadie, M. J.: Paroxysmal positional giddiness, Med. J. Aust. 54:1169, 1967.
78. McNally, W. J.: The assessment of vertigo, Minnesota Med. 50:1003, 1967.
79. Ryan, G. M. S., and Cope, S.: Cervical vertigo, Lancet 2:1355, 1955.
80. McKenzie, K. G.: One aspect of the post-traumatic syndrome in cranio-cerebral injuries, Trans. Amer. Neurol. Ass. 69:103, 1943.
81. Denny-Brown, D.: The sequelae of war head injuries, New Eng. J. Med. 227:771, 1942.
82. Hutchinson, E. G., and Yates, P. O.: The cervical portion of the vertebral artery, Brain 79:319, 1956.
83. Bergan, J. J., Levy, J. S., Trippel, O. H., and Juragi, M.: Vascular implications of vertigo, Arch. Otolaryng. 85:292, 1967.
84. Reivich, M., Holling, H. E., Roberts, B., and Toole, J. F.: Reversal of blood flow through the vertebral artery and its effect on cerebral circulation, New Eng. J. Med. 265:878, 1961.
85. Tissington Tatlow, W. F., and Bammer, H. G.: Syndrome of vertebral artery compression, Neurology 7:331, 1957.
86. Biemond, A.: Thrombosis of the basilar

artery and the vascularization of the brain stem, Brain 74:300, 1951.

87. Cawthorne, T., and Hinchcliffe, R.: Positional nystagmus of the cerebral type as evidence of subtentorial metastases, Brain 84:415, 1961.

88. Snell, F. B.: Some otic complications of streptomycin therapy, Mil. Surgeon 102:202, 1948.

89. Ford, F. R.: Clinical classification of vestibular disorders, Bull. Hopkins Hosp. 87:299, 1950.

90. Glorig, A., and Fowler, E. P.: Tests for labyrinth function following streptomycin therapy, Ann. Otol. 56:379, 1947.

91. Barr, B., Floberg, L. E., Hamberger, A. C., and Koch, H. J.: Otological aspects of streptomycin therapy, Acta Otolaryng. (supp. 75), p. 5, 1949.

92. Hawkins, J. E.: The ototoxicity of kanamycin, Amer. Otol. 68:698, 1959.

93. Lindsay, J. R., Proctor, L. R., and Work, W. P.: Histopathologic inner ear changes in deafness due to neomycin, Trans. Amer. Laryng. Rhinol. Otol. Soc. p. 259, 1960.

94. Brain, W. R.: Vertigo of central origin, Proc. Roy. Soc. Med. 55:361, 1962.

95. Krieg, W. J. S.: Functional Neuroanatomy, Philadelphia, Blakiston, 1942.

96. Bard, P., et al.: Quoted by Fulton (57).

35

Dehydration, Fluid and Electrolyte Imbalances

CYRIL M. MacBRYDE

DEFINITION

Dehydration may be defined as that bodily state resulting from excessive loss of fluid. It is implied that such loss is sufficient to endanger or actually to impair functions for which certain amounts of fluid are necessary. The life of the organism depends upon adequate performance by the body fluids of their essential functions of transportation of nutrient and excretory materials and of temperature and chemical regulation. It is important to remember that dehydration always signifies loss not only of water but of electrolyte, and that, therefore, the term dehydration is incomplete. Likewise, it is apparent that dehydration cannot be corrected by replacement of water alone; electrolyte also must be replaced.

The body fluids constitute what Claude Bernard called "the internal environment" of the body.[1] He showed that in mammals the amounts and the constituents of the body fluids varied within relatively fixed limits, variations beyond these limits endangering life. Cannon[2] designated the coordinated physiologic processes that maintain a healthful internal environment as *mechanisms of homeostasis*. When one or more of the regulatory functions breaks down, or when the body is prevented from employing its usual restorative measures, fluid may be lost in excessive amounts. Loss of fluid, which is itself the homeostatic agent of greatest importance, and is the medium in which a number of important regulators exist and are transported, may have serious consequences. In this chapter will be considered the ways in which dehydration may occur and how the body is affected thereby.

DEHYDRATION AS A SYMPTOM

The clinical picture of dehydration is usually easy to recognize. In mild or moderate dehydration, thirst, fatigue, anorexia, nausea and oliguria are observed. With more advanced degrees of dehydration the patient usually complains of extreme thirst, weakness and rapid weight loss. If the fluid loss has been extreme, the patient may be faint, prostrated or in coma, and may suffer from the severe dyspnea (Kussmaul breathing) of acidosis. Physical examination reveals dry mucous membranes; dry, inelastic loose skin; low blood pressure and soft eyeballs, and, often, the expired air smells of acetone. Fever may be present solely as the result of dehydration. Frequently the history reveals one or more influences leading to failure of fluid absorption or to excess fluid loss. Less often, the causes of the dehydration may be obscure, especially when it has been gradual in development. Sudden loss of fluid (as from hemorrhage) does not permit time for the development of dry skin and mucous membranes, but is characterized by weakness, thirst, low blood pressure, and clinical evidences of shock.

Clinically, three stages or degrees of dehydration may be distinguished: (1) simple dehydration with dry skin and mucous membranes, weight loss, etc.; (2) more advanced fluid loss with dry skin, etc., plus a fall in blood pressure and other evidence of loss of plasma volume—weakness, faintness, fever, weak pulse, shock, coma; (3) the previous manifestations plus signs of renal failure (uremia, acidosis). Severe renal failure may prevent recovery even when water and electrolytes are restored.

Central Nervous System Effects

Simple dehydration (pure water loss) results in only mild and inconstant circulatory changes (mild or moderate decrease in cardiac output and prolongation of circulation time, slight fall in blood pressure). However, mental confusion has been noted frequently. The dehydration, blood hypertonicity, and hypernatremia may terminate in delirium, coma, and respiratory paralysis.

When 12 per cent of the body water has been lost, the victim can no longer swallow; when 15 to 25 per cent has been lost, death usually results. In great heat, death comes much more quickly, from loss of temperature control and an explosive rise in deep body temperature.

Circulatory Effects

In most clinical conditions, there is concomitant loss of water and salt, although often not in the proportions in which they exist in extracellular fluid. When salt loss predominates, the circulatory collapse may be striking, since the differential osmotic pressure of extracellular fluid depends primarily upon sodium and chloride. When Na and Cl concentration in extracellular fluid drops, extracellular water moves into the cells. The Na loss is followed by a loss in circulating plasma proteins with further decrease in plasma volume; there is hemoconcentration and increased viscosity of the blood, fall in cardiac output, drop in blood pressure, and prolongation of circulation time.

In severe salt deficiency with decrease in plasma volume, low cardiac output, and consequent compensatory vasoconstriction there is increasing pallor. The pulse becomes rapid. The blood pressure falls, causing faintness. There may be fatigue, lassitude, headache, and cold sweating. Muscular cramps in the extremities often occur. Abdominal cramps, nausea, and vomiting may appear. The circulatory failure may affect the brain sufficiently to cause stupor or coma, and the kidneys sufficiently to cause renal failure. When the loss is primarily of water, thirst is striking; when salt loss predominates, thirst is mild or absent. The cause of the "shock" state may be confusing to diagnose. Diagnosis may be made by demonstrating the absence of Cl in the urine and a low Na in the plasma. Rapid improvement following treatment with intravenous saline solution confirms the diagnosis of salt depletion.

Renal Effects

Oliguria is the first response to dehydration. It is water that is retained chiefly when the loss is primarily of water; NaCl is retained more actively than normally when the loss is of both water and NaCl, or when there is primarily a NaCl deficit. The urine may fall to only 100 ml. or 200 ml. per day from the normal 1,000 ml. or more. The specific gravity may rise to as high as 1.040 from the normal 1.020 or lower. Extreme oliguria or complete anuria are accompanied by increasing signs of renal failure, plus the accompanying evidences of dehydration upon the circulation, the central nervous system, etc.

Renal insufficiency with oliguria and azotemia is a common sequel of sodium depletion, since the circulatory collapse may be manifested largely by failure of the renal circulation. Salt limitation plus vigorous diuresis, may lower extracellular electrolyte sufficiently to endanger life through renal failure.[55]

WATER BALANCE

The amount of water in the body depends upon the *water balance*, the intake normally equalling the output when the body is in a state of equilibrium. Dehydration occurs when there is a *negative water balance*, resulting from failure of intake to keep pace with a normal output, or from excessive fluid loss in the presence of a normal intake, or from both diminished absorption and accelerated loss.

The normal route of entry for fluid is the gastrointestinal tract, whereas the routes of exit are the kidneys, the lungs, the sweat glands, and the breasts (milk), only a small amount usually being excreted in the stool. Therapeutically, fluid may be introduced into the body through the veins, subcutaneous tissue, peritoneal cavity, or bone marrow. As the result of trauma, fluid may be lost from the blood vessels, the lymph vessels, and the tissue spaces in wounds, burns, etc. Excessive loss may therefore occur through both normal and abnormal channels.

Clothing and environmental and body temperature cause such fluctuations in the proportion of water intake lost through skin and lungs (totaling from 30 to 50 per cent under moderate conditions, but increasing to 90 per cent or more with high temperature, violent exercise, etc.) that *change in urine volume* when water intake is fixed does not dependably measure changes in water balance. Daily variations in body weight, however, closely reflect changes in total water content of the body. Sudden considerable gain or loss in weight indicates change in water and sodium content primarily.

CAUSES OF DEHYDRATION

Disturbance involving one or more of the routes by which fluid is taken in or lost may lead to dehydration of greater or less degree, depending upon the severity of the disorder and upon the number of routes involved. Often several factors are simultaneously operative in the production of dehydration. Thus, vomiting usually implies not only loss of fluid but failure of intake. Often these two factors leading to dehydration are accompanied by a third, diarrhea. Conditions leading to dehydration include:

1. Failure of fluid intake (unavailable, nausea, psychic disorders, etc.)
2. Failure of absorption (diarrhea, intestinal disorders, etc.)
3. Loss from gastrointestinal tract (vomiting, diarrhea, fistula)
4. Excess renal excretion due to renal factors (failure of tubular reabsorption)
5. Excess renal excretion due to prerenal factors (disturbed body-fluid chemistry)
6. Excessive perspiration or vaporization
7. Loss from wounds, burns, etc. (hemorrhage, transudation of intestinal fluid and serum).

Even the simpler forms of body-fluid disturbance involve a number of physiologic and chemical relationships. When water is not ingested, water deficit develops because of continued loss through lungs, skin, and kidneys. When the body is deprived of water, the sodium, chloride, and water output falls to a minimum as dehydration advances and the concentration in the serum of Na^+ and Cl^- rises with the developing hemoconcentration. Maintenance of the normal total ionic concentration in the extracellular fluid requires renal removal of an equivalent quantity of electrolyte. Should renal function be normal, the kidneys may be able to increase the output of solids while reabsorbing water at a maximal rate, but if there is renal impairment, the urine volume may continue high or even increase (the specific gravity being relatively fixed at a low level) and the dehydration may thus be further exaggerated. For another example, vomiting may result in loss not only of fluid but of considerable amounts of hydrochloric acid in the gastric secretion, whereas in some cases vomiting results in great loss of the alkaline duodenal content. Such alterations in the acid or base content of the body fluids require adjustments between the various compartments in fluid and electrolyte content and demand compensatory activity by the kidneys. A better understanding of these relationships is possible if we review the anatomy and the physiology of the body fluids.

ANATOMY OF THE BODY FLUIDS

The structure of the body is largely fluid, variously confined within cell walls, the walls of vessels, or in the tissue spaces. The body fluids exist in three forms (Fig. 35-1): (1) blood plasma; (2) interstitial fluid; and (3) intracellular fluid. Together, the blood plasma and the interstitial fluid (including lymph) constitute the *extracellular fluid*. The extracellular fluid constitutes the immediate environment of the organism, in which its cells and tissues exist. The interstitial fluid, which lies between the blood and the lymph vessels and the tissue cells, constitutes the organ of transfer of necessary metabolites between the cells and the vascular system. The blood plasma provides contact with the gastrointestinal tract, the lungs, the kidneys, and the skin, so that together the interstitial fluid and the plasma form a fluid structural system for transportation of nutrient and waste substances.

Of the total weight of the body, normally 50 to 70 per cent is in fluid form. Forty to fifty per cent of the body weight is present as intracellular fluid and 15 to 20 per cent as extracellular fluid. Three-quarters of the extracellular fluid is interstitial and one-quarter is intravascular.*

Normal women have a higher body fat content and lower water content than normal men: average water content for women is approximately 50 per cent; for men about 60 per cent. With advancing age in both sexes, even without obesity, there is more fat, less muscle and therefore less water content.

In obese persons, the body weight is nearer to 45 per cent water, in very lean

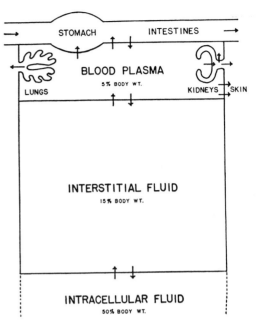

FIG. 35-1. Composition of extracellular fluid. (Gamble, J. L.: Chemical Anatomy, Physiology and Pathology of Extracellular Fluid, Boston, The Harvard Medical School)

persons nearer to 70 per cent water. Adipose tissue, of all tissues, is lowest in water content; skeletal muscle is highest.

Newborn babies have approximately 77 per cent of body weight as fluid and 23 per cent as solid. In the infant, 48 per cent of body weight is accounted for by cellular fluid, 29 per cent by extracellular fluid. Thus, the newborn baby has nearly twice as much extracellular fluid as the adult in proportion to body weight.[36]

The baby has a much more rapid fluid turnover than the adult, because (1) he is a rapidly growing individual with a high metabolic rate, and (2) because his body surface area (including the intestinal surface area) is two to three times that of an adult in proportion to weight. A baby with no water intake will lose a volume of fluid equal to its extracellular fluid volume in about 5 days, whereas it will take an adult about 10 days to lose fluid equal to his extracellular fluid volume. Babies and small children are therefore much more vulnerable than adults to water and electrolyte disorders.[36]

The body fluids have several dimensions, including volume, composition, and position. The extracellular fluid is available to us for

---

* Studies have indicated that the figures now in common use for the body content of water may be too high. The use of inulin, deuterium (heavy water), and antipyrine have permitted the simultaneous measurement of the extracellular compartment, of total body water, and by difference, the intracellular compartment. Such studies have given figures of 53 per cent (instead of 70 per cent of body weight) for total body fluid, 37 per cent (instead of 50 per cent) for intracellular fluid, and 16 per cent (instead of 20 per cent) for extracellular fluid.[4,5,6,7,32]

From measurements of body water by antipyrine and of body fat by specific gravity in the same persons, one may calculate the water content of lean body mass (fat-free tissue). This figure was found to be quite constant, averaging 71.8 per cent. Thus, it is evident that the proportion of water depends upon the amount of fat—the more fat, the lower the percentage of water.

study; the cellular fluid is not—therefore we focus our attention on the extracellular fluid. It may vary in volume, being excessive or deficient. It may reveal deficits or excesses of various components. In some disease states the *position* of the extracellular fluid becomes abnormal: for example, a disproportionately large percentage of the extracellular fluid may shift from the plasma into the interstitial compartment. Movement of the extracellular fluid takes place chiefly through the heart, the blood vessels, and the lymph channels.

The factors governing the structure of the intracellular and the extracellular fluids and the distribution of body water are chiefly concerned with the passage through the cell membrane of the two chief cations, sodium and potassium. Like other constituents of the body, water is in a dynamic state and is being constantly exchanged between the various compartments. Most of the cation of the intracellular fluid is potassium (for example, in muscle and in blood cells). Sodium is the chief cation of the extracellular fluid (for example, in the interstitial fluid and in the blood serum).

Potassium, the chief intracellular cation, exists in a state of dynamic equilibrium with the potassium of the extracellular fluids. The mechanism of maintenance of the much higher concentration of potassium within the cells as compared with that in the serum is not yet well understood. It is reasonable to believe that the oxidative energy of the cells has much to do with maintenance of this equilibrium.

It has long been known that the cell membranes are freely permeable to water, oxygen, carbon dioxide, urea, and other nutrient and excretory products. Until recently it was believed that they are relatively impermeable to sodium and potassium. Recent studies have led to new concepts and a clearer understanding of water and electrolyte physiology. Use of heavy water and of radioactive isotopes of sodium and potassium have shown that the cells *are permeable* to sodium and potassium, but that this permeability is slow compared with that of water.[4] When heavy water was injected intravenously, equilibrium with total body water was established in 120 minutes. When radioactive sodium was injected, equilibrium with extracellular sodium was attained in 60 minutes, but not with total body sodium until 24 hours. Radioactive potassium requires 15 hours before reaching equilibrium with cellular potassium.

In spite of great fluctuations in the intake of salt and water, in health there is normally great constancy of the serum sodium concentration, the range being 132 to 142 mEq./L. The constancy of the serum sodium concentration is the consequence of the fact that the salts of sodium comprise the major osmotically active solutes in the serum and that a number of physiologic mechanisms operate to maintain in health a total solute concentration in the serum within the narrow limits of 285 to 295 mOsm./L. of water.

The osmotic activity of the serum proteins is of prime importance in the distribution of extracellular fluid between the intravascular and the interstitial compartments, but protein normally contributes little to the solute activity of serum. The normal serum protein content of 60 to 70 Gm./L. amounts to only about 1 mOsm./L. because of the large molecular weight of the serum proteins (about 60,000 for serum albumin).

Maintenance of the constancy of the total solute activity of the serum is a function of the interlocking system, which may be thought of broadly as the *thirst-neurohypophysial-renal-adrenal axis*, the operations of which will be discussed below in the section on Physiology of the Body Fluids. With the *concentration* of the serum sodium thus regulated, normally the *volume* of the extracellular fluid is dictated by the *quantity* of sodium it contains. For this reason, the clinical state of hydration, largely determined by extracellular fluid volume, is in most situations largely a direct function of the extracellular content of sodium.

Cell Osmolality

Water usually, according to the fundamental rules of osmotic activity, moves into the area of higher osmolality. In the past it has been thought that the osmolality of the interstitial fluid in contact with cell walls was the same as that within the cells. Newer information indicates that normally *the cells are hypertonic* to the fluid in which they are immersed. We may still keep the concept that cell fluid and intercellular fluid *are in equilibrium* across the semipermeable membrane of the cell wall, **but** we must add the idea that there is a gradient *normally* (not always) maintained by a constant active extrusion of water by the cells. A "water pump" mechanism removes water and preserves the normal tonicity of the cell. Our previous information concerning osmal influences upon movement of solutes and water through the cell membrane remains valid. "Sick" cells, unable to extrude water, enlarge and suffer derangement of interior structure and function ("cloudy swelling" under the microscope). This may result from excess water uptake from hypo-osmal intercellular fluid, from failure of the water pump, or both. Toxic effects upon cells can halt the water pump. Removal of noxious influences or restoration of normal intercellular osmolality can lead to recovery of the cells; persistence will lead to cell death.

Although most of the body cells are relatively inaccessible for osmolality studies, **red blood cells** are easily available and, in the absence of hematologic disorder, yield much information (Ref. 35, pp. 76–78). When there is water excess, water enters the cells in general including the red blood cells; the same occurs when there is sodium loss—cell volume increases, and the mean corpuscular volume (MCV) of the erythrocyte becomes greater than normal. The normal MCV is 87 ± 5 cu. μ. Since the cell hemoglobin is diluted, the mean corpuscular hemoglobin concentration (MCHC) falls below the normal value of 34 ± 2 per cent.

In states of water excess or sodium loss, the MCV may be 93 to 94 cu. μ, with MCHC 32 to 33.5 per cent.

In the opposite condition, when cells lose water, the cell becomes smaller than normal and its contents more concentrated. The MCV is low and the MCHC tends to be elevated. The latter value cannot, however, exceed the maximum of 36 per cent, because erythrocytes cannot be supersaturated with hemoglobin.

Serum Osmolality

The normal serum osmolality is 285 to 295 mOsm. per kg. of serum water. Of this, normally 95 per cent is exerted by the electrolytes, chiefly sodium. Usually the osmolality of the extracellular water varies proportionately with the serum sodium concentration; however, there are exceptions. For example: **extreme hyperglycemia;** the high glucose concentration exerts a considerable osmotic effect, water is drawn into the serum and the sodium is diluted so that there is normal total effective osmolality with a *dilutional* (not necessarily depletional) *hyponatremia*.

A similar situation may occur in **chronic**

nephritis or other types of **renal failure** in critical illness, with retention of urea and other nitrogenous substances, lactic and other organic acids, etc. The osmolality may be normal, but the serum sodium low. There may or may not also be dehydration and true sodium depletion.

It should be noted that, in exchange of solutes, body cells respond to osmolality rather than to osmolarity. **Osmolality** is the osmolar concentration per unit weight of solvent (i.e., water). **Osmolarity** is the concentration per unit total volume of solution.

Osmolality and osmolarity may differ widely. For example: in **hyperlipemic subjects,** although the concentration of sodium per liter of *serum* may be abnormally low, its concentration per liter of serum *water* may be normal. In this instance, the osmotic tonicity of sodium (osmolality) is normal, but its osmolar concentration is low, because a large part of the serum volume is made up of serum lipids. The hyponatremia occurring with hyperlipemia is essentially due to *displacement*, whereas that resulting from hyperglycemia is *dilutional*. Such hyperlipemia occurs in some patients with diabetes mellitus, or with nephrosis. In these diseases, however, there may also be true sodium depletion with low osmolality (or with normal osmolality if there has been diuresis, dehydration, and relative hemoconcentration).

Low osmolality (around 274 mOsm./L.) occurs in two other conditions: water intoxication **(water excess syndrome)** from dilution and **chronic cellular hypo-osmolality,** which results from sodium depletion plus a dilutional factor caused by withdrawal of water from cells. The latter disorder is seen in chronic illness, with slow but steady cellular damage and continuous potassium loss. See further discussion of this syndrome under Hyponatremia.

Hyperosmolality occurs in many conditions in which there is dehydration. Normal persons under moderate conditions can go for many hours without fluid supply and have no osmal derangement. During water deprivation and rapid fluid loss, hyperosmolality results, developing especially rapidly in infants and young children because of their much greater proportionate fluid requirements.

Persons afflicted with **diabetes insipidus** who are deprived of water become distressingly dehydrated within a few hours; continued dehydration can cause death. The serum osmolality in the standard 6½-hour test period of withholding water rises to above 300 mOsm. per kg. of serum water, but such a test in a normal person causes no osmolal rise. Persons with diabetes insipidus with free access to water have normal serum osmolality.

Urine Osmolality

The osmolality of urine is a more accurate measure of renal tubular function than is the specific gravity, because the kidneys respond to osmolality of body fluids, not to specific gravity. Osmolality of urine in normal persons after a 14-hour fast is 850 mOsm. or higher. The greater significance and accuracy of osmolality measurement is indicated by this observation: at a specific gravity of 1.023, urine osmolality can range from 722 to 1166 mOsm. per kg. of urine water. Specific gravity is considerably influenced by the presence or absence or degree of albuminuria or glycosuria. Osmolality of urine is much less affected.

In diabetes insipidus with fluid intake unrestricted, urine specific gravity is below 1.010, and often may be 1.003 to 1.000. Urine osmolality in this condition is consistently below the normal plasma level of 290 mOsm., and frequently may be 100 mOsm. per kg. water or below.

The important role of sodium in the regulation of *cell* volume has only recently been appreciated. Since with radioactive isotopes it has been shown that cell membranes are permeable to water and to almost all the small solutes of the extracellular fluid, one may ask why the protein content of cells, through the osmotic attraction for water it exerts, does not result in a progressive swelling and lysis of all cells. The answer appears to be that the sodium ion, through its largely extracellular position, sets up a counter osmotic force which, together with the dynamic activity of the pumps steadily extruding water and sodium from cells, just balances the intracellular oncotic pressure and stabilizes the cell volume.

Later in this chapter under Physiology there is discussion of the mechanisms and effects of Na+ and K+ transport through cell membranes.

The extracellular position of sodium is not dependent upon impermeability of cell membranes to sodium, but rather to an active extrusion of the sodium that continuously diffuses into the cells. Through this active transport of sodium ions, in which all body cells are engaged, plus the important but less conspicuous cellular-extracellular exchange of potassium ions, the characteristic difference in ionic composition of cellular and extracellular fluids is maintained and the volume of the cells preserved. It is chiefly the sodium *retained* in the extracellular fluids and the sodium *extruded* from the cells (with the accompanying, usually reciprocal, potassium interchanges) which regulate the respective volumes of the two compartments.[56]

The energy for active extrusion of sodium from cells is derived from the breakdown of adenosinetriphosphate (ATP) and is associated with the activity of a specific enzyme[84] (see the discussion later in this chapter under the Physiology of Body Fluids: Sodium and Potassium Transport Into and Out of Cells).

Probably most cells accumulate potassium actively as well as extrude sodium, but whether the extrusion of sodium is coupled in any rigorous, quantitative way to the uptake of potassium remains unsettled. The ability to accumulate K and extrude Na in the presence of large amounts of Na and small amounts of K in the surrounding fluid is a fundamental characteristic of living cells.[57] When death of the cell occurs these ionic gradients are rapidly dissipated. These gradients are maintained by living cells in spite of permeability of cell walls to both ions. Therefore, the relative concentrations of Na+ and K+ ions in extracellular and cellular fluids must be the result of steady-state conditions supported by energy derived from cellular metabolism; it is not an equilibrium state resulting from the impermeability of cell membranes to one or more ions, as was thought earlier. The energy inherent in such ionic gradients has been secondarily adapted by certain specialized cells to afford nervous conduction and the excitation phase of muscular contraction.

In association with nerve impulse transmission and cardiac and skeletal muscle contraction, there is a specialized shift of sodium and potassium across the cell membrane. With stimulation, sodium moves into the cell, potassium moves out. During restitution of the resting membrane potential, the reverse occurs. These and other cells throughout the body which are concerned with moving sodium ions against osmolar forces (from low intracellular Na+ concen-

Fig. 35-2. Chemical anatomy of body fluids in terms of acid-base equivalence. (Gamble, J. L.: Chemical Anatomy, Physiology and Pathology of Extracellular Fluid, Boston, The Harvard Medical School)

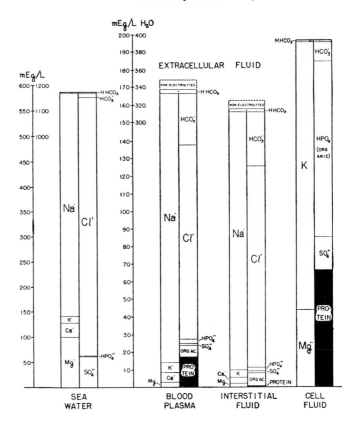

tration to extracellular relatively high concentration) and with moving potassium ions also against the gradient (from low K^+ extracellular to high intracellular) have been thought of as operating a hypothetical "sodium pump." Such a mechanism operates (according to present views) at the inner surface of the cell membrane, and the necessary energy comes from breakdown of adenosinetriphosphate. The specific enzyme involved is dependent upon Na^+ and K^+ ions for activation, and is called Na-K-ATPase (see further discussion of Na and K transport across cell membranes below, under Physiology of the Body Fluids).

Our concept of the extracellular fluid has been oversimplified, and the inulin space is not the final answer to its measurement. Sodium and chloride diffuse rapidly into collagenous connective tissue, whereas inulin and thiosulfate do not. It has been suggested that the extracellular phase, aside from the plasma in the vascular system, should be partitioned into two subphases: the *interstitial fluid*, which is an ultrafiltrate of plasma, and *connective tissue*. The inulin space defines only the plasma and the first

TABLE 35-1. DISTRIBUTION OF BODY WATER IN HYPOTHETICAL AVERAGE YOUNG ADULT MALE*

	ML./KG. BODY WEIGHT	PER CENT TOTAL	70-KG. MAN
Total body water	600 ml.	100%	42 Kg.
Intracellular	330	55	23
Extracellular	270	45	19
Plasma	45	7.5	3.2
Interstitial lymph	120	20.0	8.4
Dense connective cartilage	45	7.5	3.2
Inaccessible bone	45	7.5	3.2
Transcellular	15	2.5	1.1

* Edelman, I. S., and Liebman, J.: Amer. J. Med. 27: 256, 1959.

of these two subphases, whereas sodium and chloride diffuse rapidly through both subphases before entering more slowly the true intracellular fluid. Not only do sodium and chloride enter the intracellular fluid, but they also cross cell barriers into special fluid pools and other depots. Such pools called *transcellular fluids* include fluids in the gastrointestinal tract, in serous and synovial cavities, in the lower urinary tract, in cerebrospinal fluid, and in bile.[4,33] Bone also acts as a sodium and potassium reservoir.[51]

Water balance depends upon control of the amounts of fluid in each of the fluid compartments. Circulation of the blood requires a fairly constant volume in the vascular compartment. The volume of cell fluid to permit proper tissue metabolism must be quite constant. The usual volume of interstitial fluid is apparently ideal, but wide variations may occur without great disturbance of its functions. Water loss by vaporization and perspiration for heat regulation and by urinary excretion of waste products is at the expense of interstitial fluid. Water exchange essentially consists of loss and replacement of extracellular water, chiefly interstitial water. Plasma-volume fluctuations occur, but permissible variations are relatively limited. Cell-volume changes also occur, but these alterations can only be slight.

The chemical structure of the various compartments of the body fluids is illustrated diagrammatically in Figure 35-2.

By circulation of the blood through *the lungs*, gaseous exchange with the external environment is accomplished. The red blood cells constitute the special vehicle for transportation of oxygen and carbon dioxide between lungs and tissues, this being made possible by the reversible affinity of hemoglobin for these two substances. Water is lost from the lungs through the exhalation of vapor.

Intimate contact of body fluids with the *gastrointestinal tract* provides for the absorption of water and nutrient substances into cells and tissue spaces, and thence for transport by the vascular system, and likewise permits excretion into the intestinal tract by the same routes.

Most important of all in maintaining the constancy of structure of the extracellular fluids are *the kidneys*, which are capable of regulating not only the amount of water that leaves the body by the renal route, but the kinds and the amounts of substances in solution in that water. Thus, the chemical components of the blood plasma and the interstitial fluid are maintained within homeostatic limits largely by renal regulation.[41,46,47,49,50]

The skin, through perspiration and evaporation, is concerned with control of water balance and the excretion of certain metabolites. *Insensible perspiration* consists of the water lost invisibly from the skin without loss of salts. *Sweat* contains excretory products (urea, etc.), sodium, and chloride and other salts, and is perceptible or visible. The epidermis or outermost layer of the skin is continuously active as a factor inhibiting water loss from blood vessels and tissues by the pressure and the covering it affords. The corneal layer of the epidermis, which is of microscopic thickness except in the palms and the soles, is the layer of greatest importance in the inhibition of water loss by diffusion from the underlying tissues. When the protective skin covering is removed by burns or other injury, large quantities of water and electrolytes and of blood proteins may be lost. Thus the "dead," keratinous, ever-desquamating, thin corneum has, nevertheless, an important role in the maintenance of normal water and electrolyte balance.

PHYSIOLOGY OF THE BODY FLUIDS

The functions served by the body fluids are closely interrelated, but may be divided as follows:

1. Transportation
   (a) of oxygen and CO_2
   (b) of nutrient materials such as amino acids, glucose, fats, vitamins, minerals, etc.
   (c) of hormones and chemical regulators
   (d) of excretory products such as urea, etc.
2. Temperature regulation
   (a) by shifting the blood to the surface for cooling, or to the interior to prevent heat loss
   (b) by perspiration and evaporation of moisture from the skin surface
3. Osmotic pressure regulation
   (a) plasma-protein effects
   (b) electrolyte effects
4. Acid-base balance regulation
   (a) through respiratory control of carbonic acid
   (b) through renal chemical control.

In addition to the simple function of *transportation*, the aqueous medium in which the tissues and the cells exist provides stable physical and chemical conditions. *Temperature, the hydrogen-ion concentration,* and *osmotic pressure* are regulated by the extracellular fluid, and the influences of these factors are exerted in the fluid and through the fluid upon the tissues.

The concentration of sodium in the extracellular fluid is kept quite constant, although there is a slow, continuous interchange of water and of sodium from the extracellular fluid through cell walls.

Water alone will not enter the cells unless there is a decrease in the concentration of extracellular sodium; otherwise the cells would be hypotonic in relation to the extracellular fluid. Water alone, likewise, cannot leave the cell unless the concentration of extracellular sodium rises. Therefore, the state of hydration of the cells depends primarily upon the *concentration of sodium ion in the extracellular fluid.* A major function of the kidney is to regulate the concentration of sodium in the extracellular fluid.

The water and salt intake, the regulatory activity of the kidney, and the osmotic pressures acting across semipermeable membranes plus the dynamic activity of the water and sodium "pumps," all operate to maintain a constant internal environment. The degree of hydration and the distribution of body water are usually so well-regulated that the osmotic pressure of the fluids is kept quite constant.[4-7]

The *volume,* as well as the osmolality and the pH of body fluids, is maintained within certain limits to permit adequate performance of the various physiologic functions listed. The volume fluctuations in the several fluid compartments which are compatible with health differ considerably: interstitial volumes can vary *widely,* intravascular volumes *moderately,* and cell volumes relatively *little.* There are volume-regulatory mechanisms that are apparently separate and independent of osmoreceptors and of changes in the osmolality of the body fluids. Knowledge of the location of sensitive indicators of volume and their mode of operation is incomplete.[8] "Volume-receptors" have been described within the cranium and in vascular structures within the thorax. After disturbances of osmolality, the mechanisms operating to restore normal fluid volumes are better understood. However, when the changes are isomolar, the processes involved in the correction of aberrations in fluid volume are less clear. Following hemorrhage, for example, even in the absence of the intake of fluid, restoration of intravascular volume soon begins. If water is administered as isotonic glucose, a prompt water diuresis ensues, since glucose is not freely permeable through cell walls, and thus attracts water into the intravascular compartment. However, if water is administered as isotonic NaCl solution, there is no immediate effect upon water excretion. The volume of the body fluids is increased, body weight increases, and there is every evidence of a positive water balance. Over a period of several days there is a delayed response to the expanded fluid volume, diuresis occurs at a moderate rate over a span of days, and during these days there is a negative water balance, so that at the end of the period of adjustment, the previous normal fluid volumes and body weight are restored.

The juxtaglomerular apparatus of the kidney is a volume receptor. A fall in the pressure within the afferent renal arterioles leads to the secretion of renin, the formation of angiotensin II, and promotes the secretion of aldosterone.[68]

The body fluids constitute the system enabling transport

—of oxygen supply to tissues and of CO_2 output } through the lungs

—of nutrient supply from areas of absorption (chiefly small intestine) to the tissues

—of hormones and chemical regulators (especially to central nervous system and the kidneys)

—of electrolytes and proteins for osmotic regulation

—of constituents for acid-base regulation (to lungs, kidneys, GI tract, etc.)

—of waste products for excretion (through lungs, kidneys, GI tract)

—of nutrients, hormones, and chemical regulators to the brain and higher nerve centers, enabling over-all control.

The anatomical channels and **mechanisms** furnishing the means of transportation are the blood circulatory and lymphatic systems.

Normally there is wide variation in the amount of fluid taken into the body and excreted daily, but the total intake equals the total output with great constancy. Such equilibrium holds true over a period of a few days, not necessarily for each 24-hour day. This is necessarily so, since otherwise fluid would either accumulate in the body or dehydration would occur. By control of the amounts of fluid absorbed and excreted, stability of the volume of extracellular fluid is established, and thus *constancy of transport* is maintained.

Water and Salt: Supply and Deprivation

Water Requirement. The water intake is derived from several sources: (1) drinking water; (2) water in food; (3) water formed in combustion of food; (4) water formed in combustion of body substance. The amount of water consumed as such is usually only about one-third of the total water intake. The average normal person drinks from 1 to 1.5 liters of liquid daily, except when subjected to active exercise or high temperature, under which conditions the amount drunk may be increased severalfold. Foods furnish water because most of them are high in water content: meat, about 70 per cent; milk, 87 per cent; and certain vegetables and fruits (cucumbers, watermelon), over 95 per cent. An ordinary diet yields in combustion about 12 ml. of water per 100 calories. The total amount of water required is roughly parallel to the energy metabolism, being approximately 1 ml. per calorie. Thus, a sedentary man may need only 1,500 ml. daily, whereas a physically active man of the same size and weight may require 3,000 ml.

Water Output. Under normal temperate conditions there are certain usual proportions between water intake and its disposal by the various routes, as shown by these average daily figures of the usual ranges for an adult:

Urine	1,000-1,500 ml.
Feces	50- 200
Skin (insensible perspiration)	450-1,050
Sweat	100- 500
Lungs	250- 350
Total per 24 hours	1,850-3,600 ml.

Water Deprivation. When the body is deprived of water for any reason, dehydration with a fall in the volume of extracellular fluid occurs, insensible perspiration diminishes, and the urine volume greatly and rapidly decreases. The decrease in the urine volume is presumably due to activity of the posterior pituitary antidiuretic hormone. Conservation of water occurs through increased tubular reabsorption until the urine volume becomes minimal and its concentration becomes maximal. Glomerular filtration may fall at this point because of the reduction in blood volume and because of the rise in the colloid osmotic pressure of the plasma. Hemoconcentration occurs. The blood urea rises. As dehydration advances, water is lost out of proportion to salt, which is preferentially absorbed. The concentrations of sodium and chloride in the extracellular fluids rise and draw water from the cells. The cells also yield some potassium, which permits further escape of cellular water. Loss of 10 per cent of body water is disabling to man.[36,42,48]

Sodium Deprivation. One cannot in a

short period of days or weeks by using only **dietary restriction** seriously deplete the body sodium, because the urinary output of Na and Cl decreases so promptly. The results of sodium loss through excessive sweating, vomiting, diarrhea, etc., depend upon the amount of water simultaneously lost.[52,54] Loss of both water and salt in hypotonic solution, as in **sweat,** has immediate effects of a primary loss of salt, if water is taken in freely during the sweating. **Sweat contains about half the salt per liter (about 75 mEq. of Na)** as compared with that present in the plasma, so that much salt may be lost during heavy sweating. Sweating greatly accelerates the dehydration of water deprivation, further augmenting the rise of sodium and chloride in the serum. If sufficient water is taken in, of course, the concentration of serum Na and Cl may rapidly fall to normal or subnormal levels as a consequence of salt loss from excessive sweating. If, however, little or no water is taken in, loss of *sweat* (which is hypotonic—that is, contains more water proportionately than plasma) has primarily the effect of *water depletion*. Loss of gastrointestinal and digestive secretions, which are isotonic, should presumably deplete sodium and water in equivalent proportions. If water only is ingested, some of the water is absorbed and the remainder is discharged in the vomitus, fistular discharge or stool, carrying salt with it to make it isotonic. These conditions therefore produce salt depletion primarily. In such states, the volume of fluid lost usually exceeds the volume ingested, and there is therefore a large deficit of water associated with the salt depletion. Whenever decompression and lavage of the gastrointestinal tract are carried out (as in the treatment of intestinal obstruction), normal saline solution should be employed rather than water, in order to reduce the secretory activity of the digestive glands and of the alimentary canal to a minimum and thus prevent salt loss.

Sodium Excess. Salt taken without sufficient water during dehydration will exaggerate thirst and water loss. Sodium chloride taken in excess of body needs at any time will promote diuresis, providing that the renal mechanisms for excreting salt and water are unimpaired. However, should the ability of the kidney to eliminate salt and water be limited for any reason (circulatory failure, renal damage, hormonal disorder, etc.), overhydration and edema may result. Whenever the ratio of salt to water is greater in the ingesta than in extracellular fluid, the volume of the latter expands at the expense of intracellular fluid. Diuresis results, and the intensity of the increased water and salt output depends upon the volume and the salt concentration of the ingesta. The same processes are of course operative if the water and the salt are given parenterally. Diuresis results because of the decreased rate of reabsorption of water by the renal tubules, the osmotic effect of the high salt concentration in the glomerular filtrate tending to hold water in the tubules for excretion. The rate of glomerular filtration further increases the degree of diuresis, since it is increased more by hypertonic saline than by an equal amount of water. This is apparently the result of the greater increase in the extracellular fluid volume caused by the higher salt concentration in the blood, which draws water from the cells.

Thirst is the desire to ingest liquids. It probably should not be regarded as a simple sensation, due to dryness of the mucous membranes of the mouth and pharynx. Such dryness, which may result from many causes (mouth breathing, inhibition of salivary secretion by atropine, etc.) can, if not associated with body fluid aberration, be corrected simply by keeping the membranes moist, and the so-called thirst disappears.

True thirst is a more widely perceived sensation, more like hunger; it may or may not be associated with dryness of the oropharyngeal membranes. Thirst occurs when (1) cellular dehydration is present, or (2) when extracellular fluid volume is decreased, or (3) when certain hypothalamic centers are stimulated. It seems likely that the cells in the hypothalamic center are sensitive to the relative osmolality of the fluid reaching them, become relatively dehydrated, and relay impulses to higher centers interpreted as thirst. Studies in man suggest that when cell volume of the tissues generally is reduced by 1 or 2 per cent thirst appears.[58,59]

Studies suggesting that there is a "thirst center" in the hypothalamus are based upon observations such as these on animals[60]: (1) injection of a very small amount of hypertonic NaCl into a particular area of the hypothalamus caused intense polydipsia; isotonic NaCl solution produced no such response; (2) electric stimulation of the same area produced water ingestion; destruction of the area by electrocoagulation caused hypodipsia.

Although thirst *usually* indicates a true

physiological need for water, it is not an accurate indicator of the water *content* of the body. Thus, (1) extracellular fluid volume may be excessive, but if the effective osmolality of the fluid is high (causing cellular dehydration), thirst occurs; also (2) if extracellular fluid volume is low but the osmolality is in normal relation to that of the cells (no cellular dehydration), there will be no thirst.

Inappropriate thirst may be observed in the syndrome of hyponatremia. Here there is reduced vascular volume, which results in the stimulus to drink water; such a response does not defend the osmolality of the body fluids. In patients with hepatic cirrhosis, serum proteins may be low and blood volume high; abdominal paracentesis may lead to prompt thirst, and fluid ingestion would further distort extracellular fluid changes in the same direction. Presumably, in these instances, reduction in volume of the extracellular fluid causes cellular dehydration and activates the sensation of thirst.

It is reasonable to suppose that the factors concerned in thirst and the influences upon water balance through the control of the secretion of the antidiuretic hormone of the pituitary are part of the same regulatory mechanism. Wolf's[58,59] calculations of osmometric changes of 1 to 2 per cent cellular dehydration necessary to produce thirst are about the same as those found by Verney as resulting in secretion of ADH.[61] If one compares the effects of giving isosmolal solutions of NaCl (20 per cent) and urea (40 per cent) intravenously, thirst is much greater and water intake is much higher after the NaCl. The cellular membranes are permeable to urea, but relatively impermeable to the Na^+ and Cl^- ions, so that the *effective* hypertonicity is the most important factor, rather than the total osmolality. Other ions that do not traverse cell membranes freely have similar effects: intake of hypertonic amounts of any such solutes causes thirst. The thirst results in increased water intake, which leads to decrease in the abnormally high solute concentration. Similarly, hypertonicity of extracellular fluids results in increased ADH secretion; renal loss of water is diminished and there is relative fluid retention, which favors reduction of the hypertonicity.

Apparently the concentration of solutes in the body fluids, as well as the volume of the body fluids, determines the desire for water.[58-60] It may be that the stimulus to thirst depends upon the water content of the cells (*cellular dehydration*), and that the cells of the mucosa of the tongue, the mouth, and the pharynx are often, to the affected person, the most sensitive but not the only indicators. When the body is depleted of sodium chloride, there may be little thirst despite extreme dehydration. On the other hand, increasing the salt content of the body will cause thirst promptly, even when the total body-water content is already adequate or excessive. Severe thirst may occur in such instances apparently as a central sensation with no dryness of the mucous membranes. The rise in sodium content of the extracellular fluid causes cellular dehydration. The establishment of normal osmotic relationships after aberration in either direction is apt to terminate the sensation of thirst. Thirst occurs normally whenever the extracellular fluid volume is appreciably diminished, by whatever route whether through water deprivation, perspiration, increased renal or intestinal loss, hemorrhage, massive loss of serum into burns, etc.[45] When extracellular fluid volume falls, some water is given up *from the cellular compartment*, and this loss no doubt is the stimulus to the sensation of thirst.

It seems particularly significant that, in the experiments of Andersson[60] in which he demonstrated the presence of a thirst center in the hypothalamus, stimuli that would induce thirst would in many instances also elicit antidiuresis. The nuclei of the anterior hypothalamus which are now known to be the source of antidiuretic hormone[62] must overlap the thirst center. Verney[63] has produced evidence that the osmoreceptors may also be localized in the same nuclei. Thus, thirst center, osmoreceptor, and source of antidiuretic hormone are closely integrated anatomically as well as functionally.[56]

Thirst plays a primary role in the operations of the *thirst-neurohypophysial-renal axis* to maintain constancy of the solute concentration (particularly sodium) of the extracellular fluid. Usually, unless some circumstance prevents it, water intake keeps pace with water loss or promptly makes up for it. Whenever fluid loss is accelerated, intake is increased. In health this response is automatic and is dependent upon the sensation of thirst.

When the sensorium is clouded or the patient is in coma, the physiologic mechanisms to produce thirst may be present, but the sensation cannot be perceived. Obligatory fluid losses may proceed to dangerous or fatal levels of dehydration if the subject is unable to perceive the thirst signal or is unable for any reason to respond to it by appropriate intake of water.

TEMPERATURE REGULATION AND PERSPIRATION

The body in a cool environment loses heat chiefly through three processes: **radiation,** accounting for about 60 per cent of the total lost; **vaporization** (20 to 27 per cent), and **convection** (12 to 15 per cent). When the environment is warm, the proportions of heat loss by the various mechanisms are greatly changed, because radiation and convection become relatively ineffective. When the external temperature is 95° F. or above, evaporation from the skin surface becomes essentially the only effective way to eliminate heat. This process is facilitated by heavy sweating. Water loss through the skin (normally for an adult averaging 500 to 1500 ml. per day in a 70° F. environment—depending upon exercise, clothing, etc.) can be increased to 3 or 4 L. per day or more at moderate environmental temperatures. At high environmental temperatures and with heavy exercise, water loss through the skin may reach 10 to 12 L. daily.

When the temperature of the air is high or when body temperature is elevated by fever, *perspiration* may be greatly increased. However, under normal conditions, exercise is the chief factor leading to increased water loss as sweat. The *evaporation of water* from the body surface constitutes the most important mechanism by which body water influences body temperature. When body or environmental temperature is high, or when work is done and there is no condition to interfere with the ingestion or absorption of water, thirst provides the stimulus and spontaneously the intake is greatly increased, providing adequate fluid for this mode of temperature regulation. Usually less water is excreted in the urine (and feces) under these circumstances, and more through the lungs, so that water balance figures might be as follows:

Urine	500 ml.
Feces	50
Sweat	4,000
Lungs	500
Total	5,050 ml.

Cardiovascular Factors. To promote elimination of heat and water through the skin, a larger than normal volume of intravascular fluids is diverted to the blood vessels supplying the skin. To serve the purposes of heat elimination, a large increase in the minute volume of blood circulating through the skin occurs by reflex. An unacclimatized man forced to work in the heat has a great burden imposed upon his cardiovascular system.

Adrenocortical Factors. Hormones produced by the adrenal cortex regulate in some degree the amounts of sodium, chloride, potassium and water retained by the renal tubules or excreted in the urine. There is an adrenocortical control of the sodium and chloride of sweat also. Normally the concentration of sodium in the sweat is about one-third to one-half of that of the plasma. The administration of desoxycorticosterone or of adrenocorticotropic hormone *reduces* the salt content of sweat, as it does that of urine.[9] When the subject was put to work in a hot room and excessive sweating became apparent, there were indications suggestive of increased ACTH and adrenocortical activity: lowered concentration of the NaCl in the sweat, negative nitrogen balance and high urinary uric acid excretion. Under these circumstances with a severe stress calling for salt retention, the administration of desoxycorticosterone (or the restoration of a positive NaCl balance by giving salt) restored nitrogen equilibrium to normal. This is apparently another instance of the pituitary-adrenal system's role in responses to stress and maintenance of homeostasis. Such evidence suggests that acclimatization to heat (and possibly adaptation to strenuous muscular exertion) may consist partly in adrenocortical stimulation via pituitary ACTH, with resultant salt conservation.[37,40,50]

In the acute or early phase of excitation by pituitary ACTH of adrenocortical activity there is increase in secretion of several steroids of the adrenal cortex, including the most highly potent mineralocorticoid, aldosterone. In the later or persistent phase of adjustment, the salt lost through the sweat glands may be decreased by as much as 95 per cent by aldosterone action, without participation of ACTH or of other hormones of the adrenal cortex.[64]

Neurogenic control of sweating is well-recognized, but excessive sweating from this cause is seldom so prolonged as to affect materially total water balance—except when the organism is totally deprived of water.

Sweating associated with exercise, fever, or high environmental temperature may cause extreme dehydration if for any reason the water intake is not correspondingly increased. The usual normal loss of approximately 0.5 Gm. of NaCl through sweat per day may reach 5 to 10 Gm. or more. Extreme exertion in hot environments may cause the loss of 10 or 12 liters of water per day through the skin. Acclimatization may reduce the sweat Na concentration from a normal level of around 75 mEq. to 2 to 5 mEq. per liter.

The movement of air over the skin, as determined by clothing and wind, accelerates water loss. High humidity increases sweating. High air temperature and low humidity increase insensible water loss. As much as 10 liters may be lost through the skin in a few hours on a desert.

Should some factor prevent adequate water intake, it is obvious that water balance could not be maintained during heavy perspiration, and dehydration (reduction in extracellular fluid) would soon occur. Even when conservative measures, such as diminution of the urine output (increased tubular reabsorption), are brought into play, excessive perspiration in the presence of normal or decreased water intake would soon result in a serious deficit in body fluid.

Increase in water intake alone will not compensate for excessive fluid loss by perspiration, because not only is water so lost, but also electrolyte. Increase of water intake alone results in further loss of both water and NaCl, both by perspiration and through urine. Because of the lowered amounts of total Na and Cl in the cells and the extracellular fluid, the amounts of water in all compartments are reduced to maintain normal physiologic relationships. Adding more water without increasing the Na and Cl intake simply increases the rate of NaCl loss, since the water cannot be retained in the absence of adequate electrolyte, but takes some electrolyte with it when excreted.

Acclimatization. A process of adaptation called "acclimatization to heat" occurs when man is exposed to an environment hotter than that to which he is accustomed. When completed, acclimatization results in a remarkable increase in capacity to live and work in a hot environment without distressing symptoms. The period of time required for adaptation varies from a few days up to about 20 days, being longer for

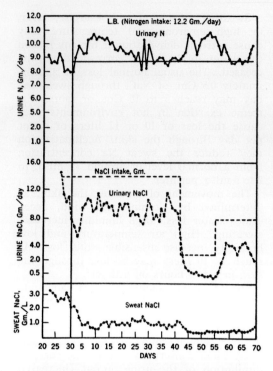

Fig. 35-3. Metabolic pattern of acclimatization to humid heat and of adjustments that occur upon sudden salt privation. (Mechanism of acclimatization to heat, Advances Intern. Med. 3:373-394; Conn[9,64])

higher temperatures. On the first day of exposure to heat, a normal subject attempting to complete a given work load may collapse with a high rectal temperature and evidence of heat prostration or heat stroke; the same subject, after exposure to the same amount of heat with a lighter work load over a period of 6 or 7 days, will be able to perform the original task easily, without cardiovascular difficulties and with a much lower rectal temperature.

The acclimatized man develops his ability to work in the hot environment without serious untoward effects through certain physiologic changes. These changes are primarily of two types: (1) alteration in cardiovascular function, and (2) modification of sweat gland activity.

Initially upon exposure to heat or after strenuous exercise or both, there is an acute diversion of blood to the periphery through reflex action, a great increase in the volume of blood circulating through the skin, and thus an acceleration of the rate of heat and water loss. This is a temporary compensatory mechanism operating in all normal persons when the heat or work are not prolonged. However, if work in the heat is continued and adaptation is successfully accomplished, more persistent changes occur: increased plasma and extracellular fluid volumes, increased peripheral circulation, and often an increase in resting cardiac output.

The fully acclimatized man produces a somewhat larger volume of sweat during performance of a standard work load than does an unacclimatized person. In dry heat this extra water loss through the skin helps eliminate heat from the body by vaporization. In moist heat, however, this advantage is lost, since much of the sweat drips off the body and is of no value in eliminating heat. However, in either case, a large sweat volume carries with it a relatively large amount of sodium chloride. The second important mechanism in acclimatization consists in a great reduction in the concentration of sodium chloride in sweat.

Conn[64] studied men performing a standard work load in a "tropical climate room" (temperature 90° F.; relative humidity 80 per cent to 90 per cent). Sweat volume was 5 to 7 liters per day. A typical response during acclimatization was a decrease in the salt concentration of sweat from an initial 3 Gm. per liter to less than 1.0 Gm. per liter by the tenth day, a saving of 10 to 14 Gm. of salt daily.

Men who continued at work in the heat, under the conditions described, had a negative nitrogen balance for the first 10 to 20 days, and showed other evidences of excitation of the pituitary-adrenal axis with liberation of several of the hormones of the adrenal cortex, not mineralocorticoids only. In the first few days of exposure to heat there is intense salt conservation both by the kidneys and by the sweat glands. However, after the first few days under conditions of large sweat volume and average salt intake, the sweat glands continue to be very efficient in salt conservation, but the renal excretion of sodium actually rises (escapes) to attain sodium equilibrium. When the early phase of negative nitrogen balance disappears, low concentrations of sodium in sweat persist as an indicator of continued and intense salt conservation by the sweat glands. Secretion of the specific adrenocortical mineralocorticoid, *aldoster-*

one, accounts for the greatly reduced NaCl content of the sweat. The maintenance of continued augmented aldosterone secretion is independent of pituitary ACTH activity and is not accompanied by a general increase in the secretion of the other adrenocortical hormones. There is thus seen to be an important difference in the physiologic processes of NaCl conservation during exposure to heat between **two clearly defined phases:** (1) during the early phase (lasting 10 to 20 days under the conditions of Conn's studies) there is acute stress with excitation of the *pituitary-adrenal axis;* (2) during the persistent phase of acclimatization which follows thereafter, the sweat glands take over the primary role under the influence of independent *aldosterone* secretion (Fig. 35-3).

Under normal conditions the renal mechanisms of salt conservation play by far the major role, but with heavy sweating the major salt-saving function of the body is turned over to the sweat glands.

In physically fit persons, work in a hot environment sufficient to elevate body core temperature on each of several successive days leads to adaptation with dramatic reduction of strain. For example, in one study the subject developed on the first day a rectal temperature of 104°F., skin temperature of 99°, pulse of 180; after adaptation these figures were 101°, 96°, and a pulse rate of 140 per minute.[56]

Acclimatization results in a new lower threshold for the onset of sweating, and thereby induces maintenance of lower skin temperature, although the total amount of sweating may not be much increased. Lessened circulatory burden is a consequence of the ability to maintain the necessary thermal gradient between body core and skin without as great an elevation in core temperature.

Whether the lowered threshold for sweating is the result of a resetting of the regulatory mechanism in the hypothalamus, increased patency of cutaneous vessels, or lowered threshold for response of receptors in the skin is not known.

Water and salt requirements vary with the extent of losses. Some men can produce sweat at the rate of 3 liters per hour for brief periods, up to 1 liter per hour for 8 hours, and as much as 0.5 liter per hour for a 24 hour period. Frequent ingestion of water sufficient to satisfy thirst has demonstrable advantages over restricted or postponed water intake. Before acclimatization, 2 to 4 Gm. of NaCl is required for each liter of sweat. Dietary intake usually provides 10 Gm. or more of NaCl daily—enough to meet ordinary requirements of sweating.

Apparently the normal person receives adequate warning of incipient heat injury through developing faintness, dizziness, or fatigue. When workers engaged in very hot industrial jobs are free to rest at intervals as need is felt, heat injury seldom occurs. Persons working in hot environments should be instructed concerning proper increases of NaCl and fluid intake—to prevent dehydration, and not to wait until symptoms are evident.

Persons with impaired circulatory reserve may be unable to respond to the great demand for mobilization of fluid necessary in adjustment to high environmental temperature. *Circulatory failure* may be precipitated by such a stress.

Persons with adrenocortical insufficiency tend to have abnormally high concentrations of salt in sweat and are less able to adjust to high environmental temperatures. One of the salt-conserving mechanisms available to persons with normal adrenocortical function is reduction of the NaCl in sweat. Salt depletion of the body from any cause results in increased adrenal cortical secretion and reduction in the NaCl concentration in sweat.[9,64,66,67]

It is significant that, during the second phase of acclimatization, reduction of NaCl intake from liberal to very low levels induces a stress response similar to that observed upon first exposure to work in the heat (Fig. 35-3). Renal conservation of salt again becomes intense and there is a negative nitrogen balance.

Another important aspect of the physiologic processes of adjustment to heat and heavy sweating is concerned with the ability of an acclimatizing man to maneuver himself into a state of positive sodium balance.[64] Upon initial exposure to work in the heat there are very large losses of sodium in sweat. The precipitous fall in sweat sodium plus the drop in urinary sodium which then occur result in a period of active retention of sodium which persists until the total amount restored exceeds that initially lost. The added NaCl plus added water cause expansion of the extracellular fluid volume, which permits long-term cardiovascular adjustment to heat, an essential part of successful acclimatization.

The aldosterone-sweat gland system can reduce salt losses from the skin by as much as 95 per cent; all forms of temperature regulation in hot climates would fail without action of this system in maintaining or even augmenting the volume of the extracellular fluid. Aldosterone plays an essential role in bringing about the cutaneous, renal, and cardiovascular adjustments necessary for man's survival in hot climates.

Summary. One may summarize a working hypothesis concerning the sequential processes involved in the physiology of acclimatization as follows: in the initial response to exposure to heat (with a moderate work load and average salt intake) there is heavy sweating with consequent contraction of the extracellular fluid and plasma volumes because of the large amount of NaCl lost in the sweat. There is a reflex diversion of a larger than normal proportion of the intravascular volume to the skin. This diversion results in decreased renal plasma flow; decreased pressure or volume in the afferent renal arterioles stimulates the juxtaglomerular apparatus (this apparatus serving as one site of the vascular volume receptors) and aldosterone secretion is stimulated through the renin-angiotensin system. Because of decreased glomerular filtration rate or increased aldosterone activity upon the renal tubules, or both, urinary sodium may fall virtually to zero. Reduction of the concentration of NaCl in sweat becomes evident about 12 to 24 hours later. Within a few days there is escape from the intense restriction of renal NaCl output; renal salt output rises and tends to fluctuate with NaCl intake. However, the excretion of NaCl in the sweat remains very low, permitting a positive NaCl balance and fluid retention, with gradual expansion of the extracellular fluid volume until a new level of sodium balance and a new fluid equilibrium is established compatible with the acclimatized state.

Untoward Effects of Heat. When the protective mechanisms are able to operate adequately, health may be maintained despite strenuous exertion in a hot environment.

Failure to adjust adequately to heat may occur quickly as in (1) cardiovascular failure or (2) heat stroke; after more prolonged heat stress, as in (3) heat prostration or (4) heat cramps.

Factors that may account for inability to accommodate to heat include: (1) lack of water intake, (2) lack of NaCl intake, (3) adrenocortical deficiency (especially of aldosterone secretion), (4) impaired cardiovascular system, central or peripheral, (5) renal failure, (6) central nervous system disorders (of temperature regulation, of ADH secretion or affecting renal salt conservation).

The state ultimately reached by prolonged perspiration in the absence of adequate replacement of salt and water is called *heat exhaustion* or *heat prostration*. It is characterized by evidence of hypovolemia: low cardiac output, low central venous pressure, peripheral vasoconstriction. Signs of inadequate blood supply to vital organs may occur: heart failure, stupor or coma, renal failure. The patient is dehydrated and may be in shock. The skin is cool, moist, pale, sometimes cyanotic. Often there are muscular and abdominal cramps. The blood pressure is low, and the pulse is weak. Restoration to normal is accomplished by treatment of the shock and replacement of NaCl and water.

Heat cramps occur in persons engaged in strenuous activity at high environmental temperature and result from extreme loss of NaCl through sweat while the water intake is kept very high. The shock-like symptoms of heat prostration are less evident, although the two conditions merge. Loss of salt may reach 20 Gm. daily. The hypotonic body fluids cause intracellular overhydration and, through abnormal diffusion conditions in the muscles, cause severe muscular spasms and pain, particularly in the arms and the legs. The Na and Cl concentrations in the serum are low, and the urinary NaCl output diminishes greatly. In heat prostration the salt and water loss are more proportionate, so that the serum electrolytes are less evidently reduced and the changes tend further to be masked by anhydremia, with hemoconcentration, but the plasma volume falls and the circulation fails.

Cardiovascular failure may be precipitated even in normal persons by exposure to extreme heat; persons with previous cardiovascular impairment, either central or peripheral, are especially susceptible. The acute diversion of blood to the periphery is responsible for the early signs of vascular collapse: rapid pulse, decreased stroke volume, sometimes decreased minute output, severe postural hypotension, fainting or coma, sometimes convulsions. Often there is evidence of vascular engorgement, such as flushing of the face, neck, and chest, injection of the sclerae, edema of nasal mucous membranes, edema of hands and feet.

The heart may fail quickly when there is reduced coronary flow from the conditions described above. The heart may fail later because of inability to cope with the increased work demanded by acclimatization (see discussion above under Acclimatization).

Heat prostration must be distinguished from *sunstroke* or *heat stroke*, also apt to occur in hot weather. The latter, however, is characterized by loss of temperature control and high fever, reaching as high as 110°F., not necessarily accompanied by dehydration. The pulse is full, blood pressure normal or high, skin hot and flushed. Headache and vertigo are common, and convulsions, coma, and death may occur. Ice-water tub baths and the administration of NaCl and water parenterally help to restore temperature control. Apparently both the mechanisms for heat production and heat elimination are involved in the production of heat stroke. Inability to lower the rate of metabolism in response to a sudden rise in environmental temperature seems particularly apt to occur in persons with arteriosclerosis and impaired cardiac reserve. Increased peripheral circulation is suddenly required to facilitate heat loss and a greater burden is thrown upon the heart, so that death may occur either from heart failure or from the hyperpyrexia itself. Diminution or cessation of sweating before the onset of acute symptoms may be observed, and is characteristic, indicating a breakdown in the mechanism of heat elimination. Persons exposed to excessive sunlight or to extremely high temperature may of course suffer from both dehydration and loss of temperature control. Loss of body fluid removes safety factors in temperature control and predisposes to heat prostration or sunstroke.

Considerable amounts of NaCl may be lost in the perspiration. The average NaCl loss by this route is about 5 per cent of the intake, or about 0.5 Gm. daily. Under conditions of very heavy sweating this may be increased to many grams (from 5 to 10 or more). If this salt lack is not made up by adequate NaCl intake, water alone being taken, weakness, vomiting, diarrhea, mus-

cular cramps, convulsions, and other signs of salt deficit may occur. This is *water intoxication*, primarily due to cellular overhydration, occurring as the result of reduced osmotic pressure of the blood. *Salt hunger* is a definite sensation which usually leads animals and man to correct this lack if NaCl is available. The mechanism of salt hunger is not yet well-understood, but apparently it depends upon the salt concentration of the extracellular fluid reaching the taste buds.[6]

OSMOTIC PRESSURE AND ELECTROLYTE REGULATION

Circulation of the extracellular fluid depends partly upon the hydrostatic pressure produced by the heart and partly upon the difference in protein content between blood plasma and interstitial fluid. The work of the heart sustains a higher hydrostatic pressure on the arterial side of the capillary bed, and, as a result of this pressure, fluid steadily moves into the interstitial spaces. On the venous side of the capillary bed the plasma proteins provide an osmotic differential which is unopposed and fluid returns to the venous capillaries and the veins.

UNITS OF MEASUREMENT

The desirability of expressing chemical measurements in truly comparable terms has been emphasized by Gamble,[3] and the following discussion on units of measurement is quoted from him:

In studying the chemical structure of extracellular fluid, measurements of its components must obviously be stated in terms of chemical equivalence. Only in this way can their relative magnitudes and inter-relationships be correctly displayed. The suitable term is milliequivalents per liter. This value is obtained by dividing milligrams per liter by atomic weight and multiplying by valence.

Conversion from milligrams per 100 ml. to milliequivalents per liter for the individual ions is as follows:

	mg. per 100 ml.
Na·	$\times 10 \div 23$
K·	$\times 10 \div 39$
Ca··	$\times 10 \div 40 \times 2$
Mg··	$\times 10 \div 24 \times 2$
Cl′	$\times 10 \div 35$
HPO_4″ (mg. P)	$\times 10 \div 31 \times 1.8$
SO_4″ (mg. S)	$\times 10 \div 32 \times 2$

The valence of HPO_4 is taken as 1.8 because, at the normal pH of extracellular fluid, 20 per cent of the concentration of this radical carries one equivalent of base, (BH_2PO_4), and 80 per cent two equivalents, (B_2HPO_4); B representing univalent base. Base equivalence per unit of (HPO_4) is therefore $0.2 + (0.8 \times 2) = 1.8$. The double valency sign is to this small extent inaccurate.

For the concentrations of carbonic acid $(H.HCO_3)$ and of bicarbonate $(B.HCO_3)$ convention prescribes the cumbersome statements: volume per cent CO_2 as carbonic acid and volume per cent CO_2 as bicarbonate. These volume per cent values are converted to milliequivalents per liter by dividing by 2.22.

The base equivalence of protein as milliequivalents per liter is obtained by multiplying grams protein per 100 ml. by the Van Slyke factor, 2.43.

In studying the osmotic features of extracellular fluid, measurements of its components are stated in terms of ionic concentration. In other words valence is disregarded. The suitable term is milliosmols per liter (milligrams per liter divided by atomic weight). The milliosmolar and milliequivalence values for the univalent ions are obviously identical. The chemical equivalence of the divalent ions is twice their milliosmolar value. The term milliosmolar is used instead of millimolar to make clear the additive osmotic effect of individual ions; e.g., the milliosmolar value of a solution of sodium chloride is twice its millimolar value.[3]

Chemical Structure of Body Fluids. Blood plasma and interstitial fluid resemble each other closely, except for the presence in plasma of the considerable amount of protein, whereas in interstitial fluid there is a very small quantity of this nondiffusible component (see the two middle diagrams, Fig. 35-2). This difference requires adjustment of the concentrations of the diffusible ions in order to preserve total cation-anion equivalence (Donnan equilibrium) within the interstitial fluid. The diagram of the interstitial fluid reveals that the base equivalence of plasma protein has been replaced by a balanced reduction of cation (note the shorter Na· column), and an increase in diffusible anion (note the longer HCO_3' and Cl' columns). This results in a total of equivalents in interstitial fluid which is less than that in plasma—in other words, the concentration of electrolytes is less. The total of equivalents in plasma stands above that in interstitial fluid by approximately the base equivalence of plasma protein (16 mEq./L.). Owing to its multivalency, the *chemical* equivalence of protein is about 8 times its concentration value.

The difference in *osmotic values* is approximately 2 milliosmols per liter—this being dependent upon the actual difference in ion concentration without regard to valence. The small difference of 2 milliosmols is of great importance in promoting normal extracellular fluid circulation (Fig. 35-2). If the level of the serum albumin falls below normal levels, fluid may not be returned to the vascular system at a rate sufficient to prevent abnormal extravascular fluid accumulation. If protein is present in extravascular areas in amounts in excess of the very low level normally present in interstitial fluid, such important clinical states as *ascites, edema, pericardial effusion,* etc., may result (see Chap. 36). A total value for the nonelectrolytes is placed across the top of the diagrams. The nonelectrolytes include the nutrient substances, such as glucose and amino acids, and the waste products of protein metabolism, such as urea. "The nonelectrolytes demand only expeditious conveyance. The electrolytes constitute a chemical framework on which rests the stability of the physical properties of extracellular fluid. Their transport is in terms of this requirement. This is the meaning of the large prominence of the electrolytes."[3]

In Figure 35-2 the values may be read on the left of the ordinate. The figures on the right give the total of equivalence (the sum of the values in both columns). The values given are those **per liter of water**—the space occupied by protein being (for this purpose) disregarded.

Note that Figure 35-2 shows that the plasma contains more total milliequivalents per liter of the various ions than interstitial fluid; that is, the plasma is somewhat more concentrated. Likewise, the cell fluid is more concentrated than the plasma.

Even during good health there are of course numerous minor variations in the electrolyte values. Since water and other substances enter and leave the extracellular fluid irregularly, and since renal adjustments require some time, large deviations may occur in the presence of disease. Recovery is permitted by the elasticity of the electrolyte system.

Cell fluid differs greatly from extracellular fluid (Fig. 35-2). Cell membranes are normally and at rest freely permeable to potassium and chloride ions, but less permeable to sodium ions. Under stimulation, cell-wall permeability may change very briefly, permitting rapid influx of Na^+ ions and rapid egress of K^+ ions. Activity of the "sodium pump" mechanism (discussed more fully later in this section) restores the extracellular : intracellular ionic concentrations and balance to normal.

In the cell, potassium constitutes the largest base component, whereas $PO_4^=$ and $SO_4^=$ are the largest anions or acid radicals. Although the interstitial and the intracellular fluids are osmotically balanced and are separated only by a thin sheet of protoplasm, their ionic patterns differ entirely.

The osmolality of the extracellular fluid (plasma) is almost entirely due to monovalent salts, which ionize into two ions each. The total osmolality, therefore, is cations $(+)$ plus anions $(-) = 2 \times 155 = 310$ mOsm./L.

For purposes of comparison and only as a rough approximation, the higher osmolality of cell fluid is given as exceeding 420 mOsm./L.

As yet data concerning composition of cell fluid are scanty and incomplete. The average composition of muscle cell fluid has been inferred from various indirect measurements to be approximately as follows:

	mEq./L.
Na^+	10
K^+	150
Mg^{++}	40
HCO_3^-	10
Cl^-	15–20
$PO_4^=$ and $SO_4^=$	150
Protein	40
TOTAL approximately	420+

It seems likely that cells of the various special organs and tissues will be found to have various compositions related to their unique functions.

Bone. The composition of bone is unique as compared to other tissues; only about 20 per cent is water and only about 35 per cent of the solids is protein. The remainder of the solid phase of bone is a latticework of inorganic salts. Of the total body sodium, 30 to 45 per cent is in bone, about 15 per cent in the extracellular phase. The largest part of the sodium present in bone is part of the crystal structure of bone, and 30 to 40 per cent of this is exchangeable with an isotope of sodium in 24 hours. Potassium is also present in bone and is exchangeable, but in much smaller amounts.

When sodium or potassium deficits occur, they may be shared by bone. Both Na^+ and K^+ of bone apparently are exchanged with H^+ ions in either direction as part of the mechanism opposing distortion of acid-base relationships.

High NaCl intake increases Na storage in bone; hyponatremia leads to mobilization of Na from bone. Since it has been shown that large quantities of sodium may enter or leave bone, it seems evident that exchanges of ions do not necessarily represent extracellular-intracellular shifts, but may result from exchanges between extracellular fluid and bone solids.[51]

Lymph and Lymphatics. Whenever there is an increase in the vascular hydrostatic pressure or in the protein content of the interstitial fluid (tending to cause an increase in the net transfer of fluid from the plasma to the interstitial space) the lymph vessels operate to reduce unphysiologic expansion of the interstitial fluid volume. Normally, the volume of lymph reaching the plasma through the lymphatic vessels in an adult is about 1.5 ml. per kg. body weight per hour, or a total of about 2,400 ml. per day. A considerable amount of protein escapes from the arterial capillaries by transudation from the plasma into the interstitial fluid. The lymphatic capillaries are far more permeable than the blood capillaries and constitute the special channels by which such protein is returned to the plasma. When for any reason the lymphatic capillaries cannot function normally to remove fluid, protein, and crystalloids from the interstitial fluid, local accumulations of such fluid may occur, or generalized edema.

The protein content of human leg lymph is normally 0.5 to 0.7 per cent. The lymph flowing from the thoracic duct, since it comes largely from the intestine and liver, varies with the digestive processes and ranges in protein content from 2 to 4.5 per cent.

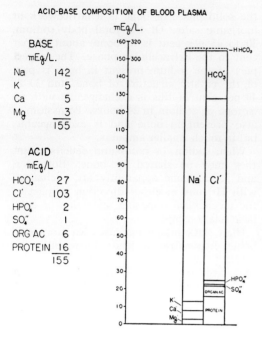

ACID-BASE COMPOSITION OF BLOOD PLASMA

mEq/L.

BASE
mEq/L.

Na	142
K	5
Ca	5
Mg	3
	155

ACID
mEq/L

HCO₃	27
Cl'	103
HPO₄	2
SO₄	1
ORG AC	6
PROTEIN	16
	155

FIG. 35-4. The relative magnitudes of the various factors of the acid-base structure of the plasma. (Gamble, J. L.: Chemical Anatomy, Physiology and Pathology of Extracellular Fluid, Boston, The Harvard Medical School)

The Blood Plasma. In Figure 35-4 are given the normal values for the components of the electrolyte structure of blood plasma. The blood plasma is the most readily accessible portion of the extracellular fluid, and by studying changes in it one can judge the effectiveness of the regulatory mechanisms. The kidneys are the chief regulatory organs, controlling the concentration in the plasma of all its components except two, the carbonic acid and the protein. The carbonic-acid content is under respiratory control. Plasma-protein content depends upon amino-acid supply to the site of plasma-protein manufacture (apparently the liver), normality and adequacy of such manufacture, and upon abnormal protein losses (if any) through kidneys, ascitic fluid, etc.

The total ionic concentration is determined by the sum of the cation values, since the adjustable part of the ionic structure is the anion HCO_3^-. The total ionic concentration is not changed when other anion values are altered, since reciprocal alterations of HCO_3^- occur. Nearly all of the base (cation) is sodium, and therefore

the efficiency of the renal control of this one electrolyte element is paramount in the maintenance of stability of the osmotic value of the extracellular fluid.

The intake of water and of sodium is variable, and their supply to the body is not regularly related; therefore, renal control is constantly in operation. However, the kidney requires time to establish osmotic equality between intracellular and extracellular fluid. Fortunately, a rapid supplementary form of control is available. An immediate prerenal adjustment takes place, depending upon the obligatory extracellular position of sodium, and consisting simply in the transfer of water from one compartment to the other as necessary to produce osmotic equilibrium. For example, if NaCl is taken in excess (beyond isotonic limits in proportion to the water ingested), water moves from intracellular to extracellular fluid. The increased volume of the extracellular fluid is then reduced by the kidney at leisure. If the contrary takes place and there is a sudden large loss of extracellular electrolyte, water shifts from the extracellular position into the cells, the excessive intracellular-fluid volume being later reduced by excretion through the kidneys. Although either water or salt depletion alone may cause the same degree of contraction in total extracellular volume, the contraction of plasma volume is greater after salt loss. Loss of salt is more deleterious to the circulation than water withdrawal. Salt depletion causes intracellular overhydration, whereas water depletion causes cellular dehydration. Thus, changes in volume of the two compartments may take place to compensate for alterations in total ion content, thereby permitting maintenance of osmotic equilibrium. The requirements of osmotic balance may be satisfied temporarily by such shifts between the two compartments. It must be recognized, however, that the effects of loss of salt and loss of water, which usually occur together and proportionately, are opposite in character when separate or disproportionate. Salt loss leads to hypotonicity in both compartments and water loss to hypertonicity.

SODIUM AND POTASSIUM TRANSPORT
INTO AND OUT OF CELLS

Practically every kind of energy expenditure by all cells, including that involved in active transport of ions across membranes, is associated with the breakdown of adenosinetriphosphate (ATP). Active outward transport of sodium from most cells requires the presence of potassium at the site toward which sodium is moved (outside the membrane), suggesting a coupling between the active transport of Na+ and K+ ions in opposite directions.[80]

Recent evidence supports the concept that an enzyme, sodium-potassium-activated adenosinetriphosphatase (Na-K-ATPase), is intimately involved in the active transport of electrolytes across biologic membranes.[84] Such an active enzyme system has been demonstrated in many cells and tissues, including intestinal mucosa,[81,82] cell membranes of kidney tubules,[83] glandular tissues, nerve cells, skeletal and cardiac muscle.[84] Demonstration of the enzyme on cell membranes or their intracellular extensions (where the hypothetical sodium "pump" is assumed to be located) has provided additional support for the hypothesis that it is involved in active ion transport.

Although the Na+ and K+ interchange across cell membranes is highly significant at many body locations, we have particularly cited previously the renal tubular cells be-cause of their major position in controlling fluid balance, electrolyte balance, and acid-base balance.

The mucosa of the gastrointestinal tract is cited too, because its cells are also greatly concerned with maintaining these balances within normal physiologic limits. When GI function is deranged and the GI mucosal cells cannot operate normally, serious disorders may become evident in these balances[79] (see Fig. 35-5).

In muscle and nerve, the unequal intracellular and extracellular distribution of cations gives rise to a difference in potential across the intervening membrane that sets up the conditions preparatory for the excitation phenomenon. In the resting nerve the interior of the nerve cell body is negative in electrical potential with respect to the exterior. The cell membrane is said to be polarized. At rest, the external surface of the membrane is positive with respect to the interior of the fiber. With stimulation, during the action potential, the membrane potential becomes reversed in sign, the interior becoming positive, exterior negative. Stim-

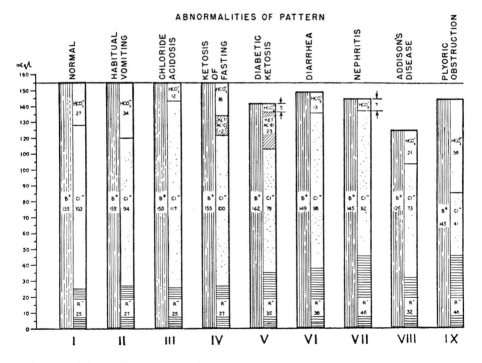

Fig. 35-5. Eight different types of abnormal patterns in the blood plasma compared with the normal pattern. The numbers within the columns give the concentrations in milliequivalents per liter. (Newburgh, L. H., and Leaf, A.: Significance of the Body Fluids in Clinical Medicine, Springfield, Ill., Thomas, p. 32)

ulation of a nerve causes Na⁺ ions to enter the cell, and K⁺ ions to leave.

In muscle cells, a similar mechanism operates: stimulation lowers the potential across the sarcolemmal membrane and a rapid influx of sodium ions into the cell occurs. The result of this inflow is reversal of potential, and the interior becomes positive to the exterior. This change of polarity constitutes the action potential. The resting potential is restored by the flow of potassium ions out of the cell.

During the action potential, the ion transfers across cell membranes have provided an immediate source of energy for conduction of further impulses. The cell involved has, as a result of this activity, gained a little sodium and lost a little potassium.

A slower process, requiring metabolic energy from within the cell, takes place *during the recovery phase* and restoration to the resting state. The energy is derived from the breakdown of ATP, involves action of the enzyme Na-K-ATPase, and results in the *extrusion of Na⁺ ions* from the cell and the *reciprocal uptake of K⁺ ions* by the cell. This mechanism (known familiarly as "the sodium pump") maintains the normal concentrations of the ions in the two compartments, extracellular and intracellular, and maintains the whole body total ionic balance between the compartments. Sodium and chloride become situated primarily in extracellular fluid, potassium primarily inside the cell membranes. The distribution of these ions results in the normal resting potential across the cell membrane, the outer surface being positive, the interior negative.

From these considerations it seems evident that Na⁺ and K⁺ transport across cell membranes affects many organs and tissues in important ways. Because of the critical role played by electrolytes in conduction along nerve fibers and in muscle, these have been especially studied.

If the Na⁺ concentration in which a neurone is immersed is decreased, the action potential is reduced. In a sodium-free solution, the action potential soon fails completely.

Potassium ions may have a dual role in neuromuscular transmission and muscular contraction:

1. K⁺ ions may be concerned with *neuromuscular transmission*. K salts given intra-arterially act selectively on the motor endplate, producing electrical responses and muscle contraction similar to that produced by acetylcholine.

2. The *excitability* and other properties of muscle appear to depend to some extent upon the relative concentrations of K⁺ ions within and outside the muscle cells.

Muscle activity is seriously impaired whenever potassium in the blood is extremely high or abnormally low. When *potassium depletion* occurs, (in potassium-losing nephritis, in prolonged diuresis, from vomiting or diarrhea, in hyperadrenocorticism, in hyperaldosteronism, etc.), there may be severe muscular weakness or episodes of paralysis. In such disorders, the K within the cells may be much below normal and the K in the extracellular fluid may approach zero. For production of the action potential and for operation of the sodium pump, some K⁺ ions must be present outside the cell membrane and an adequate supply of K⁺ ions must be present within the cell.

In *familial periodic paralysis* there is, in contrast to the previous group of disorders, no depletion of body potassium, but there is a shift of K from extracellular fluids into cells not deficient in K, with a fall in serum potassium. During an attack, stimulation of the motor nerve or direct stimulation of muscle elicits no response.

Hyperkalemic states known to be associated with muscular weakness and paralysis include many conditions in which there is severe sodium depletion and K retention. Hyperkalemia occurs with K retention in advanced renal disease, etc. In *adynamia episodica hereditaria* there is no renal K retention, but high K excretion during an attack. Apparently the elevated serum and urinary K result from loss of K from cells and movement of K⁺ ions to the extracellular position.

Studies on the ionic affinities of the enzyme system involved with Na⁺ and K⁺ transport across cell membranes are suggestive, when regarded in relation to the various conditions mentioned previously in which muscle weakness occurs both with high and low extracellular K⁺, and with high and low intracellular K⁺. Increase in the Na⁺ in an incubation mixture, with constant Mg⁺⁺ and K⁺, is followed by an increase in enzymatic activity up to a point beyond which no further stimulation is obtained. However, progressive increases in K⁺ concentration first stimulate and then inhibit the Na-K-ATPase activity. The concentrations of K⁺ that cause inhibition show a direct relation to the concentration of Na⁺ in the medium, suggesting that K⁺ at higher concentrations competes with Na⁺ for the enzyme. Indeed, kinetic analysis of the effects of Na^+ and K^+ on the enzyme[85] suggests that there is one site where the affinity for Na^+ is six to eight times higher than for K^+, and another site with high affinity for K^+ and a very low affinity for Na^+. Maximum activity requires Na^+ at one site and K^+ at a second. Studies with intact cells have revealed that ATP breakdown and ion transport require Na^+ on the inside of the membrane and K^+ on the outside, thus corroborating the evidence supplied by studies of enzyme kinetics.

Later in this chapter we discuss more completely the various clinical causes and signs and symptoms of potassium aberrations. See, in relation to ion transport mechanisms treated here, the sections under Clinical Signs of Potassium Deficiency, and Potassium Intoxication; Hyperkalemia. In reference particularly to the effects of potassium disorders on **cardiac muscle** and on the electrocardiogram there discussed, it should be noted here that cardiac glycosides are potent inhibitors of both active ion transport and Na-K-ATPase in many organs.[86] Low serum K potentiates the effect of digitalis glycosides. Digitalis intoxication in digitalized patients may be precipitated by potassium losses leading to hypokalemia. Studies suggest that the digitalis glycosides inhibit the $(Na^+ + K^+)$-stimulated ATPase by displacing K^+ from its attachment to the enzyme system. Other evidence[87] indicates that digitalis glycosides exert inhibition in an allosteric manner, rather than by direct competition with K^+.

Of great interest, of course, is the relationship of *adrenal cortex hormones* to the enzyme system and the cation transport mechanism under discussion. Adrenalectomy causes a fall in the enzyme in the kidney, but apparently not in other tissues. Activity is restored by corticosterone, but not by aldosterone.[84] Further clarification is needed of this doubtless highly important interrelationship.

FLUID REGULATORY SYSTEMS

For purposes of discussion it is helpful to group the chief organ-systems regulating fluid balance as follows:

1. Skin
2. Renal
3. Neurohormonal
4. Gastrointestinal
5. Respiratory.

All are closely interrelated. Neurohormonal effects are chiefly upon the kidney tubules, but also influence the skin and GI tract in their disposition of solutes and water.

The role of the skin has been considered previously under Temperature Regulation. In the following section we will consider the other four organ-systems controlling salt and water metabolism, beginning with the kidneys, usually the most powerful.

RENAL REGULATION OF BODY FLUIDS

The *concentrations* of sodium and of the other solutes in the extracellular fluid are normally determined chiefly by the amount of water conserved or rejected by the kidneys and by the amounts of the various solutes selectively excreted or reabsorbed by renal tubular action.

The urinary output of water and solutes varies with (1) **the solute load,** and (2) **activities of the renal tubules,** which are subject to a number of influences, as discussed later in this section.

The average daily solute load in an adult is about 1200 mOsm. The solute load is highly variable, fluctuating with the intake of the various solutes and with metabolic conditions. With high intake the load may be increased, or with augmented supply from tissues, as with fever, tissue destruction, or accelerated protein metabolism. On a diet principally of glucose, the solute load may be as low as 300 mOsm. On an average diet, it is about 1,200 mOsm. A higher water intake (response to thirst) and higher urinary water and solute excretion are normally provided when needed.

The preceding statements regarding obligatory urinary volumes apply to normal kidneys. With progressive degrees of impairment of renal function, the ability to excrete a concentrated urine (hyperosmolar to plasma) decreases. A stage may be reached with advanced renal disease at which the average solute load keeps the kidneys in a state of constant osmotic diuresis. In such circumstances, the obligatory water loss by this route is greatly increased and the urine volume is relatively large.

In addition to the effect of the solute load, the presence or absence of antidiuretic hormone (ADH) is extremely important in determining the amount of water conserved or rejected by the kidney. Under normal circumstances, the ADH mechanism exerts greater control over urinary volume than does solute load.

Receptors to small changes in the osmotic pressure of the extracellular fluid are located in the hypothalamus. The antidiuretic hormone is produced in the hypothalamus and stored in the posterior pituitary gland, awaiting release in response to proper stimuli.

When the blood reaching the osmore-ceptors is of normal tonicity, there is a small steady secretion of ADH. A rise in tonicity causes increased ADH secretion, and renal tubular resorption of water is increased; the plasma becomes more dilute and the hyper-osmolar state is corrected.

Ingestion of water without salt causes a decrease in the effective osmolality of the extracellular fluid and suppression of ADH secretion. The kidney responds by "water diuresis"—increased volume of dilute urine—and thus defends the rather narrow limits of permissible variation in osmolality of body fluids.

Renal regulation consists essentially in *selective reabsorption* of water and solute substances from the glomerular filtrate by the tubules. Urine formation seems to be the result of simple filtration by the glo-meruli, followed by modification of the composition of the glomerular filtrate by tubular absorption and tubular excretion.

The *glomerular filtrate* normally contains the same amount of water and the same concentration of contained substances (except for protein) as does the plasma. Under normal conditions the absorption of some substances by the renal tubules is practically complete; others are only partially absorbed. The tubules are capable of adding certain substances to the urine. The distal tubules are the site of ammonia formation and the final adjustment of urinary pH. According to studies of glomerular filtration with inulin, approximately 125 ml. per minute of filtrate, amounting to 180 liters in 24 hours, are produced. Urine volume usually does not exceed two liters; therefore, almost all of the water of the filtrate must be reabsorbed. With this huge amount of water must be reabsorbed all the important constituents of the plasma, such as Na and Cl. The renal NaCl excretion (actually lost in the urine) amounts to about 95 per cent of the intake normally, and for the normal adult ranges from 6 to 15 Gm. daily. Gamble[3] has calculated that by weight the quantity of Na and Cl together reabsorbed may amount to a kilogram or more per 24 hours. Normally nearly all of the water, Na, and Cl (99 per cent) and the glucose filtered through the glomeruli are reabsorbed by the tubules, but about 60 per cent of the urea, 18 per cent of

the SO_4, 12 per cent of the HPO_4, and 8 per cent of the K are excreted, reabsorption being less active for these substances.

The total daily urinary solute excretion averages normally about 30 to 40 Gm. It varies considerably both as to total amount and as to constituents, depending upon intake of various salts and foods and upon fever, increased destruction of tissue, rate of protein metabolism, etc. Representative average normal figures per liter of urine might be: urea 20 Gm., NaCl 8 Gm., K about 2 Gm., P about 2 Gm., S about 1.5 Gm., uric acid 0.6 Gm., and ammonia 0.6 Gm. The kidney allows excretion of a more dilute urine when the solute load is large; the larger the solute load, the nearer the urinary osmolality approaches that of plasma. With heavy solute loads, the specific gravity of the urine will approach the isosmolar level of approximately 1.010. Many substances, such as NaCl, Na_2SO_4, urea, sucrose, and mannitol will therefore act as osmotic diuretics. Ingestion or parenteral administration of hypertonic salt solutions thus causes diuresis and dehydration.

Normally the greatest variable in daily water loss is sensible perspiration, the output by this route varying from zero to many liters. To preserve water balance two compensatory mechanisms operate: (1) adjustment of water intake as regulated by thirst, and (2) adjustment of water output as regulated by the kidneys. Renal control may vary the concentration through a range varying from four times the concentration of plasma to about one-sixth that of plasma (1400 mOsm./L. to 50 mOsm./L.).

In the absence of renal impairment, the rate of water output by the kidneys depends upon two control systems: (1) defense of the osmolality of the body fluids, and (2) defense of the volume of the body fluids.

The defense of osmolality depends upon the response of the distal renal tubules to the antidiuretic hormone and to the rate of excretion of solutes in the urine.

Volume changes definitely call forth homeostatic protective responses. A drop in extracellular fluid volume causes thirst and results in restriction of renal water loss. The physiologic mechanisms resulting in these defensive responses are not known. It has been suggested that one mechanism may be the increased *aldosterone* secretion known to result from hemorrhage, dehydration, etc. Previously it had been postulated that the major volume receptors that control salt excretion are probably located in the walls of arteries. A well-documented reflex mechanism with a "volume receptor" leads to aldosterone secretion. The pathway is entirely outside the central nervous system and the connecting links are all humoral. The receptor is in the wall of the afferent arteriole of the glomerulus. It consists of or activates a small group of cells called the juxtaglomerular apparatus; they secrete renin. A *decrease* in stretch of the afferent arteriole activates renin secretion. Renin acts in the blood stream on protein precursors made in the liver which can be split to yield an active polypeptide called angiotensin II. This is the same material previously known to be a potent vasoconstrictor. Small amounts of angiotensin infused into the adrenal artery cause stimulation of secretion of the salt-retaining hormone aldosterone by the cells of the zona glomerulosa of the adrenal cortex. Such stimulation can occur with amounts of angiotensin too small to affect peripheral vascular tone. ACTH can stimulate the adrenal to produce aldosterone, but is much more potent in causing glucocorticoid (cortisone and cortisol) secretion. *Angiotensin is a relatively specific stimulant for aldosterone secretion.*[68]

The various constituents of the glomerular filtrate are acted upon in a number of different ways by the tubule cells. The mechanisms of the differential treatment of all the materials contained in the filtrate are as yet incompletely understood. It seems evident that active work is performed by the tubule cells, because they bring about movements opposite to those exerted through osmotic forces. Through work done by the tubule cells (1) water can be moved from a region of higher concentration to one of lower concentration; (2) solutes can be moved from a region of lower concentration to one of higher concentration.[47,49]

As concerns water, about 85 per cent of the glomerular filtrate is reabsorbed iso-osmotically. Work is involved, however, in conserving the remainder of the water, since it must be absorbed against the osmotic gradient. As the water reaches the lower tubule cells the concentration of the solutes becomes very high, but the tubules still must continue their valiant task of conserving body water and preventing dehydration. It is evident that impairment of renal function may be reflected quickly and most significantly in deranged fluid balance.

Urea is the urinary constituent chiefly responsible for the necessity of work by the renal tubules, since it is present in the urine in the largest amounts and in the highest concentration. If a man excreted 1 liter of urine it might normally contain about 15 Gm. of urea, the original glomerular filtrate having contained 30 Gm. in 180 liters. Hence, in this instance, the urea concentration of the urine is 90 times that of the plasma or the original plasma filtrate.

About 150 Gm. of glucose enter the upper ends of the tubules in 24 hours, all but 1 or 2 Gm. being reabsorbed.

The serum sodium and chloride concentrations are kept within rather narrow limits, despite wide fluctuations in the intake of sodium chloride and water, through the work of the renal tubules. If sodium is present in excess, the urine will become higher in sodium concentration than the plasma. However, should water be present in excess, the urine becomes dilute. If sodium conservation is needed, the total volume of the urine may remain the same, but the urine sodium concentration becomes less than that of the plasma.

Water and salts are reabsorbed principally in the proximal portion of the tubules, so that here the approximately 180 liters of water and 1 to 1.5 kGm. of NaCl are restored to the body. In the distal tubules more fluid is absorbed, further concentration of the urine takes place, and the final adjustments of the urinary pH are made, according to whatever the requirements may be at the time in preservation of the body's acid-base balance.

The remarkable exactitude and the delicacy of these renal functions are evident when one considers that, should the renal tubules be so little impaired as one per cent in their water-retaining ability (through intrinsic renal disease, through hormonal control or otherwise), 1.8 liters in excess of normal might be lost each day in the urine, and dehydration would result.

Neurohormonal Regulation of Fluid Balance

The renal control of fluid balance is to a large degree under hormonal influence. The hormonal influence is exerted in the activity of the distal renal tubular cells and is concerned with the amount of water reabsorbed by the tubules and with the amounts of certain solutes, particularly sodium and potassium, which are reabsorbed or excreted.

Two types of hormones affect renal tubular control of water and solutes: (1) The neurohypophysial hormone, apparently produced primarily in certain cell groups in the anterior hypothalamus and produced or stored in the posterior lobe (pars nervosa) of the pituitary. It is called *vasopressin,* or *antidiuretic hormone* and for brevity and convenience, ADH. It is a polypeptide consisting of only eight amino acids. It exerts a major controlling influence on water reabsorption. (2) Certain steroid hormones produced in the cortex of the adrenal gland. There are several of these mineralocorticoids, of which *aldosterone* is by far the most potent in promoting sodium retention and potassium excretion.

Antidiuretic Hormone Effects. In the distal renal tubules there is free permeability of the tubular membrane to water only under the influence of ADH; in the absence of this hormone only very small amounts of water can be absorbed and the tubular fluid passing on to be excreted as urine remains voluminous and dilute. The most striking example of this influence is observed in the disease *diabetes insipidus,* in which the power of the tubules to reabsorb water is greatly impaired and the renal water loss per day, instead of the normal 1.5 or 2 liters, may be 10 to 20 liters. Relief of this disorder is possible by administration of antidiuretic hormone. A diuretic influence is apparently exerted by the anterior lobe of the pituitary and the thyroid gland and is normally balanced by the posterior pituitary antidiuretic factor.[10] Urine-concentration tests indicate that patients with diabetes insipidus receiving a limited intake of fluid will continue to secrete urine of low specific gravity, with resultant dehydration and loss of body weight. In any case in which such a response is obtained, the diagnosis of organic damage of the supraoptico-hypophysial tract should be suspected. The normal antidiuretic effect, exerted through the neurohormonal control maintained through the supraoptic nuclei and the posterior lobe of the pituitary gland, is lost when the tract is injured bilaterally.

Water deprivation or dehydration from any cause resulting in a rise in plasma tonicity in normal persons results in ADH secretion, increased renal resorption of water, and decreased urine volume. Response to the hypertonicity of the plasma depends upon:

1. Integrity of the osmoreceptors
2. Integrity of the neurohypophysial sys-

tem for production of the antidiuretic hormone
3. Response of the renal tubules to ADH.

Renal tubular response may be inadequate because:

1. The amount of ADH produced or reaching the renal tubules is insufficient, or
2. The number of functional tubules is inadequate.

Thus, the lack of ADH may be simulated to some degree by severe renal impairment. Renal damage as a cause of severe polyuria is usually indicated by a number of other findings in the history, physical examination, and laboratory studies. Deficiency of ADH is distinguished from renal polyuria by specific tests (as discussed below) and diabetes insipidus is well-controlled by ADH therapy, but polyuria of renal insufficiency is not responsive to such treatment.

Dehydration or increased osmotic pressure of the blood brings about increased secretion of ADH, and increased amounts of ADH have been detected in the body fluids in such states.[11] In the hypothalamus there are "osmoreceptors," which are sensitive to fluctuations of electrolyte concentration of the plasma.[12] Thus release of ADH is controlled by changes in the electrolyte concentration, a rise causing posterior pituitary stimulation (antidiuresis), a fall causing inhibition (relative diuresis).

The osmoreceptors are groups of cells in the hypothalamus which lie in or close to the supraoptic nuclei. These osmoreceptors set up nerve impulses that stimulate secretory cells in the hypothalamus to produce ADH and stimulate the neurohypophysis (posterior lobe of the pituitary) to release stored ADH. At normal tonicity of the plasma, the receptors discharge steadily and maintain a steady secretion of ADH. If hypertonicity due to a rise in electrolyte ion concentration occurs, both the receptor impulse discharge and the ADH secretion are increased; conversely, hypotonicity reduces both the stimulus to produce and the release of ADH.

Hypertonic solutions of **urea** do not stimulate the osmoreceptors and cause no release of ADH. An elevated blood urea normally leads to increased urea excretion through increased urine volume. The nonresponsiveness of the receptors to urea prevents ADH release, which would reduce urine volume and hamper lowering of blood urea. The osmoreceptors fail to respond to high blood urea concentrations because, although urea increases the osmolality of the extracellular fluid, it diffuses freely into cells, raising cell osmolality also.

Glucose does not freely enter cells; hyperglycemia increases the relative extracellular hyperosmolality and stimulates the osmoreceptors; thus, ADH may be released. This effect is not sufficient to significantly diminish the polyuria characteristic of diabetes mellitus.

Secretion of ADH has been induced in man and animals by electrical stimulation of the hypothalamus and its components. Numerous centrally acting stimuli, such as noise, pain, or fright, may increase the secretory activity of the neurohypophysis. Certain drugs such as nicotine, acetylcholine, and alcohol inhibit secretion of ADH.

ADH renders the cells of the distal portions of the nephron permeable to water, thus permitting the passive diffusion of tubular water along an osmotic gradient across the cells and into peritubular vessels.

In the syndrome of "inappropriate ADH secretion" there are two typical changes: hypo-osmolality of the plasma and hypertonicity of the urine. Serum chloride and sodium values are low because of excessive retention of water. These changes are not characteristic of the majority of patients with *idopathic periodic edema*; therefore, if ADH secretion occurs in this syndrome, it must be associated with increased aldosterone secretion, which causes Na and Cl retention.[90]

Evidence indicates that ADH acts directly upon the renal tubules, with stimulation of these cells to absorb more water from the lumen of the tubule. Thus, water is retained and urine volume is reduced.

In diabetes insipidus, the degree of polyuria varies directly as the nitrogen excretion, which indicates that the kidneys in this disease cannot concentrate urea any better than they can salt. The antidiuretic hormone checks the excretion of water by re-establishing normal absorption in the tubules. The rate of elimination of Na and Cl is not changed by the activity of the hormone. If a normal kidney is already excreting a maximally concentrated urine, the action of additional ADH is not detectable. Thus it is possible, with the hormone, to inhibit a water diuresis, but not a diuresis induced by salt or urea, because the kidney is concentrating the salt or urea to its maximum ability.

If ADH is administered to a normal subject, the effect depends upon the amount of water available for excretion. If water is withheld, the volume of urine is not altered. If, however, water is given, the usual diuresis is prevented by the ADH, the urine volume is much less than would normally be the case and the specific gravity of the urine remains relatively high. Since ADH does not alter the excretion of salt and other solutes, *water intoxication* may result in normal persons given ADH and allowed large amounts of water.

The specific gravity of urine depends largely upon the concentrations of salts and of urea. In diabetes insipidus, the volume of the urine tends to remain very high and its specific gravity very low, as long as fluid intake keeps pace with the water loss. Prolonged water deprivation may limit the output somewhat and raise the specific gravity. Injection of ADH in proper amounts will restore output and specific gravity to normal. If urinary specific gravity is low and volume high because of renal impairment, ADH cannot restore normal conditions.

Hickey and Hare have introduced a test to measure the ability to liberate the antidiuretic principle. Hypertonic chloride solution is given intravenously during water diuresis. If the diuresis is inhibited, the hypothalamic-hypophysial system is presumed to be normal. If there is no inhibition of diuresis, the diagnosis of diabetes insipidus may be made—because hypertonic salt in the body fluids normally calls for water retention through secretion of the antidiuretic hormone.

The simple "concentration test" of renal function depends largely upon the stimulus of water deprivation to promote release of ADH. After 12 hours of nocturnal deprivation of water, at least one of three hourly urine specimens should have a specific gravity of 1.023 or above (Fishberg). If the specific gravity is lower, renal disease is suspected. Progressive diminution of concentrating ability occurs with increasing renal impairment, until the base line is 1.010. This level is reached in the common forms of renal disease (arteriosclerosis, glomerulonephritis) when the urea clearance is reduced to about 15 per cent of normal, the glomerular filtration rate is only about 20 ml. per minute (compared to the normal 125 ml.), the tubular secretory capacity is 20 per cent of normal, and the number of nephrons has been reduced by about 40 per cent.

Similar large urinary volume with fixed low specific gravity, often causing dehydration, may occur whenever the number of tubules is greatly reduced (polycystic renal disease, hydronephrosis, etc.).

The cells of the distal convoluted tubules do a minimum of osmotic work when the urinary specific gravity is 1.010, because at this point the osmotic concentrations of the fluids at the two cell faces (tubule fluid and interstitial fluid) are approximately equal.[13]

Adrenocortical Hormone Effects. The rate of tubular resorption of sodium, chloride, and water is in some degree under the endocrine influence of the *adrenal cortex*. The cortisone group of steroids promotes retention of Na, Cl, and water and loss of K. Deoxycorticosterone is some 30 to 50 times as effective in this respect. Aldosterone is effective in even smaller amounts, being some 25 times as potent as deoxycorticosterone in influencing electrolyte and water metabolism.[39,40,75] When the adrenal cortical principles concerned with sodium metabolism are secreted in inadequate amounts, sodium, chloride, and water are excreted to a highly abnormal degree, and dehydration develops. The clinical picture of the crisis of Addison's disease, with its evidences of prostration, dehydration, low serum Na and Cl, high serum K, and low blood pressure, is in large part due to renal loss of base and water.[37]

We studied adrenal function by measuring urinary 17-OH corticosteroids and 17-ketosteroids in five patients over periods of one to three months in order to determine the importance of the adrenal in the physiologic conservation of salt (Daughaday and MacBryde[14]). We found no indications of increased pituitary adrenocorticotropic hormone (ACTH) activity, or of increased adrenocortical secretion of glucocorticoids, or of androgens after salt deprivation.

Nevertheless sodium was conserved after salt deprivation and it seemed likely that the adrenal cortex played a part in the salt-conservation mechanism. We suggested that: (1) there is an adrenal cortical salt-retaining hormone, the release of which is independent of ACTH, and that (2) an "idiorenal" mechanism or renal-adrenal influence might affect adrenal steroid activity and be concerned with renal tubular sodium reabsorption.[14]

Conn and his co-workers,[9] at about the same time, were studying the salt-conserving mechanisms set into operation by heavy sweating; they also concluded that an adrenocortical hormone then not yet identified reduced salt losses partly through the kidneys, but largely through the sweat glands.

Since then the powerful salt-conserving hormone has been found and identified as aldosterone.[39] It exerts a major controlling influence on the amounts of salt excreted in the urine and in sweat.[64,75] Aldosterone is largely or usually secreted independently of ACTH activity. Aldosterone secretion is increased by (1) restricted sodium intake; sodium losses; (2) increased potassium intake; (3) reduction in extracellular fluid; (4) muscular activity; (5) the upright posture; (6) trauma, surgical stress; (7) emotional tension.

When operating physiologically, aldosterone helps to restore effective circulatory volume. In some pathologic states the effective circulatory volume may be decreased by loss of fluid from the circulation into extravascular compartments with resultant production of edema, ascites, etc. The loss of *effective* circulatory volume may cause increased production of aldosterone, although the total body fluid and NaCl content may already be excessive. In a number of pathologic states such secondary *hyperaldosteronism* is known to occur. Among these are (1) congestive heart failure; (2) the nephrotic syndrome; (3) cirrhosis of the liver with ascites; (4) idiopathic hypoproteinemia; (5) renal disease; and (6) idiopathic periodic edema.[75,90] In many of these conditions there may be sequestration of blood in the venous system and decrease in arterial flow. The volume receptors may not distinguish between decreased volume and decreased pressure; therefore, a fall in blood pressure caused by decreased cardiac output or lower peripheral resistance would also lead to salt and water retention.[68]

GASTROINTESTINAL INFLUENCES ON FLUID AND ELECTROLYTE BALANCE

The normal route for intake of food, fluids, and electrolytes is by mouth, with absorption taking place chiefly in the small intestine. Certain parallels exist between gastrointestinal and renal functions in their influences upon fluid and electrolyte metabolism. Among these are the following:

1. A large volume of fluid is necessary for the normal performance of the functions in both organ systems. The fluid is presented to a special organ of the body, having in

solution or suspension a number of essential metabolites. In both cases (GI and renal), most of the water and metabolites is reabsorbed.

For a person weighing about 70 kg. (154 lbs.), some 8.0 to 8.5 liters of fluid enters the upper GI tract per day. (This seems quite remarkable when one remembers that such a person has a plasma volume of only about 3.5 liters). About 7 liters of this consists of digestive fluids, and about 1.5 liters is taken orally. Approximately 8.0 liters of this fluid is reabsorbed in the small intestine, only about 500 ml. reaching the ileocecal valve.

In the 500 ml. reaching the colon, normally the Na concentration is about 120 mEq. per liter, the K concentration about 10 mEq. per liter. Per 24 hours, therefore, about 60 mEq. of sodium and 5 mEq. of potassium reach the colon.

Most of the secretions in the upper gastro-intestinal tract, with the exception of saliva (which is hypo-osmotic), are isosmotic with plasma. Transport operates in both directions—from plasma to gut lumen (secretion) and from gut lumen to plasma (reabsorption).

In the colon, the pattern of sodium and potassium concentration is reversed. The volume of fluid in the stool per day is usually about 100 ml. with a Na concentration of 25 to 50 mEq. per liter and K concentration of 80 to 132 mEq. per liter. Normally, therefore, the losses of electrolyte in the stool are negligible, being in the order of less than 5 mEq. of sodium and 10 to 20 mEq. of potassium. Normally only 1 or 2 per cent of daily Na excretion is by stool, and about 10 per cent of K excretion.

2. A second similarity in these two systems is that transport mechanisms much alike operate in the active movement of electrolytes across the biologic membranes involved. Water seems passively to follow the movement of solutes.

From the gut lumen into the cell, sodium can enter by passive diffusion through water-filled pores and also by facilitated diffusion via a carrier-mediated mechanism. This carrier-mediated mechanism by which sodium enters cells is apparently enhanced by presence of sugars and amino acids in the intestinal lumen. Intracellular sodium moves to the serosal border where an active mechanism (active transport or "sodium pump") extrudes the Na^+ ion from the cell.

3. A third similarity is that either of these organ systems may be deranged so that a large proportion of the fluid entering them is lost, rather than being mostly reabsorbed. Slight to extreme dehydration may result, with mild to severe depletion of electrolytes.

4. Disorders of gastrointestinal function (again resembling renal disturbances in many respects) may cause acid-base imbalances. If pyloric obstruction results in massive vomiting with high gastric HCl loss, Cl^- deficit may occur, with alkalosis resulting.

Diarrhea, with loss of fluid of 2 liters to 6 liters or more per day plus loss of base, may cause acidosis and severe dehydration, resembling in many respects, clinically and in body chemistry, the acidosis of diabetes (see, later in this chapter, under Acidosis and Dehydration).

RESPIRATORY INFLUENCES ON BODY FLUID

Man lives at many latitudes and longitudes and at various altitudes, making it necessary that he be able to adjust to many different combinations of "climates," to various temperatures and humidities, and to various oxygen concentrations of the air that surrounds him. One of the mechanisms of homeostasis, by which he preserves the constancy of his internal environment, is to adjust the temperature and water content of inspired air to that best suited to the capacities of the epithelial cells and capillaries surrounding the pulmonary alveoli.

The temperature of the environmental atmosphere may be $-20°F$ or below to above $100°F$; its relative humidity may be from 0 per cent to 100 per cent. Usually, inspired air is dryer and cooler than the optimums of 100 per cent saturation and $37.5°C$ for the alveoli. Therefore, the usual effect of the respiratory mucous membranes is to warm and humidify inspired air as it approaches air : cell membrane interphase.

Since air is usually warmed and moistened as it is breathed in and out, it removes from the body some heat and some water. At rest, the water loss is quite small, about 80 to 225 ml. per 24 hours. With moderate activity, water loss through the expired air may be 250 to 350 ml. With much physical exertion, with fever, with accelerated or deepened respiration from any cause, with high environmental temperature and very dry inspired air, etc., water loss through respiration may be several times as high.

Ordinarily, water loss through respiration is low or negligible, but under special conditions it may be high and become significant, especially if it occurs simultaneously with accelerated losses through other routes and with restricted intake.

An essential difference is, of course, evident if the dehydration occurs through respiratory loss only. There is no accompanying electrolyte loss, as is always the case if the fluid loss is through the skin, kidneys, or gastrointestinal tract. The pathophysiology is like that of *water deprivation*.

Important factors affecting water loss through expired air include:

1. Humidity of inspired air.

2. Humidity of expired air. This may be greatly influenced by the integrity and efficiency of the mucous membranes of the upper respiratory tract.

3. Rate of air exchange. In the average healthy normal adult male at rest the amount of air inspired or expired per breath (tidal volume) is approximately 500 ml. The breathing rate is about 12 to 14 per minute, so that the total air breathed in and out is about 6 to 7 liters per minute. Both rate of respiration and depth, with increased tidal volume, may be increased by exercise, fever, hot environment, etc., with increased air exchange and increased water loss.

Expired air normally is not saturated with water vapor. Normal persons in one recent study[88] showed that when completely dry air was breathed in, the expired air contained 26 mg. per liter of water. When air containing 21 mg. per liter was inspired, expired air contained 31 mg. per liter. Thus, when there was no moisture in the inspired air, there was a loss of 26 mg. per liter; when the inspired air was relatively humid, there was a loss of only 10 mg. per liter. Under basal conditions, therefore, the loss would be 225 ml. of water per 24 hours breathing dry air, and 88 ml. breathing humid air.

Higher humidification of inspired air (to 31.1 mg. per liter) with a nebulizer resulted in expired air moisture of 33.5 mg. per liter, and a loss of only 2.4 mg. per liter. The net water loss from the respiratory tract decreased in a linear fashion as the absolute humidity of the inspired air increased.

These investigators demonstrated that use of various types of devices to warm and humidify inspired air can greatly reduce water losses through expired air, and can prevent drying of mucous membranes and pulmonary complications after *anesthesia, surgery, tracheostomy, treatment in an oxygen tent*, etc.

As air passes upward and outward in expiration, it travels in reverse order through the gradients, usually less warm and less humid progressively, until it meets the air of the outside atmosphere. There is condensation in the upper cooler trachea and nose during expiration. The condensed water is, under normal conditions, absorbed through the mucosa. The expired air on average contains about 27.7 mg. per liter of water, at a relative humidity of about 75 per cent at temperature of 32°C.

Nebulizers, with or without oxygen tents, are not entirely satisfactory in providing humidification of inspired air. Metal rebreathing chambers are more effective as heat and moisture exchangers. The higher heat capacity of the metal relative to air results in transfer of heat and moisture from the expired air to the inspired air. By such devices, the normal respiratory water loss can be reduced by one-half.[88]

TYPES OF DEHYDRATION

Dehydration may be classified into three general types:

1. Conditions in which the water deficit exceeds the salt deficit:

2. Conditions in which the salt deficit exceeds the water deficit;

3. Conditions in which the water and salt deficits are present in approximately balanced or isotonic proportions.

PATHOGENESIS OF DEHYDRATION

I. Water Deficit Predominating

1. Lack of water intake: too ill, too weak, mentally obtunded, nausea, etc. Water loss proceeds through excretion via skin, lungs, etc.

2. Excessive sweating

3. Extensive skin damage from burns

4. Diabetes insipidus

5. Solute diuresis: this may occur if ill persons are given, either orally or parenterally, excessively concentrated food and fluids. There is inadequate water intake in proportion to the solutes provided; the solutes remove excessive water in the urine.

II. Salt Deficit Predominating

1. Adrenocortical deficiency

2. Renal salt-wasting diseases

3. Cerebral salt-wasting diseases:

In some cases of cerebrovascular accidents, acute encephalitis, bulbar poliomyelitis, and brain tumors, excretion of large quantities of salt may occur despite hyponatremia.

CHART OF FLUID BALANCE

		INTAKE				OUTPUT			
Day & Time	Body Wt.	Oral	Parenteral	Urine	Vomitus	Diarrhea	Insens. Loss	Sweat	Blood

FIG. 35-6. Form for clinical record of factors in fluid balance. One should enter volume estimates or actual measurements. Accurate record should be kept of oral and parenteral fluids used in treatment, and of urine and other losses.

The etiology is not clear. One theory is that there is derangement of neurogenic centers controlling renal tubular salt reabsorption. Some patients with this syndrome seem to have *inappropriate secretion of ADH;* the sequence seems to start with retention of water, then the resulting expansion of body fluids requires excretion of salt.[69] Although these patients have salt loss, if fluid intake has been relatively high the signs and symptoms may be those of water intoxication. Therapy may require restoration of serum sodium by water restriction as well as by salt administration.

4. Diabetic acidosis (in some cases; in others water loss exceeds salt loss)
5. Low sodium diet plus diuresis.

III. Isotonic or Balanced Salt and Water Deficit. When there is simple loss of fluid from the gastrointestinal tract, the loss is balanced or isotonic. However, in many clinical conditions the fluid balance status of the patient is also influenced by other factors, especially if the disorder has persisted for some length of time (many hours or days). Thus,

1. Gastrointestinal fluid losses with cessation of intake are accompanied by loss of water from skin, lungs and kidneys: the net effect is of water loss in excess of salt loss.
2. Gastrointestinal losses replaced by water result in net salt loss in excess of water loss.
3. Hemorrhage produces an initial balanced loss; prompt thirst often occurs. If water is provided without salt, and renal losses of salt proceed, there is a net salt deficit.

IV. Multiple Pathogenesis. In the classification just given, the primary causes of the various chief types of dehydration have been

separately listed: as dehydration occurs clinically, however, there are usually combinations of two or more pathogenic mechanisms, although often one may predominate. A patient with *diabetes mellitus,* for example, may develop ketosis and have dehydration with great loss of Na^+ and Cl^-, but may also have vomiting, failure of water intake, and fever with excessive sweating from an infection.

Burns can lead to two types of deficits: isotonic extracellular fluid loss by transudation, and water loss without electrolyte from increased evaporation from damaged epithelium. The transudation from blood capillaries and lymph vessels causes protein loss also; therefore, replacement of water and salt alone may not be adequate; plasma or whole blood may be required.

The untreated burn subject has initially a balanced loss of salt and water from transudation; evaporation effect is soon added, making water loss predominate. If, however, water is ingested without electrolyte, salt deficit may become the chief problem.

DETERMINATION OF THE NATURE OF DEFICITS

In each case in which dehydration is suspected, evaluation of information from the history, the physical examination, and laboratory tests will help in the analysis.

THE HISTORY may reveal abnormal factors influencing fluid intake and output, environmental temperature, etc. A knowledge of body weight before the present illness is of great help: sudden loss is usually due to fluid deficit and the amount of weight loss is of help in computing the extent of the deficit. A knowledge of the blood pressure before dehydration is very helpful: an apparently normal blood pressure may actually be hypotensive in a person known previously to have hypertension.

In problems of fluid balance it is of great

help to measure whenever possible all fluid accessions and losses, or to estimate them as closely as possible, and to record them on a special balance sheet. As treatment is administered, the character and amount of fluids is entered on the chart (Fig. 35-6).

THE PHYSICAL EXAMINATION yields important information concerning the effects of water and electrolyte deficits and permits rough estimates of the type and degree of aberrations. One notes the state of consciousness, the color, moisture, texture and turgor of the skin and mucous membranes, the blood pressure, the peripheral arterial pulsations, the temperature and color of the extremities, etc. Deep, rapid respirations suggest acidosis, and in ketosis an acetone odor may be detected on the breath. Alkalosis may be indicated by positive Chvostek and Trousseau signs. Low blood pressure, weak peripheral arterial pulsations, tachycardia and pallor or cyanosis are suggestive of vascular collapse and impaired peripheral blood flow. Such evidences of seriously affected peripheral circulation imply large fluid deficits and extreme dehydration.

LABORATORY DATA. Among the most valuable laboratory aids in the analysis of fluid and electrolyte disorders are:

Hematocrit, Hemoglobin, and Total Serum Proteins. These values are helpful in the estimation of the extent of contraction of plasma volume. When proportionately elevated they indicate hemoconcentration due to fluid deficit.

With expanded plasma volume, relative hemodilution may cause these values to be proportionately lowered.

Corpuscular Values of Erythrocytes. Cell shrinkage due to dehydration causes low mean corpuscular volume (MCV). Overhydration causes swelling of cells, and the MCV is high.

The mean corpuscular hemoglobin concentration (MCHC) is high if cells are dehydrated, and low if they are overhydrated, as compared to normal cells.

MCV normally is 87 ± 5 cu. μ.

MCHC normally is 34 ± 2 per cent.

These values may be deranged in hematologic disorders; only in the absence of such conditions can these indices be solely indicative of changes affecting the hydration of body cells in general.

Serum Osmolality. When studying hydration states, this value per kilogram of serum water gives more definitive information than the serum sodium concentration. The normal value is 285 to 295 mOsm. Lower values indicate a hypotonic serum, higher levels a hypertonic serum, as compared to normal. Serum sodium values usually—but not always—are altered in the same directions as changes in serum osmolality.

Serum sodium concentration normally ranges from 132 to 142 mEq. per liter. The serum sodium may be high, low, or normal in concentration during dehydration, depending upon the relative amount of water lost from the plasma. When hyponatremia is associated with dehydration, it suggests great deficit in extracellular fluid volume. In such circumstances there is also great loss of sodium from the body, as indicated by subnormal concentration in contracted volume.

The serum sodium concentration yields no direct information concerning total sodium stores (nor about the volume of total body fluid) but indicates only that there is a disturbance in the ratio of sodium to water.

HYPERNATREMIA

Elevated serum sodium suggests water loss in excess of salt loss. It may be accompanied by other laboratory evidences of dehydration and hemoconcentration. When normal hydration is restored, the serum Na may be normal or low, the latter indicating depletion of total body sodium.

HYPONATREMIA

Hyponatremia with dehydration and significant contraction of fluid volume implies that diuresis has not occurred as it normally does to protect the normal effective osmolality of the body fluids. The absence of such diuresis indicates that fluid volume has been sufficiently reduced to cause secretion of ADH; there must be great contraction of *extracellular fluid volume* to function as an adequate stimulus to promote the secretion of ADH. (One recalls that the *usual* effective stimulus results from an increase in osmolality of the extracellular fluid, with consequent cellular dehydration.)

Hyponatremia with Hyperglycemia. At normal glucose concentrations, the glucose has relatively little effect upon the total osmolality of the extracellular fluid. If, however, hyperglycemia is considerable, glucose increases the osmolality of the extracellular fluid to a significant degree, water is drawn from the cells into the extracellular compartment, and the serum sodium concentration is in consequence decreased. The total effective plasma osmolality may be within normal limits when there is hyperglycemia, and hyponatremia and dehydration.

One may calculate the effective tonicity as suggested by Welt.[70] *Method:* Subtract 100 from the patient's blood concentration of glucose in milligrams per cent; multiply by 10 to convert to milligrams per liter; divide by 180, the molecular weight of glucose. The figure derived indicates the *excess* of glucose in millimols or milliosmols per liter. Divide by 2 (since 1mM of the sodium salts concerned provides 2 mOsm.). Add the figure derived to the serum sodium concentration as determined at the same time. The sum will indicate the effective osmolality or tonicity of the plasma at the time. If it is between 132 and 142 it may be considered normal (part of the usual osmolar effect of sodium is, in the presence of excess glucose, significantly exerted by glucose).

Example.

Given:

Serum Na^+ = 115 mEq. or mOsm. per liter
Blood glucose = 880 mg. per cent

$$\frac{(880 - 100) \times 10}{180} =$$

43.7 mOsm. glucose per liter

$$\frac{43.7}{2} = 21.8$$

$$115 + 21.8 = 136.8 \text{ mOsm. per liter}$$

In this example the tonicity is within normal limits despite the great reduction in the concentration of sodium in the serum.

Hyponatremia with Hyperlipemia. The concentration of serum sodium and other electrolytes is ordinarily expressed per unit volume of serum. It would be more precise to express such concentrations per unit volume of *serum water.* Normally the value for serum water is so large and constant (90 to 93 per cent) that the error is not significant. However, in hyperlipemia the serum lipids occupy a larger volume and the percentage of serum that is water may be drastically reduced to as low as 70 to 80 per cent.[71] An average concentration of sodium of 138 mEq. per liter in a serum with water content of 93 per cent equals 148.4 mEq. per liter of serum *water.* If the same concentration were present in the *water* of a lipemic serum containing only 80 per cent water, the concentration per liter of *serum* would be 148.4 × 0.80 = 118.7 mEq. Thus, a very low serum sodium may be present with no decrease in the effective osmolality of the extracellular fluid.

Hyponatremia with Chronic Cellular Hypoosmolality. This syndrome occurs in many chronic illnesses in which malnutrition and cellular destruction have been persistent. Conditions in which it has been reported include tuberculosis, carcinoma, nephritis, hepatic cirrhosis, etc. The primary step in the pathogenesis is loss of K^+ from cells. Osmolality of the cells decreases, water moves into the extracellular fluid, serum sodium falls to 120 mEq. per liter or lower. Serum K is normal, as is the blood urea nitrogen. Hypoproteinemia is usually present. The MCV is low, the MCHC is high.

The serum osmalality and the cell osmolality, both abnormally low, become set at a new equilibrium, giving the name sometimes used: *new steady state.* When complications are absent, there is no total excess or deficiency of body water—no dehydration.

This condition, in which the hyponatremia is asymptomatic and which does not respond to attempts to correct the electrolyte abnormality, must be distinguished from hyponatremic states from a number of other causes that are *correctable,* including *many with dehydration,* one of which is adrenocortical deficiency.

Hyponatremia with Water Excess. Serum sodium levels may be low and all serum constituents present in low concentration when (1) excess water is *taken* into the body or when (2) excess water is *retained.* The latter can occur with **inappropriate secretion of ADH** (in some patients after trauma or surgery, or with cerebral lesions or lung carcinoma, etc.).

Hyponatremia from these causes is not due to deficit of sodium; it is a dilutional effect. There is no loss of body water, no dehydration—body water is present in excess. The consequences may be distinguished from other hyponatremic states by the history and physical findings and by certain characteristic laboratory evidence: low serum osmolality (274 mOsm. per liter or below), low serum sodium (below 130 mEq. per liter, sometimes lower than 115 mEq.), serum potassium normal or low, blood urea nitrogen normal or low, hemoglobin and hematocrit low; red blood cell volume (MCV) high, mean corpuscular hemoglobin concentration (MCHC) low, because the erythrocytes and other body cells are swollen and dilute. Water has moved into the previously relatively hypertonic cells; they become hypotonic compared to normal cells and many of their functions become impaired. Clinical evidences of this very dangerous syndrome of overhydration may develop rapidly, called *water intoxication.* If not quickly corrected, this disorder may have serious results. Weakness, apathy, and drowsiness are early symptoms. Sometimes there is anorexia, nausea and vomiting, delirium, psychotic behavior, and incoordination or extreme muscle weakness. Convulsions are a frequent symptom of severe overhydration; coma and death may occur.

Serum potassium concentration normally ranges from 3.5 to 5.3 mEq. per liter. The total quantity of potassium in the extracellular fluids is so small that relatively slight shifts of K into or out of cells cause significant changes in serum K concentration. For example, at a serum K level of 4 mEq., the total K in the extracellular fluids might be 64 mEq. (4 mg. $\times$ 16 liters). There might occur a 25 per cent loss of extracellular K to 48 mEq., but if this were accompanied by a 25 per cent contraction of extracellular volume to 12 liters, the serum K would still be 4 mEq. per liter. If fluid were taken without K, the extracellular compartment might be re-expanded from 12 to 16 liters, still containing only 48 mEq. of K, the concentration now being only 3 mEq. per liter.

Blood urea nitrogen normally ranges from 8 to 18 mg. per cent. The level of the serum BUN depends upon the rate of formation and the rate of excretion; the rate of excretion depends upon the glomerular filtration rate and the amount that diffuses back through the tubules. When urea is not being formed at an accelerated rate and there is no renal damage affecting excretion or absorption, the serum BUN reflects the adequacy of hydration. In serious dehydration, the BUN may be elevated both because of inadequate filtration due to reduced renal blood flow and because of diminished excretion by the tubules into the urine, practically all of the water and the urea being reabsorbed.

The urine provides much information concerning the state of hydration and the status of renal function. The volume of urine, its osmolality, and its concentration provide significant data. A highly concentrated urine implies adequate kidney function in the presence of a powerful antidiuretic stimulus (or actual severe fluid deficit). A high volume of urine with low osmolality and with low specific gravity suggests lack of ADH (diabetes insipidus) or extensive renal disease with great impairment of tubular reabsorption of water. Analysis of the urine for electrolytes may be informative: significant natriuresis in the presence of hyponatremia suggests a salt-wasting disease. Potassium losses in the urine suggest cellular dehydration. Routine urinalysis may reveal albuminuria and other changes suggestive of renal impairment, or of glycosuria, ketosis and dehydration.

Assessment of Fluid and Electrolyte Deficits

Water deficit is suggested by thirst, dry mucous membranes, loss of skin turgor, etc. Biochemical evidences include all of the signs of hemoconcentration: elevated hematocrit, hemoglobin, and electrolyte values. *Overhydration* occurs if salt-free fluids are given in excess during renal shutdown. The clinical signs are restlessness, apprehension, muscle cramps, and sometimes the convulsions of water-intoxication. Low serum Na is the cardinal biochemical finding.

Sodium and Chloride Deficits. Deficits of sodium usually are accompanied by deficits of other extracellular ions, especially chloride, and of extracellular water. History of conditions causing renal sodium loss (chronic glomerulonephritis, low-sodium diet plus excessive diuresis, diabetic acidosis, adrenocortical deficiency) are suggestive. Abnormal loss of gastrointestinal fluids should arouse suspicion. The clinical signs are primarily those of decreased cardiac output and peripheral vasoconstriction: cyanosis, cold, clammy skin, rapid thready pulse, hypotension, and severe oliguria. Biochemical signs are those of decreased plasma volume and hemoconcentration plus, in severe cases, evidence of renal failure: elevated blood urea nitrogen and phosphorus, lowered CO_2 combining-power. The serum Na may be low, as may the serum Cl, but these determinations may be within normal limits if there is hemoconcentration. They may become low after establishment of normal hydration. *Sodium excess* is accompanied nearly always by excess water retention in the body and edema. The serum sodium is apt to be within normal limits except during periods of water transfer.

Potassium derangements are discussed below under Intracellular Effects of Dehydration. It is essential to remember that intracellular K deficit may be present not only when serum K concentration is low, but sometimes with normal or elevated serum K.

Bicarbonate and Anion-Cation Balance.

The pH of the blood and of the extracellular fluid is determined by the ratio of the bicarbonate and other buffer anions (summed as "buffer base") to the concentration of carbonic acid. Since the latter is regulated by gas exchange in the lungs and the former by metabolic and renal transfers, abnormalities in the anion-cation balance may occur from either primary *respiratory*, or primary *metabolic* disorders. Secondary or compensatory changes may occur in the other half of the system, however, so that biochemical findings will not always indicate which change is primary: clinical evidence is necessary to permit proper interpretation of the laboratory data.

ACID-BASE BALANCE AND WATER BALANCE

The mechanisms that make possible selective resorption by the tubules are not understood. The average normal diet is predominantly "acid-ash" in character, requiring an excess of excretion of acid over base, so that the normal pH of plasma (7.4) may be maintained. This is accomplished by (1) direct saving of base by secretion of acid urine and by (2) substitution of ammonium for plasma base to cover acid radicals as they enter the urine.

The enormous degree of base-conservation constantly taking place is revealed by simply measuring the urinary pH, which is usually between 5 and 7. It must be remembered that urine at pH 6.4 is ten times as acid as blood plasma at 7.4, whereas urine at pH 5.4 is one hundred times as acid. Thus, the acidity of the urine indicates the excretion of large amounts of acid and a corresponding saving of large amounts of base. The most acid urine the kidney can form is pH 4.5. Thus, only negligible quantities of strong acids such as sulfuric or hydrochloric can be excreted as free titratable acid. Such strong acids are neutralized by Na^+ or K^+ in the plasma, but through renal tubular activity may be excreted through combination with ammonium ions.

Saving of base by excretion of acid urine (usually about pH 6) is made possible by (1) excretion of certain weak organic acids (such as citric acid) without the base linked to the acid ions in the plasma, by (2) excretion of HPO_4^- as monobasic phosphate rather than as dibasic phosphate as it exists in the plasma, and by (3) conservation of base by failure to excrete bicarbonate in the urine. It is reabsorbed by the tubules, the

sodium retained, and the CO_2 excreted by the lungs.

Respiratory Regulation. The relatively enormous amount (about 2 lb. daily) of the most abundant end product of metabolism, carbonic acid, is removed by the lungs without expenditure of base. The bicarbonate buffer system is particularly effective in permitting rapid readjustments of pH. Saving of base takes place by the interaction of bicarbonate with the relatively strong acids formed as a result of metabolic activity in the tissues (hydrochloric, sulfuric, phosphoric, and lactic acids); the excess of carbonic acid is removed (as carbon dioxide) through the lungs. Carbon dioxide is constantly being formed through oxidative processes in the body and (as carbonic acid) it can quickly combine with excess amounts of alkali to form bicarbonate. Thus, the respiratory protective mechanisms guard against either acidosis or alkalosis and protect the body against loss of electrolytes and water.

"Respiratory acidosis" may occur, with a slight increase in the CO_2 combining power of the plasma, when CO_2 is retained in excess (in asphyxia, emphysema, morphine narcosis, etc.). "Respiratory alkalosis" may occur from a decrease in blood carbonic acid due to hyperventilation (in hysteria, encephalitis, at high altitudes, etc.). These primarily respiratory deviations in acid-base balance are not associated with any considerable abnormalities in water balance. Note that the CO_2 content of the plasma is high in respiratory acidosis and low in metabolic or renal acidosis; it is low in respiratory alkalosis and high in metabolic or renal alkalosis.

Renal regulation. The *renal protective mechanisms* are more often deranged and are therefore of the greatest clinical importance. The three chief modes of conserving base are:

1. The three renal mechanisms that permit the excretion of acid urine, ensure the return of base (chiefly sodium) to the body, and preserve the stability of plasma pH at approximately 7.4. Through them the base is not normally excreted (a) as B_2HPO_4, or (b) as $BHCO_3$ to any significant extent, or (c) with the organic acids. Not only is base conserved, but water also, since if these acids took base out with them into the urine, corresponding amounts of water would be excreted.

2. The ammonium-forming ability of the distal renal tubules which permits the saving

of Na+ ions, NH₄+ ions being substituted for them in combination with acid radicals, the ammonium compounds then being excreted in the urine. Likewise, the renal tubules are able to substitute H+ ions for base ions.

3. The resorptive powers of the renal tubules are the means through which enormous quantities of sodium (and of water) are returned to the plasma.

These *base-sparing* mechanisms are also *water-sparing*, and the buffer systems are defenses not only against *acidosis* but against *dehydration*.[32,41,42,43,46]

If one assumes that 180 liters of plasma are filtered through the glomeruli per 24 hours and that each liter contains 27 mEq. of bicarbonate, one finds that 4,860 mEq., or nearly one pound, (expressed as sodium bicarbonate) is delivered into the tubules daily. Normally only 1 or 2 mEq. escape into the urine each day—the resorption by the renal tubules is practically 100 per cent.

The renal stabilization of body fluid bicarbonate rests upon (1) the renal conservation just described, and upon (2) mechanisms that promote the elimination of acid ions without the base they bind in the blood and permit restoration of that base to the body as bicarbonate.[46,47]

Under certain much less frequent conditions the buffer systems may be brought into play to combat the reverse condition, *alkalosis*. When base is ingested in excessive amounts (for example, sodium bicarbonate in relieving indigestion or treating peptic ulcer), or when chloride is lost (vomiting), an alkaline urine containing considerable amounts of bicarbonate may be excreted. Either acidosis or alkalosis tends to cause diuresis, because the kidney acts promptly to rectify any disturbance in acid-base equilibrium. Therefore, all of the buffering and protective systems guarding the acid-base balance also defend body water.

ACIDOSIS AND DEHYDRATION

Acidosis may be defined as reduction in body base. It is usually measured by determining the CO_2 combining-power of the plasma, the normal range being between 55 and 65 volumes per cent (25 to 29 mEq. per liter). Values below 25 mEq. per liter indicate loss of base. Actual measurement of the plasma hydrogen ion concentration may reveal *acidemia*, a true fall in pH resulting from uncompensated loss of base.

A number of conditions leading to acidosis

TABLE 35-2. VOLUME OF DIGESTIVE SECRETIONS PER 24 HOURS PRODUCED BY ADULT OF AVERAGE SIZE

Saliva	1,500 ml.
Gastric secretions	2,500
Bile	500
Pancreatic juice	700
Secretion of the intestinal mucosa	3,000
Total digestive secretions	8,200 ml.

and dehydration may occur. These include:

1. Excess acid ingestion
2. Inadequate base intake
3. Loss of base (vomiting, fistula, diarrhea)
4. Renal failure (acid retention and base loss)
5. Inadequate carbohydrate combustion.

It is apparent that, if an excess of acid ions is ingested, base will be required to combine with it and provide for its excretion, and that the base reserve may thus be seriously depleted and considerable amounts of water lost.

If the base supply is curtailed, a deficit may soon develop, because some base is being lost constantly, the average normal sodium excretion in the urine being about 4 Gm. daily.

Gastrointestinal Loss of Base. Very large amounts of base are secreted into the intestine in the alkaline pancreatic secretion, the bile, and the duodenal mucosal secretion (Table 35-2). Normally, practically all the fluid and the base secreted into the intestine are reabsorbed. Any disorder interfering with resorption of this base and water will cause dehydration. The tendency to such dehydration will be increased by the relative chloride excess and resultant increase in chloride and water output through the kidneys. The importance of conserving this fluid and base is emphasized when one observes that the digestive secretions may total 8,200 ml. daily in a person whose blood-plasma volume is 3,500 ml.

The development of severe dehydration and electrolyte depletion from diarrhea caused by various types of dysenteries, food poisoning, and ulcerative colitis is frequent and well-recognized. A similar but less familiar syndrome may occur with certain colonic neoplasms, particularly *villous adenomata* of the rectum and sigmoid.[71A] Symptoms of abdominal distress may be present for months or years before copious passage of mucus occurs. There may be rapid development of severe dehydration with hyponatremia, hypokalemia, azotemia, and circulatory collapse. Most of the tumors are benign, but they may become malignant. Often the tumor is within reach of the examining finger or sigmoidoscope, but the tumors may be multiple. Water and electrolyte replacement is life-saving but is of only temporary benefit. Complete excision is necessary to halt the fluid depletion.

Severe diarrhea from other various clinical causes may produce dehydration and acidosis. A patient recently studied through illness to autopsy[79] had jejunal diverticulitis and acute enteritis. Five days after onset, upon hospital entry, the physical examination revealed clinical evidence of dehydration, acidosis, low blood-pressure and mental confusion. Serum Na was 129 mEq. per liter, K was 3.3, CO_2 was 10, Cl was 89, blood urea N was 108 mg. per cent. The clinical findings resembled in many respects those of diabetic acidosis (see Fig. 35-5). The high BUN probably resulted from loss of circulating blood volume ("shock") and consequent acute renal tubular necrosis. Death occurred 15 days after onset.

Renal failure may lead to base and water loss in several ways. *Glomerular damage* may lead to retention of $PO_4^=$ and $SO_4^=$ and other acid ions that will require base and water for disposal. *Tubular damage* may interfere with resorption of water and base. Inability to secrete a concentrated urine is characteristic of chronic nephritis. For adequate excretion of waste products the urine volume therefore necessarily becomes large and dehydration may occur at any time if for any reason the intake of water is limited. When large amounts of kidney tissue are destroyed (as in polycystic disease, hydronephrosis, etc.), the intake and output of water may be of such proportions as to suggest diabetes insipidus. In chronic nephritis, ammonium production is impaired and base is lost because this usual defense of plasma sodium is not available. This diuretic effect is at least partly responsible for the failure of edema to appear in chronic nephritis until plasma protein is greatly depleted. Thus, dehydration may occur in chronic nephritis because of retention of acids, because of loss of base, and because of impaired tubular resorption of base, with accelerated water loss.

Renal tubular acidosis is a primary genetic disorder characterized by a specific tubular defect in excretion of hydrogen ions. There is hyperchloremic acidosis and inadequate acidification of the urine. Azotemia, tubular necrosis, or gross reduction in the number of functioning renal tubules are not present. The condition should be suspected when there is acidosis, but the urine is alkaline or only slightly acid. Urine volume may be

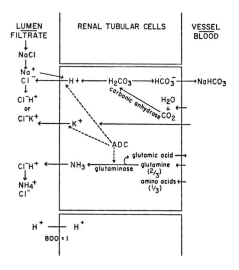

FIG. 35-7. Sites of action of adrenal cortex hormones (ADC) in renal tubular control of electrolytes. The diagram shows the processes involved in acid-base regulation as they are believed to operate in the distal renal tubular cells. The primary event is the exchange of H+ ions dissociated from carbonic acid within the tubular cell for base ions in the tubular urine. Base is thus conserved for return to body fluids (Na+ plus HCO_3^- equals $NaHCO_3$, etc.)

Note that the diffusion of ammonia into the urine is important to neutralize the H+ ions. Some free H+ ions may be excreted in the urine, but the capacity of the tubular cells to produce free acid in this way is limited to a concentration gradient of H+ ions of 800 to 1. NH_4^+ ions, formed by union of H+ ions with ammonia (two thirds from glutamine, one third from amino acids), reduce the concentration of free H+ ions, thus reducing the gradient and facilitating flow of H+ ions into the urine.

The probable sites of action of adrenal cortex hormones (ADC) are shown, indicating their importance in the tubular mechanisms involved in the exchange of hydrogen ions, potassium ions, and ammonium ions for sodium ions.[37]

copious, causing severe dehydration. There is no deficiency of carbonic anhydrase to explain the defect in H+ excretion (Fig. 35-7). Characteristic serum electrolyte findings are: low bicarbonate, phosphate, and potassium, and elevated chloride. Tubular resorption of buffer base is impaired and ammonium secretion may be decreased.

A type of renal tubular acidosis (genetic?, acquired?) has been observed in association with hepatic cirrhosis. In some of these patients it may explain hypokalemia and susceptibility (through ammonium retention) to recurrent episodes of hepatic coma.[91]

Renal protective mechanisms against acidosis. The normal pH of the body fluids (7.4) is maintained by the kidney, which keeps the plasma concentration of bicarbonate-bound base at 25 to 29 mEq. per liter, and by the respiratory system, which stabilizes the plasma carbonic acid level at 1.25 to 1.45 mEq. per liter. Stability of hydrogen ion concentration does not require fixed values for $H.HCO_3$ and $B.HCO_3$, but depends upon the maintenance of their 1:20 ratio, thus permitting flexibility in control.

The role of the kidneys in maintaining the bicarbonate concentration is a dual one, involving (1) salvage of the filtered bicarbonate and (2) restoration to the body of base utilized in neutralizing acids for renal excretion. In protecting and restoring bicarbonate, normally the renal tubules perform the amazingly efficient task of reabsorbing a pound or more of sodium bicarbonate daily, with loss of less than 0.1 per cent into the urine.

The tubular mechanisms for substituting hydrogen or ammonium ions for sodium ions in the tubular urine are of particular physiologic interest and clinical importance (Fig. 35-7).[41,46,47,78] Through substitution of these ions, acids may be excreted in free titratable form or in combination with ammonia, without loss of base. Both substitutions are performed in the distal segments of the tubules.[15]

The acidosis and dehydration of renal disease may thus be (1) partly the result of the inability of damaged renal tubules to exchange hydrogen ions and ammonium ions for base at a rate sufficient to compensate for the metabolic load, (2) partly due to failure of the tubules to absorb sodium bicarbonate, and (3) partly from retention of phosphate and sulfate with consequent displacement of bicarbonate.

Sulfonamide drugs block to some extent the renal tubular replacement of sodium ions with hydrogen ions, so that base, normally replaced by hydrogen ions and reabsorbed, is excreted in the urine. Such loss of considerable amounts of base may lead to acidosis and dehydration.

Adrenocortical activity is related to renal response to acidosis.[15,37,40,78] Not only are adrenocortical hormones necessary to adequate absorption by the tubules of sodium and water, but they are necessary for increasing the production of ammonia and titratable acidity (see Fig. 35-7). In experimental animals it has been demonstrated that (1) adrenalectomized animals normally cannot conserve sodium during induced acidosis, nor can they adequately increase ammonia and titratable acidity under such conditions; (2) the deficiency in renal response can be corrected with desoxycorticosterone or adrenal cortex extract; and (3) acidosis causes adrenocortical activation with decrease in ascorbic acid and cholesterol content of the gland. As yet a complete explanation of the adaptive response of the kidneys to acidosis is lacking, but an important part is undoubtedly played by stimulation of the adrenal cortex in some way by the acidosis, with resultant stimulation of renal tubular activity by adrenocortical hormones.

Lack of Carbohydrate Oxidation. Whenever the chief fuel, carbohydrate, is not available or for any reason cannot be utilized in adequate amounts, acidosis may develop, with resultant dehydration (Fig. 35-8). This comes about as the consequence of (1) destruction of body protoplasm with release of $PO_4^=$ and $SO_4^=$, which require base for excretion; of (2) excess Cl^-, from reduction of the base and the volume of the extracellular fluid, also requiring base for excretion; and of (3) ketone-body production due to excess oxidation of fats. These ketone bodies are excreted partly as free organic acids and partly combined with base. All of these products require an increase in the water output. The increase in the water excretion can only partly be compensated by increasing the water intake, since in the presence of diuresis a smaller than normal proportion of these substances and of water is reabsorbed by the tubules. Whenever carbohydrate is supplied or its combustion is facilitated, these processes are reversed toward normal.

Acidosis and dehydration depending upon

failure of normal carbohydrate combustion
may occur from:

1. Starvation (failure of intake)
2. Ketogenic (low-carbohydrate) diets
3. Hypoglycemia
4. Loss of carbohydrate from the gastrointestinal tract (vomiting, diarrhea,
   fistula)
5. Diabetes mellitus.

Other factors often accompany limitation
of carbohydrate combustion and increase the
severity of the acidosis and dehydration.
Among these factors are limitation of water
intake and renal failure. If there is, in addition to loss of available carbohydrate, loss
of base and fluid in the intestinal secretions
by vomiting, diarrhea, or fistula, the acidosis
and the dehydration will be much more
severe.

Diabetes mellitus constitutes a special and
a common cause of acidosis and dehydration
(Fig. 35-8). In the absence of adequate carbohydrate combustion, fat and protein become
the main sources of calories. Accelerated
combustion of fat causes production of the
ketone acids beyond the rate at which they
can be metabolized. Accumulation of the
organic ketone acids results from the accelerated fat combustion and leads to loss of
water and base. Breakdown of body protein
and lipids produces an excess of $SO_4^=$ and
$PO_4^=$, calling for more base and leading to
further water loss. The excessive drain on
the reserve of base soon becomes evident,
despite a fivefold to tenfold increase in the
rate of excretion of titratable acid and of ammonia. Soon the renal compensation fails to
keep pace, and the bicarbonate stores are

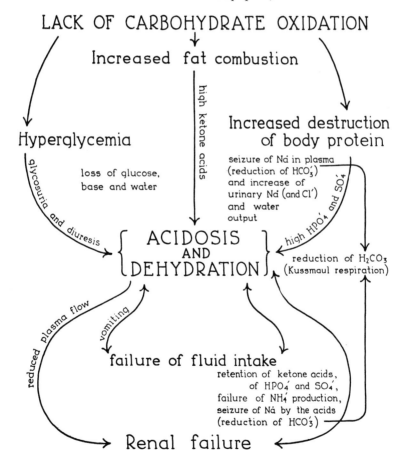

Fig. 35-8. Diagram illustrating mechanisms involved in the production of
the acidosis and dehydration of diabetic coma.

progressively depleted. The blood and other body fluids may be unable to maintain their normal slightly alkaline reaction as reserve base is depleted; acidemia occurs and death may result. The excessively high blood sugar leads to such rapid renal loss of glucose that the tubules cannot reabsorb it all, and severe glycosuria with further water loss results because of the osmotic effect of the hypertonic glucose solution in the tubules. Glucose that escapes resorption in the tubules requires for its excretion the same amount of water required by an osmotically equivalent quantity of salt. Glucose does not replace Na and Cl from the urine but, on the contrary, accelerates their excretion. Glycosuria is therefore especially dehydrating. Vomiting is a common accompaniment of diabetic acidosis, and the dehydration is thus further increased. Chloride is excreted in excess because of the reduction in extracellular-fluid volume made necessary by the reduction in sodium. The carbon dioxide combining-power of the blood plasma (normally about 60 volumes per cent, or 27 mEq. per liter) may be reduced to 20 volumes per cent (9 mEq. per liter) or less as the patient succumbs to severe diabetic acidosis and lapses into coma. Very deep and rapid "Kussmaul" respiration appears. This is characteristic of severe acidosis and results from stimulation of the respiratory center with consequent effort to expel great amounts of CO_2. The dry, inelastic skin, the dry tongue, the soft eyeballs, the weak pulse, and the low blood pressure complete the picture of the shocklike state occurring with extreme dehydration. The severe dehydration causes *renal disability* with further loss of base and retention of $SO_4^=$, $PO_4^=$ and organic acids. The renal failure may be sufficient to result in nitrogen retention and signs of uremia. Reversal of all the pathologic processes is brought about by supplying Na, Cl, and water, insulin and carbohydrate in the milder cases and in those without impairment of renal function. If the acidosis is severe or prolonged, if the patient is a small child or an elderly person, if renal function is poor, it may be of considerable benefit to supply base as sodium bicarbonate or sodium lactate as well as that furnished in physiologic NaCl solution. The intracellular ions K^+ and $PO_4^=$ should also be included in the parenteral fluids supplied, if the serum potassium is low.

ALKALOSIS AND DEHYDRATION

If dehydration occurs from vomiting that results primarily in the loss of gastric secretion (HCl), as in pyloric obstruction, alkalosis may accompany it. Signs of tetany may be present. In pernicious vomiting, after prolonged gastric drainage, or following repeated ingestion of large quantities of sodium bicarbonate, the concentration of chloride in the body fluids is reduced and that of bicarbonate is proportionately elevated. Despite the alkalosis, the urine may remain acid and contain essentially no bicarbonate. It appears that *as long as the blood chloride is depressed*, the kidney preserves bicarbonate, as if, having failed to maintain the normal proportions of the anions CL^- and HCO_3^-, total concentration at least is maintained. Only when the blood chloride is elevated to normal (and the blood K^+ also, if there has been hypokalemia), is the renal bicarbonate threshold restored to the normal range. Correction of the condition by giving intravenous physiologic NaCl solution is possible, since the body retains the Cl, excreting the excess Na and excreting HCO_3 instead of Cl in the urine until the chloride deficit has been compensated.

Metabolic alkalosis may occur as the result of great chloride loss from diuresis. This may develop acutely during treatment of acute heart failure, etc. In such a case studied recently, serum values were: Na 135 mEq. per liter, K normal, Cl 85, CO_2 47.[89] In most instances, such an electrolyte disturbance is self-limited if diuresis is halted, since adequate Cl can be supplied from the diet. If alkalosis persists, NH_4Cl therapy may be indicated.

When milder degrees of alkalosis are present (or more accurately, states of *alkali excess*), spontaneous adjustment may be very prompt. If as little as 4 Gm. of sodium bicarbonate is ingested, the urine becomes less acid promptly. Through this mechanism, either small amounts of base or very large amounts of base may be excreted. This may be accomplished even though the urinary pH may shift from the average normal of 6.0 to reactions only slightly more alkaline than that of the blood plasma. Because of the buffering action exerted by the *high carbonic acid content of alkaline urines*, much larger amounts of base can be eliminated in the urine than one might calculate. The most alkaline urine the kidney can elaborate is about pH 8.0.

Excess intake of the basic salts of sodium may cause a rise in the pH of the extracellular fluids but has little diuretic effect if renal function is normal, since the excess bicarbonate is eliminated by inhibition of its resorption in the tubules. Sodium excess in pathologic states may tend, on the contrary, to produce edema, sodium and water being retained in excess amounts, especially in circulatory or renal failure (see Chap. 36).

Whatever the cause of the alkalosis, the alkali excess must be disposed of, and the usual mode of disposal is diuresis. Alkalosis, therefore, in the absence of renal impairment, tends to produce dehydration. Alkalinizing salts such as bicarbonate or citrate promote diuresis but the effects are less pronounced than with acidifying salts, such as ammonium chloride, because distortion of the electrolyte pattern is less severe.

INTRACELLULAR EFFECTS OF DEHYDRATION

Salt loss causes intracellular overhydration, whereas water depletion causes cellular dehydration. A balanced loss of water and salt results in contraction of both extracellular and intracellular compartments. Excess fluid intake, especially with salt depletion, results in cellular overhydration and may produce the symptoms of water intoxication.

When there is considerable loss of extracellular electrolyte and water, maintenance of osmotic equilibrium may require removal not only of water but of electrolyte from the cells. Dehydration therefore causes some loss of potassium from the cells, accompanying the much larger loss of sodium from extracellular fluid. Thus, the interstitial-fluid reservoir does not completely defend the cells, since withdrawal of water and electrolyte does occur. However, since intracellular-fluid volume is two and one-half times that of extracellular fluid, the loss of fluid is proportionately smaller. Measurement of the sodium and the potassium lost, taking into consideration the relative concentrations of these two bases as they exist in the body fluids, will permit calculation of the amounts of fluid lost from each compartment.

Potassium Metabolism as Related to Acidosis, Alkalosis, and Dehydration

Since potassium is the chief cation of intracellular fluid, derangements of the electrolyte or water metabolism which are severe enough to pass beyond the first-line defenses present in the plasma and in the interstitial fluid may be evident through decrease in the K content of the cells and through alterations of the K concentration of the extracellular fluids. Under normal conditions, 98 per cent of the body potassium is intracellular. Normally, K is present in cell fluid in a concentration of about 150 mEq. per liter. This is about 35 times its concentration in the blood serum (3.5 to 5.3 mEq. per liter). Any considerable deviation from these narrow limits is apt to be associated with *disturbances in the conduction of impulses* through the nerves and in the function of muscle, both skeletal and cardiac. The *conduction system of the heart* is significantly affected by abnormal rise or fall in the serum K.

In the average normal diet, from 2 to 4 Gm. of K are ingested daily, and the renal excretion of K is so regulated that the body remains in K balance. However, when K deficit exists, K is retained, and when there is a K surplus, the excess K is excreted. It should be noted that the renal tubules have not only the ability to absorb K, but they also can actively excrete it. Renal tubular secretion of potassium may occur in severe renal insufficiency and constitutes a mechanism to prevent accumulation of potassium to toxic levels in body fluids.[16] The renal tubules can curtail urinary Na loss almost to zero under certain circumstances, but even in the presence of cellular deficiency of K and low serum K, the urinary excretion of K continues. The rate of K loss in the urine may drop with a low serum K, but there is apparently an obligatory potassium loss in the urine; no such obligatory sodium loss occurs. Approximately 40 mEq. of potassium are required daily to avoid a negative K balance from renal loss of K.

Cardiac arrhythmias may result from low serum K. A low serum K (and presumably low intracellular K) sensitizes the heart to digitalis and predisposes to digitalis intoxication. In the presence of digitalis intoxication, potassium administration may be indicated.[72] Digitalis should be administered with care to patients depleted of K (after vomiting, diuresis, etc.). Toxic doses of digitalis cause egress of K from myocardial cells and inhibit return of K into the cells. If K is given, hyperkalemia may develop. Elevated serum potassium may have serious myocardial depressant action (see below).

Muscle metabolism is profoundly disturbed whenever there is severe derangement of intracellular potassium and striking symptoms may be observed involving both (1) *somatic muscles* and (2) *the heart*.

The transfer of glucose from the extracellular fluids into cells requires potassium. Serum K may fall even if K is administered with glucose. Even small *decreases in serum K* may be especially dangerous in two groups of patients: (1) those having severe K depletion, and (2) those receiving digitalis.[73] Such patients should, to prevent the precipitation of dangerous ventricular arrhythmias, be given at least 40 mEq. of K in 5 per cent glucose per hour of treatment.

Toxic doses of digitalis cause release of potassium from the liver and interfere with the uptake of K by the cells of skeletal and cardiac muscle. Therefore, when digitalis intoxication is treated by intravenous infusions of potassium salts, there is ever present the danger of causing *hyperkalemic* cardiac arrhythmias. Apparently such a consequence can be avoided if the oral or intravenous rate of administration is slow, not exceeding 0.5 mEq. of K per minute.[74]

Since it is difficult to judge from the level of the serum K or the amount of urinary K what the state of the intracellular potassium may be, and since certain pathologic states depend primarily upon the intracellular K concentration, the clinical recognition of abnormalities of K metabolism is more difficult than the diagnosis of Na, Cl, and bicarbonate disorders.[44,52,53]

Potassium Deficiency. If deficient intake of potassium is protracted, the obligatory excretion of K proceeds, with negative K balance resulting from its continued excretion in the urine.

Dehydration and trauma to tissue will accelerate loss of K from cells and thus increase urinary K loss. Abnormal drainages of gastrointestinal fluid cause much loss of potassium (vomiting, gastrointestinal suction, drainage from fistulas, diarrhea, steatorrhea, etc.). Potassium deficiency is especially apt to be found in patients suffering from such disorders who are maintained on the usual potassium-free parenteral fluids.[17]

In diuresis, especially if associated with conditions such as those above (with K loss from cells and little or no K intake), the K loss is accelerated and deficiency is especially apt to occur.

It should be emphasized that when serum Na or Cl is low (abnormal hydration factors being eliminated), there is a body deficit of such ions. In the case of the intracellular electrolyte potassium, however, there is no such relatively simple approach to the assessment of K deficits. Deficiency of K must be suspected primarily from the clinical circumstances, since serum K may be high, normal, or low in such states, the blood level reflecting transport levels, and not necessarily tissue or cell content.

ACIDOSIS. In severe degrees of acidosis, hyperkalemia is likely to occur, but the cells may be relatively depleted of K, and the body K balance may be negative. This may be true, for example, in *diabetic acidosis*, in which there is dehydration, loss of K in the urine (hemoconcentration and loss of K from cells). Before therapy, the serum K is usually normal or elevated, but after treatment is given K excretion decreases, K moves back into the cells, the extracellular fluid volume expands, and the serum K may fall precipitously. To prevent serious K deficiency, therapy with fluids containing K may be imperative as soon as the initial *temporary hyperkalemia* has been abolished. As much as 20 Gm. of potassium may be required in the first 48 hours to make up for the negative K balance, which may have been developing for a number of days.

ALKALOSIS (if renal function is adequate) leads to transfer of sodium from the extracellular to the intracellular fluids, with displacement of K from the cells and its loss in the urine. The K balance may be negative. The serum K may be low (as it often is, if urine volume has been high) or it may be normal or elevated (high K usually occurs if there has been oliguria). Such alkalosis may occur with chloride loss (pyloric obstruction, etc.). Treatment with solutions of NaCl alone will not correct the alkalosis: one must repair the K deficit as well as the Cl deficit before the serum bicarbonate returns to normal. In general, it appears that persons depleted of K tend to develop alkalosis and that alkalosis leads to depletion of K. A renal mechanism is involved, but the details of its operation are as yet incompletely understood.[18] When K is lost from the body either through the kidneys or the gastrointestinal tract much of it is accompanied by Cl taken from the extracellular fluids. This unbalanced loss of extracellular anions is compensated for by a rise in extracellular bicarbonate. This is apparently why acute potassium deficiency is usually associated with alkalosis.[19]

ADRENOCORTICAL HORMONES exert considerable control not only over Na absorption by the renal tubules, but also over the absorption and excretion of K through the renal tubules.[37] Persons with Addison's disease tend to lose Na and retain K. The adrenocortical steroids cause retention of Na and promote the excretion of K. Overdosage with deoxycorticosterone or cortisone may cause abnormally great K loss, with low serum K and serious clinical effects. If potassium intake is deficient while K excretion is kept at a normal or accelerated rate with deoxycorticosterone, foci of necrosis may occur in the heart muscle fibers with death from heart failure. This may occur in the course of treatment of Addison's disease (Goodof and MacBryde[20]). Clinical evidence of deficiency of potassium has been observed in patients treated with ACTH (adrenocorticotrophic pituitary hormone), and with cortisone.[38] In some patients with Cushing's syndrome, hyperactivity of the adrenal cortex is accompanied by evidences of potassium deficiency.

Aldosteronism, either primary or secondary, produces high urinary output of potassium, and sodium retention. Hypokalemia, hypernatremia, and elevated CO_2 are characteristic. *The primary type,* due to an adrenocortical adenoma, causes hypertension and often is revealed when clinical evidence of hypokalemia appears after use of a diuretic to treat the elevated blood pressure. *Secondary aldosteronism* may occur with congestive heart failure, cirrhosis with ascites, the nephrotic syndrome, etc. If the cause of the excessive aldosterone production (depleted effective arterial blood volume or renal ischemia, etc.) can be removed, the hypersecretion of aldosterone will stop.

Routes of Potassium Depletion

Thus, we have discussed how depletion of potassium may occur
1. Through the urine, if intake is inadequate
2. Through tissue destruction
3. Through dehydration, diuresis, and polyuria
4. With loss of gastrointestinal fluids
5. With acidosis
6. With alkalosis
7. With adrenocortical hormone effects.

All of these are mechanisms by which there may occur actual negative potassium balance. There is in these conditions a loss of potassium from the cells and from the body, but at various stages in these various conditions the serum K may be low, normal, or even high. A normal or higher than normal serum K may occur even in the presence of a true K deficit (1) if there is dehydration with hemoconcentration or (2) if the transfer of K from intracellular fluids to the extracellular fluid is rapid.

A *low serum K* may become evident in the potassium deficiency states (1) if diuresis is promoted by the use of parenteral fluids or if dialysis is employed with fluids containing inadequate potassium; (2) if the shift of K from serum to cells is suddenly brought about: (a) by unknown factors, such as those which apparently operate at the onset of an attack of familial periodic paralysis, or (b) by movement of glucose into the cells.[21] It appears that the mechanism by which the serum K is reduced is the formation of a monopotassium salt and its deposition with hexosediphosphate during the process of glycogen formation and storage. In familial periodic paralysis an attack can be produced by the intake of a large quantity of carbohydrate. In the hyperkalemia of diabetic acidosis or of uremia, glucose and insulin therapy may lower the serum K to normal or subnormal levels. (c) By adrenocortical steroids: deoxycorticosterone, or large doses of adrenal cortex extract or of cortisone tend to cause K shift from serum into the cells.

A low serum K may occur when there is no true deficiency in the cells or total body tissues. Either (1) dilution of the blood or (2) sudden shift of K into cells may bring about such a temporary lowering of serum K.

Clinical Signs of Potassium Deficiency. A low serum K that indicates cellular deficiency of potassium usually is accompanied by a gradual diminution of strength first. The muscles become flaccid; reflexes cannot be elicited. The patient may complain of weakness only, or of a numb, dead feeling, then partial paralysis, then complete paralysis. The paralyses usually occur mainly in the extremities, ascending from the periphery toward the center. The facial and respiratory muscles often remain unaffected, but frequently respiratory paralysis may endanger life.

In potassium deficiency cardiac arrhythmias are apt to occur, especially if the patient has been receiving digitalis.[72,73,74,76] There are *electrocardiographic changes* occurring quite regularly when the serum K is below normal: depressed, broadened T waves, prolonged Q-T interval, and depression of the S-T segment. Now that the flame photometer has greatly facilitated serum K determinations, it is advisable not to depend upon the electrocardiogram alone, but if possible, to determine also the serum K. These two laboratory tests plus a careful analysis of the patient's clinical status usually clarify the pathogenesis of signs and symptoms present and indicate logical therapy (Fig. 35-9).

When serum K or intracellular K or both are low, muscles generally, including cardiac muscle, may not be able to respond to and transmit impulses normally. K+ disturbances may disrupt operation of the enzyme system involved in the active transport of cations across cell membranes.[84] Digitalis glycosides inhibit active ion transport.[86] When both low K+ and digitalis effect are operative, the subject may show **potentiation** of the digitalis action. Patients already digitalized often experience diuresis, or vomiting, or diarrhea with K loss, and consequent **digitalis intoxication** may be precipitated.

Potassium Intoxication: Hyperkalemia. Abnormal elevation of the serum potassium concentration may occur as the result of one or more of the following pathogenic mechanisms:

1. Renal failure from any cause, especially if associated with oliguria or anuria. Hyperkalemia is rare if the urine volume exceeds 500 ml. per 24 hours. The principal limiting factor in the excretion of potassium is reduction of the glomerular filtration rate.

2. Renal failure with high K intake or Na depletion, particularly when both occur simultaneously. Potassium clearance remains remarkably constant even in severe renal disease. When potassium excretion is limited, the urine volume is a significant factor. Thus, if there is oliguria and the K intake increases (for example, from the ill-advised administration of orange juice, which contains large amounts of K, or from the breakdown of red blood cells, which occurs with an incompatible transfusion), dangerous hyperkalemia may suddenly be precipitated.

3. Trauma, tissue destruction, fever, the injection of epinephrine—any stimulus adequate to cause "the alarm reaction"—may accelerate catabolic processes above the normal rates, and, if K excretion is impaired, hyperkalemia may result.

4. Dehydration. Increased tonicity of the plasma causes passage of Na into cells and of K into the extracellular fluids. Since dehydration is apt to be associated also with oliguria and with impaired renal function, the tendency toward a high serum K will progress until the dehydration and oliguria are corrected.

5. Infusion of hypertonic fluids: dehydration is increased and the shift of K from cells to plasma is facilitated.

6. Acidosis, especially with the common associated factors of dehydration, oliguria, and Na deficit.

7. Alkalosis, when complicated by dehydration and oliguria.

Clinical Signs of High Serum Potassium. The clinical signs of high serum potassium concentration closely simulate those of low potassium concentration: progressive weakness, then flaccid paralyses of the extremities, later, difficulty in phonation and respiration; often cardiac arrhythmias. Because of the clinical similarity of the symptoms occurring with abnormalities of K metabolism in either direction, it is highly desirable, whenever possible, to follow both the serum potassium and electrocardiographic changes for diagnosis and during and after treatment (Fig. 35-9).[72,73,74,76]

Abnormally high K+ ion concentration on either or both sides of cell membranes will interfere with proper functioning of many organs and tissues. Cation transport across cell membranes is disrupted in nerve and muscle, and symptoms that result from disturbance of impulse transmission may be striking.[84] Disorder of cardiac muscle func-

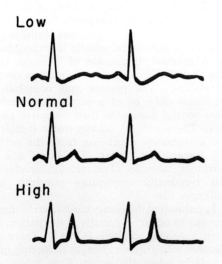

Low

Normal

High

FIG. 35-9. Changes in the electrocardiogram produced by alterations in serum potassium concentration (shown for unchanged heart rate).

tion may be a prominent manifestation. Digitalis glycosides intensify K^+ disturbances, because these drugs are potent inhibitors of both active ion transport and Na-K-ATPase activity generally. The action of these drugs may be especially evident upon cardiac muscle function because a concentration toxic to the heart is reached before the inhibitory effect is evident upon other tissues. For example, digitalis glycosides inhibit sodium reabsorption in renal tubules but are not effective diuretics in subjects without heart failure, apparently because higher concentrations are necessary for renal effects, whereas lesser concentrations exert full cardiac results.

It is important to point out that the electrocardiogram will reveal characteristic alterations, as a rule, before there are serious clinical evidences of hyperkalemia.[22] These are usually apparent whenever serum K exceeds 7 mEq. per liter. The changes in the electrocardiogram occurring with the onset and progression of potassium intoxication are usually in this order and are quite constant[22]: (1) development of tall, narrow, pointed T waves; (2) depression of the S-T segment, which tends to become a direct line from the nadir of the S to the apex of the T wave; (3) auriculoventricular block; (4) decreased amplitude and increased duration of P waves; (5) intraventricular block, with lowered R and deeper S waves; (6) prolonged Q-T interval; (7) ventricular arrhythmia; (8) sinus bradycardia; (9) disintegration of the ventricular complexes; and (10) ventricular standstill (Fig. 35-9).

Conclusions Concerning Relationships of Potassium Metabolism to Dehydration. Dehydration may cause loss of potassium in several ways. The serum potassium may be elevated or depressed in dehydration, depending upon a number of factors discussed previously. Either acidosis or alkalosis may be present in dehydration, as determined by the pathogenesis of the dehydrated state, but hyperkalemia is common in acidosis, low or normal serum K in alkalosis (except in severe oliguria). Whenever dehydration is present, disordered potassium metabolism may be expected. Whenever a derangement in potassium metabolism has occurred, abnormalities in fluid distribution have also occurred, usually with loss first of extracellular fluid with later loss of fluid from the cells and withdrawal of potassium from the cells.

DEHYDRATION AND RENAL IMPAIRMENT

Dehydration and renal dysfunction are related in two ways: (1) renal disorder may lead to water loss; (2) dehydration may cause renal failure.

1. The rate of plasma flow through the kidney, as determined by diodrast-clearance studies, is about 740 ml. per minute. The total volume of blood passing through the kidneys is therefore about 1,300 ml. per minute. This is approximately a quarter of the total cardiac output under basal physiologic conditions. About 125 ml. per minute, or approximately one-fifth of the plasma entering the kidney per unit time, is filtered by the glomeruli. Some 99 per cent or more of the glomerular filtrate is reabsorbed by the tubules. From these considerations it is apparent that rapid and efficient movement of extracellular fluid through the kidneys, with rapid renal disposal of waste products but retention of essential materials, is required for maintenance of normal fluid and electrolyte balance.

We have previously considered how derangements of renal function may interfere with water and electrolyte control. When tubular reabsorption is impaired in chronic nephritis, even to a slight degree, fluid loss is excessive and there is a tendency toward dehydration. Added to this hazard is the inability of the damaged kidney to manufacture NH_4^+ with normal rapidity. The relative failure of the ammonium mechanism causes loss of fixed base. Whenever fixed base is lost from the plasma, water must be withdrawn and excreted to preserve the normal total ionic concentration in the plasma. Thus, renal disease through impairment of both tubular function and ammonium production may cause dehydration. When, however, there is albuminuria sufficient to lower the plasma albumin, the diminished ability of the plasma to withdraw water from the interstitial fluid may combat the tendency toward fluid loss, and if the hypoproteinemia is of sufficient degree, the opposite effect of fluid retention may occur with production of edema.

Not only may renal disease produce dehydration, but serious fluid loss may occur with renal dysfunction resulting from endocrine disorders. Derangement of hormonal control of tubular water absorption produces dehydration in diabetes insipidus, and hormonal disorder causes the sodium, chloride, and water loss of Addison's disease.

2. If dehydration is severe, plasma volume may be greatly reduced and the rate of plasma flow through the kidney may fall to such a point that renal function may be seriously impaired. Extreme fluid loss of course affects all tissues and organs, but because of the very large plasma flow necessary to maintain the vital functions of the kidney, evidences of kidney failure quickly become apparent. Retention of waste products soon results in uremia, and the inability of the kidney to manufacture ammonium and to excrete acids causes acidosis. Thus, severe dehydration, if it continues for any length of time, is characterized not only by (a) signs of water loss (dry, inelastic skin, dry mucous membranes, soft eyeballs, weight loss) and (b) signs of diminished blood volume (shock, low blood pressure), but by (c) evidence of renal failure (high blood nonprotein nitrogen, high serum potassium, acidosis).

Only in very severe degrees of dehydration does renal impairment appear, however, because of the wide, elastic, and adjustable interstitial fluid compartment that protects the plasma volume. A man weighing 70 kg. has approximately 15 per cent of his body weight as interstitial fluid (10.5 liters) and 5 per cent as plasma (3.5 liters). Many liters of interstitial fluid may be lost before serious reduction occurs in plasma volume. Studies have shown that from one-third to one-half of the extracellular fluid must be removed to produce the clinical picture of dehydration.

DEHYDRATION, SALT DEPLETION AND SHOCK

The adverse effects of extensive loss of body fluid upon the circulation are well recognized. Loss of fluid is an important factor in the production of shock following various types of trauma, including burns. The loss of fluid need not be external, since large amounts of fluid accumulate in the injured region and may be unavailable to the organism, at least temporarily. When shock is associated with such segregation of fluid, intravenous saline solution may produce prompt relief.

The relative importance of (1) *trauma* and its effect upon the nervous system, the circulatory system and the skeletal muscular system, of (2) *salt depletion*, of (3) *water depletion*, and of (4) *disturbances of potassium metabolism*, in the production of shock needs clarification. In the absence of trauma, salt depletion may produce a form of collapse closely resembling traumatic shock.[23] Plasma volume, cardiac output, circulation rate and blood pressure all decline sharply, and plasma protein falls. Water depletion alone, however, fails to produce such striking effects. When water alone is lost to a degree resulting in the same decline in total extracellular-fluid volume as that produced by the salt deficit, there is no shock-like collapse. The cardiac output, plasma volume, mean arterial pressure and circulation rate may slightly decline. Usually little or no protein disappears from the plasma.

It should be noted that in the salt- and water-deprivation studies no close correlation could be established between the degree of drop in the plasma volume and the extent of the decrease in the cardiac output. Therefore, the shocklike state produced by sudden salt depletion cannot be explained by diminished plasma volume alone. Withdrawal of NaCl results in a large shift of water from the extracellular to the intracellular phase, with consequent depletion of the former and expansion of the latter. The body fluids become hypotonic and the plasma volume is decreased. The hypotonicity of the body fluids and the lowered plasma-protein content, as well as the lowered plasma volume, deserve attention.[23,42,48] The fate of the protein is not known, but it is probably segregated somewhere within the body. Current concepts picture a continuous exchange between the protein of circulating plasma and that outside the vascular spaces. Salt depletion may displace the normal equilibrium. The greater circulatory collapse produced by salt loss as compared with water loss may be related to the loss of protein from the circulation. Lowering the plasma protein may favor the disproportionate decline in plasma volume, and thus aid in producing the drop in venous return, cardiac output, and arterial blood pressure. However, such an explanation must remain hypothetical for the present. It seems quite as logical to consider that the salt depletion injures one or more parts of the cardiovascular system and thus produces shock. As extracellular salt is withdrawn, water moves (in response to osmotic forces) out of the extracellular fluid into the cells. Extracellular dehydration, intracellular overhydration and hypotonicity of both compartments, result. Potassium is lost from the cells, and either hyperkalemia or hypokalemia may occur, depending upon a number of factors discussed in the preceding section on potassium. The changes in the sodium and potassium concentration of both intracellular and extracellular fluids alter the conduction of nerve impulses and affect both the physiologic and anatomic integrity of skeletal and cardiac muscle. These changes may directly injure the cells of the heart or blood vessels, producing shock, and indirectly and only incidentally causing loss of circulating protein. That is, the protein loss may be only another evidence of vascular damage and not a contributing factor in producing the shock.

PARENTERAL FLUIDS IN THE TREATMENT OF DEHYDRATION

Although this chapter is concerned with the etiology and the pathologic physiology of dehydration as a symptom, full consideration of the subject requires some mention of attempts to restore body fluids by parenteral injection of solutions or suspensions intravenously, subcutaneously, or intraperitoneally. *Three primary aspects* of the problem deserve attention: (1) restoration of total body fluid volume to normal; (2) restoration of solutes (Na, Cl, K, etc.); (3) restoration of acid-base balance. Whether "physiologic" sodium chloride solution or some other form of fluid, such as dilute alkali, glucose solution, whole blood, plasma, etc., is selected, should depend upon the nature and the degree of the fluid loss, with consideration not only of water, but of other substances that are constituents of the lost fluids. Chemical examinations of the blood often reveal loss of water, chloride, bicarbonate, plasma protein, hemoglobin, sodium, or potassium. If one is to overcome the dehydration completely, the electrolytes should be restored along with the water. Plasma protein may be needed to re-establish normal circulation and normal interchange of substances between the blood and the intercellular fluid. To accomplish such full restoration of the fluid anatomy to normal, without too much reliance upon aid from renal activity or gastrointestinal absorption, the parenteral fluids given must be similar to normal intercellular fluid, or must at least provide the most essential mineral constituents. Sodium chloride is the most important salt because it is present in body fluids in greatest amount (Fig. 35-2). The administration of isotonic sodium chloride solution will therefore relieve many of the phenomena of dehydration. However, sodium chloride alone frequently is not capable of providing complete relief of symptoms.[24,32,35,36,70,77]

Isotonic sodium chloride solution is often

TABLE 35-3. COMPOSITION OF DARROW'S SOLUTION

GM. PER 100 ML.		MEQ. PER LITER
NaCl 0.40	Na	123
KCl 0.26	K	35
Sodium	Cl	105
lactate 0.59	Lactate	53

quite effective if renal function is relatively good, and if the dehydration has not been severe enough to cause considerable withdrawal of potassium from the cells.

When the deficit is primarily of water, one may wish to provide parenteral fluids containing no NaCl (hypernatremia already present).

When base losses exceed those of chloride, one may wish to provide much of the sodium without chloride ion.

With some of these basic considerations in mind, we may proceed to review briefly some of the most effective solutions used to replace either intracellular deficits, extracellular deficits, or both.

SOLUTIONS FOR INTRACELLULAR FLUID REPLACEMENT

When there has been a significant loss of potassium, use of solutions containing potassium may be urgently indicated.

Potassium chloride in 0.60 per cent solution with 5 per cent glucose is effective and will provide 80 mEq. per liter of K. If less NaCl is desired than that in "physiologic" saline solution, but NaCl and K are both needed, a useful solution contains 0.60 per cent KCl and 0.43 per cent NaCl, and provides 80 mEq. per liter of K and 73 mEq. per liter of Na and of Cl.[26]

Darrow[25] showed that from one-third to one-half of the extracellular fluid and of the extracellular electrolytes might be lost in severe dehydration with acidosis. He calculated that the following solution provided the most essential electrolytes and would provide an alkaline solution to combat acidosis: 0.40 Gm. NaCl, 0.26 Gm. KCl, 0.59 Gm. of sodium lactate to 100 ml. of water. The amount given was 80 ml. per kg. of body weight per 24 hours until plasma bicarbonate content and other blood chemical determinations approached normal. It was quite effective in dehydration and acidosis resulting from diarrhea in infants (Table 35-3).

A low serum sodium aggravates the untoward effects of a high serum potassium.

When the serum K is high, solutions containing K should not be given, but sodium replacement may be important, plus *methods to lower the serum K* (glucose solutions, insulin, and perhaps hemodialysis).

When the serum potassium is low and *potassium administration* is indicated, it would seem that the logical accompanying anion would be phosphate. This important intracellular ion is often deficient when K is deficient, and negative potassium balance is apt to be accompanied by a negative phosphate balance. Elkinton and Tarail[26] have suggested the use of 1 Gm. of KH_2PO_4 and 4.5 Gm. of K_2HPO_4 to 1 liter of solution (glucose, physiologic saline or protein hydrolysate) to yield a solution with pH 7.35 containing 60 mEq. of potassium per liter.

Glucose should probably be given with potassium to facilitate the transfer of K into cells. If the K deficit is severe, 75 to 150 mEq. of K per 24 hours may be administered; if mild, 30 to 50 mEq. may be adequate.

Volume of Fluids. The clinician must judge from the history, the physical findings, and the laboratory data and estimate as closely as possible the *total fluid deficit*. It may require several days to make up the total deficiency when it is severe. The daily fluid administered should include (1) maintenance fluids plus (2) fluids to supply deficit.

Maintenance for the nonsweating, nonfebrile, resting adult will require about 1,000 ml. (for water of vaporization, "insensible water loss") plus about 1,000 ml. for urinary loss, or a total of approximately 2 liters. If there is fever and sweating, one must provide an additional 0.5 to 1.5 liters daily. From 10 to 20 per cent of the body water may be lost during the development of severe dehydration. In infants, between 100 and 300 ml. of fluid per kg. of body weight may be necessary, given over a period of 12 to 48 hours. In adults, the requirements to cover maintenance plus partial deficit replacement may be 6 liters or more per 24 hours. When feasible, fluids should be given by mouth. When necessary, nasal tube administration is often successful. Subcutaneous or intravenous routes are employed when the need is urgent or there are gastroenteric disturbances. Too rapid or excessive intravenous infusion may precipitate circulatory failure and may be guarded against by frequent measurement of the venous blood pressure, which should be kept within normal limits. Isotonic fluids containing the normal electrolytes and glucose

are less likely to embarrass the circulation, but hypertonic solutions and plasma protein attract fluid into the vascular compartment and tend more rapidly to increase blood volume and blood pressure. They may produce acute circulatory failure with cardiac dilatation and pulmonary edema.

Computation of the fluid deficit will be only approximate, but may be of great importance in directing treatment. Various methods of estimation follow:[33]

1. From body weight

Example:

$$
\begin{aligned}
\text{Usual wt.} &= 70.0 \text{ Kg.} \\
\text{Present wt.} &= 67.2 \\
\text{Acute wt. loss} &= \overline{2.8} \text{ Kg.} \\
&= 2.8 \text{ liters } H_2O
\end{aligned}
$$

2. From estimated fluid losses

Example (during 2 days):

Output:

$$
\begin{aligned}
\text{Urine} &= 900 \text{ ml.} \\
H_2O \text{ vaporization} &= 3,000 \\
\text{Gastric fluid} &= \underline{2,800} \\
\text{Total} &\ \ 6,700 \text{ ml.}
\end{aligned}
$$

Intake:

$$
\begin{aligned}
\text{Oral fluids} &= 400 \text{ ml.} \\
\text{I-V fluids} &= 4,000 \\
H_2O \text{ oxidation} &= \underline{200} \\
\text{Total} &\ \ 4,600 \text{ ml.} \\
\text{Balance } H_2O &= -2.1 \text{ liters}
\end{aligned}
$$

3. From the rise in serum sodium concentration and the estimated total body water, W_1

$$\text{Deficit } H_2O = W_1 - W_2 = (0.6 \text{ wt.}) - \frac{Na_1 \times (0.6 \text{ wt.})}{Na_2}$$

Example:

$$
\begin{aligned}
\text{Given}\quad \text{Wt.}_1 &= 70 \text{ Kg.} \\
Na_1 &= 140 \text{ mEq. per liter} \\
Na_2 &= 160 \text{ mEq. per liter}
\end{aligned}
$$

Then $W_1 = 0.6 \times 70 = 42$ liters

$$W_2 = \frac{140 \times 42}{160} = 37 \text{ liters}$$

Deficit $H_2O = 42 - 37 = 5$ liters

Route and Rate of Fluid Administration. In severe dehydration intravenous infusions are often imperative to restore vital functions. To save life it may be necessary to relieve shock, and to restore as promptly as possible the blood pressure, blood volume, oxygen-carrying power, pH, and renal circulation. Initially fluids given intravenously may restore consciousness and the ability to take fluids and nourishment by mouth. Within a few hours oral alimentation may become the route of choice. This is often the case in diabetic coma. Broth and orange juice may provide adequate water, glucose, Na, Cl, and K so that it is not necessary, in many instances, to give glucose or K intravenously.

Caution to prevent hyperkalemia is imperative in administering K intravenously. Darrow, in treating infants dehydrated by diarrhea, used isotonic sodium chloride solution and dextrose, along with blood or plasma until circulatory and renal function had been restored. Then he gave subcutaneously the solution (now called Darrow's solution) containing NaCl, KCl, and sodium lactate. This solution can also be given orally, with two parts of 5 per cent dextrose in water.

When the serum K is quite low, however, glucose and NaCl solution may further lower it to dangerous levels. The use of KCl in 0.1 to 0.2 per cent solution may be very effective. The rate of K administration intravenously should not exceed a liter (2 Gm. KCl) per hour.[27,28,72,73,74]

SOLUTIONS FOR EXTRACELLULAR REPLACEMENT

1. DEXTROSE 5 PER CENT IN WATER to provide water without electrolyte. Used in simple dehydration resulting from insensible water loss in patients deprived of fluid.

2. ISOTONIC SODIUM CHLORIDE ("PHYSIOLOGIC" or "NORMAL" SALINE) SOLUTION. This 0.85 per cent NaCl solution contains 145 mEq. per liter of Na and of Cl and is therefore physiologic or isotonic with extracellular fluid only in respect to sodium, whereas the chloride is relatively high (145:100). Use of this solution, if there is no chloride deficit, may be dangerous if the kidneys are unable to excrete the chloride excess. When renal regulation is adequate, it is valuable in replacing fluid losses such as those occurring from diabetic ketosis, gastrointestinal disorders, adrenocortical deficiency, etc.

3. COMBINED SODIUM CHLORIDE AND SODIUM LACTATE SOLUTIONS. An ideal solution to correct hypotonicity when CO_2 is normal can be constructed on the basis of the 140:100 normal proportions of the Na:Cl in the serum. A mixture of 5/7 molar NaCl and 2/7 molar Na lactate will provide the Na and Cl ions in proper proportions. Thus, 700 ml. of the solution is prepared easily: combine 500 ml. of molar NaCl with 200 ml. of molar Na lactate.

Other combinations of NaCl and Na lactate[24] can be used to alter the CO_2 combining-power in either direction. A higher proportion of Na lactate may be used if the CO_2 combining-power is decreased.

4. MOLAR SODIUM LACTATE may be used when there is a severe deficit of base.

5. MOLAR SODIUM CHLORIDE is indicated when there is salt depletion with severe deficit of extracellular solute in relation to water, as evidenced by hyponatremia and hypochloremia.

6. ONE-SEVENTH MOLAR (ISOTONIC) SODIUM LACTATE is useful in certain acidotic patients, whose water requirement is normal but whose extracellular sodium is low in relation to chloride.[24]

7. ONE-SEVENTH MOLAR AMMONIUM CHLORIDE may be used when only chloride is needed, e.g., for the metabolic alkalosis resulting from loss of gastric HCl.

Choice of Fluids. When the cause of the dehydration is known, the type of fluid required is suggested by the nature of the physiologic disturbance. For example, in repeated *vomiting* from pyloric obstruction, dehydration may be accompanied by alkalosis, and the use of a solution containing bicarbonate is contraindicated, whereas chloride is greatly needed. Potassium may be needed also. After *hemorrhage*, dehydration may be extreme, but isotonic saline or lactate-Ringer's solution will be relatively ineffective. Plasma protein may restore the blood volume and relieve the shock, but whole blood, with its red cells and hemoglobin to carry oxygen and relieve anoxia of the tissues, is the only complete replacement therapy. In conditions associated with *starvation* or inability to utilize carbohydrate, glucose solution as well as electrolyte solution is necessary. Thus, dehydration with acidosis from diarrhea or loss through a fistula may require not only large amounts of water, salts, and base (such as provided in sodium lactate-Ringer's solution) but glucose as well.

In *diabetes*, especially if acidosis or coma occurs and sufficient carbohydrate cannot be ingested, glucose with insulin in large doses to accelerate carbohydrate utilization may be the only direct route to reversal of the processes resulting in the dehydration. The initially high serum K often rapidly falls during treatment of diabetic acidosis until hypokalemia becomes evident, requiring potassium replacement therapy.[29]

In diabetic acidosis, persons in the younger age groups (with good renal function—and possibly also with good hypothalamic-pituitary-adrenocortical responses to enable them to retain sodium, chloride, and water) can usually quite promptly correct even quite severe acidosis if provided with adequate amounts of isotonic NaCl and insulin.

In diabetic acidosis or in any other type of acidosis accompanied by renal inadequacy (infancy, advanced age, chronic nephritis, etc.), the capacity to reabsorb sodium may be diminished, ammonia production may be impaired, and the use of alkaline fluids with extra sodium may be beneficial.

When the blood glucose concentration is quite high, there is apparently sufficient available body glucose to allow adequate carbohydrate metabolism for some hours, even with the large doses of insulin usually necessary in the treatment of severe diabetic acidosis. Some authorities believe that dehydration and glycosuria are exaggerated by giving glucose when considerable hyperglycemia is already present and advocate avoidance of the use of glucose solutions, except when necessary to provide sufficient available carbohydrate. Others advocate the prompt use of glucose solutions in all severe diabetic acidosis.

Renal failure, with or without true uremia, often results in severe acidosis, dehydration, loss of chloride and fixed base. The severe acidosis must be relieved without help from the kidneys, too badly impaired to exercise their usual efficient functions of adjusting fluid balance and acid-base balance. The acidosis, the dehydration, and the hypochloridemia may often be relieved by "fortified" lactate-Ringer's solution. Glucose, insulin, or dialysis may be indicated to lower the serum K. Intravenous dextrose is valuable and blood may prove important in relieving the anemia so often present.

In *Addison's disease,* glucose, salt and water are needed. In *thyroid crisis,* with dehydration accompanying an extremely high metabolic rate, large amounts of glucose, as well as salt and water, are needed. In extensive *burns,* protein, as well as salt and water, is lost, and whole blood or plasma is indicated.

Dextrose solutions alone should seldom be employed in the relief of dehydration, because they may cause further diuresis and increase the dehydration. Likewise, the excessive use of hypotonic solutions is dangerous and may cause water intoxication.

Computation of Electrolyte Deficits. If the blood sodium and CO_2 combining-power are known, deficits in many conditions may be approximated by simple mathematical calculations.[33,34,35] Using 20 per cent of body weight as a rough approximation, one calculates the extracellular fluid volume; this figure is multiplied by the aberration of the serum Na from the normal 140 mEq. per liter. The product represents the degree of hypotonicity or hypertonicity of the extracellular fluid. If edema is present, the estimated edema volume is added to the estimated normal extracellular fluid volume.

EDEMA WITH HYPONATREMIA

Example:

>   Man normally weighing 70 kg.
>   Very edematous (estimate 10 liters)
>   Serum Na = 120 mEq. per liter

$$70 \times 0.2 = 14 \text{ liters extracellular fluid}$$
$$\underline{+ 10 \text{ liters edema fluid}}$$
$$24 \text{ liters total body fluid}$$

$$24 \times 20 \text{ mEq. per liter} = 480 \text{ mEq.}$$

$$\text{Na deficit} = 480 \text{ mEq.}$$

This could be administered by giving 480 ml. of molar NaCl orally or intravenously. Usually one finds that only about half of the administered Na stays in the extracellular fluid, so that in 12 to 24 hours the calculations are repeated and more Na is given if indicated.

DEHYDRATION WITH HYPERNATREMIA

Example:

>   70 kg. normal weight
> $\underline{-60 \text{ kg. present weight}}$
>   10 kg. = 10 liters fluid loss

Of this 10 liters, approximately 2 liters are extracellular fluid loss.

If serum Na = 160 mEq. per liter, $12 \times 20 = 240$ mEq. of Na must be diluted with water. This could be accomplished with $240/140 = 1.7$ liters of water, which could be given in isotonic form as 5 per cent glucose

An 8-liter deficit remains to be replaced by a solution close in composition to that of body fluid.

DEHYDRATION WITH HYPONATREMIA. Deficits of sodium may reach 50 per cent of the extracellular sodium (thus totaling as much as 1,000 mEq. in a 70 kg. adult) before death results from circulatory collapse. Ranges of deficits more commonly encountered, as in diabetic coma or pyloric obstruction, are 300 to 600 mEq. in the average adult.

If the extracellular fluid volume has been reduced and if the serum Na is low, the Na deficit consists of (1) the sodium lost with its proportional share of water, plus (2) the sodium missing from the extracellular fluid left behind (thus resulting in the lowered Na concentration).

1. Acute wt. loss of 1.5 kg. $\times$ 140 = 210 mEq. of sodium.
2. Normal wt. 70 kg. $\times$ 0.6 = 42 liters

Serum Na = 125 mEq. per liter
Deficit = 15 $\times$ 42 = 630 mEq.

Total Na deficit = 210 + 630 = 840 mEq.

ACID-BASE IMBALANCE. Deficit of sodium in excess of fixed anion (as in metabolic acidosis in diabetes, renal insufficiency, infant diarrhea, etc.): CO_2 combining-power is low in serum.

Example:
Serum CO_2 = 12 mM. per liter; 27 (normal) − 12 = 15 (deficit per liter)
14 (liters extracellular fluid volume) $\times$ 15 = 210 mM. total deficit of base; 210 mM. of base necessary to raise CO_2 to normal

Theoretically, this would require 210 ml. of molar Na lactate solution. In actual practice, 2 or 3 times this amount would probably be required, since 50 per cent or more of the Na usually enters the cells.

Chemical measurement of the bicarbonate reserve and the serum sodium, serum potassium, and chloride levels, as well as determination of the blood glucose content, and the serum protein and nonprotein nitrogen, is of great help in determining the choice and the amount of fluid replacement to be employed. *Intracellular losses* or gains of water or electrolytes cannot be measured directly with the methods now available; therefore, estimates must be based upon the history, the physical status, and laboratory tests of blood and urine. Whenever possible, frequent follow-up chemical determinations, as well as an initial diagnostic chemical study, are advisable. For example, a blood-protein level, initially apparently normal, may subsequently prove to be subnormal when hydration is restored. Acidosis may be overcorrected if excess amounts of alkaline solutions are employed, and repeated determination of the blood carbon dioxide combining power is an excellent guide to indicate how much of a solution such as lactate-Ringer's should be given, and how often repeated.

Since the concentration of the serum sodium may be an excellent guide for the regulation of replacement of this most important cation of the extracellular fluids, it should be determined before and after therapy, if the means are available, and it will often be found to yield data not deducible from CO_2 and chloride determinations.

The serum potassium concentration is of much greater importance than previously realized, as shown by a number of excellent studies. It may change quickly and should be followed, whenever possible, because the clinical signs of hypokalemia and hyperkalemia are difficult to distinguish.

The development of the flame photometer, which permits rapid and accurate determinations of serum sodium and potassium, has contributed greatly to the recent rapid advance of knowledge in this field. Rapid determination of the concentration of these cations in the blood permits accurate diagnosis and suggests the type of fluid and electrolyte therapy indicated. It also permits following the results of treatment, and the prompt adjustment of therapy to whatever changing indications may appear.

The electrocardiogram is an important adjunct to chemical measurement of the blood constituents. It is particularly useful in detecting abnormal levels of the serum potassium. The conduction of the cardiac impulse through the auriculoventricular conduction system may be impaired with serum K deviations, and the electrocardiographic tracings generally permit quite accurate deductions as to whether the serum K is high or low, often before clinical signs become evident.

DIURETICS AND DEHYDRATION

The kidneys, through mechanisms described early in this chapter, exert the most important control over the disposition of body fluid. Under certain conditions, drugs and other substances may, through increasing the urinary output, cause dehydration. In therapeutics, knowledge of diuretic agents is useful in choosing means to rid the body of excess fluid. Diuretic agents may work in either or both of two ways: (1) by increasing the rate of glomerular filtration; (2) by decreasing the rate of tubular reabsorption.

Substances acting as diuretics may be classified into four major groups,[30] as follows: (1) water and osmotic diuretics; (2) substances increasing colloidal osmotic pressure; (3) acid-forming salts; (4) inhibitors of renal tubular transport. The mechanism of action of the principal members of each group is indicated:

Water. Ingestion of large amounts of

water leads to decrease in tubular reabsorption, as the result of decrease in the secretion of the antidiuretic hormone. Water ingestion causes water diuresis.

Osmotic Diuretics. (1) Sodium Chloride. Isotonic sodium chloride administration increases blood volume and accelerates glomerular filtration.

Hypertonic sodium chloride solution increases the extracellular fluid, not only by the volume injected or ingested, but by the water withdrawn from the cells, and glomerular filtration is consequently greatly increased. In addition, the rejected sodium chloride limits resorption of water by the tubules. As a result of accelerated output of fluid into the tubules and diminished reabsorption, diuresis occurs.

In clinical edema, it should be noted, water and sodium chloride are not useful diuretics because they may be retained in the interstitial fluid, thus increasing the edema.

The frequently and often tragically demonstrated fact that no fluid intake is preferable to the ingestion of sea water was brought to our attention repeatedly during World War II. Drinking sea water causes dehydration because (1) it may cause vomiting, (2) water is pulled into the intestinal tract by the hypertonic salt solution and excessive quantities of water are excreted in the feces, and because (3) that part of the sodium chloride absorbed requires an increase in the urinary-water output.

"Salt fever," the temperature elevation caused by dehydration, may result from intravenous saline or glucose in excess.

Water intoxication, the condition resulting from excessive water ingestion, with resultant reduction in the osmotic pressure of the blood and cellular overhydration, may be promptly relieved by intravenous administration of hypertonic sodium chloride solution.

(2) Potassium salts, in contrast to those of sodium, are effective diuretics in any concentration. Potassium is the main cation of the cells of the body. When present in excess in the extracellular fluid it is filtered through the glomerulus and rejected by the tubules, taking considerable quantities of water with it.

(3) There are certain molecules, such as *urea, glucose,* and *sucrose,* which in the renal tubule require water for excretion because of their limited reabsorption.

Substances altering oncotic pressure are effective diuretics under certain conditions.

When edema is present because of low concentration of serum protein (as in nephrosis, malnutrition, chronic diarrhea, etc.), blood or plasma or albumin transfusion may prove extremely successful treatment. Plasma expanders such as dextran mobilize interstitial fluid. Acacia has a similar effect but may produce toxic results.

Acid-forming salts, such as ammonium chloride, ammonium nitrate, and calcium chloride, are powerful diuretics. The ammonium salts act by giving up the ammonium to form urea, leaving the anion to demand base from bicarbonate and to require water for excretion. Calcium similarly is freed from chloride by being excreted in the intestine or deposited in bone, and the chloride displaces bicarbonate in the extracellular fluids.

The Xanthines. Caffeine and theophylline and its derivatives (aminophylline), etc. and theobromine apparently act primarily by decreasing tubular resorption. In addition, they seem to increase the rate of glomerular filtration when it is diminished.

The Mercurials. Mercurial diuretics are among the most powerful of all diuretics. Their action is exerted through reduction in the ability of the renal tubules to absorb water. The basic mechanism of action of organic mercurials seems to be the inhibition of SH-activated enzyme systems, which are essential to provide energy for renal tubular transport. The resorption of the Cl^- ion is blocked specifically. H^+ ion transport and bicarbonate resorption are not affected. The loss of the fixed cation (chiefly Na) is secondary to the effect on the anion (Cl).

Inhibitor of Carbonic Anhydrase: Acetazolamide (Diamox). This sulfonamide depresses the rate of formation of carbonic acid by the inhibition of carbonic anhydrase, thus greatly reducing the rate of the H^+ ion and the Na^+ ion exchange in the renal tubule (see Fig. 35-7). As a result, bicarbonate resorption is incomplete, and titratable acid and ammonium disappear from the urine. The kidney elaborates an increased volume of alkaline urine.

The reabsorption of NaCl depends largely upon the process of ion exchange through which the cells of the renal tubules reabsorb sodium only in proportion to the rate at which they release hydrogen, one H^+ ion being exchanged for one Na^+ ion. The carbonic anhydrase present in the renal tubules catalyzes the formation of $H^+HCO_3^-$, which is strongly ionized, from H_2O and CO_2 (unionized); it thus promotes the liberation of H+ ions, permitting the excretion of an acid urine and reabsorption of sodium. Acetazolamide, by inhibiting carbonic anhydrase, retards tubular excretion of H+ ions and reabsorption of Na+ ions. It also increases excretion of K+ ions, which compete with H+ ions for the anions Cl^-, HCO_3^-, etc. The result is accelerated renal loss of HCO_3^-, which carries out Na+, K+, and water; there is diuresis and alkalinization of the urine.

Chlorothiazide and Hydrochlorothiazide are potent diuretic agents, which promote excretion of sodium and water by inhibiting their reabsorption by the proximal renal tubule. These compounds contain a free sulfanilamide group, but their mode of action differs from that of the carbonic anhydrase inhibitors. The diuresis produced by the thiazide diuretic drugs produces a balanced loss of sodium with its two attendant anions in approximately the proportions in the extracellular fluid; the drug acetazolamide as explained above, acts differently and causes a specific diuresis of sodium and bicarbonate. The thiazides also promote potassium excretion, and potassium depletion must be guarded against.

Aldosterone Inhibitors. An important development has been the discovery of agents that block the effect of aldosterone on the renal tubules. These compounds, the spirolactones, are derived from progesterone and are similar to aldosterone structurally. Spironolactone (Aldactone) has been extensively studied. It promotes diuresis by blocking, through competitive inhibition, the sodium-absorbing, water-retaining, and potassium-excreting effects of aldosterone on the distal renal tubules (see Fig. 35-7). The use of spironolactone is particularly indicated when potassium conservation is desired but diuresis is imperative, and when secondary hyperaldosteronism is believed to be a causative factor in edema or ascites (many cases of congestive heart failure, cirrhosis, nephrosis, idopathic edema, etc.).[75]

Triamterene does not depend upon the presence of aldosterone for its action, but otherwise resembles spironolactone in its action: in both, the primary effect is upon the distal segment of the nephron where sodium is exchanged for potassium and hydrogen ions. By reducing distal sodium resorption, they also reduce distal K+ and H+ secretion and excretion. When used alone, either of these agents is a rather weak diuretic; when used with other diuretics,

they may be quite effective. For example, when used with one of the thiazides, the natriuretic effect is additive, the thiazides acting proximal to the distal tubule, thus causing more sodium to be delivered to the site where these drugs act. Either can effectively prevent the development of hypochloremic alkalosis. Triamterene appears to have the advantage, because it does not depend upon high levels of aldosterone for its effect.[92]

Ethacrynic acid is a very potent diuretic, often able to evoke diuresis when mercurials and thiazides have failed. The drug inhibits sodium transport in most, if not all, of the ascending limb of the loop of Henle. The excretion of potassium, ammonia, and titratable acid increases during diuresis provoked by this agent, and hypokalemia and alkalosis may occur.

Furosemide, a sulfonamide derivative, is a saluretic producing a rapid, short-lived diuresis; it can be more potent than any other diuretic with the possible exception of ethacrynic acid. It acts by inhibiting sodium transport in the ascending limb of Henle's loop. Physiologically, its action resembles that of ethacrynic acid.[92]

MISCELLANEOUS DIURETICS

Digitalis is a diuretic only for persons with heart failure, and its effects upon urine flow are exerted through its action on the heart and the circulation. The mobilization of the edema fluid comes first, then the diuresis. Desiccated thyroid may promote the elimination of fluid when fluid retention is caused by low thyroid function.

Choice of a Diuretic. The promotion of diuresis when relative dehydration is desired (that is, the restoration of an overly hydrated to a normally hydrated body state) is often dramatically successful in therapy. The choice of agents is extremely important and depends largely upon the condition of the kidneys. When renal function is impaired, the mercurials, acid-forming salts, potassium salts, and urea may be dangerous.

CATHARTICS AND DEHYDRATION

Cathartics are used much too widely and physicians not infrequently see persons who intermittently produce in themselves moderate dehydration by the ingestion of preparations that increase the bulk and the liquid content of the feces. Cathartics act by one of three fundamental mechanisms, any one of which increases the water output through the fecal route. Cathartics are either irritant, bulky, or emollient in action. The *irritant preparations,* such as cascara or castor oil, cause rapid propulsion of the intestinal contents, allowing inadequate time for the usual water resorption with resultant elimination of liquid stools. *Bulky laxatives* increase the volume of the intestinal contents and thus are more physiologic in action. They may be inorganic salts that are slowly absorbed from the intestinal tract and thus hold water in the canal because of the osmotic pressure that they exert, or they may be hydrophilic colloids or indigestible fiber, which resist destruction in the alimentary canal. Examples of the saline cathartics are magnesium sulfate and sodium phosphate. Agar exerts all three types of laxative action. Agar is rich in indigestible hemicellulose, which provides bulk, is hydrophilic, and forms a mucilaginous mass that also acts as an *emollient.* Mineral oil is indigestible and unabsorbable, and acts as a *lubricant* to the fecal contents, preventing their excessive dehydration in the colon.

The saline cathartics may cause dehydration of considerable degree if taken in excessive doses. The mechanism of action of all of them is similar. During the absorption of solutes from the intestinal tract, the concentration of the salts tends to become isotonic with that in the blood serum. If the salt happens to be sodium chloride, which is easily absorbed, the salt and therefore the water, will be removed from the alimentary canal quite rapidly. However, if the solute contains ions that are slowly absorbed—for instance, the cation magnesium or the anions sulfate, phosphate, tartrate, and citrate—they are retained in the canal for a comparatively long time and thus draw water through the intestinal wall. The water leaves the extracellular fluid and enters the intestinal tract until the solution of the cathartic salt is rendered isotonic with the body fluids. The bowel becomes distended with liquid and thus the propulsion along the canal is mechanically increased and large amounts of fluid may be lost.

SUMMARY

Loss of water and electrolyte from the body or maldistribution of body water and electrolyte may produce profound disturbances of body physiology. The results of salt loss are more severe than those of water loss alone. Loss of extracellular electrolyte leads to loss of plasma volume, and is the prototype of the usual clinical conditions grouped under the term *dehydration.*

Water is in a dynamic state, and all body water is being constantly exchanged. Although sodium is the chief cation of the extracellular fluid and potassium the chief cation of the intracellular fluid, these ions are also in a dynamic state, and no part of the body is inaccessible to them. There are variations in the amount of sodium, chloride, and potassium in intracellular, as well as extracellular fluids, and a simple type of osmotic relationship is not sufficient to explain the behavior of body fluids.

The state of hydration of the cells depends primarily upon the concentration of sodium ion in the extracellular compartment. A major function of the kidney is to regulate the concentration of sodium in the extracellular fluid.

When water and salt balance are within normal limits and renal function is adequate, the regulatory processes can usually correct aberrations and preserve a relatively constant internal fluid environment. If, however, serious disturbance occurs in the water and salt balance, or in the renal regulation, it may be difficult to reverse the morbid process and dehydration may result. The symptom *dehydration,* if adequately analyzed and interpreted, may lead to detection of the cause of the water and electrolyte disturbance and its correction.

REFERENCES

1. Bernard, C.: Leçons sur les propriétés physiologiques et les altérations pathologiques des liquides de l'organisme, Paris, Baillière, 1859.
2. Cannon, W. B.: The Wisdom of the Body, New York, Norton, 1932.
3. Gamble, J. L.: Chemical Anatomy, Physiology and Pathology of Extracellular Fluid, ed. 6, Cambridge, Harvard, 1954.
   ———: Companionship of Water and Electrolytes in the Organization of Body Fluids, Stanford, Calif., Stanford Univ. Press, 1951.
4. Moore, F. D., *et al.*: Body composition; total body water and electrolytes; intravascular and extravascular phase volumes, Metabolism 5:447–467, 1956.
5. Levitt, M. F., and Gaudino, M.: Measurement of body water compartments, Amer. J. Med. 9:208–215, 1950.
6. Wilde, W. S.: Transport through biological membranes, Ann. Rev. Physiol. 17:17–36, 1955.
7. Pinson, E. A.: Water exchange and barriers as studied by the use of hydrogen isotopes, Physiol. Rev. 32:123–134, 1952.

8. Bresler, E. H.: The problem of the volume component of body fluid homeostasis, Amer. J. Med. Sci. 232:93–104, 1956.

9. Conn, J. W., and Louis, L. H.: "Salt-active" corticoids reflected in thermal sweat, J. Clin. Endocr. 10:12, 1950.

10. Heinbecker, P., and White, H. L.: The role of the pituitary gland in water balance, Ann. Surg. 110:1037, 1939.

11. Gilman, A., and Goodman, L.: The secretory response of the posterior pituitary to the need for water conservation, J. Physiol. 90:113, 1937.

12. Chambers, G. H., Melville, E. V., Hare, R. S., and Hare, K.: Amer. J. Physiol. 144:311, 1945.

13. Ray, C. T.: *in* Sodeman, W. A. (ed.): Pathologic Physiology, ed. 4, Philadelphia, Saunders, 1967.

14. Daughaday, W. H., and MacBryde, C. M.: Renal and adrenal mechanisms of salt conservation, J. Clin. Invest. 29:591–601, 1950.

15. Pitts, R. F.: Acid-base regulation by the kidneys, Amer. J. Med. 9:356–372, 1950.

16. Leaf, A., Camara, A., and Albertson, A.: Renal tubular secretion of potassium in man, J. Clin. Invest. 28:1526–1533, 1949.

17. Randall, H. T., Habif, D. V., Lockwood, J. S., and Werner, S. C.: Potassium deficiency in surgical patients, Surgery 26:341, 1949.

18. Berliner, R. W.: Renal excretion of water, sodium, potassium, calcium, and magnesium, Amer. J. Med. 9:541–559, 1950.

19. Darrow, D. C., Schwartz, R., Ianucci, J. F., and Coville, F.: The relation of serum bicarbonate concentration to muscle composition, J. Clin. Invest. 27:198, 1948.

20. Goodof, I. I., and MacBryde, C. M.: Heart failure in Addison's disease with myocardial changes of potassium deficiency, J. Clin. Endocr. 4:30–34, 1944.

21. Kolf, W. J.: Serum potassium in uremia, J. Lab. Clin. Med. 36:719–728, 1950.

22. Merrill, J. P., Levine, H. D., Somerville, W., and Smith, S.: Clinical recognition and treatment of acute potassium intoxication, Ann. Intern. Med. 33:797–830, 1950.

23. Elkinton, J. R., Danowski, T. S., and Winkler, A. W.: Hemodynamic changes in salt depletion and in dehydration, J. Clin. Invest. 25:120–129, 1946.

24. Hollander, W., and Williams, T.: Dehydration, Disease-a-Month, Chicago, Year Book Pub., Dec., 1958.

25. Darrow, D. C., Pratt, E. L., Flett, J., Jr., Gamble, A. H., and Wiese, H. F.: Disturbances of water and electrolytes in infantile diarrhea, Pediatrics 3:129, 1949.

26. Elkinton, J. R., and Tarail, R.: The present status of potassium therapy, Amer. J. Med. 9:200–207, 1950.

27. Hoffman, W. S.: Clinical physiology of potassium, J.A.M.A. 144:1157–1162, 1950.

28. Smith, F. H.: Potassium deficiency in gastrointestinal diseases, Gastroenterology, 16:73–82, 1950.

29. Danowski, T. S., Peters, J. H., Rothbun, J. C., Quashnock, J. M., and Greenman, L.: Studies in diabetic acidosis and coma, J. Clin. Invest. 28:1, 1949.

30. Goodman, L., and Gilman, A.: The Pharmacologic Basis of Therapeutics, ed. 3, New York, Macmillan, 1965.

31. Darrow, D. C.: Tissue water and electrolyte, Ann. Rev. Physiol. 6:95–122, 1944.
Darrow, D. C., and Pratt, E. L.: Fluid therapy; relation to tissue composition and expenditure of water and electrolyte, J.A.M.A. 143:365–373, 1950.

32. Weisberg, H. F.: Water, Electrolyte and Acid-Base Balance, ed. 2, Baltimore, Williams & Wilkins, 1962.

33. Elkinton, J. R., and Danowski, T. S.: The Body Fluids; Basic Physiology and Practical Therapeutics, Baltimore, Williams & Wilkins, 1955.

34. Schroeder, H. A., and Perry, H. M.: Disturbances of the internal environment and their correction, Amer. J. Clin. Path. 23:1100, 1953.

35. Goldberger, E.: Primer of Water, Electrolyte and Acid-Base Syndromes, ed. 3, Philadelphia, Lea & Febiger, 1965.

36. Snively, W. D.: Body Fluid Disturbances, New York, Grune & Stratton, 1962.

37. MacBryde, C. M.: Adrenal cortex hormones: influence on water balance and electrolyte metabolism, Missouri Med. 51:740–742, 1954.

38. ———: Significance of recent studies with ACTH and cortisone, J. Missouri Med. Ass. 47:905–909, 1950.

39. Reichstein, T.: A new adrenal hormone, Lancet 2:551, 1953.

40. Hills, A. G., *et al.*: Adrenal cortical regulation of distribution of water and electrolytes in human body, J. Clin. Invest. 32:1236–1247, 1953.

41. Gilman, A., and Brazeau, P.: The role of the kidney in the regulation of acid-base metabolism, Amer. J. Med. 15:765–770, 1953.

42. Black, D. A. K.: Body-fluid depletion, Lancet 1:305–311, 1953.

43. Leaf, A., and Newburgh, L. H.: Significance of the Body Fluids in Clinical Medicine, Springfield, Ill., Thomas, 1955.

44. Overman, R. R.: Sodium, potassium and chloride alterations in disease, Physiol. Rev. 31:285–311, 1951.

45. Adolph, E. F., Barker, J. P., and Hoy, P. A.: Multiple factors in thirst, Amer. J. Physiol. 178:538–562, 1954.

46. Pitts, R. F.: Modern concepts of acid-base regulation, A. M. A. Arch. Intern. Med. 89:864–876, 1952.

47. Mudge, G. H.: Renal mechanisms of electrolyte transport, *in* Clarke, H. T. (ed.): Ion Transport Across Membranes, New York, Academic Press, 1954.

48. Robinson, J. R., and McCance, R. A.: Water metabolism, Ann. Rev. Physiol. 14:115–142, 1952.

49. Smith, H. W.: The Kidney; Structure and Function in Health and Disease, New York, Oxford, 1951.

50. Robinson, S.: Salt conservation by kidneys and sweat glands in men, Fed. Proc. 13:119–120, 1954.

51. Bergstrom, W. H., and Wallace, W. M.: Bone as a sodium and potassium reservoir, J. Clin. Invest. 33:867–873, 1954.

52. Danowski, T. S.: Fundamental features of metabolism of sodium and potassium, Amer. J. Clin. Path. 23:1095–1099, 1953.

53. Blahd, W. H., and Bassett, S. H.: Potassium deficiency in man, Metabolism 2:218–224, 1953.

54. Black, D.: Sodium Metabolism in Health and Disease, Oxford, England, Blackwell, 1952.

55. Schroeder, H. A.: Renal failure associated with low extracellular sodium chloride; low salt syndrome, J.A.M.A. 141:117–124, 1949.

56. Leaf, A.: The clinical and physiologic significance of the serum sodium concentration, New Eng. J. Med. 267:24–30; 77–83, 1962.

57. Leaf, A., and Santos, R. F.: Physiologic mechanisms in potassium deficiency, New Eng. J. Med. 264:335–341, 1961.

58. Wolf, A. V.: Osmometric analysis of thirst in man and dog, Amer. J. Physiol. 161:75, 1950.

59. ———: Thirst, Springfield, Ill., Thomas, 1958.

60. Andersson, B.: Water and electrolyte metabolism in the goat, Acta Physiol. Scand., 28:188, 1953; 33:50, 1955; 35:312, 1956.

61. Verney, E. B.: Croonian Lecture: The antidiuretic hormone and factors which determine its release, Proc. Roy. Soc., London (Biol.) 135:25, 1947.

62. Bargmann, W., and Scharrer, E.: Site of origin of the hormones of the posterior pituitary, Amer. Sci. 39:255–259, 1951.

63. Verney, E. B.: Agents determining and influencing functions of pars nervosa of pituitary, Brit. Med. J. 2:119–123, 1948.

64. Conn, J. W.: Aldosteronism in man, J.A.M.A. 183:775–781, 871–878, 1963.

65. Belding, H. S.: Hazards to health: work in hot weather, New Eng. J. Med. 267:1052–1054, 1962.

66. Kuno, Y.: Human Perspiration, Springfield, Ill., Thomas, 1956.

67. Robinson, S., and Robinson, A. H.: Chemical composition of sweat, Physiol. Rev. 34:202, 1954.

68. Laragh, J. H., et al.: Hypotensive agents and pressor substances: effects of epinephrine, norepinephrine, angiotensin II, etc., on the secretory rate of aldosterone in man, J.A.M.A. 174:234–240, 1960.

69. Schwartz, W. B., et al.: A syndrome of renal sodium loss and hyponatremia probably resulting from inappropriate secretion of antidiuretic hormone, Amer. J. Med. 23:529, 1957.

70. Welt, L. G.: Clinical Disorders of Hydration and Acid-Base Equilibrium, ed. 2, Boston, Little, Brown, 1959.

71. Albrink, M. J., et al.: The displacement of serum water by the lipids of hyperlipemic serum, J. Clin. Invest. 34:1483, 1955.

71A. Davis, J. E., et al.: Salt and water depletion caused by villous rectosigmoid adenomas, Ann. Surg. 155:806, 1962.

72. Winsor, T.: Potassium and digitalis intoxication, Amer. Heart J. 60:151, 1960.

73. Kunin, A. S., et al.: Decrease in serum potassium and cardiac arrythmias, New Eng. J. Med. 266:228, 1962.

74. Lown, B., et al.: Digitalis, electrolytes, and surgical patient, Amer. J. Cardiol. 6:309, 1960.

75. Bartter, F. C.: The role of aldosterone in normal homeostasis and in certain disease states, Metabolism 5:369–383, 1956.

76. Friedberg, C.: Heart, Kidney and Electrolytes, New York, Grune & Stratton, 1962.

77. Maxwell, M. H., and Kleeman, C. R.: Clinical Disorders of Fluid and Electrolyte Metabolism, New York, McGraw-Hill, 1962.

78. Pitts, R. F.: Physiology of the Kidney and Body Fluids, ed. 2, Chicago, Year Book Pub., 1968.

79. Kipnis, D., Klahr, S., and McGuigan, J.: Severe diarrhea, dehydration and acidosis, Amer. J. Med. 43:452–460, 1967.

80. Garrahan, P., and Glynn, I.: Uncoupling sodium pump, Nature (London) 207:1098, 1965.

81. Berg, G., and Chapman, B.: Sodium and potassium activated ATPase of intestinal epithelium. I. Location of enzymatic activity in cell, J. Cell. Comp. Physiol. 65:361–372, 1965.

82. Hirschorn, N., Saha, J., and Rosenberg, I.: Sodium-potassium-activated ATPase in human small intestine: reversible depression in cholera and acute gastroenteritis, J. Clin. Invest. 45:1023, 1966.

83. Katz, A., and Epstein, F.: Role of sodium-potassium activated adenosine triphosphatase in reabsorption of sodium by the kidney, J. Clin. Invest. 46:1999–2011, 1967.

84. Katz, A., and Epstein, F.: Physiologic role of $Na-K-ATPase$ in the transport of cations across biologic membranes, New Eng. J. Med. 278:253–261, 1968.

85. Skou, J. C.: Further investigations on Mg^{++} + Na^{+}-activated ATPase, possibly related to active, linked transport of Na^{+} and K^{+} across cell membrane, Biochim. Biophys. Acta 42:6–23, 1960.

86. Glynn, I. M.: Action of cardiac glycosides on ion movements, Pharmacol. Rev. 16:381–407, 1964.

87. Hoffman, J. F.: Red cell membrane and transport of sodium and potassium, Amer. J. Med. 41:666–680, 1966.

88. Han, Y. H., and Lowe, H. J.: Humidification of inspired air, J.A.M.A. 205:91–94, 1968.

89. Walker, W. G.: Diuretic-induced metabolic alkalosis, J.A.M.A. 205:943, 1968.

90. Thorn, G. W.: Approach to the patient with "Idiopathic edema" or "Periodic swelling," J.A.M.A. 206:333–338, 1968.

91. Shear, L., Bonkowsky, H. L., and Gabuzda, G. J.: Renal tubular acidosis in cirrhosis: determinant of susceptibility to recurrent hepatic precoma, New Eng. J. Med. 280:1–7, 1969.

92. Bank, N.: Physiological basis of diuretic action, Ann. Rev. Med. 19:103–118, 1968.

93. Edelman, I. S., and Liebman, J.: Anatomy of body water and electrolytes, Amer. J. Med. 27:256, 1959.

94. Welt, L. C.: Water balance in health and disease, *in* Diseases of Metabolism, Duncan, G. C., (ed.) ed. 4, Philadelphia, Saunders, 1964.

95. Kleeman, C. R., and Richman, M. P.: The clinical physiology of water metabolism, New Eng. J. Med. 270:1300–1307, 1967.

96. Sharp, G., and Leaf, A.: Mechanism of action of aldosterone, Physiol. Rev. 41:593–633, 1966.

97. Gross, F.: The regulation of aldosterone secretion by the renin-angiotensin system under various conditions, Acta Endocr. (supp. 124) pp. 41–64, 1967.

36

Edema

HENRY A. SCHROEDER

Physiologic Considerations
    Vascular Factors
    Mechanisms Controlling Body Fluids
    Disturbances of Regulation of Body
       Fluids Common to Most Forms of
       Edema

**Edema Caused by Primary Transudation
of Fluids from Blood to Tissue Spaces**
    Edema Due to Changes in Capillary
       Blood Pressure
    Edema Due to Increased Permeability
       of Capillaries
    Edema Due to Decreased Osmotic
       Pressure of Plasma
    Edema Due to Decreased Tissue Pressure
    Edema of Lymph Stasis

**Edema Caused by Primary Renal Retention
of Salt and Water**
    Edema Due to Unknown Causes
    Edema Due to Multiple Factors
       Edema of Portal Venous Obstruction
       Edema of Pregnancy
       Edema of Beriberi
       Edema of Congestive Circulatory
       * Failure*
       Edema of Renal Disease

DEFINITION

Claude Bernard said:

Animals have really two environments: a *milieu extérieur* in which the organism is situated, and a *milieu intérieur* in which the tissue elements live. The living organism does not really exist in the *milieu extérieur* (the atmosphere if it breathes, salt or fresh water if that is its element) but in the liquid *milieu intérieur* formed by the circulating organic liquid which surrounds and bathes all the tissue elements; this is the lymph or plasma. . . . The *milieu intérieur* surrounding the organs, the tissues and their elements never varies, atmospheric changes cannot penetrate beyond it and it is therefore true to say that the physical conditions of environment are unchanging in a higher animal: each one is surrounded by this invariable *milieu* which is, as it were, an atmosphere proper to itself in an ever-changing cosmic environment. Here we have an organism which has enclosed itself in a kind of hot-house. The perpetual changes of external conditions cannot reach it; it is not subject to them, but is free and independent. . . . All the vital mechanisms, however varied they may be, have only one object, that of preserving constant the conditions of life in the internal environment.[1]

Edema is merely the result of expansion of the *milieu intérieur*, or the extracellular fluid of the body.

Edema is a sign common to a variety of diseases. It may be defined as any abnormal accumulation of extravascular extracellular (interstitial) fluid. The source of the fluid is the blood plasma. All edema comes from the circulating blood and its composition is similar to that of plasma, containing electrolytes (principally sodium, chloride, and bicarbonate), glucose, urea, creatinine, amino acids, and various other diffusible crystalloid substances. On the other hand, its protein content depends upon the cause of the edema, varying from the negligible quantities usually encountered in most states of chronic edema to the concentrations approaching those of plasma seen in severe local traumatic conditions.

Edema can be general or localized to a particular area or organ. When it is general, relatively large amounts of water must accumulate in the tissue spaces before swelling can be detected by physical examination. A patient's body weight may increase nearly 10 per cent before "pitting" edema becomes evident. It is obvious that diffusion of such large amounts of water and electrolytes into tissue spaces must be accompanied or preceded by the renal retention of water and electrolytes in order to maintain plasma volume. The normal ratio of plasma to extracellular fluid volume is about 1:3. If the large volume of edema fluid lost

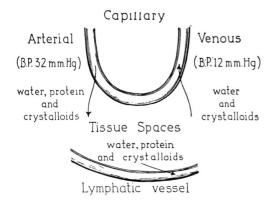

Capillary

Arterial
(B.P. 32 mm.Hg)

Venous
(B.P. 12 mm.Hg)

water, protein
and
crystalloids

water
and
crystalloids

Tissue Spaces

water, protein
and crystalloids

Lymphatic vessel

FIG. 36-1. Principal structures involved in the normal interchange of tissue fluid.

from the blood were not replaced, hypovolemia sufficient to induce severe vascular shock would occur. Small localized accumulations of edema fluid may develop without affecting the general circulation; large amounts of necessity must be accompanied by replacement, which usually means retention, and retention requires ingestion or injection.

Knowledge of the pathologic physiology of the formation of edema is incomplete. There appear to be two general groups. The first is composed of those types in which fluid from plasma primarily transudes into tissue spaces, setting in motion a mechanism for its replacement by the renal retention of salt and water and the formation of other elements lost to the circulating blood. The second comprises those types in which the primary derangement is in the renal excretion of salt and water, leading to transudation of fluid from plasma into tissue spaces. In either variety, the composition of the fluid retained may be altered in terms of concentration of electrolytes or acid-base balance. The relative amounts of fluid and electrolytes ingested and the metabolic and the renal losses apparently govern these alterations. Therefore, edema is to be considered as a derangement of water and

* For purposes of simplification in this discussion, the capillary bed is considered as a continuous network of vessels branching from arterioles and then anastomosing into larger channels on their venous ends. This is not actually the case. The capillary system must be considered as being similar to an irrigation system, with arteriovenous anastomoses, side channels, small capillary beds, and plexuses, which are constantly changing, shutting off blood from some channels and opening others. The capillary bed appears to depart from the general configuration of the arterial and venous systems, each of which resembles a river system with its watershed and tributaries.

electrolyte balance in one direction; dehydration is its counterpart, although under exceptional circumstances an edematous patient may also be dehydrated (see Table 36-1).

PHYSIOLOGIC CONSIDERATIONS

The vascular factors that lead to the formation of edema in general comprise disturbances of one or more of the normal functions governing the exchange of fluid between the intravascular and extravascular fluid compartments. These are: (1) capillary permeability, (2) capillary blood pressure, (3) colloid osmotic pressure of plasma, (4) colloid osmotic pressure of tissue fluid, (5) tissue pressure, and (6) factors influencing the formation and flow of lymph. Figure 36-1 depicts diagrammatically the principal local vascular structures involved in the normal interchange of tissue fluid.*

The general mechanisms that affect the formation of edema fluid are principally those that concern the regulation of water and electrolyte balance: (1) renal arterial and venous pressure, (2) the renal retention of electrolytes and water as influenced by extrarenal hormonal regulatory mechanisms or by intrinsic renal diseases, (3) the dietary intake of salt and water, (4) the excretion of salt and water by other than renal routes (stool, expired air, sweat, and pathologic drainage), and (5) the formation or destruction of plasma proteins.

VASCULAR FACTORS

Capillary Permeability. The area of capillary wall available for fluid interchange is extremely large. It is estimated[2] that in a man who weighs 50 kg. the area of the capillaries in his skeletal muscles alone is 6,300 m.[2] (over 1.5 acres), that their lengths total 100,000 km., and that 1 ml. of blood is exposed to a filtering surface of 0.5 to 0.7 m.[2] From animal experiments it has been determined that the capillary wall is so permeable to water and electrolytes that the entire plasma volume of a man would be filtered through his capillaries within ten seconds if there were no forces operating to retain fluid within the blood vascular system.[3] The capillary walls are permeable to all of the normal constituents of blood plasma except protein, to which they are only slightly permeable. In general, those substances that are filtered by the glomeruli of the kidney are filtered by the general capillary bed into interstitial fluid spaces. For example, inulin, which is used to measure glomerular filtration rate, also can be used to measure total interstitial fluid volume because its relatively large molecule appears to filter through capillary walls as it is filtered by glomerular capillaries. The ability of any substance to pass through capillary interstices depends probably not only on the size of its molecule but also upon its shape.

Both filtration and diffusion account for the interchange of substances between plasma and cells.[4] Capillaries, however, have diverse structures as seen by the electron microscope. Those of liver, intestine, and kidney showed pores of small size, whereas none were demonstrable in muscle, skin, connective tissue, and lung.[5] By infusion of dextran of differing molecular weights, and then measuring the amounts in lymph, it has been shown inferentially that capillaries were completely permeable to molecules of about 20 Å radius, slightly permeable to those of 30 to 40 Å radii, with some residual permeability of much larger molecules. Liver capillaries passed the largest molecules of 200 Å or greater.[6] Diffusion of lipid-soluble substances occurs directly through the capillary wall, or perhaps by active transport.[4]

Capillary Blood Pressure. The blood pressure in the capillary provides the force necessary to filter fluid through the permeable capillary walls. The driving force for filtration, therefore, comes from the heart. Blood pressure in the capillaries is controlled principally by the arterioles from which the capillaries arise. Localized arteriolar constriction will reduce blood pressure and flow in capillaries if systemic arterial pressure remains unchanged. Arteriolar dilation will lead to increased flow and pressure if systemic pressure is unchanged. However, widespread changes in arteriolar diameter are accompanied by changes in systemic blood pressure, inasmuch as the arterioles provide much of the peripheral resistance to flow and so govern the level of pressure. From these considerations, it is obvious that the force of filtration which comes from the blood pressure and the amount of fluid filtered from the blood can be altered by changes in arteriolar diameter, changes in systemic blood pressure, and changes in the total flow of blood or cardiac output.

As blood passes from arteriole to precapillary to capillary, there occurs a fall of pressure and a diminution in the amount of fluid within the capillary; further along toward the venular end restoration of fluid in the venule takes place. These changes depend upon pressure gradients. Pressure in the arteriolar limb of the capillary has been shown by direct measurements to be approximately 32 mm. Hg, whereas the pressure in the venous limb is in the neighborhood of 12 mm.[7] The average pressure in the entire capillary bed is approximately equivalent to the colloid osmotic pressure of the plasma proteins (24 mm.).[7] Owing to the gradient between the arteriolar and the venous ends of the capillary, conditions favor filtration in the arteriolar portion, and reabsorption in the venous portion.

Capillary pressure is extremely variable, depending upon arteriolar vasomotion, total flow, freedom of venous outflow, posture, temperature, neurogenic influences, and all other circulatory factors.[8] In a given capillary, at one moment, filtration may predominate, and at another, reabsorption. Although the volume of fluid entering the tissue spaces varies considerably with circulatory adjustments,[8] the total daily exchange is remarkably constant, neither dehydration nor edema developing normally.

Pressure in capillaries naturally may be altered by venous pressure. A high local or systemic venous pressure may be transmitted retrograde to venules and may alter the normal gradient. Such alterations would result in a tendency for less filtered fluid to be reabsorbed in the venular ends of the capillaries. Although systemic venous pressure measured in brachial or great veins is usually considerably lower (7 mm. Hg) than that obtained in the venular end of the capillary loop (12 mm. Hg), increases in pressure in the upright position (to 35 to 40 mm. Hg) easily could be transmitted to the venules and could influence markedly the reabsorption of fluids in the lower part of the body were it not for the many valves found in medium-sized veins. A high venous pressure, however, may be transmitted through valves if venous distention or congestion is present, and thus cause venular stasis.

Therefore, exchange of fluid between blood and tissue spaces is affected by the general level of arterial pressure as related to the state of the arterioles, the general level of venous pressure, the state of the venules and veins, which have vasomotor controls, and by the pressure-flow relationships in any given segment of the circulation. No part of the arterio-venous circulation can be considered as a passive system of tubes. When effective pressure is increased, filtration also is increased; when pressure is decreased, filtration falls.

Colloid Osmotic Pressure of Blood Plasma. Opposing the filtration force of the capillary blood pressure is the colloid osmotic pressure (oncotic pressure) of plasma—minus the colloid osmotic pressure of other tissue fluids. Both plasma and interstitial fluids have considerable oncotic pressure since they both contain approximately the same concentration of electrolytes, urea, sugar, and other diffusible materials. The principal difference between them lies in their protein content, which accounts for only about 5 per cent of the total oncotic pressure of plasma.[9] The pressure exerted by plasma protein opposes the filtration of fluids and dissolved substances and favors the reabsorption of water and of these substances. When capillary pressure is higher than plasma oncotic pressure, filtration will occur; when it is lower, reabsorption will take place.

The importance of colloid osmotic pressure in controlling fluid interchange was first demonstrated by Starling in 1896.[10] Having rendered one hind leg of a dog edematous by infiltrating it with hypertonic sodium chloride solution, Starling perfused both hind legs through the femoral arteries with defibrinated blood. The passage of blood through the edematous leg caused the edema to disappear; the returning blood was diluted by the absorbed edema fluid. Blood passing through the control leg remained unchanged. When the experiment was repeated using protein-free salt solution as the perfusing fluid, the edema fluid was not absorbed. Starling thus demonstrated that the absorption of fluid from the edematous limb was dependent upon the presence of protein in the perfusate, and concluded that the protein acted by exerting a difference of osmotic pressure within the vascular system. He later measured the osmotic pressure of the serum colloid directly and found it to be approximately 30 mm. Hg.

Subsequent measurements of the colloid osmotic pressure of human plasma have shown it to be nearer 25 mm. Hg than 30.[11] The relatively large protein molecules of the plasma exert their osmotic pull within the capillary because of their inability to pass through most capillary walls. The smaller molecules of electrolytes, urea, and sugar, although capable in solution of exerting much greater osmotic pressure, have no effect on fluid exchange as they pass freely through capillary walls. Because of the Donnan equilibrium, some of the crystalloids of the blood which do not pass freely exert an osmotic effect. The osmotic pressure exerted by plasma albumin is much greater than that exerted by globulin. One gram per cent of albumin (molecular weight about 70,000) exerts a pressure of 5.5 mm. Hg; one gram per cent of the much larger globulin is responsible for a pressure of only 1.4 mm.[12] The difference is largely due to the smaller molecular weight of albumin, because the pressure is proportional to the number of particles.

Chemical analyses of edema fluid and lymph indicate that the normal capillary endothelium acts as a semipermeable membrane, allowing the free passage of water and crystalloids and at the same time preventing the larger protein molecules of the plasma from escaping into the tissue fluid.[13] The quantitative relationship of the concentrations of protein and salt in blood and edema fluid corresponds closely to that which Donnan proved must exist in an equilibrium established across an inert semipermeable membrane. Since the capillary endothelium normally retains more than 95 per cent of the plasma protein,[8] it may be concluded that the effective colloid osmotic pressure in the body is only slightly less than estimated from measurements made in vitro.

As blood passes along the capillary and filtration of water and dissolved substances occurs, it is obvious that the protein concentration in the blood at the distal end of the capillaries must be increased. An increase in the concentration of plasma protein favors the reabsorption of water; this factor acts on the venular side.

The formation of edema fluids may be profoundly affected by changes in the colloid osmotic pressure of the plasma. Concentration of plasma protein may favor increased reabsorption of tissue fluids and produce dehydration; dilution of plasma protein favors increased filtration and decreased reabsorption of tissue fluids. The balance is probably a very delicate equilibrium, disturbed by small changes.

Colloid Osmotic Pressure of Tissue Fluid. If an appreciable quantity of protein were present in the extravascular fluid, it would tend to counteract the osmotic pressure exerted by the plasma proteins within the capillary. Although regional differences in capillary permeability exist within the body,

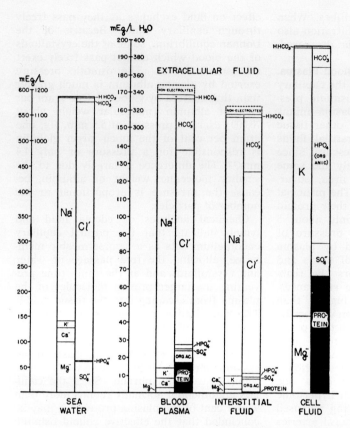

Fig. 36-2. Chemical anatomy of body fluids in terms of acid-base equivalence. (Gamble, J. L.: Chemical Anatomy, Physiology, and Pathology of Extracellular Fluid, Boston, The Harvard Medical School)

the amount of protein in the extravascular fluid is normally less than 5 per cent of that present in the blood.[8] Landis and his co-workers have presented indirect evidence that the capillary filtrate from the blood averages only 0.3 per cent protein.[14] Under normal circumstances, therefore, the colloid osmotic pressure of the tissue fluids is so small that it may be virtually ignored. It becomes significant only under conditions wherein vascular damage causes an increase in the permeability of the capillary endothelium, or when protein removal by lymphatics is disturbed, causing concentration.

Mechanical Pressure in Tissue Spaces. The space available in tissues for the accommodation of extravascular fluid is limited. When the volume of tissue fluid is increased above normal, the tissue elements must be separated and further filtration of fluid is opposed by the pressure required to cause the separation. Accurate measurements of normal tissue pressure are difficult to obtain, and the values reported by different investigators are inconsistent.[8] It is thought that the normal cutaneous tissue pressure amounts to approximately 7 mm.

Hg, whereas subcutaneous tissue pressure is appreciably less, ranging from 2 to 4 mm. Hg.[15] As the volume of interstitial fluid increases and the tissues are stretched, the tissue pressure rises appreciably.[16]

There is experimental evidence that tissue pressure is an important factor in the prevention of edema. Direct measurements in edematous patients reveal that there is always an elevation in pressure relative to the clinical status of the edema.[16] Warren, Merrill and Stead[17] have observed that when tourniquets are placed about the limbs of a dog for a period of 5 hours, plasma volume can be maintained with much less visible edema if the animal has a relatively tight skin. They conclude that the pressure of interstitial fluid (directly related to tissue tension) is a more important antifiltration factor than the volume of fluid and that the pressure exerts its effect by decreasing filtration at the arteriolar end of the capillary, increasing absorption at the venous end and augmenting the flow of lymph. Finally, it is a common clinical observation that patients who have recently lost weight or who have had previous bouts of extensive edema

TABLE 36-1. PERIPHERAL FACTORS LEADING TO
TRANSUDATION OF FLUID FROM PLASMA INTO TISSUES

TYPE OF DISTURBANCE	HYDROSTATIC PRESSURE		OSMOTIC PRESSURE		CHANGE TENDING TO RESTORE EQUILIBRIUM
	Capillary Blood Pressure	Tissue Pressure	Plasma Oncotic Pressure	Tissue Oncotic Pressure	
Equilibrium	$\dfrac{P_A + P_V}{2}$ —	P_T =	OP_P —	OP_T	....
Capillary blood pressure increased					
Arteriolar dilation	$P_A\uparrow$ —	N >	N —	N	$P_V\downarrow$ $P_T\uparrow$
Venous hypertension	$P_V\uparrow$ —	N >	N —	N	$P_T\uparrow$
Capillary permeability increased	N —	N >	N —	$\uparrow$	$P_T\uparrow$
Hypoproteinemia	N —	N >	$\downarrow$ —	N	$P_T\uparrow$
Decreased tissue pressure	N —	$\downarrow$ >	N —	N	$P_T\to N$

Symbols: P_A = Pressure at arteriolar end of capillary.
P_V = Pressure at venular end of capillary.
P_T = Tissue pressure.
OP_P = Plasma oncotic pressure.
OP_T = Tissue fluid oncotic pressure.

The dynamic formula from which this simplified one was derived is as follows:

Filtration = $P_A - OP_P - P_T + OP_T = P_T - OP_T + OP_P - P_V$ = Resorption

exhibit a striking tendency to become edematous.[18] Loss of normal tissue elasticity in such cases apparently diminishes the normal mechanical resistance to fluid accumulation. The dependent edema seen sometimes in aged persons may be accounted for by this factor.

The Flow of Lymph. As suggested in Figure 36-1, the lymphatics play an important role in controlling the interchange of fluids between capillaries and tissue spaces. Fluid within the lymphatic vessels contains appreciable quantities of protein, indicating that the walls of the lymphatics are permeable to the large protein molecules.[19] This finding is not surprising since it is well known that foreign particles, including large bacteria, are rapidly taken up by the lymphatic system when injected into various tissues of the body. That the preservation of normal intercellular fluid volume depends at least in part upon lymph flow is well demonstrated by the comprehensive studies of Drinker and his collaborators.[19] For example, such factors as venous congestion and muscular activity (which tend to increase the amount of fluid leaving the capillaries) cause an appreciable increase in the flow of lymph. Similarly, experimental procedures that lower the effective osmotic

pressure of the blood, either by injuring the capillary wall or by decreasing the concentration of protein in the plasma, cause an increased amount of fluid to escape from the capillaries into the tissue spaces and thus bring about an increase in the flow of lymph. The importance of the lymphatics is demonstrated dramatically when the normal functioning of lymphatic vessels is impaired.

Extracellular-Intracellular Relationships. The normal compositions of extracellular and intracellular fluids are shown in Figure 36-2. Cellular membranes also are semipermeable, but of a specialized variety. It is obvious that pronounced changes in extracellular osmotic pressure will influence intracellular fluids as well. The interchange of potassium, magnesium, and sodium salts may be affected by changes in concentration of extracellular fluids and may have profound effects upon cellular metabolism. Overhydration or dehydration of cells may occur. These alterations must be borne in mind during any consideration of fluid exchange and regulation.

Summary. The factors favoring filtration of fluid from plasma into tissues are: the blood pressure at the arteriolar end of the capillary minus the colloid osmotic pressure of the plasma, minus the mechanical pressure in the tissue spaces, plus the colloid osmotic pressure of the tissue fluid itself. The factors favoring reabsorption of fluid from tissues into blood are: the tissue pressure, plus the colloid osmotic pressure of plasma, minus the colloid osmotic pressure of tissue fluid, minus the blood pressure at the venous end of the capillary. During a state of equilibrium, the sum of the factors favoring filtration and the sum of those favoring reabsorption are equal. A disturbance or change in any one of these factors will lead either to increased filtration or increased reabsorption until equilibrium is again established (Table 36-1). This equation can be stated more simply: the colloid osmotic pressure of plasma, minus the colloid osmotic pressure of tissue fluid, must equal the average intracapillary pressure (half the sum of the pressure at the arteriolar end and the pressure at the venous end), minus the tissue pressure. If edema is

formed, one of these four factors is disturbed and transudation of fluid continues until there is an increase in tissue pressure great enough to overcome it, or until the disturbed factor itself is restored toward normal.

MECHANISMS CONTROLLING BODY FLUIDS

Fluid balance is normally achieved by regulatory mechanisms mediated by the kidney. The substances concerned are principally water and sodium chloride, although other electrolytes and electrolytic substances may play a part. Water is excreted in expired air, in stools, in sweat and insensible perspiration and in urine. Unless pathologic conditions are present, the amount excreted by way of expired air is quite constant, varying with the humidity of the inspired air; about 500 ml. per day are lost through this route. The stools normally contain little water, although in some pathologic condi-

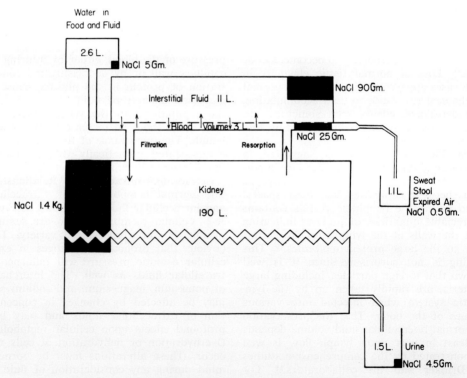

FIG. 36-3. Diagram of the total daily fluid interchange in the kidneys. The volumes are of such magnitude compared with the intake and output that relatively small absolute changes of one function without compensation by another lead to serious imbalance. Sodium chloride exchange is shown by the proportionate black squares. Bicarbonate and other anions have been ignored in the diagram for simplification, chloride being shown in terms of sodium. There is free interchange of salt and water between blood and tissue fluid.

TABLE 36-2. PRINCIPAL FACTORS FOUND OR PROPOSED FOR
REGULATING EXTRACELLULAR FLUID VOLUME

Substance Affected	Function of Circulation	Stimulus	Receptors	Mechanisms or Effects
Retention by Distal Renal Tubules				
Water	Blood volume	Reduced	Left atrium	Vasopressin
	Blood pressure	Reduced	Thyrocarotid	Vasopressin
	Osmolarity	Increased	Midbrain	Vasopressin
Salt	Blood volume	Reduced	Right atrium	Aldosterone-
	Blood pressure	Reduced	Carotid sinus	stimulating hormone(s) and ACTH
	Osmolarity	Reduced	Unknown	
Excretion by Distal Renal Tubules				
Water	Blood volume	Increased		
	Blood pressure	Increased	Unknown ? passive	(Lack of active hormones ?)
	Osmolarity	Reduced		
Salt	Blood volume	Increased	Unknown ? passive	
	Blood pressure	Increased	Unknown	(Lack of active hormones ?)
	Osmolarity	Increased	Unknown ? passive	
Intrarenal Retention or Excretion				
Water and salt	Blood pressure	Reduced	Unknown	Glomerular filtration reduced, tubular reabsorption increased
		Increased	Unknown	Glomerular filtration increased, tubular reabsorption reduced
	Osmolarity	Reduced	Unknown	Proximal tubular reabsorption of NaCl increased
		Increased	Unknown	

tions they contain so much as seriously to deplete the body and cause shock and death. Insensible perspiration depends upon the environment, as does the amount of sweat. It is not known whether the amount is controlled by other influences than environmental temperature, although sweating has a neurogenic control in part. High environmental temperatures very rapidly may deplete the body of water and of salt and thus cause hemoconcentration and diminish the volume of blood and interstitial fluid (see Chap. 35). The sodium and chloride content of sweat is apparently under hormonal control and is influenced by the activity of the adrenal cortex, the concentrations normally being about one-third that of plasma.

Renal Regulation of Water and Electrolyte Balance. The kidneys perform a marvelously exact function of regulating the water and electrolyte content of the body. To understand this mechanism, one must examine the function of the nephron and consider the several ways in which fluid and electrolyte balance may be affected. The situation in the nephron is basically similar to that in other capillaries and is governed by the same mechanisms: those of filtration and reabsorption. The complexity of the kidney as a specialized structure for excretion from the body lies principally in the addition to simple capillary filtration and venular reabsorption the structures necessary for reabsorption against osmotic pressure. The tubules perform work, the capillary bed probably does not.* Water, salts, and substances dissolved in plasma are filtered by the glomerular capillaries at a high pressure, about 75 mm. Hg. These substances then are reabsorbed by tubular epithelium back into peritubular capillary blood, some actively by

* The mucosa of the gastrointestinal tract and the tubules of sweat and of salivary glands may also perform work against osmotic pressure and be regulated by hormonal influences. Active transport in other capillaries has been suggested.

the performance of work, some passively by diffusion or by increased osmotic pressure of efferent arteriolar blood, which contains proteins concentrated by about 20 per cent. Water and salts are principally reabsorbed by the proximal tubules, the total during a day being about 190 liters and 1.4 kg., respectively. The distal tubules further concentrate the urine and adjust its pH to the needs of the body's acid-base balance. Obviously a very small change in filtration or reabsorption could have profound consequences: a 1 per cent variation would result in loss or gain of 1.9 liters of extracellular fluid—the difference between dehydration and early edema (Fig. 36-3).

It is unlikely that all of the regulatory mechanisms of such a vital function as fluid and electrolyte balance are known. However, several have been found. Powerful intrinsic intrarenal mechanisms exist; in fact, the kidney probably would perform adequately without its extrinsic nervous and hormonal influences, although it could not respond rapidly to small changes. There are direct autonomic nervous effects, and at least two hormones, one affecting retention of water and one affecting retention of sodium chloride. The subject is complex, confused, and only partially understood. It is well to examine separately the influences governing osmolarity as affecting: (1) water, (2) sodium chloride, (3) blood volume, and (4) blood pressure (Table 36-2).

Intrinsic Renal Controls. Glomerular filtration and tubular reabsorption can markedly affect water and electrolyte balances, as will be discussed. In chronic hyponatremia, for example, proximal tubules absorb excessive sodium from glomerular filtrate.[20] There are intrinsic "reflexes" maintaining renal blood flow and oxygen tension in spite of lowered perfusion pressures, the latter, however, occurring at the expense of an acid cortex.[21,22] These mechanisms are highly important and little understood.

Renin, secreted probably from juxtaglomerular cells, appears to cause release of aldosterone (and other adrenal hormones) from the adrenal cortex.[23] The stimulus for release of renin is almost always reduction in renal blood flow. The evidence strongly suggests that the effector substance formed by renin, angiotensin, stimulates the adrenal cortex of dogs[24,25] and, in vitro, of cattle,[26] as well as producing vasoconstriction (see Chapter 15). Thus arterial pressure would be raised and blood volume would tend to

be restored by the same hormone. The clinical significance of these experiments is unknown.

Hormonal Controls. Active reabsorption of water by the distal tubules is governed by the antidiuretic hormone (ADH), called vasopressin, an octapeptide formed in the paraventricular nuclei and supraoptic area, released from and stored in the posterior pituitary (neurohypophysis). Release, under control from the hypothalamic region, depends largely upon hyperosmolarity.[27] Osmoreceptors, critically sensitive to changes in the concentration of plasma electrolytes, have been demonstrated indirectly in the hypothalamus[28] and perhaps in other areas, governing secretion of vasopressin from moment to moment. Chemical structure is partly species-specific, in that hog vasopressin differs in one amino acid, lysine, from the primate and other animal ADH hormones, which have arginine. It also constricts smooth muscle of arteries and arterioles, probably through an intermediary mechanism, because it is inactive on the isolated rabbit aortic strip. Excessive amounts can be overcome by opposing influences preventing overhydration; however, no diuretic hormone has been isolated.

Active reabsorption of sodium by the distal tubules is governed mainly by aldosterone, a potent steroid formed by the zona glomerulosa of the adrenal cortex.[30] One manner of release may be through angiotensin.[32] Changes in electrolyte concentrations of adrenal perfusates have failed to show direct effects on adrenal venous contents of this hormone. Adrenocorticotropic hormone (ACTH) apparently affects it only under certain conditions and may not be its principal regulator (although prolonged use in human beings often leads to edema from salt retention). A relatively simple indole substance, structurally related to melanotonin and obtained from the area of the midbrain, "adrenoglomerulotropin," has been found to cause release[31]; its existence has been disputed.[32] Although active tubular reabsorption of sodium chloride by aldosterone can be overcome by opposing influences at a new level, preventing cellular dehydration, no natruretic hormone has been isolated or identified. However, a large part of the activity of whole adrenal extracts rests in the amorphous fraction, a fact often forgotten under the enthusiasm of dealing with pure compounds, of which the adrenal contains several.

Nervous Controls. The hormones with target sites in the kidney are apparently somewhat under nervous control. Antidiuretic hormone, released by the neurohypophysis, is affected by volume or stretch receptors in the left atrium and pulmonary veins.[33,34] Impulses are transmitted via the glossopharyngeal and vagus nerves to the medulla and thence to the hypothalamus, the exact central pathways not yet having been discovered. Both stimulatory and inhibitory fibers appear to be present. Similar receptors have been found on the arterial side, at the thyrocarotid junction. Therefore, both arterial and venous pressure may influence the release of vasopressin, so that volume, in terms of pressure, and concentration, in terms of osmolarity, are apparently mediated by nervous mechanisms in respect to water.

In respect to electrolytes, aldosterone also may be governed in part by nerves. Although the most potent stimulus to aldosterone secretion is a lowering of the intake of sodium chloride, this hormone also may be under control by both volume and pressor receptors, the former apparently situated in the right atrium, whereas the latter are perhaps in the thyrocarotid junction.[35] Afferent pathways appear to pass via the ninth and tenth cranial nerves to the hypothalamic region. Efferent influences are probably hormonal, through aldosterone-stimulating hormone(s), possibly also by release of adrenoglomerulotropin.[31] Sympathetic renal nerves also may affect sodium retention partially; when one adrenal is removed from dogs, thereby cutting part of that kidney's nerve supply, sodium and chloride are excreted differentially by the homolateral kidney.[36] The mechanism is unexplained. It must be emphasized that these nervous mechanisms appear to be of secondary physiologic importance, derangements not causing overt disease. Many clinical conditions involving disturbances are not necessarily associated with imbalances of water or electrolytes.

All vital functions are controlled by opposing influences providing readily adjustable balances under "tension." The perceptive renologist immediately will note that liberation of both antidiuretic hormone (to retain water) and aldosterone (to retain salt) is opposed by lack of release, leaving glomerular filtration rate and tubular reabsorption as the "opposing force" in the net balances of body water and salt. Teleologi-

cally speaking, these "forceless" influences leave much to be desired. A nearly perfect system would include both diuretic and natruretic components. Although suggested, neither has been identified. Furthermore, although there is some explanation of how *blood* volume is regulated, none has been proposed for the regulation of *extracellular fluid* volume, a function obviously under strong homeostatic control.

DISTURBANCES OF REGULATION OF BODY
FLUIDS COMMON TO MOST FORMS OF EDEMA

Primary transudation of fluid from blood to tissue spaces in amounts large enough to decrease effective circulating blood volume* significantly always is accompanied either by renal retention of water and electrolytes to repair the deficit or by embarrassment of the circulation. The latter circumstance occurs when the intake of fluids is limited and when available stores are depleted. The physiologic responses resulting from the initial formation of edema therefore resemble in circulatory aspects the responses to hemorrhage, differing in that red blood cells, and usually protein, are not lost. The stimulus for salt and water retention probably is common to all conditions involving loss of effective circulating blood volume, affecting the kidneys, which govern the retention, and certain other organs that govern renal regulatory mechanisms. There are several ways by which this can be accomplished.

Changes in Renal Regulatory Mechanisms. Changes in glomerular filtrate of as little as 5 per cent unaccompanied by changes in tubular reabsorption would lead to serious depletion of body fluids or to overhydration. Fortunately, reabsorption of both water and electrolytes alters normally when glomerular filtrate changes, maintaining the fluid equilibrium. A change in the amount of salt reabsorbed would lead either to excessive retention or depletion of electrolytes.

Small changes are difficult to measure accurately. Theoretically, they can result from (1) changes in filtration rate, (2) changes in renal blood flow, (3) changes in the rate of reabsorption of water and salt. Combinations are possible. A fall in glomerular filtration rate without change in the rate of reabsorption will lead to retention of fluids.

---

* The expression "effective circulating blood volume" is used in this review to denote that amount of circulating blood which is adequate to supply the needs of the body.

TABLE 36-3. SOME STIMULI FAVORING SODIUM AND WATER RETENTION
(Partly After Selkurt[42])

STIMULUS	RENAL HEMODYNAMICS			RETENTION OF ELECTROLYTES		URINE VOLUME	EFFECTIVE BLOOD VOLUME OR FLOW
	ERPF	GFR	FF	Na	Cl		
Upright position	−	−	+	+	+	−	−
Exercise	−	−	+	+	+	−	+
Sleeping	0	0	0	+	+	−	−
Sympathetic nervous stimulation	−	−	+	+	+	±	±
Loss of blood volume	−	−	+	+	+	−	−
Lowered cardiac output	−	−	+	+	+	−	−
Increased venous pressure	−	−	±	+	+	−	−
Excessive intake of salt	0	0	0	+	+	+	+
Excessive intake of water	0	0	0	±	±	+	0
DCA	±	+	?	+	+	+	+?
Aldosterone	0	0	0	+	+	−	?
Cortisone	0	0	0	±	±	±	?
Norepinephrine	−	+	+	0	0	±	+?
Vasopressin				0	0	−	?
Angiotensin	−	+	+	0	0	−	+?
Increased renal venous pressure	−	−	±	+	+	−	0
Increased ureteral pressure	−	−	±	+	+	−	0
Compression of neck	0			−	−	±	
Hypoxia		+		−	−		

Symbols: ERPF = Effective renal plasma flow.
GFR = Glomerular filtration rate.
FF = Filtration fraction.
+ = Increased.
− = Reduced.

A marked decrease in renal blood flow with less fall in filtration rate will lead to greater retention. Increased reabsorption of salt (with which water is retained) will cause retention. Which of these mechanisms operates is not known definitely; probably all of them contribute at one stage or another.

Changes in Renal Blood Flow. When insufficient blood is flowing through the kidneys, or blood is shunted away from the kidneys by some external influence, there may be insufficient filtration for excretion of fluids.[37] Under these conditions, water and salt may be retained; in themselves, they can lead to edema. Some mechanism such as this has been believed to account for the edema of congestive circulatory failure.[38] A similar situation may result when the kidneys are severely diseased, especially in nephrosclerosis and in glomerulonephritis. Insufficient blood may flow through the kidneys to form enough glomerular filtrate to rid the body of excessive water and salt, and edema may accumulate. Diseases affecting the tubules of the kidneys may also interfere with the renal excretion of salt and water by promoting either excessive or insufficient reabsorption.

Elevation of Venous Pressure. If systemic venous pressure is elevated, blood flow through the kidneys may be slowed. Retardation of blood flow may provide a longer amount of time for peritubular capillary blood to remain in contact with renal tubules. Thus, excessive reabsorption of water and salt may occur as a result of renal passive congestion.

Renal lymph flow is much larger than commonly appreciated. In the dog, Lebrie and Mayerson[39a] found an average flow about equal to the urinary volume. When venous pressure was raised, lymph flow increased about ten times, to an amount equivalent to three or four times the dog's plasma volume, protein concentration increased 50 times, and a large amount of sodium was returned to the general circulation. Increased venous pressure causes back pressure in lymphatic ducts where they enter the venous circulation.[39b] It is likely that some, if not most, of the protein normally filtered by the glomeruli re-enters the circulation via the lymphatics, and that much filtered sodium

TABLE 36-4. SOME STIMULI AFFECTING URINARY OUTPUT
(After Gauer et al.[34])

STIMULUS	CHANGE IN INTRATHORACIC CIRCULATION	CHANGE IN EXTRATHORACIC CIRCULATION	RENAL VENOUS PRESSURE	URINE FLOW
Hemorrhage	−	−	−	−
Positive pressure breathing	−	+	+	−
Inferior vena caval obstruction above renal veins	−	±	+	−
Same below renal veins	−	±	−	−
Orthostasis	−	±	+	−
Congestion of extremities by cuffs ...	−	+	−	−
Same plus 1,500 ml. blood	0?	+	0?	0
Blood transfusion	+	+	+	+
Negative pressure breathing	+	−	−	+
Head down tilt	+	−	−	+
Immersion of trunk in warm bath ...	+	−	+	+
Exposure to cold	+	−	+	+

is so retained, thus establishing a vicious circle.

Excessive Dietary Intake of Salt and Water. When large amounts of salt are ingested, the concentrating ability of the kidneys for this electrolyte may be exceeded. It has been found that man can concentrate salt roughly to 18.0 Gm. per liter of urine. Intakes greater than this result in the retention of salt, which is accompanied by retention of water. Edema and increased venous pressure have occurred as a result of excessive dietary salt intake[40]; about three to six times the normal intake is necessary. As contrasted with man, the dog can excrete large amounts of salt,[41] —about 8 times as much in proportion to body weight. However, excessive intakes of water do not lead to edema unless the kidneys are severely diseased.

Formation of Protein and Red Blood Cells. When an increase in blood volume occurs as a result of the retention of excessive fluids, which is only seen in certain forms of edema, the blood would be diluted by the retained water and salt if hematopoiesis and protein synthesis were not stimulated. Therefore, hypovolemia in which the concentrations of the constituents of the blood are normal is accompanied by an increase in the total amount of plasma proteins and the total number of red blood cells. A return to a normal blood volume must be accompanied by evidence of protein catabolism and red cell destruction, or the blood would become concentrated. The stimuli for these changes are not well-understood. Albumin and most globulins are synthesized by the liver. When,

through passive congestion, intrinsic disease, or dietary deficiency, the rate of synthesis is less than the rate of loss, plasma osmotic pressure will be lowered and the tendency to edema increased.

Stimulus for Renal Retention. Decrease of effective circulating blood volume occurs when interstitial fluid volume is increased by any of the peripheral factors leading to transudation of fluid from plasma to tissues. The common stimulus affects renal regulation of salt and water balances, causing retention of fluids to make up for the loss. The process is halted by the effects of other influences limiting the amount of edema. The total blood volume can be normal, somewhat reduced, or increased, depending upon the primary cause of the edema. This mechanism probably does not act when local accumulations of fluid collect which are too small to affect blood volume seriously. It is possible that all forms of edema, except those resulting from primary renal retention of salt and water due to excessive dietary intakes, or severe renal disease, originate in an affection of this mechanism at some point in its chain of interacting influences.

Alterations in Electrolytes. The concentration and composition of electrolytes may be disturbed seriously in edematous states. In fact, one could consider that pure isotonic edema, of itself, offers little interference with health, except for the added burden and the presumably delayed interchange of oxygen and metabolites between cell and capillary. Unfortunately, however,

TABLE 36-5. POSSIBLE COMBINATIONS OF SINGLE COMMON
ELECTROLYTE DISTURBANCES IN REFERENCE TO WHOLE BODY[43]

DESIGNATION	TOTAL BODY WATER	TOTAL BODY SALT	EXTRACELLULAR FLUIDS CONCEN- TRATION	EXTRACELLULAR FLUIDS TOTAL (BODY WT.)	EXAMPLES
Hypotonic overhydration	+	N	−	+	Water retention
Hypotonic isohydration	N	−	−	N	Salt deprivation
Hypotonic dehydration	−	−−	−	−	Adrenal insufficiency
Hypertonic overhydration	+	++	+	+	Salt water retention
Hypertonic isohydration	N	+	+	N	Salt retention
Hypertonic dehydration	−	N	+	−	Water deprivation
Isotonic overhydration	+	+	N	+	Edema
Isotonic isohydration	N	N	N	N	Normal state
Isotonic dehydration	−	−	N	−	Simple dehydration

	TOTAL BODY ACID	TOTAL BODY BASE	pH
Absolute acidosis	+	N	−
Relative acidosis	N	−	−
Absolute alkalosis	N	+	+
Relative alkalosis	−	N	+
Normal state	N	N	N

NOTE: There are 44 possible combinations of the above and 1 normal state, when one includes the relations of acid to base loss or excess, since each of the above functions can vary independently of another. When metabolic and respiratory acid-base disturbances are included, there are 81 combinations.

when serious water and salt retention is set in motion, the checks and balances that usually keep the *milieu intérieur* at an optimum concentration of salt, water, and pH may go awry. Not only may renal regulation be altered, but over- or under-production of the renal monitors may occur, leading to marked disorders of concentration and acid-base balance.[43] Since the introduction of the flame photometer in clinical practice, these disorders are being diagnosed much more frequently. In themselves, further disorders may be produced, especially in cellular concentrations of water and electrolytes which can lead to profound illness and death. Renal insufficiency may be one result.[44]

Table 36-5 lists the 44 possible combinations of changes in total body water, total body salt, total acid or base and their relations to concentrations of each. A moment of reflection will show that the subject is not as complicated as it appears on the surface. Obviously, if there is an excess of water in the body without adequate salt, extracellular fluid will be hypotonic. If total body water is then decreased in amount, dehydration will result (hypotonic dehydra-

tion). There are thus three types of edema or overhydration of the whole body, hypotonic, hypertonic, and isotonic, depending upon whether more or less salt or water is present. Only the last does not affect the integrity of the cell by disturbing the Donnan equilibrium. Likewise, acid-base imbalances may be found which can profoundly affect the cells, again from a total of too much or too little, a loss of one or the other. The electrolyte changes in dehydration are discussed in Chapter 35.

Many of these profound disturbances, which probably affect every cell in the body, are the result of eating and drinking excesses or insufficiencies of salt or water during the development of edema, while renal mechanisms are unable to make up for these mistakes. The most frequent alterations are those of hypotonicity and acidosis. Edema (overhydration) resulting from cirrhosis of the liver is especially apt to be hypotonic with respect to cells. In severe anasarca from congestive heart failure, hypotonicity often is found. When organic renal disease has caused the edema, both hypotonicity and acidosis may be present. Hypotonic overhydration, like hypertonic dehydration, is especially prone to cause renal insufficiency with respect to the excretion of water, salts, and nitrogen, and produce more edema.

Preservation of the *milieu intérieur* is vital to proper cellular function. Hypotonicity of interstitial fluid causes cellular swelling with loss of K and Mg and gain of Na by the cell. Hypertonicity induces shrinkage, but integrity of the cell membrane is disturbed in both conditions in the same direction. Acidity and alkalinity also alter the membrane's function to conserve K and Mg and to repel sodium. Basic enzymatic processes are thus changed and cellular "health" impaired. The ability of the kidneys to restore imbalances may be exceeded, leading to renal failure and death in a manner not well understood. In severe hyponatremia, for example, the kidney fails to excrete water,[44] although it is present in excess.

Of preventable nature are the iatrogenic disturbances resulting from the injection of too much salt or water into patients with limited renal function. The most common forms of edema in these are hypotonicity and acidosis, due to the prevalent use of intravenous fluids and the mistaken ideas that physiologic saline solution is a diuretic and that water given always will be excreted even when kidneys are damaged.* Intracellular excesses and losses cannot be measured at present; therefore we are forced to consider the measurable extracellular ones. Since limited renal function carries with it limited ability to adjust, we must avoid unnecessary renal work from overloading with electrolytes or water. A diseased kidney cannot make up for our own mistakes and often not for the patient's own errors in ingesting nonphysiologic amounts.

EDEMA CAUSED BY PRIMARY TRANSUDATION OF FLUIDS FROM BLOOD TO TISSUE SPACES

Edema may be caused by multiple disturbances, or it may result primarily from single factors. In the following discussion, the various types of edema will be considered in the light of their most logical explanation. It must be emphasized that

* So-called physiologic saline solution is also an acid in effect, containing 145 mEq. of sodium and 145 mEq. of chloride per liter. Extracellular fluid contains approximately 144 and 103 respectively, the balance being composed of bicarbonate and other anions. In order for saline to replace lost body fluids, about 40 mEq. of chloride must be excreted by the kidney as HCl or NH₄Cl.

all of the facts in each instance are not known, and therefore the present classification may be modified when new evidence accumulates. A general class is comprised of those forms of edema resulting from transudation of fluids due to peripheral vascular factors. The sequence of events is: first, transudation; second, loss of effective circulating blood volume, and third, restoration of blood volume by stimulation of renal regulatory mechanisms. The accumulation of edema in these conditions usually occurs gradually, small disturbances of equilibrium being followed by corrective measures in a recurring cycle until final equilibrium is attained.

EDEMA DUE TO CHANGES IN CAPILLARY BLOOD PRESSURE

Capillary pressure may be increased either by increased venous pressure or by arteriolar dilatation. The greater flow accompanying the latter may compensate for the increased filtration, many closed capillaries opening and functioning to promote reabsorption; therefore, examples of significant edema due to this are rare. States of peripheral vasodilatation (aortic insufficiency, hyperthyroidism) are not in themselves accompanied by increased interstitial fluids.

Neurologic disease affecting autonomic nervous control of vasoconstriction has been said to cause edema localized to an affected extremity or side, as seen in hemiplegia.[45] Complicating factors are the decreased lymphatic and venous flow associated with muscular inactivity. Perhaps the best example of edema caused by capillary pressure is that seen when an extremity is immersed in hot water: local and general arteriolar dilatation results. The summer edema of the ankles, especially common in women, may be partly a result of arteriolar dilatation, to which is added the increased hydrostatic pressure of the arterial blood column in the erect position (about 110 mm. Hg in the ankles), and of the venous column (about 100 mm. Hg). Although surgical sympathectomy of an extremity is not followed by edema, chemical sympathectomy by ganglionic blockade often is associated with minor degrees; both arteriolar and venular tone may be affected.

Edema of the optic disk and the brain resulting from acute and severe arterial hypertension probably represent examples of increased capillary pressure leading to transudation of plasma. Tissue pressure in the eyeball is about 25 mm. Hg; as a result, arteries and arterioles are thin-walled. When extreme vasoconstriction in the whole body occurs, these relatively weaker structures probably cannot constrict to the same degree. The result is that capillaries are forcefully engorged with blood, followed by transudation of fluid (retinal sheen), of local collections of plasma ("cottonwool" exudates) and of blood (hemorrhages).

The walls of the arteries of the brain are also thinner than are those of the rest of the body, being enclosed in a rigid skull where tissue pressure is relatively inflexible. It is possible that cerebral edema (wet brain) resulting from severe hypertension also is caused by insufficiently powerful vasoconstriction relative to the periphery. It must be pointed out that this explanation, although logical from a serious consideration of hemodynamics, is not the commonly accepted one. "Ischemia" is usually said to be the cause. Ischemia, however, directly produces edema in no other tissue.

The most common causative factor of edema is increased venous pressure, causing increased capillary pressure—especially at the venular or reabsorptive end of the capillary network. In 1926 Landis[46] demonstrated that capillary blood pressure may be measured directly by a microcannulation method. Krogh, Landis and Turner[47] studied the relation between venous pressure and the transudation of fluid from capillaries into the tissues of the human arm and showed that fluid accumulates when venous pressure is raised above 15 to 20 cm. of water. When venous pressure in the forearm was elevated above 17 cm. of water, the rate of filtration of fluid into the tissue spaces was found to be directly proportional to the increase in venous pressure. It was concluded that the increase in filtration due to elevation of venous pressure was caused by the resulting rise in capillary pressure. That a rise in venous pressure does cause an elevation of capillary pressure has been repeatedly demonstrated by direct measurements.[7,46] When venous obstruction (partial or complete) causes venous stasis and congestion, there may be added the factor of hypoxia, which leads to increased capillary permeability, and a change in the relative osmotic pressures of plasma and interstitial fluid resulting from filtration of protein into the edema. In this manner edema formation is furthered.

The simplest form of this type is the *edema of posture*. The upright position is associated with a small but definite loss of plasma volume into interstitial spaces, a concentration of protein[48] and a reduction in renal blood flow.[49,50] Therefore, pre-edema is a normal state. Swelling of the ankles is common in persons whose employment requires long periods of standing with little muscular exertion—elevator operators, for example.* When some degree of venous obstruction and cardiovascular relaxation is added, as is often the case in persons who sleep in the sitting position in busses, trains, and aircraft, edema is prone to develop but can hardly be considered pathologic.

Thrombophlebitis, phlebothrombosis (milk leg), constriction of veins by new growths, aneurysms, scarring after trauma, ligature, and other changes which *interfere with venous return* are associated with edema of the area drained by the affected veins. The ability of collateral venous channels to assume total venous flow is enormous, however; simple ligature of a single vein, even a large one, may be followed by little if any edema. Varicose veins often are accompanied by edema; dilatation of their walls renders functionless the valves that normally prevent overdistention and nullify in part the effects of hydrostatic pressure. Probably the long uninterrupted hydrostatic column from heart to foot is the principal factor concerned.

Arteriovenous aneurysms provide direct arterial pressure to the venous circulation and often are accompanied by edema, which may be surprisingly small in view of the great pressure. Arterialization of the venous wall develops; probably collateral circulation not in direct contact with the aneurysm provides most of the venous return. Reversal of the circulation by surgical anastomosis of artery to vein has succeeded in a few instances[51]; experimentally it has been performed on the coronary sinus and femoral vein with only temporary edema developing.

Pulmonary edema represents a special set of circumstances. Pressure in the pulmonary capillaries is only about 9 mm. Hg which provides a large differential between plasma

---

* Normal venous return against gravity is accomplished principally by muscular contraction, which "milks" blood upward. This exerts a very active function. The valves in the veins prevent return flow during muscular relaxation. Complete muscular rest of dependent parts therefore favors venous stasis. In the upright position the venous hydrostatic column above the foot is approximately 140 cm. of water (about 100 mm. Hg) higher than right atrial pressure when the veins are full.

TABLE 36-6. ESTIMATE OF BLOOD DISTRIBUTION IN THE VASCULAR BED
(After Bazett[53])*

AREA	VOLUME IN ml.	AREA	VOLUME IN ml.
Heart	250	Aorta	100
Pulmonary arteries	400	Systemic arteries	450
Pulmonary capillaries	60	Systemic capillaries	300
Saccular venules	140	Venules	200
Pulmonary veins	700	Systemic veins	2,050
Total pulmonary system	1,300	Total systemic vessels	3,100
Heart	250	Unaccounted 550. (Probably extra blood in reservoirs of liver and spleen.)	
	1,550		

* This table represents a rough estimate of the situation in a 30-year-old man weighing 63 kg. and 178 cm. tall, with an assumed blood volume of 5.2 liters. It will be seen that the pulmonary and systemic system account for at least 3 liters and that over 80 per cent of the blood in the peripheral circulation, excluding the capillaries, is in the venous system.

osmotic and filtration or hydrostatic pressures. In addition, pulmonary lymphatics are widespread and active. Therefore, the lungs have a built-in protection against edema, which breaks down only when high pulmonary venous and capillary pressures exceed net colloid osmotic pressure, and when alveolar edema is formed faster than the lymphatics can remove it. Pulmonary edema results, therefore, from rather extreme disturbances of one or more factors influencing fluid exchange generally. It can occur from (1) *increased capillary blood volume,* the result of a disproportion of the output of the right and left ventricles, caused by left-sided myocardial failure (as in severe arterial hypertension, aortic insufficiency, or coronary occlusion) or insufficient left ventricular filling or emptying (as in mitral stenosis or insufficiency), leading to increased pressure in pulmonary veins. A simple calculation shows that, if the left ventricle pumps continuously as little as 0.01 ml. less blood per beat than the right, over a liter will collect in the lungs in 24 hours. If the disproportion is 1.0 ml., almost 5 liters would would collect in one hour, and pulmonary venous pressure would be greatly increased. It has been estimated that pulmonary edema will develop when the lungs contain about 2 to 3 liters extra of blood. Experimental evidence that Starling's hypothesis holds for the lungs has been demonstrated in dogs.[52] Increased blood volume from massive transfusions or infusions, and arteriolar dilatation from drugs may induce it when other factors are operative. (2) *Increased capillary permeability* from the direct action of toxic gases,

poisons, and respiratory burns, leads to massive serous and bloody edema. (3) *Decreased plasma oncotic pressure* accompanying starvation, hepatic cirrhosis, or the nephrotic syndrome carries with it a tendency to pulmonary edema. (4) It is possible that *negative pressure breathing* may cause it when added to another disturbance, since positive pressure breathing favors its control.

Edema of the face may develop during severe respiratory efforts, especially in bronchial asthma and other forms of bronchial or tracheal obstruction; the effort leads to increased venous pressure. The orbital spaces are especially prone to develop fluid because of the very low tissue pressure therein; sometimes edema under the eyes is the first sign of retention of fluids. Edema localized to the upper half of the body is the cardinal sign of obstruction of the superior vena cava.

Increased venous pressure, therefore, provides one of the conditions which leads to edema, and probably constitutes the most common single factor. Systemic venous pressure can be elevated chronically in three ways: by increase in blood volume, by decrease in venous capacity (by generalized venoconstriction), and probably to a small extent by failure of cardiac filling. However, failure of cardiac filling per se does not contribute to pronounced rises, in view of the relatively small arterial blood volume as compared to the venous volume, unless other factors operate (Table 36-6). Local venous hypertension can be produced by obstructive or hydrostatic interferences with venous flow. When venous congestion is present to a significant degree, restoration of effective blood volume probably occurs, and total (but not effective) blood volume is increased.

EDEMA DUE TO INCREASED PERMEABILITY OF CAPILLARIES

The capillary endothelium normally holds within the capillaries more than 95 per cent of the protein in the plasma. If the permeability of the capillary wall increases, protein escapes into the extravascular fluid, thereby increasing its effective colloid osmotic pressure and disturbing the reabsorption-filtration equilibrium. This leads to the formation of edema, as has been demonstrated experimentally. Tainter and Hanzlik[54] have shown that the edema produced by paraphenylene diamine is due to injury of the capillary wall, resulting in escape of plasma protein. When edema is produced by acute uranium poisoning, the fluid contains a high concentration of protein, suggesting that the edema is due to capillary damage.[55] The local application of irritants to epithelial surfaces likewise produces edema in the underlying tissues. The common wheal, seen in urticaria and in various skin tests utilized in clinical practice, is in reality a form of local edema. The high protein content of the edema fluid removed from such wheals indicates that the edema formation is due, at least in part, to increased permeability of the capillaries.[56] Both heat and cold, if sufficiently severe, will cause blisters that contain a high concentration of protein.[57] Burns are characteristically followed by serous transudation. Although the edema that accompanies most acute infections is no doubt a relatively complicated phenomenon, the presence of red cells and fluid of high protein content in the tissue spaces indicates that the capillary permeability is much increased. Of particular importance is the observation by Landis[58] that *lack of oxygen*, brought on by such factors as stasis, may cause the wall of a capillary to be permeable to protein. Finally, Fishberg has concluded that the capillaries about the various serous cavities of the body are more permeable than those in subcutaneous tissues, as evidenced by the fact that the protein content of ascitic and pleural transudates is considerably higher than that of subcutaneous fluid.[59] However, it should be pointed out that the relatively high protein content of pleural and ascitic fluid may be due, not to increased capillary permeability, but rather to a relatively inefficient removal of protein by the lymphatics of the pleura and the peritoneum, as compared with those of the subcutaneous tissues, with protein concentrated as water is being reabsorbed. In addition, "tissue" pressure is low in the peritoneal cavity and is negative in the pleural spaces.

Edema is caused primarily by increased capillary permeability in conditions involving anoxia, irritation, sensitivity, trauma, capillary toxins, and certain dietary deficiency states. The edema of acute nephritis may begin in this way. Because proteins are filtered with edema fluid, reabsorption is severely hindered in proportion to the difference in concentrations of plasma and edema. Serous transudates accordingly are absorbed with difficulty and limited in extent by tissue pressure.

Enormous amounts of serous fluid may escape through capillary walls after severe burns and trauma, causing serious circulatory disturbances. Much of the resultant shock is due to mechanical loss of fluid. Renal regulatory mechanisms cannot cope with sudden losses; therefore, replacement is necessary. Saline infusions do little more than increase the amount of edema; readily filterable, they provide no osmotic difference between plasma and extravascular fluid. Protein is mandatory, therefore, and plasma transfusions are the logical means for replacement. Pressure bandages and plaster casts applied to burned or traumatized extremities before edema has fully developed often oppose the transudation of fluid by increasing tissue pressure.[60]

The edema from snake bite results from toxic action of venom upon capillaries. Such toxins increase permeability and produce transudation of protein-rich fluid. Allergic edema—whether angioneurotic, from serum sickness, from drugs, or from urticaria—is similar, although localized structures are more commonly involved. The edema of scurvy has been insufficiently studied; increased capillary fragility observed in vitamin C deficiency suggests, however, that the edema may contain protein in increased amounts.

Exudates act in a similar manner. Their high content of protein, which may be greater than that of plasma, provides the conditions for further transudation of water and electrolytes. The effects of capillary damage resulting from cellulitis, infections, and other toxic situations are opposed by localized vascular constriction and by tissue pressure.

The tense, hard, inflamed area about a local infection (boil) is a familiar example.

When protein is lost from plasma, it is probable that the mechanisms for replacement by the liver are stimulated. The formation of plasma albumin is a relatively slow process.[61] Therefore, the serious consequences of massive serous transudation cannot be nullified by renal attempts at retention of salt and water; artificial or natural replacement of the lost oncotic pressure becomes necessary. Renal retention does not restore blood volume adequately, as has been pointed out. Large amounts of protein may be stored in depots in the body; possibly depletion of these depots occurs after serous transudation.

Massive edema due to increased capillary permeability is the most serious type, because all of the factors favoring capillary reabsorption of fluid are affected, with the exception of tissue pressure. Stimulation of all the natural defenses against loss of effective circulating blood volume and loss of plasma osmotic pressure probably takes place, but until some sort of equilibrium can be established, the whole body is seriously affected. In essence, the circulatory status resembles hemorrhagic shock, except for the concentration of red blood cells which occurs.

EDEMA DUE TO DECREASED OSMOTIC PRESSURE OF PLASMA

Rapid lowering of the colloid osmotic pressure of the blood can be accomplished experimentally by bleeding animals at frequent intervals and by injecting after each bleeding only the red cells (plasmapheresis). Utilizing this method in dogs, Leiter[62] showed that chronic hypoproteinemia produced by repeated plasmapheresis caused an accumulation of extravascular fluid when the plasma protein fell to *3 per cent or less.* This observation has been confirmed a number of times.[8*]

The effect of plasma proteins in combating edema formation was demonstrated by Krogh, Landis, and Turner.[47] The amount of

* A simple method for estimating the plasma oncotic pressure is to multiply the concentration of albumin by 5.5 mm. Hg and the concentration of globulin by 1.4 mm. Hg. The total is normally 25 to 30 mm. Hg. Hypoproteinemia is said to be a factor causing edema if the total is less than 20 mm. Methods of measurement of albumin and globulin used in most clinical laboratories are not necessarily accurate, however. Edema may disappear without change in plasma proteins and may not always occur when they are low. The osmotic pressure of proteins changes with the concentration.

protein in the circulating blood was found to increase slightly in subjects standing motionless, the upright position causing protein-free fluid to be filtered into dependent tissues. The effect on filtration rate of changes in colloid osmotic pressure of the blood was studied by determining the filtration produced in the forearm by a given venous pressure while the subject stood and while he reclined. A unit rise of colloid osmotic pressure (1 cm. of water) decreased the filtration rate by 0.0027 to 0.0045 ml. per minute per 100 cc. of forearm.

Nutritional or "war" edema is probably caused primarily by disturbances in the synthesis of proteins[63] secondary to starvation, although other undescribed factors may operate. Apparently the body readjusts itself moderately well to chronic starvation; it was not uncommon to find enormous increases in edema when starved war prisoners were provided with their first good meals. Transudation of water and salt through capillaries because of low-plasma oncotic pressure can explain most of the clinical findings. Studies of starvation have shown a tendency for the renal mechanisms to retain water and salt. In one case in which hypoproteinemia apparently was associated with ceroid disease of the small intestine and liver, overloading of the circulation with concentrated salt solution revealed no renal deficiency in excretion; retention undoubtedly had been present in view of the edema. This procedure did not deplete, but rather increased, effective circulating blood volume, and the stimulus to retention was probably overcome.[64]

Hypoproteinemic edema is found in certain renal diseases, especially the nephrotic stage of glomerulonephritis. Excessive urinary losses of protein, more than 3.5 Gm. per day, probably exceed the ability of the liver to manufacture albumin. Normally, the glomerulus filters up to 30 or 40 Gm. of protein in 24 hours, almost all of which is reabsorbed by the tubules. Nephrotic glomeruli have increased permeabilities; it is not known whether decreased tubular reabsorption also plays a part, nor whether decreased hepatic synthesis contributes to the lowered plasma albumin. At any rate, low plasma colloid osmotic pressure appears to be the fundamental process concerned; blood volume is normal or low, renal retention of salt and water is highly active, and massive isosmotic edema (anasarca) usually results. Losses of essential constituents carried in plasma by albumin (lipids, vitamins, trace metals) also may contribute to the clinical state.

EDEMA DUE TO DECREASED TISSUE PRESSURE

Decreased tissue pressure may be a factor in some forms of edema. When skin and subcutaneous tissues are loose, dependent edema is sometimes noticed; this does not usually represent a pathologic condition. In aged persons and in those who have recently lost considerable weight, evening swelling of the ankles may develop, which disappears over night. Although it is difficult to separate this cause from other factors (such as the increased capillary pressure and slightly diminished oncotic pressure that may be present in such persons), clinical observations that patients recently edematous with stretched tissues gain edema more rapidly than do others with more firm tissues lend support to this conclusion. The ease of fluid formation in the pleural and peritoneal cavities, where "tissue" pressure is low or absent, is well-known.

EDEMA OF LYMPH STASIS

Lymphatic obstruction can cause edema. After radical operations for carcinoma of the breast with widespread removal of lymph nodes, swelling of the arm on the affected side may develop. After an interval, the swelling may subside partially or completely. Metastatic carcinomatosis of lymph nodes can produce the same result. Lymphangitis also may give rise to edema. Chronic osteomyelitis often is accompanied by edema of the affected part, probably due to obstruction of lymphatic channels. This process may be a contributory factor in other infections associated with cellulitis.

Filariasis in its later stages is accompanied by elephantiasis, often involving one or both legs and the genital organs. The worms become encysted in lymph nodes after hematogenous spread, and the irritation resulting from their presence is believed to interfere with the transport of lymph. Although lymphedema occurs in the initial stages, later ones are characterized by an enormous proliferation of fibrous tissue; the size of the affected extremity is partly due to fibrosis. It is believed that the scar tissue results from infection by organisms of low virulence following trauma to the edematous part. Therefore, elephantiasis may be the result of obstruction to lymph nodes and superimposed lymphangitis.

An uncommon type of lymphedema, the pathogenesis of which is little understood, is primary hereditary trophedema, or Milroy's disease. This condition is characterized by lymphedema in the legs, which is sharply demarcated at the level of a joint and which eventually involves both legs to the groin. The hereditary nature of the disease makes its recognition fairly easy.

As the lymphatics remove the small amount of protein filtered through capillaries, the fluid of lymphedema is rich in protein and its albumin fraction proportionately greater than in plasma. Naturally, tissue oncotic pressure is thus higher and its ratio to plasma greater, interfering with normal capillary reabsorption of fluids. Lymphedema is therefore difficult to remove.

EDEMA CAUSED BY PRIMARY RENAL RETENTION OF SALT AND WATER

Renal retention of salt (and therefore water) can result from (1) ingestion of more salt than normal kidneys can excrete, (2) diminution of the excretory ability for salt by renal parenchymal disease or dysfunction, so that normal intake exceeds output, and (3) stimulation of normal tubular reabsorptive mechanisms by intrinsic disease or by extrarenal hormonal influences.

Ingestion of excessive salt (20 to 30 Gm. per day) by normal subjects is accompanied by a rise in venous pressure and body weight and the appearance of minimal edema; all changes return to normal rapidly when salt is discontinued.[40] Extracellular fluid volume may be increased merely by an excess of salt accompanied by an excess of water in the body.

Certain stages of severe, often terminal, renal disease, especially arteriolar nephrosclerosis and chronic glomerulonephritis with uremia, are accompanied by edema. It is probable that this is a result of mechanical retention of salt and water due to the inability of the kidney to excrete them. Pathogenesis is not well understood, and the findings vary widely from excessive retention to excessive excretion. We may postulate that the differences occur because of the variable nature and extent of the lesions in a majority of nephrons; diminished glomerular filtration is always present, and the balance between salt and water retention and excretion depends upon the relative activity of the remaining tubules. If a majority fail to reabsorb, salt will be lost; if a majority reabsorb actively, salt will be retained and edema will appear. The wide disturbance of electrolyte balance seen in uremic states may be to some extent compensatory, because attempts to correct low sodium or chloride levels usually result in edema. Obstructive uropathies lead to edema if water and salt intake exceed output, as do primary renal diseases with diminished renal function.

Steroid substances similar to or identical with those produced by certain endocrine glands act upon the renal tubules, directly stimulating the reabsorption of salt from glomerular filtrate. Desoxycorticosterone acetate (DCA) has a strong action in this respect; testosterone, progesterone and other allied substances have it to some degree. The daily injection of DCA causes *transient* retention of salt and water, a gain in weight,[65] and in some cases, edema. Patients with adrenal insufficiency may be more prone to develop such edema than those with intact adrenals.[66] Patients treated with large doses of testosterone, estrogen, cortisone, hydrocortisone or progesterone sometimes retain salt and water and may develop mild to severe edema. Aldosterone, 9α-fluorohydrocortisone and its methyl derivative are the most potent salt-retaining substances known.

This phenomenon has provided an analogy to the edema sometimes seen in the premenstrual period. A few days before the menses (concurrent with maturation of the corpus luteum) some women have oliguria, gain weight, and notice ankle edema. As the menses begin, diuresis and weight loss occur coincidentally with the regression in the corpus luteum. The nature of the hormone causing salt retention has not been disclosed.

The edema of Cushing's syndrome may be of similar cause. Considerable endocrine imbalance, especially of the adrenal-pituitary axis, is characteristic of this group of diseases, which can be the result of tumors or hyperplasia of the adrenal cortex, or of pituitary dysfunction. Edema is not always present. The adrenal cortex secretes salt-retaining and possibly salt-losing hormones; retention may depend upon a predominance of the former. Some steroids are initially salt-retaining, then become salt-losing. Patients differ in their reactions to these substances. Stimulation of the adrenal cortex by injection of adrenocorticotropic hormone can result in considerable edema due to retention of salt;[67] the mechanism is probably through the increased reabsorption of salt due to renal stimulation by adrenal cortical hormones other than aldosterone.

The preceding examples may be considered with some reservations as edema due to primary renal retention of salt. It must be re-emphasized that all edema of any degree is accompanied by renal retention of salt initiated by the low blood volume following transudation. Primary renal edema has its seat in the kidneys alone, or in extrarenal factors stimulating the tubules directly; in other forms the renal element appears to be secondary.

EDEMA DUE TO UNKNOWN CAUSES

A variety of diseases can be accompanied by edema, the cause of which has been insufficiently studied. Speculation as to the factors involved is unrewarding until more facts are known; the mechanisms probably are to be found among those discussed, and not in some new and revolutionary concept.

Edema associated with old age, convalescence and cachexia may be caused by decreased tissue pressure, increased capillary pressure, and/or lowered oncotic pressure. Definitive studies have not been made. The sometimes massive edema of hookworm disease, which may lead to general anasarca, has as its accompaniment anemia, malnutrition, possibly lowered plasma oncotic pressure, and possibly increased capillary permeability. The edema of anemia is unexplained; increased capillary pressure due to vasodilatation, increased capillary permeability due to hypoxia, and retention of salt and water due to renal hypoxia have been considered as explanations. The edema of leukemia may have similar beginnings. The edemas of relapsing fever, of malaria and of Raynaud's disease are not understood, although portal hypertension may occur in long-standing chronic malaria. Edemas associated with dermatomyositis, disseminated lupus and Raynaud's phenomenon are not explicable at present except when renal disease is an associated factor. Hyperthyroidism is said to give rise to edema, in some instances due to increased capillary permeability, in others possibly secondary to congestive circulatory failure.

The cause of any type of edema can be fairly well understood by (1) examination of the circulatory factors, (2) examination of the renal factors, (3) measurement of the protein content of the fluid, and (4) understanding of the known mechanisms of edema formation. These procedures, direct or indirect, are available in most clinical laboratories, and require few special technics.

EDEMA DUE TO MULTIPLE FACTORS

Edema of Portal Venous Obstruction

Portal obstruction is usually the result of intrinsic hepatic disease involving the network of veins in the portal spaces of the lobules of the liver. Scarring of involved hepatic cells, constriction of venous channels, and obliteration of some of them occur as the primary disease progresses. As a result, hepatic venous resistance is increased, leading to portal venous hypertension. The venous drainage of the splanchnic bed is disturbed, therefore, and congestion of the gastrointestinal tract, the spleen, and the pancreas causes increased capillary pressure, localized to the peritoneal contents. The situation may be considered analogous to partial venous obstruction in an extremity, except that collateral circulation around the obstructed area is limited. Collateral channels are confined to the hemorrhoidal veins, the retroperitoneal plexus, the lower gastroesophageal veins, and the umbilical network through the obliterated fetal umbilical veins. Although portal hypertension provides the conditions for transudation of fluid into the walls of the intestines, where capillary vessels are continuously secreting and reabsorbing large quantities of fluid, it is possible that the increased lymphatic drainage induced by the congestion may supply the largest part of the ascitic fluid. Furthermore, the liver itself may "weep" serous exudate as a result of obstruction to lymphatic flow.

Preceding or accompanying the portal hypertension of hepatic disease is the development of abnormalities of the plasma proteins, especially reduction in the albumin content. That this is a consequence of the primary liver disease appears to be obvious, but the mechanism is not wholly explained. Therefore, decreased plasma oncotic pressure becomes a factor favoring the transudation of fluid into the peritoneal cavity and into tissue spaces.

Another factor leading to venous obstruction of a more general nature is partial *constriction of the inferior vena cava* by enlargement or contraction of the liver. The vena cava passes through a notch between the right and caudate lobes; a ligament (the vena cava ligament) crosses the vein that joins the two lobes and binds it closely to the liver. Partial vena caval obstruction of this nature would lead to little hepatic venous congestion, since the hepatic veins empty into the vena cava above this ligament; however, intrahepatic obstruction in the region of the caudate lobe might produce obstruction of hepatic veins. Therefore, venous obstruction in all subdiaphragmatic areas can result from hepatic cirrhosis; occlusion of the iliac veins leads to dependent edema, and of the renal veins, to disturbances of renal function.

The ascites and dependent edema associated with chronic hepatic disease is the result of increased capillary and decreased oncotic pressure. Other factors providing for the maintenance of ascites are the oncotic pressure of the fluid and the very low "tissue" pressure in the peritoneal cavity. The peritoneal surfaces are well-adapted to reabsorption of fluids that may contribute materially to their normal state. However, the oncotic pressure of ascitic fluid is usually much increased, not only in portal hypertension, but also in congestive circulatory failure. The electrolyte content is similar to that of plasma, but the protein content can be high, up to 5 Gm. per 100 ml. or more. Obviously, the smaller the differential is between plasma and ascitic osmotic pressures, the less readily will fluid reabsorb. Thus, peritoneal capillaries appear either to be more permeable to protein than other capillaries, or protein becomes concentrated because of failure of lymphatic reabsorption.

As emphasized before, the loss of fluid from the circulating blood requires retention of water and electrolytes in order to maintain blood volume. As in other edematous states, the kidneys are stimulated to reabsorb sodium chloride and water. Antidiuretic substance has been found in the urine of patients with cirrhosis[68]; whether this comes from the pituitary, liver, or other sources has not been determined. The renal disturbance of salt excretion, however, is similar to that found in congestive circulatory failure.[69]

Enormous amounts of protein may be lost from the circulation into ascitic fluid, contributing further to the deficiency of plasma proteins. At levels of 3 Gm. per cent, 300 Gm. would be contained in 10 liters of fluid, or considerably more than that normally present in the whole plasma volume. In actuality, a degree of plasmapheresis occurs when ascites develops, continuing the state.

The several factors that operate to promote the ascites of cirrhosis of the liver have been reviewed critically by Hyatt and

Smith,[70] to which the student is referred. From what is known, these authors believe that *portal hypertension* is not the dominant factor in marked ascites, although it is contributory. Likewise, *reduction of plasma proteins* exerts a secondary influence. Retention of sodium (presumably through *aldosterone* and other steroids) and retention of water (presumably through *antidiuretic substances*) are believed to play the major part. The diseased liver conjugates steroids poorly, and they may accumulate.

Portal hypertension can result from portal (Laennec's) cirrhosis of the liver, cholangitic or biliary cirrhosis, the invasion of trematodes or flukes into portal venous radicles, schistosomiasis, extensive carcinomatosis, and many other diseases of the liver or portal vein which result in portal venous obstruction. The presence or absence of portal hypertension is probably determined by the extent and number of venules or veins involved. Partial obstruction of the portal vein itself causes pure portal hypertension, which may not be associated with vena cava obstruction, hypoalbuminemia, or ascites.

Edema of Pregnancy

Normal pregnancy is associated with slight ankle edema, frequently during the later stages. Toxemias of pregnancy are characterized by the presence of retention of fluids. The several factors probably operating are: (1) increased capillary pressure, (2) decreased plasma oncotic pressure, and (3) renal retention of salt and water.

Increased capillary blood pressure in pregnancy can result from two conditions: direct *pressure upon pelvic veins* by the pregnant uterus and direct transmission of some arterial pressure into veins through the uterine circulation, which contains *arteriovenous anastomoses*. The pregnant uterine circulation has a large blood flow in which the normal artery-to-vein pressure gradient is less than that of most organs. Pregnancy is accompanied by an increase in circulating blood volume. The circulatory state resembles to some extent that pertaining in arteriovenous aneurysm, localized to the lower part of the body. Of equal or greater importance is the partial obstruction of the iliac veins by the large tumor, a situation that causes increased femoral venous pressure and can lead to phlebothrombosis.

Plasma oncotic pressure is not usually low in normal pregnancy, but in toxemia the albumin concentration may fall to levels contributing to edema. The minor decreases reported,[71] which may amount to 1.0 Gm. per cent of total proteins, contribute, but are not the primary factor.

The importance of positive sodium and chloride balance in the causation of water retention in both normal and toxemic pregnancies is well-established.[72,73] It is clear also that an increased excretion of sodium frequently accompanies the commonly observed postpartum diuresis.[74] There is considerable clinical and experimental evidence that the mechanism of salt retention in pregnancy is related to endocrine function. The specific hormones involved and their relative roles, however, are not known. The placenta elaborates estrogen, progesterone, DCA-like substances, and other steroids. Aldosterone in urine is increased. The fetal adrenal cortex is secreting.[75] Maternal blood volume increases, requiring formation of protein and red blood cells and retention of water and electrolytes. At term, the woman gains about 8 kg., of which 81 per cent is water requiring 720 mEq. of sodium.[76] Ability to excrete salt is functionally impaired. Taylor and his associates[77] attribute the water retention of pregnancy to the presence of excessive amounts of estrogenic substances and progesterone in the circulation. They report that estrogens and pregnandiol disappear from the urine shortly before the postpartum diuresis. They have also administered doses of estrogens and progesterone during puerperium and have observed that these drugs tend to prevent the usual postpartum loss of sodium.

In conclusion it may be stated that pregnancy edema is due to several factors, the most important of which appear to be: (1) increased intracapillary pressure in the lower extremities resulting from mechanical interference with venous return from the legs, (2) a tendency to hypoproteinemia and (3) electrolyte retention, apparently resulting from the endocrine changes that occur in both normal and toxemic pregnancies.

Edema of Beriberi

The edema associated with beriberi has been insufficiently studied to delineate the disturbances involved. However, it would appear that the plasma proteins are decreased,[78] that capillary permeability may possibly be increased and that the cardiac

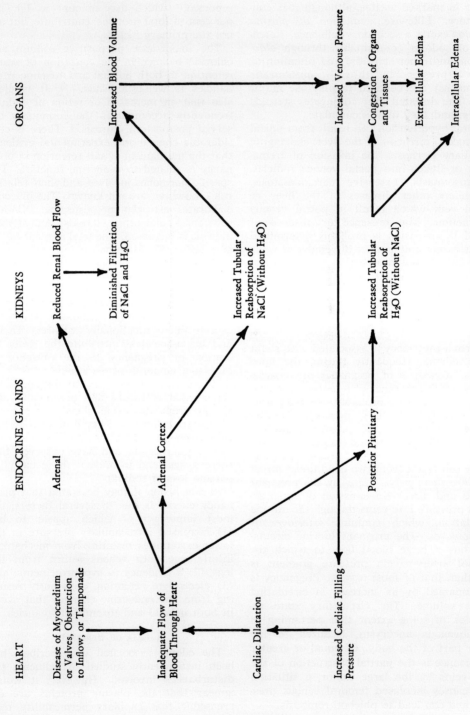

FIG. 36-4. Diagram of factors operative in producing edema of congestive circulatory failure.

disturbances leading to congestive failure may contribute to the retention of water and salt. Under some circumstances it may be difficult to distinguish between beriberi and nutritional edema except by therapeutic tests with vitamins.[79]

Decreased plasma oncotic pressure may explain the presence of the edema which accompanies chronic beriberi without cardiac insufficiency. Although there are "wet" and "dry" forms of beriberi, correlation between plasma proteins and the presence or absence of edema has not been satisfactorily determined. When deficiency of thiamine affects the cardiovascular system a characteristic chain of events is set in motion which is accompanied by tachycardia, *increased cardiac output*, cardiac enlargement and congestive failure. The pathogenesis of this condition is not clear, but a disturbance in the myocardial cells is probably present. Edema in this situation develops as a result of the congestive failure.[80] When plasma oncotic pressure is also lowered by a fall in serum albumin obviously failure will become more marked and the tendency for renal retention of salt and water will become greater. If increased capillary permeability is also present, which remains to be demonstrated conclusively, transudation will increase.

EDEMA OF CONGESTIVE CIRCULATORY FAILURE

The term congestive circulatory failure is used in this discussion rather than congestive "heart" failure, because the same sequence of events leading to edema, increased venous pressure and retention of fluids may be set in motion by noncardiac or by cardiac factors.[81] In general the primary initiating cause appears to lie in the heart. Obstruction to the inflow of blood into the heart (as in constrictive lesions involving the great veins or tricuspid stenosis) or obstruction to the outflow of blood from the heart (as in constrictive pericarditis) may reproduce peripheral signs of congestive failure exactly similar to those seen when the myocardium itself is damaged. Factors which appear to be important in the pathogenesis of the edema resulting from these causes are shown in Fig. 36-4.

Decrease in Effective Circulating Blood Volume. In almost all, if not all cases of congestive circulatory failure, the effective circulating blood volume appears to be decreased. As a result of factors arising in the heart itself or decreasing the flow of blood through the heart, the output of the heart is always *decreased* when compared to that of normal subjects, although there is some overlapping.[82] Most measurements have been made at rest; it is probable that the cardiac output in the presence of severe myocardial or valvular disease would increase much less during exertion than necessary to meet the demands of the body for oxygen. Cardiac decompensation, however, may occur in the presence of a *normal* or *high cardiac output* in such conditions as fever, beriberi, thyrotoxicosis, anemia, arteriovenous aneurysm and cor pulmonale. If there is any unitary factor at all in the development of cardiac insufficiency, it must lie in the relation between actual cardiac output and peripheral needs for blood. Therefore, in these conditions the cardiac output should be compared to the level that should be present if failure had not supervened. It has been shown that the output of the failing heart increases very little during exertion.[83] Therefore, congestive failure probably depends upon a deficit of circulating blood in relation to the body's needs.

Alterations in the Kidneys. Changes occur in the function and hemodynamics of the kidneys when congestive failure is present. Renal blood flow is markedly reduced with consequent decrease in the amount filtered by the glomerulus; as a result, filtration fraction is very high.[38] One must postulate efferent arteriolar constriction of severe degree to account for these findings. During exercise, filtration may fall to a level consistent with retention of sodium and chloride.[84] The lowered renal blood flow of itself may predispose to the retention of salt and water because of the lessened amount of filtrate formed. In normal subjects and in those without congestive failure but with a variety of renal conditions, there appears to be no correlation between glomerular filtration rate and sodium excretion.[85]

Extrarenal Influences. This mechanism does not account for all the changes seen in congestive failure, because the ability of the kidney to excrete nitrogen in many cases may be relatively unimpaired. In addition, there appears to be present a specific disturbance in the excretion of sodium and chloride by the kidney. When large amounts of hypertonic saline solution are given intravenously to cardiac patients,[64] relatively small amounts are excreted; the kidneys of normal subjects excrete the salt rather rapidly (Fig. 36-5).

This disturbance in the excretion of salt may be caused by renal venous congestion or by extrarenal hormonal influences, especially those derived from the salt-retaining hormone of the adrenal cortex. Evidence of overactivity of the adrenal cortex has been found in chronic congestive failure both by measurements of the sodium concentration of sweat[86] and by the finding of an increase in urinary aldosterone.[87] It is also true that an increased renal venous pressure will lead to diminished excretion of sodium chloride.[88,89] Abnormally small amounts of salt are excreted, however, when the venous pressure is not especially elevated and dietary restriction controls edema.[90,91]

There also may be disturbances in the excretion of water. Ingestion of water often is unaccompanied by diuresis.[92,93] Plasma sodium levels may be somewhat lower than normal, indicating dilution of body fluids. Many cardiac patients appear to have stored excess water, as judged by chloride balance studies during recovery.[91] Antidiuretic substances have been found in the urine.[94] These alterations in water balance probably are principally extrarenal in origin, acting upon the kidneys to promote excessive reabsorption of water by the tubules; diminished excretion by other routes contributes, but can hardly explain the findings.[95,96]

Increase in Total Blood Volume. Although the exact sequence of events which leads to the full-blown picture of congestive failure has not been elucidated, the same stimulus operating in other edematous states is functioning; this stimulus arises from an effective circulating blood volume or flow that is inadequate. The stimulus acts upon the kidneys to retain salt and water in the body in an attempt to re-establish effective blood flow, and therefore blood volume. The mechanism most likely concerns the volume receptors. The development of congestive failure is usually a slow process, dependent upon the *gradual accumulation of fluid*; only minor degrees occur immediately following severe myocardial infarction because there is insufficient blood in the circulation to produce edema, other than hepatic or pulmonary. The rarity with which chronic congestive failure follows a first coronary occlusion is difficult to explain. After establishment of failure, the following changes have occurred: (1) increase in total blood volume, (2) increase in body weight, (3) renal retention of salt and water, and (4) increase in venous pressure. The increase in total blood volume usually is associated with a normal hematocrit and normal or slightly low plasma proteins. However, the plasma oncotic pressure may be lower than normal, due to relative reduction in the albumin content and an increase in globulin,[97] but is not low enough to cause edema of itself. Since there is usually no great dilution of the

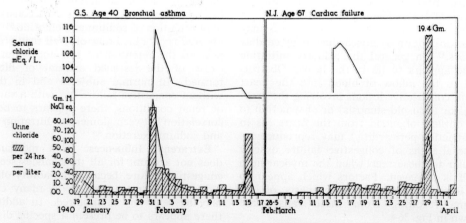

FIG. 36-5. Inability of cardiac patient to excrete sodium chloride in the urine. In the left-hand chart, data from a patient not in heart failure show that the kidney normally will excrete a large excess of chloride when hyperchloremia is artificially induced by the intravenous administration of salt solution. Data depicted in the right-hand chart indicate that in severe congestive heart failure the kidney is unable to respond to such a stimulus. In both instances the administration of a mercurial diuretic resulted in an increased excretion of chloride in the urine.[64]

blood, hematopoiesis and release from storage or synthesis of plasma proteins must have occurred. Recovery from congestive failure, as might be expected, is associated with concentration and possibly storage of plasma proteins[98] and destruction of blood.[99]

The cause of the elevated venous pressure may be twofold: first, due to the increased blood volume, most of which is on the venous side of the circulation, and second, venoconstriction, which can exert a profound influence upon total venous volume.[100,101] A third factor is that of inability of the right heart to pump the blood it receives. An examination of Table 36-6 will show that this must be of minor importance inasmuch as, exclusive of the pulmonary system and heart, over 80 per cent of the blood is normally in the veins.

Peripheral Factors. Local factors contributing to the edema of congestive failure arise from two sources: first, increased capillary blood pressure as a result of venous hypertension, and second, increased capillary permeability as a result of anoxia. The latter probably does not allow a large amount of protein to escape, since the protein content of edema fluid is usually less than 0.6 Gm. per 100 ml.—although occasionally it has been found to be as high as 1.0 Gm.[102] There appears to be little or no globulin in the fluid.

An important third factor in congestive edema is the increased flow of lymph and the marked effect of an increased venous pressure on the return of lymph to the general circulation. Although this factor was considered by Starling in 1897, its importance recently has been demonstrated experimentally in dogs by Wégria and his colleagues[39b] and clinically by Dumont and his co-workers.[106] Cannulation of the thoracic duct resulted in rapid falls in venous pressure, diminution of congestive signs and symptoms, and losses of large volumes of lymph; congestion reappeared rapidly when drainage was discontinued, before there was time for reaccumulation of much fluid. This excessive flow of lymph also was found in cirrhosis of the liver with ascites, the latter being relieved by drainage of lymph.[106] The importance of rates of lymph flow which exceed the capacity of the lymphatic ducts to carry all of the fluid thus was demonstrated in two major types of edema. Experimentally, this function also applied to pulmonary edema.[107] McMaster[103] was the first to demonstrate absence of lymph flow in the skin of patients with edema of cardiac and renal

origin, but the large contribution of visceral flow was not realized until recently.

Other Factors. The function of the liver may be altered by chronic passive congestion and may contribute to a decrease of plasma proteins; hypoxic depression of steroid conjugation may allow salt-retaining hormones to accumulate. Anorexia and malnutrition may occur, leading to further decrease. In addition, tissue pressure may be diminished after repeated attacks of edema.

Summary. The edema of congestive circulatory failure is the result of alterations in almost all of the factors leading to edema. The primary disturbance lies in or near the heart, and results in diminished effective blood flow. The renal stimulus to retention of salt and water operates. However, the peripheral factors may vary in intensity and in importance from patient to patient, depending upon a number of variable circumstances.

EDEMA OF RENAL DISEASE

All edema involves disturbances of the kidneys, and primary renal disease can cause edema. A working hypothesis divides the edemas, secondary to primary renal diseases, into two general categories: (1) those in which there is primary failure of excretion of ingested salt and (2) those involving primary failure of retaining plasma protein. The second type leads to hypoproteinemic edema, discussed elsewhere.

Several factors are believed to result in the generalized edema of acute glomerulonephritis secondary to sensitivity to Group A streptococci: (a) Increased capillary permeability, in which the glomeruli take part. (b) Inflammatory edema of the kidney itself, with resultant lowered blood flow. Protein content of edema fluid, however, is characteristic of a transudate. (c) Inflammatory excitation of tubular reabsorption of salt and water. (d) The familiar chain of events involving adrenal steroids, vasopressin, and retention of salt and water induced by lowered blood volume may or may not be operative. (e) Later, hyponatremia or congestive heart failure may contribute.[104] However, these ideas have not been proved satisfactorily.

Edema accompanying late stages of chronic glomerulonephritis, pyelonephritis, arteriolar nephrosclerosis, disseminated lupus, glomerulosclerosis, and other destructive renal diseases is probably secondary to "fixation" of intrarenal abilities to conserve or excrete water and salt. Thus, when excesses of either are ingested (or injected), the kidneys cannot respond normally, and expansion of extracellular fluid occurs, its tonicity depending upon relative amounts of each retained. When about 200,000 of the 2 million nephrons present in the normal human kidney are left, nitrogen balance may be maintained precariously. As kidneys so damaged are limited in their abilities to synthesize ammonia and excrete acids, complicating factors include acidosis and, in end stages, retention of potassium and magnesium, which may promote myocardial insufficiency. Destructive renal diseases rarely damage all nephrons alike; therefore, a wide variety of disturbances may be present, the net result of which determines the effect. Protein-losing disease from damaged *glomeruli* results in nephrotic edema; salt-losing and water-losing disease from damaged *tubules* results in dehydration and polydipsia; whereas nephrons unable to excrete excesses allow edema to accumulate. All of the other renal factors, however, may contribute, and it is difficult to separate them. Circulatory congestion from heart failure, hypoproteinemia from poor intake, lessened synthesis and urinary losses, and depletion of body sodium from overzealous treatment may play ancillary roles.

Sometimes the edema and the accompanying nitrogen retention and acidosis can be relieved partly by very careful attention to intakes of salt, water, and acids, adjusting them rigidly to the amount excreted. Kidneys thus are relieved of overwork and given a certain degree of "osmotic rest." However, this procedure requires the services of a metabolic ward, a laboratory, and a fine clinical touch; for practical purposes, it has been replaced by the use of the artificial kidney.

SUMMARY

Edema is the result of disturbances of one or several factors concerned in the normal interchange of fluid between blood and tissue spaces[105] and in the normal regulatory mechanisms of fluids and salts in the body as a whole. When the normal peripheral factors (capillary blood pressure, capillary permeability, plasma oncotic pressure, tissue pressure) are disturbed in such a way as to lead to transudation of fluid into tissue spaces, the formation of edema is initiated. The resultant loss of effective circulating blood volume affects the regulatory mechanisms of the whole body. Renal retention of salt and water to make up for the loss occurs, probably through the interaction upon the kidney of the renal monitors, aldosterone and vasopressin, or similar substances. Edema also may accompany disturbances of these regulatory mechanisms themselves, especially of the kidneys, which can cause edema without loss of effective circulating blood volume. When circulating blood volume or flow are affected primarily, as in the conditions reducing the output of the heart, the regulatory mechanisms are similarly called into play, with a resultant increase in total blood volume which leads to the formation of edema by affecting peripheral factors. Therefore, edema is a sign pointing to local disturbances affecting generally bodily functions or to general circulatory disturbances themselves. Analysis of the pathogenesis of each type is important in developing logical methods for therapy.

REFERENCES

1. Smith, H. W.: The Kidney: Structure and Function in Health and Disease, New York, Oxford University Press, 1951, Preface V.
2. Krogh, A.: Anatomy and Physiology of Capillaries, New Haven, Yale, 1922.
3. Landis, E. M.: Micro-injection studies of capillary permeability; relation between capillary pressure and rate at which fluid passes through walls of single capillaries, Amer. J. Physiol. 82: 217, 1927.
4. Pappenheimer, J. R.: Passage of molecules through capillary walls, Physiol. Rev. 33: 387, 1953.
5. Bennett, H. S., Luft, J. H., and Hampton, J. C.: Morphological classifications of vertebrate blood capillaries, Amer. J. Physiol. 196: 381, 1959.
6. Grotte, G.: Passage of dextran molecules across blood-lymph barrier, Acta Chir. Scand. (supp. 211,) pp. 1–84, 1956.
7a. Landis, E. M.: Micro-injection studies of capillary blood pressure in human skin, Heart 15: 209, 1930.
7b. ———: Capillary pressure and capillary permeability, Physiol. Rev. 14: 404, 1934.
8. Ziverfach, B. W.: Basic mechanisms in peripheral vascular homeostasis, *in* Transaction of the 3rd Josiah Macy Jr. Conference on Factors Regulating Blood Pressure, New York, Macy, 1949.
9. Van Slyke, D. D.: Factors Affecting the Distribution of Electrolytes, Water, and Gases in the Animal Body, Philadelphia, Lippincott, 1926.
10. Starling, E. H.: On the absorption of fluids

from the connective tissue spaces, J. Physiol. 19:312, 1896.

11. Claussen, F., and Schade, H.: Osmotic plasma pressure and edema, Z. Klin. Med. 100:363, 1924.

12. Govaerts, P.: Osmotic pressure of serum proteins as factor in edema and arterial hypertension, Compt. Rend. Soc. Biol. 91:116, 1924.

13. Loeb, R. F., Atchley, D. W., and Palmer, W. W.: Equilibrium condition between blood serum and serous cavity fluids, J. Gen. Physiol. 4:591, 1922.

14. Landis, E. M., Jonas, L., Angevine, M., and Erb, W.: The passage of fluid and protein through the human capillary wall during venous congestion, J. Clin. Invest. 11:717, 1932.

15. Meyer, F., and Holland, G.: Die Messung des Druckes in Geweben, Arch. Exp. Path. Pharmakol. 168:580, 1932.

16. Burch, G. E., and Sodeman, W. A.: Estimation of subcutaneous tissue pressure by direct method, J. Clin. Invest. 16:845, 1937.

17. Warren, J. V., Merrill, A. J., and Stead, E. A., Jr.: Role of extracellular fluid in maintenance of normal plasma volume, J. Clin. Invest. 22:635, 1943.

18. Harrison, T. R.: Failure of the Circulation, ed. 2, Baltimore, Wood, 1939.

19. Drinker, C. K., and Field, M. E.: Lymphatics, Lymph and Tissue Fluid, Baltimore, Williams & Wilkens, 1933.

20. Goldsmith, C., Rector, F. C., and Seldin, D. W.: Evidence for a direct effect of serum sodium concentration on sodium reabsorption, J. Clin. Invest. 41:850, 1962.

21. Schroeder, H. A., and Steele, J. M.: The behaviour of renal blood flow after partial constriction of the renal artery, J. Exp. Med. 72:707, 1940.

22. Olsen, N. S., and Schroeder, H. A.: Oxygen tension and pH of the renal cortex in acute ischemia and chronic hypertension, Amer. J. Physiol. 163:181, 1950.

23. Mulrow, P. J., Ganong, W. F., Cera, G., and Kuljian, A.: The nature of the aldosterone-stimulating factor in dog kidneys, J. Clin. Invest. 41:505, 1962.

24. Ganong, W. F., and Mulrow, P. J.: Evidence of secretion of an aldosterone-stimulating substance by the kidney, Nature 190:1115, June 17, 1961.

25. Ganong, W. F., Mulrow, P. J., and Boryczka, C. G.: Evidence for a direct effect of angiotensin-II on adrenal cortex of the dog, Proc. Soc. Exp. Biol. Med. 109:381, Feb. 1962.

26. Kaplan, N. M., and Bartter, F. C.: The effect of ACTH, renin, angiotensin-II and various precursors on biosynthesis of aldosterone by adrenal slices, J. Clin. Invest. 41:715, 1962.

27. Chambers, G. H., Melville, E. V., Hare, R. S., and Hare, K.: Regulation of the release of pituitrin by changes in the osmotic pressure of the plasma, Amer. J. Physiol. 144:311, 1945.

28. Verney, E. B.: Antidiuretic hormone and the factors which determine its release, Proc. Roy. Soc. London, (Biol.) 135:25, 1947.

30. Simpson, S. A., Tait, J. F., Wettstein, A., Neher, R., v. Euw, J., Schindler, O., and Reichstein, T.: Konstitution des aldosterons, des neuen mineralocorticoids, Experientia 10:132, 1954.

31. Farrell, G.: Adrenoglomerulotropin, Circulation 21:1009, 1960.

32. Davis, J. O.: A critical evaluation of the role of receptors in the control of aldosterone secretion and sodium excretion, in Friedberg, C. K., ed., Heart, Kidney and Electrolytes, New York, Grune & Stratton, 1962.

33. Gauer, O. H., Henry, J. P., Sieker, H. O., and Wendt, W. E.: The effect of negative pressure breathing on urine flow, J. Clin. Invest. 33:287, 1954.

34. Gauer, O. H., Henry, J. P., and Sieker, H. O.: Cardiac receptors and fluid volume control, in Friedberg, C. K., ed., Heart, Kidney and Electrolytes, New York, Grune & Stratton, 1962.

35. Bartter, F. C., and Gann, D. C.: On the hemodynamic regulation of the secretion of aldosterone, Circulation 21:1016, 1960.

36. Kriss, J. P., Futcher, P. H., and Goldman, M. L.: Unilateral adrenalectomy, unilateral splanchnic nerve resection and homolateral renal function, Amer. J. Physiol. 154:220, 1948.

37. Selkurt, E. E., Hall, P. W., and Spencer, M. P.: Influence of graded arterial pressure decrement on renal clearance of creatinine, p-aminohippurate and sodium, Amer. J. Physiol. 159:369, 1949.

38. Merrill, A. J.: Edema and decreased renal blood flow in patients with chronic congestive heart failure: evidence of "forward failure" as the primary cause of edema, J. Clin. Invest. 25:389, 1946.

39a. Lebrie, S. J., and Mayerson, H. S.: Influence of elevated venous pressure on flow and composition of renal lymph, Amer. J. Physiol. 198:1037, 1960.

39b. Wégria, R., Entrup, R. W., Jue, J., and Hughes, M.: A new factor in pathogenesis of edema of cardiac origin, Amer. J. Physiol. 213:94–100, 1967.

40. Grant, H., and Reischman, F.: The effects of the ingestion of large amounts of sodium chloride on the arterial and venous pressures of normal subjects, Amer. Heart J. 32:704, 1946.

41. Ladd, M., and Raisz, L. G.: Response of the normal dog to dietary sodium chloride, Amer. J. Physiol. 159:149, 1949.

42. Selkurt, E. E.: Sodium excretion by the mammalian kidney, Physiol. Rev. 34:287, 1954.

43. Schroeder, H. A., and Perry, H. M., Jr.: Disturbances of the internal environment and their correction, Amer. J. Clin. Path. 23:1100, 1953.

44. Schroeder, H. A.: Renal failure associated with low extracellular sodium chloride: The low salt syndrome, J.A.M.A. 141:117, 1949.

45. Weiss, S., and Ellis, L. B.: The circulatory mechanism and unilateral edema in cerebral hemiplegia, J. Clin. Invest. 9:17, 1931.

46. Landis, E. M.: The capillary pressure in frog mesentery as determined by microinjection methods, Amer. J. Physiol. 75:548, 1926.

47. Krogh, A., Landis, E. M., and Turner, A. H.: Movement of fluid through human capillary wall in relation to venous pressure and to colloid osmotic pressure of blood, J. Clin. Invest. 11:63, 1932.

48. Thompson, W. O., Thompson, P. K., and Dailey, M. E.: Effect of posture upon composition and volume of blood in man, J. Clin. Invest. 5:573, 1928.

49. Brun, C., Knudson, E. O. E., and Raaschou, F.: The influence of posture on the kidney function. II. Glomerular dynamics in the passive erect posture, Acta Med. Scand. 122:332, 1945.

50. White, H. L., and Rolf, D.: Effects of exercise and of some other influences on the renal circulation in man, Amer. J. Physiol. 152:505, 1948.

51. Beck, C. S.: Revascularization of the heart, Ann. Surg. 128:854, 1948.

52. Paine, R., Butcher, H. R., Howard, F. A., and Smith, J. R.: Observations on mechanisms of edema formation in the lungs, J. Lab. Clin. Med. 34:1544, 1949.

53. Bazett, H. C.: Transactions of the 3rd Josiah Macy, Jr. Conference on Factors Regulating Blood Pressure, p. 53, New York, Macy, 1949.

54. Tainter, M. L., and Hanzlik, P. J.: Mechanism of edema production by paraphenylenediamine, J. Pharmacol. Exp. Ther. 24:179, 1924.

55. Govaerts, P.: Pathogenie de l'œdeme au cours de l'intoxication aiguë par l'urane, Bull. Acad. Roy. Méd. Belg. 8:33, 1928.

56. Lewis, T.: Vascular reactions of skin to injury; reaction to stroking; urticaria factitia, Heart 11:119, 1924.

57. Lewis, T., and Grant, R. T.: Vascular reactions of skin to injury; liberation of a histamine-like substance in injured skin; the underlying cause of factitious urticaria and of wheals produced by burning; and observations upon nervous control of certain skin reactions, Heart 11:209, 1924.

58. Landis, E. M.: Micro-injection studies of capillary permeability; effect of lack of oxygen on permeability of capillary wall to fluid and to plasma proteins, Amer. J. Physiol. 83:528, 1928.

59. Fishberg, A. M.: Hypertension and Nephritis, ed. 4, Philadelphia, Lea & Febiger, 1939.

60. Glenn, W. W., Muus, J., and Drinker, C. K.: Observations on physiology and biochemistry of quantitative burns, J. Clin. Invest. 22:451, 1943.

61. Barnett, C. W., Jones, R. B., and Cohn, R. B.: Maintenance of normal plasma protein concentration in spite of repeated protein loss by bleeding, J. Exp. Med. 55:683, 1932.

62. Leiter, L.: Experimental nephrotic edema, Arch. Intern. Med. 48:1, 1931.

63. Kurnick, N. B.: War edema in the civilian population of Saipan, Ann. Intern. Med. 28:782, 1948.

64. Futcher, P. H., and Schroeder, H. A.: Studies on congestive heart failure. II. Impaired renal excretion of sodium chloride, Amer. J. Med. Sci. 204:52, 1942.

65. Perera, G. A.: The adrenal cortex and hypertension, Bull. N. Y. Acad. Med. 26:75, 1950.

66. Soffer, L. J.: Diseases of the Adrenals, Philadelphia, Lea & Febiger, 1946.

67. Forsham, P. H., Thorn, G. W., Prunty, F. T. G., and Hills, A. G.: Clinical studies with pituitary adrenocorticotropin, J. Clin. Endocrin. 8:15, 1948.

68. Ralli, E. P., Robson, J. S., Clarke, D., and Hoagland, C. L.: Factors influencing ascites in patients with cirrhosis of the liver, J. Clin. Invest. 24:316, 1945.

69. Farnsworth, E. B.: Electrolyte partition in patients with edema of various origins, Amer. J. Med. 4:338, 1948.

70. Hyatt, R. E., and Smith, J. R.: The mechanism of ascites, Amer. J. Med. 16:434, 1954.

71. Stander, H. J.: Williams' Obstetrics, ed. 8, New York, Appleton, 1941.

72. Freyberg, R. H., Reekie, R. D., and Folsome, C.: Study of water, sodium, and energy exchange during later part of pregnancy, Amer. J. Obstet. Gynec. 36:200, 1938.

73. Thompson, H. E., Jr., and Pommerenke, W. T.: Electrolyte and nitrogen metabolism in pregnancy, J. Nutr. 17:383, 1939.

74. Dieckmann, W. J.: Edema in pre-eclampsia and eclampsia, Amer. J. Obstet. Gynec. 41:1, 1941.

75. deAlvarez, R. R.: The retention of sodium and water in toxemia of pregnancy, in Moyer, J. H., and Fuchs, M. (eds.): Edema, Mechanisms and Management, Philadelphia, Saunders, 1960.

76. Seitchik, J.: Fluid and electrolyte metabolism in pregnancy, in Moyer, J. H., and Fuchs, M. (eds.): Edema, Mechanisms and Management, Philadelphia, Saunders, 1960.

77. Taylor, H. C., Jr., Warner, R. C., and Welsh, C. A.: Relationship of estrogens and progesterone to edema of normal and toxemic pregnancy, Amer. J. Obstet. Gynec. 45:547, 1943.

78. Brull, L., Barac, G., Brakier-Zelkoweicz, T., et al.: Les États de Carence en Belgique pendant l'Occupation Allemande de 1940-1944, p. 286, Liége, Soledi, 1945.

79. Youmans, J. B.: Some clinical aspects of dietary deficiencies, Southern Med. J. 28:843, 1935.

80. Weiss, S., and Wilkins, R. W.: Nature of cardiovascular disturbances in nutritional

deficiency states (beriberi), Ann. Intern. Med. 11:104, 1937.

81. Dock, W.: Heart failure: the relation of symptoms and signs to its severity and duration, Ann. Intern. Med. 29:11, 1948.

82. Altschule, M. D.: Physiology in Diseases of the Heart and Lungs, Cambridge, Harvard, 1949.

83. Hickam, J. B., and Cargill, W. H.: Effect of exercise on cardiac output and pulmonary arterial pressure in normal persons and in patients with cardiovascular disease and pulmonary emphysema, J. Clin. Invest. 27:10, 1948.

84. Merrill, A. J., and Cargill, W. H.: The effect of exercise on the renal plasma flow and filtration rate of normal and cardiac subjects, J. Clin. Invest. 27:272, 1948.

85. Green, D. M., Bridges, W. C., Johnson, A. D., Lehman, J. H., Gray, F., and Field, L.: Relation of glomerular fitration rate and sodium tubular rejection fraction to renal sodium excretion, Amer. J. Physiol. 160:306, 1950.

86. Highes, D. J., Turner, H. H., Moseley, A. J., and Merrill, A. J.: Mechanisms of salt and water retention in heart failure, Amer. J. Med. 7:249, 1949.

87. Luetscher, J. A., Jr., and Johnson, B. B.: Observations on the sodium-retaining corticoid (aldosterone) in the urine of children and adults in relation to sodium balance and edema, J. Clin. Invest. 33:1441, 1954.

88. Rowntree, L. G., and Fitz, R.: Studies of renal function in renal, cardiorenal and cardiac diseases, Arch. Intern. Med. 11:258, 1913.

89. Burch, G., and Reaser, P.: Rates of turnover of radiosodium in the blood and urine of normal subjects and patients with congestive heart failure, J. Clin. Invest. 26:1176, 1947.

90. Schroeder, H. A.: Studies on congestive heart failure. I. The importance of restriction of salt as compared to water, Amer. Heart J. 22:41, 1941.

91. Schroeder, H. A.: Studies on congestive circulatory failure. III. The relation of edema to urinary chlorides, Circulation 1:481, 1950.

92. Fremont-Smith, F., Dailey, M. E., and Thomas, G. W.: Dilution of blood and cerebrospinal fluid in fever, J. Clin. Invest. 6:9, 1928.

93. Fremont-Smith, F.: Mechanism of edema formation, New Eng. J. Med. 206:1286, 1932.

94. Bercu, B., Rokaw, S. N., and Massie, E.: Antidiuretic action of the urine of patients in cardiac failure, Circulation 2:409, 1950.

95. Burch, G. E.: The rates of water and heat loss from the respiratory tract of patients with congestive heart failure who were from a subtropical climate and resting in a comfortable atmosphere, Amer. Heart J. 32:88, 1946.

96. Burch, G. E.: The influence of environmental temperature and relative humidity on the rate of water loss through the skin in congestive heart failure in a subtropical climate, Amer. J. Med. Sci. 211:181, 1946.

97. Luetscher, J. A., Jr.: Electrophoretic analyses of proteins of plasma and serous effusions, J. Clin. Invest. 20:99, 1941.

98. Calvin, D. B., Decherd, G., and Hermann, G.: Plasma protein shift during diuresis, Proc. Soc. Exp. Biol. Med. 44:578, 1940.

99. Waller, J. V., Blumgart, H. L., and Volk, M. C.: Studies of the blood in congestive heart failure. With particular reference to reticulocytosis, erythrocyte fragility, bilirubinemia, urobilinogen excretion and changes in blood volume, Arch. Intern. Med. 66:1230, 1940.

100. Landis, E. M., and Hortenstine, J. C.: Functional significance of venous blood pressure, Physiol. Rev. 30:1, 1950.

101. McDowall, R. J. S.: Nervous control of blood vessels, Physiol. Rev. 15:98, 1935.

102. Bramkamp, R. G.: Protein content of subcutaneous edema fluid in heart disease, J. Clin. Invest. 14:34, 1935.

103. McMaster, P. D.: Lymphatics and lymph flow in edematous skin of human beings with cardiac and renal disease, J. Exp. Med. 65:373, 1937.

104. Daeschner, C. W.: Factors involved in the pathogenesis of renal edema: The role of aldosterone and posterior pituitary antidiuretic hormone, in Moyer, J. H., and Fuchs, M. (eds.): Edema, Mechanisms and Management, Philadelphia, Saunders, 1960.

105. Pappenheimer, J. R., and Soto-Rivera, A.: Effective osmotic pressure of plasma proteins and other quantities associated with capillary circulation in hindlimbs of cats and dogs, Amer. J. Physiol. 152:471, 1948.

106. Dumont, A. E., Clauss, R. H., Reed, G. E., and Tice, D. A.: Lymph drainage in patients with congestive heart failure, New Eng. J. Med. 269:949–952, 1963.

107. Uhley, H., Leeds, S. E., Sampson, J. J., and Friedman, M.: Some observations on the role of the lymphatics in experimental acute pulmonary edema, Circ. Res. 9:688–693, 1961.

The interested reader is referred to the following sources for more detailed data, theories and hypotheses:

Fishman, A. P. (ed.): Symposium on salt and water metabolism, Circulation 21:805, 1960.

Friedberg, C. K.: Heart, Kidney and Electrolytes, New York, Grune & Stratton, 1962.

Starr, I.: Our changing viewpoint about congestive failure, Ann. Intern. Med. 30:1, 1949.

Tobian, L.: Interrelationship of electrolytes, juxtaglomerular cells and hypertension, Physiol. Rev. 40:280, 1960.

Moyer, J. H., and Fuchs, M. (eds.): Edema, Mechanisms and Management, Philadelphia, Saunders, 1960.

Gauer, O. H., and Henry, J. P.: Circulatory basis of fluid volume control, Physiol. Rev. 43:423–481, 1963.

37

Obesity

CYRIL M. MacBRYDE

Diagnosis

Medical Importance of Obesity

Obesity and Growth

Obesity as a Symptom

The Cause of Obesity

Storage of Fat

Fat Metabolism

Hunger and Appetite

Etiology of Obesity: Pathologic Physiology
POSSIBLE FACTORS IN PATHOGENESIS
  Digestive Factors
  Absorptive Factors
  Tissue Factors
  Utilization of Energy
  Endocrine Factors
  Role of the Hypothalamus
  Influence of Heredity
  Psychologic Factors
  Social Factors

Treatment Based on Etiology

Obesity is that bodily state in which there is excessive accumulation of fat. Of "all the thousand natural shocks that flesh is heir to" none is more common, or more distressing, or ultimately more serious than its abnormal accumulation. While to the layman corpulence is primarily a cosmetic defect, making its bearer less attractive to his fellows, to the physician it is a symptom that attains the dignity and the importance of a disease.

Obesity may be defined as excess fat deposit in the body causing body weight 15 per cent or more above the optimal weight.

Adiposity may be distinguished from obesity in that the body weight may not exceed normal but the proportion of the body weight composed of fat is excessive.

Obesity is both a physical sign and a symptom. A physical sign is an anatomic abnormality which is evident to the examining physician; on this count obesity easily qualifies, as discussed in the section below on Diagnosis. A symptom is any perceptible change in the body or its functions which indicates an underlying disorder or disease; the disorder indicated by obesity is a prolonged positive energy balance which has resulted in excess storage of fat. Obesity, therefore, whether or not the patient complains of it, deserves attention and serious consideration.

DIAGNOSIS

When adiposity is sufficient, no exact methods are necessary for its determination, inspection alone being adequate. In accurate medical work, however, the diagnosis of obesity is simply the first step; one should also establish the ideal weight and the degree of obesity. One may find the approximate optimal weights according to height, sex and type of body frame by reference to Tables 37-1 to 37-4. More exact determination of the optimal weight for each person can be made by the use of a series of skeletal measurements.[1] The skeletal measurements of wrist circumference, knee circumference, shoulder width and hip width, etc., permit introduction of computations based upon the width and the depth of the body and the heaviness and the size of the skeletal framework. This permits more nearly accurate estimates of individual ideal weights than the tables based only upon height plus the rough estimate of frame caliber as "small," "medium" or "large." Such methods are satisfactory for persons of average muscular development and for those whose proportions of muscle to fat are within average normal limits. However, in two classes of cases one may be misled by using optimal weight tables or by computing ideal weight from skeletal measurements: (1) if muscle bulk is greatly above normal and the proportion of muscle to fat is high;

TABLE 37-1. DETERMINATION OF THE IDEAL WEIGHT OF BOYS

HEIGHT INCHES	5 YRS.	6 YRS.	7 YRS.	8 YRS.	9 YRS.	10 YRS.	11 YRS.	12 YRS.	13 YRS.	14 YRS.	15 YRS.	16 YRS.	17 YRS.	18 YRS.	19 YRS.
38	34	34													
39	35	35													
40	36	36													
41	38	38	38												
42	39	39	39	39											
43	41	41	41	41											
44	44	44	44	44											
45	46	46	46	46	46										
46	47	48	48	48	48										
47	49	50	50	50	50	50									
48	..	52	53	53	53	53									
49	..	55	55	55	55	55	55								
50	..	57	58	58	58	58	58	58							
51	..	..	61	61	61	61	61	61							
52	..	..	63	64	64	64	64	64	64						
53	..	..	66	67	67	67	67	68	68						
54	..	..	..	70	70	70	70	71	71	72					
55	..	..	..	72	72	73	73	74	74	74					
56	..	..	..	75	76	77	77	77	78	78	80				
57	..	..	..	..	79	80	81	81	82	83	83				
58	..	..	..	..	83	84	84	85	85	86	87				
59	..	..	..	..	..	87	88	89	89	90	90	90			
60	..	..	..	..	..	91	92	92	93	94	95	96			
61	..	..	..	..	..	..	95	96	97	99	100	103	106		
62	..	..	..	..	..	..	100	101	102	103	104	107	111	116	
63	..	..	..	..	..	..	105	106	107	108	110	113	118	123	127
64	..	..	..	..	..	..	...	109	111	113	115	117	121	126	130
65	..	..	..	..	..	..	...	114	117	118	120	122	127	131	134
66	..	..	..	..	..	..	...	...	119	122	125	128	132	136	139
67	..	..	..	..	..	..	...	...	124	128	130	134	136	139	142
68	..	..	..	..	..	..	...	...	...	134	134	137	141	143	147
69	..	..	..	..	..	..	...	...	...	137	139	143	146	149	152
70	..	..	..	..	..	..	...	...	...	143	144	145	148	151	155
71	..	..	..	..	..	..	...	...	...	148	150	151	152	154	159
72	..	..	..	..	..	..	...	...	...	...	153	155	156	158	163
73	..	..	..	..	..	..	...	...	...	...	157	160	162	164	167
74	..	..	..	..	..	..	...	...	...	...	160	164	168	170	171

Age is taken to the nearest birthday, height to the nearest inch and weight to the nearest pound. These weights are inclusive of ordinary clothing, except shoes, coats, and sweaters. (American Child Health Association, revised by Dr. Thomas D. Wood and Dr. Bird T. Baldwin)

(2) if muscle bulk is below normal and the proportion of fat to muscle exceeds normal limits. In such instances, a very muscular man may seem to weigh much more than he should, or contrariwise, a flabby person with atrophic muscles and excessive fat deposits throughout the body may have a total body weight within or even below the optimal range.

Total body weights in excess of the optimal range usually indicate an excessive fat content of the body. A more exact method of measuring the fat storage, as compared to normal, requires the determination of the specific gravity of the whole body by weighing the patient under water.[2] Since human fat has a density of 0.92, whereas the rest of the body has an average density of 1.1, it is possible to calculate the percentage of body fat when the total body density is known. A correction must be made for residual air within the lungs. This is the most accurate method yet devised for calculation of body fat content, but the difficulties involved limit its use to research laboratories. However, standards of reference have thus been provided for comparison with the results of simpler procedures.

Formulas have been devised for estimating body fat content from measurements of

TABLE 37-2. DETERMINATION OF THE IDEAL WEIGHT OF GIRLS

HEIGHT INCHES	5 YRS.	6 YRS.	7 YRS.	8 YRS.	9 YRS.	10 YRS.	11 YRS.	12 YRS.	13 YRS.	14 YRS.	15 YRS.	16 YRS.	17 YRS.	18 YRS.
38	33	33												
39	34	34												
40	36	36	36											
41	37	37	37											
42	39	39	39											
43	41	41	41	41										
44	42	42	42	42										
45	45	45	45	45	45									
46	47	47	47	48	48									
47	49	50	50	50	50	50								
48	..	52	52	52	52	53	53							
49	..	54	54	55	55	56	56							
50	..	56	56	57	58	59	61	62						
51	..	..	59	60	61	61	63	65						
52	..	..	63	64	64	64	65	67						
53	..	..	66	67	67	68	68	69	71					
54	..	..	..	69	70	70	71	71	73					
55	..	..	..	72	74	74	74	75	77	78				
56	..	..	..	..	76	78	78	79	81	83				
57	..	..	..	..	80	82	82	82	84	88	92			
58	..	..	..	..	..	84	86	86	88	93	96	101		
59	..	..	..	..	..	87	90	90	92	96	100	103	104	
60	..	..	..	..	..	91	95	95	97	101	105	108	109	111
61	..	..	..	..	..	..	99	100	101	105	108	112	113	116
62	..	..	..	..	..	..	104	105	106	109	113	115	117	118
63	..	..	..	..	..	..	...	110	110	112	116	117	119	120
64	..	..	..	..	..	..	...	114	115	117	119	120	122	123
65	..	..	..	..	..	..	...	118	120	121	122	123	125	126
66	..	..	..	..	..	..	...	...	124	124	125	128	129	130
67	..	..	..	..	..	..	...	...	128	130	131	133	133	135
68	..	..	..	..	..	..	...	...	131	133	135	136	138	138
69	..	..	..	..	..	..	...	...	...	135	137	138	140	142
70	..	..	..	..	..	..	...	...	...	136	138	140	142	144
71	..	..	..	..	..	..	...	...	...	138	140	142	144	145

Age is taken to the nearest birthday, height to the nearest inch and weight to the nearest pound. These weights are inclusive of ordinary clothing, except shoes and coats. (American Child Health Association, revised by Dr. Thomas D. Wood and Dr. Bird T. Baldwin)

skin-fold thickness over several specified areas of the body.

The total proportion of body fat has also been estimated by measurement of total body water. The most practical substance so far used in this method (based on the dilution principle) seems to be antipyrine. It is injected intravenously and after time is allowed for diffusion, the concentration of the test substance is measured in samples of the body water afforded by the blood serum. Under normal conditions total water maintains a constant relationship to lean body mass. When total body water is known, lean body mass can be calculated and the fat content of the body determined by subtracting lean body mass from total body weight.

Keys[3] has evaluated and compared the results obtained by the three methods mentioned: (1) densitometry, (2) skin-fold measurements, and (3) body water measurement. When carefully employed there is rough agreement.

Such studies have yielded a considerable amount of useful data. The human body is composed of several major components, which are largely distinct metabolically and which may show a considerable degree of independent variation. In an average

TABLE 37-3. DESIRABLE WEIGHTS FOR MEN
25 YEARS OF AGE OR OLDER

HEIGHT (with shoes on) 1-inch heels		SMALL FRAME	MEDIUM FRAME	LARGE FRAME
Feet	Inches			
5	2	112–120	118–129	126–141
5	3	115–123	121–133	129–144
5	4	118–126	124–136	132–148
5	5	121–129	127–139	135–152
5	6	124–133	130–143	138–156
5	7	128–137	134–147	142–161
5	8	132–141	138–152	147–166
5	9	136–145	142–156	151–170
5	10	140–150	146–160	155–174
5	11	144–154	150–165	159–179
6	0	148–158	154–170	164–184
6	1	152–162	158–175	168–189
6	2	156–167	162–180	173–194
6	3	160–171	167–185	178–199
6	4	164–175	172–190	182–204

(Metropolitan Life Insurance Company, Statistical Bureau)

TABLE 37-4. DESIRABLE WEIGHTS FOR WOMEN
25 YEARS OF AGE OR OLDER

HEIGHT (with shoes on) 2-inch heels		SMALL FRAME	MEDIUM FRAME	LARGE FRAME
Feet	Inches			
4	10	92– 98	96–107	104–119
4	11	94–101	98–110	106–122
5	0	96–104	101–113	109–125
5	1	99–107	104–116	112–128
5	2	102–110	107–119	115–131
5	3	105–113	110–122	118–134
5	4	108–116	113–126	121–138
5	5	111–119	116–130	125–142
5	6	114–123	120–135	129–146
5	7	118–127	124–139	133–150
5	8	122–131	128–143	137–154
5	9	126–135	132–147	141–158
5	10	130–140	136–151	145–163
5	11	134–144	140–155	149–168
6	0	138–148	144–159	153–173

(Metropolitan Life Insurance Company, Statistical Bureau)
Derived primarily from data of the Build and Blood Pressure Study, 1959, Society of Actuaries.

young man these components constitute approximately the following percentages of total body weight:

	NORMAL PER CENT
Fat	15
Extracellular water	23
Cells or "active tissue"	58
Bone mineral	4
Body weight	100

In obesity of extreme degree, the percentage of body fat may exceed 50 and even reach 70; in extreme leanness the percentage of body weight made up of fat may be lower than 10 per cent, even as low as 2 per cent.

Normal Fat Storage. Even among persons of normal weight according to the height-age-weight tables, there may be considerable differences in body fat content. This implies, of course, corresponding differences in lean body mass (presumably largely muscle).

"Normal" middle-aged men are much fatter than normal young men if body content of fat is used as the criterion of comparison, rather than height-weight-age tables. This is most clearly shown when men of equal height and weight, but of different ages, are compared.

In the group studied, the mean body fat content of 33 younger (22-29 years) men was 16.5 per cent as compared with 22.6 per cent for 33 older (48-57 years) men matched in height and weight.

The trend for older as compared with younger females was similar, with the difference that females were fatter than males at each age and relative body weight category (Keys[3]).

Women normally have more body fat than men. In the third decade the proportion in normal persons is: females 18 to 24 per cent fat, males 12 to 18 per cent. Adiposity may be considered present if the body fat content of a woman exceeds 30 per cent, of a man 25 per cent.

Problems arise in older age groups in deciding what degree of adiposity may be considered normal with increasing age. The proportion of fat to muscle increases with age in both men and women. The proportion of fat in older men and women tends to be more than 50 per cent higher than in younger persons of the same sex, height and build. They are thus relatively adipose, although they may not be obese.

No rapid clinical method is available to determine accurately the body fat content. Excess adipose tissue is usually evident, however, when physical examination reveals the muscles to be flabby. Such persons take little exercise and fatigue easily.

Persons of any age who have poor muscles are apt to be relatively adipose, although the total body weight may be normale or even subnormal, rather than excessive. More attention should be paid to *adiposity occurring without obesity*, as it may have great clinical significance.

Changing Fat Storage. The importance of actual estimation of body fat is illustrated in two alterations of the nutritional state:

1. In *prolonged undernutrition* there is a progressive loss of both fat and eventually of muscle and other "active tissue," with no change or an increase in extracellular fluid, as calculated in per cent of total body weight.

2. In *developing obesity* the weight gained consists approximately of 80 per cent pure fat and 20 per cent water; the "active tissue" percentage of the total body weight tends to show little or no change.

Fat, Active Tissue, and Basal Metabolism. An additional concept of great importance arises from the study of body content of fat and of "active tissue": computations based on active tissue indicate that most of the classic age and sex differences in basal metabolic rate are merely reflections of the body content of active tissue. The term "active tissue" here employed means all components of the total body weight except fat and water. It thus appears that younger men have higher metabolic rates per square meter of body surface than older men because of a greater proportion of metabolically active tissue and less fat. The higher rates for men as compared with women may be similarly explained.

Hydration and Body Weight. *Variations in hydration* must be taken into account when estimating the degree of corpulence from total body weight. The tables given in this chapter are predicated upon normal hydration. Dehydration may greatly reduce body weight; extracellular fluid may be reduced from the normal of about 23 per cent of body weight to as low as 10 per cent. Calculating for every liter of fluid 2.2 lbs. ("for every pint a pound"), great differences in weight may occur with no change in body content of fat or active tissue. When the body contains excess fluid, it is not always readily detectable. In undernourished persons clinical edema may not be recognizable until the excess fluid constitutes 10 per cent of the total body weight. In extreme cases extracellular fluid may account for not the normal 23 per cent, but as high as 60 per cent of total body weight. When hydrothorax, ascites, edema, etc., are present, calculations may be made, or the abnormal fluid retention must be removed, before body weight measurements may be compared with "ideal" weights in the tables.

It is very helpful when the actual fat content of the body can be computed, but for practical purposes in most cases, weighing the patient, doing a careful physical examination, and comparing the weight with the ideal weight suffice to establish the diagnosis of obesity and its degree.

Tables giving *average* weights at various ages and heights are misleading, for the optimal weight of an adult remains unchanged, but average weights increase in the middle decades. Life insurance companies have found in their statistical studies that even the minor degrees of corpulence (10 to 15 per cent above optimal weight) are accompanied by higher mortality rates. The *optimal* weight figures given in this chapter are derived from such statistical studies, which indicate that such ideal weights are important factors in longevity.

MEDICAL IMPORTANCE OF OBESITY

Incidence. Obesity, of all health defects, is the most common reason for the refusal of standard risk life insurance. In the United States estimates indicate that one fifth of the population over age 30 may be considered overweight (i.e., 10% above "ideal" weight). About 10% of our population is obese (15% over "ideal" weight). About 6.3 million persons in the country, or approximately 3 per cent of the 210 million total population, are pathologically obese (20% above "ideal" weight).

Penalty of Overweight. Dublin and Lotka[4] found that "the penalty of overweight is one-fourth to three-fourths excess in mortality." Persons who are from 5 to 14 per cent overweight have an excess mortality rate of 22 per cent; those from 15 to 24 per cent overweight, of 44 per cent; those 25 per cent or more overweight, of 74 per cent. The hazard of obesity increases with age, so that persons between 45 and 50 years of age who are 10 pounds overweight have an increase above the average death rate of 8 per cent; when 20 pounds overweight, of 18 per cent; when 30 pounds overweight, of 28 per cent; when 50 pounds overweight, of 56 per cent.

An analysis by Armstrong, Dublin, Wheatley, and Marks[4] of the causes of death among obese persons, as compared with those among persons of normal weight, revealed that deaths from degenerative diseases of the heart, the arteries and the kidneys account for the greatest proportion of the higher mortality. All types of cardiovascular-renal conditions appear to occur more frequently and with greater severity among overweight persons, including in particular heart failure, cerebral hemorrhage and thrombosis, coronary thrombosis and nephritis. More of the obese die from accidents, probably because fat people are less agile. The death rate from diabetes is almost four times as great in obese persons as in normal persons.

Barr[5] calls obesity "a stop signal, a red light of warning" and presents a lucid and stimulating review and discussion of obesity and its consequences. His adaptation and tabulation of data from the very informative insurance studies[4] are given in Table 37-5. Notice that the ratio of increase in mortality from diabetes, and from certain diseases of the liver, biliary tract, and intestines is higher among obese persons than from the much more common conditions of nephritis, cerebral hemorrhage, and coronary artery disease.

In only two of the categories listed is the mortality of the obese less than the standard for normal weight persons. The lower suicide rate is somewhat of a surprise, for although fat persons are supposed to be jolly and placid, many studies indicate a high rate of emotional disorders. A lower death rate from tuberculosis may indicate that abundant nutrition protects against it, but may mean only that few persons who have tuberculosis are overweight when they die.

Many studies have demonstrated[6] that obesity has an adverse influence upon a number of other medical disorders through (1) increasing their incidence (that is, fat people are more apt to develop the condition), (2) increasing the severity of the disease itself, (3) increasing the number and severity of the symptoms caused by the disease or (4) increasing the inci-

TABLE 37-5. RATIO OF ACTUAL TO EXPECTED DEATHS BETWEEN OVERWEIGHT PERSONS AND THOSE CONSIDERED STANDARD RISKS (100 = STANDARD RATE)

CONDITION	MEN	WOMEN
Diabetes	383	372
Cirrhosis of liver	249	147
Appendicitis	223	195
Biliary calculi	206	284
Chronic nephritis	191	212
Liver and gallbladder cancer	168	211
Cerebral hemmorhage	159	162
Coronary disease	142	175
Auto accidents	131	120
Puerperal conditions	—	162
Suicides	78	73
Tuberculosis	21	35

dence and severity of complications of the disease. Disorders influenced adversely by obesity in one or more of the four ways mentioned include diabetes, heart disease, hypertension, pulmonary emphysema, acute and chronic nephritis, arteriosclerosis, venous thrombosis and embolism, hepatic cirrhosis, appendicitis, gallbladder disease, degenerative arthritis, varicose veins, cancer and toxemias of pregnancy. Obesity causes increased fetal mortality and greater complications of obstetric delivery. Should these dangers be avoided, the fat person is still more likely than the normal person to be seriously or fatally injured, or to suffer fractures of bones. Should surgery prove necessary, the greater the adiposity the poorer the prognosis. Orthopedic difficulties are commoner among the obese, with flat feet and arthritic changes in the knees and the back occurring as frequent complications, often disabling in severity. Diaphragmatic hernia occurs more frequently in the obese and in some instances has been corrected solely by weight reduction.

Hypertension. Extensive studies have revealed that elevated blood pressure occurs in obese patients in every age group and in both sexes. There is a steady progression, both systolic and diastolic, with each increase in body weight per height of the individual. There is substantial agreement in the reports of Thompson[12] on life insurance company employees; by Master, Dublin and Marks[13] on 74,000 industrial workers, and by Levy, White, Stroud and Hillman[14] on 22,741 Army officers. The latter group found that sustained hypertension among obese persons develops at a rate 2.5 times as high as among persons of normal weight.

Obesity, Atherosclerosis, Blood Lipids, and Diet. In a study of 1,250 consecutive miscellaneous autopsies, Wilens[15] demonstrated a close association between obesity and atherosclerosis, advanced degrees of the arterial change being found twice as often among the obese as among the poorly nourished. In the age group 45 to 54 years severe generalized atherosclerosis was found in 20.2 per cent of the obese as compared with 10.9 per cent of those of average weight and with 7 per cent for the underweight. In the age group 55 to 64, the rate was 37 per cent for the obese, 17 per cent for those of average weight. In the age group 65 to 74, the rate was 45 per cent for the obese, 20 per cent for the underweight. Coronary atherosclerosis of advanced degree occurred in a distribution similar to that for generalized atherosclerosis, averaging 40.8 per cent for obese men as compared with 18.7 per cent for average-weight men.

Clinical and experimental evidence has long been accumulating that prolonged hypercholesteremia and atherosclerosis are in some way associated. The characteristic lesion of the atherosclerotic artery is the cholesterol-rich plaque (containing up to 70 per cent cholesterol). The cholesterol in the blood is carried not in simple solution but in lipoprotein complexes, the so-called "giant molecules" of Gofman. The serum cholesterol level is not altered readily by even quite large changes in the cholesterol content of the diet. However, there is a relationship between the total serum cholesterol and the total fat content of the diet. Keys[16] concluded that not the amount of dietary cholesterol, but the *total amount of fat* is the significant factor in controlling blood cholesterol levels. Low-fat diets led to a fall in blood cholesterol. Low cholesterol but high-fat diets gave high cholesterol blood levels.

Walker *et al.*[17] found that weight loss resulted in reduction of the Sf 12 to 100 lipoproteins to which Gofman attributes pathogenic significance in atherosclerosis. Gofman[18] previously had reported higher levels of these bodies in obese persons and reduction in them by low-fat, low-cholesterol diets.

This class of lipoprotein particle is found in higher than normal concentration in the plasma of patients recently recovered from coronary thrombosis; the concentration increases with age and is much higher in males under age 40 than in females, but this sex difference tends to disappear in the older age groups. These observations are in accordance with the incidence of atheromatosis with respect to age and sex.

Short[10] found that 15 per cent of those who were more than 25 per cent overweight for their height had definite electrocardiographic abnormalities. Only 8.5 per cent of persons of average weight and 2 per cent of underweight subjects showed abnormal electrocardiographic changes.

Cholesterol and probably other lipids are implicated in the problems of arterial disease, particularly of the coronary arteries. Obese persons frequently have blood cholesterol levels above normal and they are also particularly subject to coronary occlusion. It is generally agreed that:

1. Arteriosclerosis and atherosclerosis are characterized by deposition of cholesterol in the arterial walls.

2. Patients with coronary artery disease and atheroma have high blood cholesterol for their ages.

3. These conditions are common among people ingesting high fat diets, less frequent in countries where the fat intake is low.

4. Blood cholesterol can be raised or lowered by increase or decrease in the dietary intake of animal fat.

5. The ingestion of highly unsaturated fat tends to lower blood cholesterol.

The cause of the accumulation of cholesterol (particularly cholesterol esters) in the atheromatous plaques is not clear. Two main theories are proposed: (1) The filtration theory: cholesterol of the blood, present in excess or in an abnormal physicochemical state, is picked up by the arterial wall; (2) The local theory: changes in the arterial wall are primary, resulting in a local uptake of cholesterol from the plasma, or increased synthesis of cholesterol in the arterial wall.

Attempts by many investigators to relate blood lipid levels to coronary atherosclerosis have shown varying degrees of correlation with cholesterol, triglycerides, total β-lipoprotein, β-lipoprotein of Sf 0-12 and 12-400, etc. Some studies suggest that blood cholesterol elevation is as accurate a parameter as an increase in any of the other fractions. In middle age the incidence of coronary thrombosis is 3 to 6 times as high among persons with elevated blood cholesterol as when the level is normal. Correlation with β-lipoprotein cholesterol concentration seems particularly important.

Some studies indicate that triglyceride levels may be as significant, or more significant than cholesterol levels.[93,94]

Two points deserve emphasis:

1. Atherosclerosis and coronary occlusion occur in many persons who have not been shown to have any blood lipid abnormality.

2. As yet, measurement of none of the blood lipids has served satisfactorily to permit prediction of coronary thrombosis.

Whether significant prevention of atherosclerosis and its consequences will be possible by weight control or specific diet management awaits more conclusive demonstration. The evidence is already highly suggestive that weight reduction in the obese reduces the mortality from cardiovascular disease.[95]

Diets very low in fat but high in carbohydrate may lower blood cholesterol, but elevate blood triglyceride levels, presumably because of increased lipogenesis from carbohydrate.

It has been demonstrated by a number of investigators[96,97,98] that diets low in cholesterol and relatively high in polyunsaturated fats will reduce blood cholesterol and other lipid levels. Not only can the blood lipids be altered in amount and relative composition, but so can the lipids of subcutaneous fat. In a group of men[97] following such an experimental diet for 2 years, there was progressive desaturation of depot fat, the linoleic acid content rising to 24 per cent as compared with 9 per cent in those on conventional diets.

Authoritative medical committees have reviewed the evidence now available and have recommended[99,100] that physicians prescribe diets low in saturated fats, and relatively high in polyunsaturated fats for persons who have suffered atherosclerotic insults, or who are known to be susceptible or predisposed to them. Such suggestions seem justified and commendable, but probably too conservative. If we have dietary measures at hand which can prevent atherosclerosis, should we not recommend them to everyone?

Since our knowledge is limited and the conclusions to be drawn from the information now available are uncertain, should specific diet regulation be recommended for everyone as a preventive public health measure, or be confined to persons known to have atherosclerosis or to be predisposed to it (by heredity, or because of obesity, diabetes, elevated blood lipids, etc.)?

The best answer we can give at present, in view of the high incidence of atherosclerosis in the United States, the relatively high fat (especially saturated fat) diet of a high portion of persons in this country, and the long time it takes to develop atherosclerosis, seems to be this: the optimum diet for everyone should not allow excess calories and should be adequate in protein, vitamins and minerals; the fat content should supply 25 to 35 per cent of the total calories (not 45 per cent or over, as is usual), and the carbohydrate allowance should be moderate. The fats taken should be chiefly polyunsaturated as supplied in fat of fish and in vegetable oils (corn, cottonseed, soya), while foods supplying the saturated fats should be limited (meat-fats, eggs, whole milk, butter, cream, coconut oil, chocolate).

Optimal levels for blood lipids cannot be set with certainty, but these seem desirable: total lipids under 700 mg. per 100 ml., β-lipoprotein under 400 mg., cholesterol under 225 mg.

Heart, Circulation, Respiration. Obesity, dyspnea and limitation of exertion are frequently concomitant and therefore these questions have received much attention: (1) Can obesity alone cause dyspnea? (2) Does obesity per se cause heart disease? (3) Does obesity cause other disorders which may simulate heart disease? (4) Does obesity impair respiration specifically, aside from or in addition to effects it may have upon circulatory organs and function?

These questions are here considered in order:

1. Obesity can cause dyspnea, excessive fatigue and limited capacity for performing muscular work just by *increasing the body load*. In nearly all types of work, mechanical efficiency is impaired by obesity, so that a given task requires greater expenditure of energy, greater oxygen consumption, etc.

2. Obesity alone can be the cause of *pathologic changes in the heart* and of heart failure. In their study of the pathology of adiposity of the heart, Smith and Willius[7] found that the degree of cardiac enlargement in obesity is roughly proportional to the increase in body-surface area and that some of these otherwise normal enlarged hearts may fail. It is axiomatic that dilated and hypertrophied hearts

from any cause tend to fail. The eventual weakening of the cardiac musculature results from relative coronary artery insufficiency, even in the absence of occlusive arterial disease.

In many instances there is not only enlargement of the heart but "adiposity of the heart." In this condition there is an increase in the amount of subepicardial fat and of the fat lying between muscle bundles. Such fatty changes differ from the "fatty infiltration" seen in pernicious anemia, carcinoma, etc., in which droplets of fat appear within the cytoplasm of the cardiac muscle cells.

When coronary atherosclerosis occurs in association with obesity, as it so frequently does, a secondary cause of heart disease is added to the primary embarrassment of the heart muscle already operative as a consequence of the obesity per se.

Obesity has been shown, therefore, to be associated with the development of three types of true heart disease: (1) hypertrophy and dilatation; (2) fatty infiltration of heart muscle; (3) coronary atherosclerosis.

3. Obesity alone may cause dyspnea[8] since reduction in vital capacity results from *mechanical restriction* of respiratory movements by excess fat in the abdominal and thoracic walls.

In obesity, the decreased compliance of the thoracic structures produced by the encircling girdle of adipose tissue has two effects: it mechanically limits respiration, and it increases the mechanical work of breathing several fold.[103]

In obesity, because of the increased work of breathing, the oxygen costs of breathing are greatly increased. Hypoventilation may result partly from the restricted respiration and partly from the greater demand, so that respiration may not only be labored, but it may be inadequate and unable to support proper gaseous interchange in the lungs.[104] The consequences may be serious (see below).

Emphysema may result from prolonged obesity, with permanent reduction of vital capacity even after weight loss.[9,10]

4. Not only may the subcutaneous fat mass interfere with respiration, but there may be *extensive infiltration of the intercostal muscles and diaphragm by adipose tissue.*[91] Poor function of these muscles may account for serious disturbance in gaseous exchange in the lungs even in the absence of circulatory failure. Normal inspir-

ation depends entirely upon contraction of the external intercostal muscles, the levator costarum and the diaphragm. The diaphragm accounts for approximately two-thirds of the inspiratory function.

The *inadequate pulmonary ventilation* results in decrease in arterial oxygen saturation and increase in carbon dioxide retention.[92] In extreme degrees of such derangement, usually with great obesity, there may be somnolence, muscular twitching, cyanosis, secondary polycythemia, and hypertrophy and failure of the right ventricle (Pickwickian syndrome).[91,101]

Diabetes. Obesity and diabetes are interrelated in a number of ways, all of which have led to studies which have yielded information about the interlocking pathologic physiology of both conditions. For further discussion of basic concepts see discussion below under Etiology.

Here we are concerned with the medical importance of obesity as related to diabetes. We may list essential points:

1. Mortality: death from diabetes is almost four times as common among the obese.

2. Incidence: the percentage of obese persons who develop diabetes is higher than among persons not overweight, yet among all obese persons this percentage is small. However, the other way around, the correlation is very high: approximately 40 per cent of diabetics are obese when the diabetes is diagnosed, compared to a 10 per cent incidence of obesity in non-diabetics.

3. Severity: the greater the obesity, the higher the incidence of diabetes. In one series the incidence was 1.5 times normal among those 10 per cent overweight, 3 times normal if 20 per cent overweight, and 8 times normal if 25 per cent overweight.

Weight gain in overweight persons with limited carbohydrate tolerance further reduces glucose tolerance; weight reduction in the obese improves glucose tolerance.

Liver Disease. Obesity has a definite and deleterious effect upon the liver. The most significant relationship seems to be the duration rather than the degree of obesity. Zelman[19] studied liver function in 20 men who were 50 to 100 per cent overweight and not known to be suffering from any other disorder which might affect the liver. Needle biopsy revealed degenerative changes and functional tests revealed deficiencies in practically all of the patients, severe enough to be classed as of moderate degree in approximately one-half of them. Fatty infiltration and higher total metabolism with relative B-complex vitamin deficiency accompanying high carbohydrate diets were considered as probable factors in the liver derangement.

Cancer. The nature of the interrelationship is obscure, but there is widespread agreement that morbidity and mortality from cancer are increased in the presence of obesity. Hertig and Sommers[20] found a 30 per cent greater incidence of endometrial cancer in overweight women. Records of the Metropolitan Life Insurance Company covering a 14-year period reveal that incidence of deaths due to certain cancers was higher among overweight persons. Deaths from benign tumors of the uterus were higher among overweight women. Obesity not only is associated with a higher incidence of cancer, but introduces difficulties in its treatment. Hildreth[21] found that the 5-year survival rate in cancer of the cervix treated by irradiation was 37.5 per cent in women weighing over 170 lbs., but 54.6 percent in those under 170 lbs.

Psychological Consequences of Obesity. Corpulence may lead not only to the physical disorders we have discussed, but to psychologic aberrations. Fat persons may find themselves rejected by others in many life situations; they find that they are handicapped in many normal activities. Recent emphasis has been given to the psychologic factors in the *causation* of obesity; it is important also to realize that serious emotional and psychic *results* of obesity constitute some of its chief dangers.

Summary. In the preceding discussion we have reviewed some of the most significant information indicating that (1) obesity is a serious health hazard and increases the incidence and severity of many of the commonest causes of disability and death; also that (2) obesity is much commoner than it should be.

Since the *degree* and the *duration* of obesity are important factors in causing predisposition to (and establishing irreversibility of) many disorders, *prevention* of excessive weight gain is even more important than its removal.

OBESITY AND GROWTH

It has been amply demonstrated by many studies that undernourished children grow at subnormal rates.[131] The converse of this question arises: do overnourished children grow at supernormal rates? One study[106] indicates that this may be true, since greater thickness of body fat was correlated with faster growth rates and earlier maturation in children of both sexes. However, another possibility must be considered: the rapid growth and maturation and the greater fat deposit may both depend upon a growth factor other than calories alone. Nevertheless, the evidence is suggestive and supports the concept that growth and development are to a certain extent functions of nutritional influences.

Information at present available does not support the speculation that increased growth hormone might cause obesity.

Various reviews[107] of the interrelationships of nutrition and growth suggest that the well-documented increases in secular growth rate (larger recent generations) are at least in part due to better nutrition.

OBESITY AS A SYMPTOM

This brief review of the facts known concerning the consequences of corpulence emphasizes the serious nature of a condition too often neglected, or even viewed as a sign of abundant good health. Often the symptom of obesity may be only a minor complaint as far as the patient is concerned. However, the physician may discover that it deserves major consideration and, possibly, that it lies at the root of many or all of the patient's difficulties. Fortunately, the general public is becoming more conscious of the decreased efficiency accompanying overweight and its ultimate bad effects. Therefore, more frequently now than formerly the chief complaint of patients seeking medical advice is obesity. This state of affairs is desirable for three reasons: first, early recognition and treatment may prevent serious complications; second, when a patient actually complains of being overweight he has already acknowledged that he does not want to be fat, and is more apt to be co-operative in carrying out reduction therapy; third, when the case is studied early, it is easier to discover the cause of the obesity.

THE CAUSE OF OBESITY

Understanding of the reasons for and the mechanism of the deposit of excessive amounts of fat in the body will enable the physician to help his patients prevent obesity and to help get rid of it when it has occurred.

The three chief fuel-producing foodstuff groups are proteins, carbohydrates and fats. All three are to a certain extent stored in the body. However, protein and carbohydrate stores are relatively small and unimportant as energy reservoirs compared to the body stores of fat. Excessive protein storage does not occur. When protein is taken in excess of body needs, part of the excess is simply excreted, but part is converted into fat and stored as such. When too much carbohydrate is taken, all of the body glycogen reservoirs seem first to be filled, then the excess carbohydrate not utilized for fuel or stored as glycogen may be converted into fat. When prolonged fasting occurs, the fat stores may serve as a source of fuel for a long period. The glycogen stores are used up within a short time. The protein, stored chiefly in the muscles, cannot be utilized without an attack upon the very structure of the body. Fortunately, the protein is the last to go. It is evident, then, that excessive intake of fat, or of protein, or of carbohydrate will lead to excessive deposition of fat in the body. In this sense all foods are fattening, although fat itself will, of course, be stored more readily as fat. The ultimate result of a prolonged immoderate intake of food is, therefore, always the same.

A pound (453.6 grams) of fat as stored in the body is approximately the equivalent of 3,500 calories. With each gram of fat in the cells of fatty tissue there is stored only about one-tenth gram of water. Glycogen stores carry with each gram of carbohydrate some two to four grams of water. Protein does not exist as storage material—all body protein is part of active body components, such as muscle, serum proteins, hormones, enzymes, etc. As such in the body each gram of protein is associated with several grams of water. Fat is therefore the most efficiently stored of fuels.

When body fat stores are consumed to provide fuel (energy), fat is by far the most productive, yielding close to the theoretical 9 calories per gram because of the low water content; glycogen and body proteins yield not the theoretical 4 calories per gram but only 1 to 2, because of the associated water.

With a caloric deficit of about 500 calories a day, weight loss should be about a pound a week, figuring 3,500 calories (7 times 500) as about the caloric equivalent of a pound of fatty tissue. If the deficit is 1,000 calories a day, weight loss should be two pounds a week. This rate of loss is rapid enough in nearly all instances. More severe caloric restriction or the actual brief starvation sometimes practiced requires careful daily medical supervision.

A plethora of calories is the only explanation of obesity, all protestations of our corpulent patients to the contrary notwithstanding. The law of the conservation of energy applies to the human body as surely as to any other heat- and energy-producing machine. Energy, or heat as represented by the caloric equivalent of food, can be neither created nor destroyed. When the intake exceeds the output expended in work and heat, the excess will be found stored in the body tissues. In children, when the body is growing, a positive energy balance for tissue building is necessary. However, after growth is complete, the excess calories do not produce useful body tissue but detrimental adiposity. Numerous careful studies by many investigators have demonstrated conclusively that changes in body weight can be predicted accurately when all metabolic influences are known and measured. Newburgh[11] and his collaborators have published analyses of the apparently paradoxical situation in which weight is maintained temporarily in spite of low caloric intake, revealing that transient water retention is the explanation.

FAT METABOLISM AND STORAGE OF FAT

The fat absorbed from the gastrointestinal tract and the fat formed in intermediary metabolism are widely deposited in the fat depots of various tissues. The sites of greatest storage are the subcutaneous tissues, the intermuscular tissues, the omentum, the perirenal tissues, the mesentery and the pericardium.

The immediate destination of the absorbed neutral fat is the fat depots of the tissues. Here it remains until needed as a source of fuel.

The average daily fat intake of a normal adult is 70 to 120 Gm., varying greatly with total caloric intake. The fat of food consists mainly of neutral fat (triglycerides) together with small amounts of free fatty acids, lecithin and cholesterol esters. Digestion and absorption of the fats takes place chiefly in the duodenum and proximal jejunum. Formerly it was thought that triglycerides had to be completely hydrolyzed in the intestine to glycerol and three molecules of fatty acid before absorption, but present evidence indicates that such is not the case.

There are three major phases involved in the transfer of fats from the intestinal lumen to the lymphatic system: (1) the intraluminal digestive phase, during which the fat is modified physically and chemically prior to absorption; (2) cellular phase, during which the digested material passes into the intestinal mucosal cells and undergoes many physical and chemical changes, especially in preparation for (3) passage from the intestinal mucosal cells into the lymphatics.

The form in which lipids are absorbed and the rate of absorption depend upon various reactions taking place in the intestinal lumen. For optimal enzymatic activity in digestion and also for absorption, emulsification is necessary. So thorough is emulsification normally that some of the minute fat droplets pass through the intestinal wall without further preparation. Bile salts and lysolecithin are prime factors in emulsification, but protein also helps disperse the lipids. Bile salts also activate intestinal and pancreatic lipolytic enzymes, as well as playing a crucial role in absorption of all the lipids.

Most of the emulsified triglycerides are hydrolyzed to monoglycerides, diglycerides, fatty acids and glycerol. In the mucosal cells the long-chain fatty acids, monoglycerides and diglycerides are incorporated into triglycerides, which enter the intestinal lymphatics. The mucosal cells also utilize long-chain fatty acids for the synthesis of phospholipids and for the partial esterification of the absorbed cholesterol. The greater part of the absorbed lipids is carried by chylomicra (protein-stabilized particles of tri-, di-, and monoglycerides, cholesterol esters, cholesterol and phospholipids) through the lymphatics to the thoracic duct and thus into the general circulation. The distribution of fatty acids in postprandial lymph from the thoracic duct is approximately: glyceride 82 per cent, phospholipids 10 per cent, cholesterol esters 2 per cent and free fatty acids 6 per cent.

Another route is used for a smaller fraction of the products of lipid digestion: after absorption, the unesterified short-chain (12-carbon or less) fatty acids, the glycerol and the steroid hormones (estradiol, cortisol, testosterone, etc.) are transported to the liver by the portal vein.

The anatomical arrangement of the two main routes permits extrahepatic tissue, particularly fat depots, to clear the blood of chylomicra and to utilize absorbed fatty substances directly. In animal studies 60 per cent of the chylomicra may be cleared from the blood in 10 minutes, with 25 per cent of the cleared lipid being in adipose tissue, 23 per cent in muscle and 20 per cent in the liver.

Fate of Fat After Absorption. Fat may be utilized in three chief ways:

1. It is stored as neutral fat (triglycerides) in the adipose tissues.

2. It is built into the structure of all tissues. Structural lipids are as integral a part of the cell architecture as are proteins. In starvation, fat in the depots is drawn upon as a source of energy but the structural lipids are spared (until the situation becomes extreme). Among the structural lipids are:

a. Lecithin (and the related cephalins).

b. Cholesterol esters.

The lipids in these two groups are essential constituents of all cell membranes. Lecithin is a component of the medullary sheath of nerve fibers.

c. Certain specialized lipids such as the sphingomyelins and cerebrosides of the central nervous system.

d. Steroid hormones, such as those of the ovary, testis, and adrenal cortex.

3. It undergoes complete oxidation to yield energy, CO_2 and H_2O.

BLOOD LIPIDS

Normal fasting serum contains highly variable amounts of the various lipids. Cholesterol, phospholipids (fats containing phosphate esters), and triglycerides (esters of glycerol and fatty acids) constitute the principal lipids occurring in blood. The normal ranges in mg. per 100 ml. in fasting serum are:

1. Fatty acids: 250 to 500 mg. (average 300); of these approximately 80 per cent occur in triglycerides and 15 per cent are esterified with cholesterol. The remaining 5 per cent are unesterified free fatty acids presumably bound to albumin.

2. Cholesterol: 150 to 230 mg. (cholesterol esters constitute 65 to 75 per cent of the total).

3. Phospholipids: 150 to 250 mg. Phospholipids contain about 80 per cent fatty

acids, 15 to 20 per cent cephalins and 5 per cent sphingomyelins. The synthesis of phospholipids depends largely upon dietary supplies of choline. Lecithin contains choline as part of the molecule and yields choline on hydrolysis.

Total Lipids. The normal fasting total serum lipids vary from 470 to 750 mg. per 100 ml. However, determinations of total lipid are not commonly employed; studies are usually confined to estimations of cholesterol (free and esterified), phospholipids, and triglycerides including fatty acids.

Lactescence of plasma or serum is due to macroscopic aggregates of chylomicrons and low-density lipoproteins mostly from hydrolysis of triglycerides. It is especially observed in blood drawn a few hours after a high fat meal. Lactescence occurring as long as 12 hours after a meal, largely due to chylomicrons, is observed particularly in idiopathic hyperlipemia.

Physiologic hyperlipemia without lactescence is often observed in the blood of normal persons drawn 3 or 4 hours after ingestion of large amounts of fat.

Pathologic hyperlipemia occurs when carbohydrate metabolism is deficient and fats become the main source of calories (low carbohydrate diets, glycogen storage disease, diabetes mellitus, etc.).

Triglycerides and Fatty Acids. Normal fasting triglyceride varies from 0 to 250 mg. per 100 ml. Only negligible amounts of free fatty acids occur in normal fasting plasma. Total fatty acids as determined in the laboratory include triglycerides, cholesterol esters and phospholipids. Determinations of triglycerides are necessary for the differential diagnosis of the idiopathic hyperlipemias. They are usually increased in glycogen storage disease, hypercholesteremia and hyperphospholipidemia.

Phospholipid Elevation. Hyperphospholipidemia may occur in a number of conditions, including uncontrolled diabetes mellitus, nephrosis, hypothyroidism, etc. It is particularly characteristic of xanthomatous biliary cirrhosis, in which the levels may reach 800 to 3,000 mg. per 100 ml.

Cholesterol Elevation. The chief exogenous sources of this lipid are the dietary animal fats, but it is also synthesized in the body. Blood cholesterol content is increased in diabetes mellitus, arteriosclerosis and atherosclerosis, hypothyroidism, nephrosis, xanthomatosis, etc.

THE LIVER IN FAT METABOLISM

When fats are to be used, they are withdrawn (by unknown means) from the adipose tissue cells and pass to the liver. In the fasting state, unesterified fatty acids, freed from depot fat by *lipoprotein lipase* are brought to the liver for utilization. Under usual normal conditions the fat content of the liver is essentially unchanged, since the fat is metabolized as fast as it arrives.

Desaturation of fatty acids probably occurs chiefly in the liver, and phospholipids and fats deposited in the liver contain fatty acids that are more unsaturated than are fatty acids in other tissues.

Normally fat is metabolized thus:

1. The triglycerides are hydrolyzed (enzyme: liver lipase), yielding glycerol and fatty acids. The glycerol is utilized via the pathways of carbohydrate metabolism.

2. The fatty acids are oxidized to acetyl-CoA units containing 2 C each.

3. The acetyl-CoA units are completely oxidized to CO_2 and H_2O with energy liberation, or

4. The acetyl-CoA units are recombined to give acetoacetic acid (a 4 C compound). This process is called ketogenesis, since acetoacetic acid is a ketone. This is a normal step in fat metabolism, as ketones are regularly formed by the liver.

5. The liver cannot further metabolize acetoacetic acid; it is distributed to the tissues where it is completely oxidized to yield CO_2, H_2O and energy.

Ketosis occurs if the liver production of acetoacetic acid exceeds the ability of the tissues to utilize it, and ketone bodies accumulate in the blood. The maximum amount which the tissues can use is about 2.5 Gm. of fat per Kg. body weight per day (about 175 Gm. for a 70 Kg. man).

When carbohydrate supply is deficient, increased metabolism of fat may, through all of the steps above, supply energy, prevent further utilization of depleted carbohydrate stores, and thus help to maintain the blood glucose level.

FATTY LIVER. Under certain circumstances the liver cells may become abnormally loaded with excess fat. This appears to develop when (1) fat is provided in excess and glucose metabolism is deficient, or (2) the hepatic cells are unable, because of functional impairment, to normally metabolize and dispose of the fats brought to them. Since a certain minimum amount of glucose is necessary for maintenance of normal function of hepatic cells and also to preserve their anatomic integrity, and since fat metabolism is accelerated whenever glucose metabolism is deficient, (1) and (2) often occur together. However (2) may be primary when toxins, poisons, etc. damage the liver.

Neutral fat and cholesterol esters may accumulate in the liver in many conditions, especially those in which hepatic damage occurs in association with a toxic or infectious disease or prolonged nutritional disorder. Such abnormal fat deposit in the liver occurs in alcoholism, starvation, diabetes mellitus, toxemias of pregnancy, following certain poisons (phosphorus, chloroform, benzol, carbon tetrachloride), with forced fat feeding, low choline intake, etc.

Storage of Fat

The depots of body fat (adipose tissue) constitute the chief fuel reserve of the body and are composed almost exclusively of triglycerides. In contrast to the small carbohydrate reserves of about one pound, fat reserves normally are 10 to 15 per cent of body weight, amounting to 15 to 22 lb. in a 150 lb. person. This is equivalent to an energy reserve of 1000 cal. per Kg. body weight—more than a month's supply of total food energy. In obese persons, the fat reserve may be in great excess of this liberal normal safety factor, and may amount in extreme cases to hundreds of pounds.

It must be emphasized that neutral fat is not deposited in the matrix between cells or fibers. The triglycerides are stored in the cells of adipose tissue. The cytoplasm diminishes in amount as the fat accumulates, until the cell becomes a thin, cytoplasmic nucleated envelope enclosing a large fat droplet. Adipose tissue exists in a state of dynamic equilibrium with the systems regulating energy metabolism: it stores fat when present in excess of immediate metabolic needs, releasing it when required. In some manner not yet well understood, when normal fat depots are taxed to capacity by arriving fat supplies, the tissues are stimulated to grow and new cells are supplied as needed, so new adipose tissue is created to meet the demand.

The triglycerides of adipose tissue are derived from two main sources: (1) from food fat; (2) from carbohydrate.

Normally the triglycerides of the adipose tissue are in a constant state of exchange with the lipids of the plasma. The problem in obesity is to determine why the fat depots remain excessive or keep growing.

When fats are utilized as fuel, the fatty acids are broken down to carbon dioxide and water. Body fat acts as a highly efficient storehouse of energy: the capacity to store protein and carbohydrate is extremely limited, fat storage is almost unlimited. Pure fat yields 9 calories per gram in combustion, pure protein or glucose only 4 calories per gram.

When the body loses fat, however, the metabolic processes also include the loss of water: for each gram of fat stored, there is stored about 0.1 gram of water. For each gram of carbohydrate or protein lost, the water loss is much greater—some 2 to 4 grams.[129]

Fat stores are definitely in the dynamic state, less readily utilizable for calories than glycogen and glucose, but more readily available than protein. When caloric demand is brief, glucose is the chief source; when prolonged, fat becomes the chief source. The deposition and the mobilization of fat is an active metabolic process in adipose tissue.[23] Adipose tissue is supplied by a rich capillary network and is innervated by the autonomic nervous system. In the adipose tissue new fatty acids are synthesized, fatty acids are transformed to other forms of fatty acids, and glycogen also is synthesized. All of these metabolic functions are controlled by a number of hormonal and nervous influences.

Insulin plays an essential part in lipogenesis. New insight into fat metabolism is permitted by the discovery and the elucidation of the role of coenzyme A (CoA).[24,25] It seems well established that carbohydrate is converted into fat primarily by way of pyruvate, which subsequently is decarboxylated to form acetyl CoA. It appears that acetyl CoA is the major precursor of long-chain fatty acids. Thus glycolysis is the first major metabolic process involved in the conversion of carbohydrate to fat, and glycolysis is in turn dependent upon insulin. It seems that any substance which can give rise to acetyl CoA or "active acetate" can be converted to fatty acids. Adipose tissues as well as a number of other tissues have the ability to synthesize fat. When insulin is lacking, fat formation from the 2-carbon precursors, the ubiquitous "active acetate," is inhibited. It may be "too naïve to suppose that excess fat formation tends to exhaust the insulin mechanisms; however there is surely a clue herein."[26] Further discussion in the section on Etiology will emphasize the important interrelationships of fat metabolism and obesity to diabetes and hyperinsulinism.

Fats are excreted in relatively large amounts by the intestinal mucosa, to a small degree in the bile, and in minute amounts by the oil glands of the skin. In the feces, fat is normally present in three forms: soap fats (combined fatty acids), free fatty acids and neutral fat. The relative amount of each depends upon the type of fats ingested and upon the efficiency of fat digestion and absorption. In cases of diarrhea, there may be unusually large amounts of fat present in the feces, simply because of the rapid passage of food through the bowel, with poor absorption. When insufficient amounts of pancreatic lipase reach the intestine, the stools are fatty because of incomplete digestion. Absence of bile likewise results in faulty fat digestion with fatty stools.

HUNGER AND APPETITE

The terms *hunger* and *appetite* have been variously defined and are used widely with various connotations. In Chapter 21 the degree of desire for food is discussed particularly in regard to its diminution, called *anorexia*. In this chapter we are concerned with sensations of heightened desire for food, since, if gratified, excessive or too frequent hunger or appetite may lead to obesity.

As used in this chapter, *hunger* has an organic basis in the body's need for food. The need may be in the tissues, or may simply exist as hunger contractions of an empty stomach, but it can be demonstrated definitely to be due to a chemical need or a physical state. Hunger is a complex sensation and various theories have been proposed to explain it. Hunger is the principal factor controlling food intake, and consequently, body growth and nutrition. Accompanying the sensation of hunger there are frequently strong contractions of the gastric walls ("hunger contractions"). Such contractions may be inhibited and the hunger pangs relieved by filling the stomach with bulky, even inedible, non-nutritive material. Hypoglycemia usually is accompanied by hunger. Tissue need for glucose may exist when hunger is present but the blood sugar level is high or normal. (Patients with diabetes mellitus are characteristically hungry; persons who have been starved for some time may still be hungry and continue to eat after blood glucose exceeds the normal level.) It is likely that hunger due to deficiency of nutrients at the tissue level, as well as at the blood level, exists for other nutrients than glucose. The introduction of nutrients by a route other than the mouth may appease hunger and quiet hunger contractions. Animals often seek and select the specific nutrient for which need exists ("salt hunger," etc.); thus there may be various hungers depending upon the general body state and apparently controlled by one or more central mechanisms. These aspects of the problem are discussed further below under "Role of the hypothalamus and higher brain centers."

Appetite is considered primarily a psychic phenomenon, unlike hunger, which is considered essentially an organic manifestation. Appetite may be defined as the desire for food whether or not the need exists. Usually appetite accompanies hunger (desire accompanies need), but under certain circumstances this natural association may not occur, and appetite and hunger may be dissociated. Apparently, appetite is largely acquired and is dependent to a great degree upon previous experience, whereas hunger is inborn. A newborn child experiences hunger, not appetite. Conditioned stimuli and responses exert considerable control over appetite. Training and environmental influences are well known to exert profound influences upon national, local or individual desire for certain foods. Thus the psychic element in appetite is illustrated by its highly selective character. Snails or rattlesnake meat to some persons are highly desirable and even their mention may heighten appetite, but to others, even though the food may be nutritious and the person hungry, such foods may destroy appetite.

Hunger usually whets appetites. Foods usually considered unpalatable may be consumed avidly if true hunger is present. Any stimulus that increases hunger is apt also to increase appetite. When alcohol is ingested, or dilute hydrochloric acid, the flow of gastric juices is stimulated, gastric tone is raised and appetite is aroused. Often appetite is increased greatly after a few mouthfuls of food enter the stomach.

A person may be hungry and anorexic, or even nauseated at the same time. If he has an appetite, however, he welcomes food, even though he may not truly be hungry. Attractively prepared foods and pleasant food odors are powerful stimulants to appetite.

ETIOLOGY OF OBESITY

Although the immediate cause of obesity is always a positive energy balance, there are many ways in which it is conceivable that the balance may be tilted toward the positive side. Let us list these, then consider them in order:

POSSIBLE FACTORS IN THE PATHOGENESIS OF OBESITY

1. Digestive factors: is digestion more complete?
2. Absorptive factors: is absorption more efficient?
3. Tissue factors:
   A. Do tissues take up fats more readily?
   B. Do tissues fail to give up fat stores as readily as normal?
   C. Local and general tissue factors: insulin, enzymes.
4. Utilization of energy:
   A. Basal metabolic rate: is it lower?
   B. Specific dynamic action of food: is there less stimulation to increased heat production after intake of food?
   C. "Luxuskonsumption": is obesity the result of a failure to exhibit a rise in total metabolic rate following excess food intake?
   D. Total metabolism: does obesity result from conservation of energy in work, or in carrying out other normal body functions?
   E. Physical activity: does physical inactivity cause obesity?
5. Endocrine factors: role of pituitary disease, adrenal cortex, hypothyroidism, gonadal hormones, diabetes mellitus, hyperinsulinism with and without hypoglycemia, and hypoglycemia with and without hyperinsulinism.
6. Role of the hypothalamus and higher brain centers.
7. Influence of heredity.
8. Psychologic factors: mental and emotional factors influencing hunger, appetite and food intake.
9. Social factors.

Digestive Factors. Although a lack of some of the essential digestive ferments may lead to a loss from the body of calories as undigested food (for example, protein and fat loss in the feces in pancreatic disease), an excess of digestive enzymes or increased efficiency of digestion has never been demonstrated to occur in obesity. Obesity is, therefore, not explainable on the basis that the food taken into the body is more completely broken down in the gastrointestinal tract of a person who becomes corpulent than in that of a normal person.

Absorptive Factors. It is conceivable that more efficient and more complete absorption of the products of digestion might enable certain persons to gain weight without excessive intake of food. However, Neuenschwander-Lemmer[27] has compared the combustible materials in the feces with those in the food eaten, and in three obese and three normal patients found no essential differences. The utilization of the dietary constituents by the obese was no different in any way from that of the normal subjects in regard to total calories, nitrogen or fat. In this connection it is interesting to compare these figures with those obtained from a group of nine undernourished persons gaining weight rapidly upon a forced high-caloric intake. Strang, McClugage and Brownlee[28] found practically the same percentage of food ingested to be absorbed in these patients receiving forced feedings as in the obese and the normal patients in the above study. It might have been expected that less efficient absorption would be demonstrated as the result of undue strain upon digestive and absorptive mechanisms, but such was not the case. Supernormal efficiency of digestion or of absorption is, therefore, not present in obesity.

Tissue Factors. If there were a hereditary constitutional tendency of the adipose cells that enabled them to accumulate excessive amounts of fat, obesity would result. This attractive hypothesis was proposed many years ago by von Bergmann.[29] He compared obesity with growth. A child grows, storing the materials necessary for growth, even though his activity consumes great quantities of food. Thus the fat tissues of obese persons might store fat, even though the diet were inadequate to meet other body needs. This is the theory of *lipophilia*.

Hetenyi[30] carried the idea of lipophilia a step farther by postulating that fat deposited in the depots of an obese person is held there, even when needed as fuel. When the fat tissues of a normal person would release it as a source of energy, the obese person's tissues might still retain the fat.

Neither ingested nor stored fat would be readily or normally available for the energy requirements of an obese person if von Bergmann's and Hetenyi's theories should prove tenable. Increased food intake in the obese would be necessary to fill the requirements for work and heat, while fat was continuously stored. Hetenyi supported this concept by showing that when given an inadequate diet, the level of blood fats in obese persons falls more than in normal subjects. He believed that there was a delay or hindrance in the release of fat by the tissues of the obese patients.

Newburgh interpreted Hetenyi's own data as evidence against this hypothesis. He said that since obese persons have more fat in the blood when food is unrestricted, they must be either storing less or mobilizing more of it than normal persons. The lowering of the blood-fat level in obese persons by under-feeding might not mean that fat was released less rapidly from adipose tissue, but that fat that was mobilized at a normal rate was oxidized more rapidly.

If it were true that the adipose tissue cells of obese persons resist mobilization of fat in undernutrition, obese persons on restricted diets should exhibit destruction of body protein and a negative nitrogen balance. This would be true because there would be no other source of calories. Glycogen stores are rapidly exhausted in a few days of severe undernutrition. If fat were unavailable, protein would have to be utilized. However, a number of studies have shown that obese persons are *less likely to develop negative nitrogen balance* than normal subjects. Jansen[31] gave 15 medical students a diet of 1,600 calories, including 61 Gm. of protein, daily for several weeks. The average daily nitrogen loss was 2 Gm. Benedict[32] studied 12 normal subjects receiving 1,534 calories and 51 Gm. of protein daily, and noted 3 Gm. daily as the average nitrogen loss. In studying obese persons given a diet yielding 1,375 calories with 90 Gm. of protein daily, Keeton and Dickson[33] found maintenance of nitrogen balance. Even when the caloric intake is extremely low, fat stores can be mobilized sufficiently to spare body protein, as indicated by the fact that Strang, McClugage and Evans[34] found that obese persons did not lose protein when receiving only 440 calories daily and approximately 1 Gm. of protein per kilogram of ideal body weight.

Block,[35] reinvestigating the possible role of lipophilia, found that three obese subjects remained in positive nitrogen balance during a prolonged period of undernutrition. The blood lipids varied in essentially the same manner as in three normal subjects following the same diets. They at first rose, then later fell. The actual weight loss in the obese patients was in very close agreement with that predicted on the assumption that the body fat was utilized for heat production. These results indicate that the theory of lipophilia is untenable as an explanation for the usual type of obesity.

Study of blood fat and fatty acids has not uniformly revealed a greater avidity for these materials in the tissues of obese persons. When Hetenyi fed fat or injected olive oil into obese subjects, he found only a relatively slight rise in blood lipids as compared to that produced in normal persons, which might be interpreted as indicating more rapid fat deposit in the obese. However, other workers have obtained contradictory results. Obese persons commonly have a somewhat higher blood-lipid level than average normal, which certainly might not indicate increased fat storage, and might be the result of increased fat mobilization.

A possible explanation for the conflict in such studies is proposed as a result of studies by Schechter[102] who found, as did Hetenyi, a greater avidity for lipids in the adipose tissue of obese persons. The avidity was most evident in the *static phase* of obesity, less evident in the dynamic phase.

Antoniades and Gundersen[105,110] have described an enzyme in adipose tissue which releases insulin from its binding to basic protein in the plasma, thereby permitting the freed insulin to act to promote fat storage. Certain questions arise as the result of such observations: (1) Could differences in the concentrations of such an enzyme in adipose tissues account for generalized adiposity in some persons? (2) Could differences in concentrations of the enzyme explain, by its action on fat synthesis and deposition, the distribution of adipose deposits as they vary between persons and in many clinical states?

The possibility that fat cells in certain persons may react abnormally has been supported by studies of hereditary obesity in yellow mice. Radioactive carbon (C^{14}) is incorporated into their fat depots in an apparently normal manner, but the labeled fat disappeared from the tissues much more slowly than in normal mice.[36] The decrease in fat mobilization thus may be a fat cell disorder, perhaps an enzyme defect, and it can be hereditary. We have then a modern revival of the *lipophilia* theory of von Bergmann.

In the obese diabetic strain of mice, Guggenheim and Mayer[37] found that when C^{14}-labeled acetate was injected into the fasting animal, one-third less C^{14} appeared in the expired air than in normals. The incorporation of fed C^{14} acetate into fatty acids in obese mice was found to be much higher than in nonobese mice. It was concluded that the obese animals do not oxidize acetate as readily as normals and that the acetate which escapes oxidation is incorporated into fat. As a corollary to this theory, lipolysis is decreased due to impaired acetate oxidation.

The disappearance of C^{14}-labeled fat from the depots of obese rats with hypothalamic lesions proved to be just as slow as that found in yellow mice.[38] Therefore the cell defect can be acquired, and could possibly be the result of the obesity rather than its cause. The slow turnover of C^{14} in the obese diabetic mice might be due to some derangements of carbohydrate metabolism or possibly due to the large pool of fat: the abnormal composition of the animal's body. Further such studies on obese mice may yield progressive insight into the mechanisms of human obesity.

Blood lipids are usually elevated when there is a continuously greater demand for fat as fuel as the result of the lack of available carbohydrate. Hyperlipemia occurs in ether narcosis, for example, and in diabetes mellitus. Insulin in these two conditions can reduce or prevent the hyperlipemia, presumably by facilitating the combustion of carbohydrate, by decreasing fat mobilization, and by promoting fat storage. In diabetes mellitus, in malnutrition, in fasting, in certain liver disorders, and in similar conditions in which carbohydrate is lacking or cannot be utilized adequately, the blood lipids are increased and the fatty-tissue reserves are diminished.

Local factors instead of general influences controlling fat storage are known to exist, although their nature is not understood. The author has observed a number of patients who have developed the well-recognized *fat atrophy* that occurs in a relatively small percentage of patients receiving insulin repeatedly at the same subcutaneous site. There must be in certain persons local tissue responses to insulin that differ from the usual response. The author also has observed the more infrequent phenomenon of the development of *lipomata* at the site of insulin injections. Here the local-tissue effect seems to be the exact opposite, although the stimulus, insulin, is the same. In lipomatosis it seems evident that local conditions must be present that facilitate the deposit of fat. Lipomata may resist the mobilization of their contained fat, and remain unchanged during generalized weight loss and reduction in adipose tissue.

Lipodystrophy has been described in a wide variety of forms. It may affect only the face, or one-half of the face, or the legs, or all of the tissues above or below the umbilicus. The type of lipodystrophy that is most common affects women and involves the tissues above the waist. The upper half of the body, the neck and the face may be emaciated, while the girdle region, the buttocks, the hips, the thighs and the legs may be normal or obese. A number of cases of lipodystrophy have been demonstrated to be hereditary, with the exact type and location of the lesion being transmitted (van Leeuwen,[39] Nassauer-Badt[40]).

Consideration of the evident local factors influencing fat storage in such unusual conditions as lipomatosis and lipodystrophy leads to the inviting theory that the tissues in the common type of obesity may possess some such abnormal property that is generally distributed. It is known that blood, liver, pancreas and subcutaneous tissue contain various lipases. These enzymes are capable of causing profound changes locally in tissue fats under certain conditions. Little is known about the physical and the chemical conditions that activate or inhibit these enzyme systems, but they may be important in influencing fat storage. Barr[40a] feels that, since careful study by many able investigators has not revealed the cause of obesity elsewhere, better knowledge of tissue metabolism may yield the answer. He says: "It does not seem improbable that local or general conditions in the body might influence such enzyme systems and that disturbances in fat storage might occur because of their derangement; also that this might occur to a certain extent independent of the supply of fat in the food or the amount of fat or fatty acids in the blood." He feels that if the local deposits of lipomatosis can be explained by local tissue changes, the generalized adiposity in obesity may be due to the ability of the mesenchymal tissues to store and retain large amounts of fat. Such an unusual ability for the mesenchymal tissues might result from heritage, cerebral lesions or endocrine factors.

Studies of fatty tissue suggest that enzyme systems function differently in the overweight; perhaps the excess of calories over need induces changes in the storage, utilization, and mobilization mechanisms.[123] Many of these changes are reversible by weight reduction. Some studies in experimental animals suggest that in a few strains a firm storage mechanism may be hereditarily fixed and does not yield readily to dieting.[133] Bray and his co-workers have found a difference between the fatty tissue of juvenile-onset obesity cases and that of several cases of obesity caused by intracranial lesions. The juvenile forms are less able to oxidize alpha-glycerol phosphate (derived from glucose) so that it tends to go directly into triglyceride synthesis.[123b] Hirsch, Knittle, and Salans's recent work in animals and human subjects[124] indicates that the number of fat cells becomes fixed relatively early in life, that their number is related to the amount of food fed early in life, that obese adults have more and larger fat cells than do normal controls, and that these large cells are relatively resistant to the action of insulin until they lose their excessive store of fat. In these obese people, weight loss reduces the size of the fat cells but not their number. Perhaps when they are reduced in size, these cells emit some sort of chemical signal inducing a formerly obese person to eat more. A common clinical observation is that obese persons who have lost weight tend to regain it to approximately the same peak level previously attained.

These studies suggest that (1) each person has his own individually adjusted *"appestat"* mechanism, and that (2) tissue factors are perhaps related in a number of ways to fat storage and to control of appetite. Among the tissue factors may be *enzymes*. The number and size of adipocytes may be important, especially whether or not they are gorged to capacity with fat. We need to learn not only how excess calories cause existing shrunken fat cells to reload with fat, but how new formation of adipocytes is brought about.

It is notable that most of the studies so far done have been performed upon subjects already obese. Many of the observations may describe only pathophysiologic processes which are the consequences of obesity. We need studies upon non-obese subjects that will reveal to us how and why certain ones become obese, but others do not.

Utilization of Energy. Basal Metabolic Rate. If it could be demonstrated that when at rest obese persons conserve energy by lowering the rate of metabolic activity, an important influence tipping the scales toward a positive energy balance would be apparent. However, this definitely is not the case. Boothby and Sandiford[41] found that in 81 per cent of 94 obese persons the basal heat production per square meter of body surface was within 10 per cent of the normal. Strouse, Wang and Dye[42] found practically no differences in the basal metabolic rates of normal, overweight and underweight subjects. Grafe[43] studied 180 cases of extreme obesity and found a low basal metabolic rate in only three patients.

Occasionally a very low rate will be found in an obese person, but rates as low are encountered in those who are underweight. Severe hypothyroidism is not regularly accompanied by obesity.

Specific Dynamic Action. Following the intake of food, the heat production is elevated due to a "specific dynamic action" upon metabolism. This is not due to digestion or absorption, since it occurs even after the intravenous injection of glucose or amino acids. Should the metabolism of food be accomplished with less expenditure of energy, obesity might result. On the usual type of diet the total specific dynamic action in 24 hours may amount to 6 per cent of the day's energy output. Plaut's experiments[44] seemed to show a rather uniform tendency toward lowered S.D.A. in obese persons, particularly those identified as hypopituitary in type. Lauter,[45] Strang and McClugage[46] and others have been unable to confirm the demonstration of a lowered S.D.A. in obese persons. Johnston,[47] in a series of studies upon patients with definite destructive pituitary lesions, found the S.D.A. within normal limits. Protein is responsible for the greatest part of the specific dynamic action of food. Dock[48] concluded that at least 80 per cent of the effect is due to the increased heat produced by the hepatic cells during metabolic changes in protein.

While the view generally accepted at present denies that a difference in the specific heat response to food has an important role in the pathogenesis of obesity, it is difficult to reconcile Plaut's positive observations and the confirmatory results of Kestner, Knipping, Liebesny and others with the negative results of later workers. Mac-Bryde[49] reported studies indicating that the *nutritional state* might not be accompanied regularly by an alteration in the S.D.A., but that the *nutritional phase* might be accompanied by alterations in the S.D.A. During periods of weight gain, obese, normal and thin subjects had lower specific dynamic effects from a standard mixed test meal than the same subjects receiving the same meal exhibited in periods of induced weight loss. It is conceivable that heat production dependent upon liver metabolism may vary according to the disposal of amino acids, fatty acids, glucose and other products of digestion reaching the hepatic cells. During periods of storage, heat production might be low, while during periods of active utilization the specific dynamic action might be relatively high. Failure of previous workers to take into account the *phase* of nutrition, while considering the nutritional *state* only, could well account for the divergent results recorded by a number of excellent investigators. From this standpoint it is evident that one could not expect to reveal a mechanism resulting in gain of weight if the studies were done upon obese subjects actively losing weight.

It seems, therefore, that the subject of the specific dynamic action of food is not yet closed. Further studies will be necessary to determine whether other workers can confirm the author's observations that the S.D.A. may be decreased in any subject actively storing, rather than burning, a large proportion of the products of digestion.

"LUXUSKONSUMPTION." When inadequate amounts of food are taken, the basal metabolic rate may be lowered. The body possesses a means by which the combustion of body-tissue stores is retarded during severe undernutrition. Thus, in the cachexia resulting from severe anorexia nervosa, the basal metabolic rate may reach levels of minus 30 per cent, which adds to the difficulty of distinguishing such cases from Simmonds' disease. When feeding is restored toward normal, the basal metabolic rate returns toward normal values. Grafe[50] carried this concept further by postulating that in addition to the metabolic stimuli of activity and the specific dynamic action of food, the total metabolism is determined by the food intake. Excess feeding, according to this theory, could stimulate heat pro-

duction so that the surplus caloric intake would automatically be dissipated. Obesity would result from a defect in this mechanism, while thinness would develop when the luxus consumption response was too great.

It is difficult to accept these views, since they include the concept that the basal metabolic rate depends primarily upon the previous food intake. Although the basal metabolism may be altered by starvation, it has not been demonstrated that it can be elevated above normal by forced feeding. Normal human beings, as well as all mammals in the basal state, produce heat in proportion to the body-surface area without regard to previously ingested food. Wiley and Newburgh[51] showed that the surface area increases and weight is gained during superalimentation. The basal metabolic rate rises and the total caloric output increases, but the heat production still is in proportion to the surface area. It therefore seems unlikely that a rise in total metabolism prevents obesity in patients who overeat.

TOTAL METABOLISM. Numerous studies have shown that weight changes can be predicted on any diet when all metabolic factors are considered. The total metabolism of obese persons is necessarily greater than that of normal persons of the same height, age and sex. This has been shown in several ways: (1) The surface area of obese persons is greater, but the basal metabolic rate per unit of surface area is the same; therefore, the total basal heat production is greater. (2) A large proportion of the body tissue of corpulent subjects is inactive, fatty, and produces relatively little heat or energy. Therefore, to maintain the same basal metabolic rate per unit of surface area, the *active* tissues of obese persons must have a higher than normal metabolic rate. (3) Obese subjects expend more energy in performing a given amount of work; therefore, the caloric requirement is greater (Lauter[52]). (4) More work to perform a given task is necessary not only by the skeletal muscles but by the heart muscle. Cardiac work at rest may be decreased by as much as 35 per cent by weight reduction in the obese.[53] Part of the fall in total metabolism induced by weight reduction results from decreased cardiac work.

From these facts one can see that obese persons not only cannot get along on less food without losing weight, but they require more food to maintain weight than do thin persons of the same height, age and sex.

However, careful observers have recorded a number of instances in which weight was maintained for considerable lengths of time upon greatly restricted diets. For two weeks, or even longer, Newburgh and his co-workers[11] found that certain obese persons lost no weight or even gained weight upon a very low caloric intake. Diuresis then occurred, so that at the end of approximately three weeks the weight loss was just that calculated from the known caloric balance. The paradox of apparent failure to lose body fat is explained by temporary retention of water.

PHYSICAL ACTIVITY. Obese persons are significantly less active physically when compared to controls matched by age, sex, etc.[108,109] In one such study, obese women walked an average of 2.0 miles per day, nonobese women, 4.9 miles; obese men 3.7 miles, nonobese men 6.0 miles.[108] Obese children engaged in school games and sports only about one-third as much as non-obese children.[109]

There appears to be definite evidence that in the United States obesity is on the increase in all age groups—more persons now are obese than ten years ago, more then than a decade earlier, etc. Some data indicate that actual food intake is, on the average, less than in 1900. Persons of earlier decades were, however, considerably more active physically; therefore, the significant change accounting for the greater frequency of obesity today is that most of us are much more sedentary—children and teen-agers as well as adults. It is pointless to debate as a general question, however, which is more important in controlling weight, food—or exercise. Both are very important. Limiting food intake is the easiest way for most sedentary persons to promote loss or to prevent fat storage. Individuals should also seek and communities foster facilities encouraging regular, healthful, and pleasurable exercise. In the individual case, sometimes these two prime factors are both significant, sometimes only one. Neither the football player nor the paraplegic who is becoming obese can do much to alter caloric imbalance by increasing exercise. However, the man who sits at a desk all day and never even takes a walk can do a great deal.

In a study of 300 men engaged in work involving a wide range of physical activity, the voluntary food intake was studied. The lowest intake was in those engaged in light exercise. The highest intake (3,000 to 3,700 calories) was in those engaged in heavy work, but their body weights tended to remain normal. The next highest intakes (3,000 to 3,400 calories) were among those in the most sedentary occupations (supervisors, clerks, etc.) and persons in this group "were much fatter."[118,126]

Energy expenditure and body weight are well adjusted in rats doing moderately strenuous treadmill exercises. However, when the activity becomes too intense, the animals develop exhaustion, with decline in food intake and weight. If activity decreases below a certain threshold level, a commensurate decrease in food intake does not occur. In fact, if activity reaches a very low level, food intake increases again. This phenonenon of low activity apparently *causing stimulation* of appetite is a paradox—it is the opposite of what we would ordinarily expect if appetite-control mechanisms were operating normally.[118,126]

As discussed above, free-living men exhibit this phenomenon, much like the experimental animals described. Farmers take advantage of the phenomenon to fatten animals by keeping them cooped up.

The mechanism to explain this paradox is not understood. We may speculate that: (1) With very low activity there is little use of glucose by muscle and also by the hypothalamic satiety center. Therefore, satiation does not occur and the lateral feeding center is not inhibited, causing food intake to remain high or even increase, and resulting in obesity. We may also speculate that: (2) If fat is being formed in great amounts, presumably ample insulin supplies are available to promote its synthesis and storage. Possibly, the circulating insulin is actually present in hypernormal amounts. This is known to be true in hyperglycemic obese mice and in many obese persons, especially those who are prediabetic or have diabetes. Such insulin is evidently not normally operative in facilitating glucose utilization in the cells of muscle or in the nerve cells of the hypothalamic satiety center.

In many moderate or early cases of obesity, especially if physical inactivity is an obvious factor, increased exercise may lead to weight loss and better control of appetite and weight.

From such observations it is tempting to conclude that relative physical inactivity

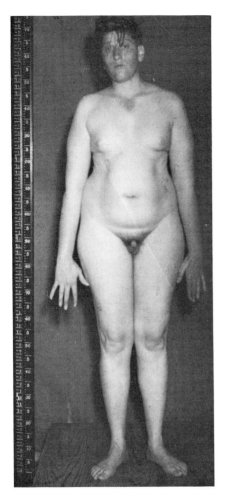

Fig. 37-1. A 24-year-old eunuchoid male with feminine distribution of fat: over breasts, hips, trochanteric regions and thighs.

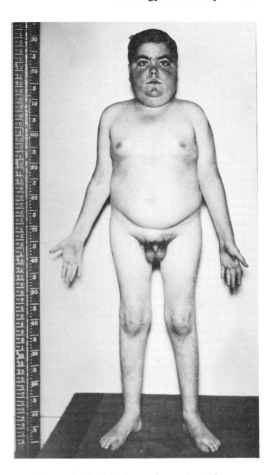

Fig. 37-2. Cushing's syndrome in a 12-year-old boy. Rubicund, plethoric face; obesity confined to face and trunk.

may be a primary factor in the etiology of the majority of cases of obesity.

However, certain considerations cast doubt upon such a sweeping generalization concerning the pathophysiology of most cases of obesity:

1. Obese persons consume more energy for the performance of each item of activity, every breath, every heartbeat, every step. The total metabolism, even with the lessened physical activity, was not significantly lower in 25 obese men.[108] Indeed, in 13 of the 25 obese men, the calculated total expenditure exceeded that of nonobese controls. Among obese women there was a calculated lower than normal total energy expenditure, as well as lower physical activity.

2. The fact that an obese person expends more energy even when "at rest" may account for his tendency to decrease overt physical exercise: therefore, inactivity may result from obesity and may perhaps not be a cause of the obesity.

Nevertheless, the role played by physical inactivity has been unduly minimized in recent years.[122] In our nation children as well as adults are more sedentary than in former generations, ride more, walk less—and are more often obese. It is probable that these facts are inter-related. Sitting requires 60 calories per hour, walking 300, swimming 500, running 900. Obviously a person who is sedentary and eats only average amounts may gain weight. If he is sedentary and eats excessively, he is apt to become obese.

Endocrine Glands. The *distribution* of body fat is largely under the control of the glands

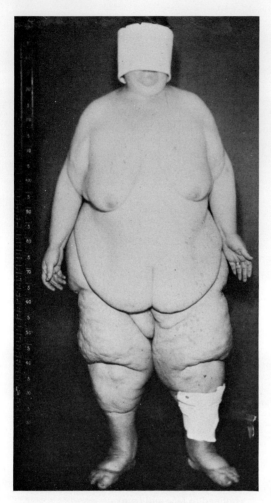

Fig. 37-3. Generalized, nodular, painful obesity sometimes called adiposis dolorosa or Dercum's disease.

of internal secretion. The simplest example of this influence is the difference between typical female adiposity and that occurring in males (Fig. 37-1). Women tend to deposit the excess fat chiefly in the region of the hips, the thighs and the buttocks, and sometimes in the mammary region, while in men the protuberant abdomen or "bay-window" distribution is characteristic. In Cushing's syndrome, one find obesity of the face, the neck and the trunk, while the extremities lose subcutaneous fat (Fig. 37-2). Virilizing tumors of the ovary or adrenal cortex may cause a normal woman to lose the rounded feminine curves of arms, legs, hips, breasts and shoulders, and to assume the angular aspects of the male. Although the distribu-

tion of body fat may depend greatly upon the endocrine makeup of the subject, the development of the obesity seldom can be attributed primarily to an endocrine disorder.

PITUITARY DISEASE. Following the report of Fröhlich[54] in 1901, in which he described an obese hypogonadal boy with a pituitary tumor, inadequate hypophysial activity was considered a cause of obesity. Cushing[55] and other workers strengthened this impression when they described obesity following hypophysectomy in animals. Smith,[56] however, demonstrated that obesity occurred only when the *hypothalamus* was injured, and not following destruction or removal of the pituitary alone.

In the earlier clinical observations and also in the experimental work the role of the pituitary was overemphasized; later, when the importance of the hypothalamus was discovered, the part played by the pituitary in the pathogenesis of obesity was too strictly minimized. Both clinical and experimental evidence suggest that (1) damage either to the pituitary or to the hypothalamus separately may cause physiologic aberrations which tend to produce obesity, and (2) normally the pituitary and the hypothalamus are integrated functionally through neural and humoral connections—thus damage to either produces changes in the other, of which obesity is a frequent consequence. As Cushing[55,57] observed, obesity commonly occurs in chromophobe adenomata which are entirely intrasellar, but the obesity is greater if there is pressure on the hypothalamus. Heinbecker *et al.*[58] found that hypothalamic lesions produced greater and quicker adiposity, but that hypophysectomy per se produced less striking weight gain. Reinecke *et al.*[59] found that hypophysectomy led to increased fat content in the rat carcass.

Clinically, as experimentally, destruction of the pituitary alone does not result in obesity, but in pituitary cachexia (Simmonds' disease). Although patients who exhibit signs of hypopituitarism and obesity are frequently encountered, in the great majority of cases it seems that the endocrine disorder is not the cause of the obesity but an associated phenomenon.

The clinical diagnosis of "pituitary obesity," formerly popular, is fortunately disappearing. A preferable term is *neurohypophysial obesity*, if there is evidence that the hypothalamus and the pituitary are involved.

The term *Fröhlich's syndrome* should be reserved for cases in which there is a known organic lesion of the pituitary-hypothalamic area with hypogonadism and obesity. The report of Fröhlich in 1901 was significant because it first related pathogenically an expanding pituitary tumor with neighborhood pressure symptoms to the obesity and genital hypoplasia exhibited by the 14-year-old male subject. *Adiposogenital dystrophy* is a useful descriptive name without diagnostic implications (Fig. 37-4). The fact that genital dystrophy accompanies the obesity may indicate that certain pathways influencing the function of the anterior pituitary may be damaged.

HYPERADRENOCORTICISM. Grafting of ACTH-secreting tumors in animals causes obesity.[109]

In hyperadrenocorticism, whether primarily due to adrenocortical hyperplasia or tumor, to pituitary-hypothalamic disorder, or to steroid administration, there is a profound alteration in metabolism of carbohydrate, protein and fat. The tissues lose protein, carbohydrate tolerance decreases, and fat deposits increase. The reason for the location of the excess fat in face, cervical hump, and central areas (trunk), while extremities become spare, is unknown. It appears that the obesity of hyperadrenocorticism or Cushing's syndrome is unique, because the tissues are depleted of protein, but at the same time fat is being deposited in excess.

In Cushing's syndrome there is a peculiar plethoric obesity confined chiefly to the head and the trunk. It is not likely that this syndrome is actually a pituitary disorder due, as originally thought, to a basophil pituitary adenoma. In many cases no such adenoma is present, and the syndrome seems to merge imperceptibly into that associated with adrenocortical hyperplasia or adrenocortical tumors. The cytoplasmic hyalinization and other changes in the pituitary basophil cells described by Crooke have apparently been found in all cases when sought. Three chief hypotheses have been offered to account for the pathogenesis of Cushing's syndrome: (1) Pituitary basophilism, either with Crooke's changes, a basophil tumor, or both, causes excess production of an adrenocorticotrophic hormone; the adrenal cortices then become hyperplastic or neoplastic and an excess production of adrenocortical hormones produces the manifestations of the disease. Some of the dysfunctions of other endocrine

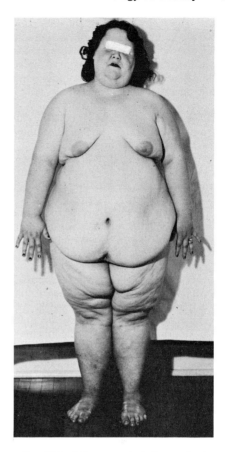

FIG. 37-4. Adiposogenital dystrophy in a 25-year-old woman. Notice the delicate facial features, the small hands and feet. There was only a small amount of breast tissue present, and menstruation was infrequent and scant.

glands may result from the primary pituitary malfunction, some from the adrenocortical hyperfunction. Heinbecker[60] has modified this concept and presents evidence that the primary disturbance is in the hypothalamus. (2) The second hypothesis states that for unknown reasons the primary disturbance arises in the adrenal cortices, with malfunction or hyperfunction expressed anatomically as hyperplasia or neoplasia. The cytologic changes in the pituitary are regarded as retrograde or degenerative in nature. (3) The third hypothesis assumes a dual etiologic process: either the pituitary or the adrenal cortex may be the primary site.

HYPOTHYROIDISM. Evidence against hypothyroidism as the usual cause of obesity has already been cited under consideration of the basal metabolic rate. Obese persons as a rule do not have the dry skin, the slow mental processes, the thin coarse hair, the hoarse voice and other accompaniments of thyroid inactivity. Myxedema is not regularly accompanied by obesity, and overweight in these patients is usually due to abnormal water retention in the body, as demonstrated by Plummer.[61]

DIABETES MELLITUS; HYPERINSULINISM. The clinical and statistical observations that diabetes is not very frequent among obese persons, but that obesity is present in a high percentage (about 40 per cent) of diabetics at the onset of the disease would seem to hold a clue: probably obesity does not "predispose to diabetes" as is so often said, but both conditions may arise from a common cause. It is probably no more accurate to think that obesity leads to diabetes than to believe that diabetes leads to obesity: neither causes the other, but both may be manifestations of the same basic endocrine and metabolic disorders.

Consideration of the interlocking pathologic physiology of the two closely related metabolic disorders, obesity and diabetes, requires a review of certain information:

1. The relative rates of lipolysis and lipogenesis depend upon the rate of glucose utilization. When glucose utilization is deficient, lipolysis exceeds lipogenesis, as in starvation, untreated diabetes, etc. When there is excess insulin and excess glucose utilization, fat formation in adipose tissue is accelerated and obesity may result.

2. Many obese diabetics have been shown to have normal or hypernormal plasma insulin levels: it would seem that certain tissues (? muscle) are refractory to insulin action, but adipose tissue is not, in such obese persons. Gundersen's observations[110] would support such a concept: proteinbound insulin of serum failed to stimulate glucose uptake by rat diaphragm; adipose tissue, however, contains an enzyme that frees the insulin. Such a situation might explain the concomitant development of diabetes and obesity: obese subjects may have difficulty in freeing insulin for nonadipose tissue and thus may have insufficient insulin action on muscle but increased insulin action in fat depots, promoting fat formation from glucose and facilitating fat storage.

3. Certain observations in many obese persons indicate hyperadrenocorticism in obesity: (a) hirsutism, amenorrhea, hypertension, colored abdominal striae, increased 17-OH and 17-KS steroid excretion (Simkin);[111] (b) decreased glucose tolerance, increased resistance to insulin, increased incidence of diabetes.

4. Insulin may be produced in excess, both because of increased food intake and because of relative insulin refractoriness of certain tissues. The excess insulin may promote accelerated lipogenesis. A number of the same biochemical reactions operate both in the adrenal cortex and in adipose tissues. Insulin produces an increase in lipids and enlargement of each. Insulin, especially in large amounts, increases adrenal glucosteroid production; these steroids in turn play an important role in stimulating increased production of insulin antagonists. A cycle may thus be set up characterized by obesity, functional hyperinsulinism (with or without diabetes) and functional hyperadrenocorticism. If the stresses thus set up are severe enough, or persist long enough, permanent insulindeficiency diabetes may result from exhaustion of the β cells of the islets of Langerhans.

5. Weight loss, induced by simple restriction of caloric intake, can reverse these processes, at least in the early stages. Obesity may disappear, glucose tolerance return to normal, and excess corticosteroid production subside.[111] The concept is suggested that obesity is not only facilitated by certain endocrine aberrations, but that obesity *causes* certain endocrine disorders. The endocrine disorders may be reversible with abolition of the obesity. It is well recognized that obesity and diabetes are closely related. Joslin[62] found that, among 1,063 diabetic patients, in 40 per cent, obesity preceded the onset of the diabetes. It is also known that patients with tumors of the islets of Langerhans often are driven to excess food intake by hypoglycemia and its associated intense hunger, and may become obese. There is a close relationship between hypoglycemia and the hunger mechanism. It seems possible that a mild degree of hypoglycemia, insufficient to produce symptoms, could be the cause of the desire for excess food. However, sugar-tolerance tests in obese persons do not give consistent results; they often show diabetic-type curves instead of flat or low curves. The work of Ogilvie, described below, may explain these apparent paradoxes. Patients who do show hypoglycemic types of sugar-tolerance curves are sometimes fat, but are usually average

or lean, so that functional hyper-insulinism may in some cases, but certainly not in all, be cited as an adequate cause for production of obesity. Obesity has been produced in rats by protamine insulin injections.[63]

Ogilvie[64] observed that, particularly in the earlier stages of adiposity in human beings, the islands of Langerhans showed marked hypertrophy. Ogilvie's studies on glucose tolerance in obese subjects are interesting, and throw light upon the probable interrelationship of these facts connecting the pancreatic islets and obesity. In one-third of his patients sugar tolerance was increased in the early stages of obesity. With advancing age it seemed that the increased or normal tolerance gave way to decreased tolerance, and ultimately this became evident in a considerable proportion of cases as clinical diabetes mellitus. Overeating may therefore be primary, and the repeated ingestion of excessive amounts of carbohydrate may exert progressively greater demands upon the islets. A functional hyperinsulinism may result and obesity develop. In those persons whose islets cannot sustain the prolonged strain, there is eventually islet-cell degeneration with production of diabetes mellitus. Subjects with a hereditary or constitutional tendency toward diabetes would thus be more apt to become diabetic as a consequence of obesity, which clinically is true and statistically is quite evident. When the islet cells have high integrity, obesity may develop and persist in consequence of chronic functional hypoglycemia.

MacKay, Barnes and Carne[65] have demonstrated that young growing normal rats eat almost twice as many calories and deposit much more body fat when offered only carbohydrate food than they do when offered only protein.

The more recent observations of Schechter[102] and others seem to confirm the classic, older studies of Ogilvie: glucose tolerance was increased in the dynamic phase of obesity, decreased in the static phase.

The obese-hyperglycemic syndrome of mice seems also to represent an endocrine imbalance characterized by excessive secretion of insulin and glucagon by the islets of Langerhans.[109]

It has not yet been demonstrated how the hypothalamic injuries described below produce obesity. There is some evidence that hypothalamic injury causes hyperphagia and that hypothalamic disorders lead to relative hypoglycemia; perhaps three types of functional hypoglycemia may lead to excessive appetite, overeating, and thus to obesity; (1) hereditary or constitutional; (2) acquired through injuries, operations, encephalitis, etc.; (3) acquired through excessive carbohydrate ingestion.

The role of carbohydrate is closely bound with psychic factors in the production of obesity. The interplay between carbohydrate craving, psychic maladjustment and obesity produces a pattern often encountered clinically in various forms.

Fasting plasma insulin levels are higher than normal in obese persons, and the insulin response to glucose is also greater in the obese. When there is diabetes and obesity, insulin levels are somewhat lower (though still higher than normal) and are inadequate in controlling the subject's blood sugar.[119]

Excessive amounts of insulin may cause obesity not only through inducing hypoglycemia and hyperphagia, but also through its specific capacity to promote storage of fat. Excessive insulin and obesity are much more frequently associated with normal blood sugars, prediabetes, and frank diabetes than with hypoglycemic disorders.

Hyperinsulinism as a diagnostic medical term is usually used to describe hypoglycemic states such as those resulting from β cell tumors of the pancreatic islets. Hyperinsulinism associated with excessive production of insulin that is relatively ineffective in lowering the blood sugar and does not cause hypoglycemia may, nevertheless, be effective in accelerating fat storage and producing obesity.

There is much evidence that factors causing the production of relatively ineffective insulin or of insulin resistance are genetically transmitted.[117,121]

The ventromedial nucleus (the satiety center in the hypothalamus) acts as a brake on the constantly active lateral "feeding" center. It also exercises a measure of control over gastric hunger contractions. A high level of glucose utilization by the cells of the medial nucleus coincides with satiety. Hunger feelings and gastric contractions occur only with states of low glucose utilization by the cells of the medial nucleus. Augmented appetite occurs with the relative hypoglycemia occurring several hours after a meal. It may also occur with low glucose utilization by the cells when blood sugar levels are normal or excessive, but the insulin supply is inadequate or ineffective.[121]

If glucose utilization in the hypothalamic

satiety center (the "glucostat" of Mayer[118]) is the chief regulator of appetite, then factors controlling glucose metabolism become of central interest in relation to food intake and obesity, especially insulin. To understand more about the pathophysiology of appetite aberrations, we need to know more about (1) factors controlling formation of insulin and its release, (2) the various actions of insulin and how it is consumed, bound, or destroyed, and (3) whether more than one kind of insulin is synthesized in the β cells of the pancreatic islets; also whether the postulated various kinds differ in types of biologic activity.[117,132]

Until recently it was believed that insulin acted only upon glucose. It is now known that insulin has actions on substrates other than glucose. It affects transport and incorporation of amino acids into muscle protein, muscle membrane potentials, lipolysis in adipose tissue, RNA synthesis, and other metabolic processes—most of these actions not yet well defined or understood. Among the tasks of investigators is to answer whether there is a common pathway through which insulin affects these apparently unrelated reactions. Since it is difficult to attribute all the effects of insulin to a single mode of action, the possibility is being explored that several kinds of insulin are produced by the β cell.[117,132]

Until recently it was believed that the glucose concentration of the blood supplying the pancreas is the only important regulator of the rate of insulin release. Other important control systems also are operative. Hyperaminoacidemia appears to be a manifestation of the insulin ineffectiveness characteristic of obesity. Furthermore, the high level of blood amino acids may provide the feedback signal to the β cell through which insulin resistance is accompanied by an appropriately augmented secretory rate of insulin.[127] In obese subjects with normal glucose tolerance, sufficient fasting hyperinsulinemia is generated to lower blood glucose concentration, and in some cases, free fatty acids to normal, but is inadequate to reduce the elevation in plasma amino acids.

THE GONADS. Castration of male human beings or other animals usually results in great weight gain. Experimentally estrogen administration causes increased storage of fat. In the commercial production of meat, estrogen is regularly administered to animals (chickens, cattle, etc.) to increase weight.

After removal of the gonads the disposi-tion is more placid and there is less tendency to muscular action. More fat but less protein is stored and the muscles are less well developed. The basal metabolic rate usually falls about 15 per cent. After the menopause, women exhibit these changes spontaneously, and similar but less evident changes are found in men past middle life. Clinically, two common types of obesity are (1) that associated with hypogonadism in young women and (2) that which develops at middle age in both men and women. The presence of gonadal secretions in adequate amounts may at least in part account for the maintenance of normal weight in the average young and vigorous man or woman.

Role of the Hypothalamus and Higher Brain Centers. Many studies[66,67] indicate that certain nuclei in the hypothalamus are essential parts, and perhaps the primary sites of the homeostatic mechanism which normally operates to match food intake to body needs. Stimulation of one of the laterally located pair of nuclei results in increase of food ingestion, whereas bilateral destruction of these nuclei results in rejection of food even to the extreme of starvation and death. A pair of medial nuclei seems to be opposite in function, for their destruction results in hyperphagia. The lateral nuclei seem to be related to hunger and facilitate the eating reflexes. The medial nuclei have been termed "satiety centers" and inhibit feeding reflexes. It is supposed that the feeding reflexes are affected by many neural connections of the hypothalamic centers with cortical, gustatory, olfactory, visual and other areas. The experimental observations have been so consistent in the many animal species that the general concept of lateral "food-drive" nuclei and medial "satiety centers" has been applied to man.

In the prefrontal area of the cerebral cortex a *higher center* has been demonstrated. In man, lesions of this region are not uncommonly associated with abnormal food intake, usually in the direction of *bulimia*. This center is connected through thalamic nuclei with the hypothalamus.

The early observations that patients with pituitary tumors frequently were obese and that operations upon the pituitaries of animals often resulted in adiposity led to the conclusion that pituitary deficiency causes obesity. Erdheim[68] as early as 1904, however, proposed that hypothalamic disorder might cause such obesity, since often at autopsy the pituitary was undamaged in cases of adiposogenital dystrophy, but evidence of extrasellar tumors or compression of the base of the brain was present. Camus, Roussy et al.[69] in a series of studies from 1913 to 1925 found that dogs with an intact hypophysis developed obesity and diabetes insipidus as a result of bilateral lesions of the tuber cinereum extending to a depth of 5 mm. in the direction of the paraventricular nuclei, and concluded that injury to the paraventricular nuclei caused the obesity. Smith's[56] observations on the rat in 1927 further established the importance of the hypothalamus in the pathogenesis of obesity: chromic acid injected into the hypothalamus caused obesity; hypophysectomy did not. Many subsequent workers showed that in this type of obesity, at least, the factors in the pathologic physiology are: a specific type of damage to the hypothalamus; this produces hyperphagia;[70] the hyperphagia results in a greater than normal rate of conversion of carbohydrates to fatty acids. A related observation of Gildea and Man[71] is that in certain patients with clinical evidence of hypothalamic dysfunction there are abnormally high blood levels of fatty acids and cholesterol. Hetherington and Ranson,[72] after a large amount of meticulous work, concluded that hypophysectomy, stalk destruction or destruction of the infundibular region in rats did not cause adiposity. Certain large bilateral symmetrical hypothalamic lesions not involving the hypophysis caused rats to become very obese. The presence of the pituitary or its absence did not influence the development of obesity so produced. Therefore, hypothalamic obesity cannot be explained by considering it to be caused indirectly by pituitary hormonal disturbance.

Heinbecker, White and Rolf[58] in work on dogs, observed that obesity results from bilateral destruction or retrograde degeneration of the paraventricular nuclei, and that hypophysectomy per se also leads to much more slowly developing, lesser degrees of adiposity, presumably due to deficiency of the pituitary tropic hormones. A role in the pathogenesis of obesity has thus been restored to the *hypopituitary state* by these workers—both in regard to deficiency of the adenohypophysis and of the posterior pituitary lobe (see below). They found that lesions of the posterior hypothalamus, caudal to the paraventricular nuclei, which interrupt fibers whose cell bodies originate

in the caudal portions of the paraventricular nuclei (resulting in retrograde degeneration of these structures), resulted in obesity. Similar lesions that did not produce the retrograde degeneration with resultant *diminution in the number of cells in the caudal portion of the paraventricular nuclei* did not produce obesity. They also found that co-existing loss of cells of the supraoptic nuclei (producing diabetes insipidus) resulted in the development of a greater obesity (75 to 110 per cent gain in 6 months as compared with 50 per cent for the paraventricular nuclear lesion alone). These workers concluded that in the dog the specific lesion resulting in obesity was the paraventricular nuclear degeneration described, and that in the presence of such a lesion *a simultaneous decrease in posterior pituitary secretion* intensified the resulting obesity.

These observations indicate that (1) hypothalamic disorder is a potent factor in producing obesity, (2) pituitary lesions may play a part, and (3) adrenocortical functional alterations may also be a factor. These investigators postulate that fibers passing caudally from the paraventricular nuclei innervate cells within the brain stem. These cells (according to the hypothesis) secrete a hormone which influences the adrenal cortex or the basophil cells of the adenohypophysis, either or both of which are concerned with the abnormal deposition of fat. These workers and others have observed that production of posterior hypothalamic lesions or transection of the infundibular stalk has resulted in loss of the basophil cells of the adenohypophysis, with concomitant evidence of functional disorders of the adenohypophysis. Low and greatly fluctuating fasting blood glucose values were produced in the dogs operated upon by White, Heinbecker and Rolf,[73] and the unstable levels were considered to be the cause of the hyperphagia occurring after hypothalamic injury.

Brooks, Lambert and Bard[74] produced obesity in 6 out of 12 monkeys following experimentally produced hypothalamic lesions. Weight was more than doubled in mature monkeys in from 8 to 10 months, after which the weight remained relatively constant. In these studies, in contrast to those just cited, the presence of an associated diabetes insipidus had no influence on the obesity, nor did the presence or absence of hypogonadism. The total caloric intake of the obese monkeys was much greater than that of their nonobese controls.

Apparently the obesity caused by hypothalamic lesions is dependent upon the interruption of descending fibers that leave the ventromedial hypothalamic nuclei and normally descend toward the brain stem.

There have been some studies of the metabolism of animals in which obesity was experimentally produced by hypothalamic injuries. Brooks et al.[74] found a greatly increased caloric intake in the monkeys operated upon. Hetherington and Ranson[72] found that (1) all of the animals operated upon became much less active than their controls, and that (2) most of the animals ate a great deal more than their controls. Some of the animals became obese without eating more than their controls, which is probably explainable by the decreased activity.

Long and his associates[75] have made excellent studies of the metabolism in hypothalamic obesity. These may be summarized as follows: (1) Animals began to eat from two to three times as much per day as they did before the production of the lesions. (2) Obesity soon developed. (3) When given only as much food as the controls, only one out of 10 animals operated upon gained more weight than its control. (4) Studies of the basal and the total oxygen consumption and of basal and postprandial respiratory quotients in paired-fed operated (nonobese) and obese operated rats showed no deviations from normal.

The conclusion of Long and his coworkers was that *"the development of obesity is apparently a consequence of increased appetite, and is not associated with any fundamental disturbance in metabolism."*

It seems clear that dysfunction of nervous elements that originate in or are mediated through certain nuclei of the hypothalamus may produce a great increase in appetite and in food intake so that obesity results. It is not yet clear how the nervous system regulates appetite, but it seems that the *hunger mechanism is under control normally*, whereas disease or destruction of certain nerve tracts releases hunger from the usual inhibitory regulation.

The nature of the change in blood constituents or tissue metabolism which acts upon the hypothalamic centers is not yet clear. Since the hypothalamus contains temperature-sensitive cells, it has been proposed by Strominger and Brobeck[76] that central action of the specific dynamic action of food might be the *effective inhibitor* of the feeding center. It is interesting to note that this concept fits well with the observations of MacBryde[49] who found in human beings, whether obese, normal or thin, that there was a *decrease in the S.D.A.* during the nutritional phase of gaining weight.

Another theory has been proposed by Mayer and Bates[77] in which the glucose available to the central nervous system is the effective mechanism. In experimental animals very small decreases in blood glucose resulted in increased feeding activity. The critical factor is considered to be the *rate of glucose utilization* by the tissues, especially by the medial hypothalamic nucleus called the satiety center (Mayer).[133] The hyperphagia of diabetes despite hyperglycemia might result from the inability of the "glucostat" tissue to utilize the glucose in the absence of adequate insulin, or if the insulin were for any reason ineffective. It seems possible that inadequate glucose or phosphates or potassium might operate as the trigger mechanism to activate the lateral "feeding nuclei"; perhaps the medial "satiety nuclei" respond to adequate levels and terminate feeding activity.

There are two theoretically possible mechanisms that might explain hyperphagia resulting from aberrations in glucose metabolism affecting hypothalamic appetite control. Either of these could operate separately, or both might operate simultaneously: (1) The cells of the hypothalamic satiety center might become relatively insensitive. (2) The insulin reaching the center might be relatively ineffective because it is bound, or blocked or chemically different.

The latter possibility is well supported by a number of observations which indicate that in many obese persons, circulating insulin concentrations are abnormally high. Blood sugar levels in such persons are normal in most instances. Many, however, are "pre-diabetic" as demonstrated by glucose tolerance tests and subsequent history. In the juvenile-onset type of diabetes the circulating insulin concentration is low. On the contrary, in the maturity-onset type of diabetes, circulating levels of insulin are high, but for reasons not now understood, the insulin is relatively ineffective upon glucose metabolism. These persons usually have mild diabetes, but it is more or less insulin resistant. They have been obese in at least 40 per cent of cases (some say 70 per cent), before diabetes was detected.

Usually it is said that obesity predisposes to diabetes and that if one is obese, his chances of developing diabetes are three times those if his weight were normal. Perhaps, however, we have been looking at this pathophysiologic mechanism wrong end to, or upside down. Possibly there is (1) ineffective insulin; then (2) hyperphagia, because of impaired glucose metabolism in the cells of the hypothalamic satiety center; (3) high insulin production apparently because of the low effectiveness of insulin; and (4) greatly augmented fat deposition resulting from the very high concentration of circulating insulin. The very high circulating insulin supply may be quite normally effective in promoting the synthesis of fatty acids and in the conversion of carbohydrate to fat and enhancement of fat storage. A person so affected becomes obese for at least two main reasons: he has lost the normal feed-back control over food intake, so that excess ingestion proceeds unchecked; and the tremendous excess of insulin facilitates formation and storage of fat (lipogenesis) and inhibits release of fat or its breakdown (lipolysis).

The problem of the specific stimuli for the hypothalamic centers regulating food intake remains unresolved. However, direct evidence[78] confirms the concept that the feeding centers exhibit special sensitivity to the hunger state. In the rat these centers take up more radioactive glucose, phosphate, or carbonate in the starved than in the fed state. These centers are unique in this regard, since other contiguous hypothalamic areas showed greater uptake during feeding rather than during starvation.

Evidence of hypothalamic disturbance in obese human beings is probably afforded by the cases having diencephalic lesions in which the obesity was previously interpreted as due to pituitary disease. Epidemic encephalitis is frequently followed by the development of obesity. The hypothalamic lesions observed as the result of encephalitis resemble in many respects those known to cause experimental adiposity.

Influence of Heredity. Obesity occurs as a familial characteristic, as demonstrated by Fellows,[79] who found adiposity occurring ten times as often in the families of fat persons as in relatives of normal or lean subjects. When both parents were obese, Gurney[80] found an incidence of adiposity in the offspring of 73 per cent; when one parent was obese, an incidence of 40 per cent; and only 9 per cent when both parents were lean.

Another study[81] disclosed the following frequencies of obesity when both, one, or neither parent was overweight, respectively: 44 per cent, 25 per cent, and 5 per cent. Hypertension, coronary artery disease and diabetes were found to be closely interrelated with obesity, and all showed high familial incidence. The gradations in frequency of this group of disorders were consistent with Mendelian laws but did not correspond with values calculated on the basis of a simple dominant or recessive gene. Since the pathologic physiology of these disorders is known to be interrelated, the etiology is probably complex. Hereditary factors may be influenced by environmental means; this is seen most clearly when one among several siblings, all obese and the offspring of obese parents, learns to control his weight.

It is possible, of course, that family habits of eating instead of a hereditary factor may produce the known high familial incidence of obesity. However, in animals it is easily demonstrable that certain strains resist fattening, while others acquire adiposity readily. The observations of Danforth[82] prove that a gene carries the obese characteristic in certain mice. Yellow male mice were mated to females of various colors. Some of the descendants were yellow, while others were not. All litter mates were kept in the same cage and had the same food offered to them. At or subsequent to sexual maturity, the yellow mice gained weight more rapidly than their litter mates. This was especially true of the yellow females. A Mendelian dominant gene carries the characters for yellowness and obesity; nonyellow mice of the same litter are not obese. In such obese animals the basal metabolic rate is said to be subnormal and the body temperature low; a hypothalamic hereditary origin of the obesity has been suggested. A hereditary obesity in mice accompanied by hyperglycemia has been described. Such animals spontaneously take a much greater amount of food than nonobese controls.

Evidence in man reveals genetic patterns of various types associated with obesity; there may be a number of different traits that may be inherited which predispose to obesity.[117]

Psychologic Factors. When it is considered that the majority of human beings maintain approximately normal body weight for many years, with relatively little variation, it is evident that food intake is usually well balanced with the caloric demands of the body. It must be supposed that *metabolic requirements regulate hunger and satiety*, so that as a rule people eat what they need and no more. As they get older and activity decreases, moderate degrees of adiposity are common. It seems likely that habits of eating continue beyond the necessity for them. Habit then becomes the regulator of food intake, and appetite becomes the servant of desire, and not of hunger. Appetite may result from the pleasant memories of the joy of eating. Appetite may be dulled or abolished by disturbed mental states, or stimulated by pleasant odors and tastes or by foods that are attractively colored or prepared.

There has always been a widespread propensity among both physicians and laity to regard obese persons, whether children or adults, simply as self-indulgent over-eaters. Commonly the corpulent are scolded; often they are made to suffer indignities by parents, siblings, spouses, friends, teachers, even doctors. Frequently they are blamed as incorrigible debauchers, practitioners of the cardinal sin of gluttony. Often they are ridiculed and made cruel objects of fun.

A study of the pathophysiologic factors operative in producing obesity shows that the explanation of excessive fat storage is not that easy; simple over-indulgence is probably an important factor in only a small minority of instances.

Obese persons are often suspicious, resentful, frequently withdrawn and depressed; no wonder, the way other people treat them. Neuroses may initiate weight gain, but it is easy to see how resultant emotional disturbances may set up a vicious circle.

The infrequency with which obesity can be attributed to organic disease, and the common occurrence of emotional disorders resulting in hyperphagia has properly received increasing recognition and emphasis. Reeve[83] found two groups, the first comprising the gaining of distant satisfactions wherein the symbolic value of the symptom, obesity, is paramount. Other students have recognized that the enlarged body may serve the patient as a fortresslike defense against a hostile world, or as a symbol of independence or prowess, or as a means to discourage suitors, to represent a wished-for

pregnancy, or to mask emotions. Reeve's second group includes those values and immediate satisfactions gained in the incorporation process, such as the sensory pleasures of food ingestion.

Obese persons in one large study showed immaturity, suspiciousness and rigidity more often than nonobese persons.[113,114] The immaturity may be expressed in failure to resist impulses, among them the impulse to eat.

When satisfactions of other types are denied, the pleasures of eating may serve in their stead. One of life's genuine delights is open to practically everyone: eating. If social, business or sexual objectives are unattainable, food may serve not only as a defense and a solace but eventually as a substitute. Although obesity is the outcome, it may not be greatly feared, or may even be welcomed. Obesity can be used as an offensive weapon as well as a defensive one. One patient gloried in her corpulence as a means of punishing her wayward husband. Another preferred to remain obese, since she could not find employment because of her great size. A child who is an invalid, or who for any other reason is the object of excessive parental solicitude, is apt to become obese.

Hamburger[84] in an excellent review finds it useful to divide patients who overeat into four groups:

1. Those for whom overeating is a response to nonspecific emotional tensions;

2. Overeating is a substitute gratification in intolerable life situations;

3. Overeating is a symptom of an underlying emotional illness, especially depression and hysteria;

4. Overeating is an addiction to food.

Brosin[85] gives excellent discussion and reviews of the work in this field. He emphasizes that psychological disorders of appetite may take various forms, resulting in anorexia and weight loss, or hyperphagia and obesity. He wisely cautions against strenuous reducing programs which fail to take into account the basic psychological conflicts in severe cases. He advises doctors to work sensitively and at length with obese patients in middle life or later, pointing out that if one takes away smoking, alcohol and finally food from a person who has few other genuine satisfactions in life, one has the obligation to put something constructive in its place.

However, as Shelton[86] has stated, it is eminently true that all or nearly all obese persons, especially women and children, are unhappy and frustrated, although this may be the psychologic result of the obesity rather than the cause of it. Short boys, excessively tall girls, adolescents with acne, bald persons, hirsute women, disfigured persons, lame persons, etc., suffer from various degrees of inferiority, frustration and unhappiness, but there is no greater incidence of obesity in these groups. On the contrary, most such unhappy states are apt to result in decreased appetite and weight loss, a common accompaniment of various neuroses, an extreme example being the so-called anorexia nervosa.

Since restriction of carbohydrate alone frequently breaks into the vicious circle of obesity caused by the carbohydrate habit, producing weight loss and improved psychic adjustment, it seems unlikely that the psychologic situation is always primary. Undoubtedly the physiologic aberration is often much more important, or of equal significance, in the etiology.

Habits of eating certain concentrated foods may be present in the absence of any deep-seated psychological abnormality. Habits of physical indolence are apparently more common in persons who become obese. Often re-education concerning diet and the establishment of new habits of diet and exercise are sufficient to establish and maintain normal weight. Helpful in the development of new habits may be: anorexigenic drugs; attractive but bulky low-calorie foods (lean meat, fruits, vegetables); antacids and avoidance of alcohol and spicy foods which cause gastric stimulation; development of interest in sports and physical activities; stimulus to become better-looking and physically more attractive; encouragement and moral support and prolonged follow-up by the physician.

Addiction to food, as to alcohol, is often a symptom of an underlying psychologic maladjustment. Psychiatric study may be needed to disclose the hidden cause of the obesity, or a history taken carefully and sympathetically will yield the necessary clues. Among children, Bruch[87] found very few patients with endocrine factors of importance causing the obesity, but many children ate excessively in response to parental encouragement, or as a means of gaining attention.[112]

The habit of carbohydrate eating, with its resultant recurrent relative hypoglycemia, may be set up in the maladjusted individual who becomes obese, so that the psychic disturbance is thus associated with excessive activity of the islets of Langerhans. Shelton[86] suggested for this common type of corpulence the descriptive term *neuropancreatic obesity*, implying that there may be a functional or organic disorder operating through the hypothalamus associated with functional hyperinsulinism.

ADDICTION TO FOOD with resultant obesity occurs often in children and adults. Neuroses or psychoses of various types are frequently involved as causes of chronic excessive ingestion of highly concentrated rich, often sweet, tasty food and drink. Among things favored by gluttonous folk primarily for their taste are candies, ice cream, pastries, soft drinks, and beer.

ADDICTION TO ALCOHOL adds to total caloric intake, and is a factor in causing obesity most often when it is only a moderate daily habit and is accompanied by a steady generous food intake. A few cocktails before meals, wine or beer with meals, etc., constitute a very easy way for a substantial caloric intake to be slipped in almost unnoticed in an easy, liquid, pleasant, sociable form. Appetite is usually stimulated by moderate amounts of alcohol; eating of a greater quantity of solid foods is increased.

There is at least one big difference that exists between a *general* addiction to food and addictions to alcohol, tobacco, certain drugs, etc. The difference is that one can live quite normally without alcohol, tobacco and drugs and can terminate such a habit completely, never being compelled to expose oneself to the dangerous agent again. To stay alive, however, the involved person must be subjected to the disturbing element, food, several times daily. He must every day be exposed to temptation and must control tendencies to relapses over months and years.

Special addictions to one or more particular foods sometimes occur, rather than a generalized compulsion toward excessive intake of all foods. Most often the foods are tasty (e.g., candies, particularly chocolate). Sweets (pies, cakes, jellies, jams, soft drinks, etc.) are often the object of the craving. Sometimes, however, the addiction is for a bland food such as bread or potatoes.

My own studies[130] in following 312 obese patients for 2 to 10 or more years reveal that, whatever the primary causes, significant weight loss occurred after treatment at some time in 75 per cent of cases. However, relapse was the rule, so that at the end of 2 to 10 years of observation and treatment, only in 8 per cent of cases could treatment be considered successful. If achievement of weight within a "normal" *range* is the chief criterion, long-term results were satisfactory in 8 per cent; if reaching and maintaining *optimal* weight is the criterion, less than half of those with "good" results could qualify. Those persons maintaining optimal weight for at least six months numbered 11 patients, 3.5 per cent of the total 312 long-term patients studied.

The most striking conclusions I drew from these studies are: (1) Short-term results usually are excellent. (2) Long-term results are very poor, because nearly all patients relapse. (3) Addiction to food seems to be by far the most frequent proximate cause of obesity; further delving into the pathophysiology reveals many different causes for the addiction. Sometimes these are primarily disturbances in physiology, but most often psychological.

Social Factors. According to a study of 110,000 persons,[113,114] obesity is seven times as frequent among women of the lowest socioeconomic level as among those of the highest level, and among men the same relationship exists, although to a much lesser degree. The elements in the environment of etiologic significance are not clear: lack of education is believed to be important. When age and socioeconomic variables were held constant, statistically significant differences in 3 out of 9 measures of mental health were observed: obese persons scored more pathologic responses than nonobese controls in measures of immaturity, suspiciousness, and rigidity.

TREATMENT BASED ON ETIOLOGY

Whenever possible, weight reduction is accomplished by specific therapy based on reversing or relieving etiologic factors. This is relatively easy in rare cases only: for example in hypothyroidism, or when an islet tumor can be removed in hyperinsulinism. Since in the common types of obesity relatively obscure physiologic disorder of appetite control is present or there is a neurosis of which obesity is only a part, treatment is difficult and often unsuccessful. It seems logical to attempt to decrease appetite at the same time a lower calorie diet is sup-

plied. This is not easy, but clinically, high protein diets seem to have this effect.[88] Simple medical psychiatry is usually necessary, so provision of diet lists alone is inadequate. Often expert psychiatric study and treatment are indicated. Other methods of treatment, as well as those mentioned, are summarized in articles,[89,90] and include the use of drugs to inhibit appetite, bulky, low-calorie diets and regulated moderate exercise.

SUMMARY

Whatever the remote causes may be, obesity is always the result of food intake in excess of bodily needs. However, certain conditions may exist that may either (1) facilitate storage of fat when the caloric intake remains constant or (2) operate to raise the intake.

Among the etiologic factors considered, certain mechanisms do not seem tenable as possible explanations of the usual type of obesity. Among these are facilitated digestion or absorption, or lipophilia of the tissues. There is no generally accepted demonstration of abnormal utilization of energy. Endocrine abnormalities may cause a decrease in the basal metabolic rate (e.g., hypothyroidism, hypopituitarism or hypogonadism) and may result in decreased muscular activity, thereby causing a tendency to gain weight. Hyperinsulinism of organic origin, with resultant hypoglycemia may cause an increased food intake. However, such endocrine abnormalities are infrequently encountered, while obesity is extremely common. Functional relative hypoglycemia seems to be seen fairly often and may lead to obesity. It occurs from overeating carbohydrate foods habitually.

Hyperinsulinism occurring with insulin resistance is frequent in obesity. Hypothalamic disorders clearly may result in obesity. Whether they do so by increasing food intake or decreasing energy output, or both, is not clear. Evidently the increase in food intake is primary as the result of hypothalamic disorders, if the results of animal studies are applicable to human beings. Hypothalamic damage seems to remove the normal inhibitory controls from the hunger mechanism. It may be that there is a connection between relative functional hypoglycemia and hypothalamic disturbance. In some clinical, as well as in some experimental instances, hypoglycemia is a feature of hypothalamic disorder. Decreased basal metabolic rate and decreased muscular activity have been observed in some cases; perhaps these mechanisms also are operative in hypothalamic obesity. Heredity seems to play a definite role and may operate both by decreasing caloric outgo and by increasing the caloric intake. Psychologic factors most often operate to increase food intake, but may cause physical inactivity also. In any case in which obesity becomes pronounced, exercise becomes more and more of a hardship. Therefore, a decrease in energy output as muscular exercise is apt to be a consequence of corpulence, and will likewise contribute to its further development.

More than one factor is usually operative in each case. The brief case histories given below are cited not because they are unusual, but because similar problems are common; as instances illustrating the concomitance of multiple etiologic influences they are typical examples.

A young woman, aged 25, came from an obese family. She had always been short, the nose and the mouth were dainty, the chin was small and pointed. The fingers tapered and the breasts were small. The menstrual periods were scanty and irregular. Her basal metabolic rate had always been low. However, her weight remained normal until she married and her husband left shortly thereafter for the Army. His allotment made it unnecessary for her to work. To console herself in his absence she lay around and read love-story magazines and ate huge quantities of ice cream and candy. She became obese rapidly, gaining 25 pounds in 3 months.

Here the groundwork was laid· a hereditary tendency toward obesity, a hypopituitary physique, moderate hypothyroidism. Yet obesity did not develop until (1) food intake increased, and (2) energy output as muscular activity was greatly diminished. The precipitating factor was psychologic: her sexual desires and other drives usually expressed in bearing and rearing children, establishing a home, etc., were frustrated; they were sublimated into eating and reading.

J. C., previously a noted professional football player, became obese at age 31, within two years after giving up the game and becoming a sedentary restaurateur. In his prime as an athlete he was 6'2", overweight by the charts at 235 lbs., very muscular, but not fat. Within 6 months after stopping active exercise he had gained 30 pounds; within two years he gained 90 pounds and exceeded 325 pounds.

His family was Italian; they loved wine, pasta, and rich foods with olive oil. Father, mother, a sister and two brothers were all overweight. His mother and her brother had mild diabetes. J. was always hungry. "You tell me I eat *too much*," he told me, "Doctor, this can't be true. Why, I've never even had *enough*."

His plasma insulin-like activity was 3 to 4 times normal. His sugar-tolerance curve was flat, like that of hyperinsulinism.

Here many factors are evident: heredity, perhaps largely involving production of excess insulin; habits of eating induced by ethnic and familial influences, and by long adjustment to the requirements of strenuous exercise; finally the sudden switch to a sedentary life, with many physiologic and psychologic implications.

Each case of obesity, therefore, deserves careful study. Proper treatment will be evident when the etiologic factors are discovered.

Whatever the pathophysiologic causes or psychologic influences may be that result in obesity, they tend to persist in the great majority of persons affected. Even with the best available medical care and prolonged encouragement and follow-up, temporary weight loss soon followed by regain of weight is the rule, so that after 3 to 5 years satisfactory results are obtained in only 5 to 10 per cent of patients.

REFERENCES

1. Shelton, E. K.: Optimal weight estimation; the method of Willoughby, Endocrinology 16:492, 1932.
2. Behnke, A. R., Jr., Feen, B. G., and Welham, W. C.: The specific gravity of healthy men; body weight ÷ volume as an index of obesity, J.A.M.A. 118:495–498, 1942.
3. Keys, A.: Obesity measurement and the composition of the body, Proceedings No. 6, Nutrition Symposium Series, National Vitamin Foundation, New York, 1953.
4a. Dublin, L. I., and Lotka, A. J.; Length of Life, New York, Ronald, 1936.
4b. Armstrong, D. B., Dublin, L. I., Wheatley, G. M., and Marks, H. H.: Obesity and its relation to health and disease, J.A.M.A. 147:1007, 1951.
4c. Dublin, L. I., and Marks, H. H.: Mortality among insurance overweights in recent years, Trans. Ass. Life Insur. Med. Dir. Amer., Oct. 11–12, 1951.
5. Barr, D. P.: Obesity, Red Light of Health, Proceedings No. 6, Nutrition Symposium Series, National Vitamin Foundation, New York, 1953.

6. Rynearson, E. H., and Gastineau, C. F.: Obesity, Springfield, Ill., Thomas, 1949.

7a. Smith, H. L., and Willius, F. A.: Adiposity of the heart; a clinical and pathologic study of one hundred and thirty-six obese patients, Arch. Intern. Med. 52:911–931, 1933.

7b. Willius, F. A.: Discussion, J.A.M.A. 101:424, 1933.

8. Prodger, S. H., and Dennig, H.: A study of the circulation in obesity, J. Clin. Invest. 11:789–806, 1932.

9. Kerr, W. J., and Lagen, J. B.: The postural syndrome related to obesity leading to postural emphysema and cardiorespiratory failure, Ann. Intern. Med. 10:569–595, 1936.

10. Short, J. J., and Johnson, H. J.: The effect of overweight on vital capacity, Proc. Life Ext. Exam. 1:36–41, 1939.

11a. Newburgh, L. H., and Johnston, M. W.: The nature of obesity, J. Clin. Invest. 8:197–213, 1930.

11b. Wiley, F. H., and Newburgh, L. H.: The doubtful nature of "Luxuskonsumption," J. Clin. Invest. 10:733–744, 1931.

11c. Newburgh, L. H.: The cause of obesity, J.A.M.A. 97:1659–1661, 1931.

11d. ———: Obesity, Arch. Intern. Med. 70:1033–1096, 1942.

12. Thompson, K. J.: Some observations on the development and course of hypertensive vascular disease. Proc. 38th Ann. Meeting, Medical Section, American Life Convention, White Sulphur Springs, 1950.

13. Master, A. M., Dublin, L. I., and Marks, H. H.: The normal blood pressure range and its clinical implications, J.A.M.A. 143:1464, 1950.

14. Levy, R. L., White, P. D., Stroud, W. D., and Hillman, C. C.: Overweight. Its prognostic significance in relation to hypertension and cardiovascular-renal disease, J.A.M.A. 131:951, 1946.

15. Wilens, A. L.: Bearing of general nutritional state on atherosclerosis, Arch. Intern. Med. 79:129, 1947.

16. Keys, A.: Symposium on Nutrition, Univ. of Buffalo Med. School, Dec. 12, 1953.

17. Walker, W. J., Lawry, E. Y., Love, D. E., Levine, S. A., and Stare, F. J.: Effect of weight reduction and caloric balance on serum lipoprotein and cholesterol levels, Amer. J. Med. 14:656–664, 1953.

18. Gofman, J. W., and Jones, H. B.: Obesity, fat metabolism and cardiovascular disease, Circulation 5:504, 1952.

19. Zelman, S.: The liver in obesity, A.M.A. Arch. Intern. Med. 90:141–156, 1952.

20. Hertig, A. T., and Sommers, S. C.: Genesis of endometrial carcinoma, Cancer 2:946, 1949.

21. Hildreth, R. C.: J. Mich. Med. Soc. 49:1175, 1950.

22. Dole, V. P., et al.: The caloric value of labile body tissue in obese subjects, J. Clin. Invest. 34:590, 1955.

23. Werthliner, E., and Shapiro, B.: The physiology of adipose tissue, Physiol. Rev. 28:451, 1948.

24. Lipmann, F.: Biosynthetic mechanisms, Harvey Lecture 44:99, 1948–49.

25. Lipmann, F.: Fat Metabolism, in Najjar, V. (ed.): A Symposium on the Clinical and Biochemical Aspects of Fat Utilization in Health and Disease, Baltimore, Johns Hopkins Press, 1954.

26. Parson, W., and Crispell, K. R.: Obesity, Disease-a-Month Series, Chicago, Yr. Bk. Pub., February 1956.

27. Neuenschwander-Lemmer, N.: Ueber Ausnutzungsversuche bei fettsüchtigen und normalen Menschen, Ztschr. f. d. ges. exper. Med. 99:395, 1936.

28. Strang, J. M., McClugage, H. B., and Brownlee, M. A.: Arch. Intern. Med. 55:958, 1935.

29. Von Bergmann, G.: Oppenheimer's Handbuch der Biochemie 4:212, 1910.

30. Hetenyi, G.: Untersuchungen über die Enstehung der Fettsucht, Deutsches Arch. f. klin. Med. 179:134–141, 1936.

31. Jansen, W. H.: Deutsches Arch. f. klin. Med. 124:1, 1917.

32. Benedict, cited by G. Lusk: Physiol. Rev. 1:523, 1921.

33. Keeton, R. W., and Dickson, D.: Excretion of nitrogen by obese patients on diets low in calories, containing varying amounts of protein, Arch. Int. Med. 51:890–902, 1933.

34. Strang, J. M., McClugage, H. B., and Evans, F. A.: The nitrogen balance during correction of obesity, Amer. J. Med. Sci. 181:336–349, 1931.

35. Block, M.: Role of lipophilia in the etiology of obesity, Proc. Soc. Exper. Biol. Med. 49:496–499, 1942.

36. Salcedo, J., and Stetten, D.: Turnover of fatty acids in congenitally obese mouse, J. Biol. Chem. 151:413, 1943.

37. Guggenheim, K., and Mayer, J.: Studies of pyruvate and acetate metabolism in the hereditary obese-diabetes syndrome of mice, J. Biol. Chem. 198:259, 1952.

38. Mankin, H., Stevenson, J., Brobeck, J., Long, C., and Stetten, D.: The turnover of body fat in obesity resulting from hypothalamus injury studied with aid of deuterium, Endocrinology 47:443, 1950.

39. van Leeuwen, H. C.: Ztschr. f. klin. Med. 123:534, 1933.

40. Nassauer-Badt, A.: Ueber partiellen symmetrischen infantilen Fettschwund und sein familiaren Vorkommen, Inaugural dissertation, Frankfurt, 1929.

40a. Barr, D. P.: The pathogenesis of obesity and lipodystrophy, New Internat. Clin. 3:135, 1941.

41. Boothby, W. M., and Sandiford, I.: Summary of the basal metabolism data on 8,614 subjects with especial reference to the normal standards for the estimation of the basal

metabolic rate, J. Biol. Chem. 54:783–803, 1922.

42. Strouse, S., Wang, C. C., and Dye, M.: Studies on the metabolism of obesity. II. Basal metabolism, Arch. Intern. Med. 34:275–281, 1924.

43. Grafe, E.: Metabolic Diseases and Their Treatment (translated by M. G. Boise), Philadelphia, Lea & Febiger, 1933.

44. Plaut, R. Deutsches Arch. f. klin. Med. 142:266, 1923.

45. Lauter, S.: Zur Genese der Fettsucht, Deutsches Arch. f. klin. Med. 150:315–365, 1926.

46. Strang, J. M., and McClugage, H. B.: Amer. J. Med. Sci. 182:49, 1931.

47. Johnston, M. W.: J. Clin. Invest. 11:437, 1932.

48. Dock, W.: Am. J. Physiol. 97:117, 1931.

49. MacBryde, C. M.: The specific dynamic action of a mixed meal and its relation to obesity, J.A.M.A. 108:589, 1937.

50. Grafe, E., and Graham, D.: Ueber die Anpassungsfähigkeit des tierischen organismus an überreichliche Nahrungszufuhr, Ztschr. f. physiol. Chem. 73:1–67, 1911.

——— and Koch, R.: Deutsches Arch. f. klin. Med. 106:564, 1912.

51. Wiley, F. H., and Newburgh, L. H.: The doubtful nature of "Luxuskonsumption," J. Clin. Invest. 10:733–744, 1931.

52. Lauter, S.: Klin. Wschr. 5:1695, 1926.

53. Master, A. M., Stricker, J., Grishman, A., and Dack, S.: Effect of undernutrition on cardiac output and cardiac work in overweight subjects, Arch. Intern. Med. 69:1010–1018, 1942.

54. Fröhlich, A.: Ein Fall von Tumor der Hypophysis Cerebri ohne Akromegalie, Wien. klin. Rundschau 15:883–886; 906–908, 1901.

55. Cushing, H.: The Pituitary Body and Its Disorders, Philadelphia, J. B. Lippincott, 1912.

56. Smith, P. E.: Harvey Lectures, 1929–30, Baltimore, Williams & Wilkins.

57. Cushing, H.: Neurohypophysial mechanisms from the clinical standpoint (Lister Memorial Lecture), Lancet 2:119, 175, 1930.

———: Papers Relating to the Pituitary Body, Hypothalamus and Parasympathetic Nervous System, Springfield, Ill., Thomas, 1932.

58. Heinbecker, P., White, H. L., and Rolf, D.: Experimental obesity in the dog, Amer. J. Physiol. 141:549–565, 1944.

59. Reinecke, R. M., Samuels, L. T., and Bauman, K. L.: Growth and metabolism of young hypophysectomized rats fed by stomach tube, Endocrinology 33:87–95, 1943.

60. Heinbecker, P.: The pathogenesis of Cushing's syndrome, Medicine 23:225–247, 1944.

61. Plummer, W. A.: Body weights in spontaneous myxedema, Tr. Am. A. Study Goiter, p. 88–98, 1940.

62. Joslin, E. P.: J.A.M.A. 76:79, 1921.

63. MacKay, E. M., and Callaway, J. W.: Proc. Soc. Exper. Biol. Med. 36:406, 1937.

64. Ogilvie, R. F.: Sugar tolerance in obese subjects: a review of sixty-five cases, Quart. J. Med. 4:345–358, 1935.

65. MacKay, E. M., Barnes, R., and Carne, H. O.: Influence of diet with high protein content upon appetite and deposition of fat, Amer. J. Physiol. 135:187–192, 1941.

66. Anand, B. K., and Brobeck, J. R.: Hypothalamic control of food intake in rats and cats, Yale J. Biol. Med. 24:123, 1951.

67. Anand, B. K., Dua, S., and Schoenberg, K.: Hypothalamic control of food intake in cats and monkeys, J. Physiol. 127:143, 1955.

68. Erdheim, J.: Ueber Hypophysengangsgeschwülste und Hirncholesteatome, Sitzungsb. d. k. Akad. d. Wissensch. Math.-naturw. Wien 113:537, 1904.

69. Camus, J., and Roussy, G.: Pituitary syndromes, Rev. Neurol. 38:622–639, 1922.

70. Brobeck, J. R., Tepperman, J., and Long, C. N. H.: Experimental hypothalamic hyperphagia in the albino rat, Yale J. Biol. Med. 15:831–853, 1943.

71. Gildea, E. F., and Man, E. B.: The hypothalamus and fat metabolism, Association Research Nerv. and Ment. Dis., Proc. (1939) 20:436–448, 1940.

72. Hetherington, A. W., and Ranson, S. W.: J. Comp. Neurol. 76:475, 1942; Endocrinology 31:30, 1942.

73. White, H. L., Heinbecker, P., and Rolf, D.: Effects of removal of anterior lobe of hypophysis on some renal functions, Amer. J. Physiol. 136:584–591, 1942.

74. Brooks, C., Lambert, E. F., and Bard, P.: Fed. Proc. 1, Part 2, p. 11, 1942.

75. Long, C. N. H., Brobeck, J. R., and Tepperman, J.: Endocrinology 30:1035, 1942.

76. Brobeck, J. R.: Physiology of appetite, Proceedings No. 6, Nutrition Symposium Series, National Vitamin Foundation, New York, 1953.

77. Mayer, J., and Bates, M. W.: Blood glucose and food intake in normal and hypophysectomized, alloxan-treated rats, Amer. J. Physiol. 168:812, 1952.

78. Larsson, S.: On the hypothalamic organisation of the nervous mechanism regulating food intake, Acta physiol. scandinav. 32: Supp. 115, 1954.

79. Fellows, H. H.: Studies of relatively normal obese individuals during and after dietary restrictions, Amer. J. Med. Sci. 181:301–312, 1931.

80. Gurney, R.: The hereditary factor in obesity, Arch. Intern. Med. 57:557, 1936.

81. Thomas, C. B., and Cohen, B. H.: Familial occurrence of hypertension, coronary artery disease, obesity and diabetes, A.M.A. Ann. Intern. Med. 42:90–127, 1955.

82. Danforth, C. H.: Hereditary adiposity in mice, J. Heredity 18:153–162, 1927.

83. Reeve, G. H.: Psychological factors in obesity, Am. J. Orthopsychiat. 12:674–679, 1942.

84. Hamburger, W. W.: Emotional aspects of obesity, Med. Clin. North America 35:483–499, 1951.

85. Brosin, H. W.: The psychology of overeating, Proceedings No. 6, Nutrition Symposium Series, National Vitamin Foundation, New York, 1953.
——: Psychiatric aspects of obesity, J.A.M.A 155:1238, 1954.

86. Shelton, E. K.: The role of carbohydrate in the production of obesity (presidential address, Association for the Study of Internal Secretions, 1944).

87. Bruch, H.: Psychiatric aspects of obesity in children, Amer. J. Psychiat. 99:752–757, 1943.

88. Fryer, J. H., et al.: A study of the interrelationship of the energy-yielding nutrients, blood glucose levels and subjective appetite in man, J. Lab. Clin. Med. 45:684, 1955.

89. MacBryde, C. M.: Treatment of Obesity, in Conn, H. F., ed.: Current Therapy, Philadelphia, Saunders, 1962.

90. MacBryde, C. M.: Obesity, in Cecil & Loeb, eds.: Textbook of Medicine, ed. 10, Philadelphia, Saunders, 1959.

91. Fadell, E. J., et al.: Fatty infiltration of respiratory muscles in the pickwickian syndrome, New Eng. J. Med. 266:861–863, 1962.

92. Said, S. I.: Abnormalities of pulmonary gas exchange in obesity, Ann. Intern. Med. 53:1121, 1960.

93. Albrink, M. J.: Lipoprotein pattern as a function of total triglyceride of serum, J. Clin. Invest. 40:536, 1961.

94. Seller, R. H., et al.: Use of I^{131} in study of lipid in coronary artery disease, Amer. J. Med. 27:231, 1959.

95. Dublin, L., and Marks, H.: Reduction in predicted mortality following weight reduction in obese persons, Proceedings No. 6, Nutrition Symposium Series, National Vitamin Foundation, p. 106–116, New York, 1953.

96. Kinsell, L.: Diets low in cholesterol and high in polyunsaturated fats, in L. Kinsell, ed.: Adipose Tissue as an Organ, New York, Grune & Stratton, 1962.

97. Dayton, S., et al.: A controlled clinical trial of a diet high in unsaturated fat, New Eng. J. Med. 266:1017–1023, 1962.

98. Goldsmith, G. A.: Serum lipids and atherosclerosis, J.A.M.A. 176:783–790, 1961.

99. Central Committee for Medical and Community Program (American Heart Association): Circulation 23:133–136, 1961.

100a. Council on Foods and Nutrition: The regulation of dietary fat, J.A.M.A. 181:411–429, 1962.

100b. Recommended Dietary Allowances, Food and Nutrition Board, National Research Council; ed. 7, Publication 1694, Washington, D.C., National Academy of Sciences, 1968.

101. Ward, W., and Kelsey, W.: The Pickwickian syndrome. A review of the literature and report of a case, J. Pediat. 61:745–750, 1962.

102. Schechter, P.: Some metabolic characteristics of essential obesity. Amer. J. Clin. Nutr. 10:433–442, 1962.

103. Naimark, A., and Cherniack, R. M.: Compliance of the respiratory system and its components in health and obesity, J. Appl. Physiol. 15:377, 1960.

104. Kaufman, B. J., Ferguson, M. H., and Cherniack, R. M.: Hypoventilation in obesity, J. Clin. Invest. 38:500, 1959.

105. Antoniades, H. N., and Gundersen, K.: Studies on the state of insulin in blood: dissociation of purified human blood insulin complexes by incubation with adipose tissue extracts in vitro, Endocrinology 68:36, 1961.

106. Garn, S. M., and Haskell, J. A.: Fat thickness and developmental status in childhood and adolescence, Amer. J. Dis. Children, 99:746–751, 1960.

107. Nutrition Reviews, 14:172, 229, 1956; 15:193, 1957; 19:36, 1961.

108. Chirico, A., and Stunkard, A. J.: Physical activity and human obesity, New Eng. J. Med. 263:935–940, 1960.

109. Mayer, J.: Obesity: Physiologic considerations, Amer. J. Clin. Nutr. 9:530–537, 1961.

110. Gundersen, K., and Antoniades, H. N.: Biological activity of insulin complexes examined by rat diaphragm tissue assay, Proc. Soc. Exp. Biol. Med. 104:411, 1960.

111. Simkin, B., and Arce, R.: Steroid excretion in obese patients with colored abdominal striae, New Eng. J. Med. 266:1031–1035, 1962.

112. Bruch, H.: The Importance of Overweight, New York, Norton, 1957.

113. Moore, M. E., Stunkard, A., and Srole, L.: Obesity, social class, and mental illness, J.A.M.A. 181:962–966, 1962.

114. Goldblatt, P., Moore, M., and Stunkard, A.: Social factors in obesity, J.A.M.A. 192:1039, 1965.

115. Karam, J. H., Grodsky, G. M., and Forsham, P. H.: Excessive insulin response to glucose in obese subjects, Diabetes 12:197, 1963.

116. Glennon, J. A., and Brech, W. J.: Serum protein-bound iodine in obesity, J. Clin. Endocrinol. 25:1673, 1965.

117. Mayer, J.: Genetic factors in human obesity, Ann. N.Y. Acad. Sci. 131:412, 1965.

118. Mayer, J.: Why people get hungry, Nutrition Today 1:2–8, 1966.

119. Perley, M., and Kipnis, D.: Plasma insulin responses to glucose and tolbutamide of normal weight and obese diabetic and nondiabetic subjects, Diabetes 15:867–874, 1966.

120. Huff, T., Horton, E., and Lebovitz, H.: Abnormal insulin secretion in myotonic dystrophy, New Eng. J. Med. 277:837; and Editorial: Insulin, how many faces? 277:877, 1967.

121. Fineberg, S. K.: Diabetes-Obesity or Obesity-Diabetes? Nutrition Today 1:16–19, 1966.

122. Bloom, W. L., and Eidex, M. F.: Inactivity as a major factor in adult obesity, Metabolism 16:679, 1967.

123a. Hollenberg, C. H., and Angel, A.: Adipose tissue metabolism and obesity, Modern Treatment 4:1083, 1967.

123b. Galton, D. J., and Bray, G. A.: Metabolism of alpha-glycerol phosphate in human adipose tissue in obesity, J. Clin. Endocrinol. 27:1573, 1967.

124a. Knittle, J. L., and Hirsch, J.: Effect of early nutrition on the development of rat epididymal fat pads: cellularity and metabolism, J. Clin. Invest. 47:2091, 1968.

124b. Hirsch, J., Knittle, J., and Salans, L.: Cell lipid content and cell number in obese and non-obese human adipose tissue, J. Clin. Invest. 45:1023, 1966.

124c. Salans, L. B., Knittle, J. H., and Hirsch, J.: The role of adipose tissue insulin sensitivity in the carbohydrate intolerance of human obesity, J. Clin. Invest. 47:153, 1968.

125. MacBryde, C. M.: Obesity, *in* Conn, H. F., and Conn, R. B., Jr., Current Diagnosis, ed. 2, Philadelphia, Saunders, 1968.

126. Mayer, J.: Overweight: Causes, Cost, and Control, Englewood Cliffs, N.J., Prentice-Hall, 1968.

127. Felig, P., Marliss, E., and Cahill, G. F.: Plasma amino acid levels and insulin secretion in obesity, New Eng. J. Med. 281:811–816, 1969.

128. Renold, A. E.: Insulin biosynthesis and secretion, New Eng. J. Med. 282:173–182, 1970.

129. Cahill, G. F.: Starvation in man, New Eng. J. Med. 282:668–675, 1970.

130. MacBryde, C. M.: Obesity: Long-term results of treatment, (unpublished manuscript).

131. Chase, H. P., and Martin, H. P., Undernutrition and child development, New Eng. J. Med. 282:933–939, 1970.

132. Williams, R. H., and Ensinck, J. W.: The Banting Memorial Lecture, 1966. Secretion, fates, and actions of insulin and related products, Diabetes 15:623, 1966.

133. Mayer, J.: Some aspects of the problem of regulation of food intake and obesity, New Eng. J. Med. 274:610, 662, 722, 1966.

38

Weight Loss and Undernutrition

CYRIL M. MacBRYDE

DEFINITIONS

Weight loss and undernutrition are physical conditions resulting from a negative nutritive balance; they occur when metabolic utilization plus excretion of one or more essential nutrients exceeds the supply.

Weight loss does not necessarily imply *malnutrition*. If the nutritive defect is of calories only while other dietary essentials are supplied in adequate amounts, stored fats only may be lost, and that may even be desirable (as in obesity). Likewise, weight loss may indicate an improvement in the physical condition when excessive amounts of fluid are eliminated (as in edema).

Undernutrition may or may not be associated with *thinness* (subnormal body weight) and is therefore not to be considered simply the opposite of obesity. When thinness without any other nutritional defect is present, the problem is primarily caloric, due to inadequate intake of or interference with the absorption or storage of energy-supplying and fat-forming foods.

There are differences in the concepts of various authorities and in their definitions of thinness and undernutrition. Some have suggested that undernutrition is indicated by body weight ten per cent or more below the optimal; others have considered true undernutrition to begin at the point when the small reserves of body protein are gone and body tissue protein is called upon to furnish calories.

Undernutrition. A broader definition is necessary for a proper concept of the problem and for good clinical practice. Let us define undernutrition as any deviation below good nutrition. Good nutrition is essential for normal growth; for normal development, maintenance and function of all body organs and tissues; for reproduction; for optimal working efficiency; for optimal calories for energy requirements; for maximal resistance to infection; and for the ability to repair injury. Undernutrition exists whenever it can be demonstrated that a nutritive deficiency is responsible for subnormal response in any of these categories.

Usually undernutrition is not simple but complex, in the sense that there is not a deficiency of a single nutrient, but several deficiencies, and these are apt to be interrelated. The terms undernutrition or malnutrition imply that the negative nutritive balance has been of sufficient degree to endanger or impair body structure or function.

One or more specific types of undernutrition may occur in the presence of normal or excessive body fat. Obesity and various types of undernutrition may therefore coexist. Obesity itself is a type of *mal* (abnormal)-nutrition.

PERSPECTIVE OF NUTRITION PROBLEMS

There is quite properly, though belatedly, a great recent upsurge in the attention paid to nutrition in the United States[46-50,62] and throughout the world.[51,52,59,63] Active workers in the field have long known that widespread malnutrition exists even in the most "advanced" and relatively "affluent" areas, despite great progress in our nutritional knowledge in the last few decades. Delivery to all people of the practical results of scientific knowledge and of technological achievements is now becoming an active concern not only of the health professions, but also of governments and of the general public.

Two obstacles have prevented good nutrition from extending to many populations and individuals—poverty, and ignorance. In many countries the poor and uneducated constitute the great majority of the population: they are often unable to purchase an optimal diet; sometimes distribution problems preclude access to the best foods; perhaps even more commonly, although proper foods may be economically and physically obtainable, they are not chosen. Many individuals, often large groups or even whole tribes will choose poor diets because of lack of information, misinformation, convenience, habit, local, religious or ethnic customs, etc. In the United States one might mistakenly think from reading nutrition manuals that we are all Anglo-Saxon in our eating habits. The truth is instead that our people are heterogeneous in racial and social backgrounds and customs; food choices differ widely in various groups and localities. Foods considered pleasing to the palate are often widely different between Spanish-Americans, Chinese-Americans, Italo-Americans, Afro-Americans, Anglo-Saxon Americans, Jewish-Americans, etc., and even among different generations of the same family. Some encourage young children to abandon milk early and to drink wine regularly at meals. Some, even with free choice in a modern supermarket select chiefly "white meat" (fat pork), greens, and cornmeal.

Even in the United States, considered highly fortunate among nations because of the economic adequacy of the great majority and because of the wide availability of education, about one person in eight is inadequately nourished. There are no nationwide surveys, but partial surveys permit this estimate. Thus, of the present U. S. population of 210 million, about 26 million persons are believed to be inadequately nourished. The majority of these are children. The commonest cause of malnutrition is poverty, in the United States as well as in many other countries.[45-50,51,52,63]

The United States has available the resources and technology to produce and distribute all nutrients necessary for all our people (plus much more for export) but this has not yet been accomplished.

About 10 per cent of the U. S. population is obese (15 per cent or more over ideal weight). This 10 per cent plus the 12 per cent estimated to be undernourished makes the startling total of about 22 per cent believed to be improperly or malnourished in our country.

Some students of nutrition estimate that 75 per cent of human beings subsist on diets providing inadequate calories and insufficient protein.[38]

MEDICAL IMPORTANCE OF WEIGHT LOSS AND UNDERNUTRITION

When the body weight originally is near the optimum and neither excess fat nor excess fluid is present, weight loss that is progressive and not easily corrected is of great importance and its study may reveal serious disease.

In Chapters 2 and 37 tables of optimal or ideal weights for various heights and ages and for both sexes are given. Usually serious degrees of thinness are apparent upon inspection only, but the tables are useful in estimating the number of pounds variation from desirable levels. It must be kept in mind that the presence of excess fluid or fat may give apparently normal or high weights in some persons with malnutrition.

When the physician is confronted with a patient who gives a definite history of progressive weight loss or shows physical evidence of it, he must search for the cause of the negative caloric balance and also for other possible associated evidences of nutritional failure. Although statistically, people of normal or somewhat subnormal body weight live longer than obese persons, patients of optimal weight seem to live longest and to enjoy the best health. The physician must not encourage his patients to keep thin, for stored calories provide a safety factor in times of stress or disease. When fashion dictates a sub-optimal weight for his patients, he should combat it and instruct in the methods of establishing the optimal weight and nutrition for each person.

States of undernourishment *without weight loss* may exhibit various evidences of *specific nature*. Such specific evidence of physical changes or functional derangement is often distinctive enough to indicate the etiology of the nutritive disorder. However, many persons consider themselves relatively well, but suffer from various *ill-defined symptoms* many of which can be traced to malnutrition. A study of 610 male industrial workers[2] revealed that 158 (approximately 25 per cent) gave evidence of suboptimal nutrition, particularly with respect to thiamine, riboflavin, ascorbic acid, calcium and phosphorus. No cases of florid or acute deficiency diseases were seen, but suboptimal nutrition and obesity were widespread among all age, income, work and ethnic groups. Dietary faults frequently observed included inadequate consumption of milk and vitamin-C-rich fruits and vegetables, and excess intake of unenriched bread and pastries, sweetened beverages and candy.

A survey of the food intake of a widely representative sample of 14,500 men, women and children in the United States in 1965[47] showed that:

1. Average diets for most sex-age groups were adequate according to Recommended Dietary Allowances (RDA) of 1968[44] for 5 of the 7 nutrients studied: protein, vitamin A value, thiamine, riboflavin, and ascorbic acid.

Calcium and iron intake were the two nutrients most often found to be below the RDA.

2. Calcium intake was below recommendations in females of all ages from 9 to over 75, averaging about 35 per cent below the RDA.

Calcium intake of males was low in teen-age boys (9 through 14) and older men (55 and over).

3. Iron intake was low (only about 50 per cent of the RDA) for all children under 3 years old.

Iron in the diet of females aged 9 to 55 averaged 36 to 39 per cent below the RDA.

4. Ascorbic acid was notably deficient in infants under 2 months and in men over 75 years.

5. Thiamine was 10 to 20 per cent below the RDA in the diets of most females.

6. Riboflavin was 10 to 20 per cent below the RDA in diets of women 20 to 75, thirty per cent below the RDA in those over 75.

7. Vitamin A value was 10 per cent below the RDA for girls and women 12-15, 18-20, and 65-74, and 20 per cent below the RDA for those over 75.

Often thorough investigation reveals that the undernutrition is the primary condition, but frequently the nutritive defect may be the presenting abnormality that leads to the discovery of other disease conditions which caused the malnutrition.

The medical significance of the discovery of a nutritive defect has three aspects:

1. The cause of a primary nutritional disorder may be detected and often may be eliminated or corrected.

2. If the disturbed nutrition is found to be secondary to some other disorder, the latter may be diagnosed and properly treated.

3. Recognition of a nutritive defect *and* another disease condition usually directs proper attention to each and improves the prognosis of both, whether or not they are causally related. Restoration of nutrition to normal exerts a favorable influence on practically all disease conditions.

WEIGHT LOSS AND UNDER-NUTRITION AS SYMPTOMS

The symptom of weight loss may not be emphasized by the patient, but unless there is an obvious explanation, it always should receive serious consideration by the physician. With or without weight loss, lack of energy, weakness and easy fatigue are usually associated symptoms of an inadequate supply of calories. When not only the energy principle (calories) but certain other essential nutrients are lacking, there may be a wide variety of symptoms, according to the specific food elements involved.

In the absence of weight loss or subnormal body weight, the evidences of undernutrition may be easily overlooked in the history or physical examination unless they happen to be striking. One of the primary purposes of this chapter is to describe the chief symptoms of malnutrition (of which weight loss is only one) and to discuss the mechanisms of their development. The protean symptomatic manifestations of nutritional deficiencies require constant alertness to permit their detection in early or mild stages. It is, of course, in these early stages that diagnosis is of the greatest importance, for by the time florid signs have appeared, correction may be difficult or irreparable damage may have been done. For example, after a compression fracture of an osteoporotic vertebra has occurred, the diagnosis of chronic protein deficiency plus prolonged calcium lack is important, but earlier diagnosis to prevent fractures is much preferable.

GROWTH: NUTRITIVE ASPECTS

During the early part of life, growth is the most striking characteristic of the organism—all the essential nutrients must be supplied in generous amounts for normal growth and development to take place. As maturity is reached, the previous necessity for a great positive balance of tissue-building elements ceases, and maintenance of tissues (with intake and expenditure equalized) is sufficient. Even structures usually considered as relatively static, such as the bones, actually have an active metabolism, losing and replacing constituents steadily. Therefore, the necessity for good nutrition does not end with the growth period. Optimal health and vigor require during the mature years not only calories for energy, but structural materials and chemical regulators of the metabolic machinery.

MATERNAL NUTRITION, FETUS AND NEWBORN

Babies whose birth weight is less than 2500 grams (5½ lbs.) are most often born to poorly nourished mothers. They have poorer chances of survival and are frequently subnormal in physical and mental development. These "low birth weight" babies include those born before completion of 37 weeks of gestation (preterm) and others who are gestationally mature but with retardation of fetal growth. Currently more than 8 per cent of all live births produce low-birth weight babies, a proportion which has been increasing annually during the past decade. Highest rates of occurrence of low birth weight are associated with being nonwhite, of low income, and in the group of youngest mothers. In the United States nearly 300,000 infants are born annually confronted with the problems attendant on low birth weight.[45,46]

Undernutrition and various other forms of malnutrition preceding and during pregnancy, especially in very young mothers, are responsible for much of the high maternal morbidity and mortality in this group. Low birth weight is especially common when the mother is very young and malnourished. Death of the infant in the neonatal period (first 4 weeks) is associated with low birth weight in one-third of all cases. Nutritional inadequacies during fetal development and in early postnatal life have long-lasting effects upon the potential for later growth and development.

Even when poverty or lack of access to proper food, or both, are not factors, malnutrition may increase dangers to mother and child. The fad of extreme slenderness is widespread, so that many women are malnourished when they become pregnant. Also, many doctors as well as patients have erred by unduly restricting caloric intake and weight gain during pregnancy. In women of normal weight prior to pregnancy, a total gradual weight gain of 20 to 25 pounds is now considered optimal.[44] Excess weight gain, as well as insufficient gain, is deleterious. In an undernourished woman, correction of her malnutrition plus provision for the needs of the pregnancy may result in an entirely appropriate total gain considerably above 25 pounds.

Severe caloric restriction inevitably causes restriction of other nutrients essential for the fetal growth process. Efforts to achieve weight reduction of obese women during pregnancy are usually unwise; the weight loss is best accomplished when the woman is not pregnant.

It is best to establish proper intake of natural foods containing all essential nutrients rather than to rely upon vitamin and mineral supplements in women preceding and during pregnancy, except for iron and folate. The amounts of these nutrients are apt to be inadequate in the diets of many women in the United States, especially for the added requirements of pregnancy. Therefore, routine supplementation with iron and folate is considered to be justified and is recommended.[45,46]

HORMONAL-NUTRITIONAL INTERRELATIONSHIPS

HORMONES → NUTRITION

These reciprocal relationships are important and complex. *Pituitary growth hormone* is anabolic, promoting nitrogen, phosphorus, potassium, sulfur and water storage in the proportions to form cells and protoplasm. *Androgens* have a similar effect, facilitating the incorporation of amino acids into proteins. *Estrogens* have protein anabolic effect, but it is considerably less marked than that of androgens. Androgens promote calcium and phosphorus reten-

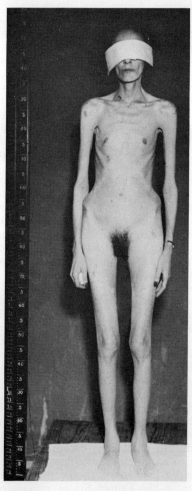

FIG. 38-1. Appearance resembling pituitary cachexia (Simmonds' disease) from severe anorexia nervosa. Woman, 33 years old, with senile aspect, emaciation, loss of hair and breast tissue and amenorrhea.

tion indirectly, their primary effect being upon the protein matrix of bone, thus laying the groundwork for calcification. The estrogens are thought to have a specific stimulating effect upon osteoblasts, and to have a greater effect upon Ca and P storage than androgens. Giving both of the two gonadal hormones has a greater effect upon bone formation than either alone.

The administration of *insulin* promotes protein and fat synthesis. In insulin lack, protein breakdown is increased and gluconeogenesis is required, both as a preliminary step in the oxidation of amino acids and as a way of forming oxaloacetate to facilitate the complete oxidation of fatty acids.

The effect of *thyroid hormone* is to stimulate cellular metabolism. Physiologic amounts are necessary for normal growth and cell activity. Excessive amounts cause abnormal acceleration of the total metabolism, with rapid consumption of energy stores and perhaps eventual use of body protein for fuel. Patients with hyperthyroidism tend to be in negative balance for all constituents of the body tissues. Appetite may be greatly increased and food intake tremendously augmented, but caloric expenditure even at bed rest may exceed attempts to keep pace with it, and there may be persistent weight loss, depletion of muscle and skeleton, loss of nitrogen and calcium, etc.

Physiologic amounts of the adrenocortical hormones are necessary for normal growth, cellular activity and energy production. The effect of excessive amounts of the *adrenal cortical steroids* is to stimulate protein breakdown and gluconeogenesis; a diabetic state may result. Sodium retention by the renal tubules is facilitated, and urinary potassium loss is increased. The adrenocortical types of steroids now are employed so widely in therapeutics that it is imperative to be familiar with signs of overdosage (moonface, edema, hypertension, glycosuria, etc.).

NUTRITION → ENDOCRINE GLANDS

In the preceding section, we have mentioned some of the chief effects of hormones on nutrition. There are also important effects of nutrition upon the endocrine glands. The synthesis of *pituitary hormones* is impaired in malnutrition, especially protein deficiency.[9] Microscopic examination of the anterior pituitary in malnourished persons has shown atrophy, and in some cases, degenerative lesions.[31] Severe malnutrition in children often causes dwarfing. The *adrenal glands* in malnourished persons are small and exhibit lipid depletion. *Thyroid* hypoactivity results from lack of pituitary thyrotropin. Decrease in *gonadal function* is among the earliest signs of malnutrition and is secondary to lack of pituitary gonadotropin. Even when careful metabolic and endocrine laboratory studies are utilized, it may be difficult to distinguish primary pituitary failure from hypopituitarism secondary to malnutrition[21a] (Fig. 38-1).

AGING AND MALNUTRITION

The processes of aging have important reciprocal interrelationships with nutrition: aging is apt to cause nutritive disorders; nutritive defects accelerate the degenerative changes usually associated with physiologic aging. Elderly persons suffer from malnourishment often because of the frequency with which economic, psychological and organic problems beset them. One must be on guard not to accept degenerative changes as the inevitable erosion of the years.[16,30,32] The nutritional status of aging persons is not dependent alone upon food, impaired digestion or absorption, etc., but also upon factors such as *stress*. In elderly persons cold, heat, emotional strain, etc., may be followed by nitrogen and other losses which may be cumulative and more difficult to replace than in younger people.[16,30,32]

Good nutrition slows and poor nutrition speeds the processes of physiologic aging. Various observations support this concept: in starvation (anorexia nervosa, etc.) the senile appearance of the subject is striking (Fig. 38-1); frequently nutritive failure in old age is mistaken for evidence of senescence itself, but often great improvement in nutrition causes an apparent rejuvenation; catabolic processes (e.g., the osteoporosis of the spine in Cushing's syndrome) may closely simulate the changes associated with aging (senile osteoporosis), etc. Even in small children, severe malnutrition (as in kwashiorkor, which means red hair) may cause dryness, scaling and pigmentation of the skin, graying of the hair, and other changes usually considered evidence of aging.

Loss of anabolic influences may cause body changes characteristic of advanced years even in the very young (e.g., progeria in certain dwarfs with pituitary failure). Loss of the anabolic influence of the sex hormones (estrogen, testosterone) may produce fatigue, muscle atrophy, osteoporosis, fine wrinkling of the skin, loss of hair, and other changes usually associated with aging. Proper use of sex hormones may greatly relieve signs of premature aging in hypogonadal persons.

CAUSE OF WEIGHT LOSS AND THINNESS

No matter how puzzling the picture may seem, there is (when hydration is normal) only a single cause of weight loss or subnormal body weight: insufficient calories are being supplied to meet the metabolic needs. It may be true either that the actual number of *calories assimilated* by the body is inadequate or that the *caloric expenditure* is excessive, or both factors may be operative, but always there is a negative caloric balance or (in the case of failure to gain) an insufficiently positive balance.

It often seems that certain persons eat more than enough to gain weight but remain thin, even when no metabolic disturbance is present and when absorption and assimilation are normal. Frequently there is a familial tendency to leanness, just as in some families obesity is common. The eating habits of families are, of course, important, and one may be able to demonstrate that certain families as a whole are "small eaters" or that the bulk of their diet is apparently great, but foods low in caloric value are consistently chosen instead of those high in caloric value.

Certain strains of animals tend to be thin while others get fat, even when both receive the same diet, so that a hereditary predisposition to leanness seems evident. In human beings the evidence is less clear, but it also seems to favor inheritance in some cases.

Local tissue factors are of some importance, probably not in the usual kinds of thinness, but undoubtedly in rare and peculiar instances of failure to deposit fat locally in certain areas. Such conditions are known as *lipodystrophy*, and the region in which little or no fat is deposited may be the upper half of the body, the legs only, or the face; or even only one side of the face, etc. The variety most frequently seen occurs in women, the upper half of the body being lean and emaciated, while from the hips down fat is deposited in normal or excessive amounts. The disorder seems to be hereditary, even the type and the location of the lesions being transmitted.

Fat atrophy occurs locally in some persons following repeated subcutaneous injections, especially of insulin.

Psychologic factors are of great importance in regulating food intake. *Appetite* is to a large degree dependent upon habit, training and emotional status. The appearance, the color, the taste, the smell and even the memory of food exert strong influences. When in emotional turmoil, most persons are apt to develop moderate or severe anorexia. When the emotional disorder is extreme, the psychoneurosis known as *anorexia nervosa* may be present, and true emaciation may result. Prolonged nervous tension with lack of appetite may be at least partially the result of overactivity of the sympathico-adrenal system, with inhibition of the parasympathetic motor system to the gastrointestinal tract, and perhaps similar inhibition of secretion of the digestive juices.

Not only excited but retarded emotional and psychological states often affect nutrition. *Depression* inhibits appetite as well as the inclination to secure or prepare proper food.

Appetite and Hunger. Appetite is the desire for food, a psychologic state which may accompany hunger, but may be present without it. Hunger is a sensation, a physiologic state related in human beings to perception of general weakness, certain sensory impulses from the alimentary tract, and perhaps to decrease in the circulating supply or utilization of blood glucose.[3,4]

Hypothalamus and Higher Nerve Center Regulation of Food Intake. Hyperphagia is induced experimentally in animals by bilateral medial lesions in the neighborhood of the ventromedial nuclei. Aphagia (complete failure of eating) occurs if lesions are produced in certain lateral hypothalamic areas. Animals becoming obese after medial lesions abruptly stop eating when lateral lesions are created.

The neural complex for the regulation of feeding seems to be analogous to the mechanisms which regulate circulation, respiration, body temperature and many other variables. That is, the control is eventually effective through the facilitation or inhibition of feeding reflexes. When feeding alone is concerned, regulation at the hypothalamic level occurs, but when other variables are introduced, such as sensation, emotion, volition, choices between foods, etc., the cerebral cortex probably contributes to the regulation.

The pathologic physiology of hunger, appetite, satiety, weight gain and weight loss, anorexia, etc., are discussed also in Chapters 21 and 37 and in recent excellent reviews.[3,4,22]

Nutritional factors are the common pathways through which the various influences on body weight and nutritive status must be exerted. Thus, the thin person who because of a neurosis cannot take enough calories differs from the thin person unable to eat because of abdominal distress caused by a peptic ulcer. In one case, the cause may be purely psychologic and in the other purely physical; or, as often happens, the psychologic and the physical elements may become closely intertwined and be present in both instances. Nevertheless, the cause of the weight loss and other symptoms of undernutrition is *inadequate food intake*, if absorption, assimilation and metabolism are normal.

Similarly, weight loss from chronic diarrhea occurs from *failure to assimilate calorigenic nutrients*, whether from a psychogenic ulcerative colitis or from tuberculous enteritis. Likewise, weight loss from prolonged fever or excessive muscular activity results from excessive *caloric expenditure*, just as it does in hyperthyroidism.

CAUSES OF SPECIFIC NUTRITIVE DEFICIENCIES

Failure to maintain adequate stores of energy-producing material such as fat may be thought of as a *general* nutritive defect, depending upon proper caloric balance. Carbohydrate, the chief usual source of calories in the average normal diet, is usually implicated, but fat also often plays an important role. Subnormal carbohydrate or fat intake causes thinness or weight loss; loss of carbohydrate as glucose in the urine (diabetes), or of fat in the stool (steatorrhea) has a similar result, etc.

Other nutritive defects may be considered more *specific:* for example, although calorie intake may be adequate, proper growth and maintenance of muscle and other tissue proteins depend upon protein intake and balance. The calorie foods cannot take the place of the tissue foods nor of other nutrients needed for many different and special functions.

Calcium, iron, iodine and the other mineral essentials; sodium, potassium, magnesium and the other electrolytes; and each of the essential vitamins must be available in certain specific amounts to maintain normal structure and function. Each of the essential nutrients may be thought of as having its own metabolism. The positive and negative phases of the metabolic cycle for each nutrient must be in such balance that adequate amounts may be utilized without production of deficits, otherwise evidences of nutritional failure will appear. Insufficient intake, excess destruction or elimination may affect one or more of the important elements in nutrition, either separately or, more often, in various characteristic combinations, depending upon their functions in the body.

As with calories, so with other nutrient essentials such as water, minerals and vitamins. Undernutrition with respect to any one of these elements results when a negative balance for that specific nutrient occurs, or when the balance is insufficiently positive to satisfy metabolic requirements.

The various types of undernutrition occur because of inadequate intake, defective absorption, impaired utilization, excessive destruction or elimination of one or more of the necessary food substances. The materials required for optimal growth and development, health and efficiency are water, certain minerals and vitamins, carbohydrate, fat and protein.

Inadequate Intake

Anorexia and Starvation. Loss of appetite and failure to ingest adequate quantities of one or more necessary foods will eventually result in malnutrition. The loss of appetite may result from any of a great number of *organic* conditions; for example, gastritis, gastric cancer, heart failure, nephritis, febrile diseases, any condition associated with severe pain, many neoplastic diseases, etc. However, anorexia often is *psychic* in origin and may be a feature of alcoholism and various neuroses or psychoses. If disinterest in food and failure to ingest an adequate diet persist, partial or complete starvation occurs. The starvation may be *general* or *specific:* in anorexia nervosa all foods are shunned, but in some simple "distastes" only one food is avoided. For example, some persons have an aversion to milk and develop calcium deficiency; others

may be vegetarians and develop anemia because of lack of protein, iron, etc.

Occult Dietary Deficiencies. Often the diet may be apparently normal, but concealed defects are present. Those who fail to ingest sufficient amounts of the proper types of foods often have easy access to them; others receive improper diets because of circumstances beyond their control.

The average undistorted diet is apt to be adequate as regards many of the food essentials without much effort as to choice of foods, but certain important nutrients may be taken in inadequate amounts. The majority of intelligent people make some attempt to utilize the modern knowledge of food values in selecting their diets. However, it has been shown that a considerable proportion of the apparently healthy normal population shows some evidences of undernutrition because many persons fail to ingest a variety of foods balanced to contain all the essential nutrients in adequate amounts. It is evident that although there are powerful physiologic demands directing our unconscious choices of foods that reinforce and assist our conscious selections, these mechanisms often fail. Man and the animals do not always instinctively select a good diet.

Poverty is the commonest cause for totally inadequate food intake. Poverty is also the usual cause of lack of variety in diet and failure to eat optimal amounts of high quality protein foods and foods that furnish important vitamins and minerals.[50,26] In most areas of the world the foods that are most readily available and least expensive are the major constituents of the diets of the poor. They primarily contain carbohydrates: corn, wheat, rice, potatoes.[63] Foods supplying fats and the "protective" nutrients (proteins, minerals, vitamins) e.g. in meat, milk, eggs, fruits, and vegetables, are in most regions more difficult to produce and distribute and are therefore more expensive. They may be available in sufficient supply to provide the Recommended Daily Allowances of all nutrients to those who can afford them; to the poor they may be obtainable infrequently or in insufficient amounts.

Ignorance is often to be blamed, for the dissemination of knowledge is far behind the advances in the available information. There is some excuse for the lay person who has had little or no opportunity to learn about proper diet. Physicians, dietitians and educators in the fields of medicine, hygiene and public health must bear the responsibility of acquiring and disseminating authentic knowledge concerning proper food selection and preparation.

Therapeutic Nutrition. The physician particularly, and his co-worker, the medical dietitian, must be careful that they do not, through ignorance or inattention, prescribe therapeutic diets that may be of value in correcting one condition but may precipitate nutritional failure because of inadequacies, excesses or imbalances.

If tube feeding is employed, or intravenous fluids, or dialysis, great care must be taken not to provoke nutritional or metabolic disorders.

The physician responsible for the care of a patient must realize that even in apparently purely mechanical conditions nutritional considerations may be of great importance. For example, immobilization of a fractured bone causes calcium and phosphorus loss and calls for attention to the intake of these elements and of vitamin D.

FOOD PREPARATION. Efforts should be made to educate physicians, educators, dietitians, nutritionists, public-health officers and the public concerning the nutritive values of foods and their proper preservation and cooking. Even if the food originally is high in vitamins and minerals, large amounts of these essential nutrients may be destroyed in *food preparation*.[17]

Minerals and salts are lost principally through peeling, washing and soaking, and discarding of cooking juices. Prolonged cooking, especially boiling, causes the greatest losses. Waste of water-soluble-vitamins also may be large; up to 50 per cent of B-complex vitamins may be lost in solution in water.[17,43]

Rice constitutes the principal staple food of many millions in the Orient. In its natural state the brown rice heads contain significant amounts of B-complex vitamins in the hulls. The rice usually eaten, however, consists of the white polished kernels remaining after the vitamin-rich covering has been removed by milling. This white milled rice when cooked contains 70 per cent water, 26 per cent carbohydrate, 2.5 per cent protein and practically no vitamins. Those who subsist upon it as their main food are apt to develop vitamin deficiencies, especially a deficiency of vitamin B_1 (thiamine) in the form of beri-beri. "Converted" rice, prepared by a different milling process, contains more thiamine and niacin. In the Philippines there is a national law that requires that milled white rice be enriched with thiamine, niacin and iron. Use of such enriched rice would prevent beri-beri. The law is not well observed or enforced and beri-beri is still common in the Philippines.

The refining of other cereals, such as wheat, with removal of the germ and of the bran layer, causes great reduction of the vitamin B content. In the United States wheat and other cereal and grain products supply about 45 per cent of the carbohydrate in the diet and about 21 per cent of the total daily calories of the average adult male. Enrichment of wheat, corn and rice products is required by law to provide standard amounts of thiamine, riboflavin, niacin, and iron.

Milk, butter, and margarine in the United States are required by law to be fortified to certain content standards of vitamins A and D.

In cooking leafy vegetables and other green and yellow varieties 20 to 30 per cent of the vitamin A value is lost. Vitamins of the B-complex and ascorbic acid are rendered inert by alkalis.

The losses of thiamine in foods from heat comparable to that of baking may be as high as 50 per cent. Even "flash" cooking at very high temperature may cause large vitamin and mineral losses. Thin white bread sheets made from whole wheat flour and water, cooked on a very hot iron sheet for only a few seconds on each side may suffer losses during baking of up to 50 per cent of the fluoride, niacin, B_6, and total pantothenate, 35 per cent of the folate, and 20 per cent of the selenium.[55] Cooking meat results in average losses of about 40 per cent of thiamine, 20 per cent of riboflavin, and 20 per cent of niacin.

Simple exposure to air causes rapid oxidation and loss of ascorbic acid from foods. Heating or cooking may result in complete inactivation of all vitamin C present. Even in rapid cooking of vegetables or fruits an average of about 40 per cent of ascorbic acid is lost. Freezing causes vitamin C losses of 30 to 40 per cent.[17,43]

Recluses getting little fresh food and subsisting largely on highly refined, overcooked, and steamed foods often develop nutritive deficiencies, especially those of thiamine, and of ascorbic acid.

CLIMATE AND SUNLIGHT. There is one essential nutrient not derived primarily from food. It is vitamin D. Few foods other than eggs, fish liver or fish-liver oils contain appreciable amounts of it. Most of the requirement is supplied through the chemical changes produced in cholesterol through irradiation of the skin by *sunlight.* During a large part of the year in cold or in temperate climates, sunlight and outdoor activity are so limited that vitamin-D deficits are common. This is especially the case in children, in whom, because of rapid skeletal growth, the requirement is high.

The *temperature* to which the body is exposed has much to do with its metabolic rate and the relative speed with which nutrients are utilized, stored, or excreted. The most essential nutrient of all, water, plays a primary role in the regulation of body temperature, and in the adjustment of body metabolism to environmental temperatures. The requirement for water depends largely upon the heat production by the body and upon the environmental temperature. (See Chapter 35.)

Moderate chilling accelerates metabolism and increases caloric and other nutritional requirements. High environmental temperatures also increase the metabolic rate and nutritional needs. Profound chilling of the body can greatly lower body temperature and tremendously reduce the rate of metabolism.

TRADITION AND HABIT. Probably third most common (after poverty and ignorance) as a factor in causing malnutrition among the apparently normal part of the population is traditional adherence to certain types of food. Deficient diets are often followed consistently because of individual, familial, group, racial, regional or religious habits.

The neglect of milk drinking and the excessive use of tea is common in some areas; in others the widely used beverage is coffee; in still others, wine or beer. In the United States there is overindulgence in sweetened and variously flavored "soft" drinks. These beverages are poor in nutritional value. Small children, teen-agers and young women especially need the calcium and other nutrients milk would provide.

In the Orient highly-milled white rice is traditionally the staple food of many millions. More effort is needed to teach the people how properly to supplement this almost pure carbohydrate principal nutrient.

In the United States many diets are deficient in thiamine (vitamin B_1), nicotinic acid, ascorbic acid, iron, and calcium, and recognizable clinical deficiency states often result in spite of adequate caloric intake

and the maintenance of normal body weight. Refined cereals, white bread, pastries, candy, and sugar are often taken in excess to the neglect of fruits, vegetables, milk, eggs, meat and whole-wheat products.[47,50]

Commercial Exploitation. Some habits are fostered for monetary gain. Powerful commercial exploitation through all the advertising media promotes the sale of soft drinks, candies, alcoholic beverages, etc., which are too often ingested in place of more beneficial foods. The natural desire of children for sweets is commonly over-indulged through parental ignorance and commercial pressures. Special taste-habits and a craving for intoxication arise partially from clever promotion of alcoholic drinks. Their use intrigues the young who wish to be sophisticated and debonair like the "beautiful people" seen in the advertisements. Unfortunately many social drinkers soon become problem alcoholics. Even moderate alcoholism means that an appreciable amount of the nutrient intake is supplied by the "empty calories" of ethanol. Protein and vitamin deficiencies are apt to become evident. Neuritis and liver damage are among the commonest disorders that result.

Need for Public Education. Attempts to educate the public and legislative bodies concerning means by which nutrition of all people can be improved[44-50] have been slow in achieving results in the United States and elsewhere,[51,52,59,62,63] but there has been much progress; retrospective surveys show that overt deficiency diseases such as pellagra, scurvy, and rickets are seen much less frequently now than two or three decades ago. The use of fortified milk has no doubt considerably lessened the incidence of rickets.

General progress in spreading the benefits of present and advancing nutritional knowledge will be achieved chiefly through *education.* Knowledge and understanding, not imposed legal regulations, must be the primary means of combating harmful *tradition,* bad old *habits,* and injurious new ones. Spreading accurate and practical knowledge of nutrition to the health professions and to non-medical people, particularly the young, everywhere will not only lead to wiser choice of foods and better preservation and preparation of foods, but to resistance to commercial exploitation of deleterious foods and beverages, and to greater production and better distribution of the most beneficial nutrients.

OTHER CAUSES OF INADEQUATE INTAKE

FADS. Food faddism, such as vegetarianism, etc., is not uncommon and may cause many different types of deficiencies.

PERVERTED APPETITE, PICA, GEOPHAGIA. Ingestion of abnormal substances may be an individual idiosyncrasy, a local custom, or a more wide-spread practice throughout a segment of society. The term *pica* means the eating of any foreign substance and thus includes *geophagia* (earth, dirt, or clay eating). Various forms of pica occur in emotionally or mentally disturbed persons, but pica is very common and is found most often among those with no psychiatric disorder. Lead poisoning is a frequent result of the habit some infants and small children have of gnawing paint from their cribs or from walls or putty from around windows. Iron-deficiency anemia accompanies the eating of laundry starch (often up to a pound or more a day) usually by women, especially during pregnancy, and chiefly among the poor in the southern part of the United States. Frequently starch or clay are ingested interchangeably.

Geophagia occurs throughout the world, especially among the poor and malnourished. Its cause is not understood. In some instances intense hunger from real starvation is the cause, when grass, leaves, earth, any readily available substance, will be eaten to allay hunger pangs. However, geophagia is often practiced when normal foods are available; a craving seems to exist which is unexplained.

Clay has been ingested as an antidote to poisons for hundreds of years. Modern studies show that it has high capacity as a cation-exchange substance. It will take up metals, prevent their absorption and cause their excretion, combined with clay, in the feces. The essential constituent of pure clay or kaolin is the mineral kaolinite, a hydrous aluminum silicate. When kaolin, or crude clay (containing many minerals, especially SiO_2, Al_2O_3 and CaO) is taken as an antidote, it may be effective against certain metallic poisons, such as mercuric chloride.[53]

That women, especially pregnant women, with geophagia are expressing their calcium lack and their iron-deficiency symptoms with an instinctive craving or traditional or legendary search for calcium and iron in the earth has been suggested. The earth contains calcium and may contain some iron, but if it contains much clay the absorption of the iron will be blocked. The anemia already present may be made much worse.[54]

Incidence. Eating of clay has been reported in Iran, Turkey, Morocco, Egypt, central Africa, India, South America and the United States. Analysis of a number of studies of incidence of pica (including geophagia) in the United States reveals surprisingly high figures. Starch eating is apparently more frequent in some (especially urban) areas than clay eating, but some persons eat both or either. Children in urban areas may eat newspaper and plaster.

Pica is several times as common among Negroes as among white persons. All studies of pregnant women in the poorest socio-economic groups show an incidence of pica of 40 per cent to 75 per cent.[53] Among children under 6 years in these same groups one-quarter to one-third have the habit, the highest incidence being under age 3. Men often have the habit in the United States and in other countries, but the practice seems to be much less common than among females.

Nutritional Effects of Geophagia. Achlorhydria was present in each of 60 children with geophagia studied in Texas, and in 6 of 8 geophagic dwarfs studied in Iran. Which is cause and which is effect is not clear.

Iron-deficiency anemia is common from clay-eating. Hypokalemia may result.

In 1960, eleven patients from Iranian villages who had long-standing geophagia were reported by Halsted and his colleagues.[53] They all had profound anemia, dwarfism, hypogonadism, and marked hepatosplenomegaly. The anemia was of pure iron-deficiency type and responded to appropriate treatment. Data obtained in subsequent studies suggested that the endocrine abnormalities might result primarily from zinc deficiency. Present evidence indicates that clay blocks zinc absorption. Investigations are in progress to evaluate the effect of zinc upon growth and sex development, especially in physically retarded children who have been malnourished.[55]

ALCOHOLISM. Chronic alcoholism is apt to cause nutritional disorders because (1) alcohol supplies calories without all the other necessary nutrients; (2) alcohol often precipitates nausea, vomiting, diarrhea and its use frequently causes anorexia; (3) it often results in liver damage, peptic ulcers, etc., which are then the further causes of nutritive defects; (4) it often is associated with psychiatric disturbances, neglect of proper diet, food faddism, etc.

ORGANIC DISEASE. The factors leading so-called normal people to poor food selection have been mentioned. Failure of intake of the necessary foods may also result from organic disease of many types. Affections of the mouth, the tongue and the pharynx such as dental disorders, gingivitis, glossitis, tonsillitis and ulcerations of various sorts, often cause restriction of the diet to liquids over a considerable period. Inflammatory, ulcerative, neoplastic or obstructive disease, or surgical changes involving the gastrointestinal tract may interfere with normal food intake or be accompanied by vomiting, nausea or anorexia. Loss of appetite, sometimes with nausea or vomiting, is frequent in many organic disorders, such as cardiac conditions, nephritis and intracranial disease.

PSYCHIC DISORDERS. Fatigue, nervous tension, emotional states, psychoneuroses and psychoses often affect the functions of the alimentary canal or cause loss of interest in food.

DRUG THERAPY. Many commonly used drugs may cause anorexia, nausea or vomiting (e.g., morphine, codeine, salicylates, digitalis), or diarrhea (mercurials, antibiotics, etc.) and thus interfere with nutrition. Not only may drugs interfere with intake, but absorption and utilization may suffer or excretion be accelerated.

Exaggerated needs are produced by certain medications, such as isoniazid or penicillamine, which tremendously increase the urinary excretion of vitamin B_6. The antituberculosis drug isoniazid may induce peripheral neuropathy unless B_6 is given concomitantly. Optic neuritis, which disappeared after administration of B_6, has occurred in patients given penicillamine.

Any agent causing prolonged diuresis is apt to cause potassium deficiency. Corticosteroids greatly increase urinary loss of potassium.

THERAPEUTIC DIETS. In the treatment of disease therapeutic diets are often employed, and inadvertently there may be prescribed a diet so deficient in one factor or more that a nutritive disorder results. In *peptic-ulcer* therapy, tomato juice and citrus fruits may be forbidden and vitamin-C deficit may occur. In the treatment of *diabetes*, care must be taken not to give a diet too low in the B-complex vitamins when bread and other cereals are restricted. In *allergic* conditions, milk, wheat, eggs, meat, orange juice, or

other foods may be eliminated from the diet and lack of calcium, protein, iron, vitamins, other minerals or other types of malnutrition may be produced. Therapeutic diets for weight reduction in *obesity* are apt to be deficient not only in calories but in other nutrients, and to prevent malnutrition the physician must in many instances ensure the intake of certain essentials while total calories are restricted. Thus a generous allowance of skimmed milk will provide adequate calcium and phosphorus intake, eggs and meat will provide protein and iron, and it may be advisable to supply supplements of vitamins A and D (because of restricted fats), B complex (because of restricted wheat and cereals) and C (because of limited citrus fruits).

NUTRITIONAL DISORDERS often interfere with food intake and thus may set up a vicious circle which tends to perpetuate and intensify the malnutrition, frequently making what was a simple, perhaps single nutrient deficit into a complex, multiple deficit. Thiamine deficiency and nicotinic acid deficiency are particularly known to cause anorexia and nausea. Anorexia is characteristic of pernicious anemia and other B_{12}-deficiency states.

INADEQUATE ABSORPTION OR UTILIZATION

Even though a proper amount of all the necessary nutrients is ingested, they may not be absorbed or utilized because of mechanical, chemical or bacterial dysfunction in the alimentary canal. Chronic diarrhea, from whatever cause, by reason of the excessively rapid passage through the body, may fail to permit time for proper digestion and absorption of water, salts and vitamins, as well as of some of the carbohydrate, the protein and the fat. When certain enzymes such as pancreatic lipase are lacking, food elements are lost (in this case fats, with steatorrhea). When bile is excluded from the intestine, fats and fat-soluble vitamins (A, D, E and K) are poorly digested and absorbed, and fats and insoluble calcium soaps are excreted. Such calcium loss, if prolonged, may lead to osteomalacia and result in pathologic fractures. Proteins may be inadequately digested and absorbed when gastric hydrochloric acid and pepsin are lacking. Other examples are the poor absorption of ferric iron in the absence of adequate hydrochloric acid and poor calcium absorption with deficient vitamin D.

Vitamin B_{12} is inadequately absorbed in

the absence of the intrinsic gastric factor; also B_{12} deficiency with macrocytic anemia may result from interference with its assimilation caused by other gastrointestinal disorders (see discussion further on in this chapter under vitamin B_{12}).

The malabsorption syndrome is the term now used to designate a group of related conditions described in the past as tropical sprue, nontropical sprue, celiac disease and idiopathic steatorrhea. In all of these diseases there is severe chronic diarrhea with bulky stools containing excess lipid. In children (celiac disease) there is growth failure. Affected patients lose weight, have flat glucose tolerance curves; depleted reserves of iron, folic acid and B_{12} (with microcytic or macrocytic anemia); vitamin K deficiency (with hypoprothrombinemia and hemorrhages); hypoproteinemia with edema; hypocalcemia with tetany, rickets or osteomalacia; and frequent electrolyte disturbances. The etiology is obscure—it is not clear whether the abnormalities found in the small intestine are primary. Biopsies of jejunal mucosa have shown short, blunted villi and the microvilli are sparse, blunted and fused; these changes reflect a major loss of the bowel absorptive area.

The anemia when macrocytic in type responds to B_{12} or folic acid therapy, but the anemia is often mixed in type and may be partly or primarily due to iron deficiency. Vitamin B_{12} and folic acid in acquired deficiencies cause improvement in the intestinal mucosa, but in congenital celiac disease have not reversed mucosal changes. Gluten-free diets have induced remissions in celiac disease and non-tropical sprue and alterations of villi toward the normal pattern have been observed following prolonged periods of such therapy.[37,40]

It is not clear whether the malabsorption syndrome is due primarily to a mucosal defect, a toxic or antibody immune response (to gluten, and possibly to other nutrients) or some other mechanism. However, it is evident that during the florid phase many important nutrients are lost in the stools and that during remission (with cessation of diarrhea) rapid repair of deficits begins promptly. For further discussion of this important gastrointestinal and nutritional disorder see Chapter 22.

Drug therapy with antibiotics or sulfa drugs can destroy bacteria constituting the normal flora of the intestinal tract which are engaged in synthesizing vitamin K and various members of the B complex group. Most of such synthesis occurs in the colon and it seems that a small part at least of such vitamins thus are supplied to human beings. Even a small supplement from this source may be important to persons consuming diets containing minimal amounts of the vitamin or its precursors.[26]

An excess of phosphorus in the diet will decrease calcium absorption. An excess of calcium diminishes iron absorption. Antacids decrease iron absorption and may perpetuate anemia in peptic ulcer therapy, etc. Aluminum hydroxide greatly decreases phosphorus absorption.

In spite of adequate intake and absorption, assimilation and utilization may be interfered with. Thus, in chronic alcoholism there may develop *hepatic cirrhosis* with inability to form serum albumin from the protein materials that reach the liver in adequate amounts through the circulation. Likewise, *hepatic parenchymal damage* may prevent adequate conversion of glucose to glycogen and its storage in the liver; or may hinder utilization of vitamin K and formation of prothrombin. *Bone-marrow damage* may prevent adequate utilization of protein and iron and other materials to form hemoglobin and red blood cells and other elements of the blood, such as white blood cells and platelets.

In *diabetes mellitus* glucose is adequately absorbed and present in the blood in excessive amounts, but it cannot be adequately utilized in the absence of sufficient insulin. Large amounts of glucose, as well as of sodium chloride and of water, escape from the body through the kidneys in the characteristic polyuria.

EXCESSIVE ELIMINATION OR ABNORMAL LOSS

Serious nutritional disturbance may result from excessive elimination of substances important to the body through normal channels or from losses through abnormal routes. Examples of excessive excretion through normal routes include diarrhea, the polyuria of diabetes just mentioned, diuresis, excessive sweating, the albuminuria of nephritis, the calciuria of hyperparathyroidism, the blood loss of menorrhagia, etc. Examples of losses through abnormal routes are blood loss from wounds; blood protein, salt and water loss from burns, vomiting, fistulae, etc.

Nutritional disorders frequently cause diarrhea, thus setting up a vicious circle.

Nutritive deficiencies especially apt to result in diarrhea include those of nicotinic acid (pellagra), and of protein (kwashiorkor).

INCREASED METABOLISM

In certain conditions, the total metabolism may be accelerated so as to require a much greater supply than normal of all nutrient materials. Whenever the demand is augmented but is not satisfied, or sufficient nutrients cannot be ingested or otherwise administered, undernutrition will occur.

Examples of *pathologic conditions*, in which attention must be paid to very high nutrient requirements as the result of generalized increased metabolism, are hyperthyroidism, fevers, neoplasms, cardiac decompensation, and trauma. Chronic low-grade infections such as tuberculosis, brucellosis, tonsillitis and arthritis may keep a patient underweight by accelerating the metabolism even without the production of fever. In such instances, the acceleration of metabolism apparently results from the action of toxins. Neoplastic diseases (cancer, sarcoma, leukemia, Hodgkin's disease, etc.) may cause tissue destruction locally and general toxic effects with increase in the metabolic rate and resultant weight loss. Cardiac conditions with prolonged tachycardia or decompensation may increase the total metabolism by as much as 25 per cent even when the patient is kept at bed rest.

Trauma, either accidental or surgical, may cause profound metabolic reactions accompanied by large losses of proteins, vitamins and other nutrients. Such losses have in the past been considered as inescapable and obligatory but studies indicate that vigorous nutritive efforts may prevent the negative nitrogen balance, etc., and promote quicker recovery.[20,33,43]

Physiologic conditions in which metabolic demands are unusually high are pregnancy, lactation, periods of prolonged strenuous muscular activity, and the periods of great activity and rapid growth of childhood.

PATHOLOGIC PHYSIOLOGY

When any of the above etiologic factors becomes of sufficient magnitude or persists for a sufficient period of time, the metabolic balance for one or more essential nutrients becomes negative. The nutrient is withdrawn from the body tissues normally containing it; therefore, tissues and organs depending upon the nutrient for performance of certain functions may receive it in inadequate amounts. At this stage assay of the blood (or tissues) may reveal low levels of the nutrient (for example, low ascorbic acid levels, low serum potassium concentration, etc.). Such low biochemical levels may continue for prolonged periods, but if the level drops farther, or demand for the nutrient suddenly increases, functions dependent upon the nutrient falter and anatomic manifestations may appear. For example, in *ascorbic acid* deficiency there occurs failure in the formation and maintenance of intercellular materials, increased capillary fragility and bleeding into the gums; in *potassium* deficiency there is diminution in neuromuscular irritability, paralyses of skeletal muscle, failure of heart muscle action and finally definite anatomic changes in the muscles.

The usual order of change in the pathologic physiology of nutritional disease is:
1. Negative balance of the nutrient factor, or insufficiently positive balance for growth, repair, and maintenance
2. Tissue depletion
3. Biochemical change
4. Functional alterations
5. Anatomic defects.

Further discussion of these stages of nutritive failure will be found later in this chapter in the section, Effects of Malnutrition.

EFFECTS OF DISEASE ON NUTRITION

As indicated in the previous section on etiology and pathologic physiology, various types of illness, of either organic or functional nature, may affect the intake, the absorption and the utilization or the excretion of the various necessary food elements, or may increase certain metabolic demands. For example, during fevers, or after surgery, intake of calories, protein and vitamins usually is diminished and losses may be accelerated at the very time when metabolism is increased and demands are heightened. These adverse influences upon nutrition are here recalled for the purpose of emphasizing that not only does disease affect nutrition, but as discussed below, nutrition exerts important effects upon disease.

EFFECTS OF NUTRITION ON DISEASE

When illness develops, the state of nutrition is important in determining the course of the disease. For example, the prognosis for a very poorly nourished person who de-

TABLE 38-1. THE SIX NUTRITIONAL GROUPS
AND THEIR BASIC UNITS

GROUP	UNITS
1. Water	Water
2. Electrolytes and minerals	Various electrolytes such as sodium chloride, etc., and various minerals such as calcium, iron, copper salts, etc.
3. Carbohydrate ..	Glucose (dextrose)
4. Fat	Fatty acids and esters
5. Protein	Amino acids (and small peptides)
6. Vitamins	Thiamine, riboflavin, etc.

velops tuberculosis is apt to be bad, and a patient with scurvy who requires surgical therapy for an obstructed intestine is in a precarious condition.

The physician must recognize the presence, the type and the degree of the malnutrition and treat it. At the same time he must treat any incidental or accompanying or causative specific disease. Often the outcome will depend more upon correction of the malnutrition than upon any therapy directed toward the other malady.

CLUES IN THE HISTORY

Since patients with many nutritive disorders do not exhibit characteristic physical findings until the undernourished state is far advanced, the diagnosis of undernutrition often depends upon obtaining clues in the history. One usually will not think of making any special tests for nutritional failure unless the history suggests the lack of some necessary foods in the diet or some derangement that may have prevented proper intake, absorption or utilization or may have caused excessive losses or increased metabolic requirements. If the physician asks the proper questions, the presence or the absence of the etiologic factors may be discovered. The fact that the patient is underweight or is losing weight is particularly suggestive. An adult who for some time has not included in his *daily diet* the following foods may in many instances have an undernourished state of some type, depending upon the essential foods missing: one pint of milk, one egg, 4 slices of whole-wheat bread or their equivalent, one serving of meat, two servings of vegetables, two

servings of fruit (one citrus), 3 teaspoonfuls of butter, or its equivalent in cream or fortified margarine. Inquiry in regard to the frequency with which these "protective" foods (that is, high in content of vitamins, minerals and protein) are taken will give the physician a fairly good indication of the probable existence of nutritional deficiency. Most persons who are not underweight or losing weight will be found to ingest sufficient carbohydrate, fat and minerals, with the possible exceptions of calcium and iron. The most commonly deficient elements are proteins, calories, vitamins, iron, and calcium. Thinness alone suggests simply lack of sufficient calories. Obesity does not preclude undernutrition with respect to minerals, vitamins or protein, but indicates only an excess of calories.

ESSENTIAL FOODS

Foods as we eat them, such as milk, eggs, meat, wheat and other cereals, fruits, vegetables, butter and oils, starches, etc., must be broken down into basic units before they can be absorbed and utilized. The six groups of nutrients with the basic units derived from them are listed in Table 38-1. A complete diet includes adequate amounts of all the essential nutrients in each of the six groups. Some of the required substances in this biochemical classification of the basic units that actually enter the blood for utilization are simple and some are complex. The various groups are highly interdependent in their nutritional and metabolic activity. The nutrients must be supplied not only in certain amounts but in certain proportions.

FUNCTIONS OF FOODS

The functions of the various nutrients must be adequately performed to maintain the anatomic integrity and the physiologic efficiency of the body. Therefore, not only must the nutrients be supplied and absorbed in proper quantity, but certain proportions must be maintained between them to ensure an optimum state of the cells and the tissues. For example, an increase in the salt intake requires a proportionately greater supply of water to keep the electrolyte composition of the extracellular fluid within normal limits. Likewise, an increase in the carbohydrate combustion demands an increase in the available thiamine.

The nutrient elements may be classified according to three general functions: (1)

as *structural* or supportive material (for bone, cartilage, skin, connective tissue, stroma of individual organs and cells; and for the blood plasma, the interstitial fluid and the lymph that together constitute the organ of transport, the extracellular fluid); (2) as *fuel* (for body heat, muscular activity and work, as well as for the energy for numerous complex intermediate metabolic processes), and (3) as *catalytic* substances or chemical regulators.

Each nutrient element performs more than a single function and every essential nutrient falls into more than one of the three categories. For example, by far the chief function of carbohydrate is to supply fuel, but some is used in the construction of special conjugated proteins in cartilage and some is needed in the formation of certain enzymes. Fats are used primarily for fuel, but adipose tissue furnishes some structural support: fats serve largely as fuel-storage materials. The fatty substances known as phospholipids and cerebrosides are important constituents of tissues and organs. Fats supply the essential fatty acids (linoleic and arachidonic); they carry the fat-soluble vitamins A, D, E and K and facilitate the absorption of calcium and phosphorus.

Energy is supplied by the combustion of food: from fat, 9 calories per Gm.; from protein, 4 calories per Gm.; from carbohydrate, 4 calories per Gm.; from alcohol, 7 calories per Gm. The basal metabolism (minimum heat production at rest, 12 to 14 hours after the last meal) varies with surface area, age and sex. The total metabolism includes caloric requirements for basal metabolism plus specific dynamic action of food, plus physical activity. Allowance of about 5 per cent must be made for the specific dynamic action of food: that is, an average of approximately 5 per cent of the total caloric value of the food is expended in preparing the food for use by the body and is not available for energy purposes.

Numerous careful studies have determined the energy requirements for various activities. Mental work is of little consequence in raising caloric needs—probably only a 3 to 4 per cent increment above basal levels being necessary. Physical activity raises metabolism greatly: for sitting or standing, about 10 per cent of the basal calories; for walking on the level at 3 miles per hour, about 1 calorie per hour per pound of body moved. Thus for a 70 Kg. (154 lb.) man of 1.8 square meters surface area at 40 calories per sq. m. per hour = 72 basal calories per hour plus 154 calories per hour for walking, or an increment of over 200 per cent. Heavy labor or strenuous sports may increase the energy expenditure by as much as 800 per cent to 1,500 per cent.

A sedentary 22 year old 70 Kg. (154 lb.) male clerk's daily requirement will be about 2,400 calories; a moderately active salesman, 3,000; a painter or carpenter, 3,500; a mason or sawyer, 4,500 to 6,000.

The "reference" female, like the reference male, is 22 years old. Her weight is 58 Kg. (128 lb.); with moderate activity her caloric requirement is 2,000 calories daily.[44]

Economy of energy metabolism is observed under certain conditions, nutritive balance being maintained with a very low caloric intake. The basal metabolic rate may decrease during undernutrition to minus 30 per cent or lower (Lusk[14]). Following severe illness this conservation mechanism may be of great importance. As nutrition and energy metabolism are restored to normal, the basal metabolic rate again rises to a normal level.

Carbohydrate and fat together supply about 90 per cent of the calories in the average normal diet. In the poorer types of diets, used especially in the lower economic groups, carbohydrate supplies from about 60 to 70 per cent; fat, from 20 to 25 per cent; and protein, about 5 per cent. In better diets, about 50 per cent of the total calories is derived from carbohydrate, from 35 to 40 per cent from fat, and 10 per cent or more from protein.

In 1966, 47 per cent of calories available at the retail market in the United States were from carbohydrates, 41 per cent from fats, and 12 per cent from proteins.[44] Calories per capita from alcohol average 76 daily in the United States. This includes children and other non-users; therefore intake by users is much higher.

Fats are expensive to produce, and during times of famine or of war, fat is apt to be the nutrient most seriously curtailed. In Madrid in 1941, fat furnished only about 10 per cent of the calories of the average diet and in 1942, Belgium and Finland were restricted to only about a fifth of their prewar fat consumption. In 1944, there was widespread mass starvation in Holland, with severe malnutrition, the result of prolonged consumption of only about 1,000 calories of food daily. About 20 per cent of one group studied had hunger edema, indicating protein starvation and hypoproteinemia, with consumption of body protein for caloric needs, the usual energy foods, carbohydrate and fat, being lacking.[5]

FATS

The term *lipid* includes true fats and other fatlike substances. Three types of lipids are important in nutrition.

1. Neutral fats are combinations of fatty acids and glycerol. Most of the food fats belong to this group, and most of the adipose tissue of the body is in this form.

2. Phospholipids contain phosphoric acid and a nitrogenous base in addition to the fatty acid and glycerol molecule. The phospholipids such as lecithin and cephalin are important constituents of cell protoplasm.

3. Sterols are combinations of fatty acids and sterols of high molecular weight. Cholesterol is the only sterol occurring as such in the body. It is found in practically every living tissue but especially in the brain, blood, skin and adrenal cortex. Irradiation of cholesterol or of its derivatives in the skin is believed to be the body's mode of making vitamin D. Cholesterol is apparently the "mother-substance" from which are manufactured the sex hormones and the adrenocortical hormones, which are of steroid structure.

An *essential* fatty acid is arachidonic acid or its precursor, linoleic acid. It is essential in the sense that it is not made in the body, therefore must be supplied in the diet, and is necessary for dermal integrity and growth of the human infant.

Functions of Fats. Fats are highly important components of diets for human beings because[44,56,57]:

1. They are the most concentrated form of food energy.

2. Adipose tissue of the body serves as the principal source of energy reserves, whether the fat in the cells is derived from dietary carbohydrate or fat.

3. With the exception of the central nervous system, virtually all tissues utilize fatty acids as a direct source of energy.

4. Fats supply not only components for storage in adipose tissue cells, serving functions of calorie storage, insulation and cushioning, but they furnish vital ingredients of cell and tissue structure and of metabolic machinery. Food fats must supply the essential fatty acids.

5. Fats in foods are necessary as carriers for fat-soluble nutrients, including vitamins A, D, E, and K.

6. Fats are important in the palatability they give to foods. Diets low in fat tend to be dry and unappetizing and have low satiation value. Although triglycerides are relatively tasteless, they contain absorbed flavors, and because of their texture make other foods more palatable.

Proportion and Kinds of Fat in Diet. In the United States about 41% of the average total daily calories are now supplied by fat; this has risen from about 25 per cent twenty years ago. In 20 years the total fat from animal sources has decreased from 75 to 66 per cent, while that from vegetable sources has risen from 25 to 34 per cent.[44]

In recent years the relationship of dietary fat to coronary heart disease and other manifestations of atherosclerosis has received much special attention. Epidemiologic studies in various parts of the world show an association between high intake of saturated fats and high incidence of coronary disease (e.g., in the United States and in Finland); whereas populations subsisting on diets low in fat, especially when low in saturated fatty acids, have relatively little coronary disease (e.g., among the Bantu in Africa, among working-class people in Greece, Naples, Madrid, and Japan).[57]

The best practical clinical guide discovered to date that is related to future coronary occlusion is the amount of cholesterol in the blood. A serum value of less than 200 vs. 300 mg. or more is associated with about 1:4 likelihood of heart attack. "Normal" values among middle-aged U. S. males are usually given as 150 mg. to 250 (average 230) per 100 ml. serum as compared with average of 165 in Naples and in the Bantu.[57] Serum triglycerides (plain neutral fats) are also higher in the blood of persons apt to have coronary atherosclerosis. Diets high in saturated fats raise blood cholesterol. Polyunsaturated fats lower blood cholesterol; cholesterol itself in the diet causes blood elevation. Diets constructed on these principles (low total fat, low cholesterol, high polyunsaturated fats) have caused a fall in blood triglycerides, and a decrease in blood cholesterol averaging about 15 per cent. When followed for some time, evidence is good that the incidence of coronary heart attacks can be decreased.

It has been suggested that the present fat in the United States diet is much too high, and that to reduce the frequency of atherosclerosis, diets be recommended in which fats provide only about 25 per cent of the daily caloric intake. A ratio of 1.1 polyunsaturated fats to saturated fats is advised, in contrast to the low average of 0.4 now spontaneously chosen.[44,56,57]

CARBOHYDRATE

Glucose, derived from the sugars and starches of the food, is the form of carbohydrate circulating in the blood. It provides a quick source of energy. Glucose is stored as glycogen in the liver, whence it may be released as required to maintain a circulating blood glucose level of about 100 mg. per 100 ml., and to provide for energy demands. Carbohydrate taken in excess of the body's immediate needs is converted into fat and stored in fatty tissues, where it serves as a source of fuel for future needs. As much as 200 to 300 Gm. of glycogen may be stored in the liver, and considerable amounts are also present in the muscles and in the skin. The intake of carbohydrate food among normal persons varies widely, ranging around 300 Gm. daily in the average normal adult of 70 Kg. body weight (154 lb.) whose total caloric requirement is approximately 2,500 calories daily, but ranging much higher when caloric demands are greater.

Brain and nerve cells subsist almost entirely on glucose for energy.

Carbohydrates provide the most varied and plentiful foods in the world. They give the highest energy yield per acre of land, and thus are very important for human survival. They are relatively easy to grow, (hence inexpensive), highly palatable, and store well with little deterioration. Classic examples of these staple foods include rice, corn, wheat, and potatoes.

In most of the world, over 50 per cent of calories come from carbohydrate foods. As societies become more affluent, carbohydrate intake decreases, fat consumption increases. Sixty years ago in the United States, 65 to 70 per cent of the calories consumed by the average person came from carbohydrates. Today, only 47 per cent comes from carbohydrates.

Use of sugars, syrups and candies has increased by 25 per cent in the past 60 years, while there has been a corresponding decrease in consumption of fruits and vege-

TABLE 38-2. CLASSIFICATION OF THE AMINO ACIDS

ESSENTIAL	NONESSENTIAL
Arginine	Alanine
Histidine	Aspartic acid
Isoleucine	Cystine; cysteine
Leucine	Glutamic acid
Lysine	Glycine
Methionine	Hydroxyproline
Phenylalanine	Proline
Threonine	Serine
Tryptophan	Tyrosine
Valine	

tables, which supply less concentrated carbohydrate, but more vitamins, minerals and bulk.

PROTEIN

Proteins are very complex organic compounds, containing carbon, hydrogen, oxygen, nitrogen and usually sulfur. The presence of nitrogen distinguishes protein, the average protein containing 16 per cent nitrogen. Some specialized proteins also contain iron, phosphorus, iodine, copper, or other inorganic elements.

Proteins are composed of simpler substances called *amino acids.* Analysis of protein hydrolysates has revealed 20 different amino acids widely distributed in proteins. The human body can manufacture many amino acids, but it cannot produce certain others in amounts adequate to meet body needs. Nitrogen balance and rate of growth have been used to determine whether the various amino acids are essential in the diet (i.e., cannot be made in the body in adequate amounts). Evidence indicates that for growth of rats (and probably of humans) there are 10 *essential* amino acids. However, only eight of these are needed to maintain nitrogen equilibrium in the human adult, histidine and arginine not being required (Table 38-2).

It should be emphasized that the "nonessential" amino acids are just as important in human nutrition as the essential ones. The terms are confusing, but traditional. The nonessential ones can be formed in the body from other sources; the essential ones must be furnished as such in proteins in the diet. Radioactive carbon (C^{14}) has been used to demonstrate the biogenesis of the nonessential amino acids. The C^{14} is found in tissues in the amino acids which are nonessential, while the essential amino acids contained none of the tracer fed in labeled precursors (sugar, acetic acid, CO_2).[1]

Proteins are classified as complete, partially complete or totally incomplete, or of high or low "biologic value," according to the adequacy with which they supply all the amino acids necessary for construction of body tissues. For example, the protein of milk (casein), though poor in cystine, is *complete*, because it alone can provide fully for life, growth and vigor. Gelatin, by contrast, is *incomplete*, of low biologic value (no tryptophan or valine; inadequate tyrosine and cystine) and will not support growth or maintain nitrogen equilibrium. The proteins of meat and eggs are of high biologic value.

For efficient protein synthesis, both the essential and the nonessential amino acids must be available simultaneously and in sufficient quantities. The production of proteins in the body is limited not only by the supply of essential amino acids but also by the speed and efficiency with which the so-called nonessentials are made available. The availability of the nonessential acids depends upon the proper function of the conversion mechanisms and it seems probable that some of the disturbances of protein formation, for instance in liver disease, may be the consequence of a failure in the formation of the nonessential amino acids.[11]

Proteins compose the major portion of the solid matter of muscles and glandular tissues. All cells and all body fluids (except bile and urine) contain protein. Serum proteins are of great value in the regulation of osmotic pressure and of fluid interchange. Proteins are amphoteric (may behave as either acid or alkali) and are of great importance in the regulation of acid-base balance. The hormones of the pituitary, pancreas (insulin) and thyroid (thyroxine) are proteins of specific structure and function. Enzymes (trypsin, pepsin, amylase, etc.) are protein in nature. Resistance to disease is in large part determined by protein substances called *antibodies*.

Protein constitutes about 75 per cent of the dry weight of the tissues of the body. Proteins are most important as structural material, and in the plasma and the red cells contribute to the essential properties of blood. Proteins are also necessary for the formation of enzymes and hormones and thus also furnish catalytic substances and chemical regulators. Protein materials, therefore, with the minerals (calcium and phosphorus for bone, iron for hemoglobin, etc.) constitute the metabolic machinery of the body. Of all the food essentials, protein is probably closest to the vital processes; its very meaning is derived from the Greek root meaning primary or first.

Protein requirements per kilogram of body weight are much higher under conditions of stress and during growth, pregnancy and lactation. See Table 38-4.

When protein nutrients are supplied in excess of the requirements for replacement of structural needs, they are converted into fat and stored. When caloric intake is inadequate, fat stores are used. This is also true of carbohydrate stores, which, however, being relatively scant, are quickly exhausted. Under such circumstances body protein will be used for fuel. Under conditions of complete starvation Lusk has estimated that 87 per cent of the calories will come from adipose tissue and 13 per cent from protein tissue; after fat stores are exhausted, body protein may become the chief source of calories. To maintain normal function and stores, protein intake per day should total a minimum of 0.9 gram per kilogram of body weight. This means that a 70 Kg. (154 lb.) man should consume about 65 grams of protein daily.

NITROGEN BALANCE may be maintained only if all the essential amino acids are supplied and absorbed in adequate amounts. If the daily protein intake is only 40 or 50 Gm. per day for a 70 Kg. person, it is especially important that the dietary protein be of high biologic value; with higher intakes the safety factor is much greater. Nitrogen balance can be preserved and the destruction of body protein for fuel can be avoided if adequate calories from carbohydrate and fat are available. If caloric requirements are not met by carbohydrates and fats, amino acids from ingested proteins and possibly from body proteins will be used as energy sources; amino acids available for synthesis of body proteins will be reduced.

WATER

Water (1) furnishes the vehicle for absorption of nutrients into the body; (2) constitutes the chief ingredient of the extracellular fluid, and thus provides the means of transport; (3) provides for excretion and secretion, and (4) is responsible, by evaporation from lungs and skin, for about 25 per cent of body heat loss, and so contributes to temperature regulation. When water intake is undisturbed, little attention to the intake is usually necessary. Excesses of water are easily disposed of unless some factor interferes with excretion (circulatory failure, nephritis, hypoproteinemia, etc.). Water enters the body as water and also as a constituent of other foods, both liquid and solid (the latter are in some cases actually from 70 to 80 per cent water) and as water of oxidation. The water requirements vary greatly with the temperature of the environment, with bodily exertion and heat production and with salt intake; under extreme conditions they may be as high as 10 liters per day. The minimum requirements of an average normal man in a temperate environment are usually from 1.5 to 3 liters per day. For a discussion of water and electrolyte requirements under various conditions see Chapter 35.

VITAMINS

A number of potent organic compounds occurring in minute quantities in natural foodstuffs have been designated as *vitamins;* they perform specific and vital functions in the cells and tissues of the body.[25]

The vitamins differ widely in chemical structure, natural distribution and physiologic function.

Vitamin deficiency is often not detected until after deprivation has been prolonged, since stores of vitamins may have been present and are only gradually exhausted.

Vitamins act primarily as part of enzyme systems in important metabolic reactions. *Nicotinic acid,* for example, becomes a component in two important coenzymes both concerned in glycolysis, tissue respiration, and fat synthesis.

Vitamins in many instances, perhaps in all, exert their specific activity when serving as the prosthetic group of an enzyme. *Riboflavin* enters into several enzyme systems, its broad activity thus probably accounting for the variety of symptoms resulting from its deficiency. *Thiamine* serves as a part of the enzyme cocarboxylase. *Biotin* and coenzyme R are identical.

Vitamins were at first named for their curative properties or were given a convenient letter designation more or less in the order of their discovery: vitamin A, the antiophthalmic factor, vitamin B_1, the antiberiberi factor, etc. Many of the vitamins have now been chemically identified, and the chemical names are usually to be preferred: ascorbic acid instead of vitamin C; thiamine instead of vitamin B_1, etc. However, in some instances descriptive names may be retained instead of the more awkward longer chemical names: e.g.: folic acid instead of pteroylglutamic acid.

Some of the vitamins are groups of related character, e.g., the B complex vitamins, of which some 15 have been described. They are grouped together chiefly because all are water-soluble and all can be obtained from the same sources, notably liver and yeast.

The vitamins can usefully be separated into two types: (1) water-soluble vitamins (ascorbic acid, B complex) and (2) fat-soluble vitamins (carotene, vitamins A, D, E and K).

The two types of vitamins differ in absorption, storage and excretion. Since the water-soluble vitamins are diffusible, impaired absorption is seldom encountered (except for B_{12} in pernicious anemia). However, the fat-soluble vitamins, normally absorbed with the lipids in foods, may be inadequately absorbed when fat digestion or absorption is impaired (biliary obstruction, steatorrhea, etc.).

The water-soluble factors are excreted in the urine. Even with high dosage, toxic accumulation is unlikely. Likewise, storage supplies may last only a few months. The fat-soluble factors are not excreted in the urine and storage capacity for them is much greater; overdosage and toxic accumulation is possible within a short period of time; therapeutic amounts may be supplied at long intervals because of slow destruction and excretion, the effects persisting often for many months or a year or more.

At present, the following vitamins are recognized as necessary for man: carotene and vitamin A, vitamin D, vitamin E, vitamin K, thiamine, riboflavin, niacin, pyridoxine, folic acid, vitamin B_{12}, ascorbic acid, biotin, and pantothenic acid.[44]

Human requirements are not established or defined for the following: inositol, choline, and the flavanoids (vitamin P).

MINERALS

Minerals make up a total of about 4 per cent of the body weight; of this about one-half (2 per cent of the total) is calcium; one-fourth (1 per cent of the total) is phosphorus; and the remaining 1 per cent is

TABLE 38-3. APPROXIMATE NORMAL DAILY
REQUIREMENTS

1. Water	3,000 ml.
2. Electrolytes (salts of Na, K, Mg, etc.)	10 Gm.
and minerals (calcium, 0.8 Gm.; Fe,	
12 mg., etc.)	1 Gm.
3. Carbohydrate	300 Gm.
4. Fat	120 Gm.
5. Protein	70 Gm.
6. Vitamins (vitamin A, 5,000 units; thia-	
mine, 2 mg.; riboflavin, 3 mg.; nico-	
tinic acid, 20 mg.; ascorbic acid, 60	
mg.; vitamin D, 400 units)	100 mg.

composed of potassium, sulfur, sodium, chlorine, magnesium and iron. These 8 elements are vital to the body economy.

At least 6 of the so-called "trace minerals" (found in very small amounts in the body) are also necessary: iodine, copper, manganese, cobalt, zinc, and fluorine.

The minerals serve four chief purposes in the body:

1. They compose a large part of the skeletal framework and the teeth. The bony structures are the main depots for calcium, phosphorus, magnesium, sodium, and the trace minerals.

2. They take part in the formation of many organic compounds, such as nucleoproteins and phospholipids, thus forming an integral part of all cells. Muscles hold large amounts of magnesium, potassium, phosphate and sodium.

3. They circulate in the body fluids as inorganic salts, as dissociated ions and in more or less loosely-bound combinations, playing a vital part in the control of acid-base equilibrium and water balance (Na, Cl, K, especially); neuromuscular irritability (Ca, Mg, K, Na); blood-clotting (Ca); membrane permeability (Ca); muscle contraction; and the transfer of energy (P), etc.

4. They make up essential parts of compounds of paramount importance: iron in hemoglobin, iodine in the thyroid hormone, as essential parts of enzyme systems, etc.

REQUIREMENTS OF SPECIFIC NUTRIENTS IN HEALTH AND DISEASE

IN HEALTH

The nutritional requirements for healthy normal persons under average conditions and under conditions of physiologic stress (such as increased muscular activity, pregnancy, etc.) have been fairly well defined, in terms both of the basic units and the actual natural foods as they are consumed. In terms of the basic units they are approximately as given in Table 38-3 when the energy expenditure is about 2,500 calories daily.

Recommended Daily Food Selection

The normal daily requirements for an average adult are present in an average normal diet that includes carbohydrate and fat sufficient to supply the necessary calories plus the following protective foods: one pint of milk, one egg, one serving (3 to 4 ounces) of meat, 3 teaspoonfuls (15 Gm.) of butter, 4 servings of whole-grain bread or cereal, 2 vegetables other than potato (one green) and 2 fruits, one of which is raw and one preferably citrus or tomato. Wholesome natural foods such as those mentioned should be selected, since these provide not only calories but necessary protein, vitamins and minerals.[43]

It is recommended that the food for each day be divided into 3 or 4 meals, each of varied composition, taken 4 to 6 hours apart.

Alcoholic drinks supply calories but fail to furnish other important nutritive materials. Alcohol supplies 7 calories per ml. (a 12 ounce bottle of beer furnishes 170 calories; 1 ounce of whisky, 105 calories). Use of alcoholic beverages in excess may decrease the desire for and intake of more wholesome, complete foods and may cause nutritive disorders.

High carbohydrate diets, even when supplemented with vitamin concentrates, often fail to provide the essential nutrients necessary to good health because of omission of protective foods. The common tendency to supply carbohydrate and fat (the fuel foods) to the partial exclusion of protein, salts, minerals and vitamins (the foods necessary for construction and operation of the metabolic machinery) leads to certain relatively frequent deficiencies. These are related chiefly to inadequacies of the following: calcium, iron, vitamins A and D, vitamin B complex, ascorbic acid, and proteins that contain the essential amino acids and are therefore of high biologic value. The fact that many persons prefer white bread to darker breads may lead to B-complex deficiencies. The use of "enriched bread" containing added thiamine, nicotinic acid and iron is a logical step in the

TABLE 38-4. FOOD AND NUTRITION BOARD, NATIONAL ACADEMY OF SCIENCES–NATIONAL RESEARCH COUNCIL RECOMMENDED DAILY DIETARY ALLOWANCES,[a] REVISED 1968

	Age[b] (years) From Up to	Weight (kg)	Weight (lbs)	Height (cm)	Height (in.)	kcal	Protein (gm)	Fat-Soluble Vitamins Vitamin A Activity (IU)	Vitamin D Activity (IU)	Vitamin E Activity (IU)	Water-Soluble Vitamins Ascorbic Acid (mg)	Folacin[c] (mg)	Niacin (mg equiv)[d]	Riboflavin (mg)	Thiamin (mg)	Vitamin B6 (mg)	Vitamin B12 (µg)	Calcium (g)	Phosphorus (g)	Minerals Iodine (µg)	Iron (mg)	Magnesium (mg)
INFANTS	0 – 1/6	4	9	55	22	kg × 120	kg × 2.2[e]	1,500	400	5	35	0.05	5	0.4	0.2	0.2	1.0	0.4	0.2	25	6	40
	1/6 – 1/2	7	15	63	25	kg × 110	kg × 2.0[e]	1,500	400	5	35	0.05	7	0.5	0.4	0.3	1.5	0.5	0.4	40	10	60
	1/2 – 1	9	20	72	28	kg × 100	kg × 1.8[e]	1,500	400	5	35	0.1	8	0.6	0.5	0.4	2.0	0.6	0.5	45	15	70
CHILDREN	1 – 2	12	26	81	32	1,100	25	2,000	400	10	40	0.1	8	0.6	0.6	0.5	2.0	0.7	0.7	55	15	100
	2 – 3	14	31	91	36	1,250	25	2,000	400	10	40	0.2	8	0.7	0.6	0.6	2.5	0.8	0.8	60	15	150
	3 – 4	16	35	100	39	1,400	30	2,500	400	10	40	0.2	9	0.8	0.7	0.7	3	0.8	0.8	70	10	200
	4 – 6	19	42	110	43	1,600	30	2,500	400	10	40	0.2	11	0.9	0.8	0.9	4	0.8	0.8	80	10	200
	6 – 8	23	51	121	48	2,000	35	3,500	400	15	40	0.2	13	1.1	1.0	1.0	4	0.9	0.9	100	10	250
	8 – 10	28	62	131	52	2,200	40	3,500	400	15	40	0.3	15	1.2	1.1	1.2	5	1.0	1.0	110	10	250
MALES	10 – 12	35	77	140	55	2,500	45	4,500	400	20	40	0.4	17	1.3	1.3	1.4	5	1.2	1.2	125	10	300
	12 – 14	43	95	151	59	2,700	50	5,000	400	20	45	0.4	18	1.4	1.4	1.6	5	1.4	1.4	135	18	350
	14 – 18	59	130	170	67	3,000	60	5,000	400	25	55	0.4	20	1.5	1.5	1.8	5	1.4	1.4	150	18	400
	18 – 22	67	147	175	69	2,800	60	5,000	400	30	60	0.4	18	1.6	1.4	2.0	5	0.8	0.8	140	10	400
	22 – 35	70	154	175	69	2,800	65	5,000	—	30	60	0.4	18	1.7	1.4	2.0	5	0.8	0.8	140	10	350
	35 – 55	70	154	173	68	2,600	65	5,000	—	30	60	0.4	17	1.7	1.3	2.0	5	0.8	0.8	125	10	350
	55 – 75+	70	154	171	67	2,400	65	5,000	—	30	60	0.4	14	1.7	1.2	2.0	6	0.8	0.8	110	10	350
FEMALES	10 – 12	35	77	142	56	2,250	50	4,500	400	20	40	0.4	15	1.3	1.1	1.4	5	1.2	1.2	110	18	300
	12 – 14	44	97	154	61	2,300	50	5,000	400	20	45	0.4	15	1.4	1.2	1.6	5	1.3	1.3	115	18	350
	14 – 16	52	114	157	62	2,400	55	5,000	400	25	50	0.4	16	1.4	1.2	1.8	5	1.3	1.3	120	18	350
	16 – 18	54	119	160	63	2,300	55	5,000	400	25	50	0.4	15	1.5	1.2	2.0	5	1.3	1.3	115	18	350
	18 – 22	58	128	163	64	2,000	55	5,000	400	25	55	0.4	13	1.5	1.0	2.0	5	0.8	0.8	100	18	350
	22 – 35	58	128	163	64	2,000	55	5,000	—	25	55	0.4	13	1.5	1.0	2.0	5	0.8	0.8	100	18	300
	35 – 55	58	128	160	63	1,850	55	5,000	—	25	55	0.4	13	1.5	1.0	2.0	5	0.8	0.8	90	18	300
	55 – 75+	58	128	157	62	1,700	55	5,000	—	25	55	0.4	13	1.5	1.0	2.0	6	0.8	0.8	80	10	300
PREGNANCY						+200	65	6,000	400	30	60	0.8	15	1.8	+0.1	2.5	8	+0.4	+0.4	125	18	450
LACTATION						+1,000	75	8,000	400	30	60	0.5	20	2.0	+0.5	2.5	6	+0.5	+0.5	150	18	450

a The allowance levels are intended to cover individual variations among most normal persons as they live in the United States under usual environmental stresses. The recommended allowances can be attained with a variety of common foods, providing other nutrients for which human requirements have been less well defined. See text for more-detailed discussion of allowances and of nutrients not tabulated.

b Entries on lines for age range 22-35 years represent the reference man and woman at age 22. All other entries represent allowances for the midpoint of the specified age range.

c The folacin allowances refer to dietary sources as determined by Lactobacillus casei assay. Pure forms of folacin may be effective in doses less than ¼ of the RDA.

d Niacin equivalents include dietary sources of the vitamin itself plus 1 mg equivalent for each 60 mg of dietary tryptophan.

e Assumes protein equivalent to human milk. For proteins not 100 percent utilized factors should be increased proportionately.

prevention of such deficiencies when inadequate amounts of the whole cereal foods are ingested.

Optimal intake of the necessary foods in normal persons depends upon various factors affecting metabolic demands, such as age, sex, size, muscular activity, pregnancy, lactation and growth. Table 38-4 gives the *recommended daily allowances* for specific nutrients of the Committee on Foods and Nutrition of the National Research Council. In this table the figures given allow for the various influences affecting normal persons and also allow in most instances a margin of safety of about 20 to 30 per cent. That is, these are not minimal daily requirements, but those that are considered *safe allowances*, since it is known that some persons because of individual characteristics require more than minimal or average amounts of certain nutrients, and since in many instances the approximate requirements are known, but exact limits are not.

In Table 38-4 we note the proportionally very high requirements of infants and young children which are necessary for their great activity and rapid growth. At age 6 months, the caloric requirement is about 120 cal. per Kg.; at one year about 100 cal.; at age 6 years, about 80 cal.; at age 12 years about 60 cal., as compared to a requirement of about 30 cal. per Kg. for a relatively sedentary adult. Protein and other requirements show a similar range. The child at 3 years needs about 2 Gm. of protein per Kg. of body weight, the child of 12 years about 1.5 Gm., and the adult about 1 Gm. The rapid appearance of clinical manifestations and the more serious results of nutritive disorders in the young are explained by their high requirements.

In Disease

The nutrient requirements during abnormal conditions such as in (1) primary undernutrition, (2) undernutrition secondary to disease, and (3) in malnourished states in which nutritional disturbance is an incidental accompaniment of or has caused (4) organic disease are, of course, varied and complex. Single deficiencies are uncommon. Lack of several or many food elements is detectable in most instances. When a single deficit is present, a characteristic picture of a single-deficiency disease may appear, such as scurvy due to lack of ascorbic acid, or hypochromic anemia due to lack of iron. However, usually the syndromes are partial and mixed. Under Causes of Specific Nutritive Deficiencies many of the organic, functional and psychic disturbances have been mentioned, with explanations of the ways in which such conditions interfere with nutrition. In each instance the requirements of the various nutrients, either to prevent malnutrition or to correct it, would depend upon the character, the severity and the duration of the malady.

The occurrence of disease highlights the necessity for *optimal* nutrition, not just minimal nutrition during health. Optimal nutrition implies provision of the materials essential not only for structure, fuel and chemical regulation, but for storage of reserves against unusual demands. Thus a previously thin person who because of illness becomes unable to take adequate calories may soon show signs of serious malnutrition. Likewise, a patient with poorly controlled diabetes may quickly exhaust his low supply of liver glycogen after a short period of vomiting, and also may soon become dehydrated because of the previously existing polyuria. A child with a bare minimum of vitamin-D stores may develop rickets when confined indoors because of a series of respiratory infections.

Increased Nutritional Requirements During Disease

A great increase in the demand for certain nutrients occurs in certain pathologic conditions. Some of the most important disorders will be considered as they affect the various necessary food elements:

Water and Salts. Water and electrolyte needs are considered together because they are intimately connected metabolically.

Normal requirements for water vary tremendously, especially with the temperature of the environment and the water lost by insensible evaporation and perspiration. Averages for adults range from about 1 to 3 liters per day. An approximate standard for diverse persons is 1 ml. per calorie of total daily metabolism. Much of the water is contained in prepared foods, the balance is ingested in liquids.

Sodium chloride requirements vary with many conditions, especially with water intake and output. An adequate intake of NaCl is about 5 Gm. daily, while average adult intakes usually range higher than necessary (8 to 15 Gm. daily).

The demands for salt and water will be

increased in any disease in which there is an excessive loss or inadequate intake. The most common conditions are fairly well known and involve the *loss of gastrointestinal secretions* by vomiting, diarrhea or intestinal fistulae. Another common cause of water and electrolyte loss is *excessive sweating* under conditions of increased environmental temperature or fever. In *diabetes mellitus*, water and salt loss may be chronic and mild with moderate dehydration, or acute and severe with extreme dehydration, as in diabetic acidosis or coma.

The amount of water and electrolyte that may be lost in a few hours or in a day under these conditions may reach the equivalent of several liters of isotonic saline solution. In other words, there may be loss of 4 liters of water or more, containing 36 Gm. or more of sodium chloride. The physician should be able to recognize, from the history alone, the existence, if not the degree, of such losses and should promptly be impressed, therefore, by the need for replacement. Patients will seldom know exactly how much fluid they have lost by vomiting or diarrhea, but the mere presence of these symptoms should immediately suggest the need for meeting such losses. Not only *replacement* but *correction of the cause* of gastrointestinal upset, or in diabetes the correction of the metabolic status, with abolition of the glycosuria and ketosis or acidosis, etc., is necessary to relieve permanently the salt and water deficit.

The term *dehydration* is often applied to the result of such loss of water and electrolyte, and this term is an accurate one, provided its variations are understood. Dehydration really means loss of water. The variations concern the substances that accompany this loss of water. In the type just described, the fluid depletion includes loss of salt in approximately isotonic concentration, that is, for every liter of water 9 grams of salt are lost. In other types of dehydration—as, for example, in that which follows extensive burns, pneumonia, peritonitis, or intestinal obstruction —the water lost contains not only electrolyte but also protein. Because the protein concentration in the fluid approaches that of plasma, this type of dehydration may be called plasma dehydration, and it will be discussed later under protein requirements.

Dehydration may involve loss of water primarily, with very little loss of electrolyte. This occurs when there is *no water intake,* but no vomiting, diarrhea, etc. Because water is necessary for the vital processes, it will be obtained from body stores as long as life lasts. Under these conditions the various body tissues become progressively depleted of fluid: first extracellular water is lost, then cellular water, until finally death occurs. There is a significant difference between this type of dehydration and that which follows vomiting, diarrhea, etc., because only small amounts of salts are lost. Indeed, the percentage of body solids increases, both extracellular and intracellular fluid compartments become hypertonic, and death is said to occur because of the accumulation of these substances in the body. This is the reason that water alone in *starvation plus dehydration* may greatly prolong life. From the practical point of view, it is obvious that the fluids administered in this type of dehydration must contain relatively little electrolyte in order to avoid increasing further the osmotic pressure in fluids of the body. Instead of administering normal saline solution to such patients, water in the form of glucose solution should be given, containing perhaps only 2 Gm. per liter of sodium chloride rather than 9 Gm. per liter. The small amount of electrolyte is added only because in water deprivation there is some actual loss of salt at the onset and complete replacement requires that it be included. Although deprivation of water is a basic cause for this simplest variety of dehydration, insensible loss through the skin under conditions of high environmental temperature will accelerate the progress of fluid depletion of this type.

For a detailed discussion of the requirements of water, sodium, chloride, potassium, etc., under various disease conditions causing depletion, see Chapter 35.

Energy Needs. True *increased requirements* for calories (not due to inadequate absorption or excessive excretion of nutrients) in disease occur in hyperthyroid states, in fever, in cancer and in other neoplastic diseases. A patient at rest in bed ordinarily requires about 10 to 15 calories per pound (approximately 25 to 30 calories per Kg.) of body weight, or about 1,200 to 1,800 calories for our "reference" 58 Kg. (128 lb.) woman, and 1,500 to 2,300 calories for the 70 Kg. (154 lb.) "reference" man.

The need for calories in *fever* increases at a rate of about 7 per cent per degree

Fahrenheit. Fever is often, in addition, accompanied by destructive processes that break down body tissue and cause excessive elimination of structural elements in the urine (e.g., calcium and phosphorus in osteomyelitis, nitrogen in cancer).

In *hyperthyroidism* the increase in caloric requirements results from (1) a basal metabolism that is accelerated, plus (2) an increment resulting from the purposeless hyperkinesia so common in the disease, plus (3) an inefficiency of motor activity that requires greater than normal energy expenditure for normal purposeful motion. Thus, a patient suffering from thyrotoxicosis and having a basal metabolic rate of plus 50 per cent requires more than an increase of 50 per cent in his caloric intake to maintain a normal energy balance and to prevent weight loss. His true total energy requirements while resting (in bed or chair 16 hours daily, sleeping 8 hours) may be calculated (approximately) as follows:

Patient is a man, age 35; height, 67 inches; weight, 154 pounds.

Basal caloric requirement (if normal) for 24 hours would be 1.8 sq. meters (surface area) × 39.5 cal. for 24 hours = ...	1,706 calories
Add 50 per cent due to thyrotoxicosis	853
Add 20 cal. × 16 hours for hyperkinesia	320
Add 10 cal. × 16 hours for inefficiency (though resting)	160
	3,039
Add 10 per cent for specific dynamic action of food	304
Total	3,343 calories

Since patients with hyperthyroidism usually have lost weight, the exact needs should be exceeded and 4,000 or 5,000 calories should be given to permit storage of protein, fat, carbohydrate, calcium and other essential nutrients of which these patients have been depleted.

Physiologic conditions increasing the total caloric need as well as raising specific protein, mineral and vitamin demands are *pregnancy*, *lactation* and prolonged and repeated *strenuous exertion*. Abnormally high or low environmental *temperatures* imposed by climate or industry may raise the requirement for all nutrients.

Psychologic conditions, if maniacal in type and accompanied by delirium and by hyperactivity, may raise all requirements.

Protein Needs. Although the normal person requires per day about 0.5 Gm. of protein per pound of body weight to maintain nitrogen balance (1 Gm. per Kg.), the needs are increased tremendously in certain types of disease. All protein foods vary in composition; body requirements demand that the protein be of good biologic value. Increased protein needs may be divided into two groups according to whether the loss is actual or metabolic. The *actual* increases are those which result from direct loss of protein from the body in one or more ways. These may be listed as follows: [15]

1. Loss of hemoglobin and plasma protein in hemorrhage.
2. Loss of plasma protein as such from the surface of burns and wounds.
3. Loss of plasma protein into the tissue cavities, i.e., peritonitis, empyema.
4. Loss of plasma protein into tissue, e.g., burns, pneumonia, intestinal obstruction, tissue trauma.

Metabolic loss of protein occurs by excessive destruction of tissue protein which is often called toxic destruction. This occurs in the following conditions:

1. After operation or injury, as a part of the so-called alarm reaction.
2. Infections of various kinds.
3. So-called toxic states that may follow infections long after fever and other evidence of infection have subsided.
4. The progressive cachexia associated with malignant neoplasms.
5. Immobilization or bed rest, with consequent muscle atrophy, etc.

The amount of protein lost in excess of the normal requirements may be tremendous. In terms of actual loss, as much as 50 Gm. a day has been observed to escape from the surface of burns and other wounds. In a single hemorrhage of 1 liter, 150 Gm. of hemoglobin and 50 Gm. of plasma protein are lost. When the losses are metabolic the amount may reach larger proportions. In a case of pneumonia, for example, the daily loss of nitrogen may be 40 Gm. per day, which (×6.25) means the destruction of 250 Gm. of dry tissue protein. This really means the loss of over two pounds of intact tissue protein, such as muscle.[15]

These figures explain the rapidity with which tremendous loss of weight may occur following a variety of diseases in which the loss of protein becomes excessive.

Vitamin Needs. Relatively little information is available in regard to the increased needs for various vitamins in disease. This undoubtedly will be forthcoming as further study reveals the metabolism of the various conditions. A few of the known facts may be discussed.[25,33,43]

The requirements for *thiamine* are known to be dependent upon the metabolism of glucose. By analogy, any condition in which more calories as carbohydrate are required probably also will require more thiamine. The modern industrial processing of foods often separates the vitamin B complex from its natural union with carbohydrate in whole grains and plants, so that nature's effort to ensure automatic proportional ingestion of these two nutrient elements is frequently thwarted. In the Orient, the use of polished rice led to the recognition of beriberi as a deficiency disease and to the discovery of the B vitamins. As might be expected, the intake of thiamine can with safety be greatly reduced if the diet is rich in fat but low in carbohydrate. This is explained by the fact that co-carboxylase, a thiamine complex, is needed for carbohydrate but not for fat metabolism.

In the sudden drastic alteration in metabolism occurring with rapid regulation of severe diabetes, signs of thiamine deficiency may appear (such as leg pains, reflex changes, and peculiar mental symptoms). Such symptoms are a reflection of the sudden shift from fat to carbohydrate as the chief source of energy, the need for thiamine suddenly becoming very great and exceeding the supply, and the whole process being accelerated by the frequent use of large doses of insulin.

In fevers and in hyperthyroidism there is a general increase in metabolic demands, largely supplied as a rule by increasing the carbohydrate intake. Signs of thiamine deficiency may appear if the intake of that vitamin is not also increased.

The amounts of thiamine required in the various diseases are difficult to estimate exactly, but from the practical point of view the precise need is perhaps not so important, since it is easy to meet even tremendously increased requirements by the simple expedient of giving large repeated doses. Between 0.5 and 1 mg. daily per 1,000 calories is needed for prophylaxis, while about ten times such doses given orally or parenterally are advisable if deficiency signs are apparent.

In some experimental work, *vitamin-C* requirements during infection (tuberculosis, rheumatic fever, etc.) have been shown to be considerably greater than normal. King and Menten found that resistance of guinea pigs to diphtheria toxin was decidedly increased when supplies of ascorbic acid were adequate. Guinea pigs adapt to cold environments much better when they have adequate intakes of ascorbic acid.

The requirements for vitamin C may be increased tremendously in certain surgical conditions. There is definite evidence that large amounts of ascorbic acid are utilized or destroyed in extensive inflammation and in postoperative conditions and burns. This evidence is based upon the fact that the vitamin frequently disappears from the plasma following injury, even though the tissues were saturated with it beforehand. Moreover, it has been observed that tremendous doses of ascorbic acid, i.e., one gram or more per day, may be required if the normal plasma level is to be maintained in such cases. High concentrations of ascorbic acid have been found to occur in the tissue fluids at operative sites. This may explain the low plasma ascorbic-acid levels after injury or operation. The vitamin may be mobilized when needed at the site of any area of inflammation or injury. Vitamin C is known to have an important beneficial influence upon wound healing. These observations may be related and may provide another example of protective activities of the body.

EFFECTS OF MALNUTRITION

The effects of malnutrition may long be concealed, with little or no physical evidence, and with symptoms so ill-defined that the subject may not seek advice, or may simply be considered a psychoneurotic even after advice is sought and some medical investigation has been undertaken. The detection of undernourished states should, of course, be early, before florid signs of nutritional failure appear.

FIVE STAGES OF NUTRITIVE FAILURE

Five successive stages of nutritional failure may be distinguished:

1. Negative Balance. In this early stage demand is so great that supply cannot keep pace, or supply is deficient, or both factors are operative in regard to one or more nutrient factors.

2. Tissue Depletion. In this stage, first the stores are used up, then the normal supplies of the nutrient in the cells and the tissues and the fluids are drawn upon. The fact that the body carries as a rule certain protective reserves allows tissue depletion to proceed for considerable periods before other more evident effects become manifest. Tissue depletion may be advanced before symptoms develop.

3. Biochemical Disturbances. When abnormalities in the tissues and the fluids reach a certain point, there may be measurable chemical changes in the blood and the tissues. For example, after the tissue protein has been greatly depleted, the amounts and the types of serum proteins begin to change, the usual alteration consisting of a considerable fall in total serum protein, affecting chiefly the albumin fraction, with a smaller relative decrease in the serum globulin.

Measurements of the body water content may be accomplished by various dilution methods, using antipyrine, deuterium oxide, etc. In undernutrition there is (in the absence of dehydration) an increase in the percentage of body weight as extracellular fluid. There seems to be replacement of fat and cellular structures with water.

Electrolytes (Na, K, Cl, bicarbonate) in the blood may be determined, but possible alterations in the blood volume must be kept in mind, since dilution or concentration will alter serum or plasma levels. In Chapter 35 a detailed discussion of dehydration and electrolyte disorders is given; in Chapter 36 excess body fluid and edema is discussed.

Vitamin A and its provitamin carotene are found in the blood, and levels vary with intake and liver stores. The vitamin circulates in the fasting state chiefly (80 per cent) as the alcohol form. The elevation after oral intake is due largely to an increase in the ester form, which disappears in about 24 hours.

In some instances a low level of ascorbic acid in the blood is discovered before signs of vitamin-C deficiency have occurred. A deficiency of prothrombin, as indicated by a lengthened prothrombin time, may indicate lack of vitamin K. When the blood pyruvic-acid level is elevated, thiamine may be depleted.

Determination of the amounts of calcium, phosphorus and alkaline phosphatase is useful in detecting disturbances of nutrition affecting the bones. Thus, in rickets, the calcium or phosphorus levels may be low and the phosphatase level elevated. In tetany associated with rickets, the calcium level is low, the phosphatase high; but in idiopathic or hypoparathyroid tetany, the serum calcium is low, phosphate high and phosphatase normal, because the bones are not affected. Thus endocrine disorders may sometimes be distinguished from vitamin-D or calcium malnutrition.

Measurement of the serum iron and the hemoglobin content of blood may reveal iron deficiency. Determination of the protein-bound iodine content of serum reflects the status of iodine and thyroid-gland metabolism.

These are some of the chemical tests which have proved helpful in revealing early stages of malnutrition. Present chemical technics are as a rule inadequate to detect nutritional deficiency before functional or anatomic evidence of malnutrition has occurred. However, progress in this direction has been rapid, and certain newer tests seem promising.

4. Functional Changes. When the operation of the body's functions becomes impeded, the patient is apt to become aware of the disturbance, but neither the subject nor the physician may at first recognize the cause. The first two stages, tissue depletion and biochemical disturbances, may have been operating over a considerable period of time. The first symptoms may be characteristic—such as paresthesiae or leg pains in thiamine deficiency, or sore gums in scurvy—but they may be obscure and confusing: for example, dyspnea and edema may at first suggest heart failure rather than its occasional cause, anemia; or a badly disturbed mental state may suggest an organic brain disease rather than pellagra. Aching legs in children have often been called growing pains when they were really the sign of rickets.

Fatigue, lack of energy, faintness, dizziness, a tendency to collapse on prolonged standing, backache, legache, chilliness and numbness were prominent symptoms of functional nature observed among the starved population of Holland during World War II. Pulse rates often fell to 40 per minute and systolic blood pressures to 80 mm. of mercury. Body temperatures of 95° F. indicated the low vitality.

5. Anatomic Lesions. It is as a rule difficult to separate functional from anatomic

TABLE 38-5. EFFECTS OF MALNUTRITION

FACTOR LACKING	FOODS LACKING	RESULTS
Calories	Carbohydrates, fats	Thinness, lack of energy, failure to grow
Protein	Eggs, meat, milk, wheat, corn, rice, peas, beans	Muscle wasting, hypoproteinemia, anemia, edema, osteoporosis, fractures of bone
Calcium	Milk	Defective bones and teeth, rickets; osteomalacia and tetany in pregnancy
Vitamin A	Green vegetables, carrots, tomatoes, milk, eggs, butter, fish-liver oils, sweet potatoes	Xerosis of conjunctiva and cornea, nightblindness, follicular hyperkeratosis
Vitamin B_1 (thiamine)	Whole cereals, milk, meat (especially liver and pork)	Beriberi, polyneuritis, anorexia, constipation
Vitamin B_2 (riboflavin)	Milk, eggs, liver, green vegetables	Cheilosis, glossitis, ocular disorders
Nicotinic acid (niacin)	Milk, lean meat, liver	Pellagra, stomatitis, glossitis, dermatitis, mental symptoms
Vitamin B_{12} (cyanocobalamin)	Muscle meats, eggs, wheat germ, liver	Hyperchromic macrocytic anemia
Folic acid	Leafy vegetables, liver	Macrocytic anemia, glossitis, diarrhea
Vitamin C (ascorbic acid)	Oranges, lemons, grapefruit, tomatoes	Scurvy, capillary fragility, hemorrhages, anemia
Vitamin D (calciferol)	Fish, fish-liver oils, milk, eggs, liver (sunlight)	Rickets, osteomalacia
Vitamin K	Green leaves: spinach, cabbage, kale, cauliflower; also egg yolk, liver; *plus* exclusion of bile from intestinal tract, or intestinal lesions, or liver disease	Prothrombin deficiency; hemorrhages resulting from prolonged bleeding and clotting time
Iodine	Fish, iodized salt	Goiter; functional thyroid disorders; cretinism in offspring
Iron	Meat, liver, eggs, beans, prunes, peas, wheat, oatmeal, spinach	Hypochromic anemia, especially during growth, menstruation, or pregnancy; blood loss

changes, and, of course, they are not separate, but really part of the same process. However, functional disturbances may be present for a long time before actual physical manifestations of malnutrition appear. The commonest physical evidence is weight loss. This may at first be slight and slow, but if the cause is not removed and the nutrition corrected, it may progress to emaciation. The fat padding is lost first and later the muscles waste. Pallor may appear; there may be hemorrhages into the skin, edema of the legs, dermatitis, collapse of vertebrae, etc. Certain special types of anatomic examination may help to identify the disorder as nutritional: for example,

x-ray films of bones for osteoporosis and rickets, and study of the number and the type of the red blood cells in anemia. The chief clinical syndromes and the chief anatomic evidences occurring in various deficiency states are given in Table 38-5.

Occasionally one sees a more or less pure single-deficiency state, but more often the deficiency is multiple and the clinical picture presented is a complex of several deficiency states: e.g., weight loss, occurring with scurvy and rickets, or fatigue and thinness plus anemia, dermatitis, polyneuritis, cheilosis, etc.

Extreme undernutrition may result in death. Less severe degrees of nutritional failure may cause extreme emaciation, loss of practically all body fat, muscle atrophy and extreme weakness that may continue for years. The skin becomes dry and rough, inelastic and wrinkled; the hair becomes dry, brittle and gray, and breaks and falls out; teeth may become carious and may loosen and fall out. The gums may soften, bleed and atrophy. There are signs of pituitary, thyroid and gonadal failure in many extreme cases, so that the final physical appearance is very similar to that seen as the result of complete pituitary failure (Simmonds' disease). (See Fig. 38-1.)

CLINICAL MANIFESTATIONS OF MALNUTRITION

When undernutrition occurs it is apt to be concealed or barely evident in the beginning and even after long periods, if mild in degree. The mild or early states of nutritive failure do not produce any weight loss in many instances, and since weight loss is mistakenly apt to be (to both patient and physician) a sine qua non of undernutrition, the condition is often allowed to go unrecognized. Malnutrition should always be suspected and looked for even in the absence of presenting symptoms or physical signs, whenever the history indicates a negative nutritive balance. The term *subclinical* is often applied to the early and mild stages of undernutrition, corresponding to the periods of tissue depletion and biochemical change. Vague ill-health may be the first symptom of which the patient complains, with general malaise and an inability clearly to define the feeling of deviation from good health. Later it may be noted that lack of energy and easy fatigability are present.

As functional changes become more evident, anatomic changes are apt to appear and the physician can often, by physical examination and biochemical tests, identify the several types or single type of malnutrition present. The physician's effort should always, of course, be directed toward early discovery of the nutritive defect, so that irreversible damage may be prevented.

Clinically, probably the commonest nutritional defect is thinness with failure to gain or negative caloric balance with weight loss. Perhaps the disturbance next most frequent is dehydration, with negative salt and water balance, seen often after diarrhea, vomiting, etc., and in diabetes. Probably the

most common of all chronic deficiencies is that of iron, producing iron-deficiency anemia. The various vitamin deficiencies are probably next in frequency, and are usually multiple and complex. Hypoproteinemia, a striking result of protein deficit, is a late stage; when edema appears, muscle wasting and protein loss have usually been going on for some time.[11,27]

Each of the effects of malnutrition (see Table 38-5) is a symptom or pathologic state requiring some analysis and interpretation.

Loss of Weight. Does weight loss always indicate malnutrition? Obviously not, for the weight lost may represent unwanted excess salt and water and may indicate improved health—for example, after digitalization for heart failure. Likewise, weight gain in a thin person is not necessarily a good sign, for if malnutrition and hypoproteinemia were present, the gain may consist of edema fluid.

Weight loss may represent loss of excessive fat and may improve physiologic performance. Obesity may be viewed mistakenly as a sign of good health, but it may mask protein, mineral or vitamin deficiencies. Whenever normal fat stores are depleted danger is imminent; caloric reserves against stress are absent. Whenever muscle and other protein structures of the body begin to waste, weight loss is a serious symptom.

Failure to Grow. Children may fail to grow properly when deprived of essential nutrients, the most important of which for growth seem to be protein, calcium, phosphorus, iron, and vitamin D. They also need the calorie-producing foods and other vitamins for optimal growth. However, failure to grow may occur from various other causes, and possible causes that must be especially considered are hypothyroidism and lack of the pituitary growth hormone, as well as chronic infections.

Lack of Energy, Easy Fatigue, Muscular Weakness. Fatigue and weakness are typical signs of malnutrition and, in early or mild cases, often the only signs.

A diet inadequate in calories may bring about an impairment of physical efficiency within a matter of days.[12]

In prolonged semistarvation, muscle strength is diminished greatly and muscle endurance is still more strikingly decreased.[8,29] In severely malnourished persons, energy expenditure above the rate of 300 calories per hour results in collapse from muscular and circulatory-respiratory failure.[21b]

Headache, sweating, vasomotor instability, dizziness, "light-headedness" or faintness may occur.

Many different types of malnutrition first become apparent through the symptoms of weakness, easy fatigue, or lethargy: lack of calories for energy, protein deficiency, thiamine deficiency, iron lack, anemia, etc.

Often the lack of energy is the result of *organic disease* which can in many ways already discussed adversely affect energy metabolism.

When a *nutritive defect* is primarily at fault a history suggestive of factors favoring malnutrition may be obtainable, or a history of weight loss and muscle atrophy or physical evidences of undernutrition may be present.

Fatigue on an organic basis must be distinguished from fatigue on a nervous basis. Fatigue and lethargy are in a high percentage of cases due to *psychic disorders* ranging from the mildest to the most severe. Dissatisfaction with life is apt to result in withdrawal from activities, loss of interest in the routine duties of the day, depression and mental and physical inactivity. If such symptoms progress they may develop into the complete withdrawal of the schizophrenic or of the severe depressive psychoses. More complete treatment of this subject is given in Chapter 29 on Nervousness and Fatigue.

Nervous Irritability. In addition to the depressive types of psychic disorders mentioned in the preceding paragraph, other psychological effects of malnutrition may occur such as irritable types of nervous tension, gum-chewing or cigarette-smoking of excessive and compulsive degree, emotional instability, etc.

Physicians who prescribe dietary reducing regimens are apt to encounter resentment and hostility among patients as well as "irritability, depression, decrease in self-initiated activity, loss of sexual drive, social introversion," etc., called the "semistarvation neurosis" as seen in a study of 36 young male volunteers.[24]

Delay in Convalescence. The duration of disability following trauma or disease is shortened significantly by adequate nutrition. Negative nitrogen balance and other manifestations of "the catabolic phase" are not considered inevitable now.[20]

Poor Wound Healing. An important role in the healing of wounds is played by the state of nutrition. Proteins, ascorbic acid, riboflavin and vitamin A are the nutrients principally involved in the healing of wounds.

Dehydration. Ordinarily dehydration may be detected early; it causes symptoms even when it has been present only a short time. In this respect it differs from carbohydrate, fat, protein, vitamin and mineral malnutrition, in which the symptoms as a rule appear comparatively late. Exhaustion, mental obtundity, dry inelastic loose skin, dry tongue and mouth, soft eyeballs, vascular hypotension, often acidosis and shock, are the usual evidences of extreme dehydration. Profound prostration will soon follow any extensive loss of water and salt that cannot quickly be repaired. For a fuller discussion of these points, see Chapter 35.

Anorexia. The common idea that an undernourished or partially starving person is apt to be ravenous for food is largely erroneous. Usually those persons who exhibit the largest appetites are husky manual workers with great caloric requirements and obese persons who do not need the calories but enjoy eating. A malnourished person as a rule has a *poor appetite* that can often be *improved* by proper nutrition. Persons who have been partially starved find it very difficult to ingest a diet anywhere near normal in the early stages of treatment, and a prolonged period of training is often necessary.[12,14]

The above considerations are important when the anorexia is the result of malnutrition alone. When the anorexia is caused by an organic or psychic disorder, and the effect of the malnutrition in depressing appetite is an additive factor, it can be seen that correction of anorexia and restoration of normal food intake may be a task of some proportions and ramifications. It is essential that the cause of the anorexia be discovered. It is only when the symptom of anorexia itself is understood in the particular case that the physician can expect to plan a therapeutic program to correct it, and thus to correct the malnutrition. (See Chap. 21.)

Impaired hepatic function has been shown to follow malnutrition. Fatty infiltration of the liver (often with hepatomegaly), develops in starvation, in pellagra, in kwashiorkor, and in many diseases of inanition, such as ulcerative colitis, tuberculosis and alcoholism. In many instances the fatty liver

TABLE 38-6. CONDITIONS AFFECTING AND
AFFECTED BY PROTEIN METABOLISM

PHYSIOLOGIC	PATHOLOGIC
Growth	Fatigue
Muscle and tissue	Convalescence
formation	Wound healing
Bone formation	Edema
Blood formation	Obesity
Pregnancy	Impaired gastroin-
Lactation	testinal absorption
Appetite and hunger	Wasting diseases
Absorption of other	Liver disease
nutrients	Kidney disease
Immunity and	
resistance	

precedes the development of hepatic cirrhosis. Lack of glucose supply with inadequate
glycogen storage renders the liver more
susceptible to toxins and interferes with
liver-cell metabolism. Lack of *choline* when
the intake is high in fat and low in protein
is known to produce liver damage. *Inositol*
acts synergistically with choline in reducing
the fat content of fatty livers in experimental animals. Experimental evidence indicates that hepatic injury (cirrhosis) results
from insufficient protein intake in association with lack of some as yet unidentified
vitamin-B factor. A decrease in the protein
content of the liver with impairment of
liver function has been shown to follow the
induction of hypo-albuminemia in dogs by
dietary means.

Protein Deficiency. Severe degrees of loss
of body protein may occur with no decrease
in the circulating blood proteins. Protein
deficiency is not synonymous with hypoproteinemia. By the time a definite fall in
the serum albumin has occurred there has
been extreme depletion of tissue protein.
At present there is no way of measuring
the various milder and intermediate stages
of protein deficiency. It is evident that the
integrity of the body-tissue proteins is
actually much more important than the
serum-protein level. Weight loss and depletion of the body's fat stores are usually apparent before protein loss. In estimating the
degree of protein deficit present one must
depend upon the indirect evidence obtained by studying the fate of protein ingested or injected into the body. Such
studies have yielded data indicating that a
tremendous decrease in tissue protein is
always present before the protein deficit is

reflected in a fall in the circulating protein
in the blood. A fall of about 30 Gm. in
tissue proteins must take place before
serum proteins decrease 1 Gm. per 100 ml.

One must consider not only the total
quantity of protein but its quality. Protein
deficiency may occur even in the presence
of the usually adequate intake of one gram
or more per kilogram of body weight, if the
protein is poor in certain essential amino
acids. Protein to be adequate in all respects for body needs must furnish all the
essential amino acids.[11,23,27,38] To ensure
this, it is recommended that proteins derived
from *animal sources* constitute at least 65
per cent of the total protein intake. When
cereal proteins furnish a large part of the
protein intake, protein synthesis may be
inadequate, since certain amino acids (lysine, etc.) may be lacking. When sufficient
calories are supplied to provide for energy
needs, the usually recommended daily allowance of one gram per kilogram of body
weight allows a safety margin of almost 100
per cent, if the proteins are of good quality.

Consideration of protein deficiencies as
they may produce or affect clinical conditions is important in various normal or
physiologic states and in certain pathologic
or disease conditions (Table 38-6).

The causes of protein deficiency, as far
as the mechanism is concerned, are the
same as for the other nutrients: inadequate
intake (either qualitatively or quantitatively); inadequate digestion, absorption or
utilization; increased metabolism and excessive excretion or loss. However, it is of
considerable importance to remember certain special features of protein metabolism:
liver disease may lead to inadequate synthesis of plasma protein; *kidney disease*
may result in severe protein loss (albuminuria), while protein losses after wounds
and burns and from hemorrhage, peritonitis or ascites may be great.

Protein deficiency is apt to result in disorders of *fluid transport* through development of hypoalbuminemia, with resultant
edema, and sometimes *ascites.*

It must not be forgotten that *hemoglobin* requires protein as well as iron for
its manufacture, and that either iron or
protein deficiency or both may cause
anemia.

A good protein matrix is necessary to
build and maintain *bone.* Adequate bone
growth in children requires not only calcium, phosphorus and vitamin D, but

proper protein. In the aged, osteoporosis may occur with deformity and fractures resulting from protein loss from the bone matrix. In Cushing's syndrome, or after prolonged administration of corticosteroids, protein is lost as well as calcium, and the bones become fragile.

The widespread misconception that protein foods are *always* harmful in kidney disease must be combated, for often recovery is possible only after restoration of a positive protein balance.

Proteins are of great importance in *defense against infections* and bacterial invasion. Investigations in acquired immunity show that antibody production is a phase of protein metabolism and that protein deficiency may impair the production of *antibodies*, with resultant loss of acquired immunity and increase in the susceptibility to infection. Protein deficiency impairs *phagocyte* formation also. Protein is likewise necessary for the production of toxins, antitoxins and antigens. Hypoproteinemia may develop rapidly in overwhelming infections and in shock, but the mechanism of its development is not understood.

KWASHIORKOR is the name applied to a syndrome caused by protein deficiency occurring primarily in tropical and subtropical areas, chiefly in children of the postweaning period (ages 1 to 3 years) in underprivileged populations. Often it occurs as the child is deprived of maternal milk and is given almost a pure carbohydrate diet, which may be quite adequate in calories. The nutritive defect appears to be primarily a deficiency of protein foods, imbalance of amino acids, and lack of accessory food factors associated with protein metabolism. Classically one finds growth failure, mental changes (apathy and irritability), weakness and atrophy of skeletal muscles, edema, dermatoses, hair loss and depigmentation, gastrointestinal symptoms (anorexia, vomiting and diarrhea), anemia and hypoalbuminemia. Adult residues include hepatic cirrhosis and a high incidence of primary hepatoma.[11,27,38]

When an extreme stage of protein deficiency is reached as the result of any process causing a negative protein balance, and hypoproteinemia, anemia and edema are present, the need for prompt analysis of the symptoms, discovery of the cause and reversal of the pathologic processes is obvious. Less obvious and more recently discovered indications for establishment of a highly positive protein balance include

acute as well as chronic *liver disease*. The tendency to hypoalbuminemia in cirrhosis of the liver has long been recognized, but only recently has attention been called to the fact that high amounts of protein as well as carbohydrate are of value in protecting liver cells against noxious agents. Such measures have proved helpful in hepatitis of various sorts, including infectious hepatitis, toxic hepatitis and subacute yellow atrophy. The sulfur-containing amino acids *methionine* and *cystine* appear to be the protein components of greatest importance in protecting the liver from toxic hepatitis.

Choline, inositol, and certain other fractions of the vitamin B complex, as well as protein, have been shown to be important in the preservation of normal liver structure and function.

IN SURGICAL CONDITIONS, attention to the protein supply is imperative because injuries and wounds cause negative balance and intake is usually greatly limited. Wound healing is adversely affected by protein deficiency.

HYPOPROTEINEMIA may be masked or concealed under two specific circumstances especially: (1) in *dehydration*, the initial serum protein determination may be normal, but the level may fall as dilution occurs when normal hydration is established, and (2) in certain conditions the rise in *serum globulin* may be sufficient to mask the fall in serum albumin, if total protein alone is measured. The term *hypoalbuminemia* is preferable to hypoproteinemia, since it is the albumin fraction that is decreased.

Because of its small molecular size, albumin is responsible for the major part of the osmotic tension of the serum proteins under ordinary conditions. The osmotic tension exerted normally by serum albumin is about five times that of serum globulin. Often the rise in serum globulin may equal or exceed the fall in serum albumin, so total protein values may be misleading. In the study of edema as related to nutritional disorders, the serum albumin level is the important factor.

Mineral Deficiencies. Mineral deficits occur as the result of a variety of abnormal conditions which may be grouped in three general classes:

1. SEVERE UNDERNUTRITION, e.g., loss of potassium, magnesium, iron, phosphorus and calcium from tissues, of sodium, chlorine

and water from the extracellular fluids; deficient intake, or excessive losses, as in sweating, polyuria, vomiting, diarrhea, etc.

2. RENAL DISEASE. In certain types of renal disease the kidneys lose much of their ability to conserve the chief base of the blood plasma and interstitial fluids, sodium; chloride and potassium losses may also occur.

3. HORMONAL DISORDERS, e.g., calcium and phosphorus loss in hyperparathyroidism; sodium and chlorine loss in adrenocortical deficiency; sodium, chlorine and potassium losses in diabetes mellitus.

SODIUM, CHLORIDE AND POTASSIUM. For discussion of water, sodium, chloride and potassium metabolism and manifestations of their derangements, see Chapters 35 (Dehydration) and 36 (Edema).

The diet is more likely to be deficient in iron than in any other mineral element. Insufficient calcium intake is next most common.[42,46,47] Mineral deficiencies most frequently seen clinically are those of calcium, iodine or iron. These minerals deserve special discussion because of the frequency and importance of the clinical manifestations associated with their lack or loss.

CALCIUM, a major mineral constituent of the body, constitutes about 1.5 to 2 per cent of the body weight of healthy mature persons. More than 99 per cent is present in bones and teeth. Active processes of bone formation and resorption constantly remove from or add to the calcium in body fluids. Calcium, in addition to its fundamental role in skeletal structure, contributes vital functions in body fluids and other tissues affecting blood coagulation, membrane permeability, neuromuscular response, muscular contractility, and myocardial function.

Unlike sodium and potassium, which are almost completely absorbed, calcium is incompletely absorbed, and the amount absorbed is enhanced when greater amounts are available in the intestine. Breast-fed infants absorb about 60 per cent of the calcium ingested; infants fed cows' milk formulas containing added carbohydrate absorb 35 to 50 per cent; adults on mixed diets containing much less calcium in proportion to total food intake absorb an average of only about 30 per cent of the calcium. Vitamin D is required for efficient absorption of calcium. Phytate, oxalate, and fatty acids of the diet form nonionized or poorly soluble calcium complexes, thus interfering with calcium absorption. Intestinal hypermotility also may reduce absorption.[42]

When skeletal stores of calcium are replete, intestinal uptake of dietary calcium is low; skeletal depletion results in accelerated uptake. Absorption rates are high in children, in pregnancy, and during lactation, apparently in response to great need at these times. Recommended daily allowances are much higher for such periods than adult maintenance requirements. (See Table 38-4). Apparently intestinal transport of calcium normally is altered in response to the state of mineralization of the skeleton, greater absorption resulting when there is demand in the bones for calcium.

Calcium intake may be inadequate whenever there is little ingestion of milk and milk products. Infants to age one year get 90 per cent of their calcium from milk; children from 1 to 8 years, 73 to 82 per cent; from 9 to 18 years, 65 to 70 per cent. Beyond age 20 milk and milk products normally furnish 50 to 55 per cent of calcium requirements. Teen-agers and many adults rebel against or neglect optimal intake of liquid milk, perhaps considering its use childish and disliking the memory of the milk forced upon them when they were children. Cheeses may be substituted in the diets of those not drinking adequate milk, as they are high in calcium content.

PHOSPHORUS. Calcium and phosphorus are appropriately considered together because of their metabolic interrelationships and because the strength and rigidity of bones and teeth depend largely upon their content of combined salts of these two mineral elements. Bone salt is an apatite similar to $CaF_2 \cdot 3\ Ca_3\ (PO_4)_2$ and $CaCO_3 \cdot CaC_2\ (PO_4)_2$. The ratio of calcium to phosphorus in bones is about 2:1. Between 70 and 80 per cent of body phosphorus is in the skeletal tissues. In addition to the important skeletal structural role of phosphorus in the inorganic form, phosphorus performs essential functions as phosphate ion in body fluids and cells, and in organic combinations in lipids, proteins, and energy-transfer enzymes. Phosphorus compounds play a central role in transformations of energy; an understanding of "high energy phosphate bonds" has been one of the major recent achievements in biochemistry. Adenosine-triphosphate and the nucleotides formed from several of the vitamins are essential in the catabolism and anabolism of carbohydrates, fats, and proteins. Nucleoproteins containing phosphorus make up a large portion of nuclear material and also occur in the cytoplasm of all cells; they are key materials in the processes of cell division, reproduction, and transmission of hereditary characteristics.

The 2:1 ratio of calcium to phosphorus in bones suggests that this might be the ideal dietary ratio, particularly during growth. However, several other considerations are important: (1) the much higher ratio of phosphorus to calcium in soft tissues (in muscle the phosphorus to calcium ratio is 15:1); (2) in ordinary diets phosphorus intake usually equals or exceeds calcium intake; (3) of the amounts ingested, a much larger proportion of phosphorus is absorbed (an average of about 70 per cent of the phosphorus as compared with about 30 per cent of the calcium). Such concepts result in recommended allowances of phosphorus equal to those of calcium, except for infants below one year of age, for whom more calcium than phosphorus is advised. (See Table 38-4.) In infants fed cows' milk hyperphosphatemia, hypocalcemia and tetany may result from the relative excess of phosphorus intake.

Even in the many adults who ingest little or no milk or milk products, if caloric intake is adequate there is little likelihood of insufficient phosphorus intake because ordinary foods contain abundant phosphorus. Although phosphorus intake is more than adequate, there may be deficient phosphorus in bone, since formation of bone salts requires appropriate amounts of calcium and Vitamin D as well.

Calcium and phosphorus deficit in adults may exist for years with gradually developing demineralization of the bones that finally may reach attention only after a vertebra has collapsed or some other bone has been fractured.

When the fault lies in deficient intake of calcium, phosphorus or vitamin D in growing children, *rickets* results; weakening of adult bones on the same pathologic basis results in the condition of poor calcification known as *osteomalacia*. If the calcium intake of the pregnant woman is inadequate, calcium for the fetal skeleton is withdrawn from her bones and osteomalacia may result. Calcium and vitamin D deprivation is a common cause of hypocalcemic tetany during infancy, pregnancy and lactation. *Osteoporosis* is the term used to describe the poor calcification and diminished strength of bony structures resulting from a defect in the formation of the bone matrix. When protein derangement occurs (disuse, malnutrition, old age, Cushing's syndrome, etc.) and the bone matrix is not normally formed or is depleted, calcification of bone may not proceed normally, or calcium and phosphorus may actually be lost from the bones and from the body, even when the intake of calcium, phosphorus and vitamin D is normal. When both mineral and protein deficiencies are present, *osteomalacia* plus *osteoporosis* may be present (e.g., senile bone changes with pathologic fractures are commonest in persons who have chronic deficits in calcium, phosphorus, and vitamin D). X-ray evidence usually shows that the anatomic process was far advanced before symptoms occurred. Occasionally aching pain in the bones may be present without fracture or malformation of the bones. A history of dislike for milk (usually with overindulgence in coffee, soft drinks, etc.) should suggest possible calcium deficiency. Large amounts of calcium and phosphorus are necessary for construction of the growing skeleton of children. In childhood, calcium and phosphorus deficit may be manifested in poor growth as well as in the deformities of rickets and in poor teeth.

The calcium or phosphorus depletion (usually both) may be caused by inadequate intake of these minerals and of vitamin D, or by losses due to pregnancy, lactation, immobilization (as in casts), hyperthyroidism or hyperparathyroidism, impaired bile secretion, chronic diarrhea (sprue and similar diseases). Hypocalcemia and osteomalacia may result from steatorrhea. Rarely is hypocalcemia due to a true nutritional calcium deficiency in adults, although low calcium intake and vitamin-D lack cause hypocalcemia and tetany in children. The level of serum calcium is primarily under the control of the parathyroid hormone. Serum calcium tends to remain normal even when intake of calcium is low and bones are much depleted of calcium.

The manifestations of calcium deficiency are evident in aberrations from normal in its control over blood clotting, the rate and the rhythm of the heart beat, the state of neuromuscular transmission of impulses and the permeability of membranes, as well as in structural abnormalities in bones and in teeth. For example, hypocalcemia may so alter membrane permeability that the volume and the pressure of the cerebrospinal fluid rise and papilledema and epileptiform convulsions occur.

FLUORIDE. Fluoride in small but widely variant amounts is present in practically all soils, water supplies, plants, and animals and therefore is a normal constituent of all diets. Highest concentrations in mammals are found in bones and teeth. Fluoride is incorporated in the structure of teeth and is necessary for maximal resistance to dental caries.[44] Many studies suggest that fluoride is important to provide optimal structure and strength of bones at all ages. Evidence is strong that older persons, especially females, have more osteoporosis in low fluoride areas. This is indicated both by decreased bone density and collapsed vertebrae.

Standardization of water supplies by addition of fluoride to bring the concentration to 1 ppm has proved to be a safe, economical, and efficient way to reduce the incidence of tooth decay—a very important nutritional public health measure in areas where natural water supplies do not contain this amount. In communities where fluoridation has been introduced, the incidence of tooth decay in children has been decreased up to 50 per cent or more. The Food and Nutrition Board recommends fluoridation of public water supplies, where needed.[44] In 1969 the Executive Council of the World Health Organization endorsed a worldwide water fluoridation program. The endorsement was signed by health authorities of 24 countries.[59]

IRON deficiency in men is uncommon, but it is frequent in women and in children. Iron is essentially a "one-way substance" that after absorption is retained and avidly conserved; upon release from cells it is stored or utilized again and again for formation of hemoglobin.[10,34]

If iron for hemoglobin formation is not available in adequate quantities, the maturation of red blood cells is retarded, the number released from the bone marrow is subnormal, and each red cell has a subnormal hemoglobin content. The characteristic manifestation of iron deficiency is hypochromic, microcytic anemia, primarily a lack of hemoglobin, although the red blood cells are often reduced in number. Accompanying the anemia there may be glossitis; cheilosis; esophagitis and indigestion with the Plummer-Vinson syndrome; brittle, flat or spoon-shaped fingernails (koilonychia); and, with very low hemoglobin, such symptoms as pallor, weakness, fatigue, dyspnea and edema.

Iron deficiency is the most widespread nutritional deficiency in the world today, in advanced as well as primitive societies.[60]

Iron deficiency is not synonymous with *iron deficiency anemia,* because deficiency of iron stores is common and exists in varying degrees up to virtual exhaustion of all iron reserves before anemia results.[10,34,60]

Two main factors distinguish the normal adult human male from the normal adult human female in regard to iron metabolism: (1) He takes in more iron, because his caloric intake is greater. The average normal diet furnishes daily iron intake of about 6 mg. per 1,000 calories. Since the average male consumes 2,800 calories daily to the average female's 2,000, his iron intake averages about 17 mg. to the female's 12 mg. Calculating 10 per cent absorption, the amounts absorbed would be 1.7 mg. vs. 1.2 mg. (2) He is apt to be in positive iron balance, storing more than he excretes, or in balance, with absorption equal to excretion.

She is apt to be in negative iron balance, because her non-menstrual losses are about 1 mg., the same as for the male, to which there are added the loss in menstruation, averaging 0.5 mg. daily. With 1.2 mg. absorbed and 1.5 mg. lost, the average daily deficit would be 0.3 mg.

The average adult male in the United States has about 50 mg. of iron per Kg. of body weight, making about 3.5 Gm. in all. Of this, 60 to 70 per cent is in hemoglobin. The rest, totaling 30 per cent to 40 per cent is held in reserve in myoglobin, cellular enzymes, and plasma, and is stored in reticuloendothelial cells. The reserve iron in a normal man is 1,000 to 1,500 mg.[60]

In the female the situation is quite different. She has a lower blood volume and a lower concentration of hemoglobin. She has less iron—only about 35 mg. per Kg. of body weight. Total iron would be 55 (Kg.) × 35 (mg.) equalling 1.9 or 2.0 Gm. Because of lower reserves, more of the female's iron is in hemoglobin, around 80 to 90 per cent. Her reserve iron totals 10 to 20 per cent of the total, ranging from 200 to 400 mg., averaging about 300 mg. The female's iron reserves are therefore in normal persons only about 20 to 30 per cent of the male's amount.

Many women with larger menstrual and pregnancy losses have no iron stores at all and therefore are especially vulnerable to iron deficiency anemia. The borderline state of iron balance is indicated by the greatly reduced or absent iron stores in two thirds of menstruating women and in the majority of pregnant women. For these groups it is desirable to increase iron intake by supplementation.[46,61]

In addition to menstruation and pregnancy there is a third situation in which the usual iron intake is frequently inadequate—that is, infancy. The newborn, full-term infant of a normally nourished mother has a high hemoglobin level which provides him with ample iron for the first few months of life, even though he has very little stored iron. The demands of growth require additional iron after the first few months. Dietary sources often fail to meet these demands. Milk, unless supplemented by iron, does not supply this need.[61]

The fall in hemoglobin during childhood coincides with the period of most intensive growth; an infant normally trebles body weight in one year. Premature infants, whose weight may increase seven-fold in one year, almost invariably have iron deficiency anemia.

In the past the "normal" hemoglobin concentrations of children from 6 months to 10 years of age have been generally accepted as being lower than those of adults. The fall in hemoglobin from 16 Gm. per 100 ml. at birth to below 12 Gm. in the first year is no longer considered a normal and physiological phenomenon; it is now believed to be evidence of iron deficiency. Three months' oral administration of iron will bring the hemoglobin in all children, including infants, up to the same level as in adult women.

The normal adult human absorbs an average of 5 to 10 per cent of iron from foods; with a dietary intake of 12 to 15 mg. absorption amounts to approximately 0.6 to 1.5 mg. daily. The amount of iron utilized for hemoglobin synthesis per day is about 20 to 25 mg. Almost one per cent of the total of the circulating red blood cells is destroyed daily. The normal adult catabolizes enough hemoglobin per day to release 20 to 25 mg. of iron. Only about 5 per cent is excreted in feces, urine, sweat, cells desquamated from the skin, etc., so that iron lost from the body totals about 1 mg. daily on the average and daily absorption tends to replace daily loss: the body tends to remain in iron balance. When iron deficiency is present, there is normally greater absorption (up to 20 per cent or more) of the dietary intake, and a positive iron balance

may persist until body stores are replenished.

The body of a normal adult contains approximately 2.5 to 5.5 Gm. of iron, depending largely upon the body weight and the circulating mass of hemoglobin. About 50 to 60 per cent of this total is found in hemoglobin; about 10 to 20 per cent in myoglobin. The important cellular enzyme portion is relatively small; the remainder is stored chiefly in organs rich in reticuloendothelial cells (liver, spleen, bone marrow).[34]

Most women enter pregnancy with inadequate iron stores. The average "iron cost" of pregnancy is 680 mg.[60,61] This exceeds considerably the usual iron in storage. Consequently, if there is no iron supplementation, the hemoglobin level falls progressively during pregnancy, and remains low long afterward. Under usual dietary conditions the iron deficit resulting from a normal pregnancy would take nearly two years to replace. Iron therapy during pregnancy is recommended.[44,61]

The modern view is that good nutrition in regard to iron requires adequate iron stores. If 90 per cent of menstruating women are to have iron stores in excess of 500 mg., it is estimated that the mean intake of women should be 18 mg. daily.[44,60,61]

At birth the child receives from the mother a somatic inheritance of about 270 mg. Children may not take in enough iron during the period of growth while the needs for iron are increasing, and thus anemia may develop. During the period of very rapid development called adolescence iron requirements are high. If intake of iron is inadequate, depletion of stores may occur and there is danger of anemia.[34,61] Women, because of blood loss at menstruation and increased demands and loss with pregnancy and childbirth, may have at times or chronically a *negative iron balance* with resultant anemia. The annual loss through menstruation averages about 300 mg.

Iron intake in adult males is, in the United States at least, more than sufficient to supply adequate iron reserves. Iron ingested is absorbed or eliminated in the stools; it is not excreted in the usual sense. Very small amounts are eliminated in the urine. These facts make it evident that iron deficiency in adult males or postmenopausal females usually means blood loss, whereas in women or children the intake may not be sufficient to balance the usual or increased demands.

Blood loss, often completely undetected by the patient or his family, and sometimes difficult to discover by the physician, is a major *pathologic* cause of iron deficiency. Peptic ulcer, esophageal varices, intestinal parasites (especially hookworms, gastrointestinal polyps, or neoplasms) and hemorrhoids are included among the pathologic causes of blood loss and consequent iron deficiency.

Women or children, of course, may have blood loss as a major cause of iron deficiency anemia, as well as men. Hookworm disease in some areas is common among children and causes dwarfing and anemia.

Infancy, childhood, adolescence, and the years of menstruation and child-bearing are the *physiologic* periods when iron needs are great, and iron deficiency may occur because absorption does not meet demands.

Blood donors can become iron deficient, if iron stores are depleted, since the donor loses 250 mg. of iron per 500 ml. of blood. As much as 10 to 50 mg. of iron per day can be mobilized from reserves for hemoglobin synthesis. Hemoglobin may be restored to normal in a few days if the donor's stores are adequate. If the donor has given blood repeatedly and too frequently, his iron stores may be exhausted. If the donor is a woman with iron reserves depleted by unusually heavy menstruation, blood regeneration may require several months, depending on iron in the diet.

In *chronic infections*, hypoferremia precedes the anemia, which is caused by impaired hemoglobin formation.[13]

IODINE intake is the principal factor determining the iodine content of the thyroid gland, the principal storehouse for iodine. The requirement for iodine is small, about 0.002 mg. daily per Kg. body weight or a total of 0.1 mg. to 0.3 mg. daily for the adult. Iodized salt is needed in many areas to insure such supply. Requirements for iodine are increased in adolescence and pregnancy.

Goiter (enlargement of the thyroid gland) results from thyroid hyperplasia due to iodine deficiency. The most urgent reason for stressing iodine as a preventive measure is not the goiter which may occur in the affected woman but the profound thyroid deficit which may result in her offspring. Cretinism occurs in the infant when the pregnant woman is so depleted of iodine that none is available for development of the thyroid of the fetus.

A normal adult thyroid gland weighs about 25 Gm. and contains 8 to 10 mg. of iodine. Normally the thyroid gland maintains an iodine concentration of about 40 mg. per 100 grams. When this concentration falls below 10 mg. per 100 grams, hyperplasia ensues and goiter may develop, with or without various types of functional thyroid disturbance (hyperthyroidism or hypothyroidism). Iodine is an important and necessary constituent of the thyroid hormone, and is thus of fundamental importance in body growth and function, exercising constant control over the rate of metabolism in all tissues.

Vitamin Deficiencies. VITAMIN A is of great nutritional importance as a growth factor. It acts as an important nutritive element in the metabolism of epithelial tissues. The normal epithelium atrophies in vitamin-A deficiency and is replaced by proliferating basal cells that become keratinized. Vitamin A is necessary in the regeneration of visual purple in the retina.

Clinical manifestations of vitamin-A deficiency are chiefly, therefore, failure to grow, xerophthalmia, dermatosis and night blindness. The precursors of vitamin A are all the carotenoid pigments commonly called carotene. The greatest source of vitamin A is food containing carotene. The skin conditions known as keratosis pilaris, ichthyosis, follicularis, etc., are probably the same or closely related, and are due to vitamin-A lack. The presence of such hyperkeratosis, usually with small pustules, especially on the extensor surfaces of the arms and legs, is especially suggestive.

THE VITAMINS OF THE B COMPLEX have such varied and important functions and the specific indications of their lack have been so fully treated elsewhere that only the chief clinical manifestations that will lead to the suspicion of nutritive failure will be recited here.

Vitamin B_1 (thiamine) exerts an important influence in carbohydrate metabolism because it is essential for the oxidation of the intermediate metabolite, pyruvic acid. Since the brain and the nerve subsist primarily upon carbohydrate, profound disturbance of cerebral and peripheral nervous-tissue function is caused by thiamine lack. Severe deficiency results in beriberi, neuritis and cardiovascular dysfunction. Anorexia is a very early and suggestive sign, also ill-defined fatigue, mental depression, irritability, and peculiar aches and paresthesiae in the legs. Thiamine requirement increases greatly with acceleration of metabolism, especially of carbohydrate.

Vitamin B₂ (riboflavin) is an important constituent of living animal cells. It enters into the formation of the prosthetic groups of several flavoprotein enzymes. Mammalian tissues have a number of different flavoprotein enzyme systems each containing a specific protein (apoenzyme) and a riboflavin-containing prosthetic group (coenzyme). These enzymes are essential in oxidative systems in living cells; thus it is axiomatic that cellular growth cannot evolve in the absence of riboflavin. Manifestations suggestive of riboflavin deficiency are cheilosis (maceration in each angle of the mouth, reddening of the lips along the line of closure, and thin, shiny, denuded mucosa); scaly, greasy desquamation in the nasolabial folds; corneal vascularization, conjunctivitis and glossitis. The requirement is 2 to 3 mg. daily.

Nicotinic acid deficiency is manifested by the lesions characteristic of pellagra: dermatitis, glossitis and stomatitis, and gastrointestinal disorders with diarrhea. The mental symptoms of pellagra may be due partly to nicotinic-acid deficiency and partly to thiamine deficiency. The human requirement for nicotinic acid is difficult to determine because part of the daily needs can be met by metabolic conversion in the tissues from the amino acid tryptophan. Deficiencies of thiamine, of riboflavin, or of pyridoxine may lead to impaired formation of nicotinic acid. The requirement is 10 to 20 mg. daily.

Vitamin B₆ (pyridoxine) is active in the body in the form of phosphorylated pyridoxal or pyridoxamine. As such, the vitamin serves as a prosthetic group in enzyme systems which are of fundamental importance in the metabolism of amino acids. In man seborrhealike skin lesions about the eyes, the nose and the mouth accompanied by glossitis and stomatitis can be produced within a few weeks by feeding a diet poor in B-complex plus daily doses of the vitamin-antagonist desoxypyridoxine.[19] Between 1951 and 1953 a number of infants in the United States developed hyperirritability and convulsions from taking a commercially distributed feeding formula which proved to be deficient in pyridoxine.[6,18] A number of other less well-defined syndromes have been described as dependent on a lack of vitamin B₆.[41] The vitamin is widely available in natural foods, and the requirement is about 1 to 2 mg. daily.

Vitamin C (ascorbic acid) is necessary for the normal development and maintenance of intercellular cement substance, ground substance and collagen in connective-tissue supporting structures, in bone matrix, tendons and cartilage, and in the smaller blood vessels. It is important in the formation of teeth and bones. It occupies an important position in cellular respiration. Vitamin-C lack retards wound healing. The needs for ascorbic acid are greatly increased in febrile diseases, hyperthyroidism and other states of accelerated metabolism. Abundant vitamin C seems to be necessary at the normoblast stage of erythrocyte development. Scurvy is now relatively rare, but less severe subclinical forms of ascorbic-acid deficiency with easy bruising, capillary fragility, appearance of petechiae, etc., are not uncommon.

Ascorbic acid facilitates the absorption of iron from the intestinal tract. The conversion of folic acid to the metabolically active form, folinic acid, requires ascorbic acid. From observations made in studies on premature and young infants, vitamin C also appears to be related to the metabolism of the two amino acids tyrosine and phenylalanine.

During infections such as tuberculosis, pneumonia, rheumatic fever, etc., additions above a normal intake are required to maintain desirable tissue levels. It seems clear that ascorbic acid is important in providing resistance to infections. An intake of 10 to 20 mg. of ascorbic acid is sufficient to protect an adult from developing overt evidence of scurvy, but higher intake is advisable to maintain desirable tissue and plasma ascorbic acid levels. The daily intakes recommended by the National Research Council (see Table 38-4) are 40 mg. for infants and children, 50 mg. for adolescents, 60 mg. for adults, and 60 mg. during pregnancy and lactation. These standards are based on observations that such requirements are necessary to maintain tissue stores near saturation and to hold plasma fasting levels near 1.0 mg. per ml.[44]

Vitamin D is essential in promoting calcium and phosphorus absorption, normal bone development, and in preventing osteomalacia and rickets. When administered in adequate amounts with sufficient ingested calcium, it is effective in treating hypocalcemia, will elevate serum calcium and prevent tetany. Aching limbs, poor growth and the typical deformities of rickets are the characteristic signs of vitamin-D deficit in childhood which should be prevented or detected earlier. When lack of vitamin D plus calcium deficiency is severe and prolonged in adults, bone deformities and pathologic fractures characteristic of osteomalacia may result. Dental growth and maintenance of sound teeth depend, among other factors, upon adequate supplies of D.

In pregnancy and lactation the vitamin-D requirements are increased, and in these states special attention to the supply of this vitamin and of adequate calcium and phosphorus is necessary.

VITAMIN-K deficiency is manifested as a tendency to hemorrhage in consequence of a lowered prothrombin content of the blood. Vitamin K is essential for the maintenance of prothrombin in the blood plasma. Prothrombin, a part of the plasma-protein complex, is one of the components of the blood which is necessary for proper coagulation. It is apparently produced in the liver. If the liver is removed or is severely damaged, the concentration of prothrombin in the blood decreases.

In the absence of vitamin K, the prothrombin level falls even if the liver is intact. Under normal conditions there are two sources of vitamin K. Vitamin K_1 is ingested with the food: since it is very widely distributed and only minimal amounts are required, dietary deficiency is rare. A second source is that supplied by the bacterial flora in the intestinal tract. Many bacteria, including members of the normal intestinal flora, produce vitamin K_2. These naturally occurring compounds are fat-soluble. In order for vitamin K to be properly absorbed (as with other fat-soluble vitamins such as A and D), it is necessary that the amount of bile in the intestine be adequate, that the intestinal absorptive surface be sufficient, and that the intestinal contents do not pass too rapidly.

Any condition which seriously interferes with intestinal absorption may be a cause of vitamin-K deficiency. However, since the requirement of the vitamin is so small, and since prothrombin activity usually must be reduced to less than one-third of normal before a bleeding tendency becomes manifest, impaired absorption alone seldom causes bleeding unless bile salts are absent from the bowel.

If there is faulty absorption plus impaired liver function, the effect in lowering prothrombin activity is additive. Some degree of liver deficiency is common in biliary tract disease. Often surgery is necessary in such conditions. Preoperative determination of prothrombin activity is important to prevent postoperative bleeding. Treatment with vitamin K may be indicated.

When bleeding results from low plasma prothrombin activity, the hemorrhage usually occurs at a site of local trauma due to accidental injury, surgery, or pre-existing disease. Ecchymoses into the skin are apt to occur first, rather than the petechiae that occur as initial signs of vitamin-C deficiency. Vitamin K is essential in facilitating prothrombin formation by the liver, but the vitamin does not make up part of the prothrombin molecule. Bile salts are not absolutely essential to vitamin-K absorption, but greatly aid it. Only small amounts of the vitamin are stored, and deficiency may be apparent in one week after its intake or absorption ceases. It is believed that the normal human adult need not take this vitamin in his diet since it is synthesized by bacteria in the intestine. The facts that clinical evidence of avitaminosis K are found in the newborn (before the bacterial flora becomes established), and in adults when there is destruction of intestinal organisms by antibiotic or sulfonamides are in consonance with this view.

Prothrombin deficiency occurs in many conditions with impaired liver function, with biliary fistulas, biliary obstruction (obstructive jaundice), sprue, steatorrhea, ulcerative colitis, during severe infections, as a toxic effect of certain drugs (sulfonamides, salicylates).

Hemorrhagic disease of the newborn and the bleeding occurring with obstructive jaundice (inadequate absorption of the fat-soluble vitamin K) may be relieved or prevented with vitamin K.

When vitamin K is given in the fat-soluble form (menadione), in the presence of obstructive jaundice or a biliary fistula, bile salts should also be given to facilitate its absorption. Water-soluble quinones with vitamin-K activity are available to use if fat absorption is impaired.

The vitamin may be given prophylactically to the mother before delivery or to babies during the first week of life to prevent prothrombin deficiency in the newborn.

When liver parenchymal involvement prevents utilization of vitamin K in the formation of prothrombin, the hypoprothrombinemia may be irreversible if the liver damage cannot be repaired.

OTHER B-COMPLEX NUTRITIONAL FACTORS

Vitamin B$_{12}$ (Cyanocobalamin). This red, crystalline compound containing cobalt, phosphorus and nitrogen is the "EMF" (erythrocyte maturation factor) or the "extrinsic factor." Classic addisonian pernicious anemia is a *conditioned deficiency disease* caused by lack of a specific mucoprotein substance secreted by the normal gastric mucosa known as the "intrinsic factor" of Castle. Since the extrinsic and the intrinsic factors are ineffective when either is given alone in pernicious anemia, Castle originally postulated that the two interacted in some way to produce the antianemia factor which is present in liver. This view is untenable now that cyanocobalamin is known to be both the extrinsic factor and the liver principle.[35]

Absorption of B$_{12}$ is facilitated by intrinsic factor, but is limited even in normal persons. The preferred route for administration of cyanocobalamin is intramuscular since huge doses (over 100 times as much) are required orally unless it is combined with a source of intrinsic factor. Absorption is mainly from the ileum. Ability to absorb B$_{12}$ is decreased by extensive gastrointestinal resections, bowel anastomoses, idiopathic steatorrhea, etc., and in the elderly. The vitamin occurs almost exclusively in foods of animal origin (especially kidney, liver, muscle meats and milk) in the form of a protein complex. Proteolytic enzymes release it in the upper gastrointestinal tract. It is synthesized by many bacteria, among which *Streptomyces griseus, Streptomyces aureofaciens* and *Bacillus subtilis* are commercial sources. Herbivorous animals obtain B$_{12}$ from micro-organisms in the rumen and it is probable that these organisms are the main sources of the vitamin in animal tissues. Omnivorous animals like man ingest vitamin B$_{12}$ in foods of animal origin (meat, milk, eggs, cheese).

Vitamin B$_{12}$ is highly effective in the treatment of pernicious anemia, producing satisfactory clinical and hematologic response and preventing the progress of neurologic lesions. It is thus obviously a nutritive factor of importance, but its place in normal nutrition is uncertain. It is essential for normal functioning of all cells, particularly of bone marrow, the gastrointestinal system, and the nervous system. It facilitates reduction reactions and participates in transfer of methyl groups. Vitamin B$_{12}$ is involved in protein, fat, and carbohydrate metabolism, but its chief importance in mammalian tissues seems to be in nucleic and folic acid metabolism. See discussion below under Folic Acid.

In addisonian pernicious anemia, the gastric mucosal atrophy is probably due to an hereditary genetic defect. *Total gastrectomy, gastritis, gastric cancer,* etc., operate through a similar mechanism in producing macrocytic anemia in some instances of these conditions. Occasionally in *pregnancy,* gastric acidity and intrinsic factor secretion are progressively inhibited until after delivery. The presence of the broad fish tapeworm in the upper intestine in some way interferes with the action of intrinsic factor sufficiently, in persons with apparently minimal amounts of this enzyme, to produce macrocytic anemia.

Extreme and prolonged B$_{12}$ deficiency produces the clinical picture of pernicious anemia, the manifestations usually appearing in this order.[28] (1) Inflammation, followed by atrophy of tongue, oral mucosa and mucous membranes of the gastrointestinal tract. (2) Macrocytic anemia with megaloblastic bone marrow. The red cells are large and have only about half the normal life (60 days instead of 120). Therefore serum bilirubin is elevated somewhat. White cells and platelets are formed at slow rates. (3) Degeneration of the peripheral nerves, the posterior and the lateral columns of the spinal cord, the cerebrum and the cerebellum.

Nutritional Macrocytic Anemia. Diets extremely low in animal protein may directly fail to provide sufficient vitamin B$_{12}$. Patients with nutritional macrocytic anemia do not respond to B$_{12}$ unless the bone marrow is megaloblastic. In the United States inadequate intake is rare as a cause of macrocytic anemia; faulty absorption and assimilation may occur with intestinal dysfunctions. The deficit in nutritional macrocytic anemia is more often *folic acid deficiency* than B$_{12}$ deficiency and often there is associated lack of *ascorbic acid.*

Pernicious and related macrocytic anemias exhibit low levels of serum vitamin B$_{12}$ and respond to the administration of B$_{12}$ itself or to B$_{12}$ in the form of highly refined liver extract. Combined system disease of the spinal cord is virtually confined to patients with achylia gastrica. Lingual and gastrointestinal disturbances are common to all of the macrocytic anemias, but vary in severity in different clinical syndromes. The blood and the bone marrow pictures overlap completely. When the anemia results from inadequate intake or intestinal dysfunction, various other evidences of associated or secondary nutritional disorders are apt to be present. In pernicious anemia, the diet is not ordinarily strikingly defective until the anemia is severe; the nutritive derangement is then the result of the illness, not its cause.

Folic Acid. The terms *pteroylglutamates* and *folic acid* are currently applied to a group of compounds included among the B-complex factors. Knowledge of the pteroylglutamate content of foods is very incomplete, but it is known that fresh green leafy vegetables, cauliflower, kidney and liver are rich sources.

Ascorbic acid facilitates the conversion of folic acid to folinic acid, its metabolically active form. Studies of the growth requirements of bacteria and of the histochemical changes in man and animals resulting from deficiencies of vitamin B_{12} or of folic acid reveal that profound and widespread derangements of nucleic acid metabolism are involved. The rapidly dividing cells of the body are among the first affected: the production of red cells and leucocytes in the bone marrow; the reproduction of the cells of the intestinal mucosa. Both folic acid and B_{12} are concerned with early stages of the synthesis of purines and pyrimidines, which together with ribose sugars and phosphoric acid, form the master molecules of both nuclear deoxyribonucleic acid (DNA) and cytoplasmic ribonucleic acid (RNA).[35]

Folic acid deficiency can be both a cause and a result of intestinal malabsorption. When the condition is an acquired deficiency disease, as in tropical sprue, therapy with folic acid may reverse the atrophic changes in the small intestine. When the defect is primary in the intestine, as seems to be the case in celiac disease, folic acid fails to correct the intestinal disorder, but a gluten-free diet may be successful. See the discussion earlier in this chapter on the malabsorption syndrome. Intestinal resections, strictures and blind loops cause loss of absorptive surface and there may also be detrimental effects exerted by bacterial growth through competing for folic acid or by causing injury to the absorptive surface of the intestine. Vitamin B_{12}, fats, calcium, iron, etc. may also be poorly absorbed. Folic acid, unlike B_{12}, is readily absorbed under normal conditions, from the upper part of the small intestine.

Maternal and infantile deficiencies of folic acid probably result from increased demand when intake is inadequate. In liver cirrhosis the metabolic conversion of folic to folinic acid may be disturbed.

Folic acids appears to be necessary for the transformation of megaloblasts into red blood cells; it is not, however, the maturation factor present in liver extract, nor is it the extrinsic factor. Folic acid usually causes remission in pernicious anemia, but response may be incomplete and relapse may occur during treatment; furthermore, neurologic lesions may progress during therapy. On the other hand, folic acid produces a satisfactory remission in sprue, tropical macrocytic anemia, "refractory megaloblastic anemia," the macrocytic anemia occurring in some cases of hepatic cirrhosis, the macrocytic anemia of pregnancy, and the megaloblastic anemia of infancy.

Some work indicates that B_{12} may be necessary to make available the naturally occurring pteroylglutamates. The role of folic acid in human nutrition needs much further clarification.

Choline, a constituent of lecithin, occurs in many foods, both animal and vegetable: liver, heart, kidney, sweetbreads, brain, egg yolk, nuts, roots and green leafy vegetables.

Choline is an essential component of acetylcholine and of the phospholipids. With methionine, cystine and creatine, it performs an important function in the general metabolic process of transmethylation. It promotes growth, facilitates fat transport, aids protein metabolism, and indirectly is important in promoting normal carbohydrate metabolism. Lack of choline produces in certain experimental animals liver changes similar to Laennec's cirrhosis in man. Choline has been used with favorable results in treating human hepatic cirrhosis, presumably by mobilization of fatty acids from the excess fat deposits in the liver. Its exact position in human nutrition has not yet been determined.

Inositol. A number of studies indicate that inositol acts synergistically with choline in reducing abnormal hepatic fat deposits in experimental animals. In view of its lipotropic activity, it is probably significant that inositol is a constituent of certain phospholipids. Little is known of the nutritional value of inositol in man.

In diabetes mellitus inositol excretion in the urine is high. Apparently it competes with glucose for resorption by the renal tubular cells. In diabetes mellitus, and in healthy persons during glycosuria from intravenous infusions of glucose, the reabsorption mechanism is inhibited and large amounts of inositol appear in the urine.[7] Whether this is harmful is not known. These facts and its high content in heart muscle suggest that it may play a role in human nutrition.

Vitamins: Relationship of Adequate vs. Supernormal Intake to Health and Vigor. There is no evidence to support the view that a *higher than adequate normal* intake of any or all vitamins will improve health or energy production or will facilitate growth or resistance to infection. However, when one or more vitamin deficiencies exist, the effect of supplying the factors lacking is strikingly beneficial.

Hypervitaminosis. Not only is excessive vitamin intake valueless in enhancing health, but it may cause serious deleterious effects. Such results from vitamin overdosage have been reported in human beings taking massive amounts of vitamins A or D.

Hypervitaminosis A has caused hard, tender lumps in the extremities and cortical thickening of underlying bones. Additional findings in some patients include fissures of the lips, loss of hair, dry skin, jaundice and hepatomegaly.

Hypervitaminosis D causes bone resorption and metastatic calcification occurs. There is hypercalcemia, hyperphosphatemia, and hypercalciuria. Calcium is deposited in the kidneys especially, as nephrocalcinosis or renal lithiasis; renal failure with uremia may result.

MALNUTRITION AS CAUSE OF DEATH

Death from malnutrition may be manifest, or obscure. That is, when the patient has obviously been suffering from a severe nutritive deficit (perhaps not susceptible of correction, such as anorexia or vomiting from carcinoma of the stomach), it is sometimes impossible to avoid death from starvation, and its cause is clearly apparent. However, the starvation may not be apparent when the cause is not so obvious: for example, in protein deficiency due to chronic nephritis, or in cerebral and peripheral nerve disturbance due to thiamine deficiency. When attention is directed primarily to only one aspect of a problem—for example, the surgical removal of a toxic goiter—death may occur because of failure to recognize and provide for the associated nutritional disturbances. The physician's responsibility consists in recognizing the nutritional aspects of all types of disease and in perceiving the abnormal practices and situations that may lead to malnutrition, so that these factors may be corrected before nutritive defects occur.

SUMMARY

The early detection of the processes leading to weight loss and undernutrition is a task of paramount importance to the physician, the nutritionist and the public-health officer. In analyzing and interpreting the symptoms indicative of malnutrition, the physician has a complex problem, since the symptoms often suggest other etiologies and frequently are vague and, as a rule, multiple in origin, due to the lack of several nutrients. An understanding of the influences leading to nutritive failure, plus knowledge of the essential nutrients and of the indications of their lack, as discussed in this chapter, will prepare the physician to appreciate the significance of symptoms due to malnutrition.

REFERENCES

1a. Albanese, A.: Protein and amino acid requirements of man, *in* Albanese, A., ed.: Protein and Amino Acid Requirements of Mammals, New York, Academic Press, 1950.
1b. Evaluation of Protein Quality. Publication 1100, National Academy of Sciences, National Research Council, Washington, D. C., 1963.
2. Babcock, M., et al.: Nutritional status of industrial workers, Milbank Mem. Fund Quart. 32:323, 1954.
3. Mayer, J.: Physiology of hunger, appetite and satiety, *in* Wohl, M. G., and Goodhart, R. S., eds.: Modern Nutrition in Health and Disease, ed. 4, Philadelphia, Lea & Febiger, 1968.
4. Brosin, H. W.: The psychology of appetite, *in* Wohl, M. G., and Goodhart, R. S., eds.: Modern Nutrition in Health and Disease, ed. 4, Philadelphia, Lea & Febiger, 1968.
5. Burger, G. C. E., Sandstead, H. R., and Drummond, J.: Starvation in western Holland: 1945, Lancet 2:282, 1945.
6. Coursin, D. B.: Convulsive seizures in infants with pyridoxine-deficient diets, J.A.M.A. 154:406, 1954.
7. Daughaday, W., and Larner, J.: The renal excretion of inositol in normal and diabetic human beings, J. Clin. Invest. 33:326, 1954.
8. Davidson, C. S., et al.: A nutritional survey of starvation in a group of young men, J. Lab. Clin. Med. 31:721, 1946.

9. Ershoff, B. H.: Nutrition and the anterior pituitary, Vitamins and Hormones 10:79, 1952.

10. Bothwell, T. H., and Finch, C. A.: Iron Metabolism, Boston, Little, Brown, 1962.

11. Albanese, A., and Orto, L. O.: Proteins and amino acids, in Wohl, M. G., and Goodhart, R. S., eds.: Modern Nutrition in Health and Disease, ed. 4, Philadelphia, Lea & Febiger, 1968.

12. Keys, A., Brozek, J., et al.: The Biology of Human Starvation, Minneapolis, Univ. of Minn., 1950.

13. Krammer, A., Cartwright, G. E., and Wintrobe, M. M.: The anemia of infection, Blood 9:183–188, 1954.

14. Lusk, G.: Physiological effects of undernutrition, Physiol. Rev. 1:523, 1921.

15. MacBryde, C. M., and Elman, R.: Nutritional Requirements in Acute and Chronic Disease, Advances in Internal Medicine, New York, Interscience, 1946.

16. MacBryde, C. M.: Aging, malnutrition and hormones, J. Clin. Nutrition 1:469, 1953.

17. Church, C. F., and Church, H. N. (eds.): Food Values of Portions Commonly Used, ed. 11, Philadelphia, J. B. Lippincott, 1970.

18. Molony, C. J., and Parmelee, A. H.: Convulsions in young infants from B_6 deficiency, J.A.M.A. 154:405, 1954.

19. Mueller, J. F., and Vilter, R. W.: Pyridoxine deficiency in human beings, J. Clin. Invest. 29:193–201, 1950.

20. Pareira, M., Conrad, E., Hicks, W., and Elman, R.: Therapeutic nutrition with tube feeding, J.A.M.A. 156:810–816, 1954.

21a. Perloff, W., et al.: The starvation state and functional hypopituitarism, J.A.M.A. 155:1307–1313, 1954.

21b. Pollack, H., et al.: Calories expended in military activities, Bull. U. S. Army Med. Dept. 74:110, 1944.

22. Rowland, C. V.: Anorexia and Obesity, an issue of International Psychiatry Clinics, 1969.

23. Rose, W. C.: Amino acid requirement of man, Fed. Proc. Am. Soc. Exper. Biol. 8:546, 1949.

24. Schiele, B., and Brozek, J.: Experimental neurosis resulting from semi-starvation in man, Psychosom. Med. 10:31, 1948.

25. Sebrell, W. H., and Harris, R. S., eds.: The Vitamins, ed. 2, New York, Academic Press, 1967.

26. Smith, D. T.: Disturbance of normal bacterial ecology by the administration of antibiotics, with the development of new clinical syndromes, Ann. Int. Med. 37:1135, 1952.

27. McCance, R. A., and Widowson, E. M.: Calorie Deficiencies and Protein Deficiencies, Boston, Little, Brown, 1969.

28. Vilter, R. W.: Vitamin B_{12}, in Wohl, M. G., and Goodhart, R. S., eds.: Modern Nutrition in Health and Disease, ed. 4, Philadelphia, Lea & Febiger, 1968.

29. Wilson, M. W., et al.: Influence of various levels of thiamine intake on physiologic response, J. Am. Dietet. Ass. 25:221, 1949.

30. Medicine in Old Age, Proceedings of Conference at Royal College of Physicians, London, J. A. Agate, ed., Philadelphia, Lippincott, 1966.

31. Zubiran, S., and Gomez-Mont, F.: Endocrine disturbances in chronic human malnutrition, Vitamins and Hormones 11:97, 1953; Zubiran, S., Gomez-Mont, F., and Laguna, J.: Endocrine disturbances and their dietetic background in undernourished in Mexico, Ann. Int. Med. 42:1259, 1955.

32. Watkin, D. M.: Nutrition in the Aged, Chapter 40 in Wohl and Goodhart.[33]

33. Wohl, M., and Goodhart, R.: Modern Nutrition in Health and Disease, ed. 4, Philadelphia, Lea & Febiger, 1968.

34. Moore, C. V.: Iron, Chapter 11 in Wohl and Goodhart.[33]

35. Castle, W. B.: Disorders of the Blood, in Sodeman, W., ed.: Pathologic Physiology, ed. 4, Philadelphia, Saunders, 1967.

36. Best, C. H., and Lucas, C. C.: Choline Malnutrition, in Jolliffe, N., ed.: Clinical Nutrition, New York, Hoeber-Harper, 1962.

37. Gardner, F. H., and Strauss, E. W.: Disorders related to disturbed absorption of the small bowel, Advances in Internal Medicine 10:137, 1960.

38. Brock, J., and Hansen, J.: Protein Deficiency, in Jolliffe, N.: Clinical Nutrition, ed. 2, New York, Hoeber-Harper, 1962.

39. Jolliffe, N.: Clinical Nutrition, ed. 2, pp. 1–87, New York, Hoeber-Harper, 1962.

40. Current Concepts in Intestinal Absorption and Malabsorption, (Symposium), M. H. Floch, ed., Am. J. Clin. Nutrition 22:239–351, 1969.

41. Frimpter, G. W., et al.: Vitamin B_6 dependency syndromes, Am. J. Clin. Nutrition 22:794–805, 1969.

42. Hegsted, D. M.: Present knowledge of calcium, phosphorus and magnesium, Nutrition Reviews 26:65–70, 1968.

43. Mitchell, H., Rynbergen, H., Anderson, L., and Dibble, M.: Cooper's Nutrition in Health and Disease, ed. 15, Philadelphia, Lippincott, 1968.

44. Recommended Dietary Allowances: Food and Nutrition Board, National Research Council, National Academy of Sciences, ed. 7, Publication 1694, Washington, D. C., 1968.

45. Shank, R. E.: A Chink in Our Armor, Nutrition Today (in press), 1970.

46. Nutrition in Human Reproduction: Report of the Committee on Maternal Nutrition, Food and Nutrition Board, National Research Council (in press), 1970.

47. Food Intake and Nutritive Value of Diets in the United States, Agricultural Research Service, U. S. Department of Agriculture, March, 1969.

48. Friend, B.: Nutrients in U. S. food supply; a review of trends, Am. J. Clin. Nutr. 20:907, 1967.

49. U. S. Department of Agriculture: National Food Situation, 122:3, 1967.

50. Report of White House Conference on Food, Nutrition and Health, Dec. 2-4, 1969; J. Mayer, chairman, Washington, D. C., issued January 2, 1970.

51. Joint FAO-WHO Expert Committee on Protein Requirements, WHO Tech. Rep. Ser. No. 301, Rome, 1965.

52. Food and Agriculture Organization of the United Nations: Requirements of Vitamin A, Thiamine, Riboflavin and Niacin, WHO Tech. Rep. Ser. No. 362, Rome, 1967.

53. Halsted, J. A.: Geophagia in man: its nature and nutritional effects, Am. J. Clin. Nutr. 21:1384–1393, 1968.

54. Minnich, V., et al: Pica in Turkey. Effect of clay upon iron absorption, Am. J. Clin. Nutr. 21:78, 1968.

55. Ronaghy, H., et al: Controlled zinc supplementation for malnourished schoolboys: a pilot experiment, Am. J. Clin. Nutr. 22:1279–1289, 1969.

56. Mead, J. F.: Present knowledge of fat, *in* Present Knowledge of Nutrition, ed. 3, Nutrition Foundation, New York, 1967.

57. Keys, A.: The peripatetic nutritionist, Nutrition Today, 1:19–23, 1966, and 2:14–19, 1967.

58. Shaw, J. H.: Present knowledge of fluoride, *in* Present Knowledge of Nutrition, New York, 1967.

59. Report from Executive Council, World Health Organization, re water fluoridation program, J.A.M.A. 208:1198, 1969.

60. Finch, Clement A.: Iron metabolism, Nutrition Today, 4:2–7, 1969.

61. Council on Foods and Nutrition of the American Medical Association: Iron Deficiency in the United States, J.A.M.A. 203:407–412, 1968.

62. Nutrition and Human Needs; Hearings, U. S. Senate. Part 3: The National Nutrition Survey, Washington, D. C., January, 1969.

63. Proceedings of the 7th World Nutrition Congress, 5 vols., Pergamon, 1968.

39

Pigmentation of the Skin

HAROLD JEGHERS and LEON M. EDELSTEIN

FACTORS INVOLVED IN NORMAL SKIN PIGMENTATION

The living human skin normally contains pigments responsible for skin color. Abnormal skin pigmentation can be appreciated only when the range and the many modifying factors of normal skin coloration are thoroughly understood. Consequently, a considerable portion of our presentation of skin pigmentation will be devoted to the normal skin color.

METHODS OF ANALYSIS OF SKIN COLOR

At the very beginning of his examination, the doctor discovers much of importance

The authors acknowledge the contributions of Edward A. Edwards, co-author of this chapter in the early editions, and Herbert Mescon, co-author for the 4th Edition.

merely by noting the color of his patient's skin. In optical terms, we say that the eye has been stimulated by light reflected from the skin. When properly interpreted, the message carried by this reflected light can prove helpful in appraising the clinical status of the patient.

Observation of skin color of patients admitted to a hospital at night should be repeated later in bright daylight. Many hospital rooms and wards are too dark, even during the day. Examination must be done in good daylight to permit proper inspection of the body surface.

Light impinging on the skin is not simply reflected from the very surface. The human skin is translucent. Light penetrates the various layers of the epidermis, the dermis, and even the more superficial strata of the subcutaneous tissue (Fig. 39-1). We may think of these layers as a series of colored screens, since normally each contains some pigment. The term *pigment* is used here to denote any colored material present in the skin, whether deposited in the tissue proper or present in the blood passing through the skin—and not merely melanin, too often thought of as the only important skin pigment. This broad concept of skin pigment is necessary to understand properly normal and abnormal skin color. As the light strikes each layer of the skin, a portion is absorbed, some is transmitted, and some is reflected. Of each portion transmitted, some will be reflected from a deeper layer. Thus, each reflected portion returns to the surface modified by the pigment of the complex skin structure. The reflected light carries two varieties of information. In its aggregate, it can be appreciated as skin color. Secondly, by analysis of this reflected light, one can determine the contributions of the various pigments to the color.

The human eye is an admirable instrument for the first type of information, that is, color per se. Even this function is poorly performed at times, because of the prevalence of poor color sensitivity, as well as the rarer forms of color blindness. Moreover, it is impossible to record or to tell others the color of a skin area in any fashion that is qualitatively reproducible. This difficulty is resolved to a certain extent by the use of color comparators, such as color charts or color tops.

An entirely objective measurement and recording of color is possible through the use of the spectrophotometer, a technic first used in 1926 by Sheard, Brown, and Brunsting for the analysis of the skin color.[1,2,3,4] The highly accurate Hardy recording spectrophotometer, introduced in 1935, was used by Edwards and Duntley and their associates[5,6,7,8] and by Buckley and Grum[64,65] for additional and expanded studies not previously possible. Further simplification of this approach for use of skin reflectance has per-

mitted large-scale studies of skin color in humans.[88,89] As a result of such investigations, analysis of skin color has been placed on a rational basis and is now explainable in both quantitative and qualitative terms. The use of these instruments must still be looked upon as a research procedure and not directly utilizable for clinical practice, but much that is applicable to medicine has been learned through their use. The objective measurement of color is expressed in terms synonymous with those used by physicists. Thus, the physicist expresses color in terms of *dominant wave length, relative brightness*, and *excitation purity* to correspond with *hue, brightness,* and *saturation.*

Lerner and his co-workers[76,77] have developed a relatively simple quantitative method for measuring skin color by photography and reflectance measurements, which is a useful additional method of study.

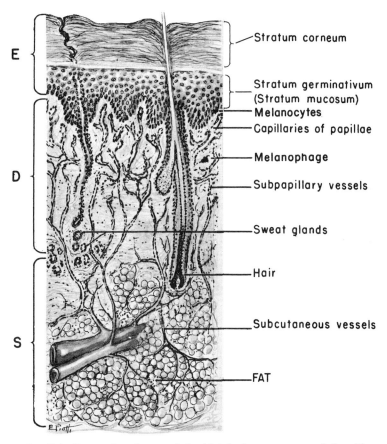

FIG. 39-1. Composite picture of the histologic appearance of the skin (semidiagrammatic). (E) The extent of the epidermis. (D) The dermis (corium). (S) The subcutaneous tissue (E. A. Edwards)

The eye is inaccurate and may fail entirely in appreciating the second variety of information contained in the skin reflectance: the identity and relative quantity of the pigments contributing to the color. It is particularly for this kind of information that spectrophotometry has been so useful. Infrared photography has been successfully used to study certain aspects of skin color changes not readily visible to the eye, e.g., vascular patterns in the skin.[94]

A material is a pigment by virtue of absorbing some particular wave lengths in the visible spectrum. A pure white substance has absorption entirely outside the visible spectrum. A substance is pure black in color because of complete absorption of all light rays within the visible spectral range. Gray color of a substance is due to partial but uniform absorption of all visible spectral rays; light gray representing less absorption than dark gray. Any color is produced by absorption of some and reflection of other light rays from the visible spectrum. The total light reflected from the skin contains the absorption bands of each pigment in the skin, identifiable by spectrophotometry. In the accompanying reproduction of curves obtained by the use of the Hardy instrument

(Figs. 39-4, 39-7–39-9, 39-11–39-14), the reflectance values of the skin, or transmission values of solutions of pigments, are shown for all wave lengths from the violet limit of visibility at 400 mμ, to the red limit at 700 mμ. Each pigment has a zone or zones characteristic of it which are known as its *absorption bands*. The finding of such bands in the curve indicates the presence of the corresponding pigments. Moreover, since the extent of light absorption is proportional to the amount of pigment present, one can give an estimate of the quantity of the pigment.[5,6]

Analysis of human skin color by means of spectrophotometry is indicative of the importance of the science of physics to medical research.[9] However, in actual practice, physicians judge skin color by total visual impression. With a proper understanding of basic science concepts, this provides considerable useful information for clinical diagnosis.

SOURCES OF SKIN COLOR

Figure 39-1 gives, in semischematic form, the characteristic histologic appearance of a section of the skin with emphasis upon the components important in skin color. On the surface of the skin is the keratinized layer (stratum corneum). Beneath this is a small

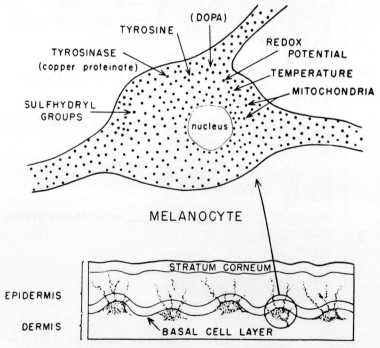

FIG. 39-2. Biochemical factors controlling melanin formation. (Fitzpatrick and Lerner: A.M.A. Arch. Derm. Syph. 69: 133)

clear layer, which represents the stratum lucidum (present only in the palms and soles) and the stratum granulosum. Above the dermis and beneath the clear layer is the stratum germinativum (stratum mucosum). Collectively, these various layers are called the *epidermis*. The stratum germinativum is composed of a small basal cell layer, and a larger prickle cell layer. Melanocytes exist in the basal layer of the epidermis (Fig. 39-2).

The basal layer of the epidermis contains conical indentations of dermis, which contain terminal capillary loops derived from the superficial subpapillary blood vessels. The dermis normally contains cells called melanophages* (which phagocytize but do not form melanin), as well as dermal melanocytes. The subcutaneous tissue contains hair follicles and shafts and fat cells, all of which play their role in skin color.

Ordinarily, melanin is present in melanocytes, located chiefly at the dermoepidermal junction, as well as in epithelial cells throughout the epidermis, including the stratum corneum. Carotene is also present in the stratum corneum.

Four pigments and the additional optical effect called *scattering* have been found to be responsible for normal skin color.[5] Whether the sweat glands contribute to color, however, is not clear. The main pigments of the dermis are oxyhemoglobin and reduced hemoglobin present in the papillary capillary projections and superficial subpapillary vascular plexuses. The pigments of the subcutaneous layer include carotene in the fat, and oxyhemoglobin and reduced hemoglobin present in the deeper vascular plexuses.

Scattering consists of a rearrangement of light as it passes through a turbid medium, whereby the reflected light shows a preponderance of the lower wave lengths (blue colors).[5] In other words, the light is rendered "more blue" or "less red." All of the skin pigments are yellow or red in hue. Spectrophotometrically, brown is a yellow of low purity. The skin is turbid, particularly in the basal layers of the epidermis. The resultant scattering offsets to some extent the otherwise extreme redness of the pig-

* The change in the terminology of pigment-producing cells was decided at the Third Conference on the Biology of Normal and Atypical Pigment Cell Growth.[50,51] Under this new terminology an adult melanin-producing cell is called a "melanocyte" instead of a "melanoblast" and a cell engulfing melanin a "melanophage" instead of a chromatophore.

ments (Plate 4) and gives a composite color, which we appreciate as "flesh color."

Scattering additionally accounts for the blue color shown by heavy masses of pigment of whatever nature, lying deeply within or beneath the skin (Plate 4). Rare exceptions occur, such as the red color of cinnabar and green color of chromate tattooing. The heavy mass of pigment absorbs almost all of the red light rays penetrating to it. The major part of the light reflected from such an area is that scattered from the turbid basal epidermis, and is therefore predominantly blue. This subject will be discussed in further detail later.

In the epidermis, **melanin** is formed by spe-

DISTRIBUTION OF MELANIN

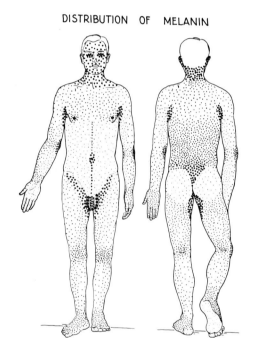

FIG. 39-3. The bodily distribution of melanin. Note primary areas of accentuation in the eyelids, the axillae, the nipples, the areolae, the nape of the neck, the umbilicus, the linear nigra, and the genito-anal region. Accentuation on the face due to sunlight exposure and at the elbows and knees due to friction. Note the small amount of melanin on the palms and soles.

With the exception of the eyelids, the ears, the axillae, the perineum, and the penis, the data were derived from spectrophotometry. The scalp was omitted from consideration. (Edwards and Duntley: Amer. J. Anat. 65:1)

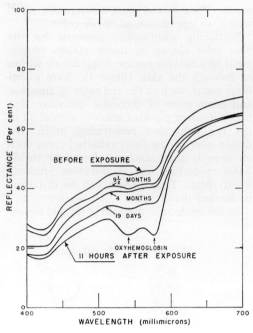

FIG. 39-4. Spectrophotometric curves of the skin after a single exposure to sunlight. Hyperemia (oxyhemoglobin bands at arrows) is maximum at 11 hours, melanin at 19 days, and melanoid at 4 months. Blood stagnation, as registered by evidence of reduced hemoglobin (blunting of oxyhemoglobin bands and depression of peak between them), persists from the early disappearance of the hyperemia for the entire duration of the experiment. (Edwards and Duntley: Science 20:235)

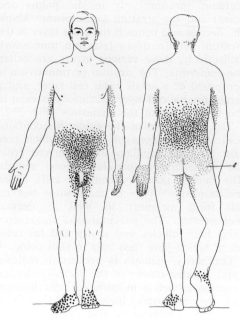

DISTRIBUTION OF VENOUS BLOOD

FIG. 39-5. The bodily distribution of predominantly venous blood. Areas not included here or in Figure 39-6 show no special predominance, except that investigation was not made of the regions noted under Figure 39-3. (Edwards and Duntley: Amer. J. Anat. 65:1)

cialized cells (melanocytes) located chiefly in the basal layer. The melanin granules are transmitted to the adjacent and overlying epidermal cells. In the process of keratinization, as the epidermal cells advance toward the surface, the pigment granules that they contain proceed with them. An occasional melanocyte also can be visualized proceeding toward the keratin layer.[71] Electronmicroscopy studies indicate that the basal melanin particles are regular and constant in form and configuration.[57] A congenital inability to form melanin is seen in albino individuals. The formation of melanin is a vital process. As the basal cells are pushed superficially in the growth of the epidermis, the cells become progressively lifeless and the granules of melanin disintegrate. In a fair-skinned person, melanin granules are not only fewer in number but smaller in size and occupy one or two lower layers of epi-

thelium. In persons of darker complexion melanin granules are larger in size and more numerous, occupying somewhat more rows of cells. Edwards and Duntley[5] noted that the disintegration of melanin gives rise to a diffuse derived pigment, which they termed *melanoid*, whose exact chemical composition or significance is still to be determined. It appears to have an absorption band in the visible violet at 400 mμ and to give the skin a yellowish sallow appearance if present in excess. Others[78] feel that melanin in fine particulate form occurring in the stratum corneum, in conjunction with strong hemoglobin absorption bands in the 400- to 420-mμ range, could account for the changes noted in the skin reflectance curve in this range.

Although present in the skin in particulate form, melanin behaves spectrophotometrically as though in solution. It shows its greatest absorption in the ultraviolet; yet it has strong absorption in the visible spectrum too, with fair transmission only toward the red. Examined in various dilutions, its color ranges from a brown when diluted, to yellow, orange, and finally orange-red when concentrated.

The basic or primary melanin formation of an individual is unrelated to exposure to sunlight and follows a definite pattern (Fig. 39-3). Szabo has painstakingly studied the melanocyte population in different regions of the body,[70] and in different layers of the skin. He has demonstrated that there is a normal population of dermal melanocytes which can be stimulated with ultraviolet irradiation and that their response is similar to that of basal melanocytes.

Melanin is a powerful pigment, and when much is present, as after tanning, or in the dark races, it effectively obscures the other pigments in the skin. In such people, observations of color change are possible only in regions primarily poor in melanin, as in palms, soles, and certain mucous membranes.[78]

Melanin may give rise to blue effects, through scattering, when massed deep in the dermis. Normally this occurs in the eyelids and axillae, in which the material is present in dermal melanophages (chromatophores) or in a hairy area which has been shaved, as in the male cheek, where melanin is present in the deep-lying hair bulbs.

Melanin appears to be the main pigment of the hair, although some additional pigments have been discovered recently. Pheomelanin is a yellow granular alkaline soluble pigment found in red hair.[66] At present it seems that pheomelanin is a combination of the melanin polymer with cysteine.[90] Variations in hair color correspond to differences noted in varying dilutions of melanin.

Oxyhemoglobin and Reduced Hemoglobin. The constant perfusion of the cutaneous and subcutaneous tissues by blood compels one to consider the pigments of the blood as cutaneous pigments. The vessels penetrated by light and thus contributing to skin color are arranged in three beds: (1) vessels of the dermal papillae, mainly capillaries; (2) the subpapillary plexus, made up predominantly of veins; and (3) the subcutaneous vessels, in which only the large veins are prominent visually. The subpapillary venous plexus presents the largest surface area of the three vascular beds. The subcutaneous veins show up mainly as blue, through the phenomenon of scattering. It is apparent, then, that the blood pigments exert their effect on skin color chiefly by their presence in the papillary and subpapillary networks.

What are the pigments involved? Those of

DISTRIBUTION OF ARTERIAL BLOOD

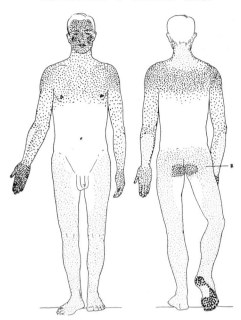

FIG. 39-6. The bodily distribution of predominantly arterial blood. Areas not included here or in Figure 39-5 show no special predominance, except that investigation was not made of the regions noted under Figure 39-3. (Edwards and Duntley: Amer. J. Anat. 65:1)

the blood plasma, yellow in color, but usually quite pale, are without much effect on normal skin color. **Hemoglobin** constitutes the important pigment material. Hemoglobin exists in the red cells in both the reduced and the oxidized form. Each has a distinct absorption spectrum and color. Oxyhemoglobin, the more brilliantly red of the two, is especially characterized in the spectrum by absorption bands at 542 and 576 mμ. Reduced hemoglobin is darker and less red, or (one might say) more blue. Its curve shows a single band at 556, replacing the twin bands of oxyhemoglobin. The proportion of hemoglobin which is oxidized varies with the class of vessel under scrutiny. Thus, in arteries, the quantity of oxidized hemoglobin is from 90 to 95 per cent; in the veins it is about 50 per cent; whereas in the capillaries the value lies between the arterial and venous levels. The subpapillary venous plexus has a larger surface area than the papillary capillary network. This is the main reason why the oxyhemoglobin bands in most areas of the skin are considerably replaced by those of reduced hemoglobin. In some areas, the fine veins are unusually prominent, whereas the capillaries are poorly developed. Such areas of venous preponderance are to be found in the lower trunk and on the dorsa of the feet (Fig. 39-5). In certain areas, on the contrary, the arterial flow and capillary perfusion are comparatively great, with a corresponding prominence of oxyhemoglobin. This is especially true in the head and neck, the palms, the soles, and in the skin over the ischial tuberosities. To the eye, these areas are considerably redder than the surrounding skin (Fig. 39-6).

The over-all contribution of hemoglobin to skin color will vary with the total quantity of that material, as in anemia or polycythemia. *Rapid changes in skin color are entirely due to changes in vessel caliber, in blood flow, and the degree of hemoglobin oxidation* (Fig. 39-7). Arterial dilation results in an increased capillary perfusion, with reddening of the skin, because of the presence of more hemoglobin, whereas arterial constriction or obstruction induces the opposite effect—a pale skin, because of a re-

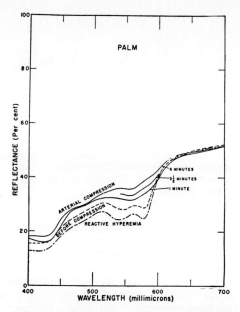

FIG. 39-7. The effects of ischemia in changing the appearance of the palm. A manometer cuff on the arm was quickly inflated above systolic pressure. In 1 minute, the curve has lost its evidence of oxyhemoglobin, and the general shape of the curve shows this to be due mainly to an increase in the reduced form.

As ischemia continues, the 3½- and 6-minute curves show less and less absorption by reduced hemoglobin, indicating a progressive diminution of blood in the skin. Vasoconstriction of cutaneous vessels may be responsible. In these relatively bloodless curves, the absorption band of carotene at 482 mμ, previously obscured, now becomes evident. Upon deflation of the cuff, reactive hyperemia is evidenced by the greatly increased absorption, with strong evidence of oxyhemoglobin. (Edwards)

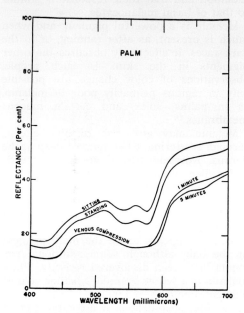

FIG. 39-8. Venous distention in the skin in response to posture and to venous compression. The palm becomes darker with the subject standing and the hand dependent. The increased absorption is caused by the presence of more hemoglobin, but the slight blunting of the twin bands of oxyhemoglobin and the general shape of the curve show this to be due mainly to an increase in the reduced form.

Compression of the arm by a manometer cuff inflated below diastolic pressure gives a further increase in the amount of reduced hemoglobin present. With continued compression, the amount of reduced hemoglobin increases for about 5 minutes, at which time the veins seem to have reached their limit of distensibility. The portion of the curve shown reveals further reduction of the hemoglobin present, but no increase in total amount. Fatigue of the veins with further distensibility undoubtedly would occur with greatly prolonged compression. The absorption band at 660 mμ in the 5-minute curve is unexplained. (E. A. Edwards)

PLATE 4

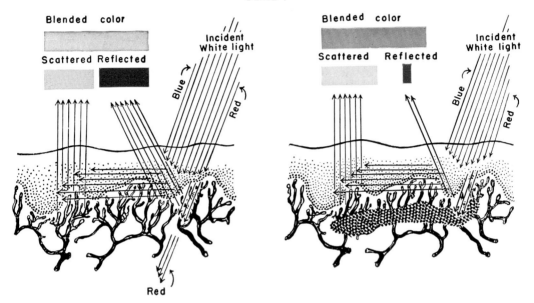

(*Left*) Incident white light (composed of spectral rays—violet, indigo, blue, green, yellow, orange and red) strikes the skin with differential absorption, transmission and reflectance at each layer. Note the reflection of some red rays from the hemoglobin in papillary capillaries and the transmission of other red rays through living tissue to give the red color of transillumination. The turbidity of the lower layers of the epidermis scatters the blue rays back to the surface. The composite of reflected red and scattered blue light blended gives to normal skin its "flesh-color" appearance.

(*Right*) The large mass of pigment present in the dermis (corium) absorbs most of the red spectral light rays, permitting reflection or transmission of only a small portion of them. Blue spectral light rays are scattered not only from deeper layers of the epidermis (as is true normally) but also from the pigment mass, resulting in a marked increase in the amount of blue light returned to the skin surface. The composite of the increased scattered blue light and minimal reflected red light gives the skin over the pigment mass a blue color. The mass in the dermis represents any of the types of pigment described in the text under Scattering Phenomenon, Blue Coloration. (Courtesy of Edward A. Edwards)

duction in the quantity of hemoglobin viewed, and a diminution in the degree of its oxidation. The capillaries are probably not capable of change in caliber independent of such changes in the arteries or veins. Interference with venous outflow depends upon posture, venous constriction, or obstruction. Under these circumstances, both the quantity and ratio of reduced hemoglobin are increased (Fig. 39-8). A comparison of visual analysis of vascular change with spectrophotometric examination demonstrates that the eye appreciates quite well the increase in quantity and ratio of reduced hemoglobin under these circumstances.

An obstruction to venous outflow may exist simultaneously with either arterial constriction or dilation, adding the bluer hue of reduced hemoglobin to the paleness of the arterial constriction or to the ruddiness of arterial dilation.

Cyanosis is appreciated when reduced

hemoglobin is present in concentrations of 5 Gm. or more per 100 ml. of blood. Cyanosis may be general (because of insufficient aeration) or local (because of obstruction to the venous flow).

An intensely red skin does not necessarily mean arterial dilation and increased capillary flow. The hands and feet occasionally may be cold, but still bright red, with evidence of highly oxygenated hemoglobin. Such findings suggest the lack of utilization of oxygen by the tissues. This is seen when the part is subjected to *extreme cold*, because very little oxygen exchange takes place at low temperature levels. It may be that lowered tissue utilization of oxygen when it exists in other conditions, such as lowered metabolism, may influence skin color. In other instances, such a change would appear to depend upon the opening of the normal arteriovenous communications of the hands or feet. Of course, it may be seen also in the presence of abnormal arteriovenous fistulae as well, especially when the fistulae are multiple and small.

Carotene is the yellow pigment of the sub-

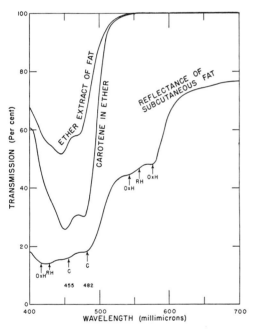

FIG. 39-9. The reflectance of the removed subcutaneous fat from a cadaver, compared with the transmission of its ether extract and with a known solution of carotene in ether. The absorption of carotene at 455 and 482 mμ are evident in all three curves. Only the band at 482 mμ is pronounced in the curves of living skin. Absorption bands of hemoglobin are noted in the fat specimen. Some of the pigment has been oxidized by exposure to the air. (Edwards and Duntley: Amer. J. Anat. 65:1)

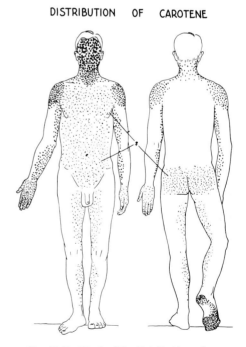

FIG. 39-10. The bodily distribution of carotene. With the exception of the regions listed under Fig. 39-3, which were not examined, the unshaded areas were particularly poor in carotene. (Edwards and Duntley: Amer. J. Anat. 65:1)

cutaneous fat. The term is used here to include a group of related carotenoids. It is found likewise in the cornified superficial layer of the epidermis and in the sebaceous glands, and also in the blood plasma[5] in a slight and variable amount.

Carotene shows absorption bands at 455 and 482 mμ (Fig. 39-9). Its color in concentrated form is a golden yellow. Spectrophotometric analysis of skin color has shown that carotene is an important normal skin color component. It shows regional variations in quantity closely resembling the pattern of arterial preponderance (Fig. 39-10). Carotene, being lipid soluble, is present maximally in lipid-rich subcutaneous areas (buttock and breast) and in those areas where surface lipid is high either from sebum secretion (face) or from lipids released in areas of most active keratinization, i.e., palms and soles.

The human subject obtains carotene mainly through the ingestion of fruits and vegetables. Intestinal absorption of carotene requires the presence of dietary fat and bile acids. In the liver, enzymatic conversion to vitamin A takes place. Excess carotene is either destroyed metabolically or excreted in sebum and possibly, to some minor degree, in the urine.

More than 30 pigments constitute the lipochrome or carotenoid group of pigments widespread in nature in plants and some animal substances. The majority have a yellow color; others are yellow to red in hue. Only four of these (alpha-carotene, beta-carotene, gamma-carotene, and cryptoxanthine) have provitamin A activity, and these collectively or separately are the ones commonly known as carotene, and are the carotenoid pigments most important in skin color in man.

NORMAL SWEAT AND SEBUM. These have not

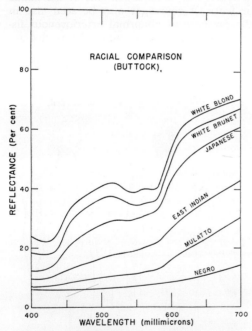

FIG. 39-11. Comparison of readings from the buttocks of males of different racial groups. This area was chosen as one in which pigment content would be minimally disturbed by exposure to sunlight. The curves vary only in their melanin content. Note how readily the oxyhemoglobin and carotene absorption bands can be seen in the spectral reflection curve in the white blond, and their obliteration by the increased melanin in the skin of those more heavily pigmented. (Edwards and Duntley: Amer. J. Anat. 65:1)

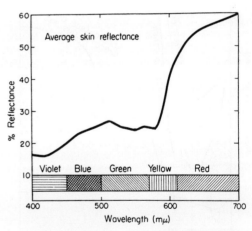

FIG. 39-12. Reflectance curve; average skin left cheek. Note the dips at approximately 415, 542, and 575 mμ. These are due to oxyhemoglobin. They are blunted when there is more reduced hemoglobin, which has a band at 555 mμ. The absorption slope from 465 to 510 mμ is due to carotenoids, which have a maximal absorption band at 480 mμ. In general, more red and yellow are reflected, and less green, blue, and violet. This explains the visual appearance of normal skin. (Buckley, W. R., and Grum, F.: Reflection spectrophotometry; use in evaluation of skin pigmentary disturbances, Arch. Derm. 83:249-261)

been found to affect skin color appreciably. When allowed to accumulate excessively, the secretion may obscure the skin's surface. However, sebum contains a little carotene, and when intake of this substance is unusually high, areas of much sebaceous secretion may appear to be yellow. This accounts, in part, for the characteristic localization of the yellow color to the greasy portion of the face in carotenemia.

PATTERNS OF NORMAL SKIN COLOR

BASIC PATTERN AND INDIVIDUAL VARIATION

Classifications of patterns of skin pigmentation are to be mentioned in reference to race, sex, and age. It is important to emphasize, however, that the particular skin colors of any two individuals falling into the same category as far as these factors are concerned, always will show some difference. It is often unsafe to make deductions of variation in color by comparing one subject with another. It is much safer to compare differences in color of one area with another in the same person, or of the same area at different times. The spectrophotometric reflectance of normal skin of the cheek and the explanation for its red-yellow rather than blue-violet visual appearance is given in Figure 39-12.

Age. It is apparent that skin color is considerably influenced by age. Darkening of the areas of primary melanin occurs in both sexes with puberty. In general, the skin darkens with age. At times a distinct melanosis is seen in senile individuals. This seems to be due to a progressive increase in melanin deposit. Evidence suggests that the younger skin also shows a more active circulation and a greater quantity of carotene. Definitive spectrophotometric analyses of age changes in skin color are not available.

The regional distribution of the pigments has been portrayed individually (Figs. 39-3, 39-5, 39-6, 39-10). It is apparent that different regions of the body vary in skin color because of their particular content of the pigments. Differences in thickness of the skin are also of undoubted importance, because a heavy epidermis will cause more scattering. Thickening of the cornified epidermis may add greater quantity of carotene, and possibly melanin. Areas in which the stratum corneum is thinnest, such as mucous membrane surfaces, accentuate the hemoglobin pigments.

Rapid variations in color, because of changes in blood vessel caliber and flow, are particularly marked in the hands, the feet, and the face. One should attempt to approximate basal conditions before giving much weight to changes in color in these regions.

RACIAL VARIATIONS

Spectrophotometry has confirmed histologic evidence that variations in the content of melanin are alone responsible for the differences in color of the various races.[15,78]

Gates and Zimmerman[52] have correlated racial coloration with melanin in the epidermis, but not with the sparse amounts of the pigment in the melanophages of the dermis. Shizume and Lerner[53] have found approximately the same level of pituitary melanocyte-stimulating hormone in Negroes as in whites. There are racial differences in melanogenesis before and after ultraviolet light stimulation as demonstrated by ultrastructural studies.[91,92,93]

The colors of the skins of the races can be arranged in a series conforming to the graduations of color in solutions of melanin of varying strength[5] (Fig. 39-11). No evidence has been found to support the theory (which is occasionally stated) that the pigmentation of the dark races is due to pigment not normally found in "the white race," or to an increase of the ordinary pigments other than melanin.

The heavy melanin deposit of the dark races, especially of the Negro, considerably obscures the other pigments.[78] Nevertheless, regions of the body with the least melanin deposit, such as the palms and soles, still may furnish valuable information regarding skin color.

SEX DIFFERENCES AND THE EFFECTS OF THE SEX HORMONES

Spectrophotometry indicates that the ruddier appearance of the male is caused by the presence in the skin of more blood (hemoglobin) and melanin than in the female. Contrariwise, the female possesses more carotene than does the male.

The regional patterns of pigment distribution differ somewhat between the two sexes. Females show stronger areas of primary melanization in the nape of the neck, the linea nigra, and axilla than do males. The contrast in amount of melanin deposit, between areas richly supplied and those poorly supplied, is more marked in the female than in the male. The buttocks of the female shows a slight arterial preponderance, rather than a venous one as in the male. Finally, females show good evidence of carotene in the breast, abdomen, and buttocks, regions which are poor in carotene in the male.

Study of castrated men and ovariectomized women gives evidence that much of the sex difference in color is genetic and not subject to complete disappearance, or reversal, upon removal of the gonads. This is not to gainsay that the gonads affect skin color considerably through their internal secretions. It is noteworthy that reactions to these sex hormones take place in the entire skin of the human, rather than in specialized zones as in other animals. A possible exception is the areolar hyperpigmentation resulting from direct application of estrogen cream.

Effects of Castration in the Male. From visual observations, it was believed that the pale sallow skin of the male castrate was due to a deficiency in melanin, but spectrophotometry indicates that melanin produc-

tion in the castrate or eunuchoid individual is only slightly diminished.

The factor mainly responsible for the abnormal color of the castrate is a pronounced reduction in cutaneous blood flow, the hemoglobin being reduced in quantity and in the degree of oxidation. Areas characterized by a large venous bed showed evidence of venous dilation and stagnation, with a real increase in reduced hemoglobin.

Carotene is substantially increased in the skin of the castrate, and could be a factor in giving the sallow appearance to these individuals.

All of the changes enumerated can be reversed by the administration of male sex hormone.

The Hormonal Control of Skin Color in the Female. The effects of the sex hormones are well-shown in the female by the changes after ovariectomy, as well as those incident to the menstrual cycle.

As in the male, removal of the gonads causes a diminution in superficial cutaneous

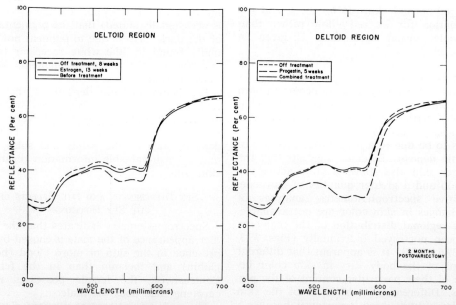

FIG. 39-13. Spectrophotometric curves of the deltoid region of an ovariectomized subject. On the left, the pretreatment curve is low in hemoglobin content, and with dominance of the reduced form. After treatment with estrogen, the curve shows a real increase in oxyhemoglobin. With cessation of treatment, the curve reverts to its pretreatment character.

On the right, the administration of progestin produces a marked increase in oxyhemoglobin. The combined use of progestin and estrogen diminishes the hemoglobin content, causing the curve to revert to its off-treatment level. (Edwards and Duntley: Amer. J. Obstet Gynec. 57:501) blood flow, with a lowered amount of hemoglobin and a relative increase in its reduced form (Fig. 39-13). Administration of estrogen is followed by an increased blood flow and an increase in oxyhemoglobin. Progestin increases the degree of oxidation of hemoglobin, but does not consistently increase the total hemoglobin present. The simultaneous administration of both products gives the

paradoxical result of a diminution of the quantity of hemoglobin, with a predominance of the reduced form. The spectrophotometric evidence available fails to show any changes in melanin attributable to variations in estrogen or progestin levels. However, there have been reports of chloasma resulting from progestational oral contraceptives.[87]

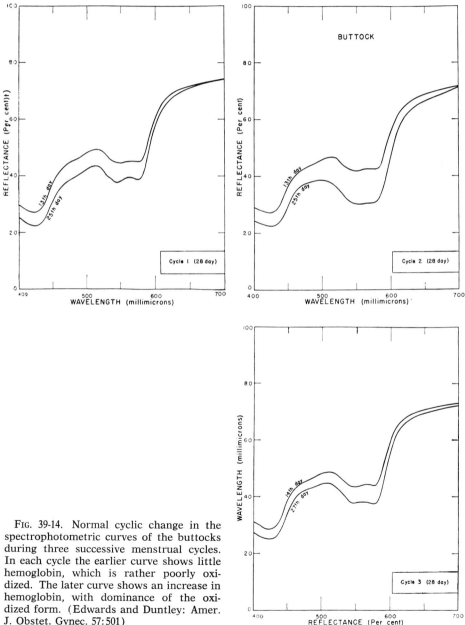

Fig. 39-14. Normal cyclic change in the spectrophotometric curves of the buttocks during three successive menstrual cycles. In each cycle the earlier curve shows little hemoglobin, which is rather poorly oxidized. The later curve shows an increase in hemoglobin, with dominance of the oxidized form. (Edwards and Duntley: Amer. J. Obstet. Gynec. 57:501)

Normal Pigmentation of the Skin

Skin color in health is produced by a composite of the four following pigments in normal amounts

  CAROTENE

  MELANIN

  OXYHEMOGLOBIN

  REDUCED HEMOGLOBIN

plus the optical effect of

  SCATTERING PHENOMENON

due to turbidity of normal epidermis

Increased Pigmentation of the Skin

  YELLOW PIGMENTATIONS (see Table 39–2)

  HEMOGLOBIN PIGMENTATIONS (see Table 39–3)

  MELANIN PIGMENTATIONS (see Table 39–4)

  METALLIC PIGMENTATIONS (see Table 39–5)

  EXAGGERATED SCATTERING PHENOMENON produced by excess of normal or presence of abnormal pigments in the corium (Table 39–6)

  MISCELLANEOUS PIGMENTATIONS

Decreased Pigmentation of the Skin

  DIMINISHED AMOUNT OF HEMOGLOBIN (ANEMIA)

  DECREASED OR ABSENT MELANIN

  EDEMA OF THE SKIN

  DIMINISHED BLOOD FLOW TO THE SKIN

  SCAR TISSUE

  MACERATED OR DESQUAMATING SKIN

It will be recalled that, contrary to the situation in the male, the output of the sex hormones in the female fluctuates widely in different times of the menstrual cycle. Early, before ovulation, neither estrogen nor progestin is present in appreciable quantity. At this time the woman's skin resembles that of the ovariectomized subject. After midcycle there is greatly increased superficial blood flow, with a maximum in the premenstrual period. This is consistent with the high estrogen production of the proliferative stage, during ovulation, and the immediate postovulatory period. Progestin is produced in the presecretory phase leading up to the premenstrual period, and the combined effect of the two hormones finally lowers the cutaneous circulation to the level observed at the beginning of the cycle (Fig. 39-14).

SKIN COLOR CHANGES AFTER EXPOSURE TO SUNLIGHT

These depend as much on blood vessel effect as on melanin synthesis. Edwards and Duntley[7] followed these changes after a single heavy exposure (Fig. 39-4). The initial hyperemia and redness increased to a maximum 11 hours after exposure. An increase in melanin was apparent in two days and reached its maximum on the nineteenth day. The early hyperemia was followed by a venous enlargement and stasis, which contributed considerably to the darkness of the tanned skin.

Since all persons are customarily exposed to sunlight, with much variation in the potency of actinic rays as well as in the area of skin exposed, the effect of sunlight exposure always must be considered by physicians in their evaluation of skin color.

Fortunately, the changes in skin color resulting from exposure to sunlight produce a surface pattern area that usually can be recognized (e.g., shape of the bathing suit, sleeve length, neckline, etc.).

Findlay[80] has shown that vasoconstriction and vasodilation affect production of melanin by ultraviolet light. This may in part explain the difference in skin color described previously because of hormonal influence on blood flow. It has not generally been appreciated that longer wave ultraviolet light and even ordinary artificial light may play an appreciable role in melanin darkening and production.[81,82]

INCREASED PIGMENTATION OF THE SKIN

Increased pigmentation of the skin may involve hemoglobin, melanin, or carotene, physiologically normal pigments (but present in excess amounts) or other pigments of endogenous or exogenous origin. Table 39-1 contains a classification of increased pigmentation of the skin based on material presented by Jeghers[10] in detail elsewhere. The reader is referred to this source for more complete clinical descriptions and for a detailed bibliography on this subject.

By curious coincidence, almost all of the causes of increased skin pigmentation not due to hemoglobin, melanin, or metallic pigmentation produce a yellow color and can be grouped together under the designation "yellow pigmentation."[10] The most important ones and their clinical characteristics are listed in Table 39-2.[10] These possibilities should be investigated in any patient presenting a predominantly yellow color of the skin.

Jaundice is the most common cause of a yellow skin color. A small amount of bilirubin, usually 0.3 to 1.0 mg. per 100 ml. of serum, is normally present in the blood. However, this small amount is not detectable even spectrophotometrically in normal skin color. The serum bilirubin must reach 2 to 4 mg. before jaundice is clinically detectable. Elevation of serum bilirubin without visible icterus is often called "latent jaundice." It is believed that when jaundice is developing, tissue staining, detectable upon clinical observation, lags behind plasma staining as indicated by elevations of the serum bilirubin, whereas the reverse is often true when jaundice is subsiding.[10] Even if deep, jaundice is readily overlooked in most types of artificial light. Only bright daylight is satisfactory for clinical observation of skin and eye color. In jaundice the color change is usually detected most readily and earliest in the sclerae and bulbar conjunctivae.

Bilirubin is the important pigment causing the yellow skin color recognized as jaundice. Watson and associates[11,12] show clearly that *biliverdin*, an oxidation product of bilirubin, is often present in jaundiced persons and gives a green tint to the yellow skin when the biliverdin content exceeds 0.3 mg. per 100 ml. of serum. Occasionally the greenish cast is strikingly evident.[95]

Biliverdinemia is a feature of regurgitation jaundice, and when marked is almost always indicative of neoplastic obstruction of the biliary tract. A lesser degree is common in liver disease. It occurs occasionally in benign biliary obstructions. It is significant that biliverdinemia is not observed on a purely hemolytic basis.[12] This fact, along with the pallor of anemia, may explain the characteristic pure lemon yellow of chronic hemolytic jaundice. Persons who are chronically jaundiced may develop a bronze color suggestive of the addition of some degree of melanosis,

in addition to their yellowish-green skin color.

Elastic tissue has been called *bilirubinophilic* because of its great affinity for bilirubin. It is believed that the characteristic distribution of jaundice, with its accentuation in the sclerae, bulbar conjunctivae, mucous membranes, and certain portions of the skin in the upper part of the body, reflects the greater amount of elastic tissue which these areas contain.[96] Meakins[13] has shown clearly that jaundice cannot be detected in an edematous skin.

Clinically, carotenemia results when an excess of carotene (carotenoid pigments) stains the serum and skin. The term *carotenoderma* sometimes is used to indicate excess tissue staining with carotene.[10,14] The color of carotenemia is best detected where the skin has a heavy layer of stratum corneum (palms and soles) and areas of the face (forehead, nose, and cheeks), which are rich in sebaceous gland activity. It is absent in the sclerae, bulbar conjunctivae, and mucous membranes of the mouth.[79] A reliable bedside test for its detection is by comparison of the physician's palm, if normal in color, with the palm of a person suspected of being carotenemic.

Carotenemia results from prolonged excess ingestion of foods rich in carotene; its use as medication; lowered body metabolism (e.g., myxedema, Simmonds' disease, etc.), which hinders conversion of carotene to vitamin A in the liver; diminution of androgenic hormonal activity (e.g., the male castrate), and possibly to some minor degree with renal failure. A mild degree is physiologic in the normal skin color of women as compared with men.[5] Carotenemia was at one time common in diabetic patients, probably because of the high lipochromic diet formerly used, although some thought it due to diminished conversion of carotene to vitamin A in the liver. Theoretically liver disease can cause carotenemia by preventing the conversion of carotene to vitamin A, which takes place in this organ, but if liver disease is severe, the yellow color of carotenemia would be masked if jaundice were present. Carotenemia per se is harmless and gradually disappears when excess intake or underlying metabolic cause is corrected. The various circumstances under which carotenemia is of clinical interest are given in Table 39-2. The exact role of the xanthophylls, as a group, in contributing to normal

TABLE 39-2. DIFFERENTIAL CHARACTERISTICS

CLINICAL CONDITION	PIGMENT RESPONSIBLE	SKIN COLOR	CHARACTERISTIC LOCALIZATION
Carotenemia	Carotene	Canary yellow Lemon yellow Orange yellow	Palms, soles, alae nasi; occasionally diffuse Absent in sclerae and mucous membrane
Jaundice (hemolytic) ..	Bilirubin	Lemon yellow with pallor	*Sclerae, mucous membrane, and diffuse skin
Jaundice (hepatic and obstructive)	Bilirubin and biliverdin	Light yellow, dark yellow, orange, saffron or yellowish-green	*Sclerae, mucous membrane and diffuse skin
Myxedema	Carotene	Sallow yellow, old ivory tint	Palms, soles and face
Ingestion quinacrine hydrochloride	Quinacrine hydrochloride	Yellow to greenish-yellow	Diffuse skin—accentuated in exposed portion and body folds; minimal or absent in sclerae and mucous membrane
Chronic uremia	Urine chromogens Carotene (?) Diminished hemoglobin	Yellowish—pallor Yellowish—tan Buckwheat tint	Accentuated in skin exposed to light; absent in sclerae and mucous membrane
Industrial staining	Various yellow chemicals	Yellows of various hues	On exposed skin (face, hands, ankles and hair); absent in sclerae or mucous membrane
Picric acid ingestion (simulated jaundice)	Picric acid and breakdown derivatives	Yellow	Sclerae, mucous membrane and diffuse skin
Generalized xanthomatoses of skin	Cholesterol and cholesterol esters	Golden yellow Chamois yellow	Patchy on skin even when diffuse; none in sclerae or mucous membrane
Local discolorations of old ecchymosis, Cullen's sign, Grey-Turner's sign, etc.	Bilirubin and derivatives	Initially blue due to scattering phenomenon; later greenish-yellow to yellow	At site of trauma; Cullen's sign at umbilicus or in abdominal scars; Grey-Turner's sign on left flank
Lycopenemia	Lycopene	Orange yellow	Skin diffusely involved; most marked on palms and dorsa of hands, forearms, face and soles

* "Scleral" staining, particularly with bilirubin, is nearly always primarily in the conjunctiva.

OF YELLOW PIGMENTATIONS OF THE SKIN

COMPARATIVE RANGE OF INTENSITY OF SKIN COLOR*	MECHANISM OF PRODUCTION	SPECIFIC AIDS TO DIAGNOSIS	COMMENT
X to XX	Excess ingestion of carotenoid foods. Low B.M.R.(?) Diminished liver function(?)	Three-layer test of serum	Carotenemia is often a factor in skin color in Simmonds' disease and in the male castrate
X to XXX	Hemolysis of blood with bilirubin retention	Quantitative test for bilirubin; lack of bile in urine	Modified by pallor of anemia
X to XXXX	Regurgitation of bile pigments into blood	Quantitative tests for bilirubin and biliverdin; bile in urine	Melanosis may develop when jaundice is chronic
X	Diminished metabolism impairs utilization of carotene	Low B.M.R.; normal serum bilirubin	Skin color modified by myxedematous condition of skin and anemia
X to XXX	Direct staining of epidermis of skin	History; specific urine tests for the medication	Blue spots due to scattering phenomenon, due to pigment deposited in corium or in cartilage noted rarely
X	Retention of urinary chromogen with deposition in tissues; oxidized to yellow color on exposed surfaces	Blood chemistries and urinalysis	Melanosis stimulated in some instances
X to XXXX	External staining of exposed skin and hair	Occupational history	Some yellow chemicals produce liver damage and true jaundice as well as staining skin directly
X to XX	Picric acid and derivatives deposited in skin and mucous membrane	Urine orange to red in color; specific tests of urine for picrates; history	May also occur with use of picric acid ointments
X to XX	Deposition of lipoids in skin	Biopsy of skin shows local lipoids	Characteristic color seen best in the common xanthomata palpebrarum
X to XXX	Breakdown of blood or hemorrhagic fluid in tissues	Clinical observation only	Depends on local formations of bilirubin, biliverdin, and derived pigments
X to XX	Excess ingestion of tomatoes	History; increased serum carotenoids with spectrophotometric confirmation of lycopene	Specific histologic and histochemical changes in liver

* X indicates skin color is barely detectable clinically. XX, XXX, XXXX indicate increasingly marked change in skin color.

or abnormal yellow color of the skin is not clear.[64] Elevated levels have been noted in hypothyroidism, nephrotic syndrome, and hyperlipemic xanthomatoses. The spectral absorption curve for xanthophyll is somewhat similar to that of B-carotene. *Lycopene*, the familiar orange-red pigment of tomatoes, is a carotenoid pigment, which, when ingested in excess, may produce a pigmentary syndrome known as lycopenemia.[67,140] It differs from carotenemia in the source of the carotenoid pigment, the presence of elevated lycopene levels in the serum, a deeper orange skin color, and specific histologic changes in the liver.

Medication. Quinacrine hydrochloride, a drug utilized at times in the therapy of amebiasis, tapeworm infestation, and malaria, is an example of medication which may produce a striking yellow skin pigmentation after a week or so of continuous use. It produces a diffuse yellow skin color as a result of direct staining of tissues, usually easily distinguished from jaundice by absence or minimal staining of the sclerae.[10] Rarely, pigmentary changes in the deeper layers of the skin or mucous membrane may be produced by such drugs, and may cause a blue color because of the scattering phenomenon.[15,83]

Yellow pigmentation of the teeth induced by tetracycline had been reported in a high percentage of young children who received this antibiotic for control of pulmonary infections associated with cystic fibrosis.[85] The offspring of a woman who received tetracycline therapy for cystic acne during pregnancy also showed yellow-brown pigmentation of the teeth.[86]

Patients with chronic uremia often manifest a skin color that has a distinct pale yellow or yellowish-tan hue.[10] The pallor can be explained readily by the severe anemia so common in this condition. The yellowish skin discoloration has been attributed to retention in the skin of chromogens ordinarily excreted in the urine and responsible for its normal amber or yellow color. Excretion of a pale urine is characteristic of long-standing renal failure. The oxidative influence of light on the skin tends to accentuate the yellowish color on the exposed portions of the skin. Retention of carotenoid pigments also has been postulated as a cause for a yellowish skin color in uremia but is not generally accepted. At times chronic uremia appears to lead to an increase in melanin pigmentation. Malnutrition and trauma from scratching may be important causes of this melanosis.

A large number of yellow chemicals used in industry can stain externally the exposed portions of the skin and even the hair a distinct yellow color. This characteristic color distribution, absence of staining of mucous membranes, bulbar conjunctivae and sclerae, and the occupational history make the diagnosis easy. Such persons are often referred to as "industrial canaries." The yellow color in certain instances is accentuated upon exposure to light.[10]

The importance of knowing about this condition lies in the fact that exposure to some of these industrial chemicals also may damage the liver with resultant true jaundice and thus confuse the clinical problem.

Ingestion of picric acid or its absorption from ointments applied to open wounds can simulate jaundice closely by the ability of this yellow chemical to stain both the skin and mucous membranes.[10] Simulation of jaundice in this fashion was apparently a common means of malingering by soldiers in some armies during World War I. This substance is toxic and occasionally produces liver disease with true jaundice. In a similar manner, the metabolic stimulant dinitrophenol, formerly used extensively for weight reduction, can stain tissues yellow. Because its toxic effects are now well-known, one rarely sees it used at present. Fluorescein sodium, used in the detection of gastrointestinal bleeding, may cause a slight yellow staining of the skin which persists for several hours[97] and disappears as the dye is excreted into the urine and stool.

Xanthomas are yellow and usually localized. Occasionally, xanthomatosis produces diffuse skin infiltration with a resultant yellowish-orange type of skin discoloration.

There are a number of dermatologic disorders characterized by yellow color of a local lesion.[16,17] They are not likely to be confused with the type of skin discoloration discussed in this section.

Blood diffused through the subcutaneous tissues in the nature of an ecchymosis, hematoma, suffusion, etc., causes at first a purplish-blue or blue discoloration from the exaggerated "scattering" effect. As the blood pigments break down, bilirubin, biliverdin, and other similar pigments are formed. Therefore, diffuse blood in tissues can produce localized areas of yellowish discoloration (bilirubin) or yellowish-green discoloration (bilirubin and biliverdin). Cullen's sign consists of this type of discoloration about

TABLE 39-3. CLASSIFICATION OF HEMOGLOBIN PIGMENTATIONS

TYPE	SKIN COLOR PRODUCED	CLINICAL SIGNIFICANCE
Predominance of reduced hemoglobin	Varies from purplish-blue to heliotrope	Clinically recognized as cyanosis
Predominance of oxyhemoglobin	Red	Color characteristic of blush, flush, erythema, inflammation, arteriolar dilation, etc.
Increased amount of hemoglobin	Reddish-blue	Caused by polycythemia vera; blood contains normal amount of oxygenated hemoglobin as well as increased amounts of reduced hemoglobin
Methemoglobinemia	Chocolate blue	Various causes, see Ref. 19
Sulfhemoglobinemia	Lead or mauve-blue	Various causes, see Ref. 19
Carboxyhemoglobinemia	Cherry red	Carbon monoxide poisoning
Cyanhemoglobinemia	Bright red	Seen as bright red spots in persons dead from hydrocyanic poison
Nitricoxidehemoglobinemia	Bright red	Seen on exposure to nitrate explosion in closed space

the umbilicus or scars in the abdominal wall and is highly suggestive of ruptured tubular pregnancy or of hemorrhagic pancreatitis.[10] Grey-Turner's sign is a similar discoloration in the left flank and suggests hemorrhagic pancreatitis[10] or retroperitoneal hematoma, as from ruptured aneurysm.

The lesions of urticaria pigmentosa may give a yellow color.[16] At times, freckles look yellowish-tan. The skin at times in the male castrate and in subsiding suntan may manifest a sallow, yellow appearance.[5,7] However, ordinarily melanin does not produce a striking yellow skin color. Its closest approximation is to give a yellowish-brown or tan.

HEMOGLOBIN PIGMENTATION

As explained previously, reduced hemoglobin and oxyhemoglobin in the small blood vessels of the superficial and especially of the deeper subpapillary plexuses play an important role in normal skin color. Many deviations from this normal pattern are seen in clinical practice as a result of changes in the nature of hemoglobin from normal. These conditions are tabulated in Table 39-3.[10]

All of the hemoglobin pigmentations have in common the feature that the color change is detected most readily upon clinical observation in the portions of the body in which the keratinized layer of the epidermis is thinnest or absent and stratum mucosum is most superficial. These are the lips, the palpebral conjunctivae, the fingernails, and the mucous membranes of the mouth. Abnormal hemoglobin colors are accentuated in the areas shown in Figure 39-6 in which oxyhemoglobin is normally predominant. Abnormal hemoglobin colors also are conditioned by the physiologic factors governing circulation in the superficial capillaries. Patients with carcinoid syndrome may have a periodic bright red to reddish-purple flush, which may be in the "blush areas" or generalized. It is probably the result of vasodilation or vasodilation with stasis.

Melanin pigment in skin, if sufficient in amount, may effectively screen out the specific absorption pattern of any hemoglobin color change and prevent its clinical recognition. A representative example is the difficulty of detecting erythema or cyanosis in the skin of a Negro.

The palms and the soles, the fingernails, the lips, and the palpebral conjunctivae should be inspected for hemoglobin color change in the darker racial groups because of the minimal or absent melanization in these areas.

Cyanosis results when the reduced hemoglobin in blood reaches 5 Gm. per cent. Apparently this is an average value, since Comroe and Botelho[18] have shown by the use of an oximeter for standardization that even trained observers (anesthetists, cardiologists, etc.) vary greatly in the ease with which they detect its presence by clinical observation in experimental subjects exposed to progressively increased degrees of anoxia. The blue color of cyanosis varies in tone and hue from deep purplish-blue to heliotrope and is influenced by numerous clinical factors. The purplish-blue hue is likely to be seen when carbon dioxide retention (which dilates vessels) accompanies anoxia. Cyanosis due to suffocation is a representative example. A false impression of cyanosis occasionally may be gained by inspection of the lips. The vermilion border may be quite blue because of dermal melanin in dark skinned people, particularly of Mediterranean origin. For a detailed discussion of the mechanism of cyanosis see Chapter 20.

Predominance of oxyhemoglobin explains almost all clinical situations characterized by a red skin color. In most instances the explanation is simply an increase in number or dilation of the superficial skin vessels, or an increase in rapidity of superficial skin blood flow, so that the red color of oxyhemoglobin dominates the total skin color to a greater degree than normal. Examples are the red-flushed skin of fever, emotion, alcoholism, and various erythemas. At times, increases in the size and number of superficial capillaries are responsible (e.g., inflammation). Also at times, the skin is bright red because oxygen absorption by tissues is impaired because of low temperature. The tongue looks beefy red in a deficiency glossitis because of desquamation of the superficial, opaque, whitish, avascular filiform papillae (analogous to the stratum corneum of the epidermis), with resultant more superficial position of capillaries just below the lingual mucosa and in the papillary projections.

Patients with true polycythemia appear to have a flushed, slightly cyanotic appearance, which is called *erythremia*. It represents the full effect of the red oxyhemoglobin tinted with the blue of an increased amount of reduced hemoglobin because of incapacity in this condition for oxygenating the hemoglobin increment. Peripheral capillary stasis further exaggerates these color changes.

Persons exposed to *carbon monoxide* fumes develop carboxyhemoglobinemia with a peculiar cherry-red color quite unlike the red of oxyhemoglobin. It disappears within half an hour after cessation of the exposure. In cases with fatal issue, the color persists. The bright red skin spots occasionally seen with cyanhemoglobinemia due to hydrocyanic poison also persist after death. The normal pink skin color of oxyhemoglobin disappears after death, and instead one notes the bluish blotches and mottling of unoxy-genated hemoglobin in dependent areas, to which the blood moves because of gravity.

Whereas a clinically recognizable cyanosis requires the presence in the blood of 5 Gm. of reduced hemoglobin per 100 ml. of blood, a comparable skin color results from 1.5 Gm. of methemoglobin and less than 0.5 Gm. of sulfhemoglobin.[19] Methemoglobinemia produces a chocolate-blue skin color and sulfhemoglobinemia a mauve-blue one. Because of the small amount of these abnormal hemoglobin pigments necessary to produce cyanosis, individuals so affected are often quite comfortable and without symptoms, in contrast with the distress frequently noted when true cyanosis is present. This is especially true if the underlying condition is benign, as in idiopathic methemoglobinemia.

Although cyanosis ordinarily is related to hemoglobin changes in red cells, it may also occur after hemolysis, in which methemoglobin and metalbumin are present in the plasma.[19]

MELANIN PIGMENTATIONS (MELANOSIS)

Melanosis is a term commonly used to denote increased melanin pigmentation of the skin. Inasmuch as this pigment is an important component of skin color normally, it becomes clinically significant only when increased or markedly decreased in amount. Any increase in the degree of melanization is relative, since the degree of melanization normal for a person of one complexion or racial group may be abnormal for another.

Melanin pigmentation in any individual can be judged best by contrasting it with its previous intensity (sometimes readily done from old photographs), by comparing one area of the body to another, and by comparison with other members of the same family of like basic complexion. Frequently the relatives have noticed and commented on a change in the person's complexion.

Fitzpatrick, Seiji, and McGugan[68] have proposed a clinically useful classification of disturbances in human melanin pigmentation caused by decreased or increased amounts. Table 39-4 contains this classification. Inasmuch as all normal persons have melanocytes in their skins, everyone has the potential for developing melanosis if affected with any of the systemic diseases listed in this classification. Only the albino with his generalized defect of melanin formation in the skin remains immune.

Metabolism of Melanin. Melanin is a normal endogenous body pigment. Over the years, many of the older controversial aspects of the mechanism of its formation and its biochemistry have become clarified. The reader is referred to the important papers by Lerner and Fitzpatrick,[21] Fitzpatrick and Lerner,[54] Lorincz,[62] Lerner,[63] Okun, Edelstein, Or, et al.[141] and Fitzpatrick and associates[98] for a more detailed discussion of the metabolism of melanin and for a complete bibliography.

Aside from the metabolism of melanin, however, there have been several recent advances in the field of pigment cell biology which may enlarge the spectrum of the tyrosine (tyrosinase?)-phenol oxidase system in the melanocyte. Demopoulos has shown that the melanoma obtains a greater portion of its energy from the tyrosine-phenol oxidase system rather than from glycolysis or the

cytochrome oxidase system,[99,102] and this phenol oxidase system may be linked to ATP generation.[142] In these studies the copper oxidase, tyrosinase, seemed to be the enzyme involved. However, recent studies of Okun, Edelstein and associates[141,107,108] indicate that a peroxidase, not tyrosinase, may be the key enzyme in initiating melanin synthesis from tyrosine. On the other hand, tyrosinase appeared to be a substrate specific dopa-oxidase, with no significant ability to utilize tyrosine in melanin synthesis. Thus, peroxidase may be involved in an alternate ATP-energy-generating system not unlike that described by Demopoulos. In addition, the ability of peroxidase to oxidize tyrosine to melanin raises the possibility that this enzyme also may have a role in catecholamine formation, since the

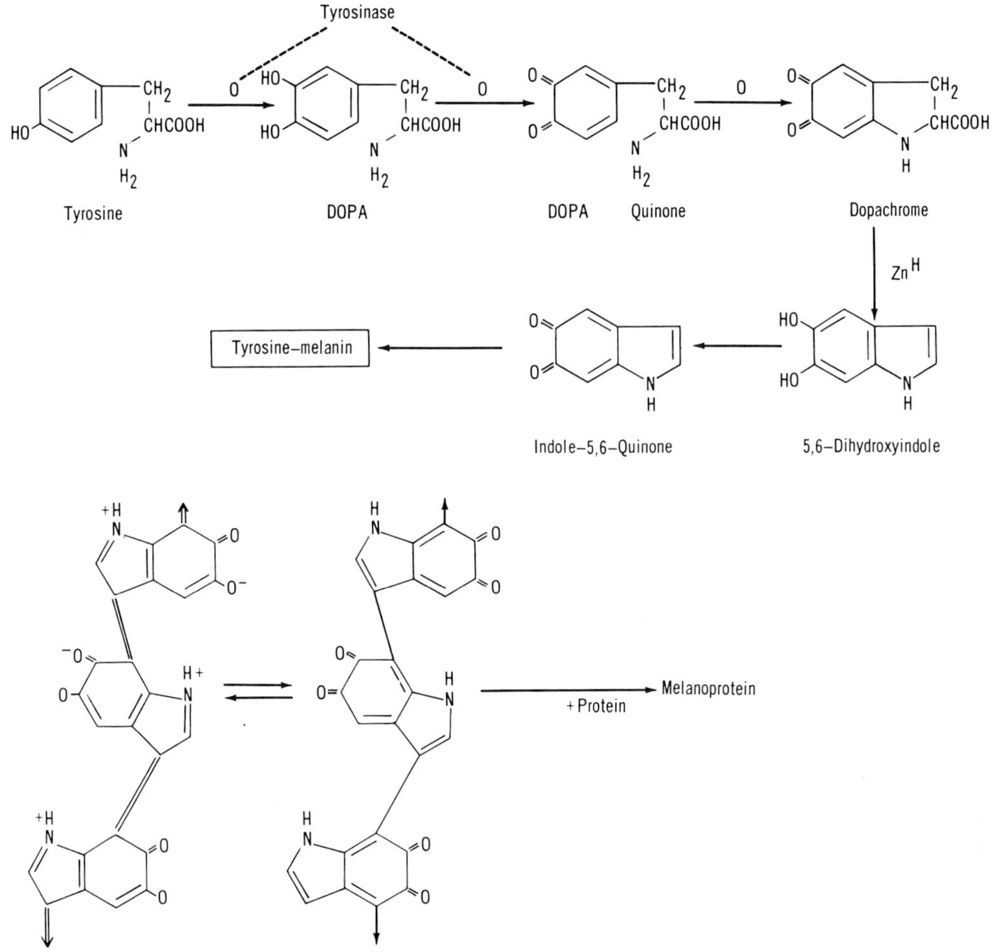

FIG. 39-15. Biosynthesis of tryosine melanin. (Fitzpatrick, T. B., Seiji, M., and McGugan, A. D.: Medical progress: melanin pigmentation, New Eng. J. Med. 265: 328, 374 and 430)

oxidation of tyrosine to DOPA is the common initial step in both melanin and catecholamine biosynthesis. Thus, peroxidase may be the enzyme involved in the synthesis of visceral *neuro*-melanin seen in brain,[103,103a,104,104a] liver, heart, adrenal and testis, and gastrointestinal tract (melanosis coli). Such knowledge should lead to a better understanding of the physiologic and pathophysiologic role of tyrosinase and peroxidase in cell growth and function, and possibly may shed additional light on subcellular factors controlling skin color.

Melanin is formed by specialized cells called melanocytes, located at the epidermo-dermal junction and derived embryologically from the neural crest region[20,21,54,68] (Figs. 39-2 and 39-16). Melanin also is formed in the hair bulb, mucous membrane, uveal tract, retina, and the leptomeninges.

Under certain stimuli, to be discussed later, melanocytes normally in clear-cell form enlarge, become dendritic, and form melanin, which accumulates as microscopic granules

in palisade cells of the basal layer of the epidermis, and is present in decreasing amounts in each outward layer of the rest of the epidermis. The number of melanin granules plays a greater role in the degree of intensity of the skin color than does the size of the individual granule. It is conceivable that dermal melanocytes may be more numerous in the regions of the eyelids and axillae to account in part for the greater darkness of the skin noted in these areas in some persons.[91-93] Melanin is absent in the epidermis of albinos, present in the least amount in blonds, somewhat more in brunets, and still more in the darker racial groups.[10]

Melanin in humans is formed from the amino acid tyrosine, which acts as the physiologic substrate in a complex enzymatic action. Lerner and Fitzpatrick[21] reviewed the evidence for the present belief that the enyzme tyrosinase (a copper-protein complex) is a single enzyme with two activities: catalyzation of the oxidation of the amino-

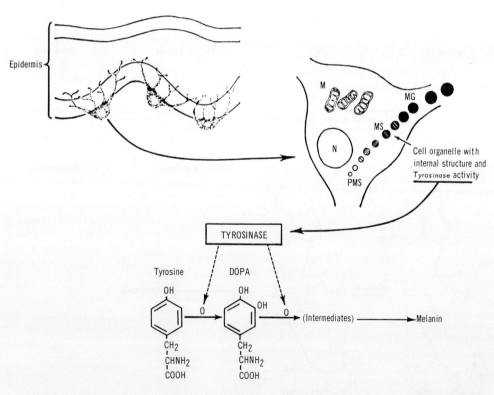

FIG. 39-16. Melanogenesis in human skin as seen in the light microscope and the electron microscope and at the molecular level. (M) Mitochondria; (N) Nucleus; (PMS) Promelanosomes; (MS) Melanosomes; (MG) Melanin granules. (Fitzpatrick, T. B., Seiji, M., and McGugan, A. D.: Medical progress: melanin pigmentation, New Eng. J. Med. 265:328, 374 and 430)

acid tyrosine to DOPA and the oxidation of DOPA in turn to melanin. It is important to emphasize that a complex series of chemical reactions constitutes the intermediate stages of this reaction, and thus the formation of melanin is subject to a variety of controlling factors other than the basic enzymatic reaction itself. These reactions as schematized by Fitzpatrick et al.[68] are shown in Figures 39-15 and 39-16.

The metabolic requirements for tyrosine are satisfied largely by conversion of phenylalanine to tyrosine by enzymatic action in the liver. Dietary tyrosine ordinarily plays a minor role (Fig. 39-19).

The paths of excretion of melanin include (1) from the skin by desquamation, and (2) by drainage through the lymphatics, to the blood stream, and excretion through the kidney. The amount in the urine is at times grossly visible (melanuria), a condition most likely to result from extensive metastases from melanotic tumors.

Lerner and Fitzpatrick[21] list the many biochemical factors regulating the formation of melanin. Some substances (e.g., DOPA) catalyze the tyrosine-tyrosinase reaction. Other substances (e.g., sulfhydryl compounds) inhibit tyrosinase by their ability to bind the copper necessary for this enzymatic action, or by their ability to inhibit the oxidation reaction directly (e.g., reducing agents such as ascorbic acid).[109] If the sulfhydryl groups are oxidized, the inactivated copper is released with increased tyrosinase reaction. A pH higher than the optimal range prolongs the induction period of tyrosine oxidation, whereas at lower values of pH, tyrosinase activity is reduced. The tyrosine-tyrosinase reaction increases with limited rise in temperature. The redox (oxidation-reduction) potential, if high, is associated with a long tyrosine induction period. The amount of the physiologic substrate tyrosine is naturally important. Lastly, oxidation is important; melanin is light-colored in reduced form and darker (black) in oxidized form. Fitzpatrick and associates,[54,68] have presented these facts in diagrams (Figs. 39-2, 39-15 and 39-16).

Screening by Melanin. Melanin in the skin protects against excessive exposure to sunlight or other sources of ultraviolet rays. It may prevent harmful effects. Some understanding of the mechanism of screening by melanin has been advanced recently by Seiji[143] and others. The proposed mechanism by which melanin functions as a photoprotective polymer is complex. However, the screening effect is concerned with its ability to absorb radiation, attenuate it by scattering, dissipate the energy as heat, and act as a stable free radical in the process. By means of this, melanin may act as a biological electron exchange polymer protecting the cells and tissues against reducing or oxidizing conditions, which might release reactive free radicals, thus causing alterations in cell metabolism. In addition, melanin in its usual perinuclear position then may absorb high-energy photons and create harmless free radicals within the polymer; it thus may protect a radiosensitive nucleus and its functional DNA.[111]

External (Physical) Causes. In many instances of melanosis, the factor responsible is the external application of a physical agent to the skin.[22]

Because of the ubiquity of exposure to sunlight, melanosis due to ordinary exposure is accepted as a component of normal skin color and called *tan.* Only when the exposure is excessive is the increase of melanization likely to be noticed. Tanning has no clinical significance unless confused with melanosis due to internal causes. Exposure to some artificial source of ultraviolet radiation acts in the same way as does exposure to natural sunlight. Persons with light complexions (blond) tan less readily and to a lesser degree than those with dark complexions (brunet).

Melanin resulting from ultraviolet exposure is deposited only in the epidermis and never in the dermis, and therefore is of a brownish hue.[22] The mechanism by which ultraviolet irradiation stimulates melanosis is complex and is believed to include[21,23] (1) catalyzing the oxidation of tyrosine to DOPA so that the DOPA so formed can catalyze tyrosine-tyrosinase enzyme reaction (Fig. 39-15), (2) oxidation of melanin already present in the skin, (3) diminishing the concentration of sulfhydryl groups in the epidermis which normally are the natural inhibitors of tyrosinase, (4) decreasing the redox potential of the skin, and (5) elevating the temperature of the skin either directly or by producing an erythema.[21,23]

The skins of albinos and the vitiliginous areas of otherwise normal skins manifest erythema and serious burning upon exposure to ultraviolet radiation because of failure of melanization in skin with these defects.

The skin may be *photosensitized* to actinic rays by application of certain substances

TABLE 39-4. DISTURBANCES OF HUMAN MELANIN PIGMENTATION*

TYPE	DECREASED PIGMENTATION WHITE (OR LIGHTER THAN NORMAL)	INCREASED PIGMENTATION	
		BROWN OR BLACK	GRAY, SLATE, OR BLUE†
GENETIC OR NEVOID	ALBINISM, oculocutaneous‡ Albinism, localized cutaneous Vitiligo (may be diffuse) Phenylketonuria (hair & iris) Infantile Fanconi's syndrome (hair)	Neurofibromatosis (*café au lait*) Polyostotic fibrous dysplasia (Albright's syndrome) Ephelides (freckling) Xeroderma pigmentosum Acanthosis nigricans (juvenile type) GAUCHER'S DISEASE‡ NIEMANN-PICK DISEASE‡	Oculodermal melanocytosis (nevus of Ota) Dermal melanocytosis (Mongolian spot)
METABOLIC		HEMOCHROMATOSIS‡ HEPATOLENTICULAR DISEASE‡ (Wilson's disease) PORPHYRIA‡ (congenital & cutanea tarda)	HEMOCHROMATOSIS‡
NUTRITIONAL	Kwashiorkor (hair)	Kwashiorkor Pellagra (may be diffuse) Sprue (may be diffuse)	Chronic nutritional insufficiency
ENDOCRINE	HYPOPITUITARISM‡ Addison's disease (vitiligoid)	ACTH- and MSH-PRODUCING PITUITARY TUMORS‡ ACTH THERAPY‡ Pregnancy (may be diffuse) ADDISON'S DISEASE‡ Estrogen therapy (nipple)	
CHEMICAL	Arsenical intoxication Hydroquinone, monobenzyl ether Chloroquin & hydroxychloroquin (hair) Guanonitrofurazone Chemical burns (with loss of melanocytes)	ARSENICAL INTOXICATION‡ BUSULFAN‡ Photochemical (drugs, tar)	Fixed drug eruption Quinacrine toxicity
PHYSICAL	Thermal burns (with loss of melanocytes) Trauma (with loss of melanocytes)	Ultraviolet light Heat Alpha, beta, & gamma radiation Trauma (for example, chronic pruritus)	
INFECTIONS & INFLAMMATIONS	Pinta Leprosy§ Fungous infections§ Postinflammatory§ (atopic dermatitis, drug eruptions, & so forth) Vogt-Koyanagi syndrome	Postinflammatory (dermatitis, exanthems, drug eruptions)	Pinta (exposed areas)

* This classification includes disorders of interest to physicians in general; many pigmentary disorders not listed are of special interest to the dermatologist.
† Gray, slate, or blue color results from the presence of *dermal* melanocytes, or phagocytized melanin in dermis.
‡ Small capital type indicates that pigmentary change is diffuse, not spotty, and there are no identifiable borders.
§ Usually *partial* loss of pigmentation; viewed with the Wood's light, the lesions are not chalk white, as in vitiligo.
Fitzpatrick, T. B., Seiji, M., and McGugan, A. D.: Medical progress: melanin pigmentation, New Eng. J. Med. 265:328.

TABLE 39-4. DISTURBANCES OF HUMAN MELANIN PIGMENTATION (*Continued*)

TYPE	DECREASED PIGMENTATION WHITE (OR LIGHTER THAN NORMAL)	INCREASED PIGMENTATION	
		BROWN OR BLACK	GRAY, SLATE, OR BLUE†
NEOPLASMS	Leukoderma acquisitum centrifugum (halo nevus) In sites of melanoma after disappearance (therapeutic or spontaneous) of tumor	Urticaria pigmentosa Adenocarcinoma with acanthosis nigricans	MALIGNANT MELANOMA,‡ advanced (generalized dermal pigmentation syndrome, with melanuria)
MISCELLANEOUS	Scleroderma§ (circumscribed & systemic types) Canities (hair) Alopecia areata (hair)	SCLERODERMA, SYSTEMIC‡ CHRONIC HEPATIC INSUFFICIENCY‡ WHIPPLE'S SYNDROME‡ Melasma (chloasma)	

externally, and possibly by their presence internally. After sensitization, marked melanosis may develop with only very limited exposure to sunlight. The deposition of melanin pigment in such induced hypersensitive states occurs in the upper dermis as well as the epidermis, with a resultant grayish-brown color.[22] This type of pigmentation may persist much longer than the ordinary melanosis due to actinic rays. Dihydroxyacetone is a topical agent able to produce a bronze appearance of the skin to simulate suntan. It apparently combines with material in the outer keratin layer, and is removed as the keratin is normally shed in a few days. The pigmented compound has not been characterized chemically, but it is definitely not melanin. It does not have the protective activity against sunburning that melanin possesses.

The alpha rays of *thorium-x* and to a lesser degree beta and gamma *roentgen* and *radium* rays stimulate melanization. In dark brunets, this may occur without a preceding erythema, although usually it follows an erythema.[22]

The application of *heat* to the skin in any form sufficient to produce prolonged or repeated erythema leads to melanosis of the areas so exposed. The classic clinical example is the reticular pattern of melanin pigmentation which follows *erythema caloricum* because of repeated application of hot water bottles to the abdomen for pain. Melanosis from heat is attributed to an increase in the rate of sulfhydryl oxidation, which releases bound copper, and to an increase in the tyrosinase reaction, as well as

direct acceleration of the enzymatic oxidation of tyrosine.[21]

Application of any of these physical agents to a degree sufficient to destroy skin (second and third degree burns) destroys the melanocytes, so that the resultant scar tissue has less pigment (both melanin and hemoglobin) than normal, and by contrast appears whiter or less pigmented than normal skin.

Irritation of the skin by application of caustic *chemicals* may produce melanin through the production of severe erythema.

Mechanical irritation of the skin, if long continued, may produce local erythema and eventually melanosis. Classic examples clinically are melanized areas in the groin from a truss and in the axillae from crutches.

An interesting example of melanosis predominantly of external origin, commonly seen in every hospital receiving indigent and neglected patients, is so-called *vagabonds' disease* or *beggars' melanosis*.[10] The pigmentation characteristically is more marked on covered than on exposed portions of the body and is especially noticeable over areas in which clothes chafe. Lack of bathing, failure to remove dirty clothes, and presence of body pediculi with resulting irritation, increase in heat in body folds, and scratching are the main factors. However, such persons are usually malnourished, so that internal factors may contribute to the melanization.

Severe pruritus is common in chronic uremia, chronic obstructive jaundice, and Hodgkin's disease. It is likely that continual *scratching* by patients with these diseases acts as a form of constant mechanical irritation and contributes to the melanosis occasionally seen in these conditions.

It is characteristic of all forms of melanosis due to external physical agents that the degree of melanization gradually diminishes when the exciting factor is removed.

Internal (Systemic) Causes. The types of melanosis of chief importance in clinical practice are those that result from internal causes. No attempt will be made here to discuss all of the dermatologic disorders with melanosis, although some may be of systemic origin. Beerman and Colburn[73] have reviewed them concisely and Cowan[72] has reviewed the ocular pigmentary disturbances. This chapter is concerned primarily with mechanisms of melanosis in conditions that are of prime interest in internal medicine (Table 39-4). The following several paragraphs will attempt to group and explain present concepts of such mechanisms according to the basic physiologic disturbances responsible,[21] rather than to discuss them purely from the viewpoint of their presence in a wide variety of apparently unrelated diseases. In most instances, the origin of melanosis involves nutritional, endocrine, nervous, or dermal causes, or some combination of these.

MELANOSIS OF NUTRITIONAL ORIGIN. There seems little doubt that many instances of melanosis can be explained on the basis of a metabolic disturbance of nutritional origin. At the end of World War II,[21,25,26] it was noted that pigmentation was common in persons held for long periods in prison or concentration camps under starvation regimens. The mechanism of the melanosis here is difficult to evaluate, since nutritional deficiency in humans is invariably of complex origin. An interesting speculation has centered about the possibility that the predominantly vegetable diets of these starved people contained proportionally less sulfhydryl amino acids (cystine and methionine), which normally inhibit melanin formation, than the amino-acid melanin precursors phenylalanine and tyrosine.[21]

In addition, there is a strong possibility that the malnutrition may have been associated with deficiency of certain factors in the diet or that inadequacy of total caloric content may have secondarily produced abnormalities of endocrine function.

Melanosis is common in pellagra (niacin deficiency) and occurs both with the low-grade chronic variety and following the subsidence of an acute pellagrous dermatitis.

The mechanism for this melanosis[21] is considered to be similar to that which follows the various types of erythematous reactions due to physical agents, as described previously. This is probably true for the type following the acute phase of pellagrous erythema. In low-grade chronic pellagra, hyperkeratosis and pigmentation of pressure areas without much erythema are at times prominent features. Release of sulfhydryl inhibition of melanin formation may be a factor.

Pigmentation is at times a prominent feature in scurvy (vitamin-C deficiency). Both melanosis and hemosiderosis (due to purpura in the skin) must be considered to explain changes in skin color in this disorder.[21] General malnutrition might also play an important role in some instances.

Although extremely rare in the United States,[10] melanin pigmentation has been noted in the skin of patients with vitamin-A deficiency. It exhibits a peculiar localization to the site of the hyperkeratotic follicular lesion so characteristic of this disease.

Lerner and Fitzpatrick[21] attribute the pigmentation in all three of these vitamin deficiencies to the release in the epidermis of normal sulfhydryl inhibition of tyrosinase, with the reason for the production of the decrease in sulfhydryl group different in each of them. In pellagra, the mechanism is that characteristic for any postinflammatory variety; in vitamin-A deficiency, diversion of sulfhydryl for increased keratin formation; and in scurvy, deposition of iron and copper in the skin as a result of the hemorrhagic tendency.

MELANOSIS OF HORMONAL ORIGIN

Pituitary and Adrenal. The generally accepted clinical impression that the endocrine system plays a major role in the control of melanin metabolism finds increasing experimental and scientific support in the medical literature.[69,74,75] The pituitary gland seems to play the dominant role, followed in importance by the adrenals, leaving estrogen and progesterone and other endocrine substances a lesser but not well-established significance.

The often confirmed observations of the darkly pigmented appearance of the acromegalic and the characteristic pallor of hypopituitarism (Simmonds' disease) give firm clinical support to the idea that the pituitary gland in humans is concerned in some way with melanin metabolism. The concept of a separate melanophore hormone, produced in the pars intermedia of the pituitary gland, has been accepted for lower forms of animal life.[10]

The presence of *melanocyte-stimulating hormone* (M.S.H.) in man is now well-documented.[69] This concept received renewed interest with reports of melanosis developing in a white male receiving ACTH (pituitary adrenocorticotropin); the pituitary extract was found to contain a significant amount of melanophore hormone (intermedin).[21,30] Such contamination could explain pigmentation reported from use of other pituitary preparations.[21] Previous evidence suggested that melanocyte-stimulating hormone (M.S.H.), present as a contaminant, was responsible in earlier reports of increased melanin pigmentation with ACTH preparations. Lerner and McGuire[77] showed that chemically pure ACTH in very large doses has skin-darkening properties.

Lerner and associates[63,69] in excellent reviews discuss the polypeptide nature and separate identity of α- and β-melanocyte-stimulating hormones (M.S.H.) secreted by the intermediate lobe of the pituitary. The reader is referred to these papers for a detailed background of this subject. This secretion has been described for many years as *intermedin, melanophore-dilating principle, melanophore hormone,* etc., and generally is accepted as significant in the pigmentation of fish and amphibia. Recent studies have now determined the presence of M.S.H. in human blood and urine. The highly active biologic effect of M.S.H. in humans is indicated by the ability of a few micrograms to influence melanocytes in humans, with a prompt detectable increase in skin pigmentation, then with diminution to previous skin color a few weeks after cessation of its use.[61]

The pattern of secretion and activity of M.S.H. resembles that of other pituitary hormones, as Calkins[31] had postulated previously. Thus, the level of its urinary excretion is raised when adrenal cortical activity is low, as in Addison's disease or after adrenalectomy. Of interest was the observation of a greatly increased M.S.H. production during pregnancy,[53,61] a period when melanization of the eyelids, the nipples, and the aerolae of the breast is increased and the linea nigra of the abdomen appears. The level of M.S.H. production is low in panhypopituitarism, which correlates with the pale skin color associated with this disorder.

Several products of the adrenal are antagonistic to the action of M.S.H. Epinephrine and norepinephrine have an inhibiting action and appear to block its action on the melanocyte. This is in accord with clinical observation that, in instances of Addison's disease in which the adrenal medulla is destroyed along with the cortex, the cutaneous pigmentation is greater than with the presence of only cortical insufficiency. Cortisone and hydrocortisone diminish melanin production,[61] possibly through inhibition of M.S.H. production.

Hall, McCracken, and Thorn[49] have studied skin pigmentation in relation to adrenal cortical function by means of the Hardy spectrophotometer. They found that a great diminution in cutaneous blood flow accompanied the melanization of Addison's disease or surgical adrenalectomy.

Recently there have been reports of M.S.H.-like and ACTH-like peptides produced by various malignant tumors of the lung (including oat-cell and carcinoid types), and of the pancreas (including undifferentiated carcinoma and islet-cell tumors), suggesting possibly a genetic expression of biosynthetic pathways not found in normal cells of these organs. Thus, when general hyperpigmentation is found in association with adrenal cortical hyperactivity (i.e., Cushing's syndrome), the physician should search for possible extrapituitary sites of malignant neoplastic secretion of these hormonelike peptides.[112] Occasionally, in Cushing's syndrome, diffuse depigmentation of the hands and feet has been seen and is thought to be related to high serum cortisol levels, resulting in decreased synthesis of M.S.H. by the pituitary.[144]

Cortisone caused a lowering of melanin skin content in patients with intact adrenals. Darkening of the skin with use of ACTH apparently depends upon increase in cutaneous blood flow as well as melanin formation. The latter effect may be due to some other product of the pituitary accompanying the ACTH as a contaminant[49]; possibly M.S.H.

The almost invariable presence of melanosis in Addison's disease has served to center considerable attention on the relation of the adrenal glands to melanin metabolism. A voluminous literature[10,21] attests to the various theories and extensive research concerning this problem.

It is believed generally that the adrenal hormones inhibit melanization under certain circumstances, as evidenced by the striking hyperpigmentation which occurs in animals following adrenalectomy, or in humans following surgical removal of adrenal cortex or the destruction or atrophy of the adrenal gland from disease.[21]

The various theories[10,21,32,33] to explain melanosis in Addison's disease include: (1) loss of sympathetic nervous inhibition of melanization occasioned by failure of the adrenal stimulation; (2) failure of the diseased adrenal gland to utilize the precursor of epinephrine, which results in its conversion to melanin; (3) diminished storage in the adrenals of vitamin C, which normally has an inhibiting effect on melanin formation; (4) depression of blood level of sodium from adrenal cortical failure, with resultant increased oxidation of ascorbic acid and diminution of its concentration, leading, in turn, to loss of its inhibitory influence on melanin formation; (5) through the possible influence of the adrenal gland in regulating the metabolism of sulfhydryl compounds, with resultant decrease in their concentration in the skin and loss of their inhibiting effect on melanin formation[21]; and (6) loss of control of melanogenesis by a pituitary-adrenal axis, in which normally the adrenal hormones inhibit release of M.S.H. or its peripheral action on melanocytes.[21,31,53,61]

This latter idea best explains the known facts and was discussed in more detail previously. Figure 39-17, from the paper by

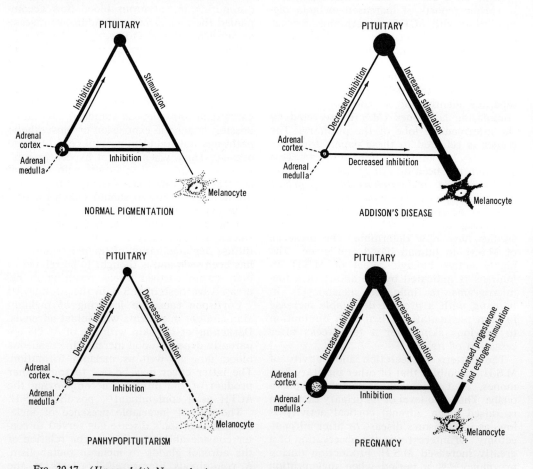

Fig. 39-17. (*Upper left*) Normal pigmentation. Hydrocortisone inhibits the output of MSH by the pituitary gland. Noradrenaline and adrenaline inhibit the action of MSH on the pigment-forming cells. (*Upper right*) Addison's disease. MSH output is increased because hydrocortisone inhibition of the pituitary is decreased. If the adrenal medulla is destroyed, the inhibition of MSH by adrenaline and noradrenaline is removed. (*Lower left*) Panhypopituitarism. MSH output is decreased because of decrease in pituitary function. (*Lower right*) Pregnancy. MSH output, progesterone, and estrogens are increased. Progesterone may have a direct MSH-like action. (Lerner, Shizume and Bunding: J. Clin. Endocr. 14:1463)

Lerner, Shizume, and Bunding,[61] clearly presents this concept in a diagrammatic fashion.

Both clinical observations and laboratory studies have established clearly that primary adrenal cortical insufficiency causes melanosis, whereas adrenal cortical insufficiency secondary to hypopituitarism does so only rarely.[10,21,35,61]

It is interesting to note that a syndrome consisting of melanosis associated with atrophic bronchitis and generalized cytologic dysplasia has been reported in patients on busulfan therapy for chronic granulocytic leukemia. Pigmentation was comparable to that of adrenocortical deficiency, but urinary steroid secretion was normal.[113]

The frequent observation of vitiligo in Addison's disease, with deep melanosis and marked patchy depigmentation irregularly distributed, is striking.

GONADS

We have mentioned already the influence of the gonads in determining the color of the skin in the normal male and female, the deviations from normal which occur in castrated men and ovariectomized women, and the reversibility of each of these with the appropriate sex hormone therapy. The gonads normally control skin color, not only through their influence on melanization, but also the skin content of hemoglobin, carotene, and melanoid.[5,6,8]

Oral administration of estrogen in women prior to the menopause has been reported as increasing the degree of melanization in the nipples, aerolae, and linea nigra.[27] Similar hyperpigmentation is said not to develop when estrogens are used after the menopause, perhaps because of diminished functional activity of the pituitary gland at this time of life. Application of estrogen-containing ointment to the skin has been reported as producing areas of increased melanization. The influence of estrogen and progesterone on human melanization requires more study for final clarification.

Melanosis of some degree occurs in almost every pregnancy. It is manifested as pigmentation of the face, accentuation of the areas of primary melanization (namely, the nipples and areolae, the linea nigra, and the vulvar areas) as well as by a generalized increase.[10,27] Occasionally the facial pigment is accentuated over the cheeks, the bridge of the nose, and the forehead in a pattern known as chloasma gravidarum[10] or more recently called melasma gravidarum or simply melasma. "Mask of pregnancy" is another term. The probable factors involved in melanosis of pregnancy are presented in graphic form in Figure 39-17. As a general rule, termination of pregnancy leads to a marked diminution in the degree of the pigmentation, but leaves some sequelae in the form of permanent residue in the nipples, the areolae, the linea nigra, and elsewhere. These are commonly accepted as presumptive clinical evidence of a past pregnancy.[10]

Oral contraceptive drugs containing both estrogens and progestins occasionally may produce melasma. Upon cessation of their use, the pigmentation may persist longer than that seen with pregnancy.[114]

Further influence of the gonads is noted in the darkening of primary areas of melanization in both sexes at puberty and the interesting observation that benign melanomas rarely become malignant before puberty.[28]

Numerous examples of in-vitro and in-vivo experiments in animals are on record which demonstrate the influence of the sex hormones on melanin metabolism.[10,21,29] Arrhenoblastoma, the masculinizing tumor of the ovary, has been reported as producing darkening of the skin. Apparently both estrogens and androgens increase melanin skin pigmentation. However, the biochemical nature of this action is still obscure.

THYROID

There is also the possibility that the thyroid gland is concerned with melanin metabolism, as suggested by the common occurrence of melanosis in hyperthyroidism—especially when chronic.[10] Lerner[63] has surveyed the present status of this endocrine gland in relation to melanin pigmentation.

It is of considerable interest that the precursor of melanin, tyrosine, is chemically quite similar to the thyroid hormones, thyroxine, and di-iodotyrosine.

MELANOSIS OF NERVOUS ORIGIN. There are a number of clinical and a few experimental observations that strongly suggest that melanization of the skin in humans may be subject (at least in some degree) to neurogenic control.[10,21] It is believed by some that imbalance in the activity of the autonomic nervous system may be important, with skin pigmentation being stimulated by parasympathetic predominance and inhibited by sympathetic predominance. Further evidence for the role of the nervous system in pigmentation is the occasional occurrence of vitiligo along the distribution of a cutaneous nerve. Similarly, repigmentation of a vitiliginous limb has been observed following accidental severing of that nerve, whereas the vitiligo of the contralateral limb remained the same.

Lerner and Fitzpatrick,[21] although unable to explain the mechanism, indicate the possible role of certain neurogenic factors in controlling melanogenesis in the human skin. They cite in support of this belief experiments reported by Haxthausen wherein normally pigmented skin gradually depigmented when grafted to an area of vitiligo, whereas vitiliginous skin gradually repigmented when grafted to normal skin. They also comment on the fact that the pigmentation of acanthosis nigricans, which in adults may be due to an abdominal visceral carcinoma (especially of the stomach), often develops when the lesion involves the celiac plexus or chromaffin system.

Melanosis is common in neurofibromatosis.[10] The congenital neurocutaneous syndrome of melanosis of the skin and central nervous system and the tendency for a skin pigment spot to localize over a spina bifida occulta are examples of the curious association of nervous lesions with melanosis.[10] Other types have been described.[10,21,63] Meningeal melanosis may occur in patients with giant pigmented nevi. A cerebral melanoma should be suspected if signs of an intracranial space-occupying lesion become evident.[115] Free melanin or melanin-containing cells have been noted in the cerebrospinal fluid in these two situations.

MELANOSIS WITH SKIN DISEASE. A variety of skin diseases are known to produce melanosis.[20] Any dermatologic disorder which produces an inflammatory response may be followed by melanosis, for reasons previously discussed.

It is likely that certain systemic diseases with end-organ response in the skin may produce melanosis by changes in skin metabolism of a localized nature. *Arsenic* apparently produces melanosis by its deposition in the skin with resultant binding of epidermal sulfhydryl substances, which results in removal of the inhibition of the tyrosinase enzyme.[21] Arsenic also may act to produce skin inflammation. The melanosis seen with scleroderma and dermatomyositis probably results from local changes in the skin which occur in these conditions.

The reader is referred elsewhere for fur-

ther information on skin pigmentation in dermatologic diseases.[20,24,73]

CLINICAL PICTURE IN MELANOSIS

Melanin normally present in the skin is not of uniform intensity over the entire body, but is accentuated in certain areas called primary zones (Fig. 39-3). These include the eyelids, the axillae, the nipples, the areolae, the umbilicus, the linea nigra, the genital region, the nape of the neck, and the anal region. In women the nape of the neck, the linea nigra, and the axillae are more heavily melanized than these areas in the male. Szabo[70] has shown marked variations in the number of melanocytes in the epidermis in different regions of the body.

Likewise, the pattern of melanosis is not one of uniform increase in intensity over the entire skin but is subject to accentuation in certain areas, which vary with the disease responsible or with exposure to external factors influencing melanin metabolism.

Although derived from the Greek meaning *black*, melanin in the epidermis ordinarily produces a yellowish-tan, tan, or brown color, but may occasionally appear black. When melanin is present in melanophages in the upper dermis without much in the epidermis, it produces a slate-gray color; when present deep in the dermis a blue color occurs, because of the scattering phenomenon.[5,10,20]

In most instances the abnormal melanosis shows accentuation in the groin, the axillae, under the breasts, between the buttocks, in skin folds, etc.—all areas of higher than average skin temperature. It is well-known that increased temperature accentuates melanin formation. Friction from belts, trusses, buttons, waist bands, garters, areas of chafing, etc., may likewise predispose to local areas of accentuation. Still another pattern is for the accentuation to occur in the normally accentuated primary zones of melanization, such as the nipples, the areolae, the linea nigra, the genital areas, and the anal areas. Another common pattern is preponderant melanosis of portions of the skin exposed to sunlight. Pigmentation of the face may be uniform or accentuated in areas as in the "mask of pregnacy." At times the eyelids become heavily melanized. The hair may rarely participate by darkening, but cases of Addison's disease have been observed with prematurely white hair. Not uncommon is the development of melanization of the mucous membranes of the oral cavity and, at times, of the eye and of the vagina. Even the nail bed may show melanosis.

With a few exceptions (e.g., acanthosis nigricans, arsenic poisoning, etc.), the melanoses of internal origin generally have a similar histologic picture, consisting of an increase in the number and density of melanin particles (melanosomes). For the most part, therefore, a skin biopsy in melanosis tells only that the pigment is melanin, as was usually surmised from the history and clinical inspection.

A few diseases produce a melanotic skin picture which, upon clinical inspection, is characteristic of or at least suggestive of the basic systemic disease responsible. These include the "rain drop" appearance and hyperkeratosis of arsenic poisoning; the wrinkled, velvety, and often papillomatous pigmentation of the neck, axillae, and groin seen in acanthosis nigricans; the ocular pingueculae and melanosis of Gaucher's disease; the blue cartilaginous areas of the ears and nose, the sclerae, and ear drums, of ochronosis; the facial mask and nipple-areolae accentuation of pregnancy, chloasma uterinum, and estrogen therapy of young women; the perifollicular skin and ocular localization of vitamin-A deficiency, etc.

As a general rule, however, the pattern of melanosis without an increase in the number of melanocytes is not distinctive of the underlying disease. The degree and pattern of melanosis from the same disease may vary greatly from one person to the next, including, at times, the ordinarily distinctive ones mentioned previously. The melanosis of certain localized hyperpigmented lesions is often distinctive enough to be readily recognized on clinical inspection (e.g., neurofibromatosis, Albright's syndrome, xeroderma pigmentosum, Peutz-Jeghers syndrome, etc.). In reference to xeroderma pigmentosum, it has been found recently that the dermal fibroblasts of these patients are unable to repair their own DNA after ultraviolet radiation (with resultant thymine dimer formation) when compared with dermal fibroblasts of normal skin. These studies were carried out by use of techniques of tissue culture and autoradiography.[116]

Freckles (ephelides) are the most common of this variety of melanosis. The pigmentation is in the form of clearly demarcated yellowish-brown to tan areas, varying in size and shape but predominantly small and most prevalent on the exposed parts of the body. They are absent in infancy, appear in childhood, never occur on the palms, soles, or inside the mouth, are more prominent in summer, and tend to fade in late adult life. The tendency to develop freckles is an inherited dominant characteristic. Except for occasional confusion with melanosis due to disease, their main significance is cosmetic.

Except possibly albinos, all persons have the potential of developing a melanotic neoplasm. Aside from the color of the local lesion and its metastases, persons with this condition in an advanced stage often have melanuria and may rarely develop a generalized darkening of the skin due to release from the tumor of precursors of melanin which are oxidized to this pigment in the epidermis.[55] This is one of the few instances in which melanin not produced locally by melanocytes can darken the skin[21]; it likewise occurs in ochronosis, in which an intermediate product of the catabolism of tyrosine, namely homogentisic acid, accumulates in the extracellular fluid and is deposited and darkens in cartilage, an area in which melanocytes do not occur.[10,21,54]

Mongolian spots (aggregates of dermal melanocytes) are blue in color and most commonly are located over the sacral areas, but may occasionally occur elsewhere. They are most common in certain of the darker races, but are seen infrequently in white babies. Such spots persist for a variable number of years after birth and eventually disappear.[10,35]

The common pigmented nevus varies from flesh color, to brown, to blue-black, depending upon the amount and depth of pigment-laden nevus cells.

The tendency for the skin pigmentation in Albright's syndrome to occur in unilateral, irregularly marginated patchy areas in roughly the same body location as the bone lesion is a distinctive clinical pattern. Also easily recognizable are the smoothly marginated *café-au-lait*[117] spots and axillary freckling[118] so commonly associated with neurofibromatosis. Such clean differentiation by visible skin patterns may not always be possible. Sometimes skin biopsies in melanotic conditions are helpful. Recent studies have shown that the melanotic macules in Albright's syndrome and in neurofibromatosis may be distinguished clearly by means of histological examination of split-skin preparations of basal melanocytes which show giant melanosomes in the latter condition. This is not generally seen in Albright's syndrome.[119]

The pigmentation pattern characteristically associated with the generalized form of intestinal polyposis (Peutz-Jeghers syndrome) occurs as small melanin spots distributed in an acral fashion inside and about the mouth, on the face, more prominent on the lower than the upper lip, and occasionally on the fingers and toes.[48] This pigmentation has thus far not been associated with polyposis limited to the stomach, the large bowel, or the rectum.

Melanin Pigmentation of Mucous Membranes. Histologic observations have shown that melanin-producing cells (melanocytes) are present in the oral mucosa of most white persons. Grossly visible melanized areas in the mouth (melanoplakia) are normally unusual in white persons of light complexion, are occasionally noted in those of dark complexion, and are very frequently observed in Negroes. Therefore, melanoplakia has the most diagnostic significance if seen in a person of light complexion or if it develops in a person in whom the mouth is known to have been clear of melanin spots by previous examination. In the darker racial groups, melanosis of the tongue rather than of the buccal mucosa proper may be suggestive of disease. The melanocytes in the mouth are subject to the same internal stimuli as those in the skin, so that melanoplakia occurs frequently in diseases that produce marked melanosis of the skin (Table 39-4). It is possible that the melanocytes in the oral mucosa may react to local physical factors in the mouth very much as do those of skin. Heat, chemical irritation, and friction may be important in this regard.[10,36,37] Also, benign and malignant tumors can arise from these oral melanocytes.[120]

Another dark pigment, to be distinguished from melanin, can be found in oral tissues. Hemosiderin may be present, usually due to trauma, but rarely as an oral manifestation of Shamberg's disease.[121]

It is of interest that melanocytes have also been demonstrated in the conjunctiva. At times, diseases that produce skin melanosis also result in an external ocular melanosis. However, this is less frequent than melanoplakia.

Melanocytes are also present in the nail bed, as indicated by the occasional occurrence of melanization here in Negroes[38] and its rare occurrence in white persons who have certain of the systemic diseases that produce severe melanosis.

METALLIC PIGMENTATION

Under certain conditions, abnormal skin color results from the deposition in skin of a group of pigments (not normally present), which have in common the fact that all are metallic. The various skin pigmentations resulting can be classified as metallic pigmentation and are presented in tabular form in Table 39-5.[10]

Most metallic pigments responsible for skin pigmentation are exogenous in origin. The important exception is hemosiderin, an iron-containing pigment, which results from local or general destruction of blood or from some defect in endogenous iron metabolism. The term *hemosiderosis* has been used in a general sense to depict deposition of this substance in body tissue.[10] In the skin it localizes in the superficial corium and if present leads to pigmentation, not only directly but also by stimulating melanin formation.

Hemochromatosis. Basically this condition is characterized by a defect in endogenous metabolism of iron with deposition of hemosiderin in certain visceral and endocrine organs as well as the skin. The mechanism for skin pigmentation is not entirely clear, but appears to involve deposition of hemosiderin in the corium and of melanin in the deep epidermis. The former pigment causes a bluish-black, slate, or lead color, whereas melanin is responsible for a brownish hue. The classic *bronze color* occasionally seen in this disease appears to depend on the combination of these two skin pigments. Copper is also deposited in the skin. The presence of iron and copper in the skin could bind the sulfhydryl substances and increase the degree of melanization by releasing inhibition of tyrosinase.[21] Likewise, deposition of hemosiderin in endocrine organs with resultant functional changes is characteristic of hemochromatosis, as witnessed by the almost constant pancreatic involvement causing diabetes mellitus. The gonads, pituitary, and adrenals are commonly involved, which could account, in part, for some of the melanosis. Cirrhosis also could be a factor.

Exogenous Hemosiderosis. Here the disease results from injection of an excess of blood in the form of repeated transfusions.[39] The excess hemosiderin resulting from the breakdown of this blood is deposited in the skin and organs and produces skin pigmentation in a manner similar to hemochromatosis.

To some degree, repeated hemolysis of internal origin leads to hemosiderin deposition, but probably only rarely is it sufficiently

TABLE 39-5. CLASSIFICATION OF THE METALLIC PIGMENTATIONS

Type	Pigment Responsible	Where Deposited	Skin Color	Circumstances for Its Causation	Clinical Significance
Hemochromatosis	Melanin and hemosiderin	Generalized in epidermis and corium	Tan; slate gray; bronze	Endogenous defect in iron metabolism, melanin stimulated by local action of hemosiderin in skin	Skin pigmentation characteristic of this disease and rarely absent; usually both melanin and hemosiderin are present
Hemosiderosis of skin from chronic hemolysis	Hemosiderin; melanin secondary	Generalized in corium	Tan; slate gray; bronze	As a result of repeated blood transfusion, especially if excess hemolysis occurs	Quite rare; suspect with use of many blood transfusions
Hemosiderosis of the lower legs	Hemosiderin; melanin secondary	Deeper epidermis and corium of legs	Brownish, copper hue, sepia	Limited to legs below knee and above shoe line; because of hydrostatic pressure increase in legs plus local capillary or blood hemolytic factor	Seen most commonly in venous stasis of leg veins, leg trauma, sickle-cell disease, chronic purpuric eruptions, congenital hemolytic jaundice, Mediterranean anemia, Gaucher's disease, Cushing's syndrome and some rare dermatologic disorders (see Ref. 10)
Argyria	Silver	Generalized in corium	Gray to blue	Deposited in skin regardless of route of entry to body; color exaggerated by exposure to the sun	Chiefly of cosmetic importance; closely simulates cyanosis
Bismuthia	Bismuth	Generalized in corium	Gray to blue	Deposition in skin over diffuse area	A rare cause of generalized skin pigmentation
Bismuth line	Bismuth sulfide	Gums near teeth	Black	Deposited in gums of persons receiving bismuth, especially if tartar deposits on teeth are present	Diagnostic of bismuth treatment, location limited to the mouth (rule out lead exposure)
Chrysiasis	Gold	Upper corium predominantly	Gray, grayish-blue to bluish-green	May follow prolonged use of gold therapy; concentrated in areas exposed to the sun	Cosmetic; gold more toxic than silver
Hydrargyria	Mercury	Epidermis and corium of local areas	Brown or slate gray (Red-cinnabar)	Of local origin; produced by rubbing mercury creams on skin, especially the face and neck	Chiefly cosmetic; simulates systemic causes of facial pigmentation; rare sensitization
Lead line	Lead sulfide	Gums near teeth	Black	Deposition in gums of lead sulfide; local mechanism is similar to bismuth line	Lead does not pigment the skin; lead line in gums is diagnostic of lead poisoning
Iron pigmentation	Basic ferric acetate	Corium	Brown	Produced by tattoo of corium; when iron salts are used on skin lesion lacking epidermal covering	Local areas only; of cosmetic importance
Chromium	Chromium oxide	Corium	Green	Tattoos	Local areas only; of cosmetic importance; rare sensitization

marked to account for skin pigmentation. These cases are difficult to evaluate since many also receive transfusions of blood.

Hemosiderosis of the Lower Legs. Extravasation of blood in the skin of the lower legs, particularly if repeated or of chronic duration, leads to deposition of hemosiderin in the corium and stimulation of melanin formation with production of a tan, brown, copper, or sepia skin color.[10] This type of pigmentation is limited to the area below the knees and above the upper level at which the shoe exerts a protective pressure and is more marked anteriorly than posteriorly. The pigmentation may be diffuse or localized to small areas, particularly about ulcers or areas of trauma. The most characteristic example seen clinically is the pigmentation noted in association with varicose veins, especially if ulceration occurs. Hemorrhagic diathesis, venous stasis in the leg veins, increased capillary fragility and changes in tissue pressure are all predisposing factors.[10] Some of the more common diseases responsible are listed in Table 39-5. Because of the many local causes of hemosiderosis in the legs, this area should never be used for biopsy study for hemochromatosis. Tan colored spots, localized mainly over the anterior tibial region, are common in diabetes.[122] Upon histologic examination, these spots show moderate telangiectasia of dermal vessels and hemosiderin deposits in dermal macrophages; thus, the skin pigmentation is associated with a chronic vasculitis, yet is possibly related to trauma or diabetic alteration of small arteries or arterioles in the dermis and subcutaneous tissue.[123]

Metal Ions in the Skin. Any silver compound that enters the body, regardless of the route of administration, results in deposition of silver in the corium of the skin; when a sufficient threshold is reached, it becomes clinically visible and is known as argyria. Exposure to sunlight greatly accentuates the color; such darkening upon exposure to light facilitates diagnosis. Although some degree of melanization may result, the main color is from the silver itself, which, because of its location in the corium, produces a slate-gray, lead, or bluish-gray skin tint. Clinically, argyria is of importance because of the disagreeable skin discoloration and the ease with which it is confused with cyanosis.

Chrysiasis (from gold) and bismuthia (from bismuth) occur rarely and simulate argyria in the mode of production and the clinical appearance. As a general rule, bis-

muth produces a dark line on the gum similar to that produced by lead.

Mercury preparations, if rubbed into the skin, produce a local area of discoloration. Metallic iron can tattoo the skin if it reaches the corium through a defect in the epidermis but cannot act systemically to influence skin color. The red and green colors of tattoos are due to mercury (cinnabar) and chromium, respectively.

EXAGGERATED SCATTERING PHENOMENON: BLUE COLORATION

As previously explained, normal "flesh" color of the skin is dependent upon the fact that "scattering" adds a blue component to offset the predominant red color reflected from the hemoglobin (Plate 4). It has been mentioned also that the same phenomenon explains the blue color seen over a heavy mass of pigment of whatever nature.

Scattering accounts for the blue color of a surprisingly wide variety of conditions encountered in medical practice.[10] The blue color of a large superficial subcutaneous vein is perhaps the best-known example. The mass of blood within the lumen of the vein, although dark red in color by reflected light if seen outside of the body (Plate 4), acts as a deep pigment substance to absorb the light reaching it. The light reflected from the tissues overlying the blood mass is scattered in the turbid vein wall and the deep part of the epidermis, to emerge as a blue color.

The tattoo artist produces a blue color in the skin by the use of black ink, the degree of blue produced being proportional to the amount of black ink and depth in the dermis at which the needle deposits the particles. The blue color of the skin which results from road accidents in which dark-colored dirt is scraped into the skin, and that which results from powder marks from explosion are other examples. A curious type of blue atrophic skin spots is seen in drug addicts who flame the hypodermic needle for sterilization purposes; injections produce blue tattoo marks by depositing carbon soot particles in the dermis or subcutaneous tissues. At times hypodermic injections of medication do the same thing. Similar spots have been noted from the bites of pubic pediculi.

The blue sclerae associated with fragilitas ossium are explained by the greater transparency of the sclerae in this condition which allows white light to penetrate to the pigmented coat of the eye with resultant absorption there, and greater preponderance

TABLE 39-6. CLASSIFICATION OF DERMAL PIGMENTATION
(Apparent Blueness: Due to Scattering Phenomenon)

Genetic	Blue nevus Mongolian spot (abnormally placed melanocytes in the dermis) Nevus of Ota Racial (in the eyelids, axillae, and nails of certain normal individuals) Incontinentia pigmenti
Chemical	Mercury (contained in face creams) Heavy metal intoxication (silver, bismuth, gold, lead) Carbon particles (tattoo, accidental pencil implant, drug addicts) Fixed drug eruption
Nutritional	Chronic malnutrition (splotchy, slate-gray pigmentation noted in prisoners of war, and experimental human starvation)
Metabolic	Hemochromatosis (due to hemosiderin particles in the dermis) Ochronosis (polymerized homogentisic acid in the dermis)
Neoplastic	Primary melanoma arising from blue nevus and nevus of Ota Metastatic malignant melanoma nodule in the dermis Malignant melanoma with melanuria and dermal pigmentation Pigmented basal-cell carcinoma Glomus tumor Hemangioma and hemangiosarcoma Neurofibromatosis*
Infectious and inflammatory . .	Pinta Chronic inflammatory dermatoses Pediculosis pubis (maculae ceruleae)
Circulatory	Purpura and hemosiderosis Cyanosis Methemoglobinemia Sulfhemoglobinemia

Classification from Fitzpatrick, Montgomery, and Lerner: J. Invest. Derm. 22:163.

* Presently considered as genetic in origin (see Table 39-4)

in the reflected light of rays scattered in the sclera itself. Greater transparency of the sclerae at birth may account for their tendency to blueness in the newborn. Rarely, individuals are born with their melanocytes located in the deep dermis instead of the lower epidermis over part or even most of their skin. Such persons exhibit a striking blue skin color in such areas. This unusual condition is only of cosmetic importance, since the skin is otherwise normal. A more common variety is the so-called *mongolian spot*, localized commonly but not exclusively over the sacral area at birth. It is due to a collection of functioning dermal melanocytes in this area which tend to lose their activity as the child develops, with gradual return of normal skin color. The blue phase of *pinta* has been demonstrated as due to deposition of melanin in the dermis. The blue color of the ears and nose, or even the skin, in *ochronosis* is due to pigment deposited in the

cartilage of the ear or nose, or at times deep in the skin.[9,10] During World War II, use of *quinacrine* hydrochloride for malaria rarely was noted to produce areas of blue color over the nose, fingernails, palate, etc., apparently the result of deposition of this substance or stimulation of some other pigment deep in the dermis.[15] A syndrome mimicking ochronosis has been described after prolonged local use of a preparation containing *resorcin*[84] in treatment of a chronic leg ulcer. The patient had dark urine containing black resorcin polymers.

There are other types of drug-induced bluish scatter pigmentation. A remarkable example is that caused by deposition in the skin of polymers of the oxidation products of *chlorpromazine*. Occasionally a patient on long-term therapy with chlorpromazine may have widespread deposition of the pigment: in the deep dermis, in the reticuloendothelial system, in parenchymal cells of liver, myocardium, kidney, brain, and lung. The pigment is actually brown, but because of the scattering effect, the skin has a purple color and affected persons have been referred to as "purple people."[124] Formation of melanin in the skin may be provoked by this drug, as suggested by Van Woert.[125] He has demonstrated in vitro that there is great increase in tyrosinase activity induced by phenothiazine compounds.[126]

The blue or purplish color of a deep ecchymosis due to a collection of pigment mass (free blood) in the subcutaneous tissue is another example.

The blue color of hematomas and the blue appearance of the umbilicus or of thin abdominal scars when the peritoneal cavity contains free blood are still other examples.

Fitzpatrick, Montgomery, and Lerner[55] discuss other disorders that produce a dermal pigmentation capable of producing a blue skin color as a result of the scattering phenomenon. The excellent classification proposed by these authors is given in Table 39-6.

The bluish discoloration occasionally noted about the eyelids and in the axillae may be because these areas in some normal people contain melanin in the dermis as well as the epidermis. The blue sheen of the shaven cheek or axillae of a person with dark hair results from "scattering" because of the darkly pigmented hair shafts in the deep dermis.[5,10] The reader is referred elsewhere[10] for references to the literature on this subject and for a key to available published colored plates. Those not familiar with this form of skin color will profit greatly by a study of such colored illustrations.

MISCELLANEOUS PIGMENTATIONS

There are a few conditions capable of producing abnormal pigments not readily classified in one of the preceding groups. Most of these are of academic interest and only rarely affect skin color to a degree to be of clinical importance. A few which come to mind are hematin in malaria, methemalbumin, porphyrins, etc. In the group would fall also the skin discolorations produced by the injection or ingestion of colored medicinal or testing substances. These are all self-evident and will not be discussed.

DECREASED SKIN PIGMENTATION

Most commonly, abnormal skin color reflects an increase of normal pigments or the presence of abnormal pigments. However, abnormal skin color at times may result from the diminution of the amount of one or more of the normal pigments or modification of their appearance by some anatomic or physiologic factor. Such changes may be just as indicative of disease as increase in skin pigmentation and fit usually into one of the following categories.

ANEMIA

The degree of pallor produced by anemia is ordinarily proportional to the hemoglobin content of the blood. As with any color values affected by amounts or chemical types of hemoglobin, the pallor of anemia is most readily detected in nonmelanized areas (i.e., the lips, the palpebral conjunctivae, and the transparent fingernails). Skin color in anemic patients varies for reasons other than diminution of hemoglobin alone. *Hemolytic anemia* may produce a combination of pallor and jaundice, as exemplified by the lemon-yellow pallor of severe pernicious anemia. Certain anemias may be associated with the skin deposition of hemosiderin. Vitiligo is not uncommon in anemia. Modern descriptions of hypochromic anemia in adolescent girls no longer include a greenish-yellow pallor. Melanin skin pigmentation occurs in refractory normochromic anemias, some cases of idiopathic microcytic hypochromic anemia, and pernicious anemia, as well as certain erythroblastic types of anemia. It may hide skin pallor and be associated at times with a spotty type of melanin pigmentation of the oral mucosa. The yellow pallor of certain hemolytic anemias may be modified by the presence of hemoglobinemia and methemoglobinemia.

DECREASE IN MELANIN PIGMENTATION

The great attention ordinarily paid in clinical practice to increased melanin pigmentation of the skin has overshadowed to a considerable degree the appreciation that there are many biochemical factors that inhibit melanin formation rather than increase it, leading to a decrease in skin pigmentation. Lerner and Fitzpatrick[21] have reviewed the many inhibitors of melanin formation. Most of these are of importance in vitro or in vivo in animals. Some, however, have been shown to be significant as melanin inhibitors in humans, and others appear theoretically possible. The implications of this phase of melanin metabolism have received little attention in regard to its relation to skin color in disease.

Albinism results not as formerly believed

from the inherited absence of melanocytes in the skin and the eyes, but rather the inability of the melanocytes to convert tyrosine to melanin, the defect being genetically controlled.[54] Melanocytes are said to be present in albino skin in numbers comparable to those in normal white skin.[56] There is no lack of the substrate tyrosine. The defect is therefore an inherited enzymatic abnormality. This has been pictorially presented by Fitzpatrick et al. (Fig. 39-18).[68] Albinism can occur in any racial group. The entire skin, eyes, and hair of such persons are completely lacking in melanin. The skin appears to be pale or a whitish-pink, the hair white, and the irides pink in color.

Partial albinism also occurs. It is controlled by a dominant gene, with lack of pigment being limited to part of the skin or hair, but with the eyes (as a rule) being normally pigmented.[40] This type can be confused easily with vitiligo. History will usually reveal that in albinism the lesion has been present since birth.

Another genetic disease of the melanocyte causing cutaneous hypopigmentation or depigmentation is the Chediak-Higashi syndrome. This is concerned with a hereditary gigantism of cytoplasmic organelles and involves not only melanosomes but also lysosomes of circulating leukocytes, especially granulocytes. Thus it seems that the disease is one of general membrane alteration rather than just a problem in the synthesis of an enzyme (tyrosinase). These patients typically have blond hair, pale skin, and photophobia due to decreased uveal pigment. They have anemia and leukopenia and are highly prone to infection. If the child lives to the age of 10 or so, he frequently develops a lymphoma-like terminal illness. The disease is inherited as a single autosomal recessive trait. The detailed membrane biochemistry has not been elucidated as yet.[127]

There are other forms of "partial albinism," such as piebaldism and Waardenberg's syndrome, in which a white forelock is present. These may be associated with other neurocutaneous genetic defects.

Vitiligo (leukoderma) represents an acquired loss of melanin pigmentation in one or more areas of the skin. It is readily recognized by its patchy distribution and, although extensive in some persons, almost never covers the entire body. It is more noticeable in persons normally heavily melanized (e.g., Negroes) and at times is readily overlooked in light blonds. Paradoxically, patches of vitiligo not uncommonly occur in the midst of skin areas of hyperpigmentation due to systemic diseases, or they may be seen adjacent to hyperpigmented patches.

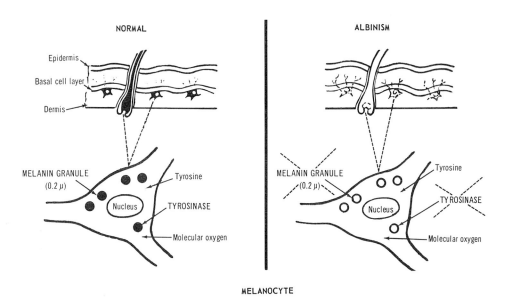

Fig. 39-18. The biochemical lesion in albinism. Note presence of "amelanated melanin granules," probably due to inability of tyrosinase mechanism. (Fitzpatrick, T. B., Seiji, M., and McGugan, A. D.: Medical progress: melanin pigmentation, New Eng. J. Med. 265:328, 374 and 430)

Vitiligo may result from (1) a variety of skin diseases that anatomically involve the melanocytes, (2) systemic disturbances that inhibit melanin formation biochemically, (3) nervous influence, and (4) autoimmune antibody formation.[128] It has been proposed that vitiligo involves autoantibodies directed against the melanocyte, melanosome, or melanin itself, but studies to determine these possibilities have not been definitive as yet.

The reader is referred to reviews for a discussion of mechanisms responsible for vitiligo.[63,129]

A common form of vitiligo occurs in persons otherwise healthy; it appears to be functional in nature, simulating in many ways the pattern of alopecia areata. This type may disappear as readily as it develops or may persist indefinitely; it may change in location with recurrence, or recur in identical areas.

Vitiligo occurs not infrequently in *Addison's disease*, depigmentation and pigmentation being intermingled in irregular patches.

Vitiligo is common in *hyperthyroidism* and may be due to increased sympathetic activity in this disease,[10] or to increased conversion of the melanin precursor tyrosine to thyroxine.[21] Areas of vitiligo have been noted in a Negro patient who was being treated with thiouracil.[41] This drug is known to act as an inhibitor of melanin in vitro by combining with the copper of the copper-tyrosinase complex. Thiouracil taken orally resulted in normal urine color in a patient with marked melanuria associated with metastatic melanoma.[42]

There is a sevenfold increase in the incidence of vitiligo in older patients with *diabetes mellitus* as compared with that in the general population.[130] Vitiligo is also common with *pernicious anemia*.[131] Because of this known association, an investigation of B_{12} absorption was done by the Schilling test in a large group of patients with vitiligo. There was definitely subnormal absorption (less than 3 per cent, as compared to normal 8 to 10 per cent) in 20 per cent of these patients.[132] Recent appearance of unexplained vitiligo should alert the physician to the possible presence of an associated systemic disease. Especially to be considered are Addison's disease, hyperthyroidism, diabetes mellitus, and pernicious anemia.

Chemical Depigmentation

An occupational vitiligo has been described in which depigmentation occurred in areas in contact with rubber-wear containing p-benzylhydroquinone.[43] Apparently this substance acts as a melanin inhibitor not only in vitro but also locally by penetration when applied to human skin. The vitiliginous areas usually remelanized slowly with cessation of application of this chemical to the skin. Hydroquinone added to diets of certain experimental animals has produced depigmentation of the hair, with return of hair pigmentation on a normal diet.[44]

Studies by Lerner and Fitzpatrick[58] indicate that monobenzyl ether of hydroquinone in ointment can be used locally to lighten hyperpigmented skin areas such as freckles, lentigo lesions, melasma of pregnancy, etc. Occasionally, marked contact-type dermatitis from this substance has been reported. More recently it has been noted that hydroquinone itself can be used effectively with lower incidence of skin sensitization. This substance can diminish the pigmentation of the normal skin of Negroes as well as hyperpigmentation of skin in white persons but does not affect normal white skin color nor the color of the eyes and hair. Applied to the skin of a pregnant Negress to produce depigmentation, it caused no change in skin color of her fetus in utero, a point verified at the time of delivery. This substance apparently acts through the ability of hydroquinone to interfere with enzyme reactions. Regeneration of skin color may require two or more months after cessation of its use. Newer depigmenting compounds have been reviewed recently.[133,134]

CHEMICAL REPIGMENTATION IN VITILIGO

Some interesting studies of therapeutic interest with regard to vitiligo have centered on the observation that 8-methoxypsoralen, used systemically, followed by exposure to solar or artificial ultraviolet radiation, may bring about remelanization.[59,60] Some investigations have suggested that a psoralen-tanned skin has a twofold protection against the sun, because in addition to increased basal melanogenesis, there may be prolonged presence of melanin in the stratum corneum.[135-137]

It is apparent that function of melanocytes in some areas of normal skin can be inhibited metabolically by one mechanism with formation of vitiligo, while simultaneously those in other areas are stimulated, with resultant melanosis.

NEVI AND DEPIGMENTATION

A vitiliginous area may develop about a nevus producing the "halo nevi." Ultrastructural studies of the biology of this tumor reveal degeneration of both basal melanocytes and nevus cells with invasion by a large number of lymphocyte-like cells. This would be compatible with an auto-immune process.[138]

Generalized Diminution of Melanin Pigment of the Skin. A number of systemic disorders produce a generalized decrease in melanization of the skin which may become clinically recognizable as pallor.

Paleness of the skin is characteristic of the male castrate. This is only in part due to diminished melanization.

Lack or diminution of melanin skin pigmentation has been noted commonly in Simmonds' disease,[34] a disorder attributable to a destructive process of the anterior lobe of the pituitary gland. This clinical finding is of great differential value in distinguishing between true Addison's disease and its simulation by secondary adrenal failure due to hypopituitarism.[10,21,34] Hypothyroidism is characterized by pallor, even in the absence of edema or anemia. There is poor circulation to the skin and decrease in melanization.

Comment has been made that children with the rare disease phenylketonuria have pale or light-colored skin, which fails to tan upon exposure to sunlight. It is due to an inborn error of metabolism in which the essential amino acid phenylalanine cannot be converted into tyrosine. In vitro, phenylalanine exerts an inhibitory effect on tyrosinase. Dietary restriction of phenylalanine in these cases results in increase of pigmentation toward normal.[68] This concept has been admirably schematized by Fitzpatrick and his associates (Fig. 39-19). Dietary source of tyrosine alone may not be adequate for melanin synthesis.[21,54]

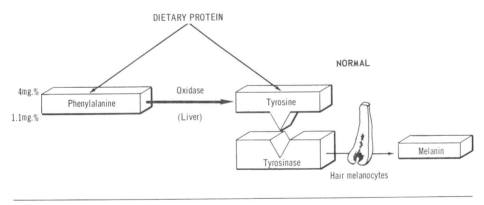

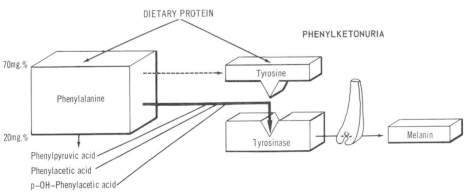

FIG. 39-19. Pathogenesis of decreased melanin pigmentation in phenylketonuria. Inhibition of tyrosine-tyrosinase mechanism by phenylalanine and other aromatic metabolites. (Fitzpatrick, T. B., Seiji, M., and McGugan, A. D.: Medical progress: melanin pigmentation, New Eng. J. Med. 265:328, 374, and 430)

Edema of the skin diminishes the intensity of melanin pigmentation as well as the color of hemoglobin.[10]

Negro babies have a rather light skin color at birth and show a progressive degree of melanogenesis, until a peak is reached in the sixth to eighth postnatal week.[47]

Depigmentation of many test animals, including cattle, results from the use of copper-deficient diets.[21] The counterpart of this in humans has not been reported but is theoretically possible. As previously mentioned, copper is necessary for the tyrosine-tyrosinase enzyme reaction.[21]

Diets deficient in the filtrate factors of the vitamin-B complex readily produce depigmentation of the hair in many test animals.[21] Gray hair and skin depigmentation have been reported in children on vitamin deficient diets, with return to normal pigmentation after adequate treatment.[45]

A number of studies indicate that the pigmentation of Addison's disease has been markedly diminished in intensity by the administration of ascorbic acid in large doses.[10] Ascorbic acid inhibits melanin formation and may also act to reduce the amount of melanin already present in the skin.[21,54]

EDEMA OF THE SKIN

Edema of the skin is associated with pallor. The structural elements of the integument are rendered more distant from each other, separated, as they are, by fluid. Light penetrating the skin path thus meets a diminished quantity of pigment. Fewer rays are absorbed and more are reflected; the skin therefore appears paler than normal. To this effect may be added the changes in the transmissibility of the tissues and perhaps significant reactions of the blood vessels, which may aid in producing the whiteness of the skin.

The characteristic white pallor of edematous skin is best shown in a child with nephrosis. Pallor is striking even though the red blood cell count may be almost normal.

Edema also hides melanin, as shown by the apparent partial loss of pigmentation noted in a subject with Addison's disease made edematous by deoxycorticosterone therapy.[10]

Jaundice cannot be detected in skin edematous prior to its onset. Unilateral body edema may occur as a trophic phenomenon in certain types of cerebrovascular disease. If jaundice then occurs in such a person, it may be limited unilaterally to the nonedematous side.[46] This explains the mechanism of unilateral jaundice.

The characteristic white color of an intracutaneous skin wheal is another example of the ability of fluid in the skin to raise it away from elements that cause color, or to dilute or separate them. The result is apparent depigmentation; the skin may be very pale.

It is evident that edema of the skin may influence its color strikingly. Therefore, one must use caution in evaluating skin color in edematous areas.

DIMINISHED BLOOD FLOW TO THE SKIN

One notes a striking pallor of the skin, if, for any reason, blood flow to the capillaries of the papillary projections and the superficial subpapillary plexuses is temporarily diminished. This serves to minimize the hemoglobin component of normal skin color. This is seen during syncope, early in Stokes-Adams syndrome, early in arterial emboli or other types of arterial obstruction, in peripheral circulatory constriction, etc.

Some persons (even though their hemoglobin content is normal) appear pale because of the inadequacy of the papillary and subpapillary vascular network or the flow of blood through these areas. That the pallor of the skin of a castrate results in part from such inadequate blood flow has already been discussed.

Inadequate blood flow in the tissues, if persistent, leads to stasis cyanosis, often mottled, so that one notes blotchy blue areas against a pale background. The characteristic ashen-gray color of peripheral circulatory constriction (shock) can be attributed to the combination of the pallor of poor capillary circulation of the skin combined with some degree of cyanosis of peripheral stasis origin.

SCAR TISSUE

Scar tissue when new is vascular and pink, when completely formed and healed is avascular and white. The white color is indicative in part of the minimal amount of melanin and hemoglobin pigment which it contains. Its optical characteristics resemble edematous tissue, and it even more strikingly reflects white light—with little differential absorption or reflection of the light rays within the visible spectrum.

MACERATED OR DESQUAMATING SKIN

Areas of the skin with these changes, similar to scar tissue, appear to have less than the normal amount of pigmentation and are white in color.

The coated tongue looks white because the filiform papillae, which have thickened and become opaque, along with debris collected between them, hide the deeper pigments and reflect white light without differential light ray absorption. With desquamation of the white filiform papillae, the mucosa with its prominent capillary projections is exposed, and one then sees the red color of a smooth atrophic tongue.

VALUE OF COLORED ILLUSTRATIONS IN MEDICAL EDUCATION

The old proverb that "one picture tells more than a thousand words" is even more true when changed to read "one *colored* picture, etc." Word descriptions of color of the skin have distinct limitations. Most helpful in teaching students the color appearance of the skin in disease is actual observation of patients. Unfortunately, patients suitable for depicting a particular condition are available only sporadically in any given institution. Next most useful would be movies, lantern slides, and photographs in color. The great expense of preparation has limited the number of colored photographs or illustrations published in monographs and medical journals, and those that have been printed are widely scattered. There is considerable educational value in systematically studying those available in the literature. For this purpose the reader is referred elsewhere[10] for a guide to many of the colored plates available in the journal literature depicting abnormalities in the color of the skin in disease. Other good color illustrations can be found by perusal of standard texts and systems of medicine. See Chapter 7 on Sore Tongue and Sore Mouth in this book.

SUMMARY

Careful inspection of the color of the skin and mucous membranes (plus the use of the spectrophotometer when possible) yields significant information in a large number of disorders.

The normal skin color depends upon various factors, chief among which are: the proportion of the light which is reflected and that which penetrates, and the depth of penetration; the amounts and proportions of the various pigments (melanin, oxyhemoglobin and reduced hemoglobin, carotene); and the phenomenon of scattering.

In health, skin coloration varies greatly between races and greatly among persons of the same race; with age and sex, with tanning from sunlight, with relative vascularity of the skin and vasomotor phenomena (flushing, vasoconstriction, etc.), and in different regions of the body. An understanding of the factors influencing normal skin coloration is necessary to permit interpretation of possible deviations from normal.

Abnormally increased pigmentation can be classified as due to (1) increased yellow components, (2) increased hemoglobin pigment of various types, (3) increased melanin, (4) increased content of metal deposits, or (5) effects of certain chemicals and drugs. Recognition of the specific cause of the abnormal increase may be of great diagnostic value and observation of alterations in the degree of pigmentation may allow deductions concerning the results of therapy, the prognosis, etc., in many conditions.

Decreased skin pigmentation occurs in partial or complete albinism, in vitiligo, in anemia, in certain endocrine states, in edema, and in skin with diminished blood supply. Proper interpretation of the pathologic physiology resulting in such losses of skin coloration is of great medical importance.

This chapter summarizes present knowledge concerning normal and abnormal skin pigments, methods of recognizing and measuring them, and the mechanisms and significance of abnormalities and alterations in skin coloration.

REFERENCES

1. Sheard, D., and Brown, G. E.: The spectrophotometric analysis of the color of the skin, Arch. Intern. Med. 38:816, 1926.
2. Sheard, C., and Brunsting, L. A.: Color of skin as analyzed by spectrophotometric methods; I. Apparatus and procedures, J. Clin. Invest. 7:559–574, 1929.
3. Brunsting, L. A., and Sheard, C.: Color of skin as analyzed by spectrophotometric methods; II. Role of pigmentation, J. Clin. Invest. 7:575–592, 1929.
4. ———: Color of skin as analyzed by spectrophotometric methods; III. Role of superficial blood, J. Clin. Invest. 7:793–813, 1929.
5. Edwards, E. A., and Duntley, S. Q.: Pigments and color of living human skin, Amer. J. Anat. 65:1–33, 1939.

6. Edwards, E. A., Hamilton, J. B., Duntley, S. Q., and Hubert, G.: Cutaneous vascular and pigmentary changes in castrate and eunuchoid men, Endocrinology, 28:119–128, 1941.

7. Edwards, E. A., and Duntley, S. Q.: Analysis of skin pigment changes after exposure to sunlight, Science 90:235–237, 1939.

8. ——: Cutaneous vascular changes in women in reference to the menstrual cycle and ovariectomy, Amer. J. Obstet. Gynec. 57:501–509, 1949.

9. Jeghers, H.: Skin color in health and disease, Med. Physics 2:984–988, 1950.

10. ——: Pigmentation of the skin, New Eng. J. Med. 231:88–100, 122–136 and 181–189, 1944.

11. Watson, C. J.: Bile pigments, New Eng. J. Med. 227:665 and 705, 1942.

12. Larson, E. A., Evans, G. T., and Watson, C. J.: A study of the serum biliverdin concentration in various types of jaundice, J. Lab. Clin. Med. 32:481–488, 1947.

13. Meakins, J. C.: Distribution of jaundice in circulatory failure, J. Clin. Invest. 4:135–148, 1927.

14. Jeghers, H.: Skin changes of nutritional origin, New Eng. J. Med. 228:678 and 714, 1943.

15. Lutterloh, C. H., and Shallenberger, P. L.: Unusual pigmentation developing after prolonged suppressive therapy with quinacrine hydrochloride, Arch. Derm. Syph. 53:349, 1946 (see colored plate).

16. Weidman, F. D.: Pathology of yellowing dermatoses; 1. Non-xanthomatous (jaundice, carotinemia, blood pigmentation, melanin, colloid degeneration and elastic degeneration), Arch. Derm. Syph. 24:954, 1931.

17. Montgomery, H.: Cutaneous manifestations of diseases of lipoid metabolism, Med. Clin. N. Amer. 24:1249, 1940.

18. Comroe, J. H., Jr., and Botelho, S.: Unreliability of cyanosis in recognition of arterial anoxemia, Amer. J. Med. Sci. 214:1, 1947.

19. Finch, C. A.: Methemoglobinemia and sulfhemoglobinemia, New Eng. J. Med. 239:470, 1948.

20. Becker, S. W., and Obermayer, M. E.: Modern Dermatology and Syphilology, ed. 2, Philadelphia, Lippincott, 1940.

21. Lerner, A. B., and Fitzpatrick, T. B.: Biochemistry of melanin formation, Physiol. Rev. 30:91, 1950.

22. Becker, S. W.: Skin: Melanin pigmentation produced by physical agents, Med. Physics 1:1430–1433, 1944.

23. Fitzpatrick, T. B., Lerner, A. B., Calkins, E., and Summerson, W. H.: Mammalian tyrosinase; melanin formation by ultraviolet irradiation, Arch. Derm. Syph. 59:620, 1949.

24. Becker, S. W.: Pigmentary diseases of the skin, Clinics 3:886, 1944.

25. Keys, A.: Caloric undernutrition and starvation, with notes on protein deficiency, J.A.M.A. 138:500, 1948.

26. Burger, G., Sandstead, H., and Drummond, J.: Starvation in western Holland, Lancet 2:282, 1945.

27. Davis, M., Boynton, J., Ferguson, J., and Rothman, S.: Studies on pigmentation of endocrine origin, J. Clin. Endocr. 5:138, 1945.

28. Pack, G. T., and LeFevre, R.: Age and sex distributions and incidence of neoplastic diseases at Memorial Hospital, New York City, with comments on "cancer ages," J. Cancer Res. 14:167, 1930.

29. Hamilton, J. B.: Influence of the endocrine status upon pigmentation in man and in mammals, *in* The Biology of Melanomas, vol. 4, p. 341, New York Academy of Sciences, 1948.

30. Sprague, R. G., Power, M. H., Mason, H. L., Albert, A., Mathieson, D. R., Hench, P. S., Kendall, E. C., Slocumb, D. H., and Polley, H.: Observations on the physiologic effects of cortisone and ACTH in man, Arch. Intern. Med. 85:199, 1950.

31. Calkins, E., quoted by Lerner and Fitzpatrick, Ref. 21.

32. Lea, A. J.: Influence of sodium chloride on the formation of melanin, Nature 155:428, 1945.

33. Sodeman, W. A.: Addison's disease, Amer. J. Med. Sci. 198:118, 1939.

34. Sheehan, H. L., and Summers, V. K.: The syndrome of hypopituitarism, Quart. J. Med. 18:319, 1949.

35. MacFarlane, E.: The sacral spot in Bengal, Science 95:431, 1942.

36. Monash, S.: Normal pigmentation of oral mucosa, Arch. Derm. Syph. 26:139, 1932.

37. Laidlow, G. F., and Cahn, L. R.: Melanoblasts in gum, J. Dent. Res. 12:534, 1932.

38. Monash, S.: Normal pigmentation in nails of Negro, Arch. Derm. Syph. 25:876, 1932.

39. Schwartz, S. O., and Blumenthal, S. A.: Exogenous hemochromatosis resulting from blood transfusions, Blood 3:617, 1948.

40. Macklin, M. T.: Genetic aspects of pigment cell growth in man, *in* The Biology of Melanomas, vol. 4, p. 144, New York Academy of Sciences, 1948.

41. Hellerstein, H. K., quoted by Lerner and Fitzpatrick, Ref. 21.

42. White, A. G.: Effect of tyrosine, tryptophane and thiouracil on melanuria, J. Lab. Clin. Med. 32 (pt. 2):1254, 1947.

43. Oliver, E. A., Schwartz, L., and Warren, L. H.: Occupational leukoderma, Arch. Derm. Syph. 42:993, 1940.

44. Martin, G. J., and Ansbacker, S.: Confirmatory evidence of the cromotrichial activity of *p*-aminobenzoic acid, J. Biol. Chem. 138:441, 1941.

45. Gillman, T., and Gillman, J.: Powdered stomach in the treatment of fatty liver and other manifestations of infantile pellagra, Arch. Intern. Med. 76:63, 1945.

46. Page, I. H.: Ipsolateral edema and contra-

lateral jaundice associated with hemiplegia and cardiac decompensation, Amer. J. Med. Sci. 177:273, 1929.

47. Zimmerman, A. A., and Cornbleet, T.: The development of epidermal pigmentation in the Negro fetus, J. Invest. Derm. 11:383, 1948.

48. Jeghers, H., McKusick, V. A., and Katz, K. H.: Generalized intestinal polyposis and melanin spots of the oral mucosa, lips and digits, New Eng. J. Med. 241:993 and 1031, 1949.

49. Hall, T. C., McCracken, B. H., and Thorn, G. W.: Skin pigmentation in relation to adrenal cortical function, J. Clin. Endocr. 13:243, 1953.

50. Gordon, M.: Pigment Cell Growth: Proceedings of the Third Conference on the Biology of Normal and Atypical Pigment Cell Growth, New York, Academic Press, 1953.

51. Fitzpatrick, T. B., and Lerner, A. B.: Terminology of pigment cells, Science 117:640, 1953.

52. Gates, R. R., and Zimmerman, A. A.: Comparison of skin color with melanin content, J. Invest. Derm. 21:339, 1953.

53. Shizume, K., and Lerner, A. B.: Determination of melanocyte stimulating hormone in urine and blood, J. Clin. Endocr. 14:1491, 1954.

54. Fitzpatrick, T. B., and Lerner, A. B.: Biochemical basis of human melanin pigmentation, A.M.A. Arch. Derm. Syph. 69:133, 1954.

55. Fitzpatrick, T. B., Montgomery, H., and Lerner, A. B.: Pathogenesis of generalized dermal pigmentation secondary to malignant melanoma and melanuria, J. Invest. Derm. 22:163, 1954.

56. Becker, S. W., Jr., Fitzpatrick, T. B., and Montgomery, H.: Human melanogenesis: Cytology of human pigment cells, A.M.A. Arch. Derm. Syph. 65:511, 1952.

57. Kenney, J. A., Jr.: Skin pigmentation: A review of recent advances in knowledge and therapy, J. Nat. Med. Ass. 45:106, 1953.

58. Lerner, A. B., and Fitzpatrick, T. B.: Treatment of melanin hyperpigmentation, J.A.M.A. 152:577, 1953.

59. Lerner, A. B., Denton, C. R., and Fitzpatrick, T. B.: Clinical and experimental studies with 8-methoxypsoralen in vitiligo, J. Invest. Derm. 20:299, 1953.

60. Kanof, N. B.: Melanin formation in vitiliginous skin under the influence of external applications of 8-methoxypsoralen, J. Invest. Derm. 24:5, 1955.

61. Lerner, A. B., Shizume, K., and Bunding, I.: The mechanism of endocrine control of melanin pigmentation, J. Clin. Endocr. 14:1463, 1954.

62. Lorincz, A. L.: Pigmentation, in Rothman, S. (ed.):Physiology and Biochemistry of the Skin, chap. 22, pp. 515–563, Chicago, Univ. Chicago Press, 1954.

63. Lerner, A. B.: Melanin pigmentation, Amer. J. Med. 19:902, 1955.

64. Buckley, W. R., and Grum, F.: Reflection spectrophotometry: Use in evaluation of skin pigmentary disturbances, Arch. Derm. 83:249, 1961.

65. ———: Reflection spectrophotometry: II. Effect of quinacrine on skin color, Arch. Derm. 83:249–261, 1961.

66. Fitzpatrick, T. B., Brunet, P., and Kukita, A.: The nature of hair pigment, in The Biology of Hair Growth, New York, Academic Press, 1958.

67. Reich, P., Schwachman, H., and Craig, J. M.: Lycopenemia: A variant of carotenemia, New Eng. J. Med. 262:263, 1960.

68. Fitzpatrick, T. B., Seiji, M., and McGugan, A. D.: Medical progress: Melanin pigmentation, New Eng. J. Med. 265:328, 374 and 430, 1961.

69. Lerner, A. B., and McGuire, J. S.: Effect of alpha- and beta-melanocyte stimulating hormones on the skin color of man, Nature 189:176, 1961.

70. Szabo, G.: Quantitative histological investigation on melanocyte system of human epidermis, in Gordon, M. (ed.): Pigment Cell Biology, pp. 44–125, New York, Academic Press, 1959.

71. Birbeck, M. S. C., Breathnach, A. S., and Everall, J. D.: An electronmicroscope study of basal melanocytes and high level clear cells (Langerhans cells) in vitiligo, J. Invest. Derm. 37:51, 1961.

72. Cowan, A.: Ocular pigment and pigmentation; 18th annual de Shweinitz lecture, A.M.A. Arch. Ophthal. 55:161–173, 1956.

73. Beerman, H., and Colburn, H. L.: Some aspects of pigmentation of the skin, Amer. J. Med. Sci. 231:451–475, 1956.

74. Deutsch, S., and Mescon, H.: Melanin pigmentation and its endocrine control, New Eng. J. Med. 257:222–226, 1957; 268–272, 1957.

75. Lerner, A. B.: Hormonal control of pigmentation, Ann. Rev. Med. 11:187–194, 1960.

76. Lerner, A. B., and McGuire, J. S.: Effect of alpha- and beta-melanocyte stimulating hormones on the skin color of man, Nature 189:176–179, 1961.

77. ———: Melanocyte-stimulating hormone and adrenocorticotrophic hormone: Their relationship to pigmentation, New Eng. J. Med. 270:539–546, 1964.

78. Buckley, W. R., and Grum, F.: Reflection spectrophotometry. III. Absorption characteristics and color of human skin, Arch. Derm. 89:110–116, 1964.

79. Abrahamson, I. A., and Abrahamson, I. A.: Hypercarotenemia, Arch. Derm. 68:4–7, 1962.

80. Findlay, G. H.: Cutaneous vasoconstrictors, primary pigmentation and the grey-blue reaction, Brit. J. Derm. 73:238–243, 1961.

81. Pathak, M. A., Riley, F. C., and Fitzpatrick, T. B.: Melanogenesis in human skin following exposure to long-wave ultraviolet and visible light, J. Invest. Derm. 39:435–443, 1962.

82. Monash, S.: Immediate pigmentation in sunlight and artificial light, Arch. Derm. 87: 686–690, 1963.

83. Tuffanelli, D., Abraham, R. K., and Dubois, E.: Pigmentation from antimalarial therapy: Its possible relationship to the ocular lesions, Arch. Derm. 88: 419–426, 1963.

84. Thomas, A. E., and Gisburn, A.: Exogenous ochronosis and myxedema from resorcinol, Brit. J. Derm. 73: 378–381, 1961.

85. Sternberg, T. H., and Bierman, S. M.: Unique syndromes involving the skin induced by drugs, food additives and environmental contaminants, Arch. Derm. 88: 779–788, 1963.

86. Madison, J. F.: Tetracycline pigmentation of teeth, Arch. Derm. 88: 58–59, 1963.

87. Esoda, E. C. J.: Chloasma from progestational oral contraceptives, Arch. Derm. 87: 486, 1963.

88. Weiner, J. S.: A spectrophotometer for measurement of skin color, Man 253: 152, 1951.

89. Weiner, J. S., Harrison, G. A., Singer, R., and Jopp, W.: Skin color in Southern Africa, Hum. Biol. 36: 294, 1964.

90. Prota, G., and Nicolaus, R. A.: On the biogenesis of phaeomelanins, in Montagna, W., and Hu, F. (eds.): Advances in Biology of Skin, vol. 8, chap. XX, pp. 323–328, Pergamon Press, London, 1967.

91. Szabo, G., Gerald, A., Pathak, M. A., and Fitzpatrick, T. B.: Racial differences in human pigmentation of the ultrastructural level, J. Cell Biol. 39: 132a–133a, 1968; also Abstract #325, 8th Annual Meeting of Amer. Soc. for Cell Biol.

92. Szabo, G., Gerald, A., Fitzpatrick, T. B., and Pathak, M. A.: Racial differences in melanogenesis before and after ultraviolet stimulation and electronmicroscope study, J. Invest. Derm. 50: 268, 1968; also Abstract #1, Proc. Meeting by Soc. for Invest. Derm.

93. Szabo, G., Gerald, A., Pathak, M. A., and Fitzpatrick, T. B.: Melanosomes behave differently in different races, Nature 222: 1081, 1968 (letter to the editor).

94. Gibson, H. L., Buckley, W. R., and Whitmore, K. E.: New vistas in infrared photography for biological surveys, J. Biol. Photog. Ass. 33: 1, 1965.

95. Fenech, F. F., Bannister, W. H., and Greech, J. L.: Hepatitis with biliverdinaemia in association with indomethacin therapy, Brit. Med. J. 3: 155, 1967.

96. Gordonson, L. L.: Scleral icterus, New Eng. J. Med. 271: 913, 1964 (letter to the editor).

97. Pittman, F. E.: The fluorescein string test: An analysis of its use and relationship to barium studies of the upper gastrointestinal tract in 122 cases of gastrointestinal tract hemorrhage, Ann. Intern. Med. 60: 418, 1964.

98. Fitzpatrick, T. B., Miyamoto, M., and Ishikawa, K.: The evolution of concepts of melanin biology, in Montagna, W., and Hu, F. (eds.): Advances in Biology of Skin, vol. 8, chap. 1, pp. 1–30, Pergamon Press, London, 1967.

99. Demopoulos, H. B.: Effects of reducing the phenylalanine uptake of patients with advanced malignant melanomas, Cancer 19: 65, 1964.

100. Demopoulos, H. B., Gerving, M. A., and Bagdoyan, H.: Selective inhibition of growth and respiration of melanomas by tyrosinase inhibitors, J. Nat. Cancer Inst. 35: 823, 1965.

101. Demopoulos, H. B., and Kaley, G.: Selective inhibition of respiration of pigmented S91 mouse melanomas by phenyl lactate, and the possible related effects on growth, J. Nat. Cancer Inst. 30: 611, 1963.

102. Demopoulos, H. B.: Effects of low phenylalanine-tyrosine diets on S91 mouse melanomas, J. Nat. Cancer Inst. 37: 185, 1966.

103. Van Woert, M. H., Prassad, K. N., and Borg, D. C.: Spectroscopic studies of substantia nigra pigment in human subjects, J. Neurochem. 14: 707–716, 1967.

103a. Van Woert, M. H., and Bowers, M. G., Jr.: Aromatic amino acid metabolism during L-DOPA therapy of Parkinson's disease, in Barbeau, A., and McDowell, F. H. (eds.): L-DOPA and Parkinsonism, Proc. of Laurentian Research Conference on L-DOPA, Montreal, Canada, 1969, Philadelphia, F. A. Davis, 1970.

104. Cotzias, G. C., Van Woert, M. H., and Schiffer, L. M.: Aromatic amino acids and modification of parkinsonism, New Eng. J. Med. 276: 374–379, 1967.

104a. Van Woert, M. H.: Reduced nicotinamide-adenine dinucleotide oxidation by melanin: Inhibition by phenothiazines (33275), Proc. Soc. Exp. Biol. Med., 129: 165–171, 1968.

105. Okun, M. R.: Histogenesis of melanocytes, J. Invest. Derm. 44: 285–299, 1965.

106. Okun, M. R., Edelstein, L. M., et al.: The histochemical tyrosine: Reaction for tyrosine and its use in localizing tyrosinase activity in mast cells, J. Invest. Derm. 53: 39, 1969.

107. Okun, M. R., Edelstein, L. M., Or, N., Hamada, G., and Donnellan, B.: The role of peroxidase vs. the role of tyrosinase in enzymatic conversion of tyrosine to melanin in melanocytes, mast cells, and eosinophils: An autoradiographic-histochemical study, J. Invest. Derm. 55: 1-12, 1970.

108. Okun, M. R. Edelstein, L. M., Or, N., Hamada, G., and Donnellan, B.: Histochemical studies of conversion of tyrosine and dopa to melanin mediated by mammalian peroxidase, Life Sci. 9: 491–505, 1970.

109. Mason, H. S., Ingram, D. J. E., and Allen, B.: The free radical property of melanin, Arch. Biochem. 86: 225, 1968.

110. Mason, H. S.: The structure of melanin, in Montagna, W., and Hu, F. (eds.): Advances in Biology of Skin, vol. 8, chap. XVII, pp. 293–312, Pergamon Press, London, 1967.

111. Pathak, M. A.: Photobiology of melanogenesis: Biological aspects, *in* Montagna, W., and Hu, F. (eds.): Advances in Biology of Skin, vol. 8, chap. XXV, pp. 397–420, Pergamon Press, London, 1967.

112. Hallwright, G. P., North, K. A. K., and Reid, J. D.: Pigmentation and Cushing's syndrome due to malignant tumor of the pancreas, J. Clin. Endocr. 24:496, 1964.

113. Ward, H. N., Konikov, N., and Reinhard, E. H.: Cytologic dysplasia occurring after busulfan (Myleran®) therapy, Ann. Intern. Med. 63:654, 1965.

114. Resnick, S.: Melasma induced by oral contraceptive drugs, J.A.M.A. 199:9, 1967.

115. Morris, L. L., and Danta, G.: Malignant cerebral melanoma complicating giant pigment naevus: A case report, J. Neurol., Neurosurg. Psychiat. 31:628–632, 1968.

116. Reed, W. B., Landing, B., Sugarman, G., Cleaver, M. E., and Melnyk, J.: Xeroderma pigmentosum: Clinical and laboratory investigation of its basic defect, J.A.M.A. 207: 2073, 1967.

117. Crowe, F. W., and Schull, W. J.: Diagnostic importance of cafe-au-lait spot in neurofibromatosis, Arch. Intern. Med. 91:758, 1953.

118. Crowe, F. W.: Axillary freckling as a diagnostic aid in neurofibromatosis, Ann. Intern. Med. 61:1142, 1964.

119. Benedict, P. H., Szabo, G., Fitzpatrick, T. B., and Sinesi, S. J.: Melanotic macules in Albright's syndrome and in neurofibromatosis, J.A.M.A. 205:618, 1968.

120. Dummett, C. O., and Barens, G.: Pigmentation of the oral tissues: A review of the literature, J. Periodont. 38:369–378, 1967.

121. Harris, D. C.: Oral manifestations associated with Shamberg's disease, Oral Surg., Oral Med., Oral Path. 19:304–308, 1965.

122. Danowski, T. S., Sabeh, G., Sarver, M. E., Shelkrat, J., and Fisher, E. R.: Shin spots and diabetes mellitus, Amer. J. Med. Sci. 251:570, 1966.

123. Fisher, E. R., and Danowski, T. S.: Histologic, histochemical, and microscopic features of the shin spots of diabetes mellitus, Amer. J. Clin. Path. 50:547–554, 1968.

124. Nahum, L. H.: The purple people syndrome, Conn. Med. 29:332, 1965.

125. Van Woert, M. H.: Isolation of chlorpromazine pigments in man, Nature (London) 219: 1054–1056, 1968.

126. ———: Activation of tyrosinase by chlorpromazine, Reilly, V. (ed.): Proc. 7th Int. Pigment Cell Conf., Seattle, Wash., New York, Appleton Century Crofts, Inc., 1970.

127. Weary, E. P., and Bender, A. S.: Chediak-Higashi syndrome with severe cutaneous involvement, Arch. Intern. Med. 119:381, 1967.

128. Bor, S., Feiwel, M., and Chavarin, I.: Vitiligo and its aetiological relationship to organ-specific autoimmune disease, Brit. J. Derm. 81:83, 1969.

129. Charcot-Turner, M. L., and Lerner, A. B.: Physiologic changes in vitiligo, Arch. Derm. 91:390, 1965.

130. Dawber, R. P. R.: Vitiligo in mature-onset diabetes mellitus, Brit. J. Derm. 80:275, 1968.

131. Allison, J. R., Jr., and Curtis, A. C.: Vitiligo and pernicious anemia, Arch. Derm. Syph. 72:407, 1955.

132. Bleifeld, W., and Gehrmann, G.: Vitamin B_{12} absorption in vitiligo, German Med. Monthly 12:273, 1967.

133. Bleehan, S. S., Pathak, M. A., Hori, Y., and Fitzpatrick, T. B.: Depigmentation of skin with 4-isopropylcatechol, mercaptoamines and other compounds, J. Invest. Derm. 50: 103, 1968.

134. Frenk, E., Pathak, M. A., Szabo, G., and Fitzpatrick, T. B.: Selective action of mercaptoethylamines on melanocytes in mammalian skin, Arch. Derm. 97:465, 1968.

135. Becker, S. W., Jr.: Psoralen phototherapeutic agents, J.A.M.A. 202:422, 1967.

136. Pathak, M. A.: Mechanism of psoralen photosensitization and in vivo biological action spectrum of 8-methoxypsoralen, J. Invest. Derm. 37:397, 1961.

137. Pathak, M. A., and Fitzpatrick, T. B.: Relationship of molecular configuration to activity of furocoumarins which increase cutaneous responses following long wave ultraviolet radiation, J. Invest. Derm. 32:255, 1969.

138. Swanson, J. L., Wayte, D. M., and Helwig, E. G.: Ultrastructure of halo nevi, J. Invest. Derm. 50:435, 1968.

139. Gold, A. P., and Freeman, J. M.: Depigmented nevi: The earliest sign of tuberous sclerosis, Pediatrics 35:1003, 1965.

140. Hughes, J. D., and Wooten, R. L.: The orange people, J.A.M.A. 197:730, 1966.

141. Okun, M. R., Edelstein, L. M., Hamada, G., Burnett, J., Blumental, G., and Or, N.: Peroxidatic tyrosinase activity in mast cells, eosinophils and melanoma cells, *in* Reilly, V. (ed.): Proc. 7th Int. Pigment Cell Conf., Seattle, Wash., New York, Appleton Century Crofts, Inc., 1970.

142. Demopoulos, H., Regan, M. A. G., and Regan, D.: The vital respiratory role of tyrosinase in pigmented melanomas, *in* Reilly, V. (ed.): Proc. 7th Int. Pigment Cell Conf., Seattle, Wash., New York, Appleton Century Crofts, Inc., 1970.

143. Seiji, M.: Subcellular particles and melanin formation in melanocytes, *in* Montagna, W., and Hu, F. (eds.): Advances in Biology of Skin, vol. 8, London, Pergamon Press, 1967, pp. 189–222.

144. Brooks, V. E. H., and Richards, R.: Depigmentation in Cushing's syndrome, Arch. Intern. Med. 117:677, 1966.

40

Itching (Pruritus)

ARTHUR L. SHAPIRO

MECHANISM OF ITCHING

Two hundred years ago, itching (pruritus) was defined as "an unpleasant cutaneous sensation which provokes the desire to scratch," and this simple definition is still the best. The sensation arises in free nerve endings of richly ramifying axons in the epidermis or in the corresponding epithelial layer of the transitional mucous membranes. Itching cannot be elicited from skin areas denuded of their epidermis. The whole integument is able to receive impulses that lead to the perception of itching. There is an increased responsiveness in the external auditory canals and in the mucocutaneous junctions of the vulva, the urethra, the anus and the nostrils.

Stimulation of the nerve endings is brought about by chemical, mechanical, thermic, or electric stimuli acting from the outside as well as from the inside. If the stimulus, in addition to its effect on the nerve endings, also simultaneously acts irritatingly on epidermal cells or capillary vessel walls, an inflammatory lesion develops. At the site of this lesion, after subsidence of the itching, an increased itching excitability persists for many hours or even days, regardless of whether or not the anatomic lesion has subsided. In this state of increased excitability, the threshold for adequate stimuli is lowered and the responses are exaggerated. Furthermore, inadequate stimuli, such as light touch, light strokes, pressure, release of pressure, and temperature stimuli elicit intense itching sensations. For example, the spot of a long-forgotten insect bite starts to itch again when it is lightly rubbed or pressed upon or exposed to sudden temperature changes. This state of itching hyperexcitability was interpreted by Graham et al.[5] as being caused by a barrage of noxious impulses from the site of injury producing a segmental excitatory state in the cord.

If this reawakening of the itching sensation recurs several times in the same spot and is responded to by vigorous scratching, the itching excitability rapidly increases, and soon a vicious cycle develops consisting of increasingly violent scratching and increasingly intense itching. This development is greatly facilitated and seriously aggravated by a proliferative reaction of the epidermis in response to repeated mechanical stimulation. The classical form of this reactive epidermal thickening is called "lichenification" (Fig. 40-1), and is dealt with in the paragraph on sequels to scratching. In pathologic conditions, the itching-scratching cycle becomes a tormenting affair. It may last many hours, and the scratch paroxysm may cease only because of total somatic and psychic exhaustion of the patient.

In understanding the mechanism of itching certain fairly well-established conceptions are useful. The nerve endings mediating the pruritic sensation are made more sensitive by *capillary dilation*. Heat thus increases the symptom, whereas cold and vasoconstriction diminish it. Epinephrine and ephedrine tend to diminish pruritus through their vasoconstrictive action. In many inflammatory skin lesions, the sensibility of the itching nerve endings is heightened mainly because of hyperemia, and if such lesions are stimulated, either chemically by pathologic metabolic products or mechanically, itching and the itching-scratching cycle arise with particular ease. On the other hand, any measure that decreases arterial hyperemia and the other signs of acute inflammation is likely to decrease the sensation of pruritus which has originated with the inflammatory process. Thus, corticotropin and adrenal corticoids, the latter in systemic as well as local application, often have a dramatic antipruritic effect, merely by virtue of their anti-inflammatory action. *Tissue anoxia* due to venous stasis (tight clothing, venous varicosities) results in itching and is relieved when the blood flow becomes adequate. Ultraviolet irradiation, x-rays, or local anesthetics by their direct action on the nerve endings temporarily may decrease their sensitivity sufficiently long to interrupt the itching-scratching cycle and stop the excessive peripheral stimulation.

Itching hyperexcitability may be elicited, not only by peripheral mechanisms, but also centrally. The perception of itching has an *integrating center* in the hypothalamus and the excitability of this center can be influenced pharmacologically. The subcortical center is under a higher control in the cortex. In animal experiments, scratch movements become greatly enhanced after bilateral ablation of the frontal cortex. Psychogenic pruritus occurs in man and will be discussed later.

The foregoing considerations indicate that two factors determine whether or not in a given pathologic process itching is produced: the intensity and the quality of the itching stimulus and the itching excitability, which under pathologic conditions may be greatly enhanced by either peripheral or central influences.

Thomas Lewis and his associates advanced the theory that itching is always brought

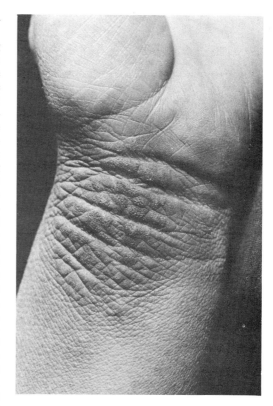

Fig. 40-1. Lichenification in neurodermatitis.

about by the release of histamine or a histamine-like substance, whatever the primary —physical or chemical—stimulus may be. According to this theory, itching and urticarial reaction ("triple response") are coordinated phenomena, both produced by mediation of released "H-substance." This theory seems to be well-founded when it is applied to itching in anaphylactic and allergic skin reactions. It cannot be accepted, however, as an explanation for pruritus without visible gross or microscopic changes, as in pregnancy, diabetes, diseases of the liver, and lymphoblastomas, because in concentrations that evoke itching, histamine also causes visible changes.

The heuristic theory of Lewis has been quite spectacularly confirmed by the advent of *antihistaminic drugs*. These drugs exert a hitherto unparalleled symptomatic effect on urticarial itching eruptions. However, in conformity with what has been said in the previous paragraph, low dosages of antihistaminics first relieve pruritus, while urticaria still remains. Also, the symptomatic effect of these drugs is constant and reliable only when itching is based upon liberation of histamine. The antipruritic effect of antihistaminics which occasionally occurs in other conditions (e.g., neurodermatitis, pruritus ani, etc.) is not based upon the antihistaminic potentialities of these drugs, but upon their side actions of general sedation or local analgesia.

Shelley and Arthur[11,12] have reported that certain proteolytic enzymes, the endopeptidases, are uniquely effective chemical stimuli for the production of pruritus in man. They have postulated that release or activation of proteases in the epidermis plays a significant role in the pathomechanism of itching. They maintain that the action of proteolytic enzymes is independent of histamine release.

IMMEDIATE STIMULI

In the present inadequate state of our knowledge we can at least list some of the factors which we now believe to provoke itching by direct or possibly indirect action at the nerve terminals. Two points must be kept in mind: (1) there may be intermediate agents (e.g., anoxia may cause release of a chemical stimulant), and (2) concomitant action of two or more modalities (e.g., chemical + temperature, or chemical 1 + chemical 2) may be necessary to produce the adequate stimulus. Various reasons for believing that some of these factors do cause pruritus are discussed under appropriate clinical headings later in this chapter.

Primary factors for which we now have some evidence include:

(1) Heat, cold, light, electrical stimuli
(2) Capillary vasodilation
(3) Anoxia
(4) Histamine
(5) Serotonin
(6) Proteolytic enzymes
(7) Bile acids
(8) Retained substances in uremia
(9) Calcium salts + uremia
(10) Certain allergens, ? with intermediate action of histamine, or by some H-substance (histamine-like in action), or by a proteolytic enzyme, etc.
(11) Certain chemicals and drugs, perhaps acting directly or through intermediate agents as suggested previously
(12) Certain cell constituents or cell products which may act directly or through an intermediate agent. These may be produced in the patient's own body or be introduced from some external source from some other organism (plant, virus, bacteria, fungus, insect, animal, etc.).

A full exploration of all the possibilities of all of the agents that may cause itching is not within the scope of this chapter. The whole subject is closely integrated with immune and protective mechanisms, autoimmune processes, etc.

All of the previously mentioned "primary factors" may be the active agents that initiate the itching, but at present it is believed that the **immediate direct stimuli** probably are (1) histamine or (2) proteolytic enzymes —or that both of these may act together.

Histamine released in the skin may explain how many of the primary factors just listed can cause itching, especially when histamine is produced as the result of an antigen-antibody reaction in the skin.

Proteolytic enzymes may be liberated in the skin or introduced into the skin through action of many of the "primary factors" listed previously.

Itch powder (Cowhage, Mucuna pruriens). The leguminous plant *Mucuna pruriens* bears on the surface of its seed pods a fine covering of tiny sharp-pointed spicules, called "itch powder" because when applied to the skin either accidentally or experimentally it provokes intense pruritus, sometimes with erythema or wheal formation, sometimes with no visible skin change. The immediate cause of the itching seems to be (1) histamine released from body cells due to a histamine-liberating action of the powder, and (2) mucunain, a proteolytic enzyme.

It has been found that, in addition to mucunain, many other proteolytic enzymes, such as papain, trypsin, plasmin, etc., produce itching after intradermal or intraepidermal administration. It is suggested[11,12] that release or activation of proteolytic enzymes, from the body's own cells or introduced from without (from bacteria, fungi, etc.), causes the itching through direct action of such an enzyme on the most superficial nerve endings in the skin.

In the sections that follow, we shall discuss the clinical aspects of itching, the chief clinical conditions in which it occurs, and the pathogenic mechanisms involved, as far as they are understood at present.

ANALYSIS OF ITCHING AS A SYMPTOM

DIAGNOSTIC EVALUATION OF ITCHING

Whether or not a cutaneous disorder elicits itching depends more on the nature of the etiologic agent than on the nature of the morphologic elements. For this reason, the value of the itching symptom in determination of etiology is considerable, particularly in the differential diagnosis of morphologically similar eruptions. For example, there is a vast variety of cutaneous manifestations of syphilis, cutaneous tuberculosis, and leprosy, but *none evokes itching*. The fact that syphilids do not cause any subjective symptom is particularly of great diagnostic value, because syphilis, the "great imitator," produces in its secondary period not only the roseola, which closely resembles toxic drug eruptions, but also lichenoid, psoriasiform, varioliform, etc., eruptions, and in its tertiary period chronic granulomatous lesions that are similar to itching lymphoblastomas. In addition to chronic infectious granulomas, the large groups of nevi and benign and malignant neoplasms of the skin also can be ruled out when itching is present.

Of course, for diagnostic evaluation, the presence or the absence of the itching sensation must be established beyond doubt. This is easy when *scratch marks* are present. But such marks are sometimes hard to differentiate from spontaneous lesions, and they are by no means always present in itching conditions. Thus, one must depend largely on the patient's statements, which are not necessarily reliable. A patient sometimes will complain of itching, although the lesion is asymptomatic, because when a lesion is elevated or has an uneven rough surface the patient often palpates that lesion, strokes it, or scratches it, and such mechanical irritation elicits a "minimal pruritus" in the nonitching lesion as well as in normal skin. Some patients will deliberately deny the itching, mainly because they feel that they have been "guilty" in scratching. Most commonly, however, the complaint of itching is exaggerated rather than understated.

To have a clear picture, it is never sufficient simply to ask the patient whether he itches or not. One also must ask the following questions: (1) Are you disturbed in your sleep by itching at night and do you wake up finding yourself scratching? (2) Can you forget about your itching in the daytime when your attention is distracted? (3) Can you stop scratching easily when you make up your mind to do so? (4) Does itching arise only in certain situations, such as warm environment, cold weather, undressing, rubbing of a piece of clothing at that spot, etc.?

We may classify the disorder as an obligate itching condition only if it definitely disturbs the patient's sleep. Otherwise the itching is a more or less accidental symptom of minor diagnostic value, because most of the inflammatory cutaneous lesions may itch occasionally as a result of increased hyperexcitability of the nerve endings. When this is the case, the patient will answer our Question 1 with "No"; Questions 2 to 4 with "Yes."

It often has been claimed that more pronounced itching at night is characteristic of one or the other skin disease, particularly of scabies; however, this is not so. Intensification of itching at night is a common feature of all conditions with obligate itching. This is partly because of the warming of the skin in bed, and partly because of the absence of the distractive perceptions of daytime activities. In addition, there seems to be a daily periodicity in the tonus of cutaneous capillaries, possibly in association with the daily periodicity of body temperature changes. A maximum of capillary dilatation seems to occur in the early evening hours when the body temperature is highest. This is assumed because the daily exacerbation of itching frequently starts a few hours before the patient goes to bed, and because increased blood flow to the skin intensifies itching excitability.

In any case, for diagnostic purposes it is essential to know whether or not pruritus awakens the patient at night in order to separate obligate and facultative itching conditions.

On this basis, the following classification can be made*:

Obligate itching disorders:

1. Pediculosis, scabies and related mite infestations, insect bites, and other external injuries resulting in urticarial wheals
2. Contact dermatitis (both primarily toxic and allergic), caused by exposure to chemical or physical agents
3. Urticaria and toxic eruptions
4. Neurodermatitis, prurigo, strophulus (miliaria)
5. Pruritus due to pregnancy, hepatobiliary diseases, lymphoblastoma, malignant internal neoplasms, kidney insufficiency
6. Dermatitis herpetiformis
7. Lichen planus

* Rare cutaneous disorders, such as prurigo nodularis, urticaria pigmentosa, etc., are not included.

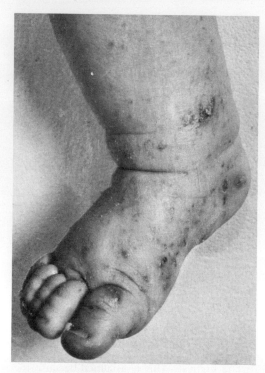

FIG. 40-2.   Scabies.   Torn-off burrows on medial aspect of heel.

Facultative itching disorders (with great variety in intensity, largely depending upon the degree of inflammation):

1. Asteatosis (xerosis, dry skin)
2. Pruritus due to diabetes
3. Psoriasis
4. Seborrheic dermatitis
5. Pityriasis rosea
6. Skin infections due to pyogenic organisms and fungi
7. Local anoxia due to varicose veins, tight clothing, etc.
8. Mechanical irritation

Non-itching disorders:

1. Developmental anomalies
2. Atrophies, degenerations and hyperplasias
3. Benign neoplasms
4. Malignant neoplasms
5. Dermotropic virus infections
6. Chronic infectious granulomas (tuberculosis, syphilis, etc.)
7. Lupus erythematodes
8. Pigmentary anomalies
9. Trophic and deficiency diseases
10. Diseases of sweat glands, sebaceous glands, hair follicles, and nails

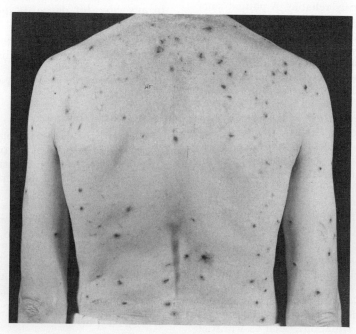

FIG. 40-3.   Neurotic excoriations.

Fig. 40-4. Eczema due to pollen. It is difficult to decide whether the punctiform lesions are dried crusts of broken vesicles or scratch marks.

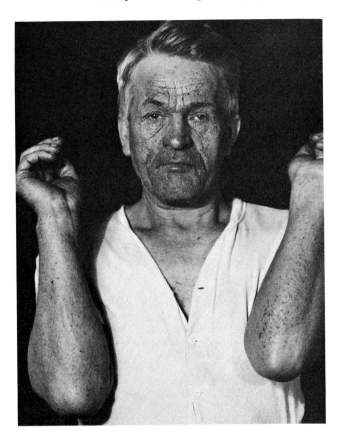

DIAGNOSTIC VALUE OF SCRATCH MARKS AND THEIR SEQUELS

Proper analysis of the complaint of itching often involves observation of the presence or the absence of scratch marks and skin changes secondary to scratching. The motor response to itching in man is carried out in different ways, namely, by scratching with the free ends of the fingernails, by rubbing with the fingertips or with the nail plates of the fingers, by rubbing one extremity with the other, by kneading movements, by pinching, and sometimes by simple pressure.

Excoriations, either punctiform or linear bloody crusts, result only from scratching with the sharp edges of the nail, and it is a notorious fact that in a great number of itching conditions such marks are not found. They are not present, or only exceptionally, in urticarial eruptions, whether of external or internal origin, nor are they found in lichen planus, and sometimes they are conspicuously absent in lichenified lesions of neurodermatitis. The nails of the neuro-dermatitis patient are often shiny, smooth, and polished as though they had been subject to careful manicuring, and this indirect sign bears witness that the patient is suffering from one of the most tormenting itching skin diseases. The patient does not "scratch"; he merely "rubs" and polishes his nails on his own skin. The eyebrows are often rubbed off, so that only a few sparse hairs remain.

In lichen planus the disproportion between severe complaints of itching and almost complete absence of scratch marks is rather characteristic. This is mentioned in order to demonstrate that the scratching technic is obviously different in different diseases.

A special technic is exerted in "prurigo of Hebra" and related conditions. The small elevated itching papules are torn off in their entirety as soon as they are formed, and only a flat bloody crust is left. In scabies, too, entire lesions are torn off—vesicles, papules and burrows, together with the sarcoptes and the ova in them (Fig. 40-2).

In neurotic excoriations the flat (normal)

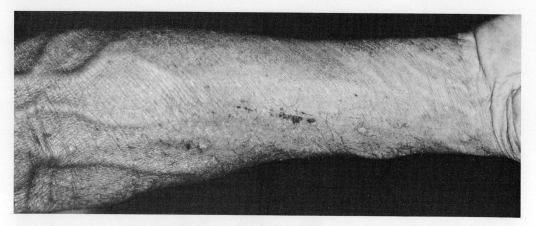

FIG. 40-5. Linear scratch marks and epidermal thickening in chronic dermatitis.

skin surface is torn off by digging or picking movements, again leaving a bloody crust (Fig. 40-3). Depending upon the depth of injury, a pitting scar may or may not result. Usually, after the crust has fallen off, a hyperpigmented spot remains for several weeks.

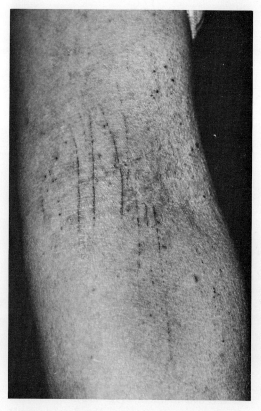

FIG. 40-6. Linear scratch marks in flexural neurodermatitis.

Punctiform scratch marks, with the tiny crusts at about equal distance from each other, may arise in normal skin, because scratching first causes a pilomotor reaction (prepapular phase of Jacquet) and continued scratching leads to the excoriation of the slightly elevated follicular surfaces.

It is often difficult to differentiate punctiform scratch marks from tiny, dried hemorrhagic vesicles (Fig. 40-4).

Long linear scratch marks (Figs. 40-5 and 40-6), often parallel because of simultaneous use of several nails, indicating uninhibited scratching, are seen mainly in pediculosis, scabies, pruritus due to pregnancy, lymphoblastomas, liver diseases, kidney insufficiency, and malignant tumors. In all of these conditions, pyogenic infections, secondary to the scratch excoriations, often occur in the form of pustules, impetigo, furuncles, lymphangitis, cellulitis, erysipelas, and acute suppurative lymphadenitis. Staphylococcic infections of the hair follicles are particularly common in pruritus due to diabetes and in exfoliative dermatitis due to arsenical poisoning.

Correct recognition of scratch marks has diagnostic significance, not only because they are objective signs of itching and scratching, but also because their characteristic localization may lead to a final diagnosis. For instance, linear scratch marks on the nape of the neck and on the upper back often lead to the discovery of head-lice infestation that otherwise would remain undetected. Scabies sometimes can be diagnosed by the localization alone of scratch marks in cases where most burrows are torn off or removed by scrubbing.

A common sequel of scratching in chronic itching conditions is the gradual **enlargement of subcutaneous lymph nodes.** Such "buboes," histologically displaying only chronic inflammatory changes, may develop insidiously, mainly in the groin and in the axillae, without any clinically manifest acute pyogenic infection. The enlarged glands are hard and indolent. The lymph node enlargement is often a source of diagnostic errors, when one endeavors to differentiate Hodgkin's disease or other lymphoblastomas from chronic dry neurodermatitis or prurigo on purely clinical grounds.

Another common consequence of chronic scratching is **lichenification,** which is represented by deepening of the normal skin lines with formation of infiltrated, slightly elevated, shiny rhomboidal fields in between the lines (Fig. 40-1). In its classical form, lichenification occurs only in dry diffuse neurodermatitis, and in circumscribed neurodermatitis, also called lichen simplex chronicus of Vidal. But similar changes, also due to epidermal thickening, are seen in chronic allergic eczema, particularly in industrial cases, in prurigo, and in lymphoblastomas. Although there is no doubt that lichenification arises from mechanical irritation, it cannot be produced experimentally, at will, by scratching. Its development requires a certain predisposition. The great readiness to develop lichenification in response to mechanical irritation is one of the most outstanding features of neurodermatitis.

Scratching or stroking not severe enough to damage the skin evokes a localized vascular response. Linear mechanical stimuli of low intensity produce a white line (dermographia alba) because of constriction of the superficial cutaneous capillary vessels. Stronger stimuli elicit vasodilation manifested by a red line (dermographia rubra). In those individuals hypersensitive to mechanical stimuli, wheal formation may follow scratching; this is known as *factitial urticaria.* In such individuals one can "write" protruding letters in the skin, and therefore the condition is also called *dermographia elevata* (Fig. 40-7). Whereas white and red dermographisms are physiologic vascular reactions, factitial urticaria is a pathologic state. It has an allergic mechanism proved because the urticarial sensitivity to mechanical stimuli can be transferred passively with the patient's serum to normal persons. Antihistaminic drugs influence favorably both the itching and whealing in this condition.

GENERALIZED PRURITUS

Pruritus Due to Tissue Anoxia

This type of pruritus has not yet been explored experimentally, and the knowledge about it is based purely on clinical observations.

Venous stasis may lead to itching in the stasic area when the superficial cutaneous veins are involved and the blood flow to the skin is slowed. The classical example is pruritus as a prominent part of the symptom complex associated with venous varicosities. It is true that the pruritus does not parallel the severity of the varicose condition. Still, there can be little doubt that the itching is of circulatory origin, because it is relieved after successful treatment of the varicosities. We have often observed prompt and complete disappearance of itching after application of a well-fitting zinc-gelatin boot. Also, it is obvious that such itching originates directly from stasis and not by interposition of inflammatory processes (stasic dermatitis), because itching is felt in areas that do not display signs of inflammation, either grossly or microscopically.

Itching due to stasis usually does not reach exasperating intensities. It is felt most intensely when the stockings are removed or, to a lesser degree, when they are put on. In daytime it may be completely forgotten, and usually it does not disturb the patient at night. In contrast with this relatively mild degree of itching, scratching is wild and often done with the nails, so that excoriations result. If the condition persists for

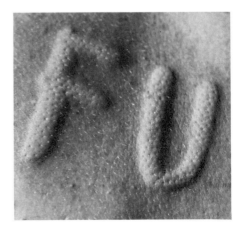

Fig. 40-7. Factitial urticaria or dermographia elevata. The letters were produced by mild stroking of the skin.

several months, diffuse thickening of the epidermis develops in consequence of chronic scratching.

For symptomatic relief of itching in stasis, local applications of icthammol pastes and ointments are used in mild cases; tar preparations are usually effective in more severe cases. These work by relieving the inflammation and diminishing the sensitivity of the nerve endings. The most effective therapy, of course, is the correction of the stasis.

It seems that even physiologically the relatively slow circulation in the lower extremities, particularly in the region of the shin bone, increases the itching susceptibility. In non-itching or moderately itching eruptions, such as psoriasis or lichen planus, lesions of the legs always itch more intensely and are scratched more than anywhere else. It is the habit of many people whose skin is perfectly normal to scratch their shins when they undress or go to bed. In a study on senile skin changes, we examined the inmates of an old-age asylum, all over 70, asking them whether or not they scratch, and if so, where. Of the 80, 45 volunteered the answer that "it feels good to scratch the shins in the evening."

This observation leads to the difficult problem of the existence of "senile pruritus." Obviously, senile degeneration and atrophy of the skin is not prurigenic, because pruritus is completely absent in cases of far-progressed senile cutaneous changes, and many cases of exasperating pruritus that are labeled as senile pruritus do not display such changes. Nevertheless, some authors claim that the administration of male sex hormone preparations is valuable in so-called *senile pruritus.* It is possible that peripheral arteriosclerosis of the cutaneous vessels with consequent local anoxemia increases itching hyperexcitability, and thus drives the patient into a vicious itching-scratching cycle, but such a mechanism has never been proved. One must think of such a possibility when there are definite signs of peripheral arteriosclerosis and when the pruritus has developed gradually. However, in most cases that are diagnosed as "senile pruritus," the pruritus has nothing to do with senility. An old man or woman may itch from the same causes as do younger patients, but these causes are less thoroughly investigated in the case of old people because of the belief that there exists an idiopathic senile pruritus. We have seen examples of so-called "senile pruritus" due to: (1) kidney insufficiency with high nonprotein nitrogen values, (2) carcinoma of the stomach, and (3) drugs. One should be particularly skeptical about accepting the diagnosis of senile pruritus when there has been a sudden onset of intense generalized itching.

Pruritus Due to Asteatosis

There is a harmony in the sensory status of the normal skin (the so-called "eudermie" of Jacquet), in which the weak physiologic impulses arising from sensory stimuli of everyday life, such as slight rubbing, slight changes in temperature and pressure, scarcely enter the consciousness and do not cause any discomfort. For the maintenance of this harmonious condition in man, a greasy cover is required on the skin surface. This cover is supplied by the sebaceous glands on most parts of the body and by lipids of scales on the palms and the soles. *Decrease in sebaceous gland activity* leads to a disturbance of the sensory status with decreased itching thresholds, i.e., by increased itching susceptibility. Physiologically, the amount of oily secretion is a function of the atmospheric temperature. It decreases with decreasing temperature, and at from 10° to 15° C. is only one-half as much as it is at 25° C. This effect of cold is the cause of *pruritus hiemalis,* popularly known as "winter itch." Of course, "dryness" of the skin—or in scientific terms "asteatosis" or "xerosis," meaning **lack of grease** on the surface—does not occur only in cold weather. Many people in moderate climates have dry skin throughout the year. The efficiency of sebaceous-gland function depends upon a great number of internal and external factors. The main internal factor is the inherited constitution of the integument, and a great influence on the sebaceous gland function is exerted by the *glands of internal secretion.* Hypogonadism is often accompanied by skin dryness, as is hypopituitarism. Some authors believe that hypothyroidism is a cause of asteatosis, although itching is not characteristic of myxedema. Either or both of two types of factors are apt to be operative in causing a deficit in the normal oily cover on the skin: (1) an inadequate supply due to constitutional deficit, endocrine imbalance, environmental effects, etc., and (2) removal of the normally supplied oily coating of the skin.

External factors, in addition to atmospheric temperature, are moisture of the air and the use of *water and soap,* with great variations of the latter's influence according to the temperature of the water, duration of the contact with water, quality of soap, technic of washing (rubbing, scrubbing, tub bath, shower bath), etc.

The low humidity common in heated rooms increases skin dryness and the tendency toward winter itch especially when this factor is combined with excessively frequent and thorough removal of skin oils in bathing. Prolonged contact with water, especially if warm or hot, immoderate use of soap, and heavy scrubbing remove protective oils and cells. Skin so affected may show no visible changes when the condition is early or mild, but may be quite pruritic. Later a true dermatitis may develop.

The asteatotic skin feels "dry" and rough on palpation and displays fine adherent scales on the surface. The characteristic sign is a superficial cracking of the horny layer in the form of a network of fine pink lines, usually in a square or a rhomboidal pattern. It is more pronounced on the extensor surfaces of the extremities, particularly on the legs, than elsewhere. In early stages there may be only a flakiness of the skin; a fine powdery "snow" of desquamation may be provoked by gentle stroking. Secondary to the dryness, a mild inflammatory reaction may develop in the form of nonsharply limited erythematous isolated patches. The itching caused by asteatosis is usually moderate, appears in spells, particularly upon undressing and when the skin is exposed to abrupt changes of the external temperature. It usually does not awaken the patient, but often makes it difficult for him to fall asleep.

The nondermatologist practitioner, unfortunately, is not sufficiently familiar with the extremely common picture of asteatosis. He may recognize the condition if there is real "chappiness" with deep rhagades, but this form, mainly occurring on the hands, is not the one that elicits pruritus.

In practice, asteatosis sometimes is mistaken for ichthyosis (which does not itch); or in other cases a desperate search is made for systemic causes of pruritus, and when no cause can be found, the case is often labeled as "senile pruritus" if the patient is over 40. It is highly desirable that asteatosis become better known in general practice because the correct diagnosis implies prompt and often dramatic relief by simple therapeutic procedures: restrictions in the use of water and soap, and massage of an indifferent lubricant into the skin. In our experience, ointment

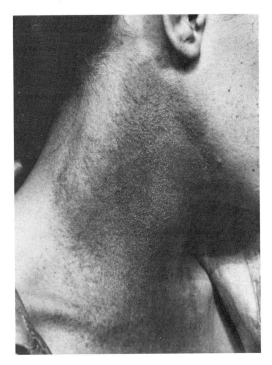

FIG. 40-8. Eczematous type of allergic reaction with intra-epidermal vesicle formation. The allergen in this case was resorcinol.

bases containing cholesterol or its derivatives, such as anhydrous lanolin or Aquaphor, are greatly superior to any other lubricant in substituting for the natural greasy cover of the skin.

HEAT, SWEAT RETENTION AND ITCHING

In many conditions associated with itching, exposure to heat, vasodilation, heavy sweating with sweat retention and irritation of the skin cause intense attacks of pruritus. **Primary miliaria (prickly heat) is a pruritic** dermatitis apparently resulting from heat plus sweat retention. It is most common in infants and is relieved by a cool environment.

ITCHING AS AN ALLERGIC MANIFESTATION

There are two types of hypersensitivity reactions of the skin, both associated with considerable itching. One is the eczematous type in which the reaction between allergen and the (hypothetical) antibody takes place in the *epidermis cells;* its typical clinical lesion is the intraepidermal vesicle (Fig. 40-8). The other is the urticarial type in

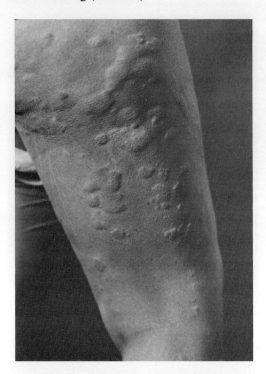

FIG. 40-9. Urticarial type of allergic reaction. This reaction is most commonly seen in hypersensitivity to drugs or foods.

pendent phenomena: (1) the anatomic (inflammatory) lesion provoked by cell injury and (2) the itching provoked by stimulation of sensory nerve endings. In allergic reactions based on histamine liberation, both phenomena are present, although the eruptions may be preceded by itching for several hours; often there may be itching with no eruption. This is the case, for instance, in

which the hypersensitivity reaction occurs in the *vessel walls of the dermis*, probably in the endothelial cells; its typical clinical lesion is the urticarial wheal (Fig. 40-9), or, in the case of lower intensities, the erythematous macule (Fig. 40-10). Roughly, it is correct that allergens acting from the outside are more likely to lead to eczematous reactions ("contact dermatitis") and allergens reaching the skin via the blood stream provoke erythematous-urticarial eruptions ("toxic erythema," "toxic eruption"). However, this is not a rule without exceptions. Drugs, such as quinine and organic arsenicals, administered internally, may lead to eczematiform reactions if allergy develops, and insect bites or sunshine cause urticarial wheals by acting from the outside.

In this connection it should be pointed out that in cutaneous allergic reactions it is not the visible lesion that "causes" itching; this is obvious from the fact that both eczematous vesicles and urticarial wheals often are preceded by itching and both last longer than the itching does. What happens is that, by the allergic tissue reaction, irritating substances are formed which cause two inde-

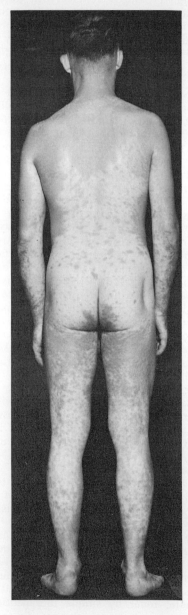

FIG. 40-10. Macular erythematous eruption caused by hypersensitivity to diphenylhydantoin.

serum sickness and in food or drug allergy, in which there may be severe general pruritus with or without an urticarial eruption. In the eczematous type of hypersensitivity, sometimes it may be that, in low concentrations, the irritating substance stimulates the itching nerve endings without causing cellular damage that would lead to visible changes.

Itching and itching eruptions due to allergens acting from the outside (leaves and flowers of plants, animal hair, an immense number of chemicals, and physical agents, such as heat, cold and light, etc.) are most intense on the uncovered parts of the body, and such regional distribution always arouses suspicion of a contact dermatitis (Fig. 40-4). If the allergen acts from the inside, the pruritus and pruritic eruption are either generalized or at least widely disseminated and, in most cases, symmetrically distributed.

PRURITUS OF PSYCHOGENIC ORIGIN

There is an itching of purely psychic origin. Merely imagining the presence of biting insects may provoke itching and scratching in centrally hyperceptive individuals. The intensity of peripherally induced itching always depends upon the central excitability. Thus it often happens that itch stimuli (for instance, a rough woolen garment) do not cause discomfort to some, but cause intolerable itching to others. On the other hand, pruritus simply due to morbid imagination must be a rare condition, since it is not encountered in true psychoses such as schizophrenia, manic-depressive insanity, or in compulsion hysteria.

Parasitophobia, a condition in which the patient tries to convince the physician that parasites are crawling on his skin, showing him small scales and dust particles, is always a sign of a severe psychosis, but it does not represent an itching disorder. The patient's complaint is not at all focused on itching; he does not claim to be compelled to scratch; his imagination is completely centered on the presence of crawling parasites.

Similarly, in **neurotic excoriations,** a common syndrome in psychoneurotic individuals, the patients hardly complain of itching. They claim that lesions like acne papules or pustules erupt on the skin; they readily admit that they feel a compulsion to "pick" on these lesions, and that it is not intolerable itching that compels them to do so (Fig. 40-3).

The psychogenic factor, however, plays a tremendous role in the development of an itching-scratching cycle. Persons suffering from neurodermatitis, most of them psychically unstable individuals, become victims of such a cycle most easily. But the development of the cycle also depends upon the degree of the increased itching susceptibility in the periphery, and if that is high, as it is for instance in Hodgkin's disease, persons with absolutely normal psyches will not be able to avoid the cycle.

In generalized pruritus that lasts more than a few days, one must be extremely cautious when diagnosing "nervous itching." Many cases of severe internal diseases, of scabies and pediculosis, and of asteatosis remain undetected because the physician, dealing with a "nervous person," thinks too readily that he has found the answer to itching in this "nervousness." Paradoxically enough, in localized itching, pruritus ani, and pruritus vulvae, the psychogenic origin is more common, or the psychogenic factor more important, than in generalized pruritus.

Emotional urticaria, also called cholinergic urticaria, is the only itching disease the psychosomatic mechanism of which is relatively well-understood. Patients suffering from this disease are, overwhelmingly, young females who break out with generalized urticaria when they get excited. They respond with urticaria to external application of heat as well as to emotional stimuli because they are *allergic to acetylcholine,* which is released in the skin in response to either emotional or heat stimuli. To local application of acetylcholine these patients display a local triple response, as though from histamine, and they break out with generalized urticaria on systemic administration of acetylcholine. When heat is applied locally, the released acetylcholine reaches the central nervous system via the blood stream and elicits there a widespread nervous impulse leading again to release of acetylcholine at the nerve endings, causing generalized urticaria. This disease represents one of the rare instances of allergy to a physiologic metabolic product.

PRURITUS DUE TO PREGNANCY

Frequently pregnant women suffer from intense generalized pruritus during the last month of pregnancy. This pruritus is often misdiagnosed as scabies and is made considerably worse by antiscabetic treatment. In the appearance of the skin there is some superficial similarity to scabies and pediculosis because of the numerous linear and punctiform scratch marks. The frequently present diffuse but uneven pigmentation (in addition to the usual pigmentation of pregnancy) and superficial pyogenic lesions constitute a picture resembling "vagabonds' disease." This diagnostic error, however, is by no means unavoidable, because the diagnosis of scabies should, whenever possible, be based on the demonstration of clinically typical burrows in typical locations, and preferably upon microscopic demonstration of the animal organisms.

The pruritus due to pregnancy is characterized by rather sudden onset and early generalization, by exasperating intense itching sensation day and night, and by sudden disappearance of the itching within the first few days after delivery. Characteristically, it is a disease of the last month of pregnancy, but occasionally it may start at any time during the last trimester. It is a pruritus appearing without accompanying cutaneous changes of the skin. The visible changes are secondary and are due to scratching, rubbing, and consecutive secondary infection. It is seen in entirely normal pregnancies in which no other signs of "toxemia" are found and in which the fetus is entirely normal. That this pruritus is caused by the pregnancy itself, probably by *metabolic products of the fetus* that are foreign to the maternal organism, is evidenced by its sudden disappearance after the baby is born and by its stereotype repetition in following pregnancies. As a matter of fact, if once a mother has been afflicted by pruritus due to pregnancy, it is highly probable that the same condition will occur in all following pregnancies.

Later in this chapter we discuss the interrelations of pruritus with hepatobiliary disease, jaundice, bile acids, etc. Present concepts suggest that high bile acid levels are at least one factor in the itching of pregnancy. Non-icteric women with pruritus during pregnancy have serum bile acid levels 30 times the normal value.[14]

For symptomatic relief of pruritus in pregnancy, generalized ultraviolet irradiations with suberythematous doses are the method of choice. Their effect is often dramatic. The patient who spent a number of sleepless nights and is completely exhausted somatically and physically will have a satisfactory night's sleep after the first irradiation. This immediate effect can almost be regarded as

having diagnostic value because no other condition responds so promptly. The usual external applications for symptomatic relief of itching, such as calamine lotion, calamine liniment, mentholated alcohol (0.25 per cent), etc., have only limited value.

In addition to the pure form of pruritus gravidarum, toxic eruptions, mainly of the erythematous and urticarial type, may appear in the last month of pregnancy and cause considerable itching. These eruptions also end abruptly after delivery, and there is little doubt that they have the same pathomechanism as has simple pruritus, originating from metabolic products of the fetus. In urticarial eruptions, the symptomatic effect of ultraviolet light is considerably less than in simple pruritus.

A less common form of itching in pregnancy is that associated with the eruption called *herpes gestationis*. The clinical picture of this eruption is identical with that of dermatitis herpetiformis, or Duhring's disease, but it is different by being clearly connected with the state of pregnancy. It appears at any time during the second half of pregnancy, disappears within a few weeks postpartum, recurs in subsequent pregnancies, but never recurs outside of the periods of gestation. The eruption is often preceded by pruritus without visible changes and only after several days do the first signs, erythematous patches, urticarial lesions, and finally the characteristic grouped vesicles and bullae appear. A characteristic sign is eosinophilia in the blood and in the blisters. The itching becomes as intolerable as it is in pruritus gravidarum. The disease is generally considered "toxic." However, this toxic state obviously must be different and more serious than that in pruritus gravidarum, because miscarriages or early death of the infant often have been reported. However, the prognosis for the mother is good. Herpes gestationis is not associated with eclampsia and never changes into pemphigus. It is not to be confused with impetigo herpetiformis, a rare lethal disease of pregnancy, the eruption of which does not itch.

DIABETIC PRURITUS

There is no simple relationship between the degree of diabetes and the symptom of itching. On the contrary, it is conspicuous that patients with mild diabetes, and particularly in the incipient phase, suffer more commonly from pruritus than those with severe forms of diabetes. Pruritus may be the very first subjective symptom of the disease, and this initial pruritus often will subside in spite of the fact that the diabetes remains uncontrolled or even becomes worse. Two patients under observation may have the same level of blood sugar, identical tolerance curves, identical sugar excretion in the urine, and still one patient will suffer from intolerable pruritus, whereas the other will not itch at all. Different degrees of acidosis do not explain this situation, because diabetic acidosis does not cause itching. The concentration of glucose in the skin (or in the epidermis) also is irrelevant; glucose when injected into the skin in high concentrations does not cause itching. Yet, there is no doubt that there is a "diabetic pruritus" in which diabetes is the causative agent, for this pruritus disappears promptly when adequate treatment is initiated, and reappears following dietary indiscretions or if the treatment becomes inadequate.

The relationship of pruritus and diabetes is complicated because diabetes provokes itching by causing dryness of the skin, and the tendency to develop this dryness shows great individual constitutional (possibly familial) variations. It also depends on the bathing habits of the patients and other external factors. It has been demonstrated that both water evaporation from the skin surface and sebaceous secretion are decreased in diabetes. Decrease of sebaceous gland secretion greatly increases itching susceptibility. As a matter of fact, diabetic pruritus can often be well-controlled by treatment of the asteatosis only, with lubricants and by restriction of the use of water and soap, without controlling the diabetes.

How diabetes causes asteatosis is not understood, and no data are available as to the variations of asteatosis with varying degrees of the metabolic disturbance. However, clinical experience shows that poorly controlled diabetes causes dehydration and that the skin may become quite dry and seems to be much less oily than normal.

It is remarkable that in juvenile diabetes, itching is uncommon, an observation that can be associated with the fact that asteatosis is rarely seen in the age group of 8 to 24 years.

Clinically, a patient who seeks the physician's advice for generalized pruritus will be particularly suspect of the presence of diabetes when his skin displays clinical signs of asteatosis, when the intensity of itching shows seemingly unexplained variations

(probably dependent upon atmospheric temperature and use of soap and water), and when scratching leads to pyogenic infections, particularly of the follicles, with a readiness that is far above the average. Otherwise the scratch marks in diabetes are not conspicuous. There might be none or a few punctiform hemorrhagic crusts. Linear scratch marks are infrequently seen. There is no particular predilectional localization of the itching, except that pruritus vulvae is apparently much more common in diabetic than in nondiabetic women.

Textbooks often enumerate diabetes among the causes of pruritus ani. However, I have not yet seen or heard of a case in which localized pruritus ani was proved to be due to diabetes. In cases of pruritus vulvae in diabetic women, the external genitalia and the vagina should be examined for monilia infection. This infection may cause pruritus vulvae.

The extended cutaneous monilia infection of intertriginous areas, involving axillae, submammary folds, umbilical fold, groin, and intergluteal folds in fat women is almost pathognomonic for diabetes. Clinically, the lesions are characterized by sharply limited, bright-red moist surfaces with overhanging scales on the edges and with irregularly arranged satellite pustules in the neighborhood. This infection causes intense itching. Diagnosis is made by microscopic and cultural demonstration of monilia.

PRURITUS, HEPATOBILIARY DISEASE AND JAUNDICE

Itching is present in about 20 to 25 per cent of jaundiced patients. That disturbance in hepatobiliary function is one of the causes of generalized pruritus is satisfactorily evidenced by the sudden disappearance of exasperating itching after cholecystectomy or operations for malignancy, after subsidence of hepatitis, etc., and by recurrence of itching with relapse of the morbid process.

A review of the literature and of 64 consecutive cases of jaundice observed in Albert Merritt Billings Hospital of the University of Chicago reveals that the presence or the absence of itching cannot be predicted from any of the standard laboratory examinations (serum bilirubin, transaminase, alkaline phosphatase, van den Bergh, blood serum cholesterol level, galactose tolerance). Likewise, upon analysis of our material, we found no correlation between pruritus and the mechanism by which the jaundice arose.

TABLE 40-1. JAUNDICE AND PRURITUS

ETIOLOGY	CASES	PRURITUS PRESENT	PER CENT
Neoplasm	9	3	33
Common duct obstruction other than neoplasm (stone, stricture, congenital malformation)	9	3	33
Infectious hepatitis ..	29	4	14
Drug poisoning (arsenic, T.N.T., cincophen)	9	4	44
Syphilis (hepatic)	1	0	0
Cirrhosis (hepatic) ...	1	0	0
Causes unknown	6	3	50
Total	64	17	26.5

Table 40-1 shows that pruritus occurs in jaundice of any sort, independent of whether it is due to malignancy, common duct stone or stricture, drugs, or infection. However, the table also shows, as far as one can draw conclusions from the relatively small number of cases, that pruritus is more frequent in icterus secondary to neoplasm, common duct stone and stricture (33 per cent), and toxic liver damage due to drugs (44 per cent) than it is in infectious hepatitis (14 per cent). This is true even though detailed analyses reveal that the serum bilirubin may be considerably higher in some of the non-itching patients with hepatitis than in some of the severely itching patients with, for instance, a stricture of the common duct.

Pruritus is obviously not dependent upon the depth of the discoloration, i.e., on the concentration of **bile pigment** in the skin. A patient with severe icterus may have no itching, whereas a patient with a mild degree of icterus, even though due to the same etiologic factor, may have severe itching. It is true that in the individual case the pruritus disappears as the jaundice decreases and, contrariwise, the itching may become more severe as the icterus deepens. However, itching also may come and go while the jaundice persists, and itching often precedes and disappears earlier than the clinical jaundice. Finally, itching also occurs in liver diseases unaccompanied by icterus. Thus it is obvious that accumulation of bile pigment in the skin is not the cause of pruritus in liver disease.

When hepatobiliary disease with or without jaundice and pruritus coexist there are

evidently chemical changes that either stimulate the nerve endings directly or alter the sensitivity of the nerve endings to external stimuli. It is not known what effect, if any, the altered blood chemistry has upon the itching center in the hypothalamus. Increase in **bile acids** has been advanced as the chemical change in the blood causing pruritus. This assumption has been substantiated by the studies of Varco,[13] who found that the pruritus due to chronic hepatic disease disappeared rapidly if external biliary drainage was established, but that itching recurred following oral administration of small quantities of bile salts.

Schoenfield[16] found pruritus with extrahepatic obstruction in 75 per cent of patients with malignant lesions and in 50 per cent of those with benign disorders. Itching occurred in 20 per cent of patients with hepatitis, and in 10 per cent of those with portal cirrhosis (associated presumably with intrahepatic cholestasis). About 75 per cent of patients with bile duct stricture or primary biliary cirrhosis have pruritus. An increase in serum bile acids is suspected as the cause of pruritus, but a parallel relationship need not exist. The concentration of bile acids in the skin is greater in patients with hepatobiliary disorders associated with pruritus than in subjects without itching, and it may exceed the concentration in the blood.

Bile acid levels apparently have some causal relationship to the itching of pregnancy. Serum bile acid levels in nonicteric pregnant women with pruritus are very high, averaging 30 times the normal value.[14]

A high concentration of bile acids in the skin seems to be associated with itching.[17] If biliary obstruction is relieved surgically, itching may be quickly alleviated or terminated.

A number of investigators have demonstrated that pruritus associated with primary biliary cirrhosis or incomplete biliary obstruction is relieved by oral administration of a basic anion exchange resin. This bile acid-sequestering resin, cholestyramine, causes increased fecal excretion of the bile acids and results in lowered serum bile acid concentration. If possible, surgical correction of extrahepatic biliary obstruction is the treatment of choice.[3,6,15]

The evidence implicating bile acids in the skin as a definite cause of at least some kinds of itching seems quite strong.

Hepatogenic pruritus is generalized in most cases. In spite of extreme intensities

FIG. 40-11. Mycosis fungoides. Intensely pruritic arciform erythematous premycotic lesion.

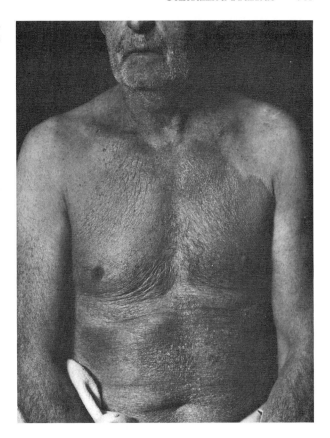

of itching, visible scratch marks and eczematization are rarely seen. Associated with itching in jaundice one occasionally sees erythematous spots and urticaria. Elevated dermographism (factitial urticaria) is common, and the elevated stripes are noticeably darker than the surrounding skin in the icteric patient. It was reported that arsphenamine icterus itches only exceptionally. In our series, 1 out of 3 cases of arsphenamine icterus was accompanied by itching.

Symptomatic relief of pruritus associated with jaundice is obtained by ultraviolet irradiations with suberythematous doses or, even more dramatically, by soft x-ray irradiations with small doses (30 to 80 roentgens). Such therapy apparently operates to produce a relative anesthesia of the nerve endings.

PRURITUS DUE TO LYMPHOBLASTOMA

This group includes myeloid and lymphatic leukemia, lymphosarcoma, mycosis fungoides, and Hodgkin's disease.

In all of these conditions, the first subjective symptom of the disease frequently is generalized pruritus, which reason alone prompts the patient to seek medical aid. This initial pruritus without visible lesions is extremely rare in myeloid leukemia, not uncommon in lymphosarcoma and in lymphatic leukemia, and extremely frequent in mycosis fungoides and in Hodgkin's disease (approximately 25 per cent of cases).

Common in all of these conditions is the frequent development of exfoliative dermatitis (generalized "erythroderma") with exasperating itching. The clinical picture is characterized by diffuse generalized erythema and lamellous scaling. Histologically, one may find all transitions between the common signs of inflammation and highly specific cellular infiltrates. Similar transitions between "toxic" and "specific" tissue changes also are seen in those nongeneralized disseminated, circumscribed, inflammatory lesions that usually precede the tumor formation, more often in mycosis fungoides and in Hodgkin's disease than in leukemia. These lesions may be simply erythematous patches (Fig. 40-11), or urticarial, vesicular, bullous, or purpuric in nature. Sometimes there may be oozing and crusting lesions, or they may simulate other dermatoses such as prurigo (Fig. 40-12), lichen planus, psoriasis, and parapsoriasis. All of these eruptions are primarily "toxic," without characteristic cellular elements, but they may later develop specific infiltrates.

Mycosis fungoides presents particularly polymorphous eruptions in the so-called premycotic stage. The single lesions are always sharply limited, and bizarre configurations, such as circinate, arciform, or arabesquelike forms are frequently seen. As long as the cutaneous infiltration of these lesions is slight, the clinical diagnosis is difficult. It is usually the exasperating itching (remaining completely uninfluenced by the usual procedures for symptomatic relief) that first awakens the suspicion that the eruption, which may simulate psoriasis or some other common dermatosis, is mycosis fungoides or one of the other lymphoblastomas. In this early phase, the diagnosis must be made by microscopic examination of a skin biopsy specimen. Later on, however, when the cutaneous infiltration is easily palpable, the clinical picture becomes more characteristic. It is a rule that plaques with definite dermal infiltration which itch intensely are manifestations of some kind of lymphoblastoma. In this situation, the symptom of itching is of paramount significance in the differentiation of lymphoblastoma from other cutaneous infiltrates, such as occur in syphilis, tuberculosis, leprosy, and deep mycotic infections, which do not itch.

In sharp contrast with premycotic lesions, the fully developed tumors of mycosis fungoides (tomatolike reddish-brown growth with rapidly developing crateriform ulcerations on the top, Figure 40-13) are not pruritic at all; neither are the cutaneous tumors in lymphatic leukemia. In Hodgkin's disease, however, all cutaneous manifestations, the diffuse infiltrative plaques as well as the nodular lesions, are equally accompanied by tormenting itching.

Cutaneous manifestations of myelogenous leukemia are rarely seen. However, in a few cases, violently itching nodular cutaneous infiltrates have been reported to be due to this blood dyscrasia.

Symptomatic relief of itching in cutaneous manifestations of lymphoblastomas can be achieved by x-ray therapy, nitrogen mustard, corticotropin, and adrenal steroids. All of these measures act indirectly by reducing the infiltrate of the primary process.

Pruritus Due to Internal Malignant Tumors

Little attention has been paid to the generalized pruritus that is caused by the pres-

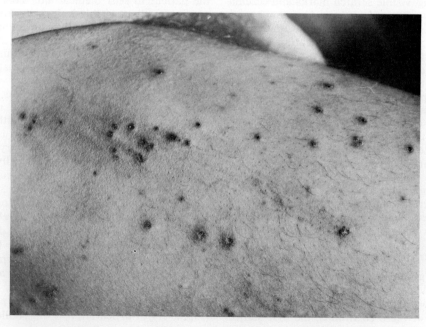

Fig. 40-12. Prurigolike eruption in lymphosarcoma. In contrast with prurigo neurotic excoriations, the edges of the lesions are infiltrated.

ence of internal malignant tumors. In the American literature this syndrome was first discussed by Becker, Kahn, and Rothman in 1942. The etiologic role of the tumor in pruritus was manifested in several cases by the disappearance of the itching after removal of the tumor and its recurrence with the reappearance of the tumor. The following unpublished case is reported as an illustration.

A 70-year old machinist was admitted to the Dermatology Clinic of Albert Merritt Billings Hospital on February 23, with the complaint of severe generalized itching of 6 months' duration. Physical examination revealed dry, scaling skin with senile atrophic changes, diffuse hyperpigmentation and numerous scratch marks. The patient was obviously in great distress because of the itching, and his family reported that for several months he spent his nights scratching and was unable to sleep. Attempts to relieve the pruritus by symptomatic treatment with routine external applications and sedatives failed completely.

Laboratory examinations revealed normocytic anemia, and 4-plus benzidin reaction in the stool. X-ray examination of the stomach showed a carcinoma of the lesser curvature near the antrum.

Subtotal gastrectomy was performed on April 9. On the second day after operation, the patient gratefully volunteered that his itching had completely disappeared. His postoperative course was uneventful. He remained under observation until September.

In malignancy, as in lymphoblastomas, the simple generalized pruritus often represents only the introductory phase to the outbreak of itching eruptions that may be prurigolike or toxic in nature. The latter eruptions may simulate erythema multiforme, dermatitis herpetiformis, acute lupus erythematodes, and may develop into exfoliative dermatitis. In most of these eruptions, as well as in simple pruritus, a great tendency to early intense diffuse hyperpigmentation is noted. This is more marked in internal malignancy than in Hodgkin's disease.

Pruritus and inflammatory eruptions have been interpreted as being due to toxic substances formed by the tumor cells, or by their decomposition products circulating in the blood stream. However, some of the itching eruptions were interpreted as being not of toxic, but of metastatic origin. It was assumed that single tumor cells transported to the skin by the blood stream are decomposed in the skin with accompanying local inflammation. Evidence of such a process was seen in cases in which metastases developed from primarily itching papular lesions. Thus, the analogy to pruritus and to itching eruptions in lymphoblastoma is close, in so far as no sharp line can be drawn between "toxic" and "metastatic" manifestations. True final neoplastic metastases of malignant tumors of the skin do not itch, even as no itching accompanies the indolent "tumors" of mycosis fungoides and of lym-

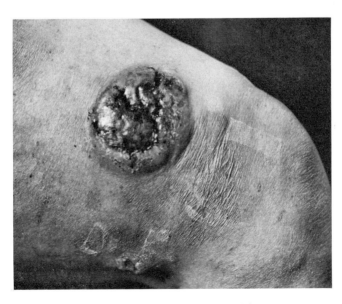

Fig. 40-13. Mycosis fungoides. Nonpruritic tumor.

phatic leukemia. One may conclude that, in these conditions, as long as there is vigorous defense in the skin against the elements of foreign growth, the cellular decomposition is sufficiently massive to result in the production of toxic substances causing itching and inflammatory reactions, whereas such events do not occur when the growth becomes uninhibited. Hodgkin's disease is a remarkable exception in so far as its cutaneous tumors, are concerned; also it is an exception in regard to its toxic manifestation, itch.

Pruritus due to internal malignant tumors seems to be rare. Over a period of seventeen years only 10 cases were reported. But there is no doubt that the number of cases would greatly and suddenly increase if more attention were paid to the syndrome by general practitioners and surgeons. Pruritus apparently may occur as a consequence of any kind of malignant tumor of any localization, mostly as a late manifestation and usually after considerable necrosis of the tumor cells has occurred. It was often reported as a terminal symptom. However, the case quoted previously, among others, demonstrates that pruritus may be an early symptom and as such may have diagnostic significance. Simple pruritus with hyperpigmentation occurs more frequently with carcinomas of the gastrointestinal tract than with growths in other locations. Itching eruptions were described also in cancers of the breast, of the bronchi, of the pancreas, the uterus, the tongue, and also in cases of sarcoma of the thyroid gland. In many of these cases, evidence was presented for the causal connection between tumor and itching eruption.

PRURITUS IN KIDNEY INSUFFICIENCY

Pruritus in kidney insufficiency is probably due to the retention of nitrogenous substances in the blood. This conclusion is drawn from the fact that itching is observed only in those cases of kidney damage in which the nonprotein nitrogen of the blood is elevated. Itching is never observed in nephritis or nephrosis unaccompanied by retention of waste products. It is not known which of the retained nitrogenous compounds is responsible for the itching. It is claimed that urea does not irritate the cutaneous sensory nerve endings of the skin if injected intradermally. A priori, one would assume that uric acid is more likely to be the itch-provoking agent. Reliable investigations, however, have not been made to clarify the mechanism of uremic pruritus.

Itching in uremia is generalized and is usually associated with a dirty yellowish-brown discoloration of the skin. Scratch marks are seen in abundance in the more severe degrees of itching. The intensity of the pruritus, however, is not proportionate to the severity of the uremia.

If the uremia can be relieved, the itching often greatly decreases or disappears. This has often been noted after therapy with adequate dialysis.[18] If secondary hyperparathyroidism complicates the renal failure, dialysis may be successful in relieving the uremia but severe pruritus may continue. Subtotal parathyroidectomy in a number of such cases has resulted in cessation of pruritus.

PRURITUS, UREMIA, AND SECONDARY HYPERPARATHYROIDISM

Persons suffering from uremia frequently develop hyperparathyroidism, the stimulus to the parathyroid glands being phosphate retention resulting from renal disease. The serum phosphorus and serum calcium are elevated, there is resorption of bone, elevated serum alkaline phosphatase, and frequent metastatic calcification. To stop this secondary hyperparathyroidism, subtotal parathyroidectomy has proved quite successful. Usually, about three and one-half of the enlarged glands are removed. Severe pruritus occurs in many patients (but not all) who have this syndrome of uremia plus excess parathyroid secretion. The pruritus has disappeared after subtotal parathyroidectomy in five out of five cases reported by one group,[19] and in nine out of nine cases reported by another group.[20] These observations strongly suggest a derangement of calcium metabolism as a likely cause of the pruritus.

The immediate stimulus to the nerve endings which causes the pruritus is not yet identified. The serum calcium falls to normal or below immediately after removal of the excess parathyroid tissue. The itching ceases in from two to seven days. Deposition of calcium salts in dermal structures may be a factor in the pruritus. In all of five cases afflicted with pruritus, uremia, and hyperparathyroidism, the calcium content of skin was abnormally high; it was not high in uremia without pruritus and without clinical hyperparathyroidism.[20] In three patients in whom postoperative disappearance of pruritus was complete, recurrence of the itching was provoked by elevation of serum calcium either by intravenous calcium or high oral calcium and vitamin D.

Thus, it appears that at least we can come to the following conclusions:

(1) In some uremic patients (not in all) certain retention products cause itching.

(2) The itching is especially apt to occur if uremia plus hypercalcemia is present.

(3) Also, excess calcium salts are present in the skin in such cases and may be the immediate cause of the pruritus.

Since hypercalcemic disorders without uremia do not cause itching, it seems likely that one or several factors in uremia predispose to production of pruritus.

Pruritus and Carcinoid Syndrome

The carcinoid syndrome has been reported in some cases[21] as being accompanied by severe pruritus; in other instances, itching has not been emphasized as a notable feature. Serotonin has been incriminated as an "itch substance" when applied locally. Also, although it causes arteries and veins to constrict, it dilates capillaries and produces the severe intermittent flushes of the carcinoid syndrome. Vasodilation in the skin greatly favors the production of pruritus, especially whenever some other predisposing factor is also active; serotonin, therefore, seems to be a likely candidate as an itch-producing agent. Serotonin causes attacks of asthma and provokes release of histamine from tissues. It could possibly induce itching by (1) direct action, (2) histamine release, and (3) vasodilation.

LOCALIZED PRURITUS

Pruritus Ani

In the discussion of pruritus ani, textbooks list a considerable number of causative factors: proctitis and colitis, high alkaline pH in the rectum and the colon, intestinal parasites, hemorrhoids, allergy to or primary irritative effect of food, antibiotics and other drugs taken orally, allergy to fecal material, fungus infection or allergic "-id" reactions to distant foci, diabetes, intestinal neoplasm, and so forth. In practice, however, although such causes occasionally are found, in the majority of cases of chronic pruritus ani, which is mainly a disease of adults, none of of these factors can be demonstrated.

In about 50 per cent of the cases of pruritus ani there is an association with neurodermatitis ("atopic eczema"). Patients with a neurodermatitis constitution have a great tendency to lichenification of the skin in response to scratching or to other forms of mechanical irritation. Neurodermatitis is often associated with eosinophilia, and a familial or individual association with asthma or hay fever ("atopy") may be present, but the cutaneous manifestation never has been proved to be due to an allergic mechanism. Since these patients are high-strung and emotionally unstable, sedative therapy is important.

In addition to patients with neurodermatitis, "idiopathic" pruritus ani may arise also in individuals of an emotionally well-balanced personality with no functional disorders. In such cases, the pruritus may start with an accidental mechanical irritation of the anus during the wiping action following a bowel movement or with irritation by hard stool particles. This irritation may be maintained by the rubbing of the anus with toilet paper during cleansing, and finally may drive the patient into a vicious cycle of itching and scratching. The perianal area often is subjected to intensive cleansing with soap and water, with removal of the normal skin oils. Use of a bland lubricant (containing lanolin, etc.) may be all that is necessary to give relief, plus restriction of use of soap and water. Application of strong drugs (antipruritics, etc.) may intensify the irritation and provoke further itching.

An auxiliary factor is venous stasis in the external hemorrhoidal ring of veins, but hemorrhoids otherwise play no part in the causation of itching. Disordered intestinal function, either constipation or diarrhea, and spasm of the anal sphincter are further auxiliary factors. Therefore, great emphasis has to be put on the regulation of bowel movements in the management of pruritus ani.

Physiologically, the anus and the perineum display a great readiness to itching, because the itching nerve endings are particularly numerous in this region (Fig. 40-14). An area

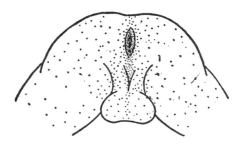

Fig. 40-14. Relative density of itching points in the male anogenital region. (Longo: Arch. de fisiol. 36:197)

of increased itching sensitivity, therefore, may easily be set up here in response to scratching.

Discussion of the alleged occasional relation of pruritus ani to suppressed emotions, particularly to psychogenic disturbances in the sexual sphere, as it has been interpreted by some psychoanalysts, is beyond the scope of this chapter. In some instances, manipulation of the genital, the perineal, and the rectal areas might be an indication of unsatisfied sexual desire. In these cases, psychiatric study may prove advisable. However, it should be emphasized that in pruritus ani highly satisfactory therapeutic results can usually be obtained with only mild sedatives and local measures directed toward elimination of external irritation.

The author is unable to confirm the numerous statements in the literature that pruritus ani is often the manifestation of a systemic organic disease. Pruritus, when due to a systemic disease, is practically always generalized.

Pruritus Vulvae

Pruritus vulvae is most commonly functional in origin, and is then frequently found in patients with neurodermatitis or in patients who display a similar syndrome of nervous exhaustion and emotional instability. Treatment in these cases is symptomatic, and emphasis is laid upon sedation.

However, local irritation as the cause of pruritus vulvae also must be investigated. Such irritating factors are: vaginal discharge of any kind; glycosuria in diabetes (by the easy fermentation of urine droplets retained on the genitals); trichomonas vaginalis infection, etc. Monilial infection of the external genitalia is common with or without diabetes, and may cause intolerable itching.

Lichen sclerosus et atrophicus, a patchy degenerative and atrophizing process, when occurring on the vulva, may cause marked pruritus, particularly in children. In the latter, pinworm infestations or gonorrheic vulvovaginitis also may cause vulvular pruritus.

When vulvar pruritus occurs during or after the menopause, it is frequently assumed that the itching is due to estrogen deficiency. As a matter of fact, replacement therapy with natural or synthetic estrogenic substances sometimes causes rapid disappearance of itching. However, the direct relationship of pruritus to the menopause never has

been proved experimentally, and strict criticism must be used in evaluating the results of estrogenic replacement therapy, because pruritus vulvae is frequently purely functional, very commonly so in the menopause, and the psychic suggestion connected with the treatment cannot be excluded. Also, almost any bland ointment may afford relief, whether containing estrogen or not. The vulvar region has often been made asteatotic (deprived of the skin's normal oily covering) by use of soap, water, etc.

The clinical appearance of pruritus vulvae varies from no visible change to eczematization with excoriations and thickening of the epithelium, up to classical lichenification. Kraurosis vulvae is similar in its initial phase. Neglected cases of pruritus vulvae with lichenification often are misdiagnosed as kraurosis, and unnecessarily extended surgical procedures are performed. One should keep in mind that in its initial phase kraurosis vulvae only can be diagnosed by histologic examination. It becomes clinically recognizable only in its atrophic phase. Also, one should remember that pruritus vulvae with lichenification is an extremely common ailment, whereas kraurosis vulvae is a rare disorder. Early microscopic diagnosis is the clue to rational therapy.

Psoriasis of the genital and anal area is highly pruritic and is manifested by sharply circumscribed, red, shiny plaques without scaling. Its diagnosis is difficult unless typical psoriatic lesions are found elsewhere.

Despite the close proximity of the vulva and the anus, itching of both areas is not usually concomitant. Both pruritus vulvae and ani have the tendency to spread to the perineum, but not further. When pruritis ani and vulvae coexist, the clinical response to treatment is usually different. Pruritus· ani tends to disappear sooner, and relapse of vulvar pruritus is more common.

Other Forms of Localized Pruritus

Localized pruritus of the external auditory canal and of the eyelids is almost exclusively a partial symptom of neurodermatitis. Occasionally itching of the ear canals is caused by fungus infection or by the irritation from a chronic discharge due to otitis media.

Localized pruritus of the nostrils is common in children suffering from intestinal parasites. The same localization of pruritus has been reported as a symptom of tumor of the brain with increased intracranial pressure. This is a remarkable localization in view of the results of animal experiments in which the nostrils were found to be sites of predilection for itching of central origin.

Localized pruritus (usually with some dermatitis, which may be mild to severe) may be provoked **by contact.** The location often furnishes the clue to the cause; causes may be animal, vegetable, mineral, chemical, etc. Some examples are: scalp, hair margins and ears (hair bleaches, dyes, and sprays); around eyes (eye cosmetics); face, especially around eyes, (frequent touch with fingernail lacquers); ear lobes (various metals in earrings); neck (wool or fur collars); wrist (metal bracelets or watchbands, synthetic plastic watchbands); legs (stockings, nylon, etc.); arms, legs (poison ivy).

The variation in human tolerance to foreign substances is extreme; some chemicals, dyes, etc. cause reactions in almost everyone; poison ivy causes no reaction in some, moderate pruritus in others, violent dermatitis in many. Nylon stockings and other synthetic clothing materials are well-tolerated by the great majority, but a few cannot tolerate certain ones of these. In a number of people, wool or certain furs cause severe itching.

SUMMARY

A detailed history is needed for evaluation of the severity of itching and of its diagnostic significance. It is helpful to differentiate obligate and facultative itching conditions. Punctiform and linear scratch marks and other sequels of scratching, such as pyogenic infections, thickening of the epithelium, lichenification, and chronic lymph node enlargement, are present in some itching disorders, but may be completely absent in others.

The nature of the immediate stimulus to the nerve endings is unknown in pruritus due to diabetes, lymphoblastomas, internal malignancies, and kidney insufficiency. In all of these conditions the degree of the pruritus does not parallel the severity of the disease. In diabetes, asteatosis of the skin is an important auxiliary factor. According to recent data, accumulation of bile acids is responsible for the pruritus in liver diseases and in obstructive disorders of the biliary tract, often associated with jaundice.

Bile acids have been implicated as a likely cause of the itching which occurs late in pregnancy in some women.

Hypercalcemia, with deposit of calcium salts in the skin, may be the mechanism producing intractable pruritus in some patients having uremia and hyperparathyroidism.

In the itching cutaneous lesions of lymphoblastomas and internal malignancies, no sharp line can be drawn between "toxic" and "metastatic" manifestations. Apparently, the products of tumor cells, either blood-borne or locally released in the skin, may cause pruritus. "Tumors" of leukemia, mycosis fungoides, and the malignant metastases do not itch, whereas the nodular lesions of Hodgkin's disease are intensely pruritic.

Psychogenic factors are important in many forms of pruritus, especially in pruritus ani and pruritus vulvae, and in so-called neurodermatitis.

Many different "primary factors" may initiate the pathogenic process that results in itching. All of these may operate to cause release in the skin of either *histamine* or one or more *proteolytic enzymes*, or both, and these may be the immediate stimuli that act on the nerve endings to provoke pruritus.

REFERENCES

1. Becker, S. W., and Obermayer, M. E.: Modern Dermatology and Syphilology, ed. 2, Philadelphia, Lippincott, 1947.
2. Becker, S. W., Kahn, D., and Rothman, S.: Cutaneous manifestations of internal malignant tumors, Arch. Derm. Syph. 45: 1069–1080, 1942.
3. Carey, J. B., and Williams, G.: Therapy for pruritus of jaundice, J.A.M.A. 176:432–435, 1961.
4. Dunbar, H. F.: Emotions and Bodily Changes, New York, Columbia, 1946.
5. Graham, D. T., Goodell, H., and Wolff, H. G.: Neural mechanisms involved in itch, "itchy skin" and tickle sensations, J. Clin. Invest. 30:37–49, 1951.
6. Hashim, S. A., and Van Itallie, T. B.: Use of bile acid sequestrant in treatment of pruritus associated with biliary cirrhosis, J. Invest. Derm. 35:253–254, 1960.
7. Jacquet, L.: Troubles de la sensibilite, *in* Besnier, Brocq and Jacquet (eds.): La Pratique Dermatologique, vol. 4, p. 330, Paris, Masson, 1904.
8. Lewis, T.: Clinical Science, Illustrated by Personal Experiences, London, Shaw, 1934.
9. Rothman, S.: Physiology and Biochemistry of the Skin, pp. 120–152, Chicago, Univ. of Chicago, 1954.
10. Shapiro, A. L., and Rothman, S.: Pruritus ani,

a clinical study, Gastroenterology 5:155–168, 1945.

11. Shelley, W. B., and Arthur, R. P.: Neurohistology and neurophysiology of itch sensation in man, Arch. Derm. 76:296–323, 1957.

12. ——: The peripheral mechanism of itch in man, Ciba Foundation Study Group, Pain and Itch, Boston, Little, Brown, 1959.

13. Varco, R. L.: Intermittent external biliary drainage for relief of pruritus in certain chronic disorders of the liver, Surgery 21:43–45, 1947.

14. Sjövall, K., and Sjövall, J.: Serum bile acids in pregnancy with pruritus, Clin. Chim. Acta 13:207–211, 1966.

15. Carey, J. B., Jr.: The pruritus of jaundice, Gen. Pract. 37:118–122, April, 1968.

16. Schoenfield, L. J.: The relationship of bile acids to pruritus in hepatobiliary disease. Presented at a conference on bile salt metabolism sponsored by the Univ. of Cincinnati

Med. Center, Cincinnati Med. Center, Sept. 28 & 29, 1967.

17. Schoenfield, L. J., Sjövall, J., and Perman, E.: Bile acids in skin of patients with pruritic hepatobiliary disease, Nature (London) 213:93, 1967.

18. Hampers, C., and Schupak, E.: Hemodialysis: The Management of the Patient with Chronic Renal Failure, p. 181, New York, Grune, 1967.

19. Hampers, C., et al.: Disappearance of "uremic" itching after subtotal parathyroidectomy, New Eng. J. Med. 279:695–697, 1968.

20. Massry, S., et al.: Intractable pruritus as a manifestation of secondary hyperparathyroidism in uremia: disappearance of itching after subtotal parathyroidectomy, New Eng. J. Med. 279:697–700, 1968.

21. Mengel, C.: Cutaneous manifestations of malignant carcinoid syndrome: severe pruritus and orange blotches, Ann. Intern. Med. 58:989–993, 1963.

Index

Page numbers in italics indicate illustrations. Page numbers followed by the letter "t" indicate tabular material.